BRADY

Paramedic Emergency Care

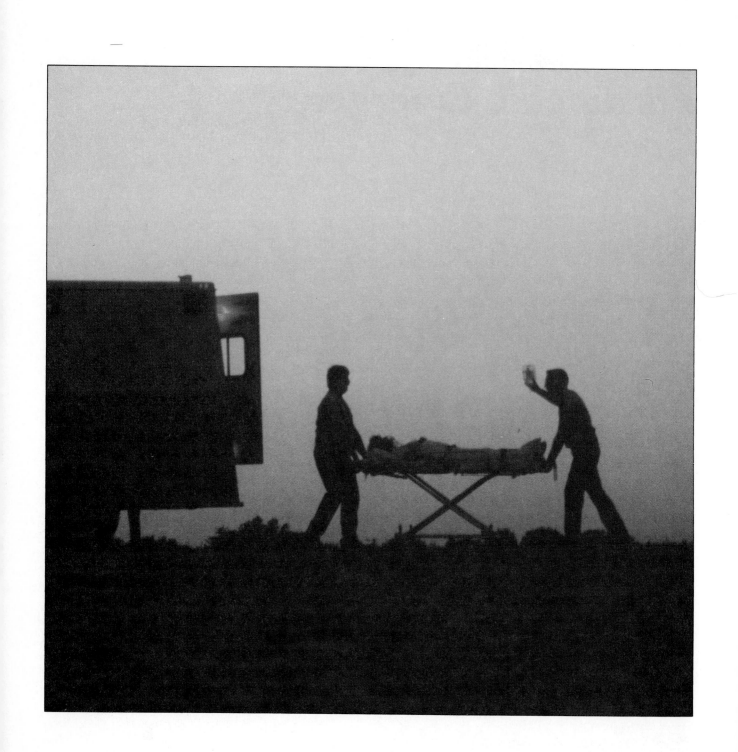

BRADY

Paramedic Emergency Care

Bryan E. Bledsoe, D.O., EMT-P
Emergency Department Physician
Baylor Medical Center
Waxahachie, Texas

Robert S. Porter, M.A., NREMT-P
Director, Central New York Emergency
Medical Service Program
Syracuse, New York

Bruce R. Shade, EMT-P
Commissioner, Cleveland Emergency Medical Services
Cleveland, Ohio

With a Foreword by
James O. Page

With Contributions From:

Richard A. Cherry, M.Ed., NREMT-P
Director of Paramedic Training
Department of Critical Care and Emergency Medicine
State University of New York Health Science Center
Syracuse, New York

Gary P. Morris, EMT-P
Deputy Fire Chief
Phoenix, Arizona Fire Department
Phoenix, Arizona

Rod Dennison, EMT-P
Emergency Medical Services Division
Texas Department of Health
Public Health Region 1
Temple, Texas

BRADY
REGENTS/PRENTICE HALL
Englewood Cliffs, New Jersey 07632

Library of Congress Cataloging-in-Publication Data

Bledsoe, Bryan E., (date)
    Paramedic emergency care Bryan E. Bledsoe, Robert S. Porter,
Bruce R. Shade, with contributions from Richard Cherry,
Gary P. Morris, Rod Dennison.
        p. cm.
    Includes index.
    ISBN 0-89303-741-9
    1. Medical emergencies.   2. Emergency medical personnel.
I. Porter, Robert S.   II. Shade, Bruce R.   III. Title.
    [DNLM: 1. Allied Health Personnel—education.   2. Emergency
Care—education. W 18 B646p]
RC86.7.B596 1991
616.02′5—dc20
DNLM/DLC
for Library of Congress   90-14196
                                                     CIP

Editorial/production supervision: Kathryn Pavelec
Interior/cover design: Linda J. Den Heyer Rosa
Cover photo: George Dodson
Interior photographer: George Dodson
Manufacturing buyers: Mary McCartney and Ed O'Dougherty
Acquisitions editor: Natalie Anderson

Prentice-Hall International (UK) Limited, *London*
Prentice-Hall of Australia Pty. Limited, *Sydney*
Prentice-Hall Canada Inc., *Toronto*
Prentice-Hall Hispanoamericana, S.A., *Mexico*
Prentice-Hall of India Private Limited, *New Delhi*
Prentice-Hall of Japan, Inc., *Tokyo*
Simon & Schuster Asia Pte. Ltd., *Singapore*
Editora Prentice-Hall do Brasil, Ltda., *Rio de Janeiro*

Art Acknowledgments:

American Heart Association, *Instructor's Manual for Advanced Cardiac Life Support, Second Edition.* Dallas, TX: American Heart Association, 1988.   Tables 20-1, 20-2, 30-4, 30-5, 30-6, 30-7, 30-8, 30-9, 30-10.

American Heart Association and American Academy of Pediatrics, *Textbook of Pediatric Advanced Life Support.* Dallas, TX: American Heart Association, 1988.   Figure 33-6; Tables 30-11, 30-12, 30-13, 30-14, 30-15, 30-16.

American Heart Association and American Academy of Pediatrics, *Textbook of Neonatal Resuscitation.* Dallas, TX: American Heart Association, 1987.   Figures 33-5, 33-7, 33-8, 33-9, 33-10, 33-11; Procedures 33-1, 33-2; Table 33-2.

Bledsoe, Bryan E., *Atlas of Paramedic Skills.* Englewood Cliffs, NJ: Prentice-Hall, Inc., 1987.   Figures 9-15, 9-16, 9-17, 10-37, 10-43, 11-29, 11-30, 11-32, 11-33, 11-35, 11-42, 12-22, 13-10, 15-19, 16-16, 16-17, 20-16, 23-6, 23-7.

Bledsoe, Bryan E., Bosker, Gideon, and Papa, Frank J., *Prehospital Emergency Pharmacology, Second Edition.* Englewood Cliffs, NJ: Prentice-Hall, Inc., 1988.   Figures 12-2, 12-3, 12-4, 12-5, 12-6, 13-4, 13-5, 13-6, 13-7, 13-15, 13-16; Tables 12-4, 13-2, 13-3, 23-1, 23-2, 23-4, 23-5, 25-1, 25-2, 25-3, 25-4, 26-1, 26-2, 30-2.

Campbell, John E., *Basic Trauma Life Support, Second Edition.* Englewood Cliffs, NJ: Prentice-Hall, Inc., 1988. Figures 14-12, 14-14, 14-22, 14-23, 14-24, 15-10, 15-15, 16-3, 16-4, 16-5, 16-7, 16-13, 16-14, 16-15, 16-16, 18-13, 18-24, 23-10; Tables 18-1, 18-2.

Grant, Harvey D., et. al., *Emergency Care, Fifth Edition.* Englewood Cliffs, NJ: Prentice-Hall, Inc., 1990.   Figures 9-2, 11-25, 21-2, 21-4, 21-7, 21-8, 23-8, 24-14, 24-15, 25-1, 26-1, 26-5, 26-9, 28-4, 28-5, 28-6, 28-7, 32-2, 32-8, 32-18, 32-19, 32-20, 32-22, 32-23, 33-3, 33-12, 33-13; Procedures 28-1, 32-1.

Huszar, Robert J., *Emergency Cardiac Care, Second Edition.* Bowie, MD: Brady Communications Company, 1982.   Figures 4-14, 4-15, 4-16, 21-12, 21-16, 21-58, 21-59, 21-60.

Martini, Frederic, *Fundamentals of Anatomy and Physiology,* ©1989, pp. 146, 150, 200, 201, 246, 316, 452, 548, 813, 817. Reprinted by permission of Prentice-Hall, Inc., Englewood Cliffs, NJ.   Figures 9-1, 9-18, 9-19, 11-2, 11-3, 15-1, 15-2, 15-3, 15-4, 15-6, 16-1, 17-1, 18-1, 20-2, 20-3, 21-1, 21-3, 21-4, 21-6, 21-9, 21-10, 22-1, 23-1, 23-2, 23-3, 24-1, 24-2, 24-10, 31-1, 31-2, 31-3, 32-4.

Schwartz, George R., Bosker, Gideon, and Grigsby, John W., *Geriatric Emergencies.* Bowie, MD: Brady Communications, 1984.   Tables 29-1, 29-2.

Shade, Bruce, et. al., *Advanced Cardiac Life Support: Certification, Preparation, and Review.* Englewood Cliffs, NJ: Brady Communications, Inc., 1988.   Figures 2-1, 11-5, 11-13, 11-22, 11-23, 11-24, 11-62, 11-63, 11-64, 11-65, 11-66, 12-7, 12-8, 12-9, 13-18, 20-15, 21-14, 21-15, 21-17, 21-18, 21-19 through 21-24, 21-33, 21-41, 21-61, 21-62, 21-63.

Walraven, Gail, *Basic Arrhythmias, Second Edition, Revised.* Englewood Cliffs, NJ: Prentice-Hall, Inc., 1986.   Figure 21-11.

Photo Acknowledgments:

The following individuals and institutions graciously provided photographs for use in *Paramedic Emergency Care:*

Acadian Ambulance Service, Inc., Lafayette, Louisiana. Figure 14-9; opening photos for Chapters 2, 4, 7, 8, 10, 12, 20.

Rod Dennison, EMT-P, Texas Department of Health, Temple, Texas.   Figures 5-5, 5-6, 5-9, 10-19.

Rusty Fowler, Chattanooga State Technical Community College, Chattanooga, Tennessee.   Figure 5-10.

Center for Emergency Medicine, Pittsburgh, Pennsylvania; and Presbyterian University Hospital, Pittsburgh, Pennsylvania.   Figures 5-8, 5-11, 5-12, 14-1, 14-16, 14-17, 14-18, 14-25, 14-26, 14-27, 14-28, 18-17, 18-18; opening photos for Chapters 5, 6, 9, 15, 17, 19, 23, 24, 25, 26, 28.

Phoenix Fire Department, Phoenix, Arizona.   Figures 6-1 through 6-7; opening photos for chapters 11, 13, 14, 16, 21.

Maryland Institute for Emergency Medical Services Systems (MIEMSS), Baltimore, Maryland.   Opening photos for Chapters 3, 27.

Scott and White Memorial Hospital and Clinic, Department of Plastic Surgery, Temple, Texas.   Figures 14-30, 18-2, 18-3, 18-4, 18-6, 18-7, 18-8, 18-9, 18-14, 18-19, 18-20, 18-21, 18-22, 18-23, 26-6, 26-7, 30-8, 30-9, 30-10; opening photo for Chapter 18.

Childbirth photography in Chapter 32 by Harriette Hartigan, ARTEMIS, 14 Short Trail, Stamford, CT, 06903.

Special Notes

To Emma, my wife of many years, who has had unbelievable patience as I completed another book. Her love and encouragement allowed me to keep going when I wanted to quit. Also, to our children, Bryan and Andrea, who make it all worthwhile.

B.E.B

To my students, who have taught me much more about prehospital emergency care and education than I have ever taught them.

R.S.P.

This book is dedicated to all the EMS providers, educators, and administrators working to make the delivery of prehospital care a true profession.

B.R.S.

Contents

5 Rescue Operations   *Rod Dennison*   **65**

6 Major Incident Response   *Gary P. Morris*   **81**

13 Emergency Pharmacology   Bryan E. Bledsoe   315

22 Endocrine and Metabolic Emergencies *Bryan E. Bledsoe* 705

23 Nervous System Emergencies *Bryan E. Bledsoe* 717

Foreword

Accuracy and coverage of the topic. Background and expertise of the authors. Timing. These are probably the most important factors in judging a textbook.

A quick look at the table of contents reveals that this text fully covers the topic. It is comprehensive and conforms to standard curricula for paramedic training. What the table of contents doesn't reveal, however, is a practical, common-sense approach to paramedic emergency care that no other text offers.

Having followed this writing project since its earliest stages, and having reviewed almost every chapter on its way to publication, my enthusiasm for the book has grown steadily. Reviewing textbook manuscripts can be real drudgery, especially when you try to do it at the end of a long workday. But this book was very different.

It's been more than 20 years since I first struggled through a paramedic training syllabus. There was no paramedic training text available, and the syllabus had been written by people who had never delivered medical care on the street. The instructors of that era spent much of their time explaining differences (between the syllabus materials and the real world) and clearing up confusion (most often in the aftermath of lectures by physicians or surgeons).

Which leads me to the second of the three criteria for judging a textbook—the background and expertise of the authors. Bryan Bledsoe, Bob Porter and Bruce Shade all have served as paramedics. Years ago, they each suffered through the adaptations of in-hospital training materials and texts. They remember their paramedic training instructors picking up the pieces after physican lectures ("What he *really* meant was . . .").

Each in his own way, Bledsoe, Porter, and Shade have created careers and presented personal examples that inspire and motivate their EMS colleagues. Bryan Bledsoe continued his formal education and was one of the first paramedics in the United States to become a physician. Bob Porter used his street experience and his education to become a national leader among EMS educators. Bruce Shade's talent and experience as a paramedic led to his position as chief administrator of one of North America's busiest urban EMS systems.

Despite their practical experience, and their demonstrated ability to communicate effectively with paramedic trainees, the coauthors sought contributions from others to cover highly specialized topics. Their contributing authors—Richard Cherry, Gary Morris and Rod Dennison—are paramedics, and each of them also brings to this text the clarity and common sense of people who write from experience rather than theory.

Timing is the other important factor in judging a textbook. This book was badly needed 20 years ago. Now that it's here, the timing is better than ever.

This textbook reinforces (and in some respects, reintroduces) the qualities that inspired many of us to commit our life's work to prehospital emergency medicine. For example, the concept that there is no pursuit, whether paid or unpaid, quite so noble as caring for others, who are in peril. Or that making a lonely and frightened elderly person feel important and dignified is a valuable use of our time.

This textbook arrives at a critical time in the short history of EMS. For reasons that are not entirely clear, many paramedics have become "high tech" but "no touch." Increasingly, complaints are heard from paramedics that their knowledge and skills are being misused on patients with minor illnesses and injuries. Newspaper reports and lawsuits increasingly describe insensitive behavior and negligent care by paramedics, and discrimination against patients who are thought to "abuse" the system.

Every organization in every field has its own culture. That culture develops over time and is most often influenced by the strongest and most negative personalities in the organization. The cultural norms that develop in the organization dictate how its people should look, talk, act and present themselves to the public.

Many segments of prehospital EMS are overdue for a cultural revolution. The expectation in too many organizations is that paramedics will be cool, curt, and unfeeling in their contacts and relationships with patients. The organizational culture in too many places has wrongly concluded that paramedics are trained and intended only to "save lives" and that any lesser assignment is wasteful and demeaning.

In too many places, continuing education and refresher training is considered a burden, and recertification exams are resented. These attitudes often reflect an organization's culture. Inherent in them is the arrogant conclusion that some paramedics already know everything they need to know, and don't want to be bothered by additional knowledge. The attitudes and the culture are badly in need of change.

If you have just purchased this book and are scheduled to begin paramedic training, and if you are planning on a career full of hot calls, exciting trauma, and back-to-back defibrillations, this would be a good time to reconsider your plans. The authors of this book would join me in urging you to take another look at EMS and what it's all about.

First, there is a lot of personal responsibility. A brief review of some of the chapters will give you an idea of what you'll be expected to know. It will be your responsibility to maintain that base of knowledge. Don't count on someone else to refresh your knowledge and skills for you. Becoming a paramedic is not an educational end-point. It must be the beginning of a continual, career length, self-motivated process of personal improvement.

There's also the last word in EMS—"service." Choosing to become a paramedic is a willing, voluntary commitment to serve others. Your patients will come in all sizes, shapes, ages, conditions, and temperaments. Some are young, but most are old. Some are rude and abusive. Many of them are ill with serious health problems of their own making.

Regardless, it is the paramedic's role to serve all patients with equal concern, skill, and attention. Inevitably, nations and their people are judged by how well they care for the ill, the infirm, and the less fortunate among them. When a paramedic concludes that a patient is unworthy of his or her best efforts, that paramedic diminishes the value of life itself.

The authors of this book have created a superb tool for educating a whole new generation of paramedics. But we can use this book to achieve more than just getting people through the course and their certification exams. We can use it to inspire every student to strive for the levels of commitment and excellence that have been exemplified by the authors.

The time has come for instructors and students alike to make an unshakable commitment to a renewed culture of caring. The process must start as the student enters the classroom and opens this book. Nurturing and enhancing the necessary knowledge, skills, abilities, and attitude must continue throughout the paramedic's career—even when the organizational culture commands mediocrity.

JAMES O. PAGE

Preface

Congratulations on your decision to further your EMS career by undertaking the course of training required for certification as an Emergency Medical Technician–Paramedic! The world of paramedic emergency care is one which you will find both challenging and rewarding. Whether you will be working as a volunteer or paid paramedic, you will find the field of advanced prehospital care very interesting.

This textbook will serve as your guide to advanced prehospital care. It is based upon the 1985 United States Department of Transportation National Paramedic Training Curriculum. The text is divided into 34 chapters, separated into 6 divisions. The first division is entitled "Prehospital Environment" and presents the basics of advanced prehospital care. The second division, "Preparatory Information," reviews the basics of emergency medical care. It also addresses the fundamentals of paramedic practice, including patient assessment, advanced airway management, shock, and emergency pharmacology. "Trauma Emergencies," the third division of the text, discusses advanced prehospital care of injuries. The trauma presentation is based upon the management principles taught in Prehospital Trauma Life Support and Basic Trauma Life Support courses. The fourth division of the book, "Medical Emergencies," is the longest and addresses paramedic level care of medical problems. Particular emphasis is placed upon cardiovascular emergencies, including interpretation of the electrocardiogram. The last two divisions address advanced prehospital care of "Obstetrical and Gynecological Emergencies" and "Psychiatric Emergencies."

Skills

Advanced prehospital skills are best learned in the classroom, laboratory, and clinical setting. The common advanced prehospital skills are presented in both the text and in the Procedure Sheets. Review these before practicing the skill.

It is important to point out that this text cannot teach skills. These are only learned under the watchful eye of a paramedic instructor.

How to Use This Textbook

Paramedic Emergency Care is designed to accompany a paramedic education program which follows the 1985 *United States Department of Transportation Emergency Medical Technician–Paramedic: National*

Standard Curriculum. The education program should include ample classroom, practical laboratory, inhospital clinical, and prehospital field experience. These educational experiences must be guided by instructors and preceptors with special training and experience in their areas of participation in your program.

It is intended that your program coordinator will assign reading from *Paramedic Emergency Care* in preparation for each classroom lecture and discussion section. The knowledge gained from reading this text will form the foundation of the information you will need in order to function effectively as a paramedic in your EMS system. Your instructors will build upon this information to strengthen your knowledge and understanding of advanced prehospital care so that you may apply it in your work. The inhospital clinical and prehospital field experiences will further refine your knowledge and skills under the watchful eyes of your preceptors.

In preparing for each classroom session, read the assigned chapter carefully. First, review the chapter objectives. They will identify what the authors feel are important concepts to be learned from the reading. Read the case study to get a feeling of why a chapter is important and how the knowledge it contains can be applied in the field. Read the content carefully while keeping the chapter objectives in mind. Lastly, re-read the chapter objectives and be sure that you are able to answer each one completely. If you aren't, re-read the section of the chapter to which the objective relates. If you still do not understand the objective or any portion of what you have read, ask your instructor to explain it at your next class session.

Ideally, you should read this entire text at least three times. The chapter should be read in preparation for the class session, the entire division should be read before the division test, and the entire text should be re-read before the course final exam. While this might seem like a lot of reading, it will improve your classroom performance and your knowledge of emergency care.

The workbook that accompanies this text can also assist in improving classroom performance. It contains information, sample test questions and exercises designed to assist learning. Its use can be very helpful in identifying the important elements of paramedic education, in exercising the knowledge of prehospital care, and in helping you self-test your knowledge.

Paramedic Emergency Care attempts to present the knowledge of emergency care in as accurate, standardized, and clear a manner as is possible. However, each EMS system is uniquely different and it is beyond the scope of this text to address all differences. You must count heavily on your instructors, the program coordinator, and ultimately the program medical director, to identify how emergency care procedures are applied in your system.

BRYAN E. BLEDSOE, D.O.
ROBERT S. PORTER
BRUCE R. SHADE

Acknowledgments

Production

The task of writing, editing, reviewing, and producing a textbook the size of **Paramedic Emergency Care** is indeed complex. Many talented people have been involved in this project.

The idea of a paramedic textbook was first discussed in the mid-1980s after release of the 1985 paramedic curriculum. Claire Merrick, formerly with Brady, finally got the project rolling by uniting the various authors and contributors. The project was later assumed by Susan Willig and Natalie Anderson when Claire left Brady. Susan and Natalie, both tremendously enthusiastic about this project and EMS, brought many great and novel ideas to EMS publishing. The format and style of this text is a reflection of their experience and expertise and will quite likely set the standard for EMS publications in the future.

After completion of the manuscript the work underwent developmental editing under the skillful direction of Ray Mullaney. Ray orchestrated a group of developmental editors who went through the 2,000 page manuscript with amazing speed and accuracy. Ray's attention to detail and experience is evident in every part of the work.

The chore of production editor was assigned to Kathryn Pavelec who took reams (literally) of manuscript, photographs, and art and produced the book in your hands. Her perseverance is deeply appreciated. She had the uncanny ability to find us, no matter where in the hospital (or world) we were located. Kathy is a true professional. This text is as much hers as it is ours.

The art and photographs came from many sources. Most of the staged photographs were by George Dodson with Lightworks Studios of Annapolis, Maryland. The new art was drafted by Network Graphics of Hauppauge, New York. Thanks to both these sources for their commitment to excellence.

Finally, the job of selling the text was handled by the Prentice-Hall Marketing Department and the Brady Telemarketing Personnel. These professionals not only sell, but also provide essential feedback from readers and instructors throughout the world.

Reviewers

The reviewers of **Paramedic Emergency Care** provided many excellent suggestions and ideas for improving the text. The quality of the reviews was outstanding and the reviews were a major aid in the preparation and revision of the manuscript. The assistance provided by these EMS experts is deeply appreciated. The reviewers include:

Jane W. Ball, R.N., Dr.P.H.
Pediatric EMS Training Coordinator
Children's Hospital National Medical Center
Washington, D.C.

Richard K. Beck, NREMT-P
Program Director/Lead Instructor
University of Alabama in Huntsville
School of Primary Medical Care
Emergency Medical Programs
Huntsville, Alabama

Richard S. Bennett, R.N., NREMT-P
Project Administrator
EMS for Children
Boise, Idaho

Marvin Birnbaum, M.D., Ph.D.
EMS Program
Clinical Science Center
University of Wisconsin
Madison, Wisconsin

Chief Kevin S. Brame
Battalion Chief
Orange County Fire Department
Orange County, California

Dena Brownstein, M.D.
Seattle Children's Hospital
Seattle, Washington

Debra Cason, R.N., M.S., EMT-P
Assistant Professor and EMS Program Director
University of Texas Southwestern Medical Center at Dallas
Dallas, Texas

Richard A. Cherry, M.Ed., NREMT-P
Director of Paramedic Training
Department of Critical Care and Emergency Medicine
SUNY Health Science Center
Syracuse, New York

Daniel J. Cobaugh, Pharm.D.
Clinical Toxicology Fellow
University of Pittsburgh School of Pharmacology
Pittsburgh, Pennsylvania

Neil Coker, EMT-P
Emergency Medical Programs
Texas Tech University Health Sciences Center
Lubbock, Texas

Judith A. Cremeens, R.N., M.Ed., CEN, NREMT-P
Assistant Professor of Emergency Medical Care
Department of Medical Services Technology
Eastern Kentucky University
Richmond, Kentucky

Ken D'Alessandro, NREMT-P
Training Officer
City of Pittsburgh EMS
Pittsburgh, Pennsylvania

Bonnie S. Dean, R.N., B.S.N., D.A.B.A.T.
Assistant Director
Pittsburgh Poison Control Center
Pittsburgh, Pennsylvania

C. Scott Dembrowski, A.A.S., NREMT-P
EMS Instructor
Columbia State Community College
Columbus, Ohio

Pamela B. doCarmo, M.S., NREMT-P
Program Head of Emergency Medical Service Technology
Northern Virginia Community College
Annandale, Virginia

Martin R. Eichelberger, M.D.
Director, Emergency Trauma Services
Children's Hospital National Medical Center
Washington, D.C.

Phil Fontanarosa, M.D.
Attending Physician and Research Director
Department of Emergency Medicine
Akron City Hospital
Akron, Ohio

Rusty R. Fowler, B.S., NREMT-P
Program Director, EMT/Paramedic Program
Chattanooga State Technical Community College
Chattanooga, Tennessee

Captain Steven K. Frye, EMT-P
Anne Arundel County Fire Department
Training and Research Division
Millersville, Maryland

Carol Goodykoontz, EMT-P
University of Texas Southwestern Medical Center
Dallas, Texas

Owen M. Grossman, M.D., F.A.A.F.P.
Assistant Professor and Associate Chairman
Department of Family Medicine
Texas Tech University Health Sciences Center
Regional Academic Health Center of the Permian Basin
Odessa, Texas

Greg L. Kennedy, A.S., B.B.A., NREMT-P
Faculty, Emergency Health Sciences
University of Southern Louisiana
Lafayette, Louisiana

Ken Koch, EMT-P
EMS Coordinator
East Central College
Union, Missouri

Alexander E. Kuehl, M.D., M.P.H.
Associate Professor
Cornell Medical College
Director, Emergency Medical Program
New York Hospital
Chairman, Education Committee, National Association of EMS
    Physicians
New York, New York

Mark Lockhart, NREMT-P
Education Coordinator
Department of Paramedic Education
Saint John's Mercy Medical Center
Saint Louis, Missouri

Paul Maniscalco, B.S., EMT-P
Deputy Chief, New York City EMS
President, National Association of Emergency Medical Technicians
New York, New York

Gregg S. Margolis, B.S., EMT-P
Coordinator, Life Support
Office of Education
Center for Emergency Medicine of Western Pennsylvania
Pittsburgh, Pennsylvania

Bill Metcalf, EMT-P
EMS Director
American College of Emergency Physicians
Irving, Texas

Linda D. Metcalf, EMT-P
Executive Director, Colorado Trauma Institute
Co-Director, Colorado Injury Prevention Research Center
Denver, Colorado

Chief Gary P. Morris, EMT-P
Deputy Fire Chief
Phoenix Fire Department
Phoenix, Arizona

Jim Moshinskie, MSHP, EMT-P
EMS Program Coordinator
Scott and White Memorial Hospital
Texas A&M College of Medicine
Temple, Texas

Kevin Parrish, R.N., EMT-P
Actronics, Inc.
Pittsburgh, Pennsylvania

Dwight A. Polk, B.A., NREMT-P
Paramedic Coordinator
University of Maryland
Baltimore, Maryland

David Potashnick, EMT-P
Paramedic Training Program
Hahnemann University
Philadelphia, Pennsylvania

Laura Randall, R.N.
Executive Director
Northern Kentucky EMS
Fort Thomas, Kentucky

Ham Robbins, R.N., EMT-P
State of Maine Emergency Medical Services
NCSEMSTC, Publications Review Committee
Augusta, Maine

Ronald Roth, M.D., F.A.C.E.P.
Assistant Professor of Medicine
Division of Emergency Medicine
University of Pittsburgh
Medical Director, Paramedic Education
Center for Emergency Medicine of Western Pennsylvania
Pittsburgh, Pennsylvania

Nels Sanddal, EMT-P
North Country Media Group
Great Falls, Montana

Andrew Stern, NREMT-P
Paramedic Supervisor
Department of EMS–Town of Colonie
Town of Colonie, New York

Douglas Stevenson, EMT-P
Houston Community College
Houston, Texas

David W. Throckmorton, M.D.
Clinical Associate Professor & Chief
Emergency Medicine Programs
University of Alabama in Huntsville
Medical Director of Emergency Services
Huntsville Hospital
Huntsville, Alabama

Patricia L. Tritt, R.N., B.S.
Swedish Medical Center
Englewood, Colorado

Michael Wainscott, M.D.
Department of Emergency Medicine
University of Texas Southwestern Medical Center
Dallas, Texas

Katherine West, R.N., M.S.Ed.
Infection Control/Emerging Concepts Inc.
Springfield, Virginia

Chief Richard Wiederhold, B.A., EMT-P
Brevard County Fire Rescue
Merritt Island, Florida

Jean B. Will, R.N., M.S.N., C.E.N., EMT-P
Executive Director
Regional EMS Training Center
Hahnemann University
Philadelphia, Pennsylvania

Mark Winstead, EMT-P
EMS Training Coordinator
Seminole County Department of Public Safety, EMS Division
Seminole County, Florida
Paramedic Program Coordinator
Seminole Community College
Sanford, Florida

Frank M. Yeiser, M.D., F.A.C.E.P.
Medical Director
Division of Emergency Medical Services
Department of Health
Commonwealth of Virginia
Richmond, Virginia

Organizations and Individuals

The authors would like to gratefully acknowledge the assistance and support of the following organizations and persons who contributed signficantly to the development of this manuscript.

Georgetown Hospital
Kenneth Potete, Administrator
Georgetown, Texas

Williamson County EMS
George Stephenson, Director
John Sneed, Training Coordinator
Georgetown, Texas

City of Annapolis Fire Department EMS
Annapolis, Maryland

Anne Arundel Medical Center Emergency Department
Annapolis, Maryland

Scott and White Memorial Hospital
Department of Plastic and Reconstructive Surgery
Charles N. Verheyden, M.D., Ph.D., F.A.C.S.
Raleigh R. White, IV, M.D., F.A.C.S.
Dennis J. Lynch, M.D., F.A.C.S.
Peter Grothaus, M.B., Ch.B., F.R.C.S.(C)
Texas A & M University College of Medicine
Temple, Texas

Scott and White Memorial Hospital
Department of Medical Photography
David Hansen
Texas A & M University College of Medicine
Temple, Texas

Maryland Institute for Emergency Medical Services Systems
Baltimore, Maryland

Center for Emergency Medicine of Western Pennsylvania
Pittsburgh, Pennsylvania

Acadian Ambulance Service, Inc.
W. Keith Simon
Lafayette, Louisiana

City of Phoenix Fire Department
Deputy Chief Gary Morris
Phoenix, Arizona

Presbyterian University Hospital
Rich Boland, EMS Coordinator
Trauma Services
Pittsburgh, Pennsylvania

Publications Committee
National Council of State EMS Training Coordinators

The following persons gave freely of their time to act as models or to provide technical support for many of the photographs used in this book:

Scott Gibson, EMT-P, Williamson County EMS

Dave Reimer, EMT-P, Williamson County EMS

Bobby Slaughter, EMT-P, Williamson County EMS

John Sneed, EMT-P, Williamson County EMS

Paul Ward, EMT, Round Rock Fire Department

Janice Ward, LVN, EMT, Georgetown Hospital

Reta Reimer, LVN, Austin MediCenter

Cyndi Gibson, Georgetown Hospital

Jana Slaughter, Georgetown Hospital

In addition, the following children served as models for various photographs in the book:

Julie Ward

Erin Ward

Melanie Slaughter

Jennifer Dean

Andrea Bledsoe

Bryan Bledsoe, II

Brian Slaughter

Special thanks go to Ronnie Taylor, EMT-P, with the City of Austin EMS, who provided excellent moulage injuries for the photography sessions.

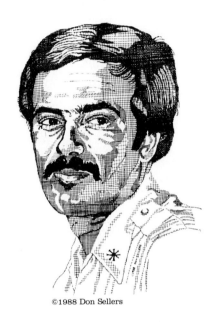

©1988 Don Sellers

This textbook is respectfully dedicated to the memory of

James Yvorra

Jim was a Deputy Chief and EMT with the Berywn Heights, Maryland, Fire Department. He was killed in January of 1988 while assisting an injured person at the scene of a motor vehicle accident in suburban Maryland. Jim was a former editor for Brady and had just finished writing his second book. In addition to his EMS work Jim was a nationally recognized expert in the field of hazardous materials incident response. Jim was a remarkable individual. His death was indicative of his dedication to helping others. It also reminds us of the inherent dangers of our profession. He will be truly missed.

About the Authors

BRYAN E. BLEDSOE, D.O., EMT-P

Dr. Bledsoe is an emergency medicine physician with special interest in prehospital care. He received a B.S. degree from the University of Texas at Arlington in Arlington, Texas and received his medical degree from the University of North Texas–Texas College of Osteopathic Medicine. His internship was at Texas Tech University in Odessa, Texas, and residency training at Scott and White Memorial Hospital–Texas A&M College of Medicine in Temple, Texas. Prior to attending medical school, Dr. Bledsoe, a Texas native, worked as an EMT, Paramedic, and Paramedic Instructor. He completed EMT training in 1974 and paramedic training in 1976 and worked for 6 years as a field paramedic in Fort Worth. In 1979 he joined the faculty of Texas College of Osteopathic Medicine and served as coordinator of EMT and Paramedic programs at the college. He is active in emergency medicine and a member of numerous professional organizations. He is on the board of medical directors for NAEMT and co-medical director for the paramedic society.

Dr. Bledsoe has authored three other EMS books published by Brady Communications including *Manual of Emergency Drugs*, *Prehospital Emergency Pharmacology*, and *Atlas of Paramedic Skills*. He is married to Emma Bledsoe. They have two children, Bryan and Andrea, and live in Arlington, Texas.

ROBERT S. PORTER, M.A., NREMT-P

Mr. Porter is the Director of the Central New York Emergency Medical Services Program, which serves an eleven-county region with a population of 1.4 million people. Mr. Porter is a Wisconsin native and received his bachelor's degree in education from the University of Wisconsin. He completed his master's degree in Health Education from Central Michigan University. Mr. Porter was certified as a Basic EMT and EMT Instructor in 1973 and was nationally registered as a paramedic in 1978. Mr. Porter has been an EMS educator since 1973 and has taught Basic EMT and paramedic programs in Wisconsin, Michigan, Louisiana, and Pennsylvania. Mr. Porter is a past chairman of the National Society of

EMT Instructors/Coordinators and is a site evaluator for accreditation of paramedic programs. He has published numerous articles in EMS periodicals and is the author of the workbook that accompanies this text.

BRUCE R. SHADE, NREMT-P

Mr. Shade is currently Commissioner for the Cleveland Emergency Medical Service in Cleveland, Ohio. Cleveland EMS is a third city service operation that responds to over 70,000 EMS calls per year. Mr. Shade has attended Cuyahoga Community College and Lakeland Community College in Cleveland, Ohio. Mr. Shade, an Ohio native, was certified as an EMT in 1972 and as a paramedic in 1976. He was educational supervisor and paramedic instructor for the city of Cleveland from 1980–1986. Mr. Shade is currently Chairperson, Society of EMT Instructor/Coordinators with the NAEMT and a member of many other professional organizations. Mr. Shade is co-author of *Advanced Cardiac Life Support: Certification, Preparation, and Review,* published by Brady Communications. In addition, he is a frequent contributor to EMS periodicals. He is married to Cheri Shade. They have two children, Katie and Christopher. He and his family live in Willoughby, Ohio.

About the Contributors

RICHARD A. CHERRY, M.Ed., NREMT-P

Mr. Cherry is Director of Paramedic Education for the SUNY Health Science Center in Syracuse, New York. He is a New York native and holds a B.A. degree in Education from Saint Bonaventure University in Olean, N.Y. and a M.Ed. degree from SUNY College in Oswego, N.Y.. He was initially certified as an EMT in 1975 and as a paramedic in 1978. He is active in instruction of BCLS, ACLS, ATLS, and PALS courses. He has published numerous articles in EMS and Emergency Medicine journals. Mr. Cherry is married to Patricia Cherry. He and his wife reside in Dewitt, N.Y.

DEPUTY CHIEF GARY P. MORRIS

Chief Morris is currently Deputy Fire Chief of the Phoenix, Arizona, Fire Department. He holds an A.A. degree in Fire Science from Phoenix College as well as a B.S. degree in Industrial Supervision from Arizona State University in Tempe, Arizona. Chief Morris was certified as an EMT in 1971 and was one of the first two EMT's with the Phoenix Fire Department to do so. He was certified as a Paramedic in 1975 during Arizona's first state-sponsored paramedic training program. Chief Morris has many publications to his credit including over 2 dozen EMS journal articles and numerous chapters in EMS and Fire Service Books. He remains active in EMS instruction with special interest in Mass Casualty response and is a popular speaker at EMS conferences. Chief Morris is the recipient of *Firehouse Magazine's* Heroism and Community Service Award, the Disabled American Veterans' Meritorious Service and Life Savings Efforts Award, as well as the Phoenix City Council's Phoenix Very Outstanding Citizen Award. Chief Morris is married to Shirley Morris, a Registered Nurse. They have four children and reside in Phoenix, Arizona.

ROD DENNISON, EMT-P

Rod Dennison is the Program Manager of the Texas Department of Health Region 1 EMS Division. Mr. Dennison is a San Antonio, Texas, native and has attended Texas A&M University, the University of Texas at Arlington, and Baylor University. He holds a B.S. degree in Education with emphasis on English and Biology. Mr. Dennison is a nationally-recognized expert in technical rope rescue and cave rescue. He has written many articles and presented several seminars on technical rope rescue and mass casualty response. He has been an EMT since 1976 and a paramedic since 1978. Mr. Dennison is single and lives in Temple, Texas.

Notice

It is the intent of the authors and publisher that this textbook be used as part of a formal paramedic education program taught by a qualified instructor and supervised by a licensed physician. The care procedures presented here represent accepted practices in the United States. They are not offered as a standard of care. Paramedic-level emergency care is to be performed *only* under the authority and guidance of a licensed physician. It is the reader's responsibility to know and follow local care protocols as provided by medical advisors directing the system to which he or she belongs. Also, it is the reader's responsibility to stay informed of emergency care procedure changes.

Notice on Drugs and Drug Dosages

Every effort has been made to ensure that the drug dosages presented in this textbook are in accordance with nationally accepted standards. When applicable, the dosages and routes are taken from the American Heart Association's Advanced Cardiac Life Support Guidelines. The American Medical Association's publication *Drug Evaluations,* and the material published in the *Physician's Desk Reference,* are followed with regard to drug dosages not covered by the American Heart Association's guidelines. It is the responsibility of the reader to be familiar with the drugs used in their system, as well as the dosages specified by the medical director. The drugs presented in this book should only be administered by direct order, either verbally or through accepted standing orders, of a licensed physician.

Notice on Gender Usage

The English language has historically given preference to the male gender. Among many words, the pronouns "he" and "his" are commonly used to describe both genders. Society evolves faster than language and the male pronouns still predominate in our speech. The authors have made great effort to treat the two genders equally, recognizing that a significant percentage of paramedics are female. However, in some instances, male pronouns have been used to describe both male and female paramedics solely for the purpose of brevity. This is not intended to offend any readers of the female gender.

Notice on Photographs

Please note that many of the photographs contained in this book are taken of actual emergency situations. As such, it is possible that they may not accurately depict current, appropriate, or advisable practices of emergency medical care. They have been included for the sole purpose of giving general insight into real-life emergency settings.

BRADY

Paramedic Emergency Care

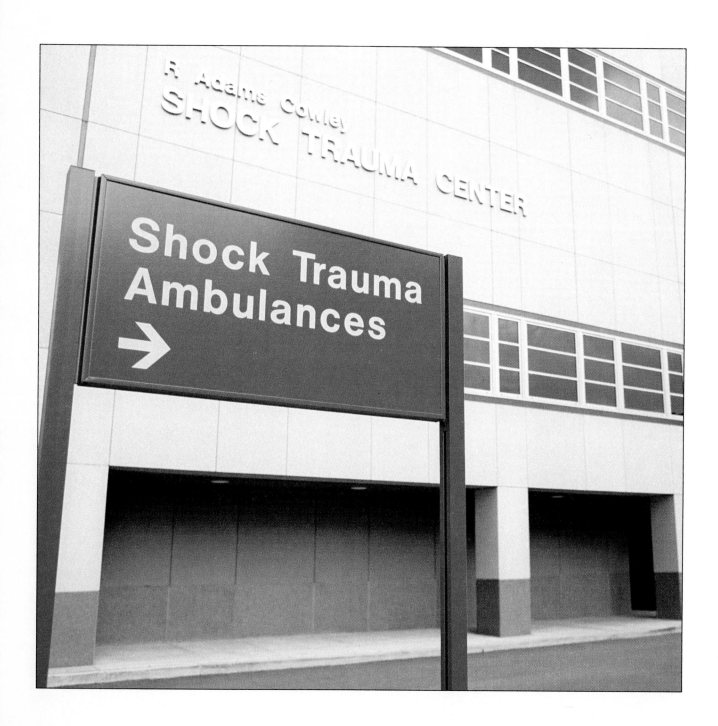

Roles and Responsibilities of the Paramedic

Objectives for Chapter 1

Upon completing this chapter, the student should be able to:

1. Define the role of the EMT-Paramedic.
2. Define and give examples of professional ethics.
3. Define and give examples of behavior that characterizes the health care professional.
4. List the duties of the EMT-Paramedic in preparation for handling emergency medical responses.
5. List the duties of the EMT-Paramedic during an emergency response.
6. List the duties of the EMT-Paramedic after an emergency response.
7. List the post-graduation responsibilities of the EMT-Paramedic.
8. State the major purposes of a national organization.
9. List some national organizations for EMS providers.
10. State the major purposes of the National Registry of Emergency Medical Technicians.
11. Describe the major benefits of subscribing to professional journals.
12. State the benefits and responsibilities of continuing education for the EMT-Paramedic.
13. Distinguish between certification, licensure, and reciprocity.

On a warm summer evening in July, 1958, two speeding cars collide at an urban intersection. Bystanders immediately recognize that the accident is serious and notify the police. The police dispatcher relays the call to patrolling officers by way of two-way radios. Three ambulance services in the vicinity hear about a "10-50 major" on their police monitors. After noting the address, the ambulance drivers race to their vehicles. The first ambulance to hit the street is owned by Nathan–Crigler Funeral home. The ambulance is truly a work of art. It is a dark blue Mercury station wagon, with a chrome mechanical siren and a fireball beacon on the roof. Most impressive, however, is what's inside. The vehicle contains a high-performance Ford engine, four-speed transmission, four-barrel carburetor, and racing suspension. As the ambulance turns onto the highway, the driver floors the accelerator. The ambulance quickly accelerates to a cruising speed of more than 100 miles per hour. Down the road the driver sees the flashing beacons of the police cars and begins to slow, down-shifting, and pulling right up to the most damaged automobile. Immediately, the driver and the attendant jump out and start looking for the most injured patient. Near the corner, they find an unconscious female with multiple facial lacerations. The attendant runs to the ambulance, grabs the stretcher, and quickly returns to the patient. The driver and the attendant grab the patient—one under the armpits, the other under the knees—and quickly lift her onto the stretcher. During the lift, the patient's head falls back and she moans lightly. She moans again as her head hits the top of the stretcher. After quickly putting her in the ambulance, both the driver and the attendant return to the front seat. The driver states, "She looks bad . . . Let's haul!," and, with a jolt, the ambulance departs for the hospital. With the road straight the driver is able to go 110 miles per hour. They soon arrive at St. Mary's hospital and deliver the

INTRODUCTION

So you want to become a paramedic! Before you begin this long but rewarding journey, it is important to understand what a paramedic is, what your future role will be, and what society will expect from you. In addition, you must understand how to maintain a professional attitude in a field that has evolved from primitive roots to the sophisticated industry known as **Emergency Medical Services** (EMS) in less than 30 years.

It's not all flashing lights and sirens. The paramedic is expected to provide not only competent emergency medical care, but also emotional support for the patient and family members. Often, you will be providing these services for people who neither understand nor appreciate what you did, and are unaware of your extensive training. But, if self-satisfaction and pride in a job well done are reward enough for you, and if you have a genuine desire to help people in need, being a paramedic can be a very fulfilling career.

As the highest-trained prehospital emergency care provider in the EMS system, the paramedic accepts the awesome responsibility for patient care. While others manage a variety of factors during an emergency medical incident, the paramedic concentrates on the care and well-being of the patient. Your willingness to accept this role during a medical emer-

■ **emergency medical services** a complex health care system that provides immediate, on-scene patient care to those suffering sudden illness or injury.

patient to a waiting stretcher. Without changing the sheets, they return the stretcher to the ambulance and head back to the accident scene. After 22 weeks, the patient finally was able to leave the hospital. The doctors had determined that nothing else could be done for her neck-down paralysis, and she was sent to a home for the crippled.

Yesterday, a similar accident happened at the same intersection. As before, bystanders immediately knew it was serious. A passerby grabbed his cellular telephone and dialed 9-1-1. The EMS dispatcher took the essential information and activated the EMS system. The first members of the EMS system to arrive were firefighters trained as EMT's. The lieutenant in charge quickly assessed the scene and requested additional equipment and personnel. Within a minute, the first ambulance arrived. The senior paramedic quickly surveyed the scene and noted that five people had been injured, two apparently seriously. He declared a Multiple-Casualty Incident and implemented the Incident Command System. The patients were triaged, and each responding ambulance had its assignment. The most critical patient was an unconscious female lying near the curb. An EMT manually stabilized the patient's spine while the paramedic performed the primary assessment. Then the secondary assessment was completed. The patient's Glasgow Coma Scale was 10, but her vital signs were stable. The paramedics quickly, but gently, completely immobilized the patient from head to toe. Oxygen was administered and an IV established. The patient was transported to a Level I trauma center, where a neurosurgeon assumed her care upon arrival.

The patient responded well. She will have to spend five weeks in cervical traction and she faces a long rehabilitation. However, she has no paralysis and the doctors expect her to recover.

gency and direct others to carry out your treatment plan is the first step in becoming a paramedic.

What will the public expect from you? Prior to the late 1960s, emergency medical services were far different from those available today. Most local fire departments had primitive rescue squads whose members had little training in emergency procedures and little or no knowledge of spinal immobilization or airway management techniques. Funeral homes operated ambulance services that offered little more than fast, horizontal transport in vehicles ill-suited for this purpose. The public did not expect much from prehospital emergency medical care, and did not receive much.

In 1966, a major research project conducted by the National Academy of Sciences-National Research Council led to the publication of a landmark paper titled "Accidental Death and Disability: The Neglected Disease of Modern Society." This historic document, commonly called the "white paper," described the inadequacies of emergency medical care in this country. It criticized both hospital emergency rooms and prehospital emergency care. It made recommendations for establishing emergency medical services systems and emergency medical technician training programs, and for upgrading ambulances. Through the efforts of the U.S. Department of Transportation Curriculum Committee, the Emergency

✱ The paramedic's primary responsibility in any emergency is patient care.

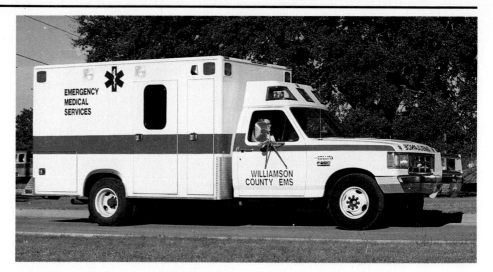

FIGURE 1-1 EMS has evolved into a comprehensive health care system providing state of the art emergency care at the scene and en-route to the hospital. The modern ambulance is truly a mobile emergency department.

Medical Technician (EMT), a professionally trained and certified basic-life-support provider, evolved. The EMT would be trained to administer oxygen and cardiopulmonary resuscitation, perform basic splinting and bandaging, and immobilize patients who had spinal cord injuries. Thus, the EMT became the first certified prehospital emergency care provider.

The innovative work of Dr. J. Frank Pantridge, a physician at the Royal Victoria Hospital in Belfast, Northern Ireland, introduced the concept of bringing advanced cardiac life support to the patient in the field. Shortly thereafter, legislation was enacted in the United States allowing specially trained EMT's to provide services that used to require a physician. Dr. Eugene Nagel, with the University of Miami School of Medicine, trained the first U.S. paramedics in Miami. Formal paramedic programs were soon organized in Los Angeles, Seattle, and Columbus, Ohio. These important developments began as bold initiatives by a few dedicated physicians who believed that prehospital emergency care would reduce preventable deaths. Today, there are more than 400 paramedic education programs in the United States.

The greatest cultural impact, however, came in 1971. The television series "Emergency," which popularized two young firefighter paramedics in weekly episodes, set the first standard for the professional paramedic. They were clean-cut, they responded promptly, they had a solution for everything, and they remained calm in the most stressful situations. The children who watched that show in the '70s are today's taxpayers. They expect the same skillful, compassionate, top-quality care that was portrayed on "Emergency." Achieving such a high level of patient care and customer service is a major challenge for the paramedic of the '90s.

Much of this chapter will deal with conceptual and highly specialized information. However, the ability to accept these concepts and apply them to one's professional conduct ultimately separates the outstanding paramedic from an average one.

PROFESSIONAL ETHICS

■ **ethics** the rules, standards, and morals governing the activities of a group or profession.

Ethics are the rules or standards that govern the conduct of members of a particular group. Physicians have long subscribed to a body of ethical standards that were developed primarily for the benefit of the patient.

The Oath of Geneva

I solemnly pledge myself to consecrate my life to the service of humanity; I will give to my teachers the respect and gratitude which is their due; I will practice my profession with conscience and dignity; the health of my patient will be my first consideration; I will respect the secrets which are confided in me; I will maintain by all the means in my power the honor and noble traditions of the medical profession; my colleagues will be my brothers; I will not permit considerations of religion, nationality, race, party, politics, or social standing to intervene between my duty and my patient; I will maintain the utmost respect for human life from the time of conception; even under threat, I will not make use of my medical knowledge contrary to the laws of humanity. I make these promises solemnly, freely and upon my honor.

FIGURE 1-2

These standards have subsequently been extended to the allied health professions. Ethics are not laws, but standards for honorable behavior designed by the group; conformity by all members is expected. As members of an **allied health** profession, paramedics must recognize a responsibility not only to their patients, but also to society, to other health professionals, and to themselves. In 1948, the World Medical Association adopted the "Oath of Geneva." (See Figure 1-2.) In 1978, the National Association of Emergency Medical Technicians adopted the EMT Oath (see Figure 1-3) and a Code of Ethics (see Figure 1-4). These documents detail the guiding principles for professional EMT service.

■ **allied health** term used to describe ancillary health care professionals, apart from physicians and nurses, such as paramedics, respiratory therapists, and physical therapists.

The EMT Oath

Be it pledged as an Emergency Medical Technician, I will honor the physical and judicial laws of God and man. I will follow that regimen which, according to my ability and judgment, I consider for the benefit of patients and abstain from whatever is deleterious and mischievous, nor shall I suggest any such counsel. Into whatever homes I enter, I will go into them for the benefit of only the sick and injured, never revealing what I see or hear in the lives of men unless required by law.

I shall also share my medical knowledge with those who may benefit from what I have learned. I will serve unselfishly and continuously in order to help make a better world for all mankind.

While I continue to keep this oath unviolated, may it be granted to me to enjoy life, and the practice of the art, respected by all men, in all times. Should I trespass or violate this oath, may the reverse be my lot. So help me God.

Adopted by The National Association of Emergency Medical Technicians, 1978

FIGURE 1-3

The EMT Code of Ethics

Professional status as an Emergency Medical Technician and Emergency Medical Technician-Paramedic is maintained and enriched by the willingness of the individual practitioner to accept and fulfill obligations to society, other medical professionals, and the profession of Emergency Medical Technician. As an Emergency Medical Technician at the basic level or an Emergency Medical Technician-Paramedic, I solemnly pledge myself to the following code of professional ethics:

A fundamental responsibility to the Emergency Medical Technician is to conserve life, to alleviate suffering, to promote health, to do no harm, and to encourage the quality and equal availability of emergency medical care.

The Emergency Medical Technician provides services based on human need, with respect for human dignity, unrestricted by consideration of nationality, race, creed, color, or status.

The Emergency Medical Technician does not use professional knowledge and skills in any enterprise detrimental to the public well being.

The Emergency Medical Technician respects and holds in confidence all information of a confidential nature obtained in the course of professional work unless required by law to divulge such information.

The Emergency Medical Technician, as a citizen, understands and upholds the law and performs the duties of citizenship; as a professional, the Emergency Medical Technician has the never-ending responsibility to work with concerned citizens and other health care professionals in promoting a high standard of emergency medical care to all people.

The Emergency Medical Technician shall maintain professional competence and demonstrate concern for the competence of other members of the Emergency Medical Services health care team.

An Emergency Medical Technician assumes responsibility in defining and upholding standards of professional practice and education.

The Emergency Medical Technician assumes responsibility for individual professional actions and judgment, both in dependent and independent emergency functions, and knows and upholds the laws which affect the practice of the Emergency Medical Technician.

An Emergency Medical Technician has the responsibility to be aware of and participate in matters of legislation affecting the Emergency Medical Technician and the Emergency Medical Services System.

The Emergency Medical Technician adheres to standards of personal ethics which reflect credit upon the profession.

Emergency Medical Technicians, or groups of Emergency Medical Technicians, who advertise professional services, do so in conformity with the dignity of the profession.

The Emergency Medical Technician has an obligation to protect the public by not delegating to a person less qualified, any service which requires the professional competence of an Emergency Medical Technician.

The Emergency Medical Technician will work harmoniously with and sustain confidence in Emergency Medical Technician associates, the nurse, the physician, and other members of the Emergency Medical Services health care team.

The Emergency Medical Technician refuses to participate in unethical procedures, and assumes the responsibility to expose incompetence or unethical conduct of others to the appropriate authority in a proper and professional manner.

The National Association of Emergency Medical Technicians

FIGURE 1-4

■ **morality** the principles of right and wrong as governed by individual conscience.

While legal guidelines obligate the paramedic to certain actions, ethical standards suggest that certain behaviors are right or wrong. The paramedic will encounter many situations that present a **moral dilemma.** For example, the paramedic must decide between a patient's rights and family members' wishes when called upon to resuscitate a terminally ill patient in cardiac arrest. Another example is that of the intoxicated, belligerent patient who has sustained a head injury, but refuses transport. The paramedic must choose between the risk of abandonment and a possible charge of false imprisonment when deciding how to best manage the patient. How paramedics act in such cases will depend mostly on their personal values and ethical convictions. Legally, a paramedic must provide for the physical well-being of the patient. Ethically, the paramedic must also care for the emotional welfare of the patient and others at the scene.

The science of EMS involves advanced technology, research, and the delivery of sophisticated prehospital emergency medical care. The art of EMS means carrying out the duties with sincerity, compassion, grace, and a respect for human dignity. The best paramedics are excellent technicians who never forget that their patients are human beings with rights and feelings. If you always place the patient's welfare above everything but your own safety, you will probably never commit an unethical act. Treating all patients as you would members of your own family is all that can be expected from you as a paramedic. The best paramedics are aware of not only their legal obligations, but also the ethical and moral responsibilities of the job.

PROFESSIONALISM

Professionalism describes the conduct or qualities that characterize a practitioner in a particular field or occupation. Health care professionals promote quality patient care and take pride in their profession; they set high goals. They earn the respect and confidence of team members by performing their duties to the best of their abilities, and by exhibiting a high level of respect for their profession. Attaining professionalism is not easy. It requires an understanding of what distinguishes the professional from the non-professional. Here are some guidelines:

Professionals place the patient first; non-professionals place their egos first. Professionals practice their skills to the point of mastery, then keep practicing them to improve and stay sharp. Non-professionals do not believe their skills will fade, and see no reason to constantly strive for improvement. Professionals understand the importance of response times; non-professionals get there when it's convenient. Professionals take refresher courses seriously, because they know they have forgotten a lot and they are eager for new information. Non-professionals believe they don't need training sessions and dislike being required to attend them. Professionals set high standards for themselves, their crew, their agency, and their system. Non-professionals aim for the minimum standard and can be counted on to take the path of least resistance. Professionals critically review their performance, always seeking a way to improve. Non-professionals look to protect themselves, to hide their inadequacies, and to place blame on others. Professionals check out all equipment prior to the emergency response. Non-professionals hope that everything will work, supplies will be in place, batteries will be charged, and oxygen levels will be adequate.

Maintaining professionalism requires effort. But, the result of that effort—the admiration and respect of one's peers—is the highest compliment a person can receive. True professionals establish excellence as their goal and never allow themselves to become satisfied with their performance. Professionalism is an attitude, not a matter of pay. It cannot be bought, rented, or faked. Although a young industry, EMS has achieved recognition as a bona fide allied health care profession. Gaining professional stature is the result of many hard-working, caring individuals who refused to compromise their standards. The paramedic must always strive to maintain that level of performance and commitment known as professionalism.

■ **professional** a person who exhibits the conduct or qualities that characterize a practitioner in a particular field or occupation.

✱ The paramedic is a health care professional.

ROLE OF THE PARAMEDIC

The role of the paramedic is diverse. It includes not only patient care, but a variety of responsibilities before, during, and after an emergency response. Prior to responding to a medical incident, preparation is the key. The paramedic must be prepared mentally, physically, and emotionally. At the very least, the paramedic is expected to maintain a high level of medical knowledge, expert recall of local treatment protocols, and a mastery of practical skills. Because the public has the right to quality patient care, these items are non-negotiable.

The physical demands of the job require ongoing training: aerobics for cardiovascular fitness; exercises for muscular strength and endurance; stretching for increased flexibility; and an understanding of the biomechanics of lifting, to prevent early retirement caused by lower-back injuries. Psychological stability is also essential to withstand the emotional strain of the job. Recognizing the effects of stress, and practicing ways to alleviate it, are the keys to long-term survival. The paramedic must also become familiar with:

- ❑ Policies and procedures of the local EMS system
- ❑ The communications system, both hardware (radios) and software (frequency utilization and communication protocols)
- ❑ Local geography, including populations during peak loads and alternative routes during rush hours
- ❑ Support agencies—what is available from neighboring departments and how to coordinate efforts and resources

Leadership is an important, but often forgotten, aspect of paramedic training. Paramedics are the prehospital team leaders. They must develop a leadership style that both suits their personalities and gets the job done. Although there are many successful styles of leadership, certain characteristics are common to all great leaders:

✳ The paramedic is the prehospital team leader.

- ❑ self-confidence
- ❑ established credibility
- ❑ inner strength
- ❑ the ability to remain in control
- ❑ the ability to communicate
- ❑ the willingness to make a decision
- ❑ the willingness to accept responsibility for the consequences of the team's actions

The successful team leader knows the members of the crew, and knows their capabilities and limitations. Ask crew members to do something they are not capable of doing, and they will question not their ability to perform, but your ability to lead. (See Figure 1-5.)

During an emergency response, the paramedic has the responsibility to:

1. Size up and assure scene security.
2. Determine the needs of the incident and communicate that information to the emergency medical dispatcher.
3. Conduct the patient assessment.
4. Assign priorities of care and develop a treatment plan.
5. Communicate the plan to crew members.

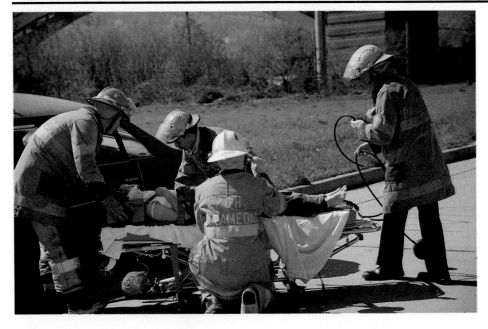

FIGURE 1-5 The paramedic is the leader of the emergency medical services team and must interact with patients, bystanders, and other rescue personnel in a professional and efficient manner.

6. Initiate basic and advanced life-support procedures, according to established standing orders. (See Figure 1-6.)
7. Assess the effects of treatment.
8. Establish contact with the medical control physician to discuss further treatment.
9. Direct and coordinate transport of the patient to the appropriate medical facility.
10. Maintain rapport with the patient, with support agencies, and with hospital personnel.

After the response, the paramedic is responsible for restocking the ambulance in preparation for the next call. The paramedic is also re-

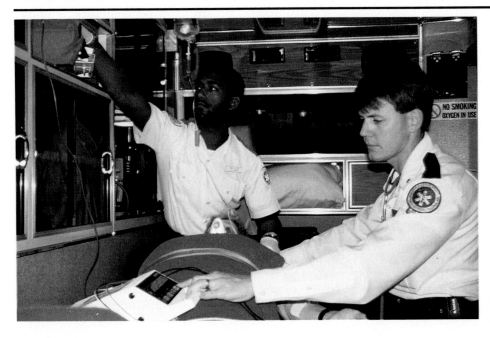

FIGURE I-6 The paramedic's primary responsibility in any emergency situation is patient care.

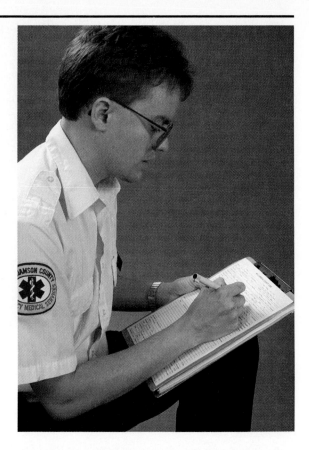

FIGURE 1-7 The responsibility of the paramedic does not end with delivery of the patient to the emergency department. Post-call documentation, re-stocking, and run critique are as important as the call itself.

sponsible for all documentation concerning the incident. The importance of accurate and complete documentation cannot be overemphasized. Proper record-keeping helps to ensure continuity of patient care from the prehospital to the hospital setting. To avoid potential legal problems and embarrassing court situations, the paramedic should record on the runsheet observations only (the patient had an odor of alcohol on his breath), not opinions (the patient was drunk). The former cannot be disputed and the latter cannot be proved. (See Figure 1-7.) Reviewing the call with crew members will improve future team performance. Finally, the paramedic team leader should check the crew members for signs of **critical-incident stress,** and assist anyone who needs help.

The role of the paramedic also includes duties not associated with emergency responses. CPR training, EMS demonstrations, seminars, teaching first-aid classes, and accident prevention programs are all responsibilities of the paramedic. In addition, educating the public to recognize a medical emergency, to initiate basic life-support procedures, and to promptly and efficiently access the EMS system is an important part of the paramedic's role.

POST-GRADUATE RESPONSIBILITIES

Upon successful completion of a course following the **National Standard Curriculum for EMT-P,** the paramedic usually will become certified. **Certification** is the process by which an agency or association grants recognition to an individual who has met its qualifications. Many states certify emergency medical technicians and paramedics. After attaining state certification, paramedics are permitted to work within an established

■ **critical incident stress** stress reaction commonly experienced by emergency personnel after a large or particularly stressful emergency response.

■ **National Standard Curriculum** paramedic training curriculm published by the United States Department of Transportation, widely used as the standard guidelines for paramedic education.

■ **certification** the process by which an agency or association grants recognition to an individual who has met its qualifications.

emergency medical services system under the direct supervision of a physician medical director.

Licensure is the process by which a governmental agency grants permission to engage in a given occupation to an applicant who has attained the degree of competency required to ensure the public's protection. For example, a state grants licenses to physicians, teachers, and barbers to perform the duties associated with those professions. Some states choose to license paramedics instead of certifying them.

Reciprocity is the process by which an agency grants automatic certification or licensure to an individual who has comparable certification or licensure from another agency. For example, some states grant reciprocity to paramedics who are certified in another state.

Maintaining certification is the responsibility of the paramedic. Each state, region, and local system may have its own policies, regulations, and procedures for certification. Paramedics cannot function without satisfying those requirements.

CONTINUING EDUCATION

Certification or licensure marks the beginning, not the end of the paramedic's education. Paramedics have an important responsibility to continue their education. Everyone is subject to the decay of knowledge and skills. Skills and knowledge, both basic and advanced, suffer from infrequent use. It is wise to remember that as call volume decreases, training must increase.

Field paramedics have many choices in continuing education for keeping up their interest and staying informed. Case reviews, videotapes, cassette lectures, inhospital rotations in patient care areas, field drills, mobile classrooms that bring educational presentations to outlying squads, self-study exercises, and periodic "teaching days," in which a variety of topics are covered in lectures and presentations, are a few of them. Administrators are limited only by their imagination and ingenuity when designing continuing education programs.

Since EMS is a relatively young industry, new technology and data emerge rapidly, and the paramedic must make a conscious effort to keep up. A variety of journals, seminars, and learning experiences are available to help. Only through continuing education and recertification requirements can the public be assured that quality patient care is being delivered. Refresher requirements vary from state to state, but the goal of this training is the same—to review previously learned materials and to receive new information.

✱ The paramedic must continually strive to stay abreast of changes in EMS.

PROFESSIONAL ORGANIZATIONS

Belonging to a professional organization is a good way to keep abreast of the latest technology. Communicating with members from other parts of the country provides an excellent opportunity to share ideas with people of similar backgrounds. Some national EMS organizations are:

National Association of Emergency Medical Technicians (NAEMT)
National Association of Search and Rescue (NASAR)
National Association of State EMS Directors (NASEMSD)
National Association of EMS Physicians (NAEMSP)

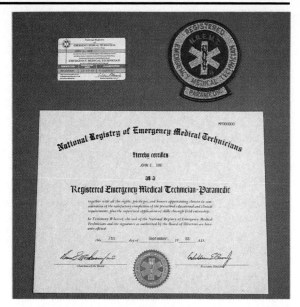

FIGURE 1-8 The National Registry of Emergency Medical Technicians develops and administers standardized testing for all levels of EMT from EMT-Basic to EMT-Paramedic. Completion of the National Registry testing may follow completion of an approved paramedic training program.

National Flight Paramedics Association (NFPA)

National Council of State EMS Training Coordinators (NCSEMSTC)

These are just some examples of organizations through which paramedics, emergency physicians, and nurses can enrich themselves and pursue their particular interests.

NATIONAL REGISTRY

The National Registry of EMT's is an agency that prepares and administers standardized testing materials for EMT-Basic, EMT-Intermediate, and EMT-Paramedic. (See Figure 1-8.) This agency assists in developing and evaluating EMT training programs, and establishes the qualifications for registration and biennial re-registration. The registry is currently the only vehicle for establishing a national minimum standard of competency, and it serves as a major tool for reciprocity. The exam provides verification at the national level of paramedic training, and sets a medical-legal standard for evaluating the competence of paramedics to deliver quality ALS patient care.

PROFESSIONAL JOURNALS

A variety of journals are available to keep the paramedic aware of the latest changes in an ever-changing industry. These journals also provide an abundant source of continuing education material, as well as an excellent opportunity for EMS professionals to write and publish articles.

SUMMARY

To become a Paramedic, you must be willing to accept the responsibility of being a leader in the prehospital phase of emergency medical care. The responsibilities include on-call emergency duties and off-duty preparation. When the emergency call comes in, you must already be prepared to respond. If you are not, it is too late.

It is important to begin your paramedic training with the understanding that you will not be spending the majority of your time in emergency medical situations. Instead, you will spend most of your time preparing yourself to do the job properly. If you can accept this reality and you are willing to undertake the responsibility of preparing for this dynamic occupation, then you are ready to begin your Paramedic education. Remember: the best paramedics are those who make a commitment to excellence.

FURTHER READING

ISERSON, K. V., et al. *Ethics in Emergency Medicine.* Baltimore: Waverly Press, 1986.

NATIONAL ACADEMY OF SCIENCES, NATIONAL RESEARCH COUNCIL. *Accidental Death and Disability: The Neglected Disease of Modern Society.* Washington, DC: U.S. Department of Health, Education, and Welfare, 1966.

PAGE, JAMES O. *The Paramedics.* Morristown, NJ: Backdraft Publications, 1979.

PAGE, JAMES O. *The Magic of 3 AM.* Solana Beach, CA: JEMS Publishing, 1986.

PANTRIDGE, J. F., and J. S. GEDDES. "A Mobile Intensive CareUnit in the Management of Myocardial Infarction." *Lancet, 2* (1967): 271–273.

U.S. DEPARTMENT OF TRANSPORTATION. *National Standard Curriculum: Emergency Medical Technician—Paramedic.* Washington, DC, 1985.

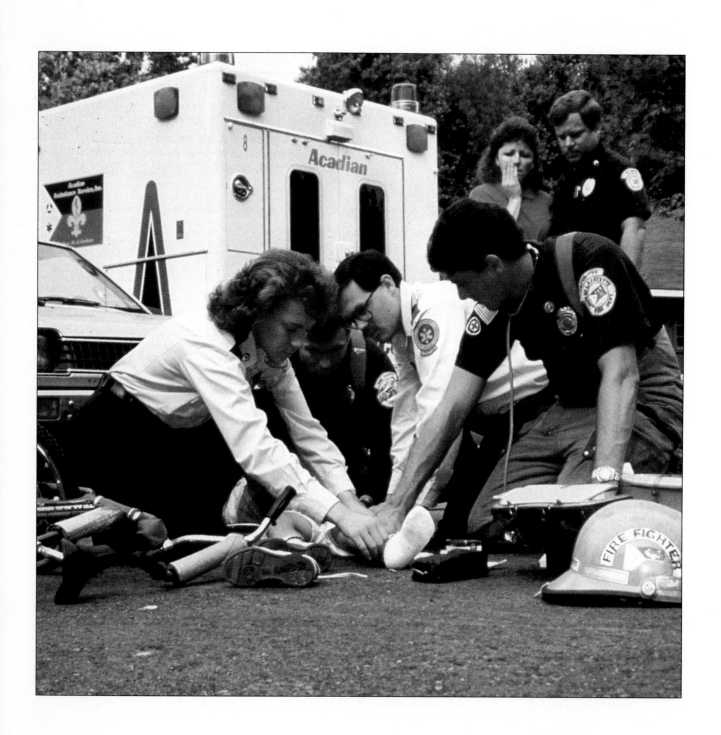

Emergency Medical Services Systems

Objectives For Chapter 2

Upon completing this chapter, the student should be able to:

1. Describe the development of the EMS system in the United States.

2. List and define the components of an EMS system.

3. Explain the oversight duties of an EMS administrative agency.

4. Discuss the responsibilities of the physician medical director regarding on-line and off-line medical control.

5. Describe public involvement in an EMS system, with regard to system access, recognition of an emergency, and initiation of basic life support.

6. Describe the components of an effective medical and organizational communications system.

7. Describe the components of emergency medical dispatching: system status management, interrogation guide-lines, response protocols, pre-arrival instructions, and dispatcher training.

8. Describe the coordination of patient transfer with ground and air transport services.

9. Describe the components of a quality assurance program.

10. Discuss the value of research in EMS.

11. Describe the categorization of receiving facilities and explain how the coordination of resources is attained.

12. List the components of mutual aid and mass-casualty planning.

13. Outline the various designs and financing methods for an EMS system.

On Saturday morning Mr. Chlopek is up as usual at 7:30 to mow the yard. He hasn't been feeling right the last few days and dreads the yard work. However, at his wife's insistence, he starts the mower and begins to mow. After making the first pass, he develops a terrible pressure in his chest. He feels as if he's been kicked in the chest. He leaves the mower running and sits down on the gasoline can. By now, he is pale and is sweating profusely. Shortly, his vision goes black and he falls to the ground.

Across the street, Mr. Webber is retrieving his morning paper and sees Mr. Chlopek collapse. Mr. Webber, a high school football coach, runs across the street. He quickly sees that his friend is in cardiac arrest. He calls for help, and starts CPR. Another neighbor arrives to help. Mr. Webber instructs him to call EMS. When he calls 9-1-1, the neighbor is shaken, and blurts out to the dispatcher, "Hurry! Bill collapsed and John is doing CPR." In his excited state, he could not recall his neighbor's address and hangs up to go help.

The dispatcher is able to determine the address through the enhanced 911 system. He then dispatches the appropriate EMS response. Within two minutes, the First Responders, who are members of the volunteer fire department, arrive. They assume care of the patient and begin two-person CPR. Within another two minutes, the EMT-I crew arrives by rescue unit. The EMTs quickly apply an automatic defibrillator, and a countershock is delivered within five minutes of the patient's collapse. Two minutes later, the paramedics arrive and assume care from the EMTs. The patient now has a pulse and is being effectively ventilated with supplemental oxygen. The paramedics place an IV, and administer 100 milligrams of lidocaine and start a lidocaine drip. They package the patient and transport him to Central Hospital.

In the emergency department, the physician quickly evaluates the patient. An ECG confirms the presence of an anterior wall myocardial infarction. The esophageal obturator airway (EOA) placed by the EMT-I's is replaced by a nasotracheal tube and the patient is transferred to the coronary care unit, where a cardiologist assumes his care. The patient does well. Two weeks after his heart attack, he undergoes a coronary artery bypass graft (bypass surgery). He is discharged 10 days later.

INTRODUCTION

■ **EMS System** a comprehensive approach to providing emergency medical services.

The **Emergency Medical Services system** is a complex health care system made up of personnel, equipment, and resources. The EMS system has several components. The prehospital component includes:

- ❏ lay persons trained in CPR
- ❏ the First Responder
- ❏ the Emergency Medical Technician
- ❏ the paramedic

The hospital component includes:

- ❏ the emergency nurse

❑ the emergency physician

❑ specialty physicians (e.g., trauma surgeons, cardiologists)

Support personnel also help the EMS system operate smoothly. In the prehospital phase, they include EMS dispatchers, law-enforcement personnel, firefighters, and other public-safety workers. In the hospital, respiratory therapists, radiologic technicians, and other specialists provide important support services. All components of the system must work together to assure quality patient care.

Usually, the first EMS person to respond to a medical emergency is the First Responder. The First Responder may be a police officer, firefighter, or lay person who has received basic emergency medical training in an approved First Responder program. The First Responder's role is to stabilize the patient until the EMT or paramedic arrives. First Responders are trained in CPR, basic airway management, and other basic skills.

The next component is the EMT. The EMT may respond in a fire department vehicle or in an ambulance. He or she should either continue the stabilization started by the First Responder, or initiate life support measures. The next component, the paramedic, should provide advanced life support care, if indicated. Several EMS systems are **"tiered"** in this order of incident response. (See Figure 2-1.) Care is handled by EMTs

■ **tiered response** a type of EMS system where BLS-level vehicles are initially dispatched to all calls unless ALS-level care is needed.

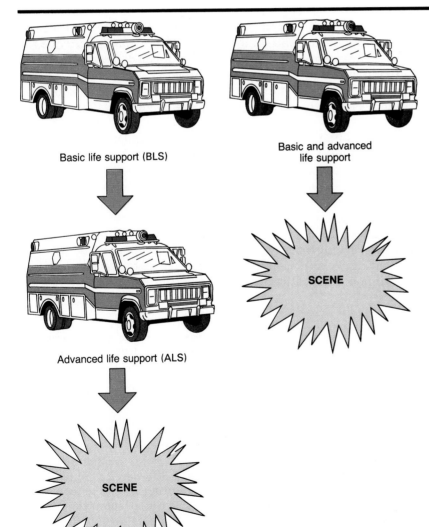

Basic life support (BLS)

Basic and advanced life support

Advanced life support (ALS)

SCENE

SCENE

FIGURE 2-1 Many systems utilize a tiered response. BLS responders arrive first. ALS care, if required, arrives later. Other systems simply dispatch an ALS vehicle on each call.

unless advanced life support is indicated. In many other EMS systems, however, paramedic personnel respond to every incident in case advanced life support care is needed.

Upon arrival at the hospital emergency department, patients are usually assigned priorities for care by a triage nurse or physician. Then the emergency department nurse and physician take over. If needed, a surgeon or other specialist will be summoned to the emergency department.

The system depends on the strength of all its components. A weakness in any one of them weakens the entire system, and patient care suffers. This chapter will address the components of the EMS system and discuss the problems with such a system.

THE HISTORY OF EMS SYSTEM DEVELOPMENT

Emergency Medical Services (EMS) is a health care system requiring the integration of several components. It is designed to provide appropriate care for all emergency patients. Until the late 1960s, few areas provided adequate prehospital emergency medical care. The prevailing thought was that care began in the hospital emergency department. Rescue techniques were crude, ambulance attendants poorly trained, and equipment minimal. There was no radio communication, and no physician involvement.

Eventually, as costs forced many mortician-operated ambulance services to withdraw, local police and fire departments had to provide this service. In many areas, volunteer groups were formed. The result was a proliferation of local, independent EMS provider agencies that could barely, if at all, communicate with each other. In addition, it was impossible to coordinate response activities on a scale larger than simple, local calls.

The publication in 1966 of "Accidental Death and Disability: the Neglected Disease of Modern Society," by the National Academy of Sciences–National Research Council, focused national attention on the problem. "The White Paper," as the report came to be called, spelled out the deficiencies in prehospital emergency medical care. It also suggested guidelines for the development of EMS systems, the training of prehospital emergency medical providers, and the upgrading of ambulances and their equipment. Although many improvements have been made since the report's publication, a surprising number of inadequate services still exist. This landmark publication set off a series of federal and private initiatives:

> **1966**—Congress passed the National Highway Safety Act, which forced the states to develop effective EMS systems or risk losing federal highway construction funds.
>
> **1971**—The White House funded nearly $9 million toward EMS demonstration projects. These projects were designed to be models for subsequent system development.
>
> **1972**—The Robert Wood Johnson Foundation provided grants for establishing regional EMS projects and communications systems.
>
> **1973**—Congress passed the Emergency Medical Services Systems Act, which provided funding in a series of projects awarded to develop regional systems. In order to be eligible for this funding, a program had to include the 15 necessary components for an EMS system that the act specified:

1. Manpower
2. Training
3. Communications
4. Transportation
5. Emergency facilities
6. Critical care units
7. Public safety agencies
8. Consumer participation
9. Access to care
10. Patient transfer
11. Standardized record-keeping
12. Public information and education
13. System review and evaluation
14. Disaster management
15. Mutual aid

Unfortunately, the designers of this legislation left out two major components: system financing and medical control. When federal funding was significantly reduced in the early 1980s, many systems faced economic disaster and had no solid plan for financial recovery. Even worse, many systems were operating without physician direction. The legislative oversights have meant a long, uphill battle for medical directors attempting to re-establish authority and accountability for medicine practiced by EMTs and paramedics in the streets. In many ways, the EMS Systems Act paved the way for system development. But in some respects, it sent EMS in the wrong direction. This act was amended in 1976 and again in 1979. A total of $215,000,000 was appropriated over a seven-year period toward the establishment of regional EMS systems.

In 1981, the passage of the Consolidated Omnibus Budget Reconciliation Act (COBRA) wiped out all federal funding for EMS, except block grant programs administered by the Department of Transportation and the Health and Human Services Administration. Only a small portion of this money, however, is available for EMS activities. These funds are given to the states, which in turn disburse the money to formally established regional systems. Since 1972, some areas have been able to effectively manage their grant monies. These areas have developed strong, efficient systems of prehospital emergency medical care. But many other areas have not. Today, in this technologically advanced country, there are still startling regional differences in the quality of prehospital care.

THE SYSTEMS APPROACH

The efficient delivery of emergency medical care requires a team effort and a systematic approach to get the best use of existing resources. There is no "best" method for providing prehospital emergency medical care in a given area. However, certain essential elements are considered "standard" for ensuring the best possible patient care in any region. Each system must develop operational policies for its components. Included among these policies are the items described below.

System Administration

An administrative agency should first be established. This agency will be responsible for managing the local system's resources, and for developing operational guidelines and standards for each component. A budget is created to operate the system and to select a qualified administrative staff. The agency should incorporate a planning board—composed of providers, representatives of the medical community, emergency physicians, and consumers—that will advise and assist the agency in setting policy. A medical director must be contracted, who will retain the ultimate authority and responsibility for all issues of patient care. The agency will designate who may function within the system. It will develop policies consistent with established state requirements. The EMS agency must develop a quality assurance program to evaluate the system's effectiveness, and to ensure that the best interest of the patient is always top priority. In short, the needs of the patient are determined, then the system is designed to meet those needs. The coordination of system components to meet the patient's needs is the responsibility of the EMS agency.

In addition to regional and municipal EMS agencies, states have EMS agencies. The state EMS agencies are typically responsible for: allocating funding to local systems; enacting legislation concerning the prehospital practice of medicine; licensing and certifying field providers; enforcing all state EMS regulations; and appointing regional advisory councils. In essence, EMS is a series of systems within a system. The integration of these systems and the cooperation of all participants result in a better quality of emergency medical care.

Medical Control

■ **medical director** a physician, who by experience or training, handles the clinical and patient care aspects of the EMS system.

The EMS system will retain a **medical director,** who will be actively involved in, and ultimately responsible for, all clinical and patient care. All prehospital medical care provided by non-physicians is considered an extension of the medical director's license. Every prehospital ambulance or rescue service must have a medical director who is responsible for that service. Prehospital care providers are designated agents of the medical director, regardless of whose employees they may be. For this reason, the medical director determines which providers may care for patients within the system. The medical director is the ultimate authority in all on-line and off-line medical control issues. (See Figure 2-2.)

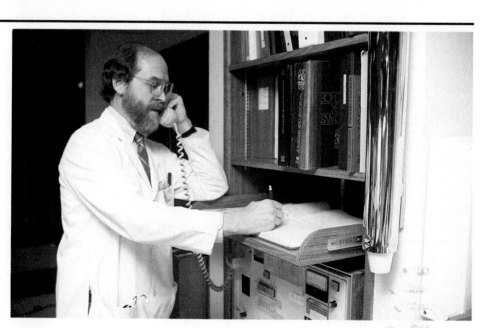

FIGURE 2-2 Medical control is an essential component of EMS. There are two aspects of medical control, direct and indirect. On-line medical control, as depicted here, provides immediate direction for on-scene care.

Direct medical control exists when prehospital providers communicate directly with a physician at a medical control or resource hospital. The physician's direction is usually based on established protocols for managing specific problems. This physician assumes responsibility and gives treatment orders for patients. Direct medical control physicians should be experienced in emergency medicine. They should have completed a training program that emphasizes system particulars, treatment protocols, and communications policies and procedures. Once they've become proficient in these areas, they should go through a formal certification process. They should also be required to ride with crews to get a feel for the realities of prehospital field medicine. Medical control communications are sometimes delegated to a mobile intensive care nurse (MICN), physician assistant (PA), or paramedic. In all circumstances, however, ultimate on-line responsibility rests with the medical control physician.

Control of a medical emergency scene should go to the individual with the most knowledge and best training in prehospital emergency stabilization and transport. When an advanced life support unit, under medical direction, is requested and dispatched to the emergency scene, a doctor/patient relationship is established by the physician providing medical control. The paramedic is responsible for the subsequent management of the patient, and acts as the medical control physician's agent unless the patient's physician is present (as in a doctor's office). If the private physician is present and assumes responsibility for the patient's care, the paramedic should defer to the physician's orders.

The ALS unit's responsibility reverts to the direct medical control physician whenever the private physician is not in attendance (in the back of the ambulance, for example). If an **intervener physician** is present and on-line medical control does not exist, the paramedic should relinquish responsibility to the physician. But first, the physician must identify himself or herself, and demonstrate a willingness to accept responsibility and to document the intervention as required by the local EMS system. If the treatment differs from established protocol, however, the physician should accompany the patient to the hospital. If an intervener physician is present and direct medical control does exist, the on-line physician is ultimately responsible. In case of disagreement between the intervener physician and the on-line physician, the paramedic must take orders from the on-line physician, and put him or her in contact with the intervening physician.

Indirect medical control includes training and education, protocol development, audit, chart review, and quality assurance. To be effective, medical control must have official and clearly defined authority, with the power to discipline, or limit the activities of, those who deviate from the established standard of care. (See Figure 2-3.)

Protocols are designed by the off-line medical control system to provide a standardized approach to common patient problems and a consistent level of medical care. When treatment is based on such protocols, the on-line physician assists prehospital personnel in interpreting the patient's complaint, understanding the findings of their evaluation, and applying the appropriate treatment protocol. Protocols will be designed around the four T's of emergency medical care:

Triage
Treatment
Transport
Transfer

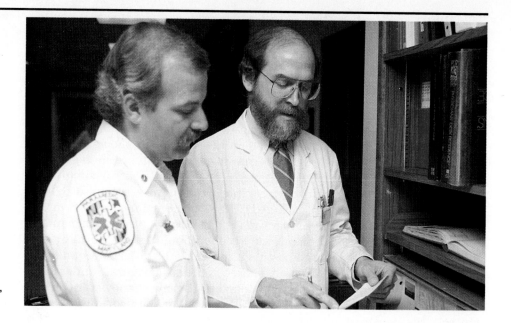

FIGURE 2-3 Indirect medical control includes training, chart review, protocol development, audit, and quality assurance.

■ **triage** the act of sorting patients by the severity of their injuries.

■ **standing orders** paramedic field interventions that are completed before contacting the direct medical control physician.

Triage guidelines help the physician make decisions involving patient flow through an EMS system. This simply means allocating the system's resources to the needs of victims. The EMS dispatcher will determine the type, level, and priority of response to the victim. The victim will then be directed to the appropriate receiving facility, which can provide definitive care, or stabilize the victim until he or she is transferred to a definitive care facility.

Treatment often includes emergency interventions by field personnel. Some procedures will be done upon a direct order from the medical control physician. Others will be **standing orders.** Treatment protocols should be kept current with new research.

Transport involves decisions about mode (air vs. ground), and the level of care during transport (ALS vs. BLS, paramedic vs. nurse, nurse vs. physician, etc.). Most plans call for taking the patient to the closest appropriate facility, as designated by the system. Transport plans are based on three factors:

1. Nature of the injury or illness
2. Condition of the patient
3. Estimated transport time

Transfer protocols cover the management of inter-hospital patient transfer. They allow for regionwide continuity of care when patients are transferred. Agreements between receiving facilities within the system ensure that the patient is admitted to a definitive care facility.

Protocols will also be established for special circumstances, such as the proper handling of "Do Not Resuscitate" orders, patients who refuse treatment, sexual abuse, abuse of children or elderly persons, initiation and termination of CPR, and intervener physicians. Although protocols standardize field procedures, they should allow the paramedic flexibility to improvise and adapt to special circumstances. Protocols establish a basis for medical care and a standard for accountability in an EMS system.

Public Information and Education

The public is an essential, yet often overlooked, component of an EMS system. An EMS system should have a plan for educating the public about recognizing an emergency, accessing the system, and initiating basic life support.

The American Heart Association (AHA) estimates that 350,000 cardiac arrests per year occur before the patient reaches the hospital. Most happen within two hours of the onset of cardiac symptoms, because many patients deny that something is wrong and delay calling for help. If the patient, a family member, friend, or bystander can recognize the emergency and intervene in time, many cases of sudden death can be prevented. Families of patients with coronary artery disease should be targeted for instruction in recognizing emergency symptoms.

The second aspect of public education is system access. Systems with Emergency 9-1-1 telephone service make access easy. The phone number should be well-publicized, and citizens should be taught how to give information to the emergency medical dispatcher. For regions with a single, seven-digit access number, the process is similar. For areas with multiple access numbers, however, the problem may be overwhelming. In any case, the public must learn how to access the system efficiently in an emergency, thereby avoiding life-threatening delays.

After recognizing that a medical emergency exists, the bystander must initiate basic life support (BLS) procedures: cardiopulmonary resuscitation (CPR). This could also include patient stabilization after major trauma and hemorrhage control. Abundant research in the last 10 years indicates a relationship between response times and the patient's ultimate recovery. Communities that have many citizens trained in BLS, plus a rapid paramedic response, have proven that a large number of patients can be successfully resuscitated. On the other hand, communities weak in prompt bystander CPR have shown a much lower rate of recovery. The role of the bystander in emergency medical care is critical to successful resuscitation of a cardiac arrest victim. The AHA estimates that 100,000–200,000 lives can be saved each year in the United States with implementation of community CPR programs and fast paramedic response.

Future public involvement may include bystander defibrillation. Research shows increasing numbers of successful first-responder defibrillation programs. With the advent of automatic external defibrillators, the technology may someday allow affordable, portable automatic defibrillators in public places—such as theaters, churches, and malls—or in the homes of cardiac patients. The public component must not be overlooked when designing or improving an EMS system.

EMS Communications

The communications network is the heart of any regional EMS system. Coordinating the components into an organized response to urgent medical situations requires a comprehensive, flexible, communications plan. The six basic components of a communications system are:

1. Citizen access
2. Single control center
3. Organizational communications capabilities
4. Medical communications capabilities
5. Hardware
6. Software

Any citizen with an urgent medical need should have a simple and reliable mechanism for accessing the EMS system. A well-publicized universal number, such as 9-1-1, provides direct citizen access to the communications center. Multiple community telephone numbers add life-threatening minutes to any emergency response system. The basic emergency telephone number, 9-1-1, available from American Telephone and Telegraph (AT&T) since 1967, is a toll-free telephone service that enables the caller to dial three digits to reach a single public safety answering point. Enhanced 9-1-1 (E-911) gives automatic location of the caller, instant routing of the call to the appropriate public emergency service (fire, EMS, police), and instant callback capabilities should the caller hang up too soon.

A single communications center that can communicate with and direct all emergency medical units in the system is best. Systems with multiple control points cannot ensure the best use of resources or the best emergency response. The EMS dispatcher should be in charge of all emergency vehicle movements in the area to maintain system readiness. Ideally, all public service agencies should be dispatched from the same communications center. The communications center should be able to reach emergency vehicles throughout a large geographical area. In some regions, repeaters and relays may be needed.

Organizational communications allow efficient and effective use of the system's resources. After the caller has successfully accessed the system, the EMS dispatcher must be able to communicate with emergency units to provide the best response, and to facilitate operations on the scene. Emergency units must also be able to communicate with each other, and with other agencies during mutual aid and disaster operations. Hospitals must be able to communicate with other hospitals in the region to assess specialty capabilities. The organizational plan enables the EMS dispatcher to effectively manage all aspects of system response, and assess the system's readiness for the next response.

Medical communications allow the paramedic to communicate with the receiving facility and, in many areas, to transmit ECG telemetry signals to the on-line physician. Hospitals must also be able to communicate with each other (usually by a land-line or microwave network) to facilitate patient transfer.

Communications hardware includes radios, consoles, pagers, transmission towers, repeaters, telephone land lines, and any other telecommunications equipment required to operate the system. Communications hardware is discussed in more detail in Chapter 4.

Software includes the radio frequencies used for various functions and the communications protocols used by the system. Radio procedures and policies consistent with FCC standards and local protocols, and back-up communications plans for disaster operations are essential.

An EMS system must have an effective, practical communications network. No one system design will meet the needs of all communities. Each regional system should design a communications network that is simple, flexible, and practical. (See Figure 2-4.)

Emergency Medical Dispatching

Emergency medical dispatching is the nerve center of an EMS program. The activities of medical dispatchers are crucial to the efficient operation of the system. Dispatch is the means for assigning and directing appropriate medical care to the victim. An emergency medical dispatching plan should include pre-established interrogation protocols, pre-assigned re-

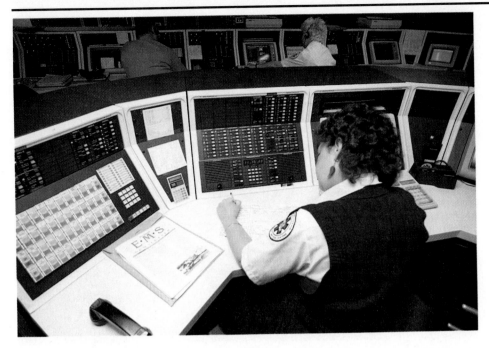

FIGURE 2-4 The ideal communications center is a single center which can communicate with and control the movement of all emergency units within the system.

sponse configurations, system status management, and pre-arrival telephone instructions. Medical direction for the emergency medical dispatcher is a responsibility of the EMS medical director. Quality assurance of the EMS dispatch program is an EMS agency responsibility.

Any effective emergency medical dispatching system has certain key components. EMS dispatchers do more than send ambulances; they make sure the system's resources are in a constant readiness to respond. System status management relies on projected call volumes and locations, not geographical or political tradition, to strategically place ambulances and crews. The system is used to reduce response times.

Another dispatch system is priority dispatching. In this system, first used by the Salt Lake City Fire Department, medical dispatchers are trained to medically interrogate a distressed caller, prioritize symptoms, select the appropriate response, and give lifesaving pre-arrival instructions. A set of medically approved protocols is used by all dispatchers. These priorities must reflect the level of appropriate response, including types of personnel, number of vehicles, and mode of response. During the interrogation, the dispatcher asks a set of standard questions to determine the level of response.

A pre-arrival instruction program by medically trained dispatchers was introduced by the Phoenix Fire Department in 1974. While emergency units are responding, the caller may initiate lifesaving first-aid techniques with the dispatcher's help. In 1985, the Seattle EMS system initiated a successful program of instructing callers in CPR. Although critics of this service point out the increased liability of priority dispatching and of treatment instruction by dispatchers, the future most likely points to the increased liability of not providing the service.

Medical dispatchers must be both medically and technically trained. Emergency Medical Dispatch (EMD) training should cover basic telecommunication skills, medical interrogation, the giving of pre-arrival instructions, and dispatch prioritization. The course should be standardized and should include certification by a governmental agency. (See Figure 2-5.)

✳ The EMS communications system must be tailored to the individual needs of the local EMS system.

✳ EMS Dispatchers must be both medically and technically trained.

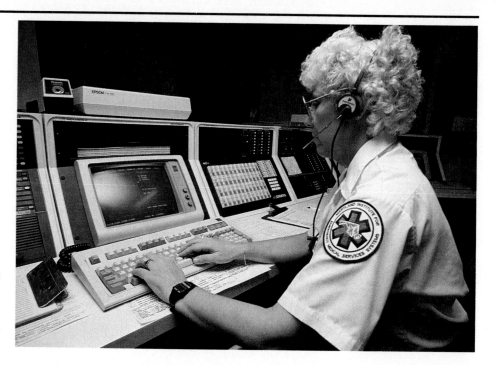

FIGURE 2-5 The EMS dispatcher of today is a skilled professional. Ideally, all EMS dispatchers should complete an approved Emergency Medical Dispatch training program. Concurrent EMT or paramedic certification is desirable.

An effective EMS dispatching system will place first responding units on the scene within four minutes following the onset of the emergency. The AHA reports that brain resuscitation will be unsuccessful if response times exceed four minutes, unless there was proper BLS intervention (CPR). While systems must be prepared for the worst-case scenario (sudden death), their design must provide for a rapid BLS response.

Many studies have suggested that definitive care (defibrillation) in sudden death victims within eight minutes can produce 43% successful outcomes with patients in ventricular fibrillation. Many systems are now using EMTs or First Responders for this definitive care. Early defibrillation programs have been extremely successful across the country in reversing sudden death mortality. The goal of emergency response is: BLS care in less than four minutes, and ALS care in less than eight minutes following the event. High-performance systems meet this standard more than 90% of the time.

An effective emergency medical dispatching program should include pre-established caller interrogation protocols, pre-determined response configurations, system status management, and pre-arrival caller instructions. It should be under full control of the physician medical director and the EMS agency.

Education and Certification

The two kinds of education programs for EMS personnel are: original education and continuing education. Original education programs are the initial training courses for prehospital providers. They involve the completion of a standardized course that meets or exceeds the United States Department of Transportation (USDOT) national curriculum for that level (EMT-Basic, EMT-I, EMT-D, EMT-P). Continuing education programs include refresher courses for recertification and periodic in-service training sessions. All education programs should have a medical director who is involved in the EMS system. The EMS agency is responsible for assuring funding for these programs.

There is a variety of prehospital certification levels for communities to choose from. In 1983, because of variations in state and regional EMS terminology, there were as many as 30 levels of prehospital care providers. Since then, the National Registry of EMTs has recognized, and the Department of Transportation has developed curricula for, three levels:

EMT-Basic. The EMT-Basic should be competent at CPR, airway management, hemorrhage control, stabilization of fractures, emergency childbirth, basic extrication, communications, and use of the pneumatic anti-shock garment. In some cases the EMT may undergo additional training in defibrillation (EMT-D).

EMT-Intermediate. The EMT-Intermediate (EMT-I) should possess all the EMT-Basic skills. In addition, he or she should be competent at advanced airway management, intravenous fluid therapy, and certain other advanced skills. (See Figure 2-6.)

EMT-Paramedic. The EMT-Paramedic should possess all the skills required of an EMT-Basic and EMT-I. In addition, he or she should be trained in advanced patient assessment, trauma management, pharmacology, cardiology, and other medical emergencies. Paramedics should successfully complete Advanced Cardiac Life Support (ACLS) and Pediatric Advanced Life Support (PALS) courses as offered by the American Heart Association. Basic Trauma Life Support (BTLS) or Prehospital Trauma Life Support (PHTLS) course completion is also desirable. (See Figure 2-7.)

The curricula for these primary education programs include classroom lectures, practical skills lab work, hospital clinical experience, and, at the advanced levels, a supervised field internship.

The training of prehospital personnel is a critical phase of EMS system design. Attitudes and values that are learned in the classroom carry over into the streets. EMS instructors should remember that the process of training is as important as the training itself. The goal is for personnel to graduate from the program with a high regard for human dignity and a passion for excellence. In addition, graduates realize that certification marks the beginning—not the end—of their education. Instructors who inspire excellence and set an example for being punctual and reliable will graduate students who value those virtues.

Patient Transportation

Patients who are transported under the direction of an emergency medical services system should be taken whenever possible to the closest appropriate medical facility. The medical control physician should have the authority to designate that facility, based on the needs of the patient and the availability of services. In some cases, the patient's need for special services—trauma, burn, pediatric, etc.—means designating a facility that is not nearby. At other times, the closest facility will be designated for stabilization of the patient while transfer is arranged. The ultimate authority for this decision, however, remains with the on-line medical control physician.

All transport vehicles, ground and air, should be licensed and locally approved. Equipment lists should be consistent with system-wide standards. In 1983, the American College of Surgeons' Committee on Trauma recommended a standard set of equipment to be carried by providers of basic life-support services. In 1988, The American College of Emergency Physicians (ACEP) published a recommended list of advanced life-support supplies and equipment to be carried on ALS units. Both sets of recommendations serve as excellent guidelines for any prehospital EMS sys-

■ **EMT-Basic** a person, currently certified, who has successfully completed the U.S. Department of Transportation (USDOT) National Standard Curriculum for EMT-Basic.

■ **EMT-Intermediate** a person, currently certified, who has successfully completed the USDOT National Standard Curriculum for EMT-I.

■ **EMT-Paramedic** a person, currently certified, who has successfully completed the USDOT National Standard Curriculum for EMT-P.

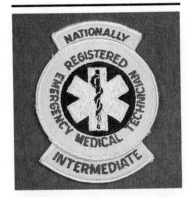

FIGURE 2-6 The EMT-Intermediate provides limited, advanced life support care typically including IV therapy and advanced airway management.

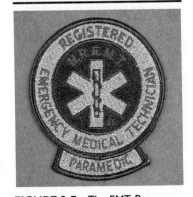

FIGURE 2-7 The EMT-Paramedic is the highest level of training for prehospital providers. He or she should be trained in all aspects of advanced prehospital care.

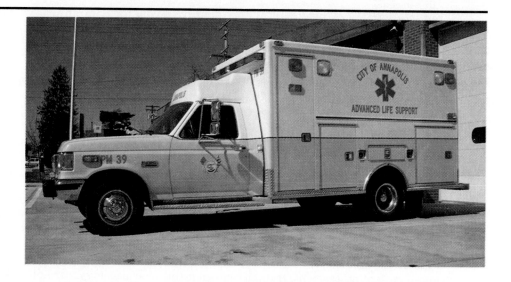

FIGURE 2-8   Type I ambulance.

tem. Regional standardization of all equipment and supplies would best facilitate interagency efforts during disaster operations.

In 1974, responding to a request from the Department of Transportation, the General Services Administration developed the KKK-A-1822 Federal Specifications for Ambulances. This first attempt at standardizing an ambulance design to permit intensive life support for patients en route to a definitive care facility, defined three basic types of ambulances:

Type I—Conventional cab and chassis on which a modular ambulance body is mounted, with no passageway between driver's and patient's compartments. (See Figure 2-8.)

Type II—Standard van, body and cab form an integral unit; most have a raised roof. (See Figure 2-9.)

Type III—Specialty van with forward cab and integral body, with passageway from driver's compartment to patient's compartment. (See Figure 2-10.)

Only these certified ambulances may display the registered "Star of Life" symbol as defined by the USDOT's National Highway Traffic Safety Administration (NHTSA). The word "AMBULANCE" should appear in mir-

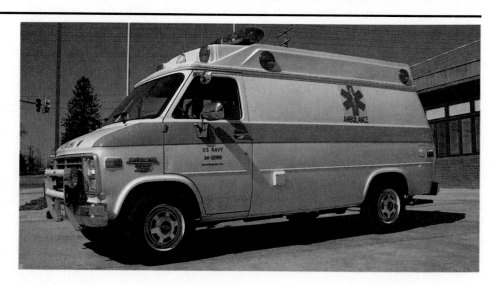

FIGURE 2-9   Type II ambulance.

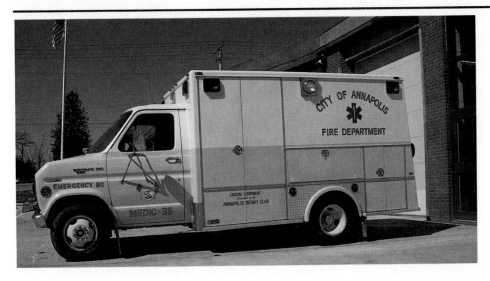

FIGURE 2-10 Type III ambulance.

ror image on the front so that other drivers can identify the ambulance in their rearview mirrors.

In 1980, revision KKK-A-1822A aimed at improving ambulance electrical systems by designing a low-amp lighting system to replace antiquated light bars and beacons. This standard helped to reduce electrical system overloads. In 1985, revision KKK-A-1822-B specified changes based on National Institute for Occupational Safety and Health (NIOSH) standards. These include reducing siren noise, high engine temperatures, and exhaust emissions, safer cot-retention systems, wider axles, hand-held spotlights, battery conditioners for longer life, and venting systems for oxygen compartments. The KKK specifications are intended to improve the safety, reliability, and function of ambulances. All ambulances purchased with federal funds during the 1970s were required to comply with these criteria. Since then, however, some states have adopted their own stricter criteria.

Patients can be transported by ground or air. The use of helicopters for medical transport was introduced during the Korean War and expanded in Vietnam. The success of these military evacuation procedures led to their use in civilian ambulance systems. In 1970, the Military Assistance to Safety and Traffic (MAST) program was established. This demonstration project set up 35 programs nationwide to test the feasibility of using military helicopters and paramedical personnel in civilian medical emergencies. Today, trauma care systems use military, law enforcement, municipal, hospital-based, and private helicopter transport services to transfer patients. (See Figures 2-11 and 2-12.) Fixed-wing aircraft are also used when patients must be transported long distances, usually more than 120 miles.

Getting the right patient to the right facility requires a transport system that includes specific patient transfer protocols coordinated by a single agency. These protocols should be based on patient severity, length of travel, and availability of resources at the facility. Since the early 1970s, trauma care systems, such as the Maryland Institute for Emergency Medical Services Systems (MIEMSS), have designated various levels of receiving facilities around the state. MIEMSS employs a single system communications center (SYSCOM) to coordinate the aeromedical transport of critical trauma patients to the appropriate facility. The state is divided into five regions, in which ground and air transport resources are strategically placed for the maximum benefit of all Maryland resi-

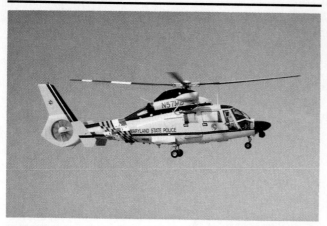

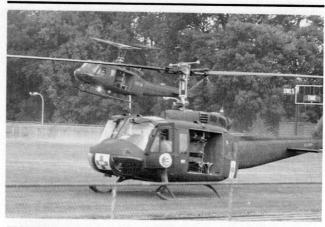

FIGURE 2-11 The helicopter has become an integral and important aspect of prehospital care. The helicopter offers smooth and rapid transport as well as a mechanism for providing specialized emergency care, once limited to the hospital, at the scene of the medical emergency.

FIGURE 2-12 The military helicopter proved its value in reducing morbidity and mortality in the Vietnam war. Military helicopters are frequently made available to assist civilian EMS systems.

dents. The Maryland system works well because it is a coordinated, well-organized operation.

Quality Assurance

An EMS system must be designed to meet the needs of the patient. Quality Assurance (QA) is simply an objective means of determining why the system works or doesn't work. The quality of an EMS system is reflected in the daily medical practices of its prehospital care providers. Ongoing monitoring and evaluation of the entire system are an essential component of any program committed to quality. In EMS, the only acceptable quality is *excellence*.

✱ A Quality Assurance (QA) program is an essential element of EMS today.

A QA program documents effectiveness—if you cannot prove quality, you do not have it. It also identifies problems (you don't know a problem exists unless someone discovers it), and selects areas that need improvement (mediocrity, complacency, and adequacy are unacceptable in EMS). A good QA program documents in writing the quality of the system. An effective Quality Assurance program demands a commitment from all participants.

The major component of any QA program is documentation. Patient care reports must be checked for completeness and adherence to system treatment protocols. Response time data should be tabulated, training logs kept up-to-date, and system audit records filed for future use.

A formal audit and review process is intended to determine system inadequacies and protocol inconsistencies. The review should be conducted by an emergency physician who is not affiliated with any provider organization in the region. Any system participant should be able to initiate a run audit. The desired data include dispatch tapes, prehospital care data, incident reports, emergency department and inpatient records, and autopsy findings. The data must be evaluated for accuracy of charting and assessment, appropriateness of treatment, patterns of error, morbidity, mortality, and need for protocol revision. Proper or improper care revealed by the audit should be promptly praised or criticized by the medical director.

The ten "musts" of a QA program are:

1. Solicit consumer feedback!
   EMS is a service. Find out how good yours is by sending comment cards to patients or their families.
2. Solicit hospital feedback!
   Were field diagnoses and treatments appropriate? You are destined to repeat your mistakes unless someone points them out.
3. Evaluate personnel in the field!
   Evaluating field personnel only on hospital-arrival condition and run charts can be misleading.
4. Evaluate instructors and instruction!
   Field personnel will emulate their instructors. Check the accuracy of course content.
5. Conduct consistent case reviews!
   Review calls consistently.
6. Make remedial training available!
   Help personnel improve performance in specific areas. Make remedial sessions easily accessible.
7. Require continuing education and make sure it's available.
   Help your personnel in their pursuit of excellence. Publish lists of training and continuing education programs in your area.
8. Staff efficiently and effectively.
   Avoid burnout (too many calls) and rustout (not enough calls) by appropriate staffing and management policies. People are the most vital resource in EMS.
9. Schedule preventive maintenance!
   Equipment and apparatus cannot fail during an emergency.
10. Reward your people publicly for excellence.
    Give recognition for a job well done as often as possible.

The cost of sloppy and inefficient EMS is seen in lost wages, more taxes, increased payments for long-term rehabilitation, and other financial consequences. Ultimately, taxpayers and insurance buyers will have to bear these burdens. The price of high-quality EMS is actually less expensive. Spending dollars on a strong quality assurance program will save money in the long run. The QA officer must be enthusiastic and must genuinely care about patient care and the EMS personnel. Good quality is a direct result of commitment.

Research

In order to provide a scientific basis for prehospital EMS, a formal ongoing **research** program is an essential component of the system. Existing and future procedures, techniques, and equipment must be evaluated scientifically. For moral, educational, medical, financial, and practical reasons, an EMS system design must include research. Unfortunately, many protocols and procedures that paramedics use today have evolved without clinical evidence of their usefulness, safety, or benefit to the patient.

Future EMS research projects must address these issues:

1. Which prehospital field interventions actually reduce morbidity and mortality?
2. Are the benefits of certain paramedic field procedures worth the potential risks?
3. What is the cost/benefit ratio of sophisticated prehospital EMS systems?
4. Is field stabilization possible, or should paramedics begin immediate transport in every case?

■ **research** diligent and scientific study, investigation, and experimentation in order to establish facts and determine their significance.

✱ EMS policies, procedures, and protocols should be based on sound medical knowledge supported by pertinent research.

Paramedics should be familiar with the components of a research project. First, a problem is identified and the reason for the study is explained. Next, a hypothesis, or the precise question to be asked, is stated. Third, a literature search is done to identify the body of published knowledge. Next, the study design is selected, with all logistics clearly outlined and all patient-consent issues examined and approved. When this preparation is completed, the study can begin. The raw data are then collected, analyzed, and correlated in a statistical application. The results are assessed and correlated with the original hypothesis. The final step is writing a cohesive, comprehensive paper for publication in a medical journal.

Paramedics are encouraged to participate in research projects. Current EMS practice must be justified by hard clinical data derived from an objective, valid program of ongoing research.

Receiving Facilities

All hospitals are not equal in emergency and support service capabilities. Hospital categorization identifies the readiness and capability of a hospital and its staff to receive and effectively treat emergency patients. Categorization originated from the realization that patients have varying degrees of illness and injury, and that receiving facilities have varying capabilities to provide initial or definitive care. A facility categorization system lets the EMS system's coordinators know in advance of specialty areas within the EMS delivery system. This knowledge expedites the transportation of emergency patients to hospitals that will provide definitive treatment, or lifesaving stabilization, until transfer can be arranged.

Once categorization has been established, regionalizing available services helps give all patients reasonable access to the appropriate level of facility. Burn, trauma, pediatric, psychiatric, perinatal, cardiac, spinal, and poison control centers, are examples of specialty-service facilities that offer high-level care for specific groups of patients. Large EMS systems should designate a resource hospital that will coordinate the system's specialty resources and ensure appropriate patient distribution.

Ideally, receiving facilities should have these capabilities: an emergency department with an emergency physician on duty at all times, surgical facilities, and a lab, blood bank, and X-ray capabilities available around the clock. Receiving facilities should also have: critical intensive care units, a documented commitment to participate in the EMS system, and a willingness to receive all emergency patients in transport, regardless of their ability to pay. And they should have the ability to provide medical audit procedures to ensure quality assurance and medical accountability, and the desire to participate in mass-casualty preparedness plans. (See Figure 2-13.)

A hospital categorization inventory is designed to match the clinical needs of emergency patients with the emergency facility best prepared to treat them. This should result in a system of regional hospitals that provide highly specialized emergency care. (See Figure 2-14.)

Mutual Aid/Mass-Casualty Preparation

No system is an island, and the resources of any region will sometimes be overwhelmed. A formalized mutual aid agreement policy will ensure that help is available when needed. Mutual aid agreements can be between neighboring departments, municipalities, systems, and even states. Cooperation among all EMS agencies must supersede geographical, political, and historical boundaries.

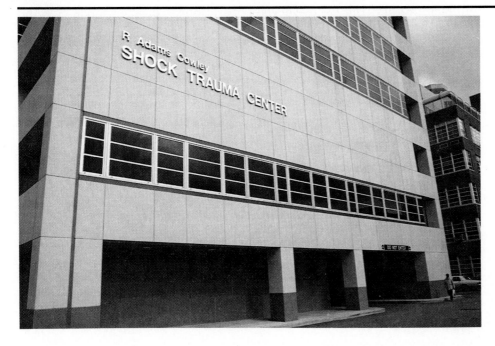

FIGURE 2-13 Hospital emergency departments have evolved along with EMS. A prime example is the R. Adams Cowley "Shock Trauma Center" in Baltimore, Maryland.

Each system should put in place a mass-casualty plan for unexpected catastrophes that may overwhelm available resources and normal operations. There should be a coordinated central management agency that identifies commanders within the framework of the incident command system and the existing mutual aid plan. The plan should integrate all EMS system components and have a flexible communications system. Frequent drills should test the plan's effectiveness and practicality. The communications, dispatch, and control systems should be capable of coordinating a system-wide response to a major medical incident without a major change in personnel, equipment, or operating protocol. Standardized apparatus, equipment, supplies, and radio hardware and software

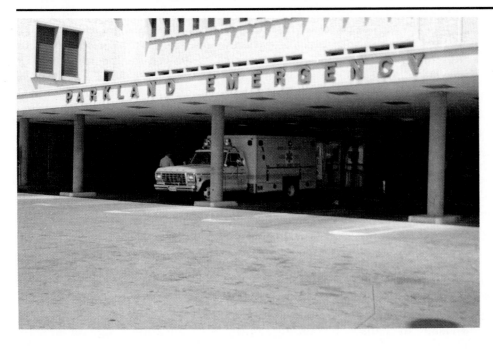

FIGURE 2-14 Hospital emergency departments should be categorized based on their ability to provide care. This categorization should be based upon staffing, physical plant, equipment, and availability of specialty care.

will facilitate shifting from everyday operations to disaster mode. Specific components of a mass-casualty plan will be discussed in Chapter 6.

System Financing

At present in the United States, there is a wide variety of EMS system design. EMS services can be hospital-based, fire department- or police department-based, municipal third service, private commercial business, volunteer, or, some combination thereof. From fully tax-subsidized municipal systems, to all-volunteer squads supported solely by contributions, major differences exist in the philosophy of EMS system finance. EMS funding can come from: tax subsidies, contributions, corporate sponsorship, subscription plans, Medicare, Medicaid, private medical and auto insurance, fund-raising activities, prepaid health care programs (HMO), and user fees.

Two new approaches are the Public Utility Model and the Failsafe Franchise. In these systems, a municipality establishes the design and standards for the contract bid, then periodically—usually every three or four years—holds wholesale competition for the market. The provider firm that wins the contract must manage services properly and efficiently throughout the contract term, or face severe penalties.

SUMMARY

An EMS system comprises a number of components, all of them crucial to providing emergency medical care for sick and injured people. The system is a continuum of care: from the EMT who conducts public education classes; to the mechanic who keeps the ambulance fleet running; to the emergency medical dispatcher who calms a distressed caller and provides life-saving instructions over the phone; to the paramedic who provides field intervention; to the emergency department physician, surgeon, and physical therapist who will see the patient through definitive care and rehabilitation. No one component, no one person, is more important than another. EMS is a total team effort.

EMS systems are designed with the patient as the highest priority. They begin with a strong administrative agency, which structures the system around the patients' needs, and grants the medical director ultimate authority in all issues of patient care. The medical director is an emergency physician who remains actively involved in all components of the system. An EMS system uses a single-number access (E-911), and a centralized communications center that handles all emergency medical emergencies in the area, and coordinates all levels of communication, organizational and medical, within the region. EMS dispatchers, who are trained and certified, control the movement of all emergency medical units within the area. They have pre-designed interrogation protocols, pre-established priority response modes, and system status management procedures, and they give pre-arrival instructions. On at least 90% of all emergency calls, the system places BLS units on the scene in four minutes, ALS units in eight minutes. Coordination of ground and air transport service follows established protocols at the communications center.

Mutual aid agreements ensure a continuum of care during peak-load periods and personnel shortages. Disaster plans are formalized, rehearsed regularly, and revised when necessary. Hospitals are categorized according to their readiness to provide essential and specialty services within the region. Personnel are trained according to the USDOT national standard curricula. An ongoing continuing education program encourages each system provider to achieve excellence. A Quality Assurance program documents the system's performance daily. An ongoing research program attempts to validate the actions of prehospital providers through scientific, clinical evaluation. Finally, the system flourishes because of a strong, stable financial plan that ensures consistent patient care of the highest quality.

FURTHER READING

American College of Emergency Physicians, Emergency Medical Services Committee: Control of Advanced Life Support at the Scene of Medical Emergencies. *Ann Emerg Med,* 13: 1984, pp. 547–548.

American College of Emergency Physicians: Prehospital Advanced Life Support Skills, Medications, and Equipment. *Ann Emerg Med.* 17: 1988, pp. 1109–1111.

CLAWSON, J. J., and DERNOCOEUR, K. B. *Principles of Emergency Medical Dispatch.* Englewood Cliffs, NJ: Prentice Hall, 1986.

Consolidated Omnibus Budget Reconciliation Act (COBRA) of 1981. Public Law 97–35. August, 1981.

COWLEY, R. A., et al. "An Economical and Proved Helicopter Program for Transporting the Emergency and Critically Injured Patient to Maryland." *J Trauma,* 13: 1973, pp. 1029–1038.

Department of Health and Human Resources: Military Assistance to Safety and Traffic: Report of Test Program, 1971.

Department of Transportation and General Services Administration: Federal Specifications—Ambulance KKK-A-1822 B-1985, Emergency Medical Care Surface Vehicle. Washington, DC, Specifications and Consumer Information Distribution Section (WFSIS).

EISENBERG, M., et al. "Paramedic Programs and Out-of-Hospital Cardiac Arrest: Factors Associated with Successful Resuscitation." *American Journal of Public Health,* 69: 1979, pp. 30–38.

EISENBERG, M. S., et al. "Emergency CPR Instruction via Telephone." *American Journal of Public Health,* 75: 1985, pp. 47–50.

"Essential Equipment for Ambulances." *Am Coll Surg Bull,* 68: 1983, pp. 36–38.

"Essentials and Guidelines of an Accredited Educational Program for the Emergency Medical Technician—Paramedic." American Medical Association, Joint Review Committee on Educational Programs for EMT-Paramedic, revised 1989.

HACKER, L. P. "Time and Its Effects on Casualties in World War II and Vietnam." *Arch Surg,* 98: 1969, pp. 39–40.

Highway Safety Program Manual, US Department of Transportation, Federal Highway Administration, National Highway Safety Bureau, 1969.

HUNT, R. C., et al. "Influence of Emergency Medical Services Systems and Prehospital Defibrillation on Survival of Sudden Cardiac Death Victims." *American Journal of Emergency Medicine,* 7: 1989, pp. 68–82.

Robert Wood Johnson Foundation Special Report on Emergency Medical Services Systems. Princeton, NJ, 1977.

KUHL, A. "National Association of EMS Physicians." *EMS Directors' Handbook.* St. Louis, MO: CV Mosby, 1989.

National Academy of Sciences, National Research Council: "Accidental Death and Disability: The Neglected Disease of Modern Society." Washington, DC, US Department of Health, Education, and Welfare, 1966.

National Association of EMS Physicians: Consensus Document on Emergency Medical Dispatching.

National Standard Curriculum for EMS Dispatchers, ed. 2, US Department of Transportation, 1983.

NIXON, R. M. President's Message of Health Care System. House of Representatives, 92nd Congress, Washington, DC: March 1972.

PAGE, J. O., et al. "Twenty Years Later." *JEMS,* 11: 1988, pp. 30–43.

Standards and Guidelines for Cardiopulmonary and Emergency Cardiac Care. *JAMA,* 255: 1986, pp. 21, 2905–2913.

STOUT, J. L. "Measuring Your System." *JEMS.* January 1983, pp. 84–91.

————. "System Status Management." *JEMS,* 1983, pp. 22–30.

————. "Ambulance System Designs." *JEMS.* January 1986, pp. 85–99.

United States Department of Transportation: National Standard Curriculum: Emergency Medical Technician—Intermediate. Washington, DC, 1985.

United States Department of Transportation: National Standard Curriculum: Emergency Medical Technician—Paramedic. Washington, DC, 1985.

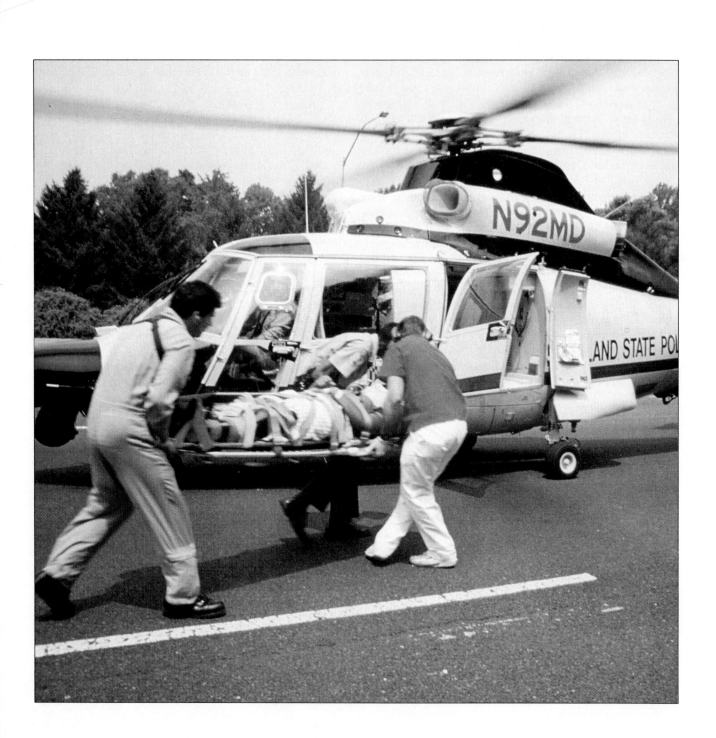

Medical–Legal Considerations of Emergency Care

Objectives for Chapter 3

Upon completing this chapter, the student should be able to:

1. Describe the two categories of law in the United States.
2. Define the following:
   - tort
   - negligence
   - assault
   - battery
   - false imprisonment
   - abandonment
   - duty to act
   - slander
   - libel
3. List and define the four components required to prove negligence in a malpractice proceeding.
4. Discuss the concept of *res ipsa loquitur.*
5. Define assault and battery and give examples of each.
6. Discuss the Medical Practice Act and its implications in prehospital care.
7. Describe the purpose and limitations of Good Samaritan Laws.
8. Describe the motor vehicle laws in your state that apply to emergency vehicles.
9. Explain what is meant by the term "delegation of authority."
10. Define a "Living Will."
11. Define "Natural Death Act."
12. Discuss the concept of "standard of care" as it applies to prehospital care.
13. Discuss consent, including:
    - implied consent
    - informed consent
14. List several methods of protecting yourself from malpractice liability.
15. Discuss the importance of the medical record.

CASE STUDY

EMS 706 is dispatched to an unknown medical emergency. The dispatcher reports that the patient is near the intersection of Highways 36 and 317 and police are also enroute. The ambulance and police officers arrive simultaneously, although from different directions. The patient is a middle-aged male, staggering near the shoulder of the road. A truck is parked nearby. The paramedics deem the scene safe and approach the patient behind the police officers. The lead police officer asks him if anything is wrong. The patient immediately turns and lunges at the officer. He is quickly subdued, thrashes around, then loses consciousness. The paramedics quickly assess airway, breathing, and circulation. They detect no other problems during this primary assessment.

Upon beginning the secondary assessment, they note a Medic-Alert bracelet that says "Diabetic." Hypoglycemia is suspected. While one crew member completes the secondary survey, the other performs a Dextrostix and notes the blood sugar to be 26 mg/dL. Per approved standing orders, an IV is established and 50 mL of 50% dextrose is administered. The patient immediately arouses. He quickly becomes fully oriented and is found to be polite and grateful. He states that he has been having some problems lately with dosing his insulin and says this is the third episode of hypoglycemia in two weeks.

The paramedics encourage him to go to the hospital for additional evaluation. The patient declines, stating that he already has scheduled a physician's appointment, and that he is late for a business meeting. The paramedics assure themselves that the patient is fully conscious and that he is oriented and capable of refusing consent. They then aseptically discontinue the IV, have the patient sign a "refusal of transport" form, and return to service.

INTRODUCTION

Legal issues are an important concern of the paramedic. As a paramedic, you will interact with the legal system frequently, and you must be familiar with all its components. In addition, you must be familiar with all laws affecting prehospital care. This chapter will address the medical-legal aspect of emergency care, with emphasis on prehospital care. (See Figure 3-1.)

LEGAL PRINCIPLES

The United States has two general categories of law, civil law and criminal law. Both are subject to principles set forth in the U.S. Constitution. **Criminal law** deals with crime and punishment. Criminal **litigation** involves legal action by a state against an offending individual. Homicide and rape are examples of criminal wrongs. **Civil law,** on the other hand, deals with non-criminal issues, such as contracts, domestic relations, and torts. Civil law involves actions filed by one individual against another. Examples of civil litigation are divorce, contract disputes, and

■ **criminal law** the division of the legal system that deals with wrongs against society or its members.

■ **litigation** the act or process of carrying on a lawsuit.

■ **civil law** the division of the legal system that deals with non-criminal issues and conflicts between two parties.

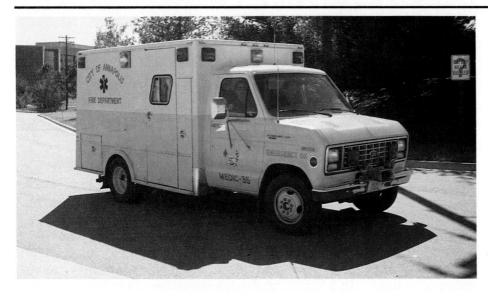

FIGURE 3-1 Each EMS response has the potential of involving EMS personnel in the legal system.

child custody. **Tort law,** a branch of civil law, deals with civil wrongs committed by one individual against another. A malpractice suit is an example of a tort.

As an EMT or paramedic, you may become involved in any aspect of the legal system. You may be called as a witness in a criminal offense. You may be asked to testify in a civil matter, such as divorce or a contract dispute. And, you could be named in malpractice litigation.

■ **tort law** a branch of civil law concerning civil wrongs between two parties.

LAWS AFFECTING EMS

Most laws that affect emergency medical services and paramedics are state laws. Although these laws often vary from state to state, they have several principles in common. This section will address common legal principles, laws, and legislation that affect the paramedic.

Medical Practice Acts and State EMS Legislation

A Medical Practice Act is state legislation that defines the scope and role of the paramedic and all prehospital workers. Often, a state will have a general medical practice act that governs all health care professionals.

Paramedics are not licensed to practice independently. Paramedics may only function under the direct supervision of a licensed physician, through a **"delegation of authority."** The term means that, as a paramedic, you are practicing under the auspices and license of the physician. This supervision may be direct—by telephonic or radio communications—or by accepted, approved standing orders. Failure to adhere to this requirement could make you criminally liable for practicing medicine without a license.

■ **delegation of authority** the granting of privileges by a physician to a non-physician to perform well-delineated skills and procedures.

✳ The paramedic may only function under the direct supervision of a licensed physician.

Most states have EMS laws that govern paramedics and set forth the requirements for certification or licensure, and recertification or relicensure. In addition, most states have laws and regulations that define the skills and procedures a paramedic may perform. It is your responsibility to fully understand the EMS laws and regulations of your state.

Good Samaritan Laws

Virtually every state has "Good Samaritan Laws," which protect from liability people who assist at the scene of a medical emergency. Many states have expanded these laws to cover prehospital personnel. Generally, a person is immune from liability for assisting at the scene of a medical emergency if he or she acts in good faith, is not negligent, acts within the scope of his or her training, and does not accept payment for his or her services. The Good Samaritan Laws of many states now protect prehospital personnel, even though they may be paid.

Motor Vehicle Laws

As with EMS laws, motor vehicle laws vary from state to state. It's important that you know the laws of your state. Generally, there are special motor vehicle laws governing the operation of emergency vehicles. These laws may apply to such considerations as speed and use of the siren and emergency lights. In addition, many municipalities have local rules and regulations for emergency vehicles. You should keep up to date on state and municipal laws where you work.

Other Laws

Many states have enacted laws to protect the public. The paramedic must abide by these laws. Most states have laws requiring a health care worker who suspects child abuse or abuse of the elderly to report the incident. Violent crimes, such as rape and shootings, should also be reported to law enforcement officials. Emergencies that threaten public health, such as animal bites, must be reported to the appropriate authority.

As a paramedic, you should be familiar with local laws and regulations governing the use of physical restraints for violent or confused patients. You should also be familiar with the regulations governing entry into restricted areas, such as military installations, nuclear power plants, and sites with hazardous materials.

RIGHT TO DIE

■ **living will** a written request to withhold heroic life support measures from a patient with a terminal condition. A living will is usually executed before the person becomes ill or injured and is used to express that person's wishes.

Many states have enacted laws governing "living wills." A **living will** is a a patient's written request that no heroic medical measures be carried out in the event of terminal illness or injury. In addition, some states have enacted "natural death acts," which are similar to living wills. They are specific requests made by a patient, after being informed of terminal illness, that he or she not be resuscitated or placed on life-sustaining equipment should his or her condition deteriorate. You should determine whether living wills or natural death requests are legal in your state.

"Do Not Resuscitate" (DNR) orders are a particular problem. Often, paramedics will be called to nursing homes or residences where they may find a patient in cardiac arrest and in need of resuscitation. As a rule, the paramedic is legally obligated to resuscitate a patient. If a physician has written a specific order to avoid resuscitation, the EMS system should not have been summoned. However, legal "living wills" and "natural death requests" should be honored. If there is any doubt, however, resuscitation should be initiated.

Occasionally, you may be requested to treat a patient as a "slow code" or "chemical code only." This is nonsense. Cardiac resuscitation is an "all-or-none" proposition. There is no such thing as treating a cardiac arrest with medications only, abandoning airway management and defibrillation. To do so amounts to negligence and must be avoided.

STANDARD OF CARE

A paramedic is expected to practice the same level of care as any other competent paramedic in the community who has equivalent training. As a rule, you are expected to perform as a "prudent person" would in a similar situation. Any deviation from this standard might open you to allegations of negligence.

✱ The paramedic is expected to practice the same level of care as any other competent paramedic in the community with equivalent training.

NEGLIGENCE AND MEDICAL LIABILITY

Negligence is defined as deviation from accepted standards of care recognized by law for the protection of others against unreasonable risks of harm. In medical care, negligence is synonymous with malpractice.

In a malpractice proceeding, the complaining party must establish and prove four particular elements in order to win a lawsuit for negligence. First, the complainant must establish that the paramedic had a duty to act. This duty may be established by a contract, such as that between a private ambulance company and a city or county. In this case, the paramedic has a legal obligation to care for the patient. Often, however, the act of voluntarily assuming care of a patient implies that there was a duty to act.

Second, the complainant must prove there was a breach of duty by the paramedic. This simply means that the paramedic's conduct was not that expected of a reasonable, competent paramedic, given the same or similar circumstances. This breach can be failing to act, acting inappropriately, or acting beyond the level of certification or training.

Third, the complainant must prove there were damages and that he or she was harmed by the actions of the paramedic. This is an essential component. A lawsuit cannot be won if the defendant's actions caused no ill effects.

Finally, the complaining party must prove that the paramedic's actions were the **proximate cause** of the damages. Proximate cause means that someone's or something's actions were the immediate cause of the problem. For example, a patient who is injured in an ambulance accident could prove that his or her injuries resulted from the accident, and the accident was the "proximate cause" of the injuries. On the other hand, a patient who suffered a heart attack while in the ambulance would have difficulty proving that the ambulance ride was the "proximate cause" of his illness.

In some cases, a complainant may invoke the doctrine of *res ipsa loquitur*, Latin for "the thing speaks for itself." The doctrine is used in cases in which it would be difficult for the complainant to prove all four elements of negligence. To support *res ipsa loquitur*, the complainant must prove that the damages would not have occurred in the absence of somebody's negligence, that the instruments causing the damages were under the defendant's control at all times, and that the patient did nothing to contribute to his or her own injury. When the doctrine of *res ipsa loquitur* is invoked, the burden of proof shifts from the plaintiff to the defendant.

■ **negligence** a deviation from an accepted standard of care. It is synonymous with malpractice in the context of medical care.

■ **proximate cause** a legal concept describing a person, who, through his or her actions, does something that produces an effect. In current usage, it usually means that a person was the immediate causative factor in a civil or criminal wrong.

■ *res ipsa loquitur* a Latin phrase meaning "the thing speaks for itself," used in negligence proceedings.

An example of a case in which *res ipsa loquitur* might be used in the prehospital setting is the defibrillation of a conscious patient who does not have cardiac disease or dysrhythmia. To prove negligence, the plaintiff's attorney would have to show that the damage would not have occurred without the defibrillation, that the defibrillator was under the paramedic's control, and that the patient did not contribute to the injury. Many cases in which *res ipsa loquitur* would be successful are settled out of court.

Unlike criminal cases, which require proof of guilt "beyond a reasonable doubt," civil cases require only proof of guilt by "preponderance of the evidence."

Areas of Potential Medical Liability

There are several areas of potential liability that you should recognize and take into account when you care for patients.

■ **consent** the granting of permission to treat, by a patient to a health care provider.

Consent. **Consent** is the granting of permission to treat. More accurately, it is the granting of permission to touch. Consent is based on the concept that every human being of adult years and sound mind has the right to determine what shall be done with his own body. Touching a patient without appropriate consent may subject you to charges of assault and battery.

✳ Patient care should always be preceded by valid patient consent.

For consent to be legally valid, it must be informed. That is, a patient must be made to understand the nature and risks of the procedures to be performed and made aware of all the risks involved. Consent must be obtained from every conscious, mentally competent adult person before treatment is started.

In the unconscious adult, consent for emergency treatment is considered implied. For example, an unconscious adult diabetic could be treated immediately under the doctrine of implied consent.

In the case of children, or mentally incompetent adults, consent must be obtained from the parent or legal guardian. If a responsible adult is not available, and a life-threatening condition exists, emergency treatment may be undertaken without formal consent. In certain cases, children or mentally incompetent adults may be "wards of the state," and the state may grant consent for treatment.

A patient can withdraw consent for treatment at any time. However, such refusal must also be informed. A common example of this problem is the unconscious hypoglycemic patient. When the patient regains consciousness after being given dextrose, he or she may refuse transport to the hospital. The patient should be encouraged—*but cannot be forced*—to go to the emergency department. He or she has regained consciousness and is now capable of making consent decisions. In these cases, advanced life support measures, such as IV fluids, should be discontinued, and the patient should complete a release-from-liability form.

■ **abandonment** the termination of a health care provider-patient relationship, without assurance that an equal or greater level of care will continue.

Abandonment. **Abandonment** is the termination of the paramedic-patient relationship without assuring a mechanism for continuation of the care. Thus, you should not initiate patient care, then arbitrarily discontinue it. In addition, you should not turn over care of a patient to personnel with less training than you have. For example, a paramedic who has initiated advanced life support care should not turn the patient over to an EMT crew for transport. Physically leaving a patient unattended may be grounds for a charge of abandonment. An example would be an elderly patient on an ambulance stretcher, who, while briefly left unattended by the paramedic, fell off the stretcher and fractured a hip. A plaintiff's attorney could charge abandonment as the breach-of-duty component in a negligence proceeding.

Refusal of Service. Many EMS runs do not result in transport of a patient to the hospital. Emergency care should always be offered a patient, no matter how minor the injury or illness appears to be. Often, the patient will refuse emergency care or transport. In such cases, the patient should be asked to sign a "release from liability" or "refusal of transport" form. If possible, the signing should be witnessed by an individual who is not part of the EMS system, such as a police officer or family member. A patient's refusal to sign the form should be documented, and witnessed, if possible, by a non-EMS individual. The refusal must be informed. That is, the patient must be informed of all possible risks of refusing care.

Assault and Battery. Failing to obtain appropriate consent could open the paramedic to allegations of assault and battery. **Assault** is defined as unlawfully placing a person in apprehension of immediate bodily harm without his or her consent. **Battery** is the unlawful touching of another individual without his or her consent. Assault and battery can be either a criminal offense, or a civil offense, or both.

■ **assault** an action that places a person in immediate fear of bodily harm.

■ **battery** the unlawful touching of a person without his or her consent.

False Imprisonment. Like assault and battery, false imprisonment is a tort that can be prevented by obtaining appropriate consent. False imprisonment is defined as intentional and unjustifiable detention. It is a particular problem with psychiatric patients. In most cases, you can avoid allegations of false imprisonment by having a law enforcement officer apprehend the patient and accompany you to the hospital. If no officer is available, you must carefully judge the risks of false imprisonment against the benefits of detaining the patient. You should determine whether medical treatment is immediately necessary, whether the patient poses a threat to himself or herself or to the public, and whether the physical facilities and equipment are available for the patient.

Libel and Slander. **Libel** is the act of injuring a person's character, name, or reputation by false or malicious writings. **Slander** is the act of injuring a person's character, name, or reputation by false or malicious spoken words. Allegations of libel can be avoided by respecting the patient's confidentiality. The medical record should be accurate and confidential. Slang and labels should be avoided. Since many states consider ambulance run reports part of the public record, you should never write anything on the run report that could be labeled as libel.

■ **libel** the act of injuring a person's character, name, or reputation by false or malicious writings.

■ **slander** the act of injuring a person's character, name, or reputation by false or malicious spoken words.

Slander can be avoided by limiting oral reporting of a patient's condition to the appropriate personnel. Many EMS systems record ambulance-hospital radio transmissions. In addition, scanners, which give the public access to EMS transmissions, are common in the United States. Information transmitted over the radio should be limited to essential matters of patient care. In most cases, the patient's name and the status of his or her insurance should not be broadcast.

Medical Liability Protection

The best protection from potential liability is practicing good prehospital care. In addition, all actions, procedures, and medications should be adequately documented on the run report. A complete, well-written run report is your best protection in a malpractice proceeding. (See Figure 3-2.)

FIGURE 3-2 Example of completed patient report form as used by the Cleveland Emergency Medical Service.

✱ The patient's report should *never* be altered.

To the court, observations and treatments not documented on the run report were not performed. Documentation has become so important that some EMS systems have started requiring paramedics to dictate their reports. These dictations are later transcribed and placed on the permanent record. (See Figure 3-4.)

The medical record should never be altered. An intentional alteration amounts to an admission of guilt by the paramedic. If a medical run report is inaccurate, a written amendment should be attached to the report. The date and time the amendment *was written*—not the date of the original report—should be noted on the paper.

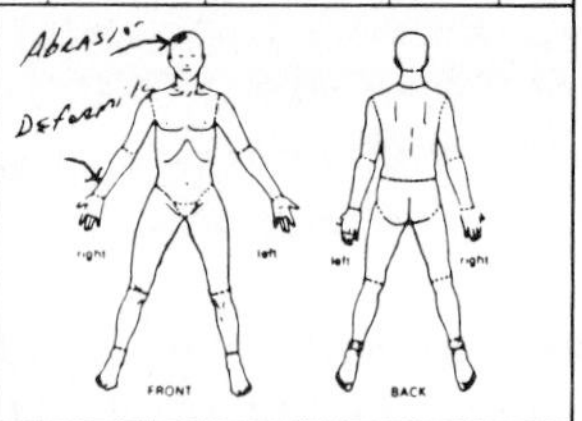

Another important step to take is the purchase of personal malpractice insurance. Malpractice insurance is one of the best investments you can make. Although many employers provide malpractice insurance, it is still a good idea to get your own coverage. Some corporate policies are inadequate. Many are written to protect the policyholder—city, county,

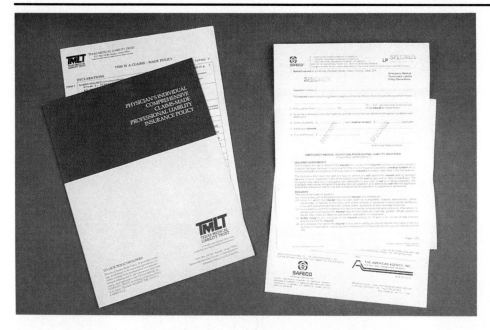

FIGURE 3-3 All prehospital personnel should consider the purchase of professional malpractice insurance. This is especially important in cases where the employer's policy may be inadequate.

private company owner—not the paramedic. These policies will not cover you off duty. Also, some cities claim governmental immunity from liability, even though such claims are controversial. The courts are increasingly striking down governmental immunity statutes. The claim of governmental immunity is not good protection. Alternative coverage should be obtained.

SUMMARY

Paramedics cannot avoid becoming involved in the legal system. The nature of the job requires interaction with law enforcement authorities. It also requires paramedics to be at scenes where they may be material witnesses to a crime or domestic dispute. The paramedic is not immune from allegations of malpractice. However, malpractice charges may be avoided by adhering to the following guidelines:

❑ Always obtain informed consent before initiating treatment.
❑ Practice only those skills and procedures a reasonable and prudent paramedic would, given the same or similar circumstances.
❑ Practice only those procedures authorized directly by the base station physician or by approved local standing orders.
❑ Prepare accurate and legible medical records that thoroughly document the entire EMS incident—from scene response to hospital emergency department.
❑ Discuss patient information with only those who need to know. Limit writings and oral reports to information essential to patient care.
  Purchase and maintain malpractice insurance and see that your employer does the same.

High-quality patient care is always your best protection.

FIGURE 3-4 Some EMS systems now require their paramedics to dictate the patient report. The dictation is transcribed later and placed on the patient's record. This saves time and allows for a more legible document.

FURTHER READING

Brody, Howard. *Ethical Decisions in Medicine.* 2nd ed. Boston: Little Brown, 1981.

George, James E. *Law and Emergency Care.* St. Louis: C. V. Mosby, 1980.

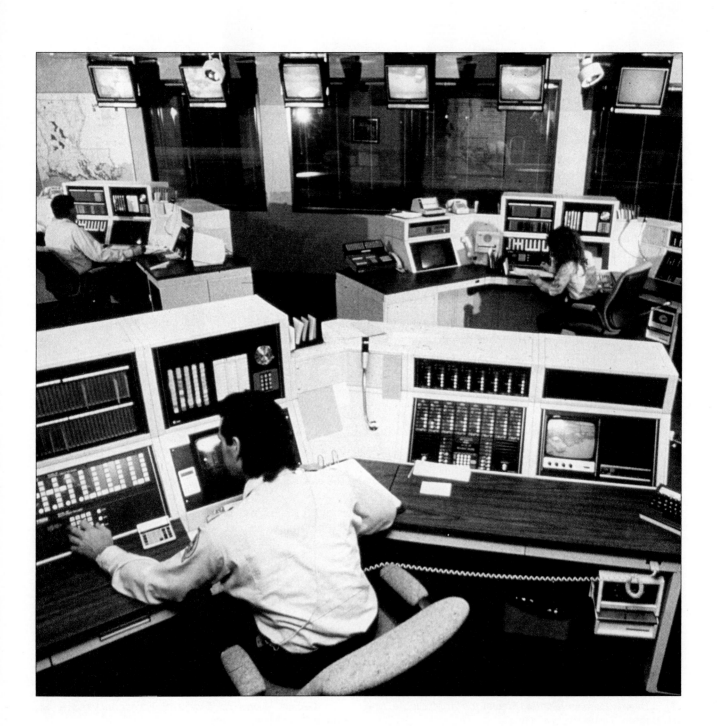

EMS Communications

Objectives for Chapter 4

Upon completing this chapter, the student should be able to:

1. Describe the sequence of an EMS event.
2. Describe the five communications phases of an EMS response.
3. Define the following:
   - base station
   - mobile two-way transmitter/receiver
   - portable radio
   - repeater
   - voting
   - remote console
   - encoder
   - decoder
4. Describe the advantages of a repeater system over a nonrepeater system.
5. List the two types of sound-wave transmission.
6. Define the following:
   - Hertz
   - band
   - biotelemetry
   - modulator
   - demodulator

7. Describe simplex, duplex, and multiplex transmissions and give an example of each.
8. Describe the 10 "Med Channels" and their usage.
9. Discuss the importance of communications equipment maintenance.
10. Describe briefly the functions and responsibilities of the Federal Communications Commission.
11. Define briefly the role of the EMS dispatcher.
12. Describe how information necessary to initiate an EMS response is obtained.
13. Describe the purpose of EMS radio codes and give examples of local radio codes.
14. List radio techniques that improve efficiency.
15. List the important components of the patient medical report and prepare and present such a report on a simulated patient.
16. Name five uses of the written EMS form.
17. Prepare an EMS form based on a simulated patient.
18. Describe the most common causes of interference in biotelemetry communications.
19. Describe the importance of written medical protocols.

CASE STUDY

On a dry, warm Sunday afternoon, a 31-year-old white male loses control of his motorcycle and strikes a highway sign. Several people witness the incident. The first bystander to reach the patient quickly returns to his automobile and calls 9-1-1 on his cellular telephone. The dispatcher takes the necessary information and dispatches an ALS ambulance and an engine company. After the units take off, the dispatcher instructs the caller in basic emergency care. The EMS unit and engine company get the call via a computer print-out of all essential information. They quickly arrive at the scene and initiate the appropriate care. Because he has a severe head injury, the paramedics perform only a limited assessment and immediately transport the patient.

As the ambulance departs, the paramedic relays the following:

Paramedic: 801 to EMS receiving.

Medical Control: Go ahead, 801.

Paramedic: We are leaving the scene of a one-person motorcycle accident on Interstate 35. We have one victim, a white male who appears to be in his 30s. He was apparently the rider of a motorcycle that went off the roadway and struck a sign. He is unconscious, with obvious facial and chest trauma. Medical history is unknown. Vital signs are: Blood pressure 110/60, Pulse 110, respirations 10. Glasgow coma scale is 3. An endotracheal tube has been placed. There is a large laceration above the right eye with an exposed skull fracture. There is also blood draining from the right ear. Pupils are dilated and minimally reactive, yet equal. Palpation of the cervical spine does not reveal any obvious deformity. A rigid C-collar is in place and the spine has been stabilized. There is no tracheal deviation. Breath sounds are symmetrical, yet diminished. There is subcutaneous emphysema on the right as well as several palpable rib fractures. The abdomen is soft and the pelvis appears stable. There may be some lower-extremity fractures. Respirations are being assisted with a demand valve using 100% oxygen. We will attempt an IV enroute. Our ETA is 10 minutes.

Medical Control: We copy, 801. Attempt an IV en route, but transport immediately. Hyperventilate the patient and notify us of any further problems.

Paramedic: We copy, EMS receiving: attempt an IV en route and hyperventilate the patient.

Medical Control: The patient will be going into Trauma 1. The trauma team will be in the ED awaiting your arrival.

Upon arrival, the patient is met by the trauma team and a neurosurgeon. Despite comprehensive care, the patient dies as a result of his head injury. However, at the family's request, the patient's organs are harvested. They are sent to cities more than 1,500 miles away and used in two transplant operations.

INTRODUCTION

Communications are a fundamental of prehospital care. All aspects of prehospital care require constant, efficient communications. In addition to using routine radio communications, the paramedic must organize and present patient information through spoken communication or in written reports.

The sequence of an EMS event illustrates the importance of communications in prehospital care:

Occurrence
Detection
Notification and response
Treatment and preparation for transport
Transport and delivery
Preparation for the next event

A typical EMS response begins with the occurrence of an accident or illness. Then, someone must detect the emergency and summon EMS. Upon receipt of essential information, the dispatcher sends the appropriate EMS unit to the scene of the emergency. At the scene, treatment will be initiated and the patient prepared for transport to the appropriate medical facility. The patient will then be transported to the hospital and care of the patient is transferred to the hospital staff. Following delivery of the patient, the medical record must be completed. Then, all equipment must be prepared for the next response. Communications play a significant role throughout.

The first link in EMS communications is notification of the EMS system. (See Figure 4-1.) Notification occurs between a party requesting help and the EMS dispatcher. In much of the country, notification is made through the public telephone system, by dialing 9-1-1 or another well-publicized emergency number. EMS can also be summoned by other means, such as radio communications from another emergency agency. The EMS dispatcher will quickly determine the nature of the emergency, the address, the cross street, and a call-back telephone number. The appropriate EMS unit is then dispatched. After the EMS unit is dispatched, many systems have a paramedic or other health care worker give the caller simple first aid instructions until the vehicle reaches the scene.

The second link in the communications sequence is notification of the appropriate EMS personnel. (See Figure 4-2.) It may occur through direct telephone link, a radio dispatch system, pagers, or computer-generated dispatch instructions. Personnel are then directed to the scene and progress is monitored throughout the response. The EMS dispatcher may also alert the hospital personnel who will receive the patient.

The third link in the system is communications between the paramedic and medical control. (See Figure 4-3.) Following their initial assessment, the paramedics contact the hospital and relay a report of the patient's condition. The paramedic may have to communicate directly with the emergency physician. Telemetry of the patient's **ECG** may be necessary.

The fourth link is direct communication with hospital personnel after arrival in the emergency department. (See Figure 4-4.) This frequently includes making a detailed verbal patient report, which may address the patient's response to ordered drugs and therapies. A detailed

■ **ECG** an electrocardiogram (ECG) is a graphic recording of the electrical activities of the heart.

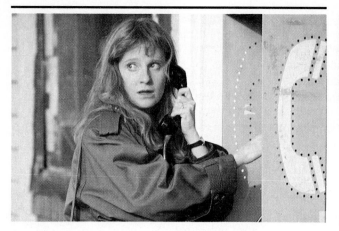

FIGURE 4-1 The first link in EMS communications is notification of the emergency. Citizen access to EMS is most efficient by having a standard emergency number for the entire system such as 9-1-1.

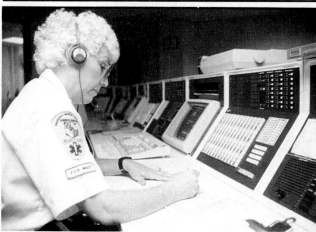

FIGURE 4-2 The second link in EMS communications is notification and dispatch of appropriate EMS personnel.

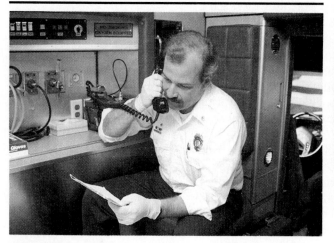

FIGURE 4-3 The third link in EMS communications is communications between the paramedic and the hospital.

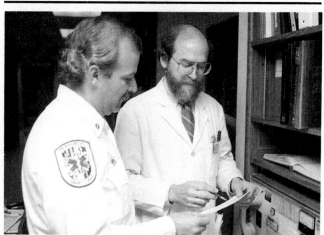

FIGURE 4-4 The fourth link in EMS communications is direct communications with the emergency department staff upon arrival.

written patient report should also be completed. In many systems, this report becomes a part of the patient's permanent medical record.

The fifth, and final, link is notification of EMS dispatch that the EMS unit is in service and available for response. The EMS unit should be restocked, cleaned, and refueled before being declared in-service.

This chapter will address the fundamentals of EMS communications required for rapid and efficient patient care.

COMMUNICATIONS SYSTEMS: TECHNICAL ASPECTS

■ **radio** an electronic device that transmits sound waves and telemetry over distances using electromagnetic waves.

Communications systems vary in complexity and cost. A simple communications system may include a self-contained desktop transmitter/receiver, a speaker, a microphone, an antenna, and a one-piece, vehicle-mounted **radio**. A complex system, on the other hand, may include remote consoles, high-power transmitters, repeater stations, satellite receivers, multiple-frequency radios, and encoders. The communications system is usually custom-designed for each EMS system.

Base Station

The base station is the principal transmitter and receiver of an EMS communications system. It is usually the most powerful radio in the system and may be controlled by remote console. The power output is typically 45 to 275 watts. The maximum allowable base station power is set by the Federal Communications Commission (FCC) and is stated on the base station license. When determining maximum allowable wattage, the FCC considers the size of the service area, as well as the surrounding geography. Some base stations are multiple-channel systems, but most can only communicate on one channel at a time. (See Figure 4-5.)

Mobile Two-Way Radios

The mobile two-way transmitter/receiver is usually a vehicular-mounted device that operates at much lower power than a base station—typically, 20–50 watts. Normal range, without a repeater system, is 10–15 miles over average terrain. Transmissions over flatlands or water will increase the range, while transmissions over mountains, through dense foliage, or in urban areas with large buildings, will decrease the range. The mobile radio may be single- or multiple-channel and may have telemetry capability. (See Figure 4-6.)

Portable Radios

Portable radios are handheld devices, with a low power output, typically 1–5 watts, that limits their range. Considerably smaller than mobile radios, they allow radio communications away from the vehicle. Portable radios may be single- or multiple-channel. Often, they must be used with a repeater system. (See Figure 4-7.)

Repeater Systems

A **repeater** is a device that receives a transmission from a low-power portable or mobile radio on one frequency, and re-transmits it at a higher power on another frequency. Repeaters are important in large geographical areas because portable and mobile radios may not have enough range to communicate with each other, or with medical or dispatch facilities.

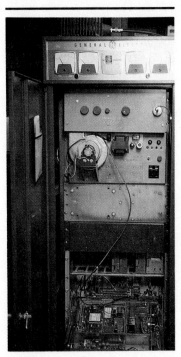

FIGURE 4-5 EMS base station.

■ **watt** a fundamental unit of electrical power.

■ **repeater** a radio base station modified to retransmit a radio broadcast so the range of the broadcast can increase.

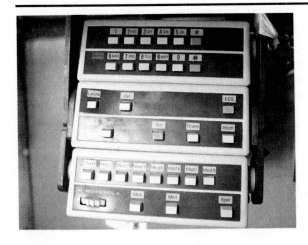

FIGURE 4-6 Control head of ambulance mounted two-way radio.

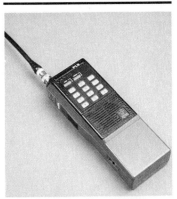

FIGURE 4-7 Portable radio commonly used in EMS communications.

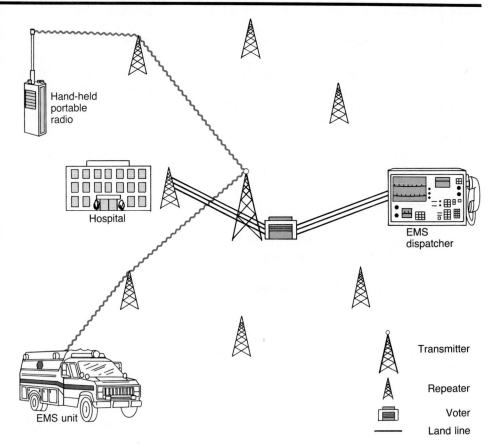

FIGURE 4-8 Example of typical EMS communications system showing the relationship of repeaters, portable radios, voter, and remote consoles.

■ **voting** a process by which the repeater station receiving the strongest incoming signal is chosen to rebroadcast that signal.

Repeaters often have tower-mounted antennas to facilitate the reception of low-power transmissions. Use of a repeater allows two users of low-power radios to hear each other, thus preventing simultaneous transmitting. Many larger EMS systems have more than one repeater. Often, when a mobile unit transmits, more than one repeater will pick up the transmission. The system is designed so that the repeater receiving the strongest signal will transmit the message. This process is called **"voting."** Some systems use repeaters mounted in the vehicle. These repeaters receive the transmission from the low-power portable radio and boost the signal for transmission to the base station. This method is used especially for transmitting remote telemetry. (See Figure 4-8.)

Remote Consoles

Generally, the base station should be placed where it will provide the widest range. It is not always possible, or desirable, to have the dispatch center at the base station. Thus, the base station can be controlled by a remote console. The remote console allows complete operation of the base station from any location. (See Figure 4-9.) This is achieved by using dedicated telephone lines or microwave transmitter links. In many cases, more than one remote may be attached to a base station.

Satellite Receivers

Satellite transmissions may be used to cover large areas. Often, repeaters are placed strategically to receive low-power portable transmissions. The

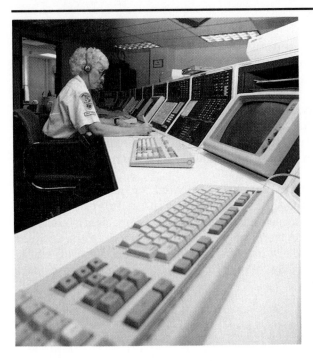

FIGURE 4-9 EMS remote console. Often it is not practical to locate the dispatch console at the transmitter site. Instead, it can be located anywhere and connected by way of telephone lines, microwave, or satellite links.

repeater then relays the information to a satellite, which, in turn, relays it to the remote base station. (See Figure 4-10.)

Encoders and Decoders

There may be a number of base stations on one frequency. This is common for channels used to transmit patient information to the hospital. Several hospitals receive and transmit on the same frequency. Thus, these hospital receivers can be activated by an **encoder.** An encoder is a device that resembles a telephone keypad. When activated by pressing the buttons, it sends specific tones over the air. (See Figure 4-11.) Each receiver has a **decoder,** which recognizes the tones and activates the remote base station. Only the sequence of tones specific for the base station will activate it. Most pagers work on the same principle.

■ **encoder** a device for generating unique codes or tones that are recognized by another radio's decoder.

■ **decoder** a device that receives and recognizes unique codes or tones sent over the air.

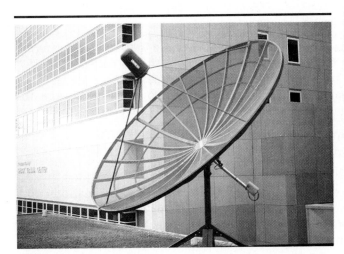

FIGURE 4-10 Satellite communications allow a tremendously increased range and versatility.

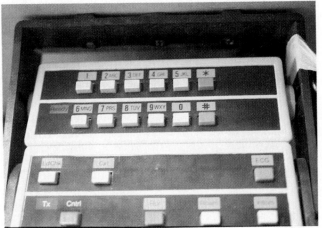

FIGURE 4-11 Typical ambulance mounted encoder. This device will allow paramedics to access hospital radios by way of electronically generated tones.

Mobile Telephones

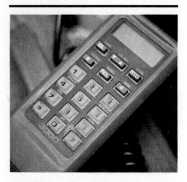

FIGURE 4-12 Cellular telephone technology has opened a whole new era in EMS communications. Now, high quality transmission of telefacsimile (FAX), computer data, and 12 lead ECGs from the ambulance to the base station is possible.

Many EMS systems are finding mobile telephones a cost-effective way to transmit essential patient information to medical control. The advantages of mobile telephones became apparent with the advent of "cellular telephones," now in operation throughout most of the United States. A cellular telephone service is divided into various regions called "cells." These cells are actually radio base stations, with which the mobile telephone communicates. When the transmission becomes out of range for one cell, it is immediately picked up by another cell with no interruption. (See Figure 4-12.)

Hospitals may have a telephone line dedicated for use by paramedics to talk with the medical control physician. Since the cellular system provides so many frequencies, accessing a line is rarely a problem. Telemetry can be performed on the same frequency by use of a demodulator. Cellular technology has opened a new era in EMS communications. Now, an ambulance can transmit 12 lead ECGs, telefacsimiles (FAX), and computer data to the dispatcher or hospital.

RADIO COMMUNICATIONS

Radios function by the transmission of sound waves over designated radio frequencies. There are two types of sound wave transmissions: amplitude modulation (AM) and frequency modulation (FM). AM transmissions have greater range because they follow the curvature of the earth. But, they are more subject to interference and are generally not acceptable for EMS use. FM transmissions are strictly "line of sight"; that is, they do not follow the curvature of the earth but travel in a straight line. However, FM transmissions are much cleaner than AM transmissions and are less subject to interference. The majority of EMS communications are via FM.

The radio frequency is designated by its number of cycles per second. One cycle per second is referred to as a **Hertz (Hz).** Prefixes are commonly added to simplify frequency description:

■ **Hertz** a measurement of radio frequency, one cycle per second.

kilohertz (KHz) = 1,000 cycles per second
megahertz (MHz) = 1,000,000 cycles per second
gigahertz (GHz) = 1,000,000,000 cycles per second

Radio communications are typically in the 100 KHz to 3,000 GHz range.

A group of radio frequencies fairly close together is called a **"band."** Such frequencies are usually assigned a special use by the Federal Communications Commission (FCC). Bands designated for EMS usage include:

■ **band** a group of radio frequencies close together on the electromagnetic spectrum.

Very High Frequency (VHF) Low Band = 30 MHz–50 MHz
Very High Frequency (VHF) High Band = 150 MHz–170 MHz
Ultra High Frequency (UHF) = 450 MHz–470 MHz

Recently, many EMS systems have expanded their communications system and now use frequencies in the 800 MHz range. This band offers even clearer communications with minimal interference. As a rule, UHF transmissions have less range than VHF transmissions, but they are less susceptible to interference.

The FCC controls all licensing and frequency allocations. It has designated 10 EMS channels for use nationwide. Eight are for paramedic/physician communications, two are reserved for EMS dispatch.

The 10 EMS channels are:

Channel	Transmit Frequency	Receive Frequency	Usage
MED 1	463.000 MHz	468.000 MHz	EMT/MD
MED 2	463.025 MHz	468.025 MHz	EMT/MD
MED 3	463.050 MHz	468.050 MHz	EMT/MD
MED 4	463.075 MHz	468.075 MHz	EMT/MD
MED 5	463.100 MHz	468.100 MHz	EMT/MD
MED 6	463.125 MHz	468.125 MHz	EMT/MD
MED 7	463.150 MHz	468.150 MHz	EMT/MD
MED 8	463.175 MHz	468.175 MHz	EMT/MD
MED 9	462.950 MHz	467.950 MHz	DISPATCH
MED 10	462.975 MHz	467.975 MHz	DISPATCH

Biotelemetry

Vital patient information, such as ECGs, can be transmitted over the radio by a process called **biotelemetry.** (See Figure 4-13.) In the ambulance, ECG voltage is converted from an electrical impulse to audio tones via a **modulator**. The audio tones are then transmitted to the hospital over the radio. At the hospital, they are converted back to electrical impulses by a demodulator and displayed on an oscilloscope, or on ECG paper, or both. Most new EMS radios have a built-in modulator and most base stations have a built-in demodulator.

Telemetry is subject to interference by such things as muscle tremor, loose electrodes, 60 Hz interference (from other electrical sources), fluctuations in transmitter power, and by the transmission of voice communications while telemetry is in progress.

■ **biotelemetry** the process of transmitting physiological data, such as an electrocardiogram, over distance, usually by radio.

■ **modulator** a device that transforms electrical energy into sound waves.

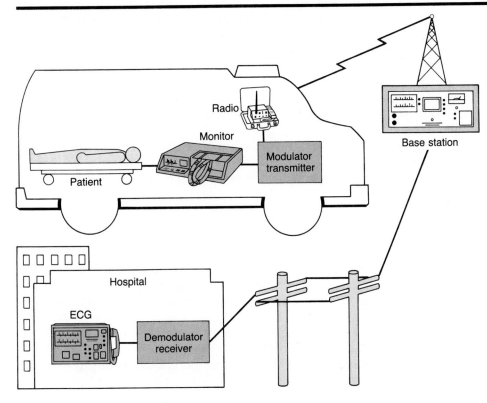

FIGURE 4-13 Biotelemetry allows the transmission of patient data, such as the ECG, from the scene to the hospital. This technology opened the door for the development of prehospital advanced life support.

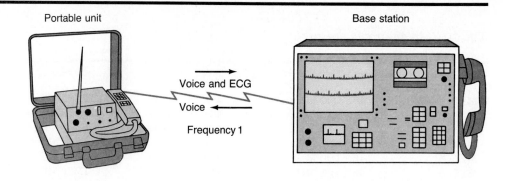

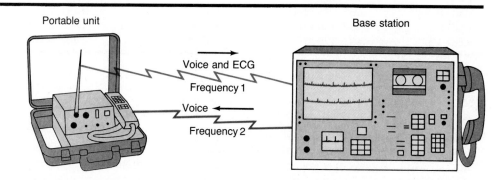

FIGURE 4-14 Simplex communications.

FIGURE 4-15 Duplex communications.

Transmission Types

■ **simplex transmissions**
method of radio transmission in which both transmission and reception occur on the same frequency.

■ **duplex transmissions**
method of radio transmission in which simultaneous transmission and reception occur using two frequencies.

■ **multiplex transmissions**
method of radio transmission in which voice and other data can be transmitted simultaneously by use of multiple frequencies.

Several types of radio transmission are possible; usage may vary from system to system. The most simple communications systems use **simplex transmissions,** (See Figure 4-14.) in which both transmission and reception occur on the same frequency. In a simplex system, transmission and reception cannot occur at the same time. A person must transmit a message, release the transmit button, and wait for a response. Most dispatch systems use simplex transmissions.

Duplex transmissions allow simultaneous two-way communications by using two frequencies. (See Figure 4-15.) This method works like telephone communications. Use of a repeater to boost signal strength is another form of duplex transmission. It allows the receipt of a transmission on one frequency, and rebroadcast of the same transmission on another. It functions as a simplex system, however, because the user must release the transmit button to hear the response. Because it transmits and receives the same message at the same time, it is classified as a duplex system.

Some systems have the capability of **multiplex communications.** Such systems make it possible to carry on a conversation with the medical control physician and transmit telemetry at the same time. (See Figure 4-16.)

EQUIPMENT MAINTENANCE

Communications equipment is expensive and fragile. It must be protected from harsh environments and dusty or wet conditions. Dropping a radio is a common cause of equipment damage that can usually be avoided by careful handling.

Regular cleaning of radio equipment will improve the radio's physical appearance and life expectancy. Clean exterior surfaces with a slightly damp rag and very mild detergent. Do not use cleaning solvents. (See Figure 4-17.)

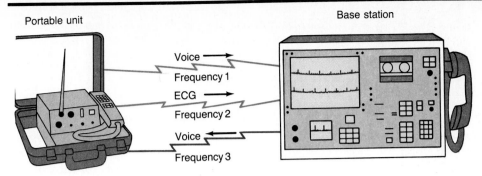

Portable unit

Base station

Voice →
Frequency 1

ECG →
Frequency 2

Voice ←
Frequency 3

FIGURE 4-16 Multiplex communications.

Malfunctioning radio equipment should be repaired by a qualified technician. Preventive maintenance will reduce breakdowns and increase the radio's service life.

Most portable radios and ambulance-based defibrillator/monitors are powered by rechargeable batteries. These batteries are very expensive and must be carefully maintained. Fresh, recharged batteries should be placed daily in the radio and defibrillator/monitor. Spare batteries should always be available. The manufacturer's recommendations for charging, cycling, and replacing batteries should be closely followed.

RULES AND OPERATING PROCEDURES

The Federal Communications Commission (FCC) is the governmental agency responsible for controlling and regulating all radios and radio communications in the United States. Its primary functions are to:

- ❑ License and allocate radio frequencies.
- ❑ Establish technical standards for radio equipment.
- ❑ License and regulate personnel who repair and operate radio equipment.
- ❑ Monitor frequencies to assure appropriate usage.
- ❑ Spot-check base stations and dispatch centers for appropriate licensing and records.

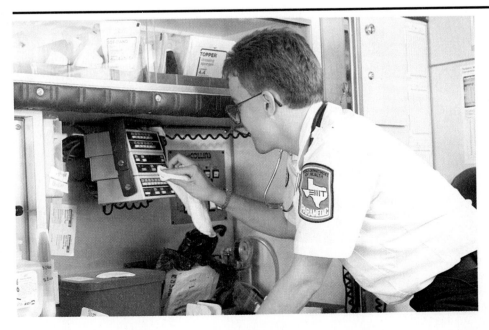

FIGURE 4-17 EMS communications equipment should be cleaned and inspected daily. Any problems detected should be immediately referred to a qualified service technician.

The FCC requires all EMS communications systems to adhere to appropriate governmental regulations and laws.

DISPATCH PROCEDURES

■ **emergency medical dispatcher** person responsible for assignment of emergency medical resources to a medical emergency.

The **emergency medical dispatcher** is a central component of the EMS system. (See Figure 4-18.) Comprehensive EMS dispatch training is based upon the EMS Dispatcher National Standard Curriculum, produced by the U. S. Department of Transportation. Major responsibilities of the EMS dispatcher are to:

❑ Obtain necessary information about the emergency, as quickly as possible.
❑ Direct the appropriate emergency vehicle to the right address.
❑ Monitor and coordinate communications among providers in the system.
❑ Instruct the caller in basic first aid measures that can be undertaken until emergency assistance arrives.
❑ Maintain written records.

Dispatchers may be dedicated solely to EMS events. Or, they may handle dispatching for an entire public safety system, including fire and law-enforcement agencies.

The dispatcher must decide which vehicles to dispatch. In the larger systems, this may be handled by **computer-aided dispatch (CAD).** To use EMS resources most efficiently, the dispatcher must know the location of all vehicles and their capabilities (ALS or BLS). The dispatcher must also determine whether rescue or other support services are required.

■ **computer-aided-dispatch** enhanced dispatch system in which computerized data is used to assist dispatchers in selection and routing of emergency equipment and resources.

The skilled dispatcher must know what information to get from a caller before dispatching an EMS vehicle. Necessary information includes:

❑ The location and nature of the emergency. The vehicle may be dispatched as soon as these facts are known.
❑ An appropriate "call back" number in case of accidental telephone disconnect.

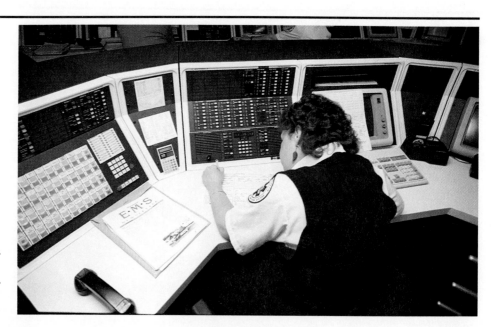

FIGURE 4-18 The EMS dispatcher has evolved into a highly trained and important member of the EMS team. In addition to technical expertise, EMS dispatchers must have knowledge of medical emergencies, local geopgraphy, and available resources.

The following example shows proper EMS dispatch:

- ❏ Call placed and answered by the EMS dispatcher.
- ❏ What is the caller's name and call-back number?
- ❏ What is the address of the event?
- ❏ What is the nature of the event?
- ❏ DISPATCH FIRST AMBULANCE
- ❏ Is the patient unconscious, not breathing, or bleeding severely?
- ❏ Is the patient trapped? Is there a fire or other hazard?
- ❏ UPDATE AMBULANCE CREW AND DISPATCH SUPPORT HELP
- ❏ Are there emergency care measures the caller can perform until the ambulance arrives?

RADIO CODES

Some EMS systems use radio codes, either alone or in combination with English. Radio codes can shorten radio air time and provide clear and concise information. They can also allow transmission of information in a format not understood by the patient, family members, or bystanders. There are, however, some disadvantages. First, the codes are useless unless everyone in the system understands them. Second, medical information is often too complex for codes. Third, several codes are infrequently used, so valuable time may be wasted looking up a code's meaning.

Some systems still use the **Ten-Code system.** Published by the Associated Public Safety Communications Officers (APCO), it is used primarily for dispatch, occasionally in EMS. Many EMS systems, however, have abandoned all codes in favor of standard English.

■ **Ten-Code system** radio code system published by the Association of Public Safety Communications Officers that uses the number "10" followed by another code number.

RADIO COMMUNICATIONS TECHNIQUES

Proper use of the radio results in efficient and professional communications. All transmissions must be clear and crisp, content concise and professional. Here are some guidelines for efficient radio usage.

1. Listen to the channel before transmitting to assure that it is not in use.
2. Press the transmit button for one second before speaking.
3. Speak at close range, approximately 2–3 inches, directly into, or across the face of, the microphone.
4. Speak slowly and clearly. Pronounce each word distinctly, avoiding words that are difficult to understand.
5. Speak in a normal pitch, keeping your voice free of emotion.
6. Be brief. Know what you are going to say before you press the transmit button.
7. Avoid codes unless they are part of your EMS system.
8. Do not waste air time with unnecessary information.
9. When transmitting information:
   - ❏ Protect the privacy of the patient. When appropriate:
     Use codes.
     Use telephone rather than radio.
     Turn off external speaker or radio.
     Don't use the patient's name.

❑ Use proper unit numbers, hospital numbers, proper names, and titles.

❑ Do not use slang or profanity.

❑ Use standard formats for transmission.

10. Use the "echo" procedure when receiving directions from the dispatcher or physician orders. Immediate repetition of the statement confirms accurate reception and understanding.

11. Always write down addresses, important dispatch communications, and physician orders.

12. When completing a transmission, obtain confirmation that your message was received and understood.

Occasionally, communications equipment will not function properly. If you are far from the base station, particularly if you have a portable radio, try to get to higher terrain to broadcast. Also, structures that contain steel and concrete can interfere with radio transmission. Simply moving outside the building or near a window will improve communications. If communications still aren't working, try the telephone.

COMMUNICATION OF MEDICAL INFORMATION

General Concepts

One of the most important skills of the paramedic is to gather essential patient information, organize it, and relay it to the medical control physician. The medical control physician will then issue appropriate orders for patient care. In many instances, written protocols are available. Written protocols are predetermined guidelines for patient care developed by the medical control board of the EMS system. Protocols may vary from system to system. Specific written protocols should be available for all major types of medical emergency. In addition, there should be protocols to deal with such situations as the obviously ill patient who refuses transportation; problems with a non-EMS physician interfering at the scene; and questions relating to "Do Not Resuscitate" (DNR) directives.

Communication of Patient Information by the Paramedic

The communication of patient information to the hospital or to the medical control physician is a fundamental component of the EMS system. Verbal communications, which may occur via radio or land line, provide the hospital with enough information on the patient's condition to prepare for care. In addition, these communications should initiate required medical orders for patient treatment in the field.

A standard format for transmission of patient assessment information allows efficient use of the medical communications system, permits the physician to quickly assimilate information about the patient's condition, and assures that medical information is complete. The format should be concise and should include:

1. Unit call name and name or number of the paramedic.
2. Description of the scene.
3. Patient's age, sex, and weight.
4. Patient's chief complaint.
5. Patient's primary problem.

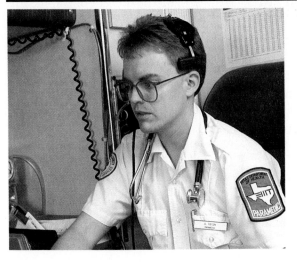

FIGURE 4-19 The patient report should be accurate, clear, and concise. Microphone systems such as that pictured allows hand-free operation so that patient care activities can continue.

6. Associated symptoms.
7. Brief history of the present illness.
8. Pertinent past medical history, including surgeries, medications, and medication allergies.
9. Physical exam findings, including:
   - ❑ Level of consciousness (AVPU system)
   - ❑ Vital signs
   - ❑ Neuro exam
   - ❑ General appearance and degree of distress
   - ❑ ECG (if applicable)
   - ❑ Trauma Index and Glasgow Coma Scale (if applicable)
   - ❑ Other pertinent observations, and significant positive and negative findings.
10. Treatment given thus far.
11. Estimated time of arrival at the hospital.
12. Name of private physician.

✱ The patient report should be accurate, clear, and concise.

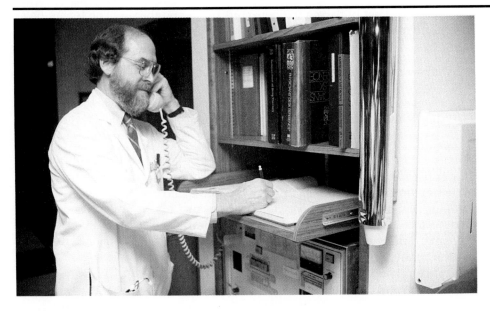

FIGURE 4-20 A clear, concise patient report will enable the emergency department staff to prepare for the needs of the patient.

Await further questions and orders from the medical control physician. When communicating from the field with the physician, the paramedic should remember to:

❑ Be accurate and complete.
❑ Provide whatever information is requested.
❑ "Echo" back the physician's orders.
❑ Question unclear or inappropriate orders.
❑ Report back when orders have been carried out and describe the patient's response.
❑ Keep the physician informed of any changes in the patient's condition.
❑ Protect patient privacy.
❑ Consult with the physician when transport of the patient is deemed unnecessary.
❑ Contact the medical control physician for advice on what course to take.

Upon arrival, verbally report essential patient information to the provider assuming care. This report should include a brief history, pertinent physical findings, treatment, and responses to that treatment.

Biotelemetry

Some systems use telemetry for every patient; others never use it. Use of telemetry alone, without field interpretation, is not appropriate. The paramedic should always verify his or her interpretation with medical control, either over the radio or after arrival at the hospital. A 15- to 20-second telemetry strip is usually sufficient. Continuous telemetry is rarely required, since it uses excessive airtime and depletes batteries.

Written Communications

The written patient report is as important as any verbal communication. From a legal standpoint, it may be more important. Most EMS systems use a standard set of forms to document prehospital care. The forms have several purposes.

❑ The written record of the patient's initial condition and care remains at the hospital after the paramedics have left.
❑ The patient report becomes a legal record of the patient's prehospital care and usually becomes a part of the patient's permanent medical record.
❑ The written record can document a patient's refusal of care and transport.

The patient report is essential for medical audits, quality control, data collection, and billing. In addition, a complete and accurate patient report form is the paramedic's best defense against malpractice. (See Figure 4-21.) EMS forms should be as complete as possible. They should show response times, vehicle numbers, personnel, weather, and patient information. Other material, such as medication flow sheets and ECG strips, should be attached. All information must be legible and the form should be signed by the paramedic.

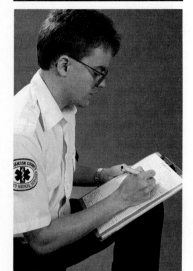

FIGURE 4-21 Post-call documentation is as important as the run itself. It should be completed promptly, accurately, and legibly.

SUMMARY

One of the most fundamental aspects of prehospital care, communications are essential to the efficient operation of an EMS system. Communications begin with the citizen accessing the EMS system, and end with the completion of the patient report and subsequent run critique. Communications must be concise, legible, and complete. They must conform to national and local protocols. The more sophisticated and advanced an EMS system becomes, the more sophisticated and advanced the communications must also become.

FURTHER READING

BLEDSOE, BRYAN E. *Atlas of Paramedic Skills*. Englewood Cliffs, NJ: Prentice Hall, 1987.

MACNEIL, CROSS, and PAUL MANISCALCO. "Cellular Technology: An EMS Overview." *Emergency Medical Services* 18, no. 7 (August 1989).

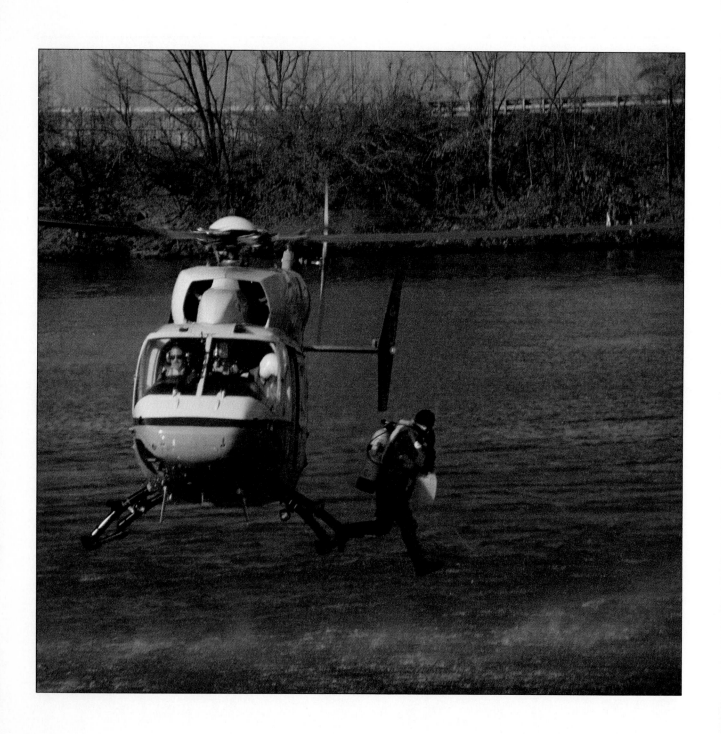

Rescue Operations

Objectives for Chapter 5

Upon completing this chapter, the student should be able to:

1. List the items required for personal safety during a rescue.
2. List the items required for patient safety during a rescue.
3. List the types of hazards that might be encountered at a rescue scene.
4. Discuss the need for written safety procedures.
5. Describe the role of the Safety Officer.
6. Describe how pre-planning contributes to the safety and efficiency of a rescue operation.
7. Define the 6 phases of a rescue.
8. Discuss the key elements of each rescue phase.
9. List the 3 types of information, in addition to hazards, a paramedic should get during scene assessment.
10. Describe why a paramedic's technical capability must be guaranteed before he or she attempts to reach an entrapped patient.
11. List the 2 key goals of patient assessment in a rescue.
12. List 5 situations in which patients may have to be moved prior to complete stabilization.

13. Name the 3 major responsibilities of a paramedic assigned to patient management during a rescue.
14. List the specialty rescue resources that should be accessible to a paramedic.
15. Discuss how prolonged time in reaching—or in disentangling, removing, and transporting—a patient will:
    a) affect patient condition
    b) necessitate management protocol modification.
16. List 3 responsibilities of the paramedic during patient disentanglement.
17. Explain the steps in patient reassessment and stabilization during removal.
18. List the 4 types of problems the paramedic will encounter during patient removal.
19. Discuss why patient removal requires a coordinated team effort.
20. Explain how the method of patient transport is determined.

Fire Unit 1204, a volunteer-operated paramedic ambulance, is dispatched to assist an injured person in a rural state park, approximately 15 miles from the station. Because of winding roads, the response takes nearly 20 minutes. Upon arrival, the paramedics are met by a park ranger, who informs them that an amateur rock climber has fallen. The site is a vertical cliff, popular with local climbers. One of the paramedics is taken by four-wheel-drive vehicle to a trail that leads to the victim. The other paramedic stays with the ambulance because the portable radio will not reach dispatch from the park.

Upon arrival at the scene, the paramedic spots the patient through binoculars. He is on a rock ledge, about 55 feet below the trail. The cliff is a straight face, and ropes will be required. The on-scene paramedic relays the patient information to the paramedic at the ambulance. He, in turn, calls dispatch and requests the vertical rescue team and the medical evacuation helicopter. Shortly after the call, arrangements are made for two members of the rescue team to be flown in with the medical evacuation helicopter. Upon arrival at the scene, the vertical rescue team is taken to the site of the emergency. After assuring scene and personal safety, the rescuers prepare their equipment for descent and access to the patient.

One of the first rescuers down is a paramedic. He performs a primary and secondary assessment. He discovers the patient is unresponsive with multiple fractures. Blood pressure and pulse, however, are stable. The patient is immobilized and an IV established. Because required rigging of the ropes will prolong the time to removal, the paramedic starts a second IV, cleans and dresses all wounds, and splints all fractures. It takes approximately 25 minutes for the entire vertical rescue team to rig the rescue and remove the patient. Finally, the patient is lifted to the trail and transported to the waiting helicopter.

INTRODUCTION

■ **rescue** to free from confinement or danger.

Rescue can be defined as the freeing of a subject from entrapment or threat of danger. Because there are so many situations that might require someone's rescue, a paramedic cannot be trained to meet them all. In fact, proficiency in more than a few rescue specialties is rare. Nonetheless, all EMS responders will eventually be called to a situation requiring rescue. Therefore, paramedics must prepare themselves for such situations *before* they arise. Each paramedic will have to make preparations that are specific to his or her training and ability, and are in conjunction with the planned responsibilities of the EMS system. (See Figure 5-1.)

Because the field of "rescue" entails so many specialties, this chapter will not present step-by-step rescue procedures or extensive lists of specialty equipment. Instead, it will provide references and offer an overview of considerations that apply to most rescue scenarios.

SAFETY

The first step in preparing for rescue response is to develop an individual protective equipment cache. This equipment is generalized because it has application in many rescue situations.

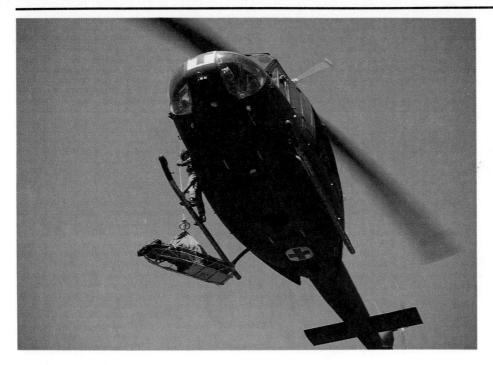

FIGURE 5-1 Rescue is a dangerous activity and safety is the number
one priority. It is impossible for an
individual paramedic to be highly
trained in all types of rescue. Instead, specialized rescue teams
should be utilized.

Paramedic Safety

All paramedics should have at least the following equipment immediately
available: (See Figure 5-2.)

Helmet. The best helmets have a 4-point, non-elastic suspension system, in contrast to the 2-point system found in construction hard hats.
Most of the 4-point suspension helmets are designed to withstand more
severe impacts than hard hats. Avoid helmets with non-removable "duck
bills" in the back because a helmet should be compact enough to wear in
tight spaces.

Eye Protection. Goggles, vented to prevent fogging, and industrial
safety glasses held by an elastic band are both adequate and should be
readily available.

Hearing Protection. From a purely technical standpoint, the best hearing protectors are the high-quality earmuff styles. However, "best" is not
just a technical consideration. Practicality, convenience, and availability
are also major concerns. The multi-baffled rubber earplugs used by the
military, and the sponge-like disposable earplugs are good choices, and
both should be readily available. They should be used by crews or patients
whenever the protection of hearing is necessary, especially if superior
hearing protectors are either unavailable or impractical.

Respiratory Protection. Surgical masks or commercial dust masks are
adequate for most occasions. These should be routine equipment on all
EMS units.

Gloves. Leather work gloves are usually best. They allow free movement of the fingers, as well as good protection. Heavy, gauntlet-style
gloves are too awkward for most rescue work.

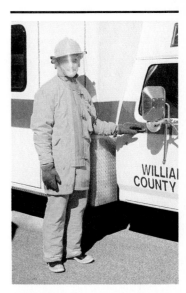

FIGURE 5-2 Each EMS unit
should contain basic safety equipment to protect both the paramedics and the patient.

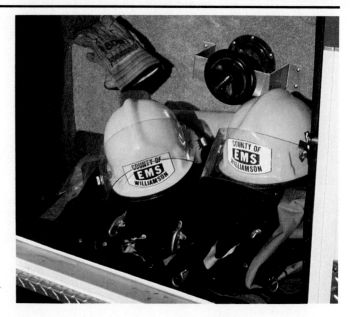

FIGURE 5-3 The quantity of safety and rescue equipment that can be carried on a standard ambulance is limited.

✱ Personal safety is your first concern in any rescue situation.

Boots. High-top, steel-toed boots with a coarse lug sole are preferred. For rescue operations, lace-up boots are more stable, provide better ankle support, and don't pull off as easily in deep mud. However, these benefits must be weighed against the call-to-call advantages of pull-on boots.

Coveralls. Coveralls add some arm and leg protection and can be put on quickly. They also protect uniform pants and shirt. They can be designed with bright colors or reflective symbols for high visibility. The insulated style is very helpful in cold weather.

Turnout Coat/Pants. Turnout gear provides the best protection against the sharp, jagged metal or glass a paramedic might find when extricating someone from vehicle wreckage or structural collapse. This equipment should be available to all paramedics.

Specialty Equipment. Hazardous-materials suits or SCBA (self-contained breathing apparatus) should only be made available to personnel who are thoroughly trained in the applications of this equipment. These items are often supplied on specialty support vehicles, such as hazardous material (Haz-Mat) response units. (See Figure 5-3.)

Patient Safety

After you ensure that responding personnel have adequate safety equipment, you should consider patient safety. Although many of the considerations for rescuer safety also apply to patients, there are several significant differences. A patient safety equipment cache should include at least the following:

Helmets. There is usually no need for patient helmets to be as heavy-duty as those of rescuers. Since patient helmets are mostly used to protect against minor hazards, less expensive, construction-type hard hats are adequate. If severe hazards are anticipated, patients should be outfitted with the same high-grade helmets that rescuers use.

Eye Protection. Vented goggles, held in place by elastic bands, are ideal. They are not as easily dislodged as safety glasses. Workshop face shields may be used.

Hearing and Respiratory Protection. The same considerations for protecting rescuers' hearing apply to patient hearing protection. Earplugs are usually adequate.

Protective Blankets. A variety of protective blankets should be available to protect patients from debris, fire, or weather. Inexpensive vinyl tarps do a good job of shielding patients from water, weather, and most debris. Aluminized rescue blankets should be available for protection from fire or heat. Commercially available wool blankets, or the less expensive variety at surplus stores, provide excellent insulation from the cold. Plastic sheeting (the kind used by landscapers) is inexpensive, durable (usually 3-4.5 millimeters thick), and comes in large rolls. Trash bags of many sizes and thicknesses are very useful. The 30- to 40-gallon trash/leaf bags are the most versatile. However, one 55-gallon-drum liner is large enough to cover a single patient and can be used as a disposable blanket, poncho, or vapor barrier.

Protective Shielding. Circumstances may call for protective equipment more substantial than blankets or plastic sheets. Shields specifically designed for litters and baskets should be available. They can either be purchased or homemade. Keep in mind that a device that shields a patient from debris or the elements may also limit rescuers' access to the patient. The more securely packaged a patient is, the more difficult monitoring and patient care become, and the more likely that changing patient conditions will be overlooked. All rescue teams should be trained to use backboards and other commonly found equipment as shields to protect patients from fire, weather, falling rock or debris, or from glass and other sharp-edged objects.

Safety Procedures

All teams should have written safety procedures that are familiar to every team member. These procedures should specify required safety equipment, particular actions required or prohibited, and any rescue-specific modifications in assignments. Contents should include sections on all types of anticipated rescue, and a statement that every operation must have a **Safety Officer.** The Safety Officer should be someone with the knowledge and authority to intervene in unsafe situations. This person makes the "go—no go" decision for the operation.

■ **safety officer** a person with the knowledge and authority to intervene in unsafe rescue situations who makes the "go-no go" decision for the rescue operation.

Pre-Plan

A major contributor to personnel safety, and a significant influence on operational success, is the rescue pre-plan. Preplanning starts with the identification of locations, structures, or activities that are likely to be the site or cause of events that would require a rescue. Effective preplanning evaluates specific hazards and identifies training and equipment needed to manage them, generates plans for efficient use of personnel and equipment, and anticipates the need for additional equipment, manpower, and expertise. (See Figure 5-4.)

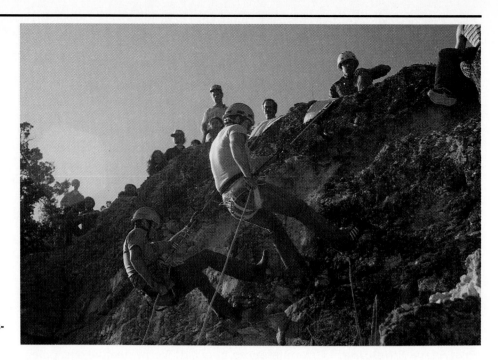

FIGURE 5-4 Dangerous rescue techniques, such as vertical rescue, should be frequently practiced to assure the utmost safety.

✱ Only personnel trained in the type of rescue needed should participate in dangerous rescue techniques.

Screening

Personnel screening is often used by search-and-rescue planners to determine the participants in the rescue process. Programs are available that identify physical capabilities of crew members. Findings of these programs could have significant impact on personnel assignments. In addition, psychological testing is recommended. It may even be desirable to screen for specific traits, such as phobias. For example, a rescuer's inordinate fear of heights or small spaces should be considered in assigning duties.

THE RESCUE OPERATION

Paramedics should know that rescue operations are composed of six general phases:

- ❏ assessment
- ❏ gaining access
- ❏ emergency care
- ❏ disentanglement
- ❏ removal
- ❏ transport

Assessment

The assessment phase of every rescue should begin during response to the scene. (See Figure 5-5.) Since most EMS calls do not require true rescue procedures, responding crews must remain alert to information that could signal the need for technical, rescue intervention. If a rescue is indicated, responders must evaluate the situation more specifically and anticipate circumstances that may require assistance. During response,

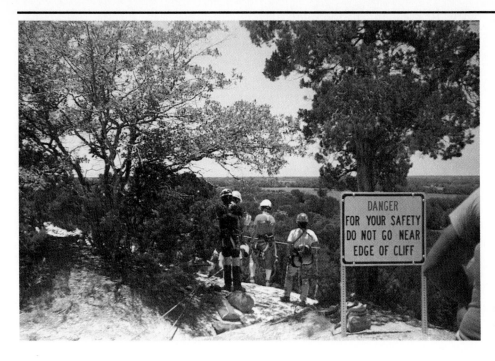

FIGURE 5-5 The first step of the rescue operation is to assess the scene so as to determine what resources and equipment will be required.

paramedics should gather several types of information, which must be clarified and reevaluated at the scene. This information includes:

Nature of the Situation. To accurately assess the need for additional personnel, medical supplies, specialized teams, or sophisticated equipment, a rapid determination of the circumstances must be made: structural collapse, vehicle extrication, high-rise rescue, water rescue, etc.

Specific Patient Location. In situations that "hide" patients—such as entrapments in vessels, cave-ins, and structural mishaps—the exact location of the patient should be determined from dispatch. If possible, a responsible, on-scene person should be requested to meet arriving crews and guide them to the patient.

In many cases, locating the patient constitutes the major portion of the rescue. Large-scale search operations are highly complex. They may require the assistance of experienced search managers, or specialists in electronic detection or search dogs.

Number of Victims. Calling for backup is a common procedure to most paramedics and dispatchers. However, initiation of mass-casualty response procedures, implementation of mutual-aid agreements, and call-out of off-duty personnel are relatively slow, unfamiliar processes. Consequently, first-in crews must quickly notify dispatch if the magnitude of the incident exceeds the capacity of responding units and routine backup. In addition, estimated severity of injuries should be reported, along with on-scene needs for advanced life support (ALS) capability. On-scene personnel can also help estimate the patient transportation needs.

At a rescue scene, medical personnel must make several other critical assessments. These include:

Scene Hazards. All threats to rescuers must be identified and dealt with. Hazards might include:

- Active fire
- Downed power lines
- Falling objects or collapse
- Structural failure
- Rock fall
- Cave-in
- Hazardous materials
    gasoline spills
    natural gas leaks
    caustics
    radioactive materials
    toxic, poisonous, or etiologic agents
- Water hazards
    broad expanses of open water
    swiftly moving water
    chemical or biological contamination
    floating debris
- Cold
- Ice
- Height
    cliffs
    high-rise structures
- Confinement
    tank cars
    vessels
    trenches
    caves
- Psychological hazards
    threats to rescuers or patients from working at heights
    being in small tight structures
    physical threat from hostile crowds
    being confronted with a large number of seriously injured or dead
        persons
- Atmospheric threats
    toxic atmosphere
    explosive atmospheres
    oxygen-displacing or oxygen-depleted atmospheres
- Urgency

Medical.   Uninjured, trapped victims give rescuers more time. Injured patients require more immediate intervention.

Environmental.   Conditions such as rain, rapidly rising water, extreme cold, heat, and high winds increase the need to expedite the rescue.

Situational.   Circumstances such as urban violence and hostage situations are becoming common. They are a profound threat to the physical and mental well-being of rescuers.

Capability of Responding Units/Need for Backup.   Responders often overestimate their capability to handle a rescue situation. They are some-

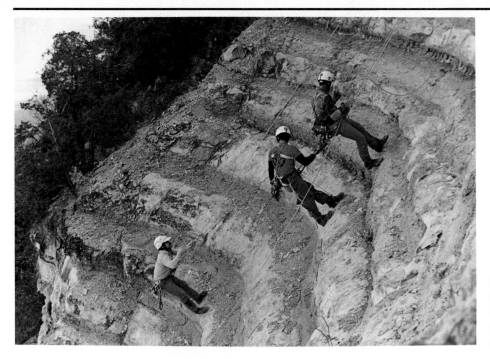

FIGURE 5-6 The second step of the rescue operation is gaining access. In specialized rescues, such as vertical rescue, this can be a long process.

times hesitant to request reserves or specialty rescue teams. Any mistake made in calling out backup manpower or specialized teams should be made on the side of overreaction. Too much, too soon can be recalled. Too little, too late can be catastrophic.

Gaining Access

The Rescue Plan.   Once a thorough assessment of the situation has been completed, the next step in the rescue is gaining access to, or direct contact with, the patient. (See Figure 5-6.) This phase is often the technical beginning of the rescue, which evolves into the disentanglement and removal phases. While gaining access, the paramedic must use appropriate safety equipment and procedures. This is the time for the paramedic and supervisory personnel to honestly evaluate the paramedic's training and ability to see which technical procedures will be needed to access the patient. Undertrained, poorly equipped, or inexperienced rescue personnel must not put their safety at risk through foolhardy, if well-intentioned, rescue attempts.

During the access phase, key medical, technical, and supervisory personnel must agree on the methods they will use to accomplish the rescue. To assure that everyone understands and supports the rescue plan, a formal briefing should be held for rescue personnel before the operation begins. Even with well-trained personnel and adequate equipment, rescue efforts are often poorly executed because team members do not understand the "big picture" or do not know what they, or their fellow rescuers, are supposed to do.

Emergency Care

After the rescue plan is set, medical personnel can begin to make patient contact. But remember: no personnel should enter an area to provide patient care unless they are protected from hazards and have the technical

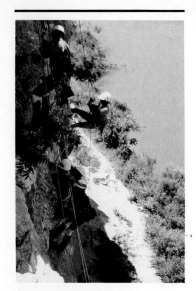

FIGURE 5-7 The third step in the rescue operation is patient assessment and emergency care. This must be modified based on the environment of the rescue.

skills to safely reach, manage, and remove patients. The interests of both rescuer and patient may be best served by a First Responder with expertise in the type of rescue under way—for example, a Haz-Mat, vertical, or swift-water expert. A paramedic who doesn't have such skills may end up having to be rescued.

In a rescue, the paramedic has three major responsibilities:

1. to start patient assessment and care as soon as possible
2. to maintain patient care procedures during disentanglement
3. to accompany the patient during removal and transport

Patient Assessment.   To the extent possible, each patient should quickly be assessed with regard to the standard primary survey (ABC and c-spine status). (See Figure 5-7.) Critical next steps are rapid, secondary assessment and medically oriented recommendations to evacuation teams.

Because a long time may pass before patients are ready for transport, their condition can change significantly during disentanglement and removal. Anticipating these changing conditions, paramedics should perform patient assessment with two goals in mind:

1. identifying and caring for existing patient problems
2. anticipating changing patient conditions and determining the assistance and equipment needed to cope with those changes

Management.   Continually evaluate risks to rescuers and patient. In many situations, the best overall patient care requires rapid basic stabilization and immediate removal. Final positive patient outcome may depend upon initial sacrifice of definitive patient care so the patient and rescuers can be removed from imminent danger. Here are some examples of such situations:

- ❑ injured, stranded window cleaners, water/radio-TV tower workers, high-rise construction workers
- ❑ victims of trench cave-ins
- ❑ persons stranded in swift-running, rising water
- ❑ victims of vehicular entrapment with associated fire
- ❑ persons overcome by life-threatening atmospheres

In all these cases, the risk of injury to the rescuers, and the possibility of making patient injuries worse by applying "definitive" patient care at the scene, could justify rapid transport of a non-stabilized patient to a safer location. This rapid movement might be required even though the transport itself will aggravate the patient's injuries.

Generally, care for the entrapped patient has the same foundation as all emergency care. This includes:

1. ABC's must be assessed, monitored, and maintained.
2. Life-threatening hemorrhage must be controlled.
3. Spinal immobilization must be accomplished.
4. Major fractures must be splinted.
5. **Packaging** in consideration of patient injuries, extrication requirements, and environmental conditions must be provided.

■ **packaging** the completion of emergency care procedures needed for transferring a patient from the scene to an ambulance.

Disentanglement

Disentanglement from such situations as wrecked vehicles, structural collapse, or cave-ins may be the most technical and time-consuming part of the rescue. (See Figure 5-8.) Paramedics assigned to patient care have three types of responsibilities during a rescue. They must:

1. assure that they have the technical expertise and gear to safely enter and function in the active rescue zone.
2. be prepared to provide prolonged patient care.
3. have knowledge of specialty-rescue resources.

Prolonged Patient Care. Specifics of patient management during a rescue are often the same as protocols and procedures used "on the street." However, some specifics may be—or should be—significantly different. Differences are based mainly on the effects of lengthy time periods required to access, disentangle, or evacuate the patient. EMS personnel are trained in rapid stabilization and transport, particularly with trauma patients. However, during a rescue mission, the desire to achieve speedy transport, as well as to obey the cherished "Golden Hour" rule, may be irrelevant. Paramedics must be able to "shift gears" mentally when circumstances prevent application of familiar Basic Trauma Life Support (BTLS) or Prehospital Trauma Life Support (PHTLS) protocols.

Even more important is the formal training of at least some personnel in managing patients whose injuries have been aggravated by prolonged lack of treatment. Procedures adopted from wilderness medical research are useful in managing a patient who has had no care for hours, or who cannot be evacuated promptly. The position papers of the Wilderness Medical Society or the Wilderness EMT course, sponsored by the National Association for Search and Rescue, can serve as guidelines for protocols that anticipate these situations. Regardless of their source, many protocols vary substantially from standard EMS procedures. A system's protocols for extended patient care must be negotiated through, and approved by, medical control. These protocols should address at least eight considerations:

1. long-term hydration management
2. repositioning of dislocations
3. cleansing and care of wounds
4. removal of impaled objects
5. pain management
6. assessment and care of head and spinal injuries
7. hypothermia management
8. termination of CPR

Paramedics should also be prepared to provide more in-depth psychological support for their patient than would normally be required. The paramedic must establish a solid rapport with the patient; constant reassuring conversation is helpful. There are several specific rules the paramedic should follow.

1. Learn and use the patient's name.
2. Be sure the patient knows your name and knows that you will not abandon him or her.

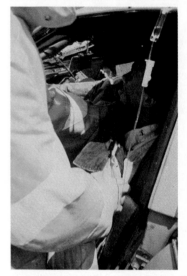

FIGURE 5-8 The fourth step in the rescue operation is disentanglement. It can be prolonged, as in the case of entrapment in autos.

3. Be sure that other team members know and use the patient's name. The term "it" (referring to the extrication process) should never be substituted for the patient's name.

4. Avoid negative comments regarding the operation or the patient's condition within earshot of the patient.

5. Explain all delays to the patient and reassure him or her if problems arise.

6. Advise extrication teams on technical aspects of the operation that could directly impact the patient's condition.

Removal and Transport

Other than during the disentanglement phase, the paramedic's technical experience is probably most important during the removal and transport stages of the rescue. (See Figure 5-9.) In critical situations, the paramedic may be required to assist rigging, **extrication,** or evacuation crews. *Most important,* the paramedic must have technical insight into the overall rescue operation to be an effective patient advocate. It is the paramedic's responsibility to make technical recommendations to the rescue teams regarding patient care.

For example, in a cliff rescue, it is not the job of the paramedic to decide which haul system to use. However, it would be the paramedic's responsibility to recommend that the rescue litter be lifted either vertically or horizontally, because patient position would affect such conditions as head trauma, lower-extremity fractures, breathing difficulty, shock, or spinal injury.

During removal, the paramedic must remain with the patient. This is also a time for reassessment. A patient who's being disentangled or extricated cannot possibly be completely evaluated or managed. However, once the disentanglement is finished—but before removal is far along—a thorough patient survey should be completed. The paramedic should reevaluate the need for:

❑ airway adjuncts
❑ oxygen delivery systems
❑ spinal immobilization
❑ IV solutions, other shock-management procedures
❑ drug administration
❑ cardiac monitor
❑ wounds dressed
❑ fractures splinted

During the physical movement of the patient, vital signs and patient responsiveness must be constantly monitored. The paramedic must frequently communicate with evacuation crews to determine the best:

Terrain. Evacuation routes must be evaluated for hazards and difficulty, both physical and technical.

Personnel. Technical experts should be assigned to equipment operation and rigging duties. The strongest team members should handle lifting and litter-carrying. Do not forget to constantly monitor team members for injury or fatigue.

Equipment. Try to get the "right tool for the right job." Making do with tools that aren't suited to the job can lead to a failed rescue. For example,

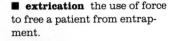
■ **extrication** the use of force to free a patient from entrapment.

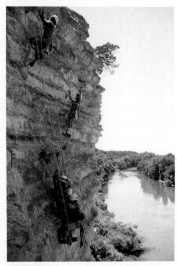
FIGURE 5-9 The fifth step in the rescue operation is removal of the patient.

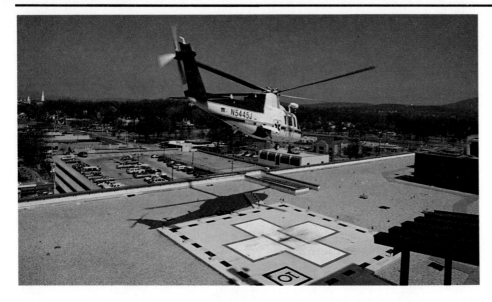

FIGURE 5-10 The sixth, and final step, in the rescue operation is transport of the patient. This can either be by helicopter or ground ambulance as the situation may warrant.

one would never choose a chicken wire Stokes basket, instead of a SKED, for a confined-space rescue.

Technique. Paramedics and rescue personnel should frequently discuss methods, and agree upon compromises between ideal patient care and technical constraints.

Transportation. **Transportation** to a medical facility should be thought out well in advance, especially if delays are predictable. Decisions regarding patient transport, whether by ground vehicle, by aircraft, or by physical carry-out, should be coordinated through, and approved by, medical control. (See Figure 5-10.)

■ **transportation** the act of moving a patient from the scene into the ambulance, or from the ambulance into the emergency department.

RESCUE RESOURCES

Although paramedics are not responsible for developing a rescue resource list, they should have ready access to such a list. No list can cover all scenarios and kinds of assistance. However, a resource list should include expertise and equipment resources for at least the following types of rescue.

❏ Transportation accidents
     automobiles
     buses
     trains
     industrial machinery
     farm and construction equipment
     aircraft
❏ Hazardous materials release (See Figure 5-11.)
❏ Structural collapse
❏ Trench cave-ins
❏ Confined space
     manmade vessels—silos, storage tanks
     mines
     natural caves

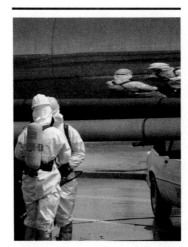

FIGURE 5-11 Hazardous materials require special training and special equipment. Most fire departments will have a Haz-Mat team.

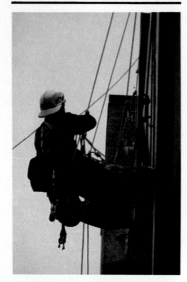

FIGURE 5-12 High angle rescue is dangerous and difficult. It should be deferred to persons trained and experienced in high angle rescue techniques.

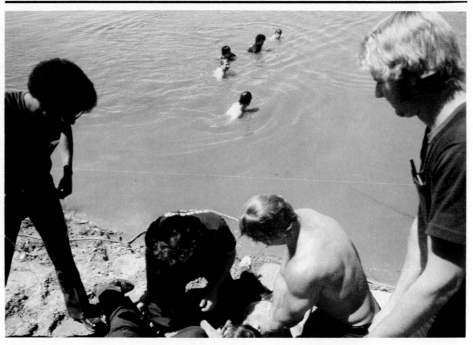

FIGURE 5-13 Water rescue can be deceptively dangerous. Paramedics should not enter the water unless they have been properly trained and have the appropriate equipment.

❑ High-angle accidents (See Figure 5-12.)
      structural—window cleaners, construction workers
      natural—cliffs and gorges
❑ Water accidents (See Figure 5-13.)
      open water (lakes, slow rivers)
      swift water
          natural white water
          floods
      underwater
      ice

SUMMARY

All rescue operations can be divided into at least six functional phases:

1. Assessment
2. Gaining access
3. Emergency Care
4. Disentanglement
5. Removal
6. Transport

All paramedics functioning in a rescue operation must be properly outfitted with protective equipment. In addition, it is imperative that they have training specific to their assigned rescue. In a rescue, the paramedic must access the scene quickly so assessment and management may begin. At times, situational threats to the rescuer or patient may dictate non-standard expeditious patient removal. However, patients should be assessed and cared for as thoroughly as conditions permit. They should be continually re-assessed and re-packaged as removal progresses.

During the operational phases of the rescue, the paramedic must provide direct patient care, and work with technical teams to assure optimal patient management. Paramedics assigned to rescue duties should have training in caring for patients who require prolonged management, because it sometimes takes a long time to locate, access, remove, or transport the patient.

The paramedic must accompany the patient throughout the removal phase, monitoring any changes in condition, and should coordinate patient transport to an appropriate medical facility.

REFERENCES

International Fire Service Training Association
  Oklahoma State University
  Stillwater, OK 74078

The American Red Cross
  National Headquarters
  18th and E. NW
  Washington D.C. 20006

Ohio Department of Natural Resources
  Division of Watercraft
  Columbus, Ohio 43224

Rescue 3
  P.O. Box 4686
  Sonora, Calif. 95370

Air Force Rescue Coordination Center
  Scott Air Force Base
  Illinois

Federal Emergency Management Agency (FEMA)
  Washington D.C.

National Institute of Occupational Safety and Health (NIOSH)
  Washington D.C.

Occupational Safety and Health Administration (OSHA)
  Washington D.C.

Department of Transportation (DOT)
  Washington D.C.

National Fire Academy
  Emmitsburg, Maryland

Environmental Protection Agency (EPA)
  Washington D.C.

National Fire Protection Association
  Batterymarch Park
  Quincy, MA 02269

ORGANIZATIONS

National Cave Rescue Commission (NCRC)
  Cave Avenue
  Huntsville, AL 35810

National Association for Search and Rescue (NASAR)
  P.O. Box 3709
  Fairfax, VA 22038

Wilderness Medical Society
  P.O. Box 3907
  Point Reyes Station, CA 94956

Mountain Rescue Association
  P.O. Box 2513
  Yakima, WA 98902-2513

The Ocean Corp.
  10840 Rockley Rd.
  Houston, TX 77099

National Association of Underwater Instructors
  P.O. Box 14650
  Montclair, CA 91763-1150

6

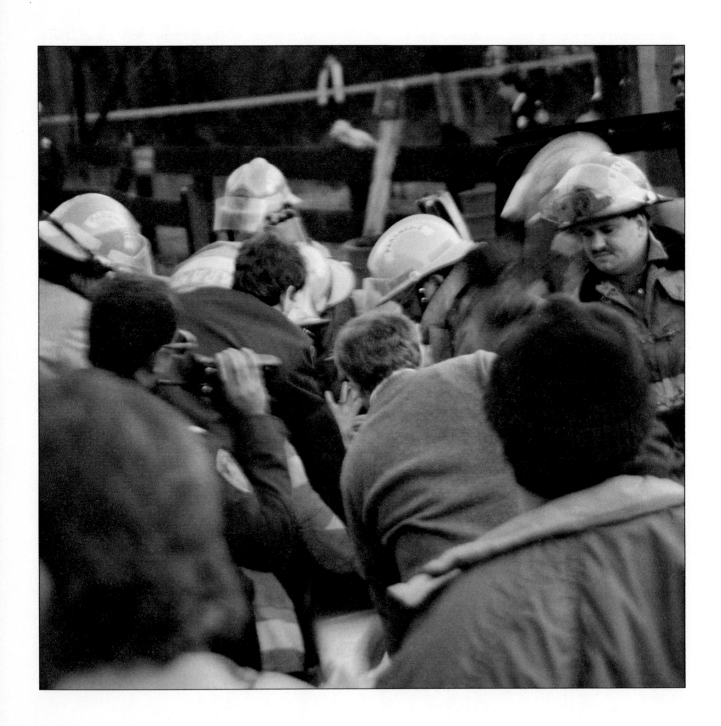

Major Incident Response

Objectives for Chapter 6

Upon completing this chapter, the student should be able to:

1. Describe the need for controlling and organizing responding rescuers at a mass-casualty incident.

2. Identify the incident commander and explain how to contact him or her.

3. Explain the responsibilities of an incident commander.

4. Describe the transfer of command process for the incident commander and sector officers.

5. Explain the communication system requirements at a mass-casualty incident, as well as tell how to use the system to direct rescuers and process information for decision making.

6. Describe the "sectors" that are used at mass-casualty incidents and explain the responsibilities of each sector.

7. Explain the need for triage and tagging at mass-casualty incidents.

8. Explain the START method of triaging patients.

9. Explain the importance of plans and procedures in responding to mass-casualty incidents.

CASE STUDY

A charter bus carrying some 40 passengers drifts off the freeway immediately north of downtown. Upon leaving the road, the bus overturns and slides down an embankment. Dispatch sends out a number of fire department and ambulance units, based on the initial report indicating a bus accident with numerous injuries.

The first unit arrives at the scene. Its initial report back to dispatch: "Unit 501 to dispatch, we're on the scene at I-77 and milepost 114. I have a charter bus over the embankment. Some occupants out of the bus. Further report to follow. Unit 501 is command."

The senior paramedic leaves his vehicle and walks around the scene, performing a quick size-up to determine what additional resources will be required. He relays, "I-77 command to dispatch. I have a bus on its side, fuel leaking. I have an estimated 40 patients, ten or 12 appear critical. Dispatch a second alarm assignment and ten ambulances. Have all units stage 100 yards north of the incident in the southbound lanes. Advise the highway patrol of a major incident, and have them close the freeway in both directions."

Fortunately, the EMS system has a prepared Multiple Casualty Incident plan, and it is immediately implemented. Appropriate personnel are directed to the scene. Later, the on-duty supervisor arrives and assumes command of the incident. Various sectors are set up to quickly and efficiently manage the victims. Incoming ambulances and rescue personnel arrive at the staging sector. From there, they are directed to triage, treatment, extrication, or the transporation sector. Throughout the response, control of the incident is in the hands of the incident commander. Although resources were severely taxed, all patients were triaged, treated, extricated, and transported to the appropriate hospital.

INTRODUCTION

During his or her career, a paramedic will respond to multiple-patient incidents. These events generally involve fewer than ten patients and a variety of injury condition levels (stable to extremely critical). Rarely will the individual paramedic experience a large-scale mass-casualty incident involving 40, 50, 100, or more patients. Even so, these major events do occur. Therefore, the paramedic must understand his or her role in mass-casualty management and how to organize rescuers who will respond to the incident.

The first EMTs arriving at a multiple-patient or major mass-casualty incident will quickly be overwhelmed. There will be far more patients than treatment personnel can handle—a situation that will persist well into the event. In addition, there will be confusion and a great deal of chaos.

The actions that the first EMTs on the scene take to organize the wave of rescuers to follow will determine the outcome of the incident. Correct actions will bring organization, efficiency, and calmness to a mess. Improper or delayed actions will create more confusion and chaos.

When a paramedic encounters a major medical event, priority must be placed upon organization of rescuers as well as on patient care. If the paramedic is unable to organize rescuers, patient care can be missed or

✱ Organization and control of rescuers is essential in any mass-casualty event.

delayed, duplication of efforts occurs, and, ultimately, patient transportation is delayed or misdirected.

INCIDENT COMMAND SYSTEM

A proven program, called the **incident command system,** has been developed over the past two decades to assist emergency services in managing a large-scale event. Originally designed to manage the huge numbers of fire fighters who were combating California's major brush fires, it was found to be extremely effective also in structural fire attack management and, more recently, in mass-casualty management.

There are a number of different incident command systems used in this country. Some are more complex than others. All, however, are spin-offs from the original California system. Each has been modified to fit local circumstances.

There are several nationally recognized standards that apply to incident command systems and mass-casualty management. This chapter will present a commonly used and uncomplicated application of the system for mass-casualty management, one that meets national standards. It will also discuss plans and standard operating procedures relating to mass-casualty management, and the paramedic's role in mass-casualty management.

The incident command system has the following benefits:

1. It provides an organizational plan that is designed to effectively manage incident needs.
2. It provides a blueprint for organizing, controlling, and coordinating the substantial **resources** that are likely to respond to a major incident.
3. It provides an organizational framework in which similar functions are grouped, and responsibilities are identified and defined.
4. It identifies and defines lines of authority.
5. It provides an orderly means to communicate and process information for decision making.

■ **incident command system** a management program designed for controlling, directing, and coordinating emergency response resources. It applies in managing fires, hazardous materials, and mass casualty incidents, as well as during other rescue operations. Major components of the system include the incident commander and a subdivided subordinate management team of sectors or divisions.

■ **resource** term applied to all personnel, vehicles, apparatus, equipment, and medical supplies that respond to an emergency incident.

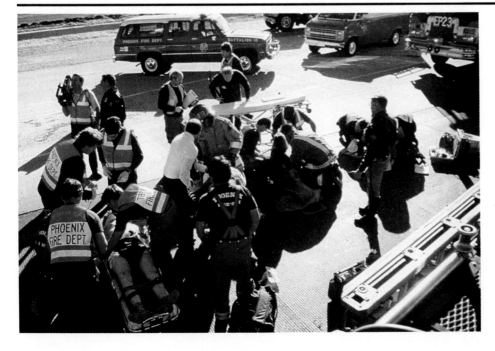

FIGURE 6-1 The Incident Command System assists in controlling and coordinating manpower and resources at a Multiple Casualty Incident (MCI).

■ transfer of command a process of transferring command responsibilities from one individual to another. Commonly a formal procedure of face-to-face communication, followed by a briefing on the situation, and then a radio announcement to a dispatch center that a certain individual has now assumed command of the incident. The transfer of command process also applies in the transfer of sector or division responsibilities.

■ incident commander the individual in charge of and responsible for all activities at an incident when the incident command system is in effect.

■ sector a component of the incident command system consisting of a group of rescuers working for a supervisor within the sector. The supervisor is commonly referred to as the sector officer.

■ division used by some agencies in place of the term "sector" to describe a group of rescuers working for a supervisor. The supervisor is commonly called a divisional officer.

■ staging the collection of vehicles at a central location for distribution as needed at a major incident scene.

6. It provides a common terminology.
7. It identifies a transfer of command process
8. It offers performance evaluation criteria.

All these benefits will be explained further in the chapter.

The cornerstone of the incident command system is the requirement that overall incident command responsibilities be fixed in one person. The system further requires that a strong, direct, and visible command mode be established as early as possible during an operation. An effective command organization must then be developed, including an orderly means of **transfer of command** to higher-ranking officers or supervisors who subsequently arrive on the scene.

The significance of having an immediate and single **incident commander** cannot be overly emphasized. If incident command is not established immediately, rescuers will take independent actions, often in conflict with one another. Within minutes, chaos may become irreversible. Similar chaos will occur if two or more people attempt to command the incident. Once command is established, the incident commander will begin to organize his or her forces by subdividing the incident into three to five (and sometimes more) components. These components are often called **sectors** or **divisions.** Each component will be assigned an officer in charge of all activities within that sector/division. Portable radios will be used to maintain communication with the incident commander. The sectors established are extrication, treatment, transportation, staging, and supply.

Since nearly all mass-casualty incidents require some form of **extrication,** followed by **treatment** and **transportation** of patients, these tasks become logical command organization components or sectors. Multiple rescue vehicle response will also require centralized **staging** of these vehicles at the scene to avoid congestion, so a **staging sector** would be required. In some situations, additional medical supplies may be needed, thus requiring a **supply sector.** Each of these five sectors becomes a component of the incident command organization. Each sector serves a group of similar functions, so there is no conflict in management objectives (i.e., more than a single sector trying to manage patient extrication and a large patient treatment area at the same time).

This subdivision is necessary for two major reasons:

1. The incident commander cannot be expected to personally direct the activities of all rescuers at a scene by physically running about the scene giving orders. This is commonly referred to as the "chicken with its head cut off" syndrome. The inefficiencies are obvious: an out-of-control leader is no leader at all.
2. Management studies have shown that a group leader (i.e., a **sector officer**) provides the close leadership and direction necessary for efficient management of rescuers with common objectives.

Each sector generally assumes a radio designation consistent with its function. Therefore, the incident command component responsible for extricating patients would be called the "extrication sector," the component treating patients would be called the "treatment sector," and so on. Such common terminology is necessary when large numbers of rescuers are involved and particularly if multiple agencies respond. Some communities, however, may alter their sector titles to fit local circumstances. For example, the extrication sector may be called the "rescue sector" and the treatment sector may be called the "**triage sector.**" Some communities may call the various components divisions (e.g., rescue division) rather than sectors. Even though these titles may be modified, task objectives remain basically the same.

These titles will be used in radio communications throughout an incident. The incident commander will assume the radio designation of "command" or some modification of that (e.g., "incident command," "I.C.," etc). When communicating with a **transportation sector,** the incident commander would use the radio call "command to transportation sector."

The use of function/task titles for the sectors and command makes it easy for rescuers to remember who's responsible for what during a stressful event. It avoids the problem of trying to remember apparatus or unit identity numbers, which change as higher ranking officers arrive and assume incident command or sector responsibilities. The titles "command" and "transportation," for instance, remain the same throughout all transfers of command and sector responsibilities.

Many communities use the incident command system on a routine basis for smaller scale medical incidents. For example, a fire department or EMS service may automatically implement the system any time three or more units are committed to a medical incident. This routine use of the system has proven to be highly successful, and such application is recommended. While this routine use might at first appear as an "overkill" use of the system, it does provide better on-scene control of rescuers. An additional benefit, frequent training, is also gained. When a major event occurs, rescuers will have been exposed to the system on numerous past occasions, so they will use it smoothly and naturally.

The Incident Commander

As noted earlier, the cornerstone of effective incident management is a single incident commander and the establishment of command by the first arriving units. The first unit on the scene must assume control of the incident and direct all initial rescue efforts. As the incident develops, and more resources arrive, command will be transferred to higher ranking officers.

Assuming command means assuming the responsibilities of command, providing the control and direction necessary, and using the radio designation "command." Normally, this is done over the radio on an assigned incident frequency, in order that other responding units know that command has been established. From this point on, all additional responding units will announce their arrival on the scene and await instructions from the incident commander. This brief arrival standby is necessary to eliminate free-lancing of rescuers, which often is in conflict with command's plan or other operations already under way at the scene. It further allows command to assess the needs before committing rescuers, which results in better application of resources. As soon as the incident commander determines the appropriate use for arriving units, he will order them to the scene and commit them to areas of need.

As the first unit on the scene, and after assuming control of the situation, the incident commander will transmit a brief radio report to **dispatch.** This accomplishes a number of objectives, including:

1. Dispatch and other units will know a unit is on the scene and in command.
2. Dispatch, as well as other responding units, knows the nature and seriousness of the incident. If it's reported to be a major incident, responding crews can begin to mentally prepare and plan their activities for arrival.

■ **sector officer** the person supervising a group of rescuers. The sector officer is subordinate to the incident commander and receives direction from the incident commander.

✱ The cornerstone of effective incident management is a single incident commander.

■ **dispatch** term used to describe the dispatch center for emergency services. Also called alarm headquarters.

3. Dispatch can automatically implement some behind-the-scenes support activities (i.e., to notify hospitals, helicopter services, etc.).

To explain how the incident command system works at a major incident, let's refer to the accident scenario at the beginning of this chapter.

As you recall, a charter bus carrying 40 passengers drifted off the freeway, overturned, and slid down an embankment. The dispatch center sent out a number of fire department and ambulance units. The first unit of that assignment arrives at the scene and reports, "Unit 501 to dispatch, we're on the scene at I-77 and milepost 114. I have a charter bus over the embankment. Some occupants out of the bus. Further report to follow. Unit 501 is command." (The term "command" remains the title of the incident commander throughout the incident—no matter how many times command responsibility is transferred to higher-ranking officers.)

A rapid evaluation follows to determine exactly what the situation is and the number of patients involved. This evaluation, or **size-up,** is different from **triage.** The size-up is a quick walk around and a quick count of patients to get a more accurate picture of the situation. Often the basic information will be obvious on arrival, and an initial report can then be given.

A second size-up can be more accurate, and a follow-up report will be given to dispatch. The initial incident commander will request additional resources as necessary to meet the demand of the incident. Experience suggests that it is generally better to request more units than you think you need. Making piecemeal requests for individual units is not good practice. When requesting additional resources for a major incident, the incident commander will establish and identify a staging area.

In fire departments, additional resources are often grouped as **alarms.** Each additional alarm brings a given number of fire units to the scene. If the initial unit on the scene was from the fire department, the typical follow-up report might be, "I-77 command to dispatch. I have a bus on its side, fuel leaking. I have an estimated 40 patients, ten or 12 appear critical. Dispatch a second alarm assignment and ten ambulances.

■ **size up** a quick assessment of a situation to determine the nature and extent of the emergency scene, and decide what resources will be needed to resolve the emergency.

■ **alarms** term used by the fire service to identify groups of fire apparatus and personnel called to assist on-scene personnel at major events. Each alarm brings a given amount of personnel and apparatus to the scene.

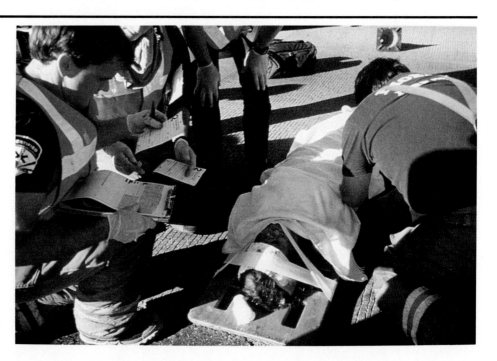

FIGURE 6-2 Triage tagging is essential in Multiple Casualty Incidents.

Have all units stage 100 yards north of the incident in the southbound lanes. Advise the highway patrol of a major incident and have them close the freeway in both directions."

The command officer will then put together a plan of action, or management strategy, that will help personnel stabilize the situation, and then extricate, treat, and transport patients.

Once an organization is developed (i.e., all sectors are in place), and more resources arrive on the scene, the incident commander will assign these resources to the various sectors based on progress reports, incident needs, and other priorities that fit with his or her strategic plan. The incident commander will continue to control, direct, organize, and coordinate all incident activities until the incident is resolved. The sector officer will implement command directions and manage all activities within his or her sector.

An important part of the incident command system is the need for a continuous monitoring and reassessment of incident needs and progress. The incident scene will remain a dynamic event, with constantly changing conditions and problems. The incident commander will stay abreast of conditions by continually seeking progress reports and other information from assisting units. The incident commander typically remains at a fixed location, generally in his vehicle. (Some communities may have a special command vehicle that responds to major events, and from which the incident commander may operate.)

Experience has proven that it is best for the commander to remain at a fixed location, or **command post.** An incident commander running about a scene has lost control of his or her responsibilities and can't be found for face-to-face communications. The command post should be close to rescue operations, at a position where the incident commander can view as much of the operation as possible, yet still be out of the way. In the bus accident scenario, the command post would be located on the freeway, above the accident site and next to the treatment area.

■ **command post** a fixed location where the incident commander is located. Typically a vehicle with radio communications, it is often staffed by a number of other agency representatives, who will provide support and coordination in the rescue effort.

Finally, as the incident winds down, the incident commander will coordinate the release of units, and ensure that hospitals and related agencies are notified that the incident has concluded. A transfer of command to the appropriate police or investigative agencies then takes place.

Transfer of Command

As additional higher-ranking officials arrive on the scene, transfer of command will take place. The mere fact that a higher-ranking official has arrived on the scene does not mean he or she has assumed command. Even though the officer might have been monitoring radio transmissions en route, the official will have missed a lot of face-to-face communication. The transfer of command is a quick and simple, yet important, process. The arriving official will report to the officer in command for a briefing, after which command will be transferred. In most incident command systems, a radio announcement is made to dispatch, alerting dispatch to the fact that command has been transferred, as in: "Command to dispatch, Battalion 4 has assumed command."

It's important to point out that the same transfer of command process takes place at the sector level. No officer should assume command of an incident or sector before he or she knows what has already taken place.

As we continue with the bus accident scenario, command has been established by the first unit on the scene. If additional crew members are aboard this unit, they will begin the triage process. It's important that rescuers rapidly assess all patients for injury priorities and stop only long enough to correct life-threatening medical problems. Shortly after the first unit arrives, additional rescuers begin to appear on the scene, and the incident commander begins to assign sector officer responsibilities.

Extrication Sector

The extrication sector is normally the first one established by the incident commander, and is assigned to the next arriving rescuers. Additional sectors follow as more rescuers appear on the scene. The **extrication sector** is responsible for the management of victims where they are found at the incident site and the delivery of those patients to the **treatment sector.** Normally the extrication sector operates within the **hazard zone** (e.g., within the aircraft or at a collapsed area). In this case, extrication activities take place in and near the bus, where personnel manage **primary treatment** (such as airway problems and severe bleeding) and movement of patients to the treatment sector.

More definitive patient care will take place in the treatment sector. Because the **extrication officer** and his or her crews operate in the wreckage area, this official is in the best position to evaluate which resources will be needed to extricate patients and deliver them to the treatment sector. This evaluation, or size-up, will be completed early in the incident, and resource needs will be reported to the incident commander. The commander will react to requests and provide available resources, obtained from the staging sector or by request to dispatch.

Once the extrication sector has been established and additional rescuers approach and enter the bus, the sector officer will begin to determine if patients should be triaged and tagged where they're found or as they arrive in the treatment sector. The criteria involved in this decision will vary from community to community. Normally, patients would be triaged where they're found, then moved to the treatment area based on life-threatening injury priorities.

Critical patients would be extricated, delivered to the treatment sector, and transported before patients with more stable injuries. In order to do this, patients need to be triaged and tagged where they are found. However, if a life-threatening hazard exists, such as an uncontrolled fuel leak or a fire condition, patients will need to be moved on a first-come, first-served basis. Triage and tagging can take place upon arrival in the treatment sector.

In the bus accident scenario, most patients will be triaged on-site prior to removal from the bus. Because of the confined space conditions within the bus, however, it may be difficult to reach some patients until wreckage, or other patients around them, is removed. Interior conditions may also mean that less-critical patients should be removed and delivered to the treatment sector first, in order to reach entrapped critical cases.

The extrication sector often operates in a significant hazard area, and the sector officer must take appropriate action to provide safety for patients and rescuers. In this scenario, a fire fighter may have to stand by with a pressurized fire hose or apply foam to the vehicle's fuel leak for fire protection. (See Figure 6-3.) The bus may have to be blocked up or otherwise secured to prevent further slippage. Rescuers may have to wear protective clothing. As more resources arrive, the incident commander will appoint a site safety sector officer to handle incident safety responsibilities.

■ **extrication sector** the component of the incident command system that is responsible for freeing victims from wreckage and managing them at an accident site.

■ **treatment sector** the title for a sector within the incident command system that is responsible for collecting and treating patients in a centralized treatment area. A sector officer is assigned as the supervisor.

■ **hazard zone** an area of rescue operations that poses a significant physical threat to rescuers.

■ **primary treatment** patient treatment that targets three life-threatening medical problems: breathing trouble, hemorrhaging, and circulation trouble.

■ **extrication officer** title of an individual who supervises all personnel and activities related to an extrication process.

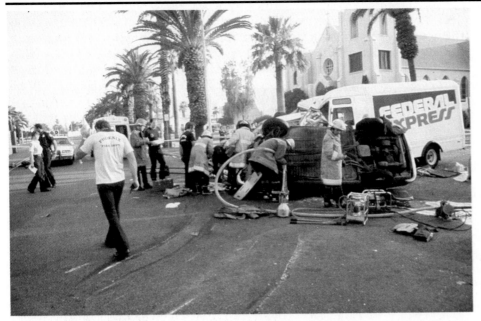

FIGURE 6-3 The Incident Command System in use. The accident is a five vehicle, nine patient accident. This photograph shows the extrication sector in operation. Rescue workers work to extricate two patients in an overturned vehicle. Protective clothing is worn and a fire hose is deployed. The extrication sector officer is at the left of the photograph with clipboard in hand.

The extrication officer will evaluate what manpower, backboards, extrication equipment, and other medical supplies will be required to extricate and move patients to the treatment sector. In some cases, paramedics will be needed to start IV lines on patients who are expected to be trapped a long time. Only a few paramedics will be needed in the extrication sector; the majority will be assigned to the treatment sector.

All resource requirements will be reported to the incident commander. This officer, in turn, will provide resources based on availability and priority needs of the entire incident (and all sectors). As more and more personnel assigned to the extrication sector arrive at the bus, the sector officer will meet and direct them to appropriate patients and extrication duties. The extrication officer will supervise all personnel assigned to his or her sector and manage all activities within that sector.

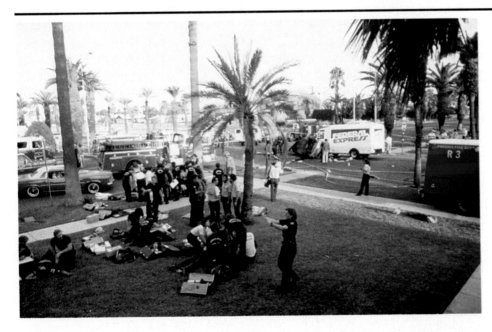

FIGURE 6-4 Overview of the incident site. The extrication sector is operating in the background and the treatment sector in the foreground.

As the first extrication crews gain access to the vehicle, they will encounter walking wounded and uninjured passengers. The extrication officer will be responsible for assembling these survivors and assessing their injuries. They will then be taken to an isolated area (separate from the extrication and treatment sectors), treated as needed, and held until appropriate transportation can be arranged. Only a few rescuers will be needed to manage and assess these survivors.

Throughout the extrication operation, the extrication officer will update the command officer on progress. (The most significant notification comes when the extrication officer reports that the last survivor has been extricated.) The extrication officer will also coordinate activities with the treatment sector officer and other agencies and sectors involved in the extrication process.

Treatment Sector

Shortly after the extrication sector is established, a treatment sector must be created. The treatment sector officer will establish an area where patients can be collected and treated. Central treatment areas permit maximum patient care in incidents that involve large numbers of patients.

In this bus accident scenario, the vehicle is just off the freeway and down an embankment. Inadequate space and sloping ground adjacent to the bus make the area impossible to use effectively as a place for patient treatment. Although somewhat more difficult to reach, the road surface makes a better treatment area. Lots of space will be available at this location for 40 patients, rescuers, and equipment. The site will also be relatively flat. The painted traffic lane stripes can provide visible dividers between critical and delayed treatment areas. The road also provides convenient access to ambulances and other specialized equipment.

The treatment officer will determine how many treatment personnel will be needed to handle all patients, as well as what medical supplies are necessary. Various rules of thumb have been proposed, but the bottom line is that a minimum of one treatment person per patient will be required. This resource requirement will be reported to command. The command officer will notify the staging officer that appropriate resources should be sent to the treatment sector. In some cases, such progress reports will lead the incident commander to call additional resources to the scene.

Paramedics should attend first to critical patients, and then to patients triaged as a delayed category. With regard to paramedic use, the majority of these **ALS**-trained personnel will be assigned to treatment sector operations. Only a few paramedics will be needed in the extrication sector, if any, and they will primarily treat trapped patients who face a long-term extrication process. Many systems award patient treatment needs such high priority that they avoid or minimize assigning paramedics to sector officer responsibilities.

The treatment area will be divided into two sections. One will treat all critical patients, while the other will treat those who have been less seriously injured. As patients arrive, the treatment sector officer or an aide will determine to which area the patient should be routed. If triage tagging has not been done prior to the patients' arrival in the treatment sector, that will take place at this time. The treatment sector officer will ensure that all patients are placed in the proper treatment area and are attended to in a timely manner. All treatment personnel will be closely supervised. The treatment officer will provide progress reports to command throughout his or her sector operation.

■ **ALS** Advanced Life Support. EMS personnel trained to use intravenous therapy, drug therapy, intubation, and defibrillation.

It is essential that the location of treatment centers be reported early to the extrication officer and the incident commander. Follow-up reports when the first patients arrive and when the last patient arrives must also be provided. Other progress reports will be given to the incident commander as essential information or situations become known.

The treatment officer's close coordination with both the extrication officer and the transportation officer will be maintained throughout the rescue effort.

Transportation Sector

As patients are treated and "packaged" for moving, the transportation sector becomes involved. This sector's officer has a real challenge: he or she will determine and obtain all transportation for the patients. The sector officer will also notify hospitals and coordinate patient allocation to those facilities. (Separate radios should be used to communicate with hospitals and with the dispatch center.) Hospitals must be alerted early, and their capacity for receiving and treating patients must be determined. Communication will flow continuously between the transportation sector officer and medical facilities regarding the number of patients, their injury conditions, hospital patient allocation, arrival times, etc.

The transportation sector will set up operations near the exit of the treatment sector area and close to the ambulance patient-loading site. This sector's officer will work closely with the treatment sector officer in determining which patients are to be transported, in what order, and to which medical facilities. It is the transportation sector officer who determines which hospital the patient will be sent to, based on hospital availability reports and patient conditions. The transportation sector officer then arranges appropriate transportation (ambulance, helicopters, etc). He or she normally communicates directly with the staging officer, so that ambulances can be sent to the treatment area as needed (generally one or two units at a time). As patients are loaded, the transportation sector officer, or an aide, will tear off the triage tag stub (if used) and alert receiving hospitals about how many patients are en route, patient priorities, the nature of their injuries (in brief and general terms), and their estimated times of arrival.

■ **transportation sector** the title for a sector within the incident command system that is responsible for obtaining and coordinating all patient transportation. A sector officer is assigned as the supervisor.

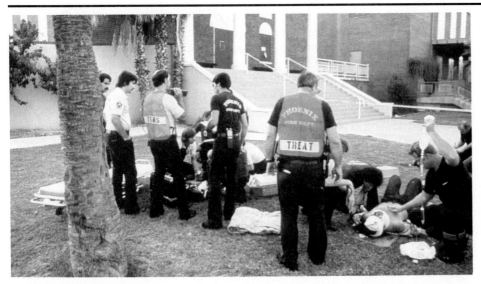

FIGURE 6-5 The Treatment Sector and Transportation Sector Officers are shown in the treatment sector. Both are wearing sector vests for easy identification. The transportation sector officer is coordinating the transport of a patient.

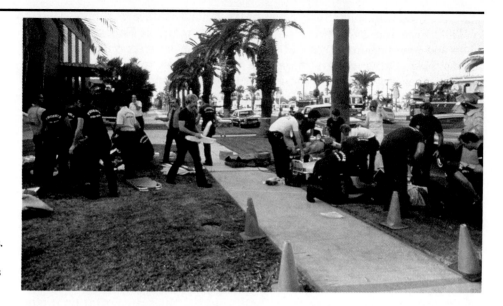

FIGURE 6-6 The sidewalk created a natural divider between the critical and delayed treatment areas. The traffic cones identify the entry point and enhanced flow of patients into the treatment area.

■ **landing zone** an area or sector designated as a landing point for helicopters.

The transportation sector officer may also be responsible for establishing a helicopter **landing zone,** if helicopters are used. This usually requires an aide with a radio (communicating on the command channel). The aide may also need an additional radio for air-to-ground radio communications, in order to provide landing instructions and coordination. Some agencies establish a separate landing zone sector officer for air transportation operations. The transportation sector officer typically employs several aides: one assigned to hospital radio communications, one to the landing zone (if helicopters are used), and one to the patient-loading area. Additional personnel may be required at larger disasters. As group leader, the sector officer supervises these aides.

The transportation sector will provide frequent progress reports to command and, in many cases, to various hospitals. Command will be advised when the sector is in operation and the first patients are transported. It's especially important that the transportation sector officer advise command and hospitals when the last patient is transported.

■ **staging sector** the component of the incident command system that is responsible for managing a staging area.

Staging Sector

As more rescuers and emergency apparatus arrive on the scene, a staging area is needed for vehicles. It's important that the area immediately around the bus remain uncongested, so that ambulances will have access to the scene. As soon as the incident commander recognizes that he's dealing with a major operation, he will establish a staging sector and assign a sector officer. An appropriately centralized staging location should be selected and announced at that time. All additional apparatus—fire, police, ambulance, or other vehicles and agencies (e.g., news media)—will report to staging.

Exceptions are made in the case of apparatus carrying specialized equipment that the incident commander has requested. Such resources will be sent directly to the scene. The staging sector will be established reasonably close to the incident, yet far enough away to minimize site congestion. The staging area will also be organized to avoid internal congestion and allow apparatus the mobility to move up to or around the incident site.

As site sectors report their resource requirements to the incident commander, that official will in turn determine which units are available. In some cases, the incident officer will request more resources from dispatch. The command officer then communicates these needs to the staging officer, who selects the appropriate units and sends them directly to the needy sectors. Within the staging sector, assignments are communicated face-to-face. The staging officer then advises the incident commander which units were sent.

To further minimize congestion at the incident site, personnel assigned to sectors will, when possible, leave the staging sector on foot and hand-carry any additional medical equipment they need to function at the incident site. In some cases, a single pick-up truck, ambulance, or other vehicle can be used to taxi large numbers of personnel and equipment from staging to the incident site.

Supply Sector

Once the size of an incident extends to the point at which routine stocks of medical supplies and equipment carried on apparatus are exhausted, a supply sector (otherwise known as "support" or "resource") will be established. Radio designation for this sector could be "supply sector." This sector is responsible for procuring and assembling the equipment and medical supplies necessary to meet the anticipated demands of the incident.

The location of the supply sector at the incident site would typically be near the treatment sector, because it generally has the greatest demand for the supply sector's services. All requests for the supply sector's services normally go through command first. However, the incident commander may find it more practical to have the extrication, treatment, and transportation sectors communicate directly with the supply sector when requesting supplies. Face-to-face communications are preferred.

Triage Sector

The command organization presented thus far assumes that triage is a continuous process, initiated by the first arriving crews and closely monitored and reevaluated throughout the extrication, treatment, and transportation process. But patient conditions change. Therefore, a person assigned solely to triage may not be required. This assumes that all personnel, especially the people operating in the extrication sector, have the adequate medical training necessary (emergency medical technician basic levels) to make triage and tagging decisions.

The local incident command system may prefer to have the incident commander designate a triage sector in addition to the extrication, treatment, and transportation sectors. This additional sector would be responsible for triage and tagging of all patients, which could take place within the extrication sector, or at the entrance to the treatment sector operations. In either case, close coordination with the sector officer will be important.

Triage and Tagging: the S.T.A.R.T. Method. START is an acronym for Simple Triage and Rapid Treatment, a method of triaging and treating patients that was developed in Newport Beach, California, in the early '80s. The START method has proved to be an excellent and rapid approach to triaging large numbers of patients, and only limited medical training is required to use the method effectively. Under the START concept, the

■ **supply sector** the title for a sector within the incident command system that is responsible for obtaining and distributing additional supplies at a major incident. A sector officer is assigned as the supervisor.

■ **triage sector** the title for a sector within the incident command system that is responsible for triaging all patients. A sector officer is assigned as the supervisor.

■ **triage** a process of sorting patients, based on severity of injury, for treatment and transportation. Critical patients are typically treated and transported before stable patients.

■ **START** the acronym for Simple Triage And Rapid Treatment. The START program describes a rapid method of triaging large numbers of patients at an emergency incident.

first rescuers to a scene clear it of any walking wounded, simply with a verbal instruction to all mobile survivors that they should walk to a described location. These patients are then moved out of the wreckage area and told to stay put. Later, arriving rescuers will further assess these patients and treat any injuries. Survivors must always be thoroughly assessed when time and resources become available, as they may have hidden serious injuries.

Once the walking wounded are out of the way, rescuers should continue their rapid triage. Patients will be triage tagged at the completion of each assessment. Each patient's triage assessment should be completed in less than 60 seconds. The three areas to be assessed are ventilation, perfusion and pulses, and neurological.

The first assessment evaluates ventilation. If it is adequate, the rescuer goes to the next item. If ventilation is inadequate, basic attempts to clear the airway, such as debris removal or repositioning the head, will be taken. Depending on the results of these corrective actions, the patient is classified as one of the following:

❑ *No respiratory effort:* **dead/non-salvageable**
❑ *Respirations above 30:* **critical/immediate**
❑ *Respirations below 30:* **delayed**

The next assessment evaluates perfusion. The rescuer quickly checks for a radial pulse. If it is detected, the patient most likely has a systolic blood pressure of at least 80 mm Hg. (It should be noted that only the detection of a radial pulse is assessed; pulse rates are not considered at this point.) Each patient falls into one of the following categories:

❑ *No radial pulse:* critical/immediate
❑ *Pulse present:* delayed

The third assessment evaluates the neurological status of the patient. Based on this assessment, the patient is placed in one of the following categories:

❑ *Unconscious:* critical/immediate
❑ *Altered level of consciousness:* critical/immediate
❑ *Altered mental process:* critical/immediate
❑ *Normal mental responses:* delayed

It should be pointed out that the first assessment that produces a "critical/immediate" category stops further triage assessment of the remaining areas. The patient is tagged "critical/immediate" at that time. Only correction of life-threatening problems, such as airway blockage or severe hemorrhaging, would be undertaken before moving to the next patient.

The START process permits a few rescuers to very rapidly triage a large number of patients. No specialized medical training is required to make these initial triage decisions. After patients are moved to the treatment area, more detailed assessments can be conducted by paramedics.

Communications

In presenting the incident command organization, we have only superficially discussed the communications aspects. Radio communications are absolutely essential. However, too much communications—or multiple rescuers operating on separate radio channels—can collapse the rescue efforts.

All rescuers and agencies assigned to the various sectors must be able to communicate with the incident commander. Therefore, all sector officers will be equipped with a radio tuned to the same frequency as the incident commander's. Other channels can be used for support activities (e.g., alerting and briefing hospitals, etc).

A great number of rescuers working on the same radio channel can also create problems, especially when some are broadcasting non-essential information. Simply put, too much communication can damage the rescue effort.

The incident command system controls chaos to a great extent. Go back to the bus accident scenario. Such an incident could easily attract 30 rescue units (fire and ambulance). Without the incident command system and the organizational structure described in this chapter, the officer in charge would then have to communicate throughout the incident with 30 people via radio. And those 30 could also be communicating among themselves. It is easy to see this as communications overload.

Remember, all personnel assigned to each sector work for and communicate only with their sector officer. In the vast majority of cases, because the sector officer is in the work area, this communication is face-to-face. Only occasionally would a member of a sector need to communicate by radio with his or her sector officer. In any case, only the five sector officers should communicate with their incident commander. It is easy to see that the incident command system minimizes radio overload, while allowing the incident commander to control and maximize the use of available resources.

Progress reporting is also essential to the incident command system. Incident command is all about decision-making. Decisions cannot be made without accurate information. Thus, sector officers should frequently update their incident commander on what is happening in each sector. If a sector has a problem meeting its objectives, needs more resources, or faces other problems, the sector officer must advise and seek help from the incident commander. Otherwise the situation will worsen. If things are going well, the incident commander must also know this. Progress reports, however, should contain only essential information. If the sector officer does not have any significant information to give the incident commander, that officer should stay off the radio.

Radio codes (e.g., 10-97) pose tremendous problems and should be avoided. These codes can create misunderstandings and confusion, as resources from outside the jurisdiction (and even from within it) may not know what a particular code really means. The use of plain English for all communications is absolutely essential.

PLANS AND PROCEDURES

Community and agency planning for disaster management is also essential. All parties likely to respond to a major incident must have compatible plans and procedures. The elimination of any "turf battles" is a must. Close coordination and cooperation will bring more efficient response to disasters and help in day-to-day operations.

The question of which emergency service should ultimately assume command of overall operations needs to be determined locally. In many cases, local ordinances and other laws make the fire department responsible for managing mass-casualty incidents; in other communities, it's the ambulance service. If multiple fire departments or ambulance companies from other jurisdictions respond, control of the situation typically belongs to the service in whose jurisdiction the incident occurred.

It's important that command responsibilities and procedures be worked out by all emergency agencies prior to any disaster. Protocols should describe how all agencies will respond, how they will function on the scene, and what their lines of authority and responsibility will be. Protocols should tell each rescuer what performance is expected.

All emergency agencies should integrate the incident command system into all their daily operations. Paramedics should consult their employers to determine whether an incident command system is being used by those employers, or at least by another local agency responsible for incident management. Appropriate plans and procedures, as well as training in the incident command system, should be available to new employees. A progressive emergency service organization will already be using the system. If a community does not yet have an incident command system, the lead agency for incident management should begin to activate the system and provide related training.

INCIDENT DUTIES

A paramedic reporting to the scene in our bus accident scenario will either work in one of the sectors or be assigned as a sector officer, although occasionally, a paramedic will serve as incident commander. Under the incident command system, after being assigned to work in a particular sector, the paramedic should report first to the sector officer for a specific assignment. He or she should then continue to report only to that sector officer. No "free-lancing" of activities is permitted. Face-to-face communication with the sector officer is essential; radio communication should be avoided. All problems, progress, and resource needs should be addressed to the sector officer. That officer will, in turn, provide progress reports and request additional resources from the incident commander.

The paramedic assigned as a sector officer must remember that he or she is a manager of rescuers and the rescue effort, and not a treatment person. Only very early in the operation, when a few rescuers are on the scene, is it justified for the sector officer to get involved in hands-on activity. Once additional resources begin to arrive, the sector officer must assume the management role. A sector officer who allows himself or herself to be pulled into a hands-on activity loses overall awareness and control of a sector's needs and responsibilities.

The sector officer must obtain a radio (preferably portable) that has a channel to communicate directly with command. He or she must receive an initial briefing from the incident commander regarding the incident's current status and the commander's plan and objectives. If a paramedic is assuming control of a sector from another paramedic, the transfer of command (for the sector) process must take place.

The objective of the sector officer is to quickly assess the situation as it relates to the responsibilities of his or her sector, and then obtain the resources necessary to fulfill those responsibilities. As rescuers arrive in a sector, the officer in charge must meet them and give them their tasks. The sector officer must closely supervise the rescuers to ensure that the sector's objectives are accomplished. Close coordination between adjacent sectors and with command will be necessary.

The sector officer must be an aggressive manager. He or she cannot assume that another person is taking care of something, or that something will naturally take care of itself. Close supervision of personnel assigned to a sector is a must. Patients must be quickly and safely extricated, treated, and transported. If you are a sector officer, it is your job to make things happen!

ESSENTIAL ITEMS

During mass-casualty incidents, there are items that can help an incident commander and sector officers perform more effectively. The first is a clipboard with pencils and paper. No one, under the stress of a major incident, can be expected to track everything from memory. The incident commander must continually be aware of, and have the ability to track, what units are assigned to various sectors, what remains in staging, and many other details. This sort of information must be written down and tracked. The same information-tracking efforts are required of sector officers. Each will need to know which units are assigned to them. The transportation sector, in particular, will need to document how many patients each hospital can take, which ambulances are transporting, etc. The need for documentation and tracking is obvious. Some communities even develop pads or worksheets that organize important information and provide reminders of what needs to be done.

Sector vests are also excellent tools in a rescue operation. These brightly colored garments identify sector officers (and aides) in a crowd of rescuers. Some vests have sector titles printed on them, which makes it easier for rescuers to quickly locate sector officers. Typically, these vests are carried in supervisor vehicles (such as battalion chief cars) or other specialized vehicles. Some agencies include a vest in all vehicles. They should be issued as early as possible during an incident.

With regard to the use of ambulances and their personnel, past experience in mass-casualty events has provided some important lessons. There will always be fewer ambulances available than patients, until well into an event. For the most part, rapid transportation of patients is of

■ **sector vest** a vest worn by sector or divisional officers and their aides to identify them as having incident management responsibilities. They are typically bright colored and bear titles.

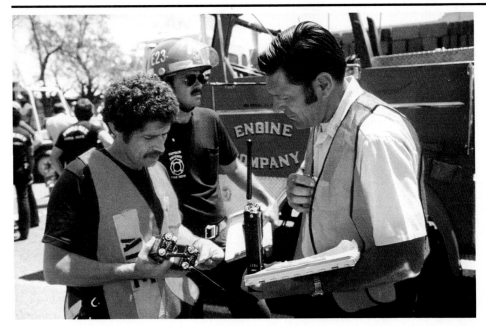

FIGURE 6-7 This photograph illustrates three major supporting tools for a MCI. The sector vests help identify sector officers. The clipboards with paper and pencils help track and coordinate resources and patients. Portable radios are absolutely essential for controlling and coordinating rescuers.

highest priority (especially during trauma-related events), so rescue personnel should quickly treat and package all patients. Multiple trips must be made to and from hospitals in order to clear a scene of all patients. The speed of patient transportation will depend on the number of ambulances available and how rapidly they can return to the scene.

It's important that ambulances and the personnel manning them be used solely for transportation, whenever possible. Other paramedics (not assigned to a transport ambulance) should treat patients on the scene and assume sector officer responsibilities. Such organization will depend on local resources, personnel training levels, and mass-casualty plans, but ambulance transportation needs must be given the highest priority.

SUMMARY

Paramedics will inevitably be involved in some form of multiple-incident response. While most of these events will involve no more than two or three vehicles—and fewer than five or six patients—the incident command system should be employed. If a major incident develops, procedures used on a day-to-day basis, such as START and the incident command system, can be immediately implemented, with all members of the response aware of their roles in the rescue.

The following is a brief review of responsibilities held by the personnel responding to a multiple-incident event:

Command Officer Responsibilities

1. Assume an effective command mode and position.
2. Transmit a brief initial situation report to the communication center.
3. Rapidly evaluate the situation.
4. Request additional resources and provide assignments as necessary.
5. Develop a management strategy or plan.
6. Delegate authority and responsibility to subordinates, in order to accomplish incident needs and objectives.
7. Assign units as required, consistent with the needs of the incident and standard operating procedures or disaster plans, then provide specific operating objectives for these units.
8. Provide continuing effective command, until relieved by a higher ranking official.
9. Review and evaluate the effectiveness of site operations through frequent progress reporting, then revise operations as required.
10. As an incident winds down, return units to service, and terminate command when appropriate.

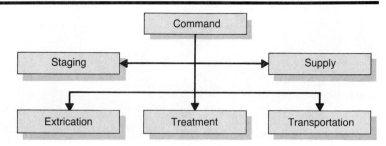

FIGURE 6-8 Organization of the Incident Command System for a large MCI.

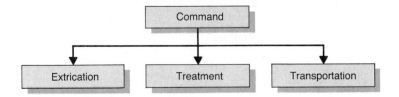

FIGURE 6-9 Organization of the Incident Command System for a small MCI.

Extrication Officer Responsibilities

1. Determine whether triage and primary treatment are to be conducted on-site or at the treatment sector.
2. Determine resources needed to extricate trapped patients and deliver them to the treatment sector.
3. Provide for site safety (very important!).
4. Determine resources needed for triage and primary treatment of patients.
5. Communicate resource requirements to command.
6. Allocate assigned resources.
7. Assign, direct, and supervise personnel and resources.
8. Collect, assemble, and assess patients with obvious minor injuries, and isolate them from the treatment and extrication sector operations.
9. Provide frequent progress reports to command.
10. Report to command when all patients have been extricated and delivered to the treatment sector.
11. Coordinate with other sectors as required.

Treatment Officer Responsibilities

1. Locate a suitable treatment sector area, and report that location to the extrication sector manager and command.
2. Evaluate resources required for patient treatment and report those needs to command.
3. Provide suitable "immediate" and "delayed" treatment areas.
4. Allocate resources.
5. Assign, direct, supervise, and coordinate personnel within the sector.
6. Report progress to command.
7. Coordinate with other sectors.

Transportation Officer Responsibilities

1. Establish ambulance staging (if command has not done so) and patient loading areas.
2. Establish and operate a helicopter landing site.
3. Work with the communication center and hospitals to obtain medical facility status and treatment capabilities.
4. Coordinate patient allocation and transportation with the treatment sector, the communication center, and hospitals.
5. Report resource requirements to command.
6. Supervise assigned personnel.
7. Coordinate with other sectors.
8. Report when the last patient has been transported.

Staging Sector Officer Responsibilities

1. Coordinate with the police department to block streets, intersections, and other access routes required for staging operations.
2. Ensure that all apparatus and vehicles are parked in an appropriate and or-

CITY OF PHOENIX, ARIZONA
FIRE DEPARTMENT
EMS MEDICAL WORKSHEET

☐ 2 + 1 MEDICAL
☐ FIRST ALARM MEDICAL

INCIDENT NO. ____________

ADDRESS ______________________________ TIME ____________

INCIDENT TYPE ____________________

1 2 3 4 5 6 7 ☐

☐ INITIAL REPORT
☐ INITIATE COMMAND
☐ PERSONNEL PROTECTION
☐ TRIAGE
☐ EXTRACTION ☐ ALL CLEAR
☐ TREATMENT
☐ TRANSPORTATION
☐ TRAFFIC / CROWD CONTROL
☐ HOSPITAL NOTIFICATION
☐ SCENE STABILIZED
☐ PROGRESS REPORTS

☐ ____________________

FIRE DEPT

EP		
EP		
EP		
E		
E		
L		
L		
R		
R		
BC		

AMBULANCE

1		
2		
3		
4		

HELICOPTER

1		
2		

COMMAND

EXTRICATION	TREATMENT	TRANSPORTATION	

PRIORITY 1	PRIORITY 2	PRIORITY 3	PRIORITY 4

PT #______ PRIORITY ______ UNIT(S) TREATING ______ UNIT TRANSPORTING ______ HOSPITAL ______ INJURY ______ NAME ______ ADDRESS ______ SEX ______ AGE ______	PT #______ PRIORITY ______ UNIT(S) TREATING ______ UNIT TRANSPORTING ______ HOSPITAL ______ INJURY ______ NAME ______ ADDRESS ______ SEX ______ AGE ______
PT #______ PRIORITY ______ UNIT(S) TREATING ______ UNIT TRANSPORTING ______ HOSPITAL ______ INJURY ______ NAME ______ ADDRESS ______ SEX ______ AGE ______	PT #______ PRIORITY ______ UNIT(S) TREATING ______ UNIT TRANSPORTING ______ HOSPITAL ______ INJURY ______ NAME ______ ADDRESS ______ SEX ______ AGE ______
PT #______ PRIORITY ______ UNIT(S) TREATING ______ UNIT TRANSPORTING ______ HOSPITAL ______ INJURY ______ NAME ______ ADDRESS ______ SEX ______ AGE ______	PT #______ PRIORITY ______ UNIT(S) TREATING ______ UNIT TRANSPORTING ______ HOSPITAL ______ INJURY ______ NAME ______ ADDRESS ______ SEX ______ AGE ______

92-45.2D REV. 8/85

FIGURE 6-10 EMS Medical Worksheet for use in the treatment sector during a MCI.

derly manner within staging, in order that they may be easily moved to the incident site.

3. Maintain a log of units available in the staging area, as well as an inventory of all specialized equipment and medical supplies that might be required at the scene.
4. Confer with command about what resources must minimally be maintained in the staging area, and coordinate requests for these resources with the communications center.
5. Assume a position that is visible and accessible to incoming and staged units. This can best be accomplished by one unit leaving its emergency lights on while all others turn their lights off upon entering the staging area. The staging officer will be located at the vehicle with its lights on. He or she should wear a sector vest.
6. Announce the location of staging to command and the communications center, so that all responding units will report to the proper staging location.

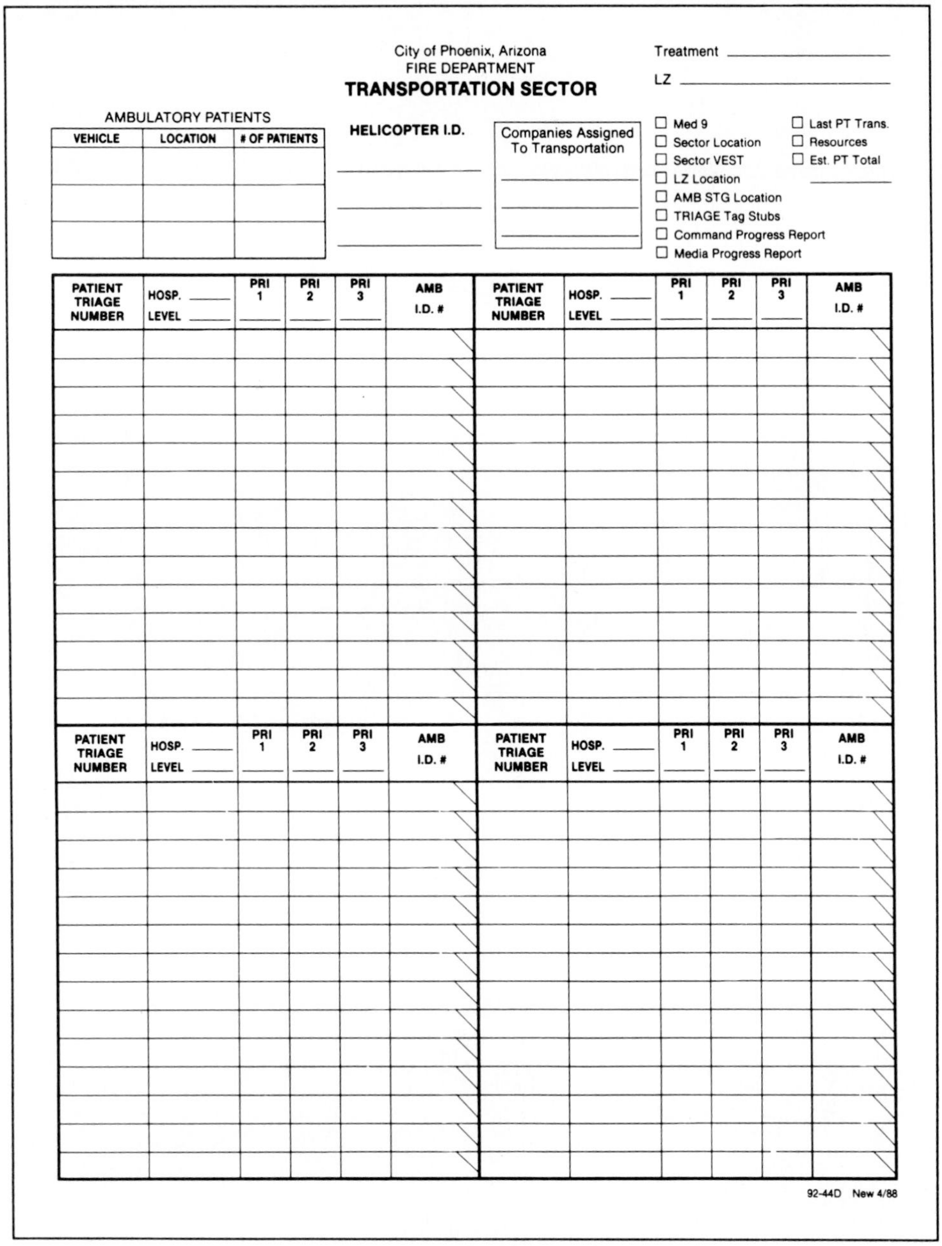

City of Phoenix, Arizona
FIRE DEPARTMENT
TRANSPORTATION SECTOR

Treatment ______
LZ ______

AMBULATORY PATIENTS

VEHICLE	LOCATION	# OF PATIENTS

HELICOPTER I.D.

Companies Assigned To Transportation

- ☐ Med 9
- ☐ Sector Location
- ☐ Sector VEST
- ☐ LZ Location
- ☐ AMB STG Location
- ☐ TRIAGE Tag Stubs
- ☐ Command Progress Report
- ☐ Media Progress Report
- ☐ Last PT Trans.
- ☐ Resources
- ☐ Est. PT Total

PATIENT TRIAGE NUMBER	HOSP. ___ LEVEL ___	PRI 1	PRI 2	PRI 3	AMB I.D. #	PATIENT TRIAGE NUMBER	HOSP. ___ LEVEL ___	PRI 1	PRI 2	PRI 3	AMB I.D. #

PATIENT TRIAGE NUMBER	HOSP. ___ LEVEL ___	PRI 1	PRI 2	PRI 3	AMB I.D. #	PATIENT TRIAGE NUMBER	HOSP. ___ LEVEL ___	PRI 1	PRI 2	PRI 3	AMB I.D. #

92-44D New 4/88

FIGURE 6-11 Example of Transportation Sector worksheet for use during a MCI.

Supply Sector Officer Responsibilities

1. Establish a suitable location for support sector operations, normally near the treatment sector.
2. Determine the medical supply and equipment needs of other sectors.
3. With the transporation sector, coordinate procurement of medical supplies from hospitals.
4. Coordinate the procurement of additional supplies not available from hospitals.
5. Report additional resource requirements to command.
6. Allocate supplies and equipment as needed.
7. Report progress to command.
8. Coordinate activities with other sectors.

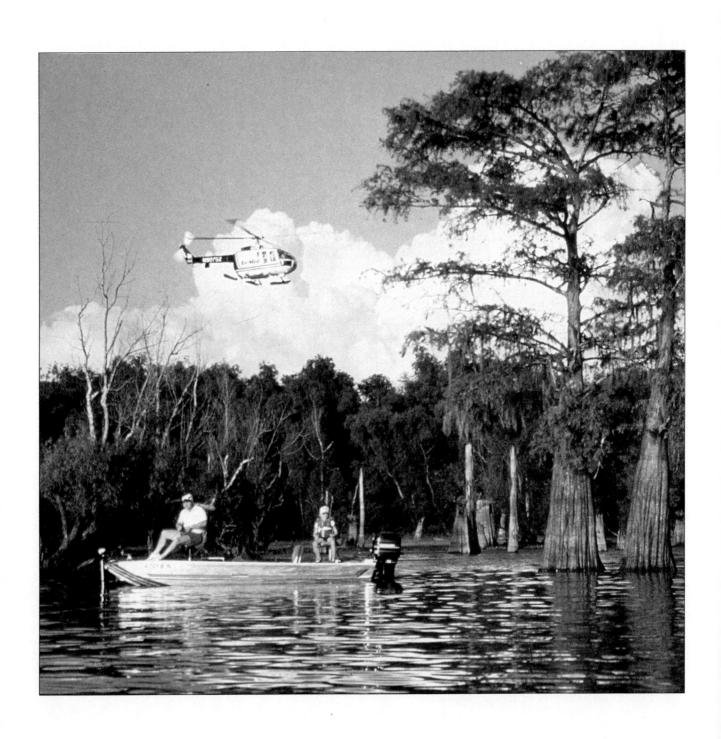

Stress Management in Emergency Services

Objectives for Chapter 7

Upon completing this chapter, the student should be able to:

1. Define the term "stress."
2. List some causes of stress.
3. Describe the three phases of the stress response.
4. Describe at least five defense mechanisms commonly used to deal with stress.
5. Describe the common physiological responses to stress.
6. Name common causes of job stress for the paramedic.
7. Describe "burnout."
8. List techniques the paramedic can use to deal with stress.
9. Describe the purpose of Critical Incident Stress Debriefing.
10. Describe the stages of the grief process.
11. Describe the needs of the dying patient, the family of the dying patient, and the EMT-P.

CASE STUDY

On November 22, Medic 16 was dispatched to a local laundromat on an "unknown medical emergency." The dispatcher advised that the call came through the police department, but had no other information. Police officers, however, were en route. On that date, Medic 16 had a crew of three. The driver, and senior paramedic, was Bill Wyncek, who had three years of EMS experience. The other paramedic was Cathy Downley, who, despite her less than one year of experience, performed like a seasoned veteran. A paramedic student, serving his field internship, was also on the unit.

Arriving at the scene, the paramedics found police officers crouched behind their cars with guns drawn. The paramedics could learn only that there was a shooting and that the suspect was still inside the laundromat. The stand-off lasted more than an hour. Police negotiators tried to reason with the suspect. It was eventually learned that the suspect had recently separated from his wife, had lost his job, and had hurt his back in a fall. The suspect became more hostile as the ordeal continued. Finally, in anger, he sprayed the police cars with automatic weapon fire. The police returned fire. Then, there was quiet. After about five minutes, the suspect appeared in the door with the pistol barrel in his mouth. He made an obscene gesture at the police and squeezed the trigger.

Police officers carefully advanced into the laundromat. They declared the scene safe and summoned the paramedics. Nothing could have prepared the crew of Medic 16 for the scene inside. The laundromat was covered with bullet holes and blood. There were three victims. One, probably the gunman's wife, was obviously dead, shot 20–30 times. The other victims were two young children, one an infant. Both were dead; both had multiple bullet holes. With nothing to be done for any of the victims—including the gunman—the paramedics returned to the ambulance, slowly and in silence. Calmly, Bill picked up the EMS microphone: "Medic 16 clear, no transport." They returned to the station. Although Bill showed no outward signs of emotion, his internal emotions were in turmoil. He had never seen a person die violently before his eyes. Beyond that, he and his wife have a baby girl, about the age of the little girl who was killed.

Fortunately, Cathy talked with supervisors about the incident. A Critical Incident Stress Debriefing was called. The paramedic student was included. It took Bill a long time to open up and describe his feelings. He was angry—at the gunman, at society in general. The meeting, and two later ones, helped Cathy, Bill, and the student deal with their emotions and feelings. All three are still in EMS.

INTRODUCTION

Stress is an inherent aspect of emergency medical services. Prehospital personnel must learn to manage stress, as well as the particular stressors that cause it. Dealing with stress in a positive manner promotes emotional and physical health and prevents "burnout." This chapter will discuss emergency medical services stress and stressors and how to manage them.

STRESS

Stress is defined as a non-specific mental or physical strain. It is always present to some degree in everyone. A **stressor** is any agent or situation that causes stress. Physical and emotional factors involved in stress include:

- ❑ Loss of something an individual values
- ❑ Bodily injury, or threat of injury
- ❑ Poor health or nutrition
- ❑ Frustration
- ❑ Ineffective coping mechanisms

The several stages of stress are:

Alarm reaction. An alarm reaction occurs at the first exposure to the stressor. The signs are increased pulse rate, pupillary dilation, and other responses of the sympathetic nervous system. If resistance to stress is diminished, the physiological and emotional response can be overwhelming.

Stage of resistance. This stage starts when the individual begins to adapt to the stress. Physiological parameters, such as pulse and blood pressure, may return to normal. As adaptation develops, resistance rises above the normal level.

Stage of exhaustion. Prolonged exposure to the same stressors leads to the exhaustion of an individual's adaption energy. The signs of the alarm reaction reappear, but they are now irreversible.

REACTIONS TO STRESS

People react to stress in several ways. One of the most common is the use of **defense mechanisms.** These are adaptive functions of the personality that help an individual adjust to stressful situations. They are in continuous use and are healthy, unless their overuse begins to distort reality. Most defense mechanisms are unconscious and automatic. Some are conscious efforts to seek relief from a particular stressor. Common defense mechanisms include:

Repression. Repression is an involuntary banishment of unacceptable ideas or impulses into the unconscious. This is characterized by unconscious forgetting of stressful events. It is important to understand that repressed conflicts do not change in quality and intensity, and that they constantly seek expression. An example of repression is simply not thinking about a particularly stressful event. However, the event may frequently enter your conscious mind or your dreams.

Regression. Regression is a return to an earlier level of emotional development. Inappropriate, childlike behavior or comments may appear.

Projection. Projecting is the act of attributing to another person or object one's own unacceptable thoughts, feelings, motives, or desires. This may appear as aggression toward others, but is actually anger with one-

■ **stress** a nonspecific mental or physical strain. It is always present to some degree in everyone.

■ **stressor** any agent or situation that causes stress.

■ **defense mechanisms** adaptive functions of the personality that help an individual adjust to stressful situations.

self. An example of projection is anger directed at a dispatcher who had little to do with the stressful event.

Rationalization. Rationalization is a common defense mechanism. Acceptable or worthwhile motives are applied to feelings, thoughts, or behavior that actually spring from other unrecognized motives. Generally an unconscious or retrospective process, rationalization is a way of "explaining" our behavior. It is often self-deceiving. An example of rationalization is stating that a suicide death "finally freed" the deceased from his or her misery.

Compensation. Compensation is a conscious or unconscious attempt to overcome real or imagined shortcomings by developing skills or traits to offset, or compensate for, those deficiencies. For example, a person with a physical disability applies increased energy to developing other abilities. This activity redirects the person's attention from his or her disability.

Reaction Formation. Reaction formation is channeling one's overt behavior or attitudes in a direction opposite to one's underlying, unacceptable impulses.

Sublimation. Sublimation is the act of diverting unacceptable, instinctual drives into socially acceptable channels.

Denial. Denial is the unconscious banishment of consciously unacceptable thoughts, feelings, wishes, or needs. It closely resembles rationalization.

Substitution. Substitution is the replacement of unattainable or unacceptable activity by activity that is attainable or acceptable. It also applies to redirection of an emotion from the original object to a more acceptable substitute.

Isolation. Isolation is the separation of an unacceptable impulse, act, or idea from its memory origin, thereby removing the associated emotional charge. In other words, isolation seeks to retain the memory, but not the feeling associated with it.

ANXIETY

■ **anxiety** an emotional state caused by stress. It is characterized by increase in sympathetic nervous system tone.

Anxiety is an emotional state caused by stress. It is a major cause for the development of coping mechanisms. Anxiety alerts a person to impending or perceived danger. Facilitated through the sympathetic nervous system, it maintains all potential resources, emotional and physical, in readiness for emergencies. Anxiety is each individual's perception of the environment around him or her. It is based on a person's psychological processes. The factors that lead to anxiety can be divided into two general categories:

1. *Internal Causes.* Internal anxiety can be caused by inner conflicts between our expectations and our current motivations. In other words, are we living up to our self-expectations?
2. *External Causes.* External causes of anxiety are those imposed by the people and events around us.

A "normal" level of anxiety varies from individual to individual. It acts as a warning system to put us on guard, so we won't be overwhelmed by sudden stimulation or immobilized in a critical situation. "Normal" anxiety is adaptive as it helps us cope with stressors by focusing our attention. It helps us increase our tolerance for stress by developing coping mechanisms and defenses.

This process is evident in emergency medical services. The first emergency response an EMT or paramedic makes is a very stressful event. The pulse rate is high, the pupils are dilated, thought processes are poorly organized, and tension is high. However, over time, the body adapts to stress. Each response becomes more and more routine. However, as long as the EMT or paramedic is "on call" for emergency response, his or her level of anxiety never returns to a non-work state. Keeping anxiety at an "on-alert" level is a coping mechanism. Because it is impossible to predict and prepare for the next problem, anxiety helps the paramedic maintain a level of readiness.

Although many reactions to anxiety and stress are positive, there are also detrimental ones. Detrimental reactions include the failure of anxiety to stimulate the appropriate coping mechanisms. Conversely, an increase in anxiety that is disproportionate to the actual danger would also be detrimental. These reactions may interfere with a rational thought process, disrupt performance, or cause physical problems.

Most of the many physiological reactions to stress are mediated by the autonomic nervous system. Stress triggers an increase in sympathetic tone, and a subsequent release of norepinephrine and epinephrine. In addition, there is an increase in corticosteroid production in the adrenal cortex. Physiological responses that can be felt include:

❑ heart palpitations
❑ difficult or rapid breathing
❑ dry mouth
❑ chest tightness or pain
❑ anorexia, nausea, vomiting, abdominal cramps, flatulence, or the classic "butterflies in the stomach"
❑ flushing, diaphoresis, or fluctuation in body temperature
❑ urgency or frequency of urination
❑ dysmenorrhea, decreased sexual drive or performance
❑ aching muscles or joints
❑ backache or headache

Effects that are not felt include:

❑ increased blood pressure and heart rate
❑ blood shunting to muscles
❑ increased blood glucose levels
❑ increased catecholamine production by the adrenal glands
❑ reduced peristalsis in the digestive tract
❑ pupillary dilation

People react differently to stress. The patient and family may react with anger, guilt, or indecisiveness. The paramedic may react with impatience, fear, or anger. It is important to remember that the patient and family are not as adept at dealing with stress as the paramedic. Because of indecisiveness, the patient and family members should not be given too many alternatives. Despite his or her emotions, the paramedic must maintain a professional attitude and remain non-judgmental.

PARAMEDIC JOB STRESS

The occupational stressors in emergency medical services include the following: (See Figure 7-1.)

Multiple Role Responsibilities. The paramedic is often a "jack of all trades." The various responsibilities may become overwhelming. This is particularly true of systems in which paramedics also function as firefighters, police officers, or safety officers.

Unfinished Tasks. The requirements of the job often leave personal and work tasks incomplete. For example, once a patient is delivered to the hospital, paramedics often lose track of the person they spent a great deal of time and energy treating. On a continuous basis, this can result in stress.

Angry or Confused Citizens. Paramedics do not see society at its best. The very people who require our help can be a source of stress, as a result of either their physical condition or their emotional response to stress.

Meeting Continuous Time Constraints. Emergency medical services, like many other occupations, place time constraints on personnel. Over time, these constraints result in stress, especially if they cannot be met.

Absence of Challenge. It is hard to believe that emergency medical services can be unchallenging. But, routine runs can get old, and, in some systems, interesting and challenging runs are rare.

Overdemand on Time, Energy, Ability, or Emotions. Emergency work often demands a great deal of time. The shifts are long and emotionally and physically demanding. In addition, overwork tends to add stress on our physical and emotional health.

Necessary Restrictions on Practice. The scope of practice of paramedics is restricted. The limits can often be frustrating, especially for personnel with previous medical experience. For example, corpsmen in the military work more independently than paramedics. When such people enter EMS, they often feel frustrated that they are not allowed to perform procedures they formerly did routinely.

Unpredictable Changes in the Workplace. No one can deny that emergency medical services work varies day to day. However, lack of stability can become stressful.

Lack of Recognition. Paramedics are often "silent heroes" who routinely do what many people feel is worthy of recognition. Continued lack of recognition can be stressful.

Limited Career Mobility. Many EMS organizations do not provide much opportunity to move up. This deficiency can cause frustration and stress. The limited opportunities for advancement should be considered before entering the profession.

Abusive Patients and Dangerous Situations. Emergency medical service is dangerous. Verbal and physical abuse by patients complicates the

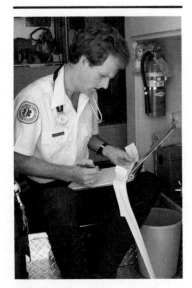

FIGURE 7-1 EMS is stressful. Paramedics must learn to deal with stress so as to avoid frustration and burnout.

matter. The paramedic should never become complacent, but must be careful not to overreact to abuse from patients or inherent dangers at the scene.

Critically Ill or Dying Patients. No matter how well-adapted a paramedic becomes, caring for critical and dying patients is often stressful. Treating these patients is frustrating, since, all too frequently, medical intervention is too late, or death is unpreventable.

BURNOUT

Burnout is an occupational hazard of emergency medical services. Burnout occurs when the coping mechanisms no longer buffer the stressors of the job. The paramedic often just "doesn't care." He or she loses interest in the job, the family, and such normal activities as sex, recreation, and the need for companionship. Patient care begins to suffer, along with the paramedic's personal and emotional health.

Burnout is best treated by prevention. Each paramedic should be routinely evaluated for burnout. Stressful assignments, such as busy stations or those with a higher incidence of critical patients, should be shared among personnel. Stressful events should be routinely followed by critical incident stress debriefing. Other mechanisms to prevent burnout are presented in the next section.

■ **burnout** burnout occurs when the coping mechanisms no longer buffer the stressors of the job. It can compromise personal health and well-being.

MANAGING STRESS

The paramedic must learn to manage stress in order to survive in emergency medical services. He or she must learn to recognize the early warning signs of anxiety. It's important to remember that some stress is valuable; it is protective and improves performance. A paramedic must learn to recognize his or her own optimal stress level and attempt to maintain it.

Paramedics must have an adequate perception of a stressful event. It is important to ask yourself these questions:

❏ Do you see what is really happening?
❏ Are you blaming yourself unjustly?
❏ Are your expectations realistic?

Try to sort events into categories of importance, urgency, and degree of actual threat.

Another method of coping with stress is to seek and use situational support. Talking about the situation with someone, as soon as possible, is a simple and effective way of coping. (See Figure 7-2.) Particularly stressful situations, involving multiple personnel, may benefit from group discussion. A good example is critical incident stress debriefing, available in many systems.

Other factors in managing stress are adequate sleep and rest; "leaving the job at work"; and balancing work and recreation. Physical activity is a good stress reliever. Try to have some friends who are not involved in EMS, as well as some who are. Learn to accept that certain things are beyond your control and cannot be changed. Above all, use adequate coping mechanisms. Determine which defense mechanisms are effective for you and adopt those most likely to reduce stress.

✱ The paramedic must learn to manage stress in order to survive in EMS.

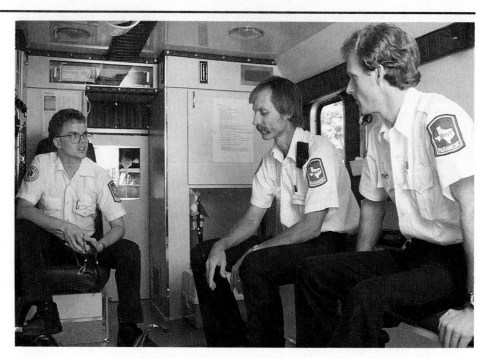

FIGURE 7-2 Informal discussions with colleagues concerning your feelings and frustrations are helpful and should be encouraged. Following particularly stressful incidents a Critical Incident Stress Debriefing may be warranted.

■ **critical incident stress debriefing** a meeting of rescue workers after a stressful event to allow an open discussion of their emotions and feelings.

CRITICAL INCIDENT STRESS DEBRIEFINGS

Critical Incident Stress Debriefings are structured group meetings that allow emergency and rescue personnel to openly discuss their feelings and other reactions after a critical incident. They are not psychotherapy or psychological treatment. They are, however, designed to reduce the impact of a critical event, and to accelerate the normal recovery of normal people who are suffering through normal, painful reactions to an abnormal event.

DEATH AND DYING

Death and dying are a part of emergency medical services. It is important to develop an appropriate personal attitude about death and the dying patient, as well as about the patient's family.

The family of a dying patient, as well as the patient, goes through a grief process initially described by Dr. Elizabeth Kubler-Ross. The grief process has several identifiable stages.

Denial and Isolation. This stage is used by most dying patients. It is healthy and acts as a mental buffer between the shock of dying and dealing with it. It happens throughout the illness. It is a temporary stage, often giving way to acceptance.

Anger. In the anger phase, the patient and the family ask, "Why me?" People are angered at the loss and may project their anger to anything and anyone. It is important to remember that this anger has little to do with the people or things present; they are often simply "targets." The anger can be difficult for the paramedic to deal with. Try not to take the patient's or the family's anger personally. Be tolerant, and don't be afraid of anger. Don't become defensive. Listen to the patient and the family.

Bargaining. Bargaining is a defense mechanism used by the dying patient to formulate some sort of "agreement," which, in the patient's mind, postpones the inevitable.

Depression. Depression is common and expected. It is a normal response to the greatest loss. In "reactive depression," the dying patient reacts to the needs of a life situation. For example, who will care for the children or take care of funeral arrangements? There is also "preparatory depression." In this state, the patient is often silent and reassurance is not meaningful.

Acceptance. Acceptance may not be a happy stage. At this point, the patient is without fear and despair, and often is devoid of feelings. The patient becomes less involved with people as he or she prepares to face death alone. At this stage, the family needs help, understanding, and support more than the patient.

It is important to recognize the needs of individuals when dealing with the dead or dying. The dying patient needs dignity and respect, sharing, communication, hope, privacy, and control. The family has needs, too. They often go through a grief process similar to the patient's. They may need to express their feelings of rage, anger, and despair. In addition, they need to reduce their feelings of guilt. The paramedic, as well, may go through some grief stages. This coping requires a lot of energy to cover feelings. It should be followed by adequate time for reflection and discussion.

Management of the Dead or Dying Patient

How the paramedic reacts to death and the dying patient reflects his or her own thoughts and beliefs. It is natural to feel uncomfortable. Don't bring up the subject of death. Let the patient do so. Don't falsely reassure the patient or the family. Do not be afraid to tell the patient that he or she is dying if asked. Use non-verbal communications, such as a gentle tone of voice, appropriate facial expression, and a reassuring touch.

If the patient is already dead, the family becomes "the patient." Comfort the family with kind deeds, such as calling neighbors, family members, or a minister. The family needs to hear the word "dead." Avoid euphemisms like "expired," "passed away," or "moved on." Recognize that the family will cope with death in much the same manner as they deal with everyday stresses.

SUMMARY

Stress is a part of emergency medical services. You should recognize that a certain level of stress is important. You should also recognize that increasing stress can seriously affect personal health and job performance. Paramedics must learn to adapt to stress and deal with it positively. They must also learn to deal with stress in other people.

FURTHER READING

MITCHELL, JEFF, and GRADY BRAY. *Emergency Services Stress: Guidelines for Preserving the Health and Careers of Emergency Services Personnel.* Englewood Cliffs, NJ: Prentice Hall, 1990.

8

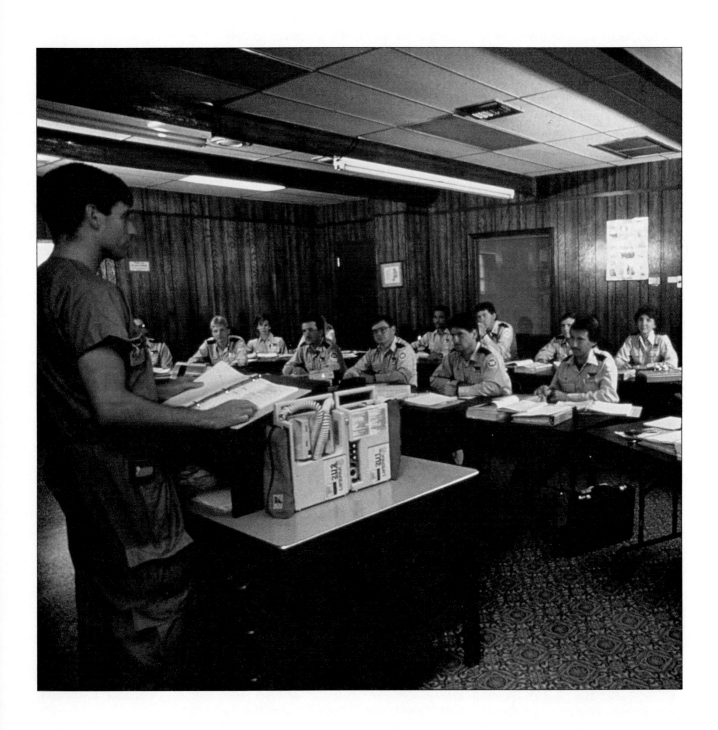

Medical Terminology

Objectives for Chapter 8

Upon completing this chapter, the student should be able to:

1. Define and use common medical terms.
2. Identify medical terms relating to anatomy.
3. Identify common medical abbreviations.
4. Identify common root words and define their meaning.
5. Identify and define common suffixes and prefixes.
6. Locate at least ten medical terms in a medical dictionary.

INTRODUCTION

■ medical terminology the language and terms of medicine, based mostly on Latin and Greek.

Medical terminology is the language of medicine. Like other fields, medicine uses specialized terms and abbreviations. To communicate effectively, those who work in medicine must speak and understand the same language. A knowledge of medical terminology will help the paramedic comprehend reading material and get more benefit from classes and lectures. Knowledge of medical terminology will also facilitate communication with physicians, nurses, and other health care personnel.

Initially, medical terminology may appear to be a foreign language—most medical terms are derived from either Greek or Latin. New terms are constantly being introduced, many of which are also derivatives of Greek or Latin.

The Greeks were the founders of modern medicine and many of their terms have remained in use. When the seat of medicine passed to ancient Rome, Latin became the universal language of medical science and remained so for many centuries.

Medical Dictionary

A medical dictionary is a good aid for the paramedic, in the classroom and on the job. Medical dictionaries not only define and spell terms, they also provide medical information. Some of the main features of a medical dictionary are pronunciation, spelling, definitions, vocabulary, subtopics, etymologies, and medical synonyms. Also included are sections on first aid, diseases, drugs, and anatomy. Phonetic spelling is usually noted in parentheses. Subtopics in the dictionary offer related words; etymologies give the derivatives of words and their Greek or Latin meanings. The word defined will be followed by a list of associated words.

Medical Terminology

■ prefix one or more syllables affixed to the beginning of a word to modify its meaning.

The three parts of a medical term are the **prefix, root word,** and the **suffix.** Not all medical terms have both a prefix and suffix, but most have one or the other. To identify the meaning of a medical term involves identifying each of its parts. For example:

■ root word a word to which a suffix, prefix, or both is affixed.

| Tonsil | + | itis | = | Tonsillitis (inflammation of the tonsils) |
| (root word) | | (inflammation) | | |

Root Words

■ suffix one or more syllables affixed to the end of a word to modify its meaning.

A root word is defined as the part of a word that conveys its essential meaning. It is distinguished from the parts that modify this meaning. Roots may be attached to other roots to form words, or prefixes and suffixes may be attached to roots to form words.

The following are some examples:

algia (pain)
caus (burn) } causalgia (burning pain)
partus (labor)   postpartum (after birth)
tropho (nourish)   hypertrophy (overnourishment)

Common Root Words	**Meaning**
abdomino-	belly or abdominal wall
acou-	to hear

Common Root Words	Meaning
acq-	water
acro-	extreme ends of a part
aden-	a gland
adip-	soft fat of animals
alb-	white
alg-	pain
all-	other, different
anc-, ang-, ank-	bend or hollow
andr-	male
angi-	blood vessel
aort-	large artery exiting from the left ventricle
arter-	artery
arth-	joint
artic-	joint
asphyxia	unconsciousness due to suffocation
asth-	short drawn breath, panting
asthenia	weakness
aud-, aur-, aus-	to hear
bio-	life
brachy-	short
branchi-	arm
bronch-	one of the major divisions of the trachea
bucc-	cheek
burs-	pouch or sac
caes-, cis-	cut
call-	hard, thick skin
calx, calca-	heel
can-	malignant tumor
caput, capitis	head
carc-	cancer
card-, cardia-	heart
carotid	great arteries of the neck
carpus	wrist
caus-, caut-	to burn
celi-	hollow or cavity, specifically the abdomen
cent-	center/centimeter/centigrade
-centesis	puncture of a cavity
ceph-	head
cerv-	neck
chol-	bile
chond-	cartilage
chrom-	color
cil-	hairlike process
cleid-	collarbone (clavicle)
cochlea	a part of the inner ear
coll-	gelatin, neck
cond-	knuckle

Common Root Words	Meaning
core	pupil
cori-	skin
corp-	the body
cry-	cold
cubitus	elbow
-cuss	shake violently
cyan-	blue
cyc-	circle
cyst	bladder, cyst
dent-	tooth
derm-	skin
digit	finger
duct	to lead or guide
edem-	swelling
embryo	fetus
enter-	intestines
eryth-	red
-esth-	sensation
eti-	cause
facil-	easy
febr-	fever
flex	to bend
foramen	opening
fract-	to break into pieces
gangl-	tumor under the skin, junction of nerve cells
gangr-	gnawing sore
gast-	stomach, belly
gen-, gon-	become, produce
gets-	carry, produce
glomerulus	plexus of capillaries
gnosis	knowledge
-gram	something written
-graph	to write
gyn-	female
hem-, -em	blood
hepat-	liver
heter-	other, different
homo-	the same
humerus	upper arm
hydr-	water
hyster-	the womb
idi-	personal, one's own
idio-	distinct
ingui-	front of body between hips and groin
lact-	milk

Common Root Words	Meaning
lev-	left side
ligament	band of fibrous tissue connecting two bones
ling-	tongue
-lith-	stone
mal-	bad
meatus	external opening
med-	middle
mega-	large
melan-, melen-	black
men-, mena-	monthly
menin-	membrane covering brain and spinal cord
morb-	disease
myel-	marrow or spinal cord
myo-	muscle
nephr-	kidney
noct-	night
nomen-, nomin-	name
oa-, oss-, ost-	bone
ocul-	eye
odon-	tooth
oo-, ov-	egg
opthalm-	eye
orch-	testes
ot-	ear
palpate	to touch
pari-, part-	to bear
pariet-	wall
path-	disease
pea-, ped-	foot
ped-	child
percuss	to strike
phag-	to eat
photo-	light
placenta	organ supplying nutrients to the fetus during gestation
pleur-	membrane surrounding lung and lining the thoracic cavity
pneum-	breathing
pod-	foot
pseud-	false
psych-	mind
ptosis	falling down
pty-	spit out
pur-, pus-, py-	pus
pyel-	pelvis (including pelvis of kidney)
pyr-	fever

Common Root Words	Meaning
quad-, quar-, quat-	four
radius	rod
ren-	kidney
reticulum	network
retina	inner nerve-containing layer of the eye
rhin-	nose
rub-	red
salpinx	tube
sang-	blood
scler-	hard
sebum	hard fat of animals
sect-, seg-	to cut
sepsis	containing growing bacteria
sept-	wall
serum	fluid formed when blood clots
sinus	cavity or hollow
somat-	body
sphincter	muscle that closes an opening when it contracts
spir-	coil
stasis	standing
stature	height
status	condition
stern-	chest
stoma	opening or mouth
sulc-	groove on surface of brain
tachy-	rapid
tact-	to touch
talus	heel
tarsus	bones of the forefoot
tel-	distance
temp-	time, or temple of the head
tendon	fibrous tissue connecting muscle to bone
tetr-	four
tom-	to cut
toxic	poisonous
trachea	windpipe
trich-	hair
ur-, urin-	urine
vagina	female genital canal
varic-	dilated vein
vertebra	bone supporting the spinal column
vertex	top of the skull
vertigo	dizziness
viscera	internal organs
viscous	sticky

Common Root Words	Meaning
xen-	foreign
xer-	dry

Prefixes and Suffixes

Prefixes. Prefixes are placed at the beginning of root words to modify a word's meaning. They are never used alone. If the root word starts with a vowel, and the prefix ends with one, then the final vowel of the prefix is dropped.

"Dys" is a prefix meaning disordered, painful, or difficult. Dysrhythmia would imply a disorder of a heart rhythm. Some other examples of prefixes are:

a (without or lack of)	apnea (without breath)
tachy (fast)	tachycardia (fast heart rate)
derma (skin)	dermatitis (inflammation of the skin)
erythro (red)	erythrocyte (red cell)

Common Prefixes

Prefix	Meaning	Example
a, an-	without, lack of	Apnea (without breath) Anemia (lack of blood)
ab-	away from	Abnormal (away from the normal)
acr-	pertaining to extremity	Acromegaly (enlargement of the bones of the distal parts)
ad-	to, toward	Adhesion (something stuck to)
aden-	pertaining to gland	Adenitis (inflammation of a gland)
ana-	up, back, again	Anastomosis (joining of two parts)
angio-	blood vessel, vessel	Angiokinetic (Pertaining to changes of blood vessels)
ante-	before, forward	Antenatal (occurring or formed before birth)
anti-	against, opposed to	Antipyretic (against fever)
arthro-	joint	Arthrodynia (pain in a joint)
auto-	self	Auto-intoxication (poisoning by a toxin generated within the body)
bi-	two	Bilateral (both sides)
blast-	germ or cell	Blastoma (a true tumor of cells)
bleph-	pertaining to eye	Bleparotomy (surgical cutting of an eyelid)
brady-	slow	Bradycardia (slow heart rate)
cardio-	pertaining to heart	Cardiography (recording of the actions of the heart)
cephal-	pertaining to head	Cephalopathy (any disease of the head or brain)
cerebro-	brain	Cerebrospinal (referring to the brain and spinal cord)
chole-	pertaining to bile	Cholelithiasis (stones in the biliary system)
circum-	around, about	Circumflex (winding around)
contra-	against, opposite	Contralateral (on the opposite side)

Common Prefixes (continued)

Prefix	Meaning	Example
cost-	pertaining to rib	Costal margin (margin of the ribs)
cyst-	pertaining to bladder	Cystitis (inflammation of the bladder or any fluid-containing sac)
derma-	skin	Dermatitis (inflammation of the skin)
di-	twice, double	Diplopia (double vision)
dia-	through, completely	Diagnosis (knowing completely)
dys-	with pain or difficulty	Dyspnea (difficulty breathing)
e-, ex-	from, out of	Excise (to cut out or remove completely or surgically)
ecto-	out from	Ectopic (out of place)
em-	in	Empyema (pus in the chest)
endo-	within	Endometrium (within the uterus)
enter-	pertaining to the intestines	Enteritis (inflammation of the intestines)
epi-	upon, on	Epidermis (the skin)
erythro-	red	Erythrocyte (red blood cell)
eu-	healthy	Eupnea (normal breathing)
exo-	outside	Exogenous (produced outside the body)
extra-	outside, in addition	Extrasystole (premature contraction of the heart)
gastr-	pertaining to the stomach	Gastritis (inflammation of the stomach)
gynec-	pertaining to women	Gynecology (study of women's diseases)
hem-, hemato-	pertaining to blood	Hemoglobin (pigment of red blood cells)
hemi-	half	Hemiplegia (paralysis of one side of the body)
hydro-	water	Hydropenia (deficiency in body water)
hyper-	over, excessive in	Hyperplasia (excessive formation)
hypo-	under, deficient in	Hypotension (low blood pressure)
hyster-	pertaining to uterus	Hysterectomy (removal of the uterus)
in-	not	Inferior (beneath; lower)
infra-	below, after	Infrascapular (below the scapula)
inter-	between	Intercostal (between the ribs)
intra-	within	Intralobar (within the lobe)
iso-	equal	Isotonic (having equal tension)
laterad-or lateral-	side	Laterodeviation (displace to one side)
leuk-	pertaining to anything white	Leukocyte (white blood cells)
macro-	large	Macroblast (abnormally large cell)
micro-	small; "one millionth part of"	Microplasia (dwarfism)
myo-, mye-	pertaining to muscle	Myoma (muscle tumor)
neo-	new	Neoplasm (new growth)
nephr-	pertaining to kidney	Nephrectomy (surgical excision of the kidney)
neuro-	nerve	Neurocanal (central canal of the spinal cord)
olig-	little	Oliguria (little production of urine)
oophor-	pertaining to ovary	Oophorectomy (surgical excision of an ovary)

Prefix	Meaning	Example
ophthal-	pertaining to eye	Exophthalmos (protruding eyeballs)
ot-	pertaining to ear	Otitis media (inflammation of the middle ear)
para-	by the side of	Parathyroids (along side of the thyroid)
patho-	disease	Pathology (study of the nature and cause of disease)
per-	through	Perforation (a breaking through)
peri-	around	Pericardium (fibroserous sac enclosing the heart)
phago-	to eat	Phagocyte (cells that eat debris)
pneumo-	air; lung	Pneumothorax (abnormal presence of air in the thorax)
poly-	many	Polycystic (containing many cysts)
post-	after, behind	Postpartum (after childbirth)
pro-	before, in front of	Prognosis (forecast as to the outcome of disease)
proct-	pertaining to rectum	Proctoscopy (inspection of the rectum)
pseudo-	false	Pseudoanemia (false anemia)
psych-	pertaining to the mind	Psychiatry (treatment of mental diseases)
pulmo-	lung	Pulmonary (involving the lungs)
py-	pertaining to pus	Pyorrhea (discharge of pus)
pyel-	pertaining to renal pelvis	Pyelitis (inflammation of the renal pelvis)
retro-	backward	Retroflexion (bending backward)
rhin-	pertaining to nose	Rhinitis (inflammation of nose)
salping-	pertaining to a tube	Salpingectomy (excision of the oviduct)
semi-	half	Semiflexion (partially flexed)
sub-	under, moderately	Subacute (moderately sharp)
supra-	above	Supraclavicular (above the clavicle)
sym-	with, together	Symphysis (grow together)
tachy-	fast	Tachycardia (fast heart rate)
trans-	across	Transfusion (pour across)
tri-	three	Tricuspid (having three cusps)
uni-	one	Unilateral (one sided)
vaso-	vessel	Vasopressor (agent that increases vascular resistance)

Suffixes. Suffixes are placed at the end of the root word or prefix to alter the meaning of a word. Pronunciation sometimes requires changing the last letter or letters of the root word when the suffix is added. Also, it may be necessary to change the last vowel. An example is the word cardiology, derived from "cardia." The word neuritis, derived from "neuro," is an example of dropping the final vowel in the root word to add a suffix that begins with a vowel.

Other examples of suffixes are:

'pnea (breathing)	dyspnea (difficulty breathing)
'ology (science of)	cardiology (science of the heart)
'cyte (cell)	leukocyte (white cell)
'rrhagia (bursting forth)	hemorrhage (burst forth of blood)

Suffix	Meaning	Example
-algia	pertains to pain	Neuralgia (pain along a nerve)
-blast	germ of immature cell	Myeoblast (bone marrow cell)
-cele	tumor, hernia	Enterocele (hernia of the intestine)
-centesis	puncturing	Thoracentesis (a procedure involving puncture and drainage of the pleural space)
-cyte	cell	Leukocyte (white cell)
-ectomy	a cutting out	Tonsillectomy
-emia	blood	Anemia
-itis	inflammation	Tonsillitis
-ostomy	creation of an opening	Gastrostomy (artificial opening into the stomach)
-lysis	destruction or loosening	Lysis (destruction or loosening of adhesions)
-oma	tumor, swelling	Neuroma (tumor of a nerve)
-osis	condition of	Psychosis (a mental disorder, characterized by disordered thinking)
-pathy	disease	Neuropathy (disease of the nervous system)
-phagia	eating	Polyphagia (excessive eating)
-phasia	speech	Aphasia (loss of speech)
-phobia	fear	Hydrophobia (fear of water)
-plasty	repair of; tying of	Nephroplasty (suturing of a kidney)
-ptosis	falling	Enteroptosis (falling of the intestine)
-rhythmia	rhythm	Tachydysrhythmia (faster than a normal rhythm)
-rrhagia	bursting forth	Hemorrhage (flowing of blood)
-rrhaphy	suture of; repair of	Herniorrhaphy (repair of a hernia)
-rrhea	flowing	Pyorrhea (discharge of pus)
-scope	instrument for examination	Bronchoscope (instrument for looking into the bronchi)
-scopy	examination with an instrument	Bronchoscopy (examination of the bronchi)
-taxia	order, arrangement of	Ataxia (failure of muscle coordination)
-trophia	nourishment	Atrophy (a wasting away of something)
-uria	to do with urine	Polyuria (excessive production of urine)

Common Abbreviations

Medical documentation tends to be lengthy and time-consuming. As a result, abbreviations become routine. The following list of abbreviations pertains to prehospital care.

Abbreviation	Meaning
$\overline{a}$	before
aa	of each
AAO X 3	Alert and oriented to person, place, and time
abd.	abdomen
Ab	abortion
a.c.	before meals

Abbreviation	Meaning
ACLS	advanced cardiac life support
adm.	administration
AF	atrial fibrillation
aq.	water
ARDS	Adult Respiratory Distress Syndrome
ASA	aspirin
ASHD	atherosclerotic heart disease
AMA	against medical advice
ant.	anterior
AP	front-to-back (anteroposterior)
A & P	anatomy and physiology
APC	Aspirin, Phenacetin, and Codeine
art.	artery
AT	atrial tachycardia
AV	atrioventricular
BBB	bundle branch block
b.i.d.	twice a day
BM	bowel movement
BP	blood pressure
BS	blood sugar, breath sounds
BSA	body surface area
BVM	bag-valve-mask
C	centigrade
$\overline{c}$	with
Ca	carcinoma, cancer
CAD	coronary artery disease, computer-assisted dispatch
Caps.	capsule
CBC	complete blood count
cc	cubic centimeter
CC or C/C	Chief complaint
CCU or MICU	coronary care unit or medical intensive care unit
CHF	congestive heart failure
Cl⁻	chloride
CM	centimeter
CNS	central nervous system
c/o	complains of
CO	carbon monoxide
CO₂	carbon dioxide
COPD	chronic obstructive pulmonary disease
CP	chest pain
CPR	cardiopulmonary resuscitation
CSF	cerebrospinal fluid
CSM	carotid sinus massage
CVA	cerebrovascular accident
CVP	central venous pressure
CXR	chest x-ray
D/C	discontinue
D & C	dilatation and curettage
DM	diabetes mellitus
DOA	dead on arrival
DOE	dyspnea on exertion

Abbreviation	Meaning
DPT	diphtheria, pertussis, and tetanus vaccine
DT's	delirium tremens
D-5-W	dextrose 5% in water
DVT	deep venous thrombosis
Dx	diagnosis
ECG, EKG	electrocardiogram
EEG	electroencephalogram
e.g.	for example
ENT	ear, nose, and throat
EOMI	extraocular movements intact
ER/ED	emergency department
ETA	estimated time of arrival
ETOH	alcohol (ethanol)
F	Fahrenheit
FH	family history
fl	fluid
fx	fracture
GB	gall bladder
GI	gastrointestinal
→	going to or leading to
Gm., g	gram
gr.	grain
GSW	gunshot wound
gtt.	drop
GU	genitourinary
GYN	gynecologic
h, hr.	hour
H/A	headache
H, (H)	hypodermic
Hb., Hgb.	hemoglobin
Hct.	hematocrit
H & H	hemoglobin & hematocrit
Hg	mercury
H & P	history and physical
hs	at bedtime
Hx	history
IC	intracardiac
ICP	intracranial pressure
ICU	intensive care unit
IM	intramuscular
inf.	inferior
IPPB	intermittent positive pressure breathing
IV	intravenous
JVD	jugular venous distention
K^+	potassium
kg	kilogram
KVO	keep vein open
L	left
L	liter
LAC	laceration
lb.	pound

Abbreviation	Meaning
LBBB	left bundle branch block
liq.	liquid
LLL	left lower lobe of the lung
LLQ	left lower quadrant of abdomen
LOC	level of consciousness
LPM	liters per minute
LR	lactated Ringer's
LUL	left upper lobe of the lung
LUQ	left upper quadrant of abdomen
m	meter
MAE	moves all extremities
MAP	mean arterial pressure
mcg.	microgram
MCL	midclavicular line
MCL	modified chest lead
mEq.	milli-equivalent
μg.	microgram
mg., mgm.	milligram
MI	myocardial infarction
MICU	mobile intensive care unit, medical intensive care unit
mL	milliliter
mm	millimeter
MS	morphine sulphate, multiple sclerosis
MVA	motor vehicle accident
Na^+	sodium
NaCl	sodium chloride
NAD	no apparent distress
$NaHCO_3$	sodium bicarbonate
NC	nasal cannula
NG tube	nasogastric tube
NPO	nothing by mouth
NKA	no known allergies
NS	normal saline
NSR	normal sinus rhythm
NTG	nitroglycerine
N/V	nausea/vomiting
O_2	oxygen
OB	obstetrics
OBS	organic brain syndrome
OD	overdose
O.D.	right eye
OR	operating room
O.S.	left eye
oz.	ounce
$\bar{p}$	after
PAT	paroxysmal atrial tachycardia
p.c.	after meals
pCO_2	carbon dioxide pressure
P.E.	physical exam, pulmonary embolism
PERL	pupils equal and reactive to light

Abbreviation	Meaning
pH	hydrogen ion concentration
PID	pelvic inflammatory disease
PND	paroxysmal nocturnal dyspnea
p.o.	by mouth
PO	postoperative or "post op"
pO_2	oxygen pressure or tension
post.	posterior
1°	primary, first degree
PRN	as needed
psi	pounds per square inch
pt.	patient
PT	physical therapy
PTA	prior to admission
PVC	premature ventricular contraction
q	every
q. h.	every hour
q.i.d.	four times a day
RBBB	right bundle branch block
RBC	red blood count
RHD	rheumatic heart disease
RL	ringer's lactate
RLL	right lower lobe of the lung
RML	right middle lobe of the lung
R/O	rule out
ROM	range of motion
RUL	right upper lobe of the lung
RUQ	right upper quadrant of abdomen
Rx	take; treatment
s̄	without
2°	secondary, second degree
SA	sino-atrial
S/S	signs/symptoms
SC, SQ	subcutaneous
SICU	surgical intensive care unit
SIDS	sudden infant death syndrome
SL	sublingual
S.O.B.	shortness of breath
ss	half
stat.	immediately
Sub. Q.	subcutaneous
S.V.T.	Supraventricular Tachycardia
sym. or Sx	symptoms
tab.	tablet
tbsp.	tablespoon
TIA	transient ischemic attack
t.i.d.	three times a day
TKO	to keep open
TPR	temperature, pulse, respiration
tsp.	teaspoon
u	unit

Abbreviation	Meaning
URI	upper respiratory infection
USP	United States Pharmacopeia
VD	venereal disease
VO	verbal order
vol.	volume
V.S.	vital signs
WBC	white blood count
WNL	within normal limits
wt.	weight
y.o.	year old
↑	increased, elevated
↓	decreased, depressed
ø	none
Ⓡ	right
Ⓛ	left
μ	micro
α	alpha
β	beta
≃	approximate
O	normal
X2	times two
ii	two
iii	three
/	per
≠	not equal
>	greater than
<	less than
?	questionable, possible
♂	male
♀	female
+	positive
−	negative
△	change

SUMMARY

By learning the lists of root words, prefixes, and suffixes in this chapter, and consulting the medical dictionary regularly, you will gain a command of medical terminology. Knowing medical terminology is essential for preparing medical records, learning new material, and communicating with other health care personnel.

This chapter has been a brief introduction to medical terminology. Paramedic personnel are encouraged to complete a course in medical terminology; several self-programmed texts are available.

FURTHER READING

Dorland's Illustrated Medical Dictionary. 26th ed. Philadelphia: W.B. SAUNDERS, 1981.

Mosby's Dictionary: Quick Reference for Emergency Responders. Saint Louis: C.V. MOSBY, 1989.

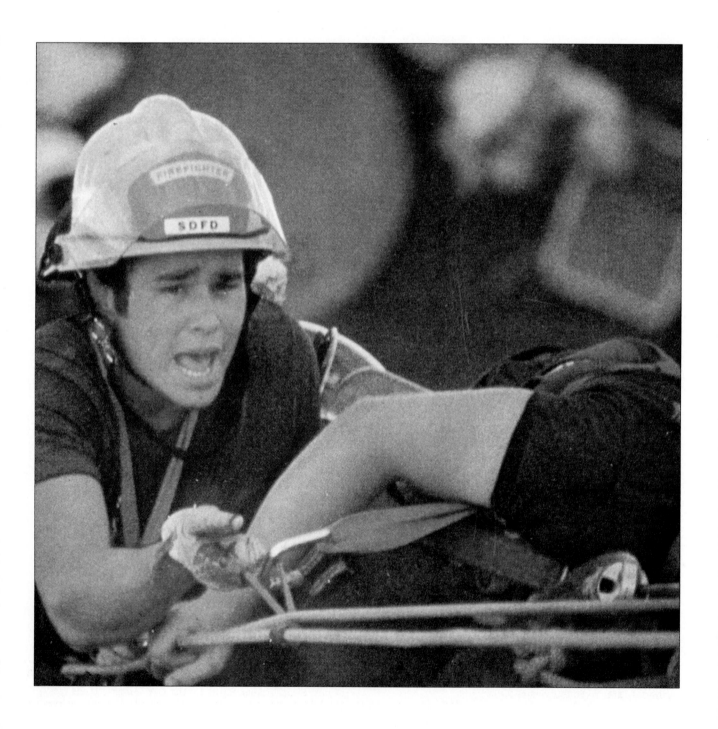

9

Anatomy and Physiology

Objectives for Chapter 9

Upon completing this chapter, the student should be able to:

1. Define the following terms:
   - anatomy
   - physiology
   - biochemistry
   - biophysics
2. Describe the hierarchy of the human body.
3. Define the following:
   - cell
   - tissue
   - organ
   - organ system
   - organism
4. List the four types of tissue.
5. List the major body organ systems and describe their functions.

6. List the topographical anatomy terms frequently used in emergency medical services and give an example of each.

7. Describe in topographical terms the location of various lines on the chest.

8. Describe the four anatomical divisions of the abdomen and list the organs within each.

9. Describe, in anatomical terms, a mark on the chest and abdomen in a way that tells the medical control physician the precise location of the lesion.

10. List the major body cavities and the important organs in each.

11. Define homeostasis, and give an example of a homeostatic response.

CASE STUDY

Saturday night begins like many other Saturdays for the crew of Medic-4. The sun has been down only 15–20 minutes when the computer printout alerts the crew to a shooting at the Zodiac Bar and Grill on the south side of town. Fortunately, the bar is only two minutes from the station. Upon arrival, the paramedics find a male victim lying in the doorway. Several police officers are present, and a crowd is gathering. The paramedics approach the patient. He is a thin male, with several bloodstains on his shirt. As they remove the victim's shirt, a police officer informs the paramedics that this is a drug-related shooting and tells them the alleged assailant and his assault rifle are in custody.

The patient is alert, yet weak. Primary survey reveals no compromise of the airway, breathing, or circulation. There are three apparent entrance wounds in the anterior chest. While Paul is obtaining vital signs, Steve, the senior paramedic, contacts medical control. He reports, "We have a 22-year-old male, with multiple gunshot wounds to the chest. There are three entrance wounds and two apparent exit wounds. The first wound enters the chest in a mid-clavicular line on the right, at the level of the third rib. The second enters in an anterior axillary line, at the level of the tenth rib on the right side. The third wound appears to be a shallow wound in the right mid-axillary line, at the sixth intercostal space; it apparently doesn't penetrate the thorax. Blood pressure is 90 by palpation. The pulse is 110 and respirations are 20. We have placed the PASG and are administering supplemental oxygen by non-rebreathing mask. We are preparing to transport the patient and will attempt an IV and secondary assessment en route. Our ETA is 4 minutes."

Dr. Johnson, the on-line medical control physician, alerts the surgical crew. Based on the paramedics' description of the wounds, the surgeons expect to find a penetrating wound to the liver and a probable pneumothorax. Within minutes, the surgical crew is opening instruments for both a thoracotomy and exploratory laparotomy. When the victim arrives at the hospital, two IVs are in place. The patient is quickly examined by Dr. Johnson and taken immediately to the operating room. The patient is in the operating room 18 minutes after the paramedics arrived at the emergency scene.

INTRODUCTION

This textbook presents a "systems approach" to medical emergencies and trauma. That is, each type of emergency is presented in the chapter corresponding to the body system most involved. For example, acute myocardial infarction is presented in the cardiovascular emergencies chapter; emphysema is presented in the respiratory emergencies chapter; and so on. Each chapter begins with the anatomy and physiology that pertain to the body system under discussion. This chapter will present the fundamentals of human anatomy and physiology, leaving detailed discussions of various body systems to later chapters.

Anatomy is the study of body structure, whereas **physiology** is the study of body functions. Two related disciplines are biochemistry and biophysics. **Biochemistry** is the study of chemical events occurring within a living organism. **Biophysics** is the application of the principles of physics to body mechanics. As a paramedic, you will be expected to understand relevant anatomy, physiology, and biochemistry. During EMT training, you learned a great deal of anatomy and physiology. As a paramedic, you will be expected to expand this knowledge in areas appropriate to advanced prehospital care.

STRUCTURE

The human body consists of a hierarchical system, ranging from the smallest structural element, the cell, to the entire organism. This section will address human anatomy as it applies to emergency medical care.

The Cell

The most elemental component of the human body is the **cell.** (See Figure 9-1.) The cell is the basic unit of life. It contains all necessary components to turn essential nutrients into energy, remove waste products, reproduce, and carry on other essential life functions. Within the cell are several specialized structures, called **organelles.** Each organelle has a specific function. Examples of organelles and other cellular structures are:

Nucleus. The nucleus contains the genetic material, DNA, and the enzymes necessary for replication of DNA. DNA must be constantly copied and transferred to the new cells.

Mitochondria. The mitochondria are the energy factories of the cells. They convert essential nutrients into energy sources, often in the form of adenosine triphosphate (ATP).

Cell Membrane. The cell membrane is a very important structure that encircles the cell and protects it from the outer environment. Vital functions of the cell membrane—which will be discussed in a later chapter—include electrolyte and fluid balance, and the transfer of enzymes, hormones, and nutrients into and out of the cell.

Cytoplasm. The substance that fills and gives shape to the cell, cytoplasm provides many biochemical functions.

Tissues

The types of cells in the body depend on their location and function. **Tissue** refers to a group of cells that perform a similar function. The four basic types of tissue are:

Epithelial Tissue. Epithelial tissue lines body surfaces and protects the body. In addition, certain types of epithelial tissue perform specialized functions, such as secretion, absorption, diffusion, and filtration. Examples of epithelial tissue are skin, mucous membranes, and the lining of the intestinal tract.

■ **anatomy** the study of body structure.

■ **physiology** the study of body function.

■ **biochemistry** the study of chemical events occurring within a living organism.

■ **biophysics** the application of the principles of physics to body mechanics.

■ **cell** the basic unit of life and the fundamental element of which an organism, such as the human body, is composed.

■ **organelles** specialized structures within the cell which provide for cellular needs.

■ **nucleus** cellular organelle which contains the genetic material (DNA).

■ **mitochondria** organelle responsible for provision of cellular energy.

■ **cell membrane** structure which surrounds the cell. It plays a major role in maintaining the internal environment of the cell.

■ **cytoplasm** material within the cell that provides for structure, support, and certain biochemical functions.

■ **tissue** a group of cells, which, together, have a common function or purpose.

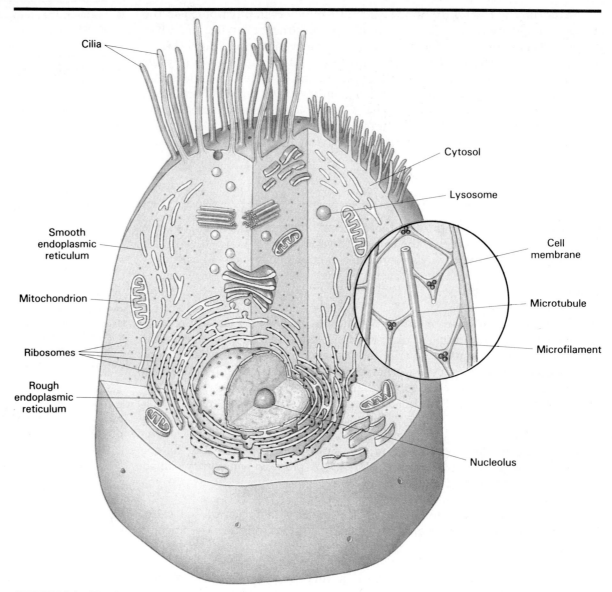

FIGURE 9-1 The Cell.

Muscle Tissue.   Muscle tissue has the capability of contraction when stimulated. The three types of muscle tissue (see Figure 9-2) are:

> **Cardiac muscle.** Cardiac muscle tissue is found only within the heart. It has the unique capability of spontaneous contraction without external stimulation.
> **Smooth muscle.** The smooth muscle is that muscle found within the intestines and encircling blood vessels. Smooth muscle is generally under the control of the involuntary, or autonomic, component of the nervous system.
> **Skeletal muscle.** Skeletal muscle is the most abundant muscle type. It allows movement and is mostly under voluntary control.

Connective Tissue.   Connective tissue is the most abundant tissue in the body. It provides support, connection, and insulation. Examples of connective tissue are bones, cartilage, fat, and blood.

Nerve Tissue.   Nerve tissue is specialized tissue that transmits electrical

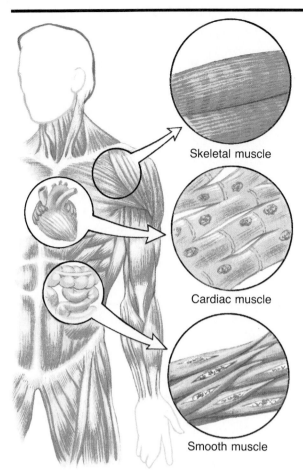

Skeletal muscle

Cardiac muscle

Smooth muscle

FIGURE 9-2 There are three types of muscle. Skeletal muscle, also called voluntary muscle, is found throughout the body. Cardiac muscle is limited to the heart. Smooth muscle, occasionally called involuntary muscle, is found in the intestines, arterioles, and bronchioles.

impulses throughout the body. Examples of nervous tissue are the brain, spinal cord, and peripheral nerves.

Organs

A group of tissues functioning together is an **organ.** For example, the pancreas consists of epithelial tissue, connective tissue, and nervous tissue. Together, these tissues perform the essential functions of the pancreas, including production of certain digestive enzymes and regulation of glucose metabolism.

■ **organ** a group of tissues with a common function.

Organ Systems

A group of organs that work together is referred to as an organ system. (See Figures 9-3 to 9-14.) Examples of organ systems are:

Cardiovascular System. The cardiovascular system consists of the heart, blood vessels, and blood. It transports nutrients and other essential elements to all parts of the body.

Respiratory System. The respiratory system consists of the lungs and associated structures. It provides oxygen to the body, while removing carbon dioxide and other waste products.

Gastrointestinal System. The gastrointestinal system consists of the mouth, esophagus, stomach, intestines, liver, pancreas, gall bladder, and rectum. It takes in complex nutrients and breaks them down into a form that can be readily used by the body. It also aids in the elimination of excess wastes.

Genito-urinary System. The genito-urinary system consists of the kidneys, ureters, bladder, and urethra. It is important in the elimination of various waste products. It also plays a major role in the regulation of water, electrolytes, blood pressure, and other essential body functions.

Reproductive System. The reproductive system allows for reproduction of the organism. In the female, it consists of the ovaries, fallopian tubes, uterus, vagina, and breasts. In the male, it consists of the testes, prostate, seminal vesicles, vas deferens, urethra, and penis.

Nervous System. The nervous system consists of the brain, spinal cord, and all peripheral nerves. It controls virtually all bodily functions and is the seat of intellect and being.

Lymphatic System. The lymphatic system is often considered a part of the cardiovascular system. It consists of the spleen, lymph nodes, lymphatic channels, and the lymph itself. It is important in fighting disease, in filtration, and in removing waste products of cellular metabolism.

Endocrine System. The endocrine system is another control system closely associated with the nervous system. It consists of the pituitary gland, pineal gland, pancreas, testes, ovaries, adrenal glands, thyroid gland, and parathyroid glands. There is well-documented evidence that other organs—such as the heart, kidney, and intestines—have endocrine functions. The endocrine system exerts its effects through the release of chemical messengers, called hormones.

Muscular System. The muscular system is responsible for movement, posture, and heat production. It consists, primarily, of the skeletal muscles.

Skeletal System. The skeletal system consists of the bones, cartilage, and associated connective tissue. It provides for support, protection, and movement.

Organism

■ **organism** a group of organ systems; the functional unit of life.

■ **homeostasis** the natural tendency of the body to maintain the internal environment relatively constant.

The sum of all cells, tissues, organs, and organ systems is the **organism.** As this book will make clear, the failure of any component, from the cellular level to the organ-system level, can cause the development of a medical emergency.

Homeostasis refers to the body's natural tendency to keep all physiological activities fairly constant. That is, whenever a change occurs in the body, the body immediately attempts to correct the change. At the cellular level, the body will strive to maintain a very constant environment, because cells do not tolerate extreme environmental changes. As an organism, the body uses each organ system to maintain its internal environment. For example, an accumulation of carbon dioxide and lactic acid occurs after exercise. The body immediately attempts to return itself to the resting state by eliminating the excess carbon dioxide, and by removing the accumulated lactic acid.

The Eye and Ear

THE EYE

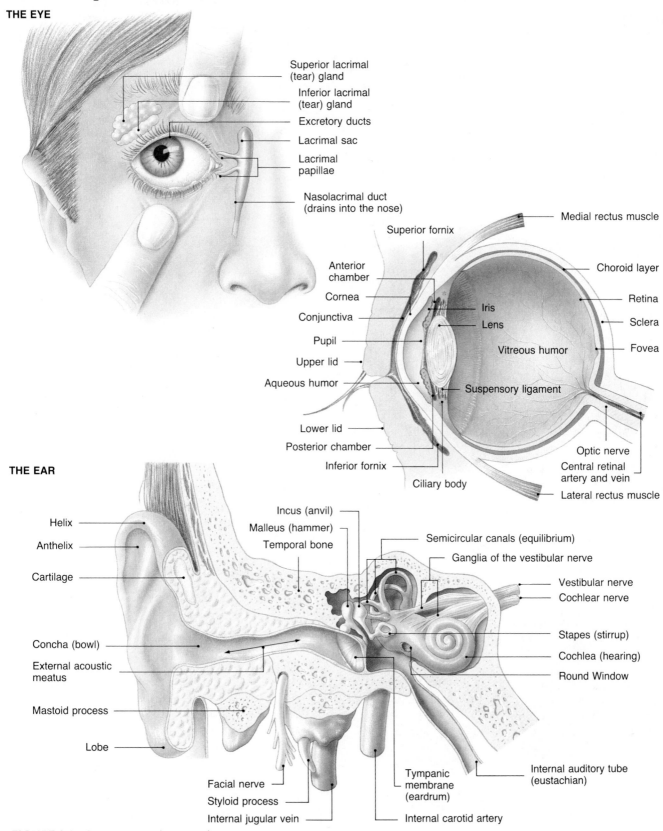

Superior lacrimal (tear) gland

Inferior lacrimal (tear) gland

Excretory ducts

Lacrimal sac

Lacrimal papillae

Nasolacrimal duct (drains into the nose)

Superior fornix

Anterior chamber

Cornea

Conjunctiva

Pupil

Upper lid

Aqueous humor

Lower lid

Posterior chamber

Inferior fornix

Ciliary body

Iris

Lens

Vitreous humor

Suspensory ligament

Medial rectus muscle

Choroid layer

Retina

Sclera

Fovea

Optic nerve

Central retinal artery and vein

Lateral rectus muscle

THE EAR

Helix

Anthelix

Cartilage

Concha (bowl)

External acoustic meatus

Mastoid process

Lobe

Incus (anvil)

Malleus (hammer)

Temporal bone

Semicircular canals (equilibrium)

Ganglia of the vestibular nerve

Vestibular nerve

Cochlear nerve

Stapes (stirrup)

Cochlea (hearing)

Round Window

Internal auditory tube (eustachian)

Facial nerve

Styloid process

Internal jugular vein

Tympanic membrane (eardrum)

Internal carotid artery

FIGURE 9-3 Special senses; the eye and ear.

Membranes

THE SKIN

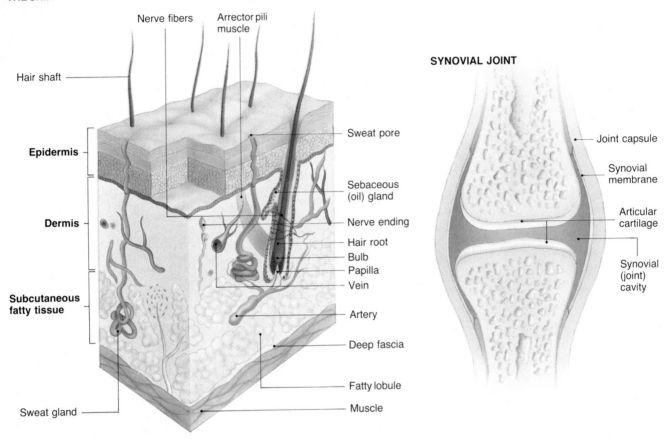

SYNOVIAL JOINT

THE PLEURA

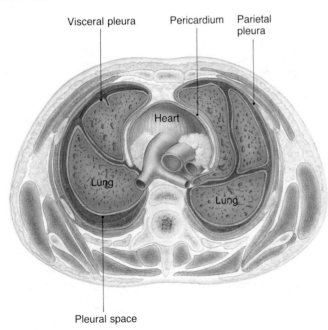

THE PERITONEUM

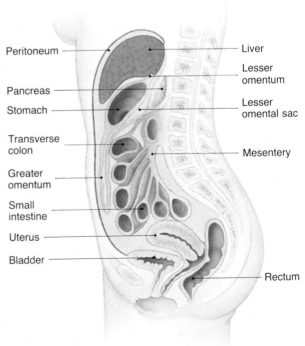

FIGURE 9-4   Membranes.

The Skeletal System

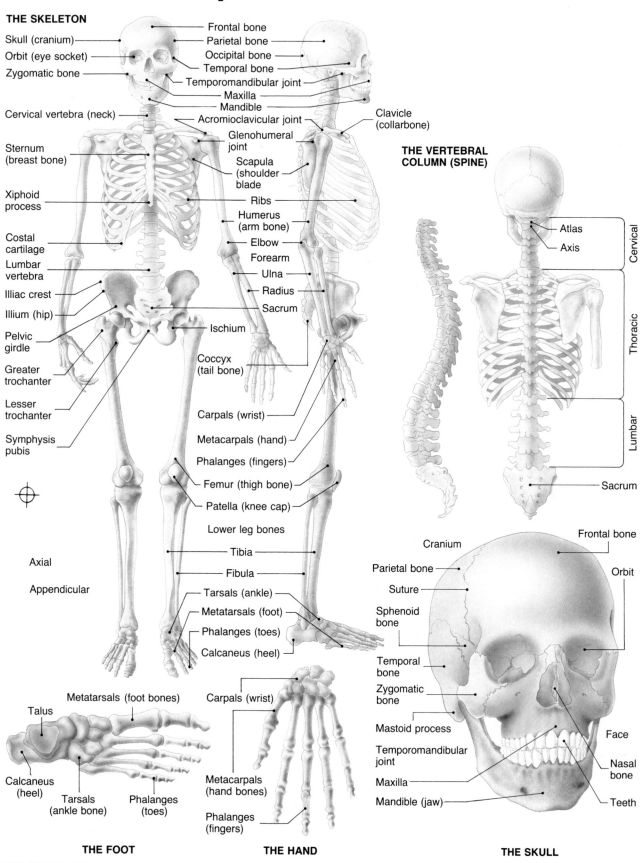

THE SKELETON

Skull (cranium)
Orbit (eye socket)
Zygomatic bone
Cervical vertebra (neck)
Sternum (breast bone)
Xiphoid process
Costal cartilage
Lumbar vertebra
Illiac crest
Illium (hip)
Pelvic girdle
Greater trochanter
Lesser trochanter
Symphysis pubis
Axial
Appendicular

Frontal bone
Parietal bone
Occipital bone
Temporal bone
Temporomandibular joint
Maxilla
Mandible
Acromioclavicular joint
Glenohumeral joint
Scapula (shoulder blade)
Ribs
Humerus (arm bone)
Elbow
Forearm
Ulna
Radius
Sacrum
Ischium
Coccyx (tail bone)
Carpals (wrist)
Metacarpals (hand)
Phalanges (fingers)
Femur (thigh bone)
Patella (knee cap)
Lower leg bones
Tibia
Fibula
Tarsals (ankle)
Metatarsals (foot)
Phalanges (toes)
Calcaneus (heel)

Clavicle (collarbone)

THE VERTEBRAL COLUMN (SPINE)

Atlas
Axis
Cervical
Thoracic
Lumbar
Sacrum

Cranium
Parietal bone
Suture
Sphenoid bone
Temporal bone
Zygomatic bone
Mastoid process
Temporomandibular joint
Maxilla
Mandible (jaw)

Frontal bone
Orbit
Face
Nasal bone
Teeth

Metatarsals (foot bones)
Talus
Calcaneus (heel)
Tarsals (ankle bone)
Phalanges (toes)

Carpals (wrist)
Metacarpals (hand bones)
Phalanges (fingers)

THE FOOT   **THE HAND**   **THE SKULL**

FIGURE 9-5   The skeletal system.

137

The Muscular System

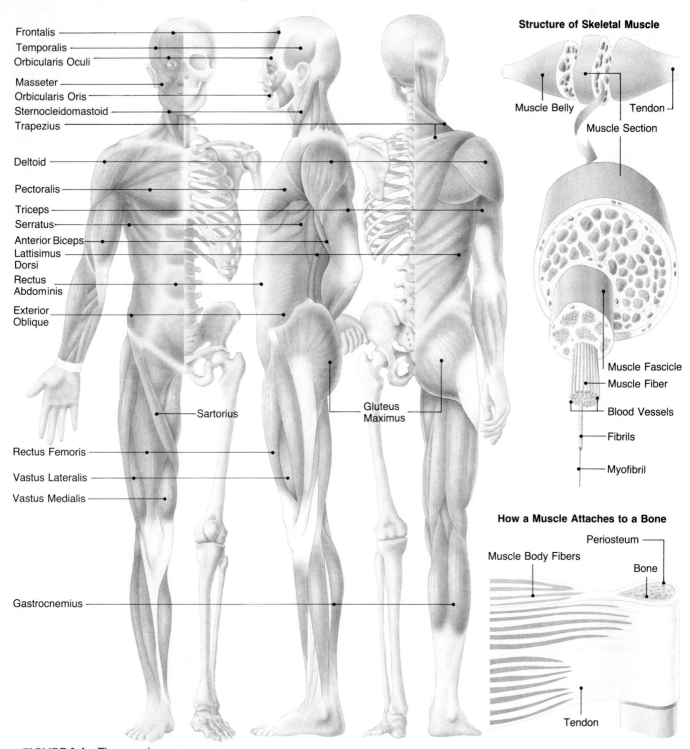

Frontalis
Temporalis
Orbicularis Oculi

Masseter
Orbicularis Oris
Sternocleidomastoid
Trapezius

Deltoid

Pectoralis

Triceps
Serratus
Anterior Biceps
Lattisimus
Dorsi
Rectus
Abdominis

Exterior
Oblique

Sartorius

Rectus Femoris

Vastus Lateralis

Vastus Medialis

Gastrocnemius

Gluteus
Maximus

Structure of Skeletal Muscle

Muscle Belly

Tendon

Muscle Section

Muscle Fascicle
Muscle Fiber

Blood Vessels

Fibrils

Myofibril

How a Muscle Attaches to a Bone

Periosteum

Bone

Muscle Body Fibers

Tendon

FIGURE 9-6   The muscular system.

The Cardiovascular System

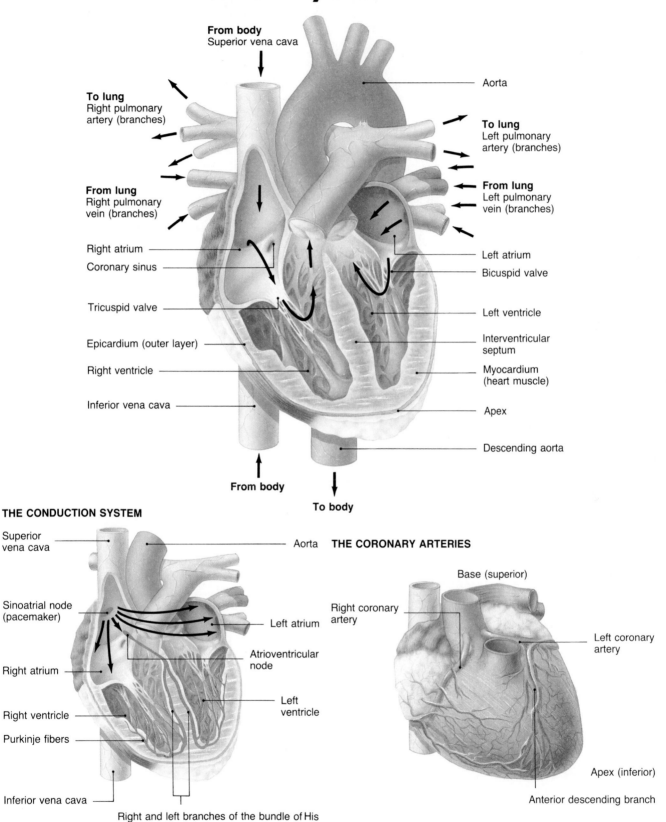

From body
Superior vena cava

Aorta

To lung
Right pulmonary
artery (branches)

To lung
Left pulmonary
artery (branches)

From lung
Right pulmonary
vein (branches)

From lung
Left pulmonary
vein (branches)

Right atrium

Coronary sinus

Left atrium

Bicuspid valve

Tricuspid valve

Left ventricle

Epicardium (outer layer)

Interventricular
septum

Right ventricle

Myocardium
(heart muscle)

Inferior vena cava

Apex

Descending aorta

From body

To body

THE CONDUCTION SYSTEM

Superior
vena cava

Aorta

THE CORONARY ARTERIES

Base (superior)

Sinoatrial node
(pacemaker)

Left atrium

Right coronary
artery

Left coronary
artery

Atrioventricular
node

Right atrium

Right ventricle

Left
ventricle

Purkinje fibers

Apex (inferior)

Inferior vena cava

Anterior descending branch

Right and left branches of the bundle of His

FIGURE 9-7 The cardiovascular system.

The Circulatory System

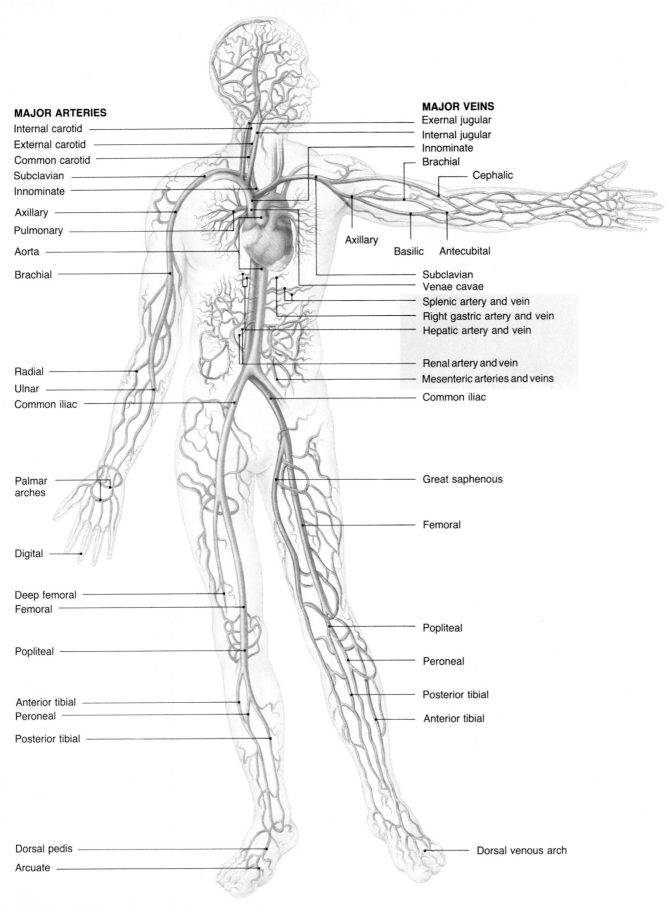

MAJOR ARTERIES

Internal carotid
External carotid
Common carotid
Subclavian
Innominate
Axillary
Pulmonary
Aorta
Brachial

Radial
Ulnar
Common iliac

Palmar
arches

Digital

Deep femoral
Femoral

Popliteal

Anterior tibial
Peroneal
Posterior tibial

Dorsal pedis
Arcuate

MAJOR VEINS

Exernal jugular
Internal jugular
Innominate
Brachial
Cephalic

Axillary

Basilic   Antecubital

Subclavian
Venae cavae
Splenic artery and vein
Right gastric artery and vein
Hepatic artery and vein

Renal artery and vein
Mesenteric arteries and veins

Common iliac

Great saphenous

Femoral

Popliteal

Peroneal

Posterior tibial

Anterior tibial

Dorsal venous arch

FIGURE 9-8 The circulatory system.

The Nervous System

THE BRAIN

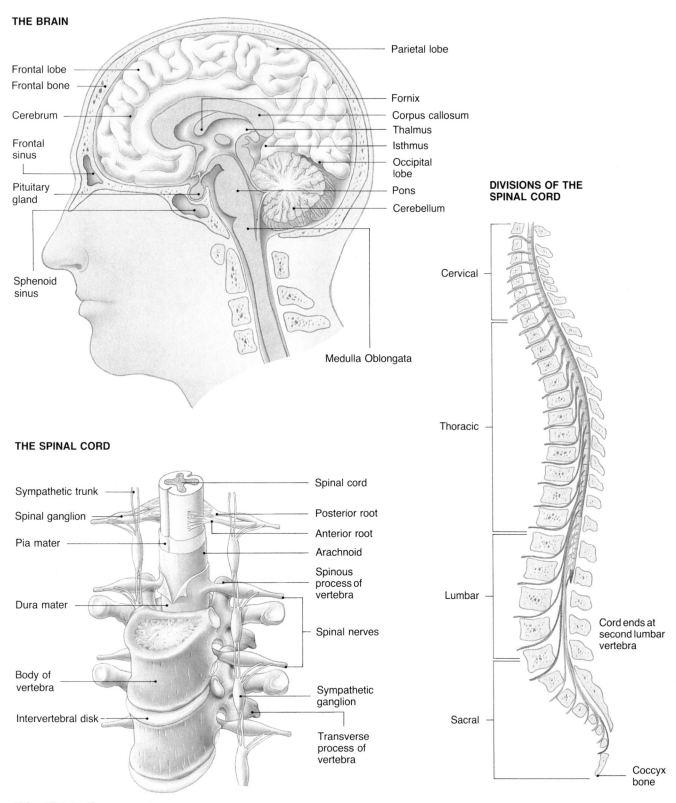

Parietal lobe

Frontal lobe

Frontal bone

Cerebrum

Frontal sinus

Pituitary gland

Sphenoid sinus

Fornix

Corpus callosum

Thalmus

Isthmus

Occipital lobe

Pons

Cerebellum

Medulla Oblongata

DIVISIONS OF THE SPINAL CORD

Cervical

Thoracic

Lumbar

Sacral

Cord ends at second lumbar vertebra

Coccyx bone

THE SPINAL CORD

Sympathetic trunk

Spinal ganglion

Pia mater

Dura mater

Body of vertebra

Intervertebral disk

Spinal cord

Posterior root

Anterior root

Arachnoid

Spinous process of vertebra

Spinal nerves

Sympathetic ganglion

Transverse process of vertebra

FIGURE 9-9   The nervous system.

Nervous System (continued)

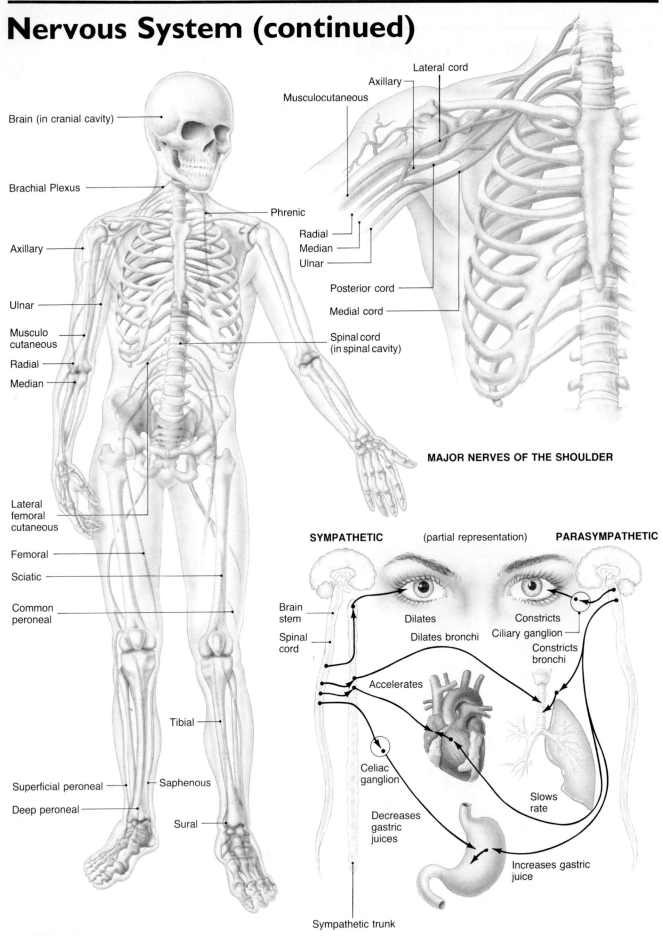

Brain (in cranial cavity)

Brachial Plexus

Axillary

Ulnar

Musculo cutaneous

Radial

Median

Lateral femoral cutaneous

Femoral

Sciatic

Common peroneal

Tibial

Superficial peroneal

Deep peroneal

Saphenous

Sural

Phrenic

Radial
Median
Ulnar

Posterior cord

Medial cord

Spinal cord (in spinal cavity)

Lateral cord

Axillary

Musculocutaneous

MAJOR NERVES OF THE SHOULDER

SYMPATHETIC (partial representation) **PARASYMPATHETIC**

Brain stem

Spinal cord

Dilates

Dilates bronchi

Accelerates

Celiac ganglion

Decreases gastric juices

Sympathetic trunk

Constricts

Ciliary ganglion

Constricts bronchi

Slows rate

Increases gastric juice

FIGURE 9-10 The nervous system (continued).

The Respiratory System

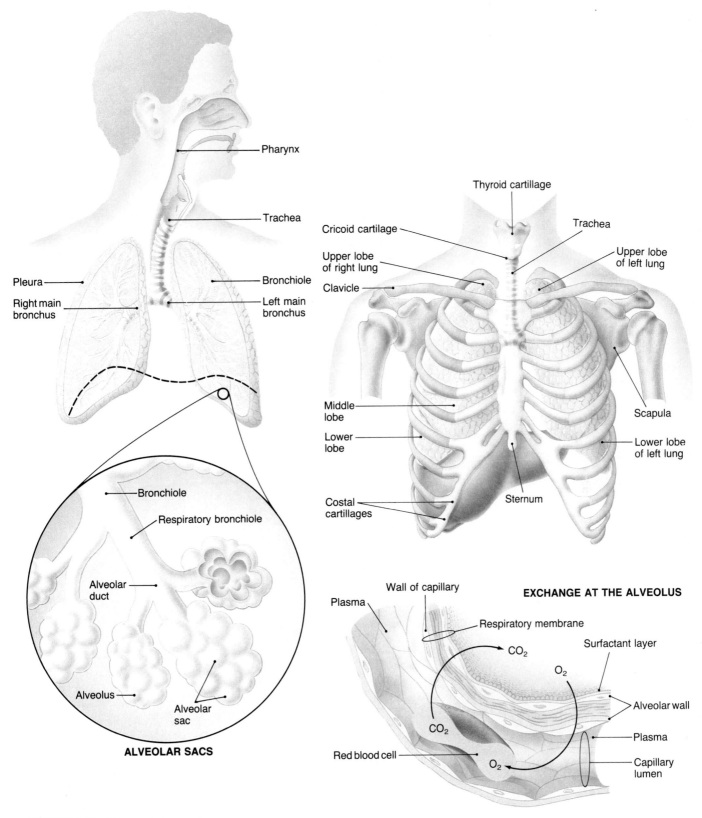

Pharynx

Trachea

Pleura

Bronchiole

Right main bronchus

Left main bronchus

Thyroid cartilage

Cricoid cartilage

Trachea

Upper lobe of right lung

Upper lobe of left lung

Clavicle

Middle lobe

Scapula

Lower lobe

Lower lobe of left lung

Costal cartilages

Sternum

ALVEOLAR SACS

Bronchiole

Respiratory bronchiole

Alveolar duct

Alveolus

Alveolar sac

EXCHANGE AT THE ALVEOLUS

Wall of capillary

Plasma

Respiratory membrane

Surfactant layer

CO_2

O_2

CO_2

Alveolar wall

Plasma

O_2

Capillary lumen

Red blood cell

FIGURE 9-11 The respiratory system.

The Digestive System

ORGANS OF THE DIGESTIVE SYSTEM

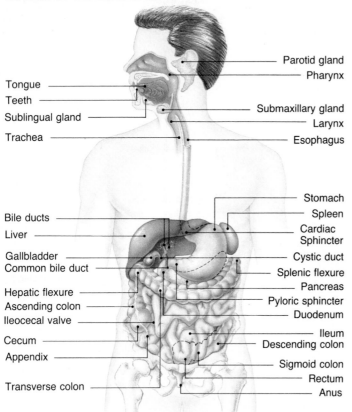

Parotid gland
Pharynx
Tongue
Teeth
Submaxillary gland
Sublingual gland
Larynx
Trachea
Esophagus

Stomach
Spleen
Bile ducts
Cardiac Sphincter
Liver
Gallbladder
Cystic duct
Common bile duct
Splenic flexure
Hepatic flexure
Pancreas
Ascending colon
Pyloric sphincter
Ileocecal valve
Duodenum
Ileum
Descending colon
Cecum
Appendix
Sigmoid colon
Rectum
Transverse colon
Anus

LIVER, STOMACH, AND PANCREAS

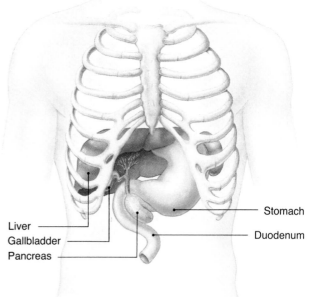

Stomach
Liver
Duodenum
Gallbladder
Pancreas

LARGE INTESTINE

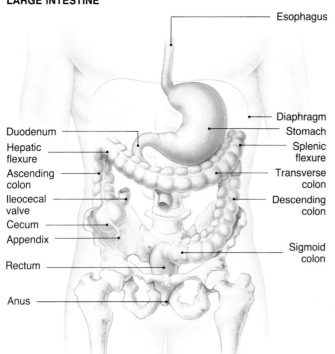

Esophagus
Diaphragm
Stomach
Duodenum
Hepatic flexure
Splenic flexure
Ascending colon
Transverse colon
Ileocecal valve
Descending colon
Cecum
Appendix
Sigmoid colon
Rectum
Anus

SMALL INTESTINE

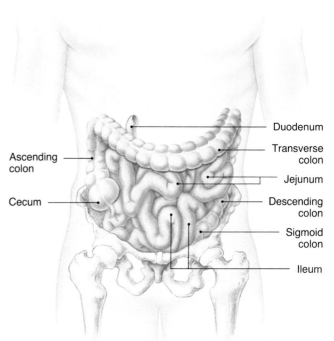

Duodenum
Transverse colon
Ascending colon
Jejunum
Cecum
Descending colon
Sigmoid colon
Ileum

FIGURE 9-12 The digestive system.

The Urinary System

ORGANS OF THE URINARY SYSTEM

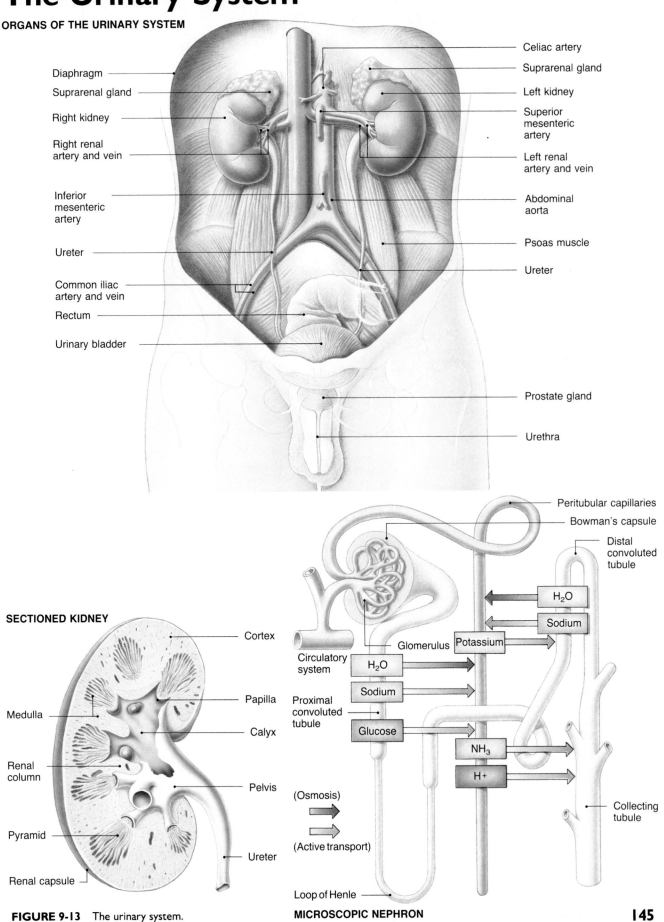

Diaphragm
Suprarenal gland
Right kidney
Right renal artery and vein
Inferior mesenteric artery
Ureter
Common iliac artery and vein
Rectum
Urinary bladder

Celiac artery
Suprarenal gland
Left kidney
Superior mesenteric artery
Left renal artery and vein
Abdominal aorta
Psoas muscle
Ureter
Prostate gland
Urethra

SECTIONED KIDNEY

Cortex
Papilla
Calyx
Pelvis
Ureter

Medulla
Renal column
Pyramid
Renal capsule

MICROSCOPIC NEPHRON

Peritubular capillaries
Bowman's capsule
Distal convoluted tubule

H_2O
Sodium
Potassium

Glomerulus
Circulatory system
H_2O
Sodium
Proximal convoluted tubule
Glucose
NH_3
$H+$

Collecting tubule

(Osmosis)

(Active transport)

Loop of Henle

FIGURE 9-13 The urinary system.

145

The Reproductive System

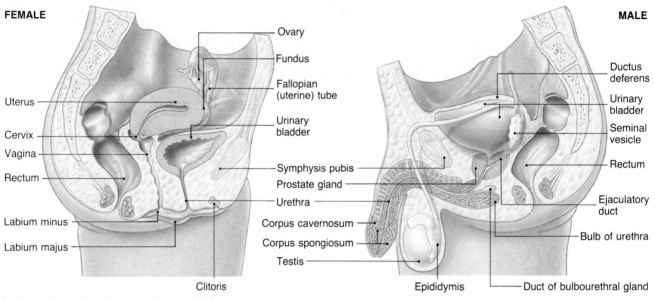

FEMALE

- Ovary
- Fundus
- Fallopian (uterine) tube
- Urinary bladder
- Symphysis pubis
- Prostate gland
- Urethra
- Corpus cavernosum
- Corpus spongiosum
- Testis

Uterus

Cervix

Vagina

Rectum

Labium minus

Labium majus

Clitoris

Labium minus (singular), Labia minora (plural)
Labium majus (singular), Labia majora (plural)

MALE

- Ductus deferens
- Urinary bladder
- Seminal vesicle
- Rectum
- Ejaculatory duct
- Bulb of urethra
- Duct of bulbourethral gland

Epididymis

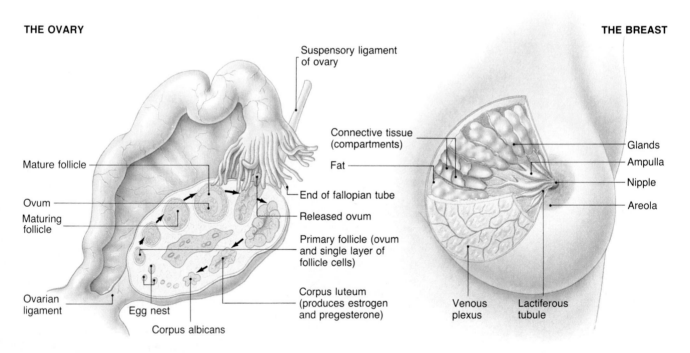

THE OVARY

- Suspensory ligament of ovary
- End of fallopian tube
- Released ovum
- Primary follicle (ovum and single layer of follicle cells)
- Corpus luteum (produces estrogen and pregesterone)

Mature follicle

Ovum

Maturing follicle

Ovarian ligament

Egg nest

Corpus albicans

THE BREAST

- Connective tissue (compartments)
- Fat
- Glands
- Ampulla
- Nipple
- Areola

Venous plexus

Lactiferous tubule

FIGURE 9-14 The reproductive system.

TOPOGRAPHICAL ANATOMY

The paramedic must be familiar with topographical anatomy. He or she will often have to describe certain illnesses and injuries to the medical control physician. Using topographical terms will help the paramedic pinpoint an injury and convey other information accurately and logically.

Anatomic Terms

General topographical terms are listed and defined, below:

Relating to Direction

anterior—toward the front of the body
ventral—toward the front of the body
posterior—toward the back of the body
dorsal—toward the back of the body
lateral—away from the midline of the body
medial—toward the midline of the body
craniad—toward the head
cephalad—toward the head
caudad—toward the tail
superior—toward the top of the body
inferior—toward the bottom of the body
superficial—toward the exterior of the body
deep—toward the interior of the body
internal—inside the body
external—outside the body
proximal—nearer the trunk of the body compared to another point
distal—farther from the trunk of the body compared to another point

Relating to Body Position

supine—lying horizontal with the face upward
prone—lying horizontal with the face downward
lateral recumbent—lying on the side
lithotomy position—lying with the face upward, the legs flexed, and the thighs abducted
Fowler's position—elevation of the head of the bed, usually 45 degrees or more, with the patient in a supine position
Semi-Fowler's position—elevation of the head of the bed, less than 45 degrees, with the patient in a supine position
Trendelenburg position—lying supine with the lower part of the body elevated above the head.

Relating to Body Movement

abduction—a movement away from the body
adduction—a movement toward the body
flexion—the act of bending
extension—the act of straightening
pronation—the act of rotating the arm, bringing the palm of the hand to a position of facing downward
supination—the act of rotating the arm, bringing the palm of the hand to a position facing upward

Topographical Anatomy of the Chest

The exterior of the chest can be described with standard anatomical lines. (See Figures 9-15, 9-16, and 9-17.) A vertical line drawn from the mid-axilla downward separates the anterior chest from the posterior chest. This is called the *mid-axillary line.* A vertical line drawn from the center of the manubrium (the top of the sternum) to the xiphoid process (the bottom of the sternum) is called the *mid-sternal line.* It separates the right anterior chest from the left anterior chest. A vertical line drawn along the spine is the *mid-spinal line,* which separates the left posterior chest from the right posterior chest. The chest can be further divided by drawing vertical lines from the mid-clavicle and mid-scapula. Further localization can be obtained by counting the intercostal spaces (the spaces between the ribs).

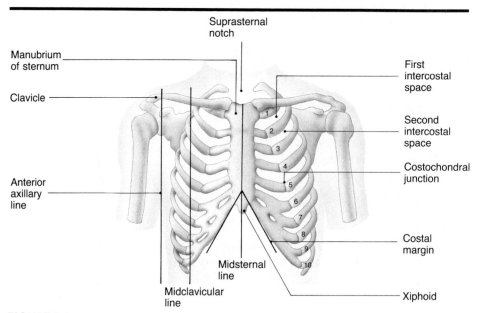

FIGURE 9-15   Topographical anatomy of the chest (anterior view).

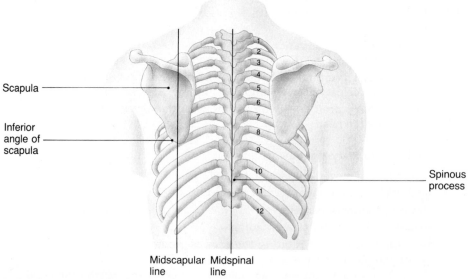

FIGURE 9-16   Topographical anatomy of the chest (posterior view).

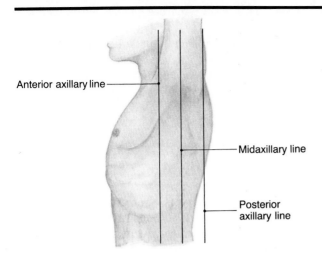

Anterior axillary line

Midaxillary line

Posterior axillary line

FIGURE 9-17 Topographical anatomy of the chest (side view).

Topographical Anatomy of the Abdomen

The abdomen is divided into four quadrants by drawing a vertical line from the xiphoid process to the symphysis pubis. This line is then halved, and a horizontal line drawn to separate the upper abdomen from the lower. The back is also part of the abdomen. It should be considered when referring to the abdomen. The point where the twelfth ribs attach to the twelfth vertebra is called the costovertebral angle (CVA). It is an important point in physical examination. The lateral aspect of the abdomen is often called the flank.

Organs contained within each abdominal quadrant include (see Figure 9-18):

❑ *Left Upper:* spleen, tail of the pancreas, stomach, left kidney, and part of the colon.

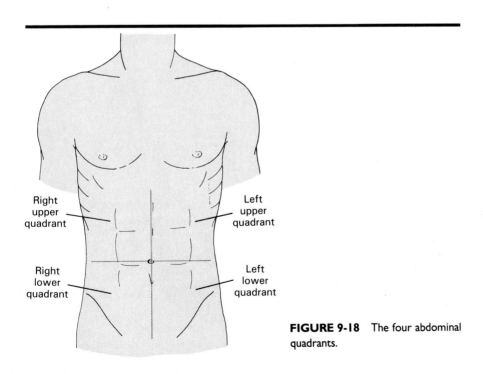

Right upper quadrant

Left upper quadrant

Right lower quadrant

Left lower quadrant

FIGURE 9-18 The four abdominal quadrants.

- *Right Upper:* liver, gall bladder, head of the pancreas, part of the duodenum, right kidney, and part of the colon.
- *Right Lower:* appendix, ascending colon, small intestine, and the right ovary and fallopian tube.
- *Left Lower:* small intestine, descending colon, and left ovary and fallopian tube.

BODY CAVITIES

The body contains several compartments, referred to as cavities. (See Figure 9-19.) The superior-most cavity is the *cranium* or *cranial vault,* which contains the brain. The *thoracic cavity* is the compartment that contains the heart, lungs, and mediastinum. It is bordered superiorly by the root of the neck, and inferiorly by the diaphragm. The *abdominal cavity* is bordered by the diaphragm superiorly, and the pelvic inlet inferiorly. It contains the liver, gall bladder, stomach, pancreas, spleen, intestines, kidneys, and adrenal glands. The *pelvic cavity* is bordered superiorly by the pelvic inlet, and inferiorly by the pelvic floor. It contains the bladder, rectum, ovaries, fallopian tubes, and uterus. There is no anatom-

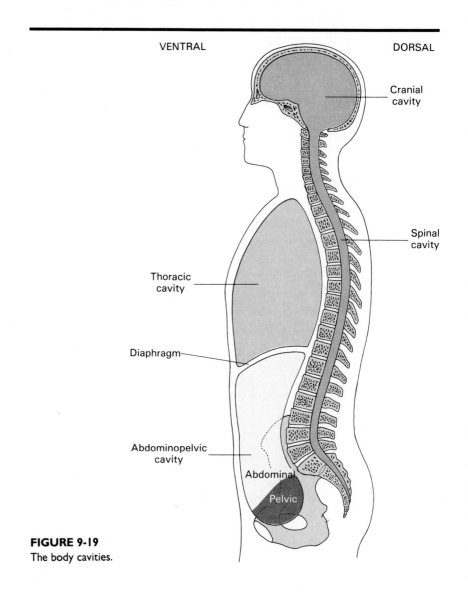

VENTRAL

DORSAL

Cranial cavity

Spinal cavity

Thoracic cavity

Diaphragm

Abdominopelvic cavity

Abdominal

Pelvic

FIGURE 9-19
The body cavities.

ical division between the abdomen and the pelvis; they are often referred to as the abdominopelvic cavity. The *spinal cavity* extends from the base of the skull, down through the spinal canal, to the sacrum. It contains the spinal cord and associated structures.

SUMMARY

This chapter has presented the fundamentals of anatomy and physiology. Detailed discussion of each body system will appear in later chapters. At regular intervals, you should review pertinent anatomy and physiology. A thorough understanding of anatomy will often allow you to predict, with reasonable accuracy, what injuries and illnesses have occurred, based on the location of the patient's injury or complaint.

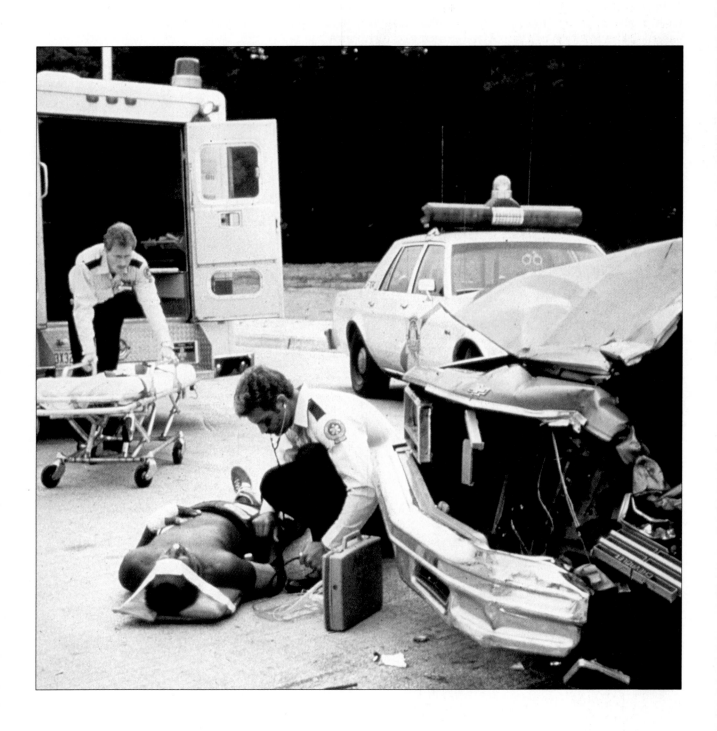

10

Advanced Patient Assessment

Objectives for Chapter 10

Upon completing this chapter, the student should be able to:

1. Identify the information gathered in each of the six phases of patient assessment.

2. List the hazards of the accident or medical emergency that must be ruled out before patient care can occur.

3. Explain the five elements of the primary assessment and the criteria for evaluating them.

4. Identify the three results of the primary assessment and actions the paramedic should take for each.

5. List by anatomical area each of the signs and symptoms examined during the secondary assessment.

6. Define the elements of the vital signs, and explain the significance of each to overall patient evaluation.

7. Describe the information needed for patient assessment that comes from evaluating the chief complaint.

8. Identify the important details gained by questioning the patient about medications, medical history, allergies, and personal physicians.

9. Demonstrate a complete patient assessment—from evaluation of dispatch information, to documentation of the call at its conclusion.

CASE STUDY

Medic Rescue Unit 21 is dispatched to the scene of a one-car accident in a residential area on a warm and sunny August day. The fire department is enroute, but is expected to arrive a few minutes after the ambulance.

At the scene, an auto is found against a utility pole whose wires are down. The gas tank is ruptured and is spilling fuel. Window glass is scattered about the scene and the auto body is severely deformed. The paramedic team parks the unit well away from the utility poles, sets up a perimeter, and ensures that bystanders are kept at a safe distance. They instruct the patient, who is slumped over the steering wheel, to remain where he is until they make sure the power is turned off and the scene secured. The fire company arrives and calls for the power to be shut off. They secure the vehicle with blocks, set up a charged line, and contain the leaking fuel.

Once the power is shut off, the crew begins the primary assessment. The patient appears unconscious, but is breathing and has a good pulse. There is a small contusion on his forehead, and the windshield is broken where his head probably hit it. A bystander explains that she saw the car swerve wildly as it traveled down the street, just before the impact. No skid marks are visible on the roadway.

The primary assessment reveals only some audible wheezes and stridor. The modified jaw thrust, applied with cervical precautions and a cervical collar, does not correct these conditions. There are no signs of injury to the chest, neck, or head, other than the forehead wound and a small welt on the patient's posterior neck. The pupils are equal and reactive.

As the secondary assessment starts, the patient begins to awaken. He asks what happened, then explains that he thought he was stung by a bee. He had a severe reaction to a bee sting last year, and has a special kit at home in case it happens again. Vitals are taken while a complete history is learned. The patient displays a blood pressure of 110/76, strong distal pulses at a rate of 90, and an oxygen saturation of 98 percent. The history is unremarkable for pre-existing conditions, other than the allergy to insect stings. The wheezing persists, and the patient complains of a lump in his throat.

Oxygen is applied by non-rebreather mask. An IV of lactated Ringer's solution is started with a 16 gauge over the needle catheter; it is run slowly. The report is given to medical command. Orders are received for 0.3 mg of epinephrine subcutaneously and 50 mg Benadryl IM. The patient is carefully monitored while the spine board is placed. Then, the patient is secured and is extricated. The wheezes disappear and the patient states that the lump in his throat is gone. He is transported uneventfully to the hospital and the receiving physician. He spends the night and is released the next morning.

INTRODUCTION

■ **patient assessment** that act of examining a patient in order to detect a medical problem.

Patient assessment is one of the most important skills performed by the paramedic. Not only does it help determine what may be wrong with the patient, it also provides a reasonable picture of what happened, how it happened, and how the patient will probably respond to care.

Patient assessment is a straightforward skill. When performed properly, it takes only a few minutes to complete. Failure to provide an appropriate patient assessment can lead to devastating results for the patient. Advanced-level patient assessment must be thorough and comprehensive, because many of the procedures and medications used in advanced prehospital care are potentially dangerous. The administration of drugs, defibrillation or cardioversion, pleural decompression, or advanced airway skills can seriously harm or kill a patient, especially if applied when not needed.

The EMS system has significant medical accountability. Any advanced procedure performed must be supported by appropriate signs, symptoms, and history from a complete patient evaluation. Post-call documentation must clearly confirm the pathology that required advanced intervention. Proper patient assessment uses sight, hearing, touch, and smell to determine and record the patient's condition. When synthesized, information discovered by the senses will give a good idea of the patient's condition and will help to expose the underlying problem(s).

For the most part, the assessment process is the same whether the patient's condition results from trauma or illness. It should consist of a review of the dispatch information, survey of the scene, primary assessment, secondary assessment, determination of the vital signs, and patient history. It should begin with an evaluation of the patient's environment, continue with an evaluation of airway, breathing, and circulatory function, and proceed to a complete evaluation of the patient. It is a process that is never really completed, because the patient must be continuously re-evaluated. Assessment is an important skill for the paramedic to master. It must be perfected through careful thought, regular practice, and honest self-evaluation.

PATIENT ASSESSMENT

The six distinctive phases in patient assessment are:

- ❑ review of the dispatch information
- ❑ survey of the scene
- ❑ primary assessment
- ❑ secondary assessment
- ❑ determination of vital signs
- ❑ patient history

While the first three steps must occur in the listed order, the last three may occur simultaneously, or in various sequences. The order should be determined by the local EMS system's operating protocols and by the patient's condition. For the purposes of this discussion, medical and trauma assessment will be presented together. In practice, however, they would be approached separately. It should also be remembered that trauma may have been precipitated by a medical problem, or vice versa. Auto accidents are often brought about by heart attack or alcohol intoxication. Medical problems may arise from previous trauma, such as head-injury-induced epilepsy, or from internal bleeding that is secondary to an earlier fall. You should always focus on what appears to be wrong with the patient, but stay alert for the unexpected.

REVIEW OF DISPATCH INFORMATION

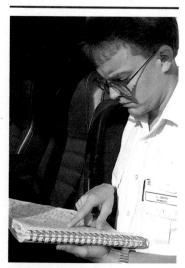

FIGURE 10-1 The first step in patient assessment is review of the dispatch information. Information provided by the dispatcher can allow you to mentally prepare for the emergency.

✱ Review the dispatch information to determine the nature and location of the emergency and to begin to plan your response and care.

Assessment of the emergency situation begins before the patient is seen and long before he or she is touched. Immediately upon receiving the dispatch information, the paramedic should begin to evaluate the situation, plan the steps of assessment, and determine the appropriate care. (See Figure 10-1.) Dispatch information provides more data than is generally recognized. The scene location can often indicate the type of medical emergency and its potential seriousness. The location of a medical or traumatic call—such as a response to a cardiologist's office, a particular stretch of roadway, or the home of a patient who frequently summons EMS—can identify the nature of the call and the care expected at the scene. The location may also suggest special considerations toward scene approach and vehicle placement. A divided highway with few turnarounds may require entering against traffic (the wrong way on a one-way street) to avoid negotiating through miles of congestion. High-speed traffic passing an accident requires effective traffic control by police and may dictate placement of the vehicle between oncoming traffic and the site of patient care. (See Figure 10-2.)

The trained dispatchers of today's modern EMS system are skilled in taking information and assessing the severity of a call. Information provided by the EMS dispatcher can often indicate what skills and equipment may be required at the scene.

The paramedic is responsible for a great deal of forethought in response to a patient's call for help. Planning the response before arrival at the scene can increase efficiency and performance. Preparing equipment beforehand ensures that it is operational and readily available. (See Figure 10-3.) There is nothing more frustrating than to arrive at an acute emergency only to find that an essential piece of equipment has failed. It's just as frustrating to leave the patient's side to retrieve a needed piece of equipment from the ambulance (or to describe the piece to a bystander so he or she may retrieve it). It's better to load more equipment onto the stretcher than may be required than to be caught short.

Use the time enroute to the scene for mental preparation. (See Figure 10-4.) The emergency response places a lot of stress on the paramedic. It may be beneficial to relax and organize a simple plan for the scene response. The person in charge of the medical response should not drive. Emergency vehicle operation deserves maximum concentration; it does not allow for distraction.

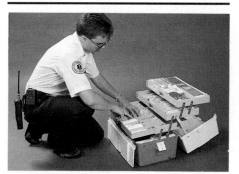

FIGURE 10-2 The response to the scene must be carefully planned to avoid any potential delays. Such factors as traffic, road conditions, and the time of day should be taken into consideration.

FIGURE 10-3 Preparing equipment for the response is almost as important as the response itself.

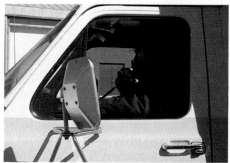

FIGURE 10-4 During the response the paramedic in charge should mentally prepare for the emergency while his partner drives.

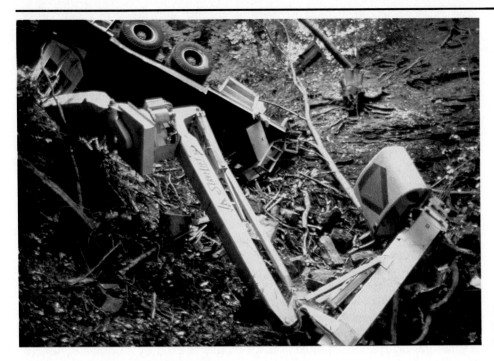

FIGURE 10-5 The initial survey of the scene can provide a great deal of information about the emergency.

SURVEY OF THE SCENE

Arrival at the scene begins the formal assessment process. (See Figure 10-5.) The paramedic can now learn more about the nature and seriousness of the call. The facial expressions of bystanders often indicate stress levels and reveal how they perceive the "emergency." The mechanism of injury or illness, as well as possible hazards, may be apparent. (The evaluation of the mechanisms of injury will be presented in Chapter 14.) The paramedic must determine the number of patients or potential patients and whether assistance is needed from police, fire, rescue, or other safety services. All these elements of the scene survey should be recognized before arrival at the patient's side.

A paramedic must be aware of the hazards of the emergency response. In many cases, these hazards may cause harm to patients and paramedics alike. An injured paramedic may be unable to assist the patient. It is essential to actively look for hazards, not just notice them. Scene hazards may be fire, structural collapse, toxic inhalation or contamination, explosion, electrocution, traffic problems, slippery surfaces, and sharp objects like broken glass or jagged metal. Although these perils are normally associated with trauma, they are often found at the settings of medical emergencies. A prime example is the dispatch to the home of a family that is complaining of headache and malaise (a generalized ill feeling), only to find the problem is secondary to a faulty heater and resultant carbon monoxide poisoning.

In hazardous conditions, adequate protective equipment for both the patient and the paramedics must be available. (See Chapter 6.) Common protective equipment should include blankets, turnout gear, self-contained breathing apparatus, helmets, gloves, and safety goggles. Paramedics who are not trained to use appropriate safety equipment should not enter the scene. In such a case, other rescuers who are protected must bring the patient to the paramedics.

If the scene is a hazardous environment, the patient should be protected as well. Blankets, hard hats, and goggles are suggested. In an active extrication, additional protection should be offered to avoid injury from the dynamic forces being used. If toxic chemicals or fumes are present, the patient should be afforded protection from further contamination, and provided with decontamination as early as possible. Certain dangers, such as furniture, lamp cords, steps, small stairways, narrow halls, and door openings, can impede safe patient "extrication" from what is considered a medical call. Spilled fluids, ice and snow, broken glass and debris, and wet embankments call for extreme care in moving the patient to the ambulance. These situations should be anticipated from the initial scene appraisal, and followed by steps to reduce the risk of injury to both rescuers and patients.

Weather conditions are not often considered hazards, but a cold evening with a low wind-chill factor and freezing rain can be dangerous for both a paramedic and patient. Such conditions may require blankets, weather barriers, and heat sources during a prolonged extrication; protection for the acute medical patient during transport from the house to the ambulance; or an alternative route from a residence to the unit to avoid slippery areas. Failure to recognize and prepare for these problems can lead to frustrating, even disastrous, experiences.

* Survey the scene to determine scene hazards, the nature and severity of injuries, the number of patients, and the need for additional resources.

Evaluation of bystanders and family members is another aspect of scene analysis. It is essential for safe, orderly, and controlled incident management. If the response is to an injury caused by a domestic altercation, the paramedic crew may be endangered by the same person who attacked the patient. An adversarial crowd may interfere with the paramedic's ability to care for the patient at the scene. If the bystanders are emotionally upset, there may be more than just the primary (ill or injured) patient to treat.

Survey of the scene also includes a visual search of the area for the patient or patients. As the paramedic approaches the incident scene, he or she should ask if there could be other passengers or persons involved in the accident, or affected by the medical problem. The paramedic must determine how many patients need transport, and where the most serious patient can be found. Evaluation of the mechanism of injury and evidence suggesting multiple patients may answer these questions. A two-car accident must include at least two drivers. Other clues, such as diaper bags, child auto seats, or twin "spider webs" on the windshield, may lead to a search for more patients than those already found. During the scene survey, a conscious effort must be made to look for articles of clothing from different age groups (infant, child, or adult), and from both sexes. What is found may suggest additional patients.

As the scene assessment is completed, the initial responding paramedic must decide whether to call for assistance. Fire suppression, rescue, police, or other services may be required. Should a paramedic confront a hazard beyond his or her training, or discover more than one seriously injured patient, he or she should immediately summon help. Doing so will speed the response and allow the responding paramedics to concentrate on patient care.

PRIMARY ASSESSMENT

■ **primary assessment** first aspect of the patient assessment designed to determine any immediate threats to the patient's life. It assesses airway, breathing, and circulation and looks for significant hemorrhage.

The **primary assessment** is intended to gather just enough information to exclude serious and immediate threats to life. (See Figure 10-6.) It should evaluate the standard ABCs of emergency care. In addition, the patient's level of responsiveness should be rapidly assessed. The components of the primary assessment should be evaluated and updated frequently throughout the response. Any change in the patient's condition from the initial primary assessment, deleterious or otherwise, should be noted and its cause sought.

The primary assessment, especially for the traumatic emergency, looks to critical anatomical areas to determine whether immediate transport or on-scene stabilization is indicated. It is designed to detect a diminished level of consciousness, uncorrectable respiratory compromise, and the signs or symptoms of impending shock. If any of these conditions are recognized, the patient should be immediately transported. Otherwise, the patient should be given care at the scene and transported in the normal manner. While less than 10% of trauma patients require rapid transport before stabilization, their survival depends upon definitive surgical intervention, which is available only at a **trauma center.** The assessing paramedic must continually anticipate, and examine the patient for, signs of deterioration. He or she must be ready to stop on-scene stabilization and transport immediately.

The primary assessment consists of the A-B-C-D-E steps of emergency care.

A = Airway (and cervical spine control)
B = Breathing
C = Cardiovascular function
D = Neurologic disability
E = Exposure and examination of the head, neck, chest and abdomen for assessment of potentially critical injuries.

The primary assessment, not including intervention, should take no longer than 90 seconds. It should be quickly and methodically executed. The paramedic must learn to focus on the priorities and not become distracted. Should the **mechanism of injury** indicate the slightest possibility of spinal injury, the victim's head and neck must be stabilized. This should be done as early as possible during the primary assessment. The slightest movement of an unstable cervical spine can cause irreparable damage, including **paraplegia, quadriplegia,** or even death. "Overcare" is the better choice in this circumstance—cervical immobilization will present little risk to the patient who doesn't need it; failure to provide it is deadly to the patient who does. Manual immobilization should be followed by mechanical stabilization. (See Chapter 15.) (The procedure may be modified for immediate transport: substitute manual immobilization of the spine to get a seated patient to the spineboard, when short spineboard application would be ideal.)

Beginning the primary assessment, the paramedic should identify himself or herself and state what he or she intends to do. (See Figure 10-7.) For example, "I'm John Doe, a paramedic from Ashwaubenon Rescue Squad. I'm here to help you." This approach establishes the paramedic's level of training, authority, and reason for being at the patient's side. It also allows the patient to refuse care. As discussed in previous chapters, care cannot be provided without either implied or informed consent. In providing this information, the paramedic can begin to establish rapport with the patient.

The paramedic should calm and reassure the patient, who must be made to feel that he or she is in good hands and that the situation is under control. The paramedic must be compassionate and must show concern for how the patient feels. All too frequently, paramedical personnel forget how significant an injury is, even a minor one, to a patient. Often, the call is routine and does not have the excitement of a cardiac arrest or major auto accident. To the patient, however, it is real and personal pain. The ill or injured victim may worry about the long-term consequences on

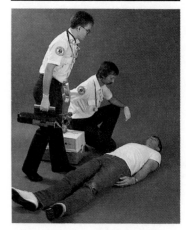

FIGURE 10-6 The first step upon arrival at the patient's side is the primary assessment.

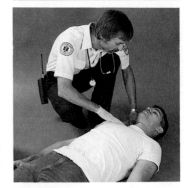

FIGURE 10-7 If the patient is conscious, identify yourself, and your level of training.

work, child care, and finances. Lacking the paramedic's training and experience, a victim may have unrealistic fears. The paramedic must understand these fears and support the patient psychologically, as well as physiologically.

A verbal response by the patient will tell a great deal about his or her condition. An organized, appropriate, and coherent statement shows that the patient has a well-perfused and oxygenated brain, as well as adequate respiratory function to support reasonable speech. Failure of the patient to respond in this manner could indicate a serious or emergent problem.

Airway and Breathing

The physical evaluation begins with the familiar ABCs. The airway and breathing are critical to a patient's survival, even short-term, and must be rapidly and carefully assessed. That assessment must be periodically repeated to ensure that the airway remains unobstructed and that breathing is adequate in both volume and rate. Since normal respiration is passive and almost imperceptible, very close examination is necessary. The volume of air moved with each respiration is only about 500 ml. A normal rate is 12–24 respirations per minute. The exchange is very quiet because airway sounds tend to be soft and unobtrusive. Any deviation from this pattern is cause for concern and further investigation.

Though airway and breathing separately make up the A and B of the ABCs, they must be evaluated together. Breathing will not occur without an airway and, conversely, confirmation that an airway exists cannot be made unless air moves through it. Airway and breathing are not easy to evaluate in the initial assessment. It takes careful and conscious effort by the paramedic to determine that the airway is clear and breathing is adequate. Look, listen, and feel to find out if the patient is indeed breathing and has an open airway.

Look. Look at the external portions of the airway; the patient's mouth and nose. (See Figure 10-8.) Note any signs of trauma, vomitus, or other mechanisms or agents that might compromise the airway. Examine for nasal flaring, fluid or objects in the airway, or for cyanotic or ashen discoloration of the lips. Observe the chest for adequate respiratory excursion. The motion should be symmetrical and smooth. There should be no **paradoxical movement** nor should one side rise and fall more than the other. Determine whether the volume of air being moved with each breath is adequate or excessive. Normal respiration occurs 12 to 20 times per minute and displaces about 500 mL of air (6–12 L/min). Smaller volumes are of concern because the first 150 mL is not really exchanged (dead space volume). With a normal respiratory volume of 500 mL, 350 mL of air reaches the **alveoli.** If the respiratory effort exchanges only 300 mL of fresh air, the air available to the alveoli is reduced from 350 mL to 150 mL. In other words, a 40% reduction in the volume of inspired air is equal to a 60% reduction in the critical air exposed to the alveoli and circulating blood.

Look also to the rate of respiration. If it drops below 12 breaths per minute, the total volume of inspired air per minute may not be enough to maintain life. An abnormally fast respiration rate (more than 24 per minute) may indicate excitement, a metabolic problem, shock, or head injury. Certain other respiratory characteristics are noteworthy in the primary assessment. Does the abdomen move with an exaggerated motion, suggesting spinal-cord injury and diaphragmatic breathing? Are accessory muscles of the neck being used to move the air, reflective of increased

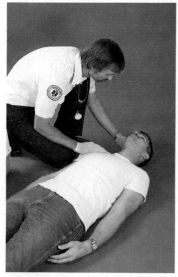

FIGURE 10-8 The first step in assuring the patient has an open airway and is breathing is to LOOK for the chest to rise and fall with respirations.

■ **paradoxical movement** moving in a fashion opposite to that expected. It is often seen in flail chest injuries where the flail segment moves in an opposite direction compared to the rest of the chest.

■ **alveolus (pl. alveoli)** one of the millions of microscopic chambers in the lung. It is where the gases of respiration are exchanged.

airway resistance? Are there **retractions** (drawing in of the tissue) between the ribs or above the clavicles, resulting from increased inspiratory effort? This action is often caused by a partial or complete airway obstruction.

Listen. Are the respirations quiet or noisy? **Apnea** is by far the quietest—and the most pathologic—respiratory pattern. Ensure that respirations are indeed present and that they're relatively quiet. (See Figure 10-9.) Evaluate any noisy respiration. **Snoring** is generally caused by gravity moving the relaxed tongue into the posterior pharynx. It can be corrected by proper head-positioning: head tilt-chin lift in the medical patient; chin lift, modified jaw thrust, or nasopharyngeal airway insertion in the trauma patient. (See Chapter 11.)

The crowing or **stridorous** respirations of laryngeal obstruction are ominous sounds. In addition to showing airway involvement, they may indicate a problem that's very difficult to correct in the field. **Wheezing,** another sound that may accompany respiration, is suggestive of lower-airway constriction and another problem that is hard to correct. Gurgling may be heard, caused by fluids in the airway, mouth, or nose. It represents a serious threat to the airway and demands immediate attention. It may also indicate congestive heart failure and the need for advanced cardiac life-support measures.

Feel. Feeling the motion of warm and humid exhalation on your cheek or the back of your hand may give you a sense of how much air the patient is moving with each breath. (See Figure 10-10.) It may be the most obvious sign that the patient is breathing at all. If, during assessment of the airway and breathing, you find anything that threatens effective respiration, you should correct it at once. As you learned in Basic Cardiac Life Support (BCLS), the brain, heart, and kidneys cannot survive long without oxygen. The airway and respiratory effort must be able to provide oxygen and rid the body of carbon dioxide effectively enough to support life. This ability must be assured before any further assessment is done or care given.

The patient who is unable to protect his or her airway (deeply unconscious and lacking a gag reflex) should be intubated with an endotracheal tube. If respirations are absent, or the volume moved with each breath is believed to be much less than 6 liters per minute, respiratory support with supplemental oxygen should be provided. This can be done via mouth-to-mask, bag-valve-mask, or by demand valve. These steps must be completed before assessment and management can continue.

Circulation

Oxygen delivered to the alveoli does little good without a mechanism to circulate it to the body's cells. Once adequate respiratory function is established, circulation should be evaluated. The carotid pulse should be palpated for general rate and character. (See Figure 10-11.) The rate should be between 50 and 120 beats per minute. The pulse should be strong and regular. Examining the skin is another step in evaluating circulation. The skin is one of the first organs to lose blood flow (due to peripheral vasoconstriction) in the face of hypovolemia or other types of shock. It may appear mottled (blotchy), cyanotic, pale, or ashen in color. It may also feel cool and clammy (moist) to the touch. This often indicates that warm, circulating blood has been shunted to more critical areas. Any of these signs indicates a serious problem with circulation.

■ **retraction** the act of drawing back or inward. (e.g., acute airway obstruction when the intercostal spaces and sternal notch retract).

■ **apnea** the absence of breathing.

■ **snoring** upper airway noise caused by the partial obstruction of the airway by the tongue or similar materials

■ **stridor** a high-pitched "crowing" sound, caused by restriction of the upper airway.

■ **wheezing** whistling type breath sound associated with narrowing or spasm of the smaller airways.

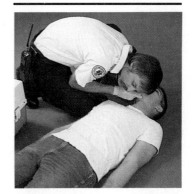

FIGURE 10-9 Next, you should listen for air movement.

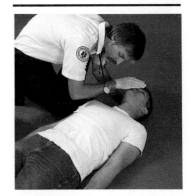

FIGURE 10-10 Next, you should feel for air movement with your hand or cheek.

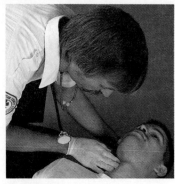

FIGURE 10-11 Palpate the carotid pulse to rapidly determine the status of the circulatory system.

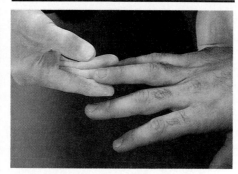

FIGURE 10-12 Perfusion can also be assessed by testing capillary refill.

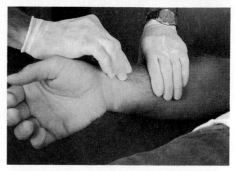

FIGURE 10-13 The presence of a radial pulse will generally indicate that the patient has a blood pressure of at least 80 mm/Hg.

■ **capillary refill** diagnositc sign for evaluating peripheral circulation. A capillary bed, such as a fingernail, is compressed. The time taken for color to return to the bed is the capillary refill time, usually 2 seconds or less.

Perfusion also may be evaluated by looking at **capillary refill.** If a portion of skin or a nail bed is compressed, it will turn white or pale (blanch). When pressure is released, the speed at which the color returns reflects the state of the peripheral circulation. (See Figure 10-12.) The pink color should return within two seconds with good circulatory function. A longer capillary refill time suggests circulatory compromise. The exception is during cold weather, when vasoconstriction may normally be present.

Various pulses can be used to approximate the patient's systolic blood pressure. As the pulse wave travels away from the heart and the central circulation, it becomes weaker. The radial pulse will normally disappear when the systolic pressure drops below 90 mmHg. (See Figure 10-13.) If the pressure drops to between 70 and 80, the femoral pulse will disappear. The carotid pulse usually remains until the systolic pressure drops below 60 mmHg.

Disability

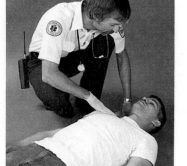

FIGURE 10-14 The patient's level of consciousness must be quickly assessed using the "AVPU" system.

Disability refers to assessment of the central nervous system (CNS) to determine any deficit. Initially, during the primary survey, the paramedic should determine the patient's level of consciousness. There are many ways to describe a patient's level of consciousness. Terms such as obtunded, semi-conscious, and confused, have different meanings for different people. Because of this, the paramedic should use the following classification system represented by the acronym AVPU. (See Figure 10-14.)

A = Alert
V = responds to Verbal stimuli
P = responds to Painful stimuli
U = Unresponsive

■ **Glasgow Coma Scale** scoring system for monitoring the neurological status of patients with head injuries.

Additional evaluation of the nervous system, including application of the **Glasgow Coma Scale,** should be performed during the Secondary Survey.

Expose and Examine

The "E" of the rapid assessment refers to exposure of the head, neck, chest, and abdomen to look for the presence of serious pathology. These regions can account for significant hemorrhage, potential respiratory compromise, and other life-threatening injuries. The paramedic should continue to examine for any significant injury that could compromise airway or respiration, or contribute significantly to hypovolemia. The head and neck should be rapidly examined for signs of severe injury and possible intracranial trauma. (See Figure 10-15.) Facial injuries should be identified as they may contribute to airway distress. The neck should be evaluated for any signs of trauma, edema, or discoloration, which could suggest future problems. The chest is examined for signs of deceleration injuries or fractures, or any instability of the chest (such as gross deformity or flail chest). (See Figure 10-16.) Potential for an open pneumothorax should be ruled out by observing for any open wounds, remembering that any penetrating open wound may have an associated exit wound.

The abdomen also merits close visual evaluation. Look again for any hint of blunt or penetrating trauma. Care should be taken to observe for any pulsating masses and any discoloration. If there is abdominal guarding, pain, or tenderness the possibility of internal bleeding should be suspected. Finally, the Primary Survey must include a quick but thorough visual exam for severe bleeding. (See Figure 10-17.) The entire body should be scanned to ensure that uncontrolled bleeding does not continue. Pay close attention to the hidden body areas, such as behind the lower back and buttocks and in the inguinal region, and to areas whose involvement is suggested by the mechanism of injury.

Primary Survey Results—Trauma Patient

After completing the primary survey, the paramedic should be able to determine whether stabilization at the scene or immediate transport, with stabilization enroute, is required. Critical trauma patients are much more likely to survive if they get to surgery within an hour of the incident. This time has become known as the **Golden Hour.** The Emergency Medical Service System is generally given 10 minutes (1/6 of the "Golden Hour") of on-scene time to assess, correct immediate life-threatening problems, and prepare for transport. Should the patient show a threat to respiratory function, central nervous system deficit, or any signs or symptoms of the development of shock, he or she should receive immediate transport to a definitive care facility, preferably offered by a trauma center. The current evaluation systems for the trauma patient help to prioritize condition and predict outcome. One example is the **Trauma Score,** which uses the outcome of the Glasgow Coma Scale. The Trauma Score also includes respiratory rate, thoracic expansion, systolic blood pressure, and capillary refill. An example of the Trauma Score is illustrated in Figure 10-18.

In evaluating primary assessment results, it is very important to keep in mind the time between the accident or medical event and the conclusion of the primary assessment. Frequently, the time between occurrence and EMS arrival is considerable, because of either delayed system entry or significant distance to the scene. If the time interval is long, and the patient is stable, the situation is probably not highly emergent. However, if EMS arrives shortly after the problem developed and the patient appears stable, the index of suspicion that something is seriously wrong must be higher.

Primary Survey Results—Medical Patient

The medical patient is often a different matter. Stabilization of the cardiac arrest patient is best accomplished at the scene. Many other medical emergencies, though less acute than cardiac arrest, still merit scene sta-

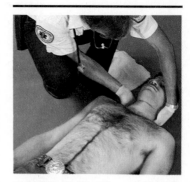

FIGURE 10-15 The neck should be gently palpated noting any deformity or tenderness.

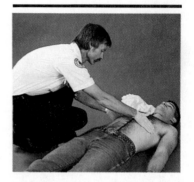

FIGURE 10-16 The chest should be briefly inspected and palpated so as to detect any open wounds or other problems which may threaten the patient's life.

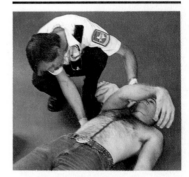

FIGURE 10-17 The posterior chest should be inspected and palpated for any possible injury.

■ **Golden Hour** the first hour following a serious accident. Studies have shown that patients who receive definitive care within the first hour have an increased chance of survival.

Revised Trauma Score

Respiratory Rate	10–29/min	4	
	>29/min	3	
	6–9/min	2	
	1–5/min	1	
	None	0	
Respiratory Expansion	Normal	1	
	Retractive	0	
Systolic Blood Pressure	>89 mmHg or greater	4	
	76–89 mmHg	3	
	50–75 mmHg	2	
	0–49 mmHg	1	
	No Pulse	0	
Capillary Refill	Normal	2	
	Delayed	1	
	None	0	
Cardiopulmonary Assessment			

Glasgow Coma Scale

Eye Opening	Spontaneous	4	
	To Voice	3	
	To Pain	2	
	None	1	
Verbal Response	Oriented	5	
	Confused	4	
	Inappropriate Words	3	
	Incomprehensible Words	2	
	None	1	
Motor Response	Obeys Command	6	
	Localizes Pain	5	
	Withdraw (Pain)	4	
	Flexion (Pain)	3	
	Extension (Pain)	2	
	None	1	
Glasgow Coma Score Total			

TOTAL GLASGOW COMA SCALE POINTS

13 – 15 = 5
9 – 12 = 4
6 – 8 = 3
4 – 5 = 1

Conversion = Approximately One-Third Total Value

Neurologic Assessment

Total Trauma Score = Cardiopulmonary + Neurologic ⟶

FIGURE 10-18 The Revised Trauma Score.

✱ The primary survey quickly assesses the patient's **A**irway, **B**reathing, **C**irculation, and neurologic **D**isability, and **E**xposes any other life-threatening conditions.

✱ At the conclusion of the primary survey, the decision is made to transport the patient immediately with care provided enroute or to provide care on-scene.

bilization rather than rapid transport. However, be aware that medical conditions can also require immediate transport. Hypovolemic shock, due to ruptured ectopic pregnancy or a dissecting or ruptured aneurysm, can rapidly result in exsanguination. The only definitive care of such cases is surgical closure of the internal wound.

The paramedic must examine the patient for subtle indications of developing problems and immediately transport the patient if scene stabilization is unlikely. If the decision has been made to care for the patient—medical or trauma—by rapid transport, the patient should be moved quickly to the ambulance, with most advanced-care procedures accomplished enroute. (See Figure 10-19.) The patient should receive high-flow oxygen via standard, non-rebreathing or partial rebreathing mask. If respiration is not adequate, the patient should be ventilated. The bag-valve-mask or demand valve (use the demand valve with caution in the chest trauma or chronic obstructive pulmonary disease patient). Advanced airway care should be considered, including placement of an endotracheal tube (or possible trans-tracheal jet insufflation device). If tension pneumothorax is suspected, pleural decompression may be requested by medical control. PASG should be considered, as should bilateral large-bore IVs, prepared to run wide-open or under pressure infu-

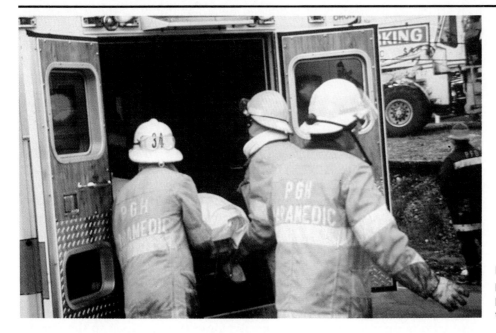

FIGURE 10-19 Patients in hypovolemic shock should be transported immediately with stabilization attempted enroute.

sion, as called for by medical control. If scene care and stabilization is chosen, then the patient should receive oxygen and other supportive measures as you begin the secondary assessment.

SECONDARY ASSESSMENT

The **secondary assessment** should be modified according to the type of patient. If the problem was trauma-related, and the patient is stable, a complete head-to-toe evaluation is merited. If the patient is a routine transport for direct hospital admission, limited evaluation may suffice. When doing assessments, paramedics tend to err on the side of too limited rather than too complete. A poor assessment will miss significant signs and symptoms; a complete assessment will rarely cause harm or significant discomfort, unless it delays transport of the severely injured patient.

The four components of physical examination are: **inspection, palpation, auscultation,** and, occasionally, **percussion.** Each of these evaluation techniques can reveal information essential to complete and accurate patient assessment.

Inspection

Inspection is the most valuable tool in appraising the patient's condition. It is non-invasive, and it is the least-endangering component of the assessment. Inspection can provide a great deal of information, which makes it easy to overlook important signs and symptoms. The physical examination, like the entire patient assessment process, must be organized and structured so as not to miss critical findings.

The paramedic is frequently the first care provider to assess the ill or injured person. Since the assessment occurs very soon after the injury, many of the classical signs and symptoms of trauma are subtle, even absent. A clear example is the discoloration of a contusion. While most emergency department personnel see the expected "black-and-bluish" color, the early arrival of the paramedic leaves no time for the injury site

■ **secondary assessment** part of the physical assessment process where detailed historical and physical findings are evaluated in order to determine the patient's medical or traumatic problem.

■ **inspection** the physical assessment skill of visually examining a patient.

■ **palpation** the physical assessment skill of examining a patient by touch.

■ **auscultation** the process of listening to sounds made by the internal organs; usually associated with the use of the stethoscope.

■ **percussion** the act of striking an object or area to elicit a sound or vibration.

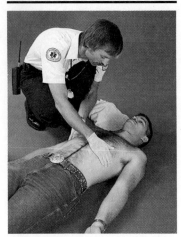

FIGURE 10-20 Palpation is an important examination technique. It is best accomplished with the pads of the fingers.

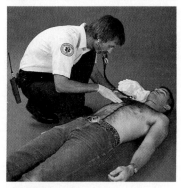

FIGURE 10-21 Auscultation is the process of listening to the body sounds, usually with a stethoscope. In prehospital care it is used primarily to evaluate the chest and to determine blood pressure.

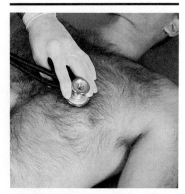

FIGURE 10-22 Hold the stethoscope diaphragm to the chest with gentle pressure.

to discolor. It is often only reddened (erythematous) at the time of the initial assessment. The paramedic must be exceptionally conscientious in evaluating the soft tissues in order to detect the early evolving injury site.

Palpation

Palpation should take place with the pads of the fingers, using the same pressure needed to feel for a pulse; gentle, not overbearing. Too much pressure will dull the examiner's perception and, in some cases, injure the patient. (See Figure 10-20.) In the case of abdominal palpation, it may be necessary to apply pressure gently by placing the fingers of the opposite hand over the sensing fingers. This method will increase the examiner's sensitivity to any masses, guarding, or other phenomenon developing within the abdomen. The paramedic must be careful to honestly sense with the fingers. Humans rely more on visual input than touch. The tendency is to "feel" with the eyes, rather than with the fingertips. Palpate for deformity, crepitus (a grating sensation), pulsing masses, and fluids. Sense for areas of warmth that might reflect injury before significant edema or discoloration has occurred. During palpation of a patient who is unresponsive or responsive only to pain, look to the face to determine response to touch. Many patients who are unable to speak respond to pain with facial expressions, or purposeful or purposeless motion.

Auscultation

Auscultation is the evaluation component that uses the stethoscope. (See Figure 10-21.) The instrument should be used sparingly in the field. When used properly, however, it provides invaluable information. A stethoscope is used primarily to determine blood pressure and assess breath sounds. The sounds heard are of very low amplitude and are difficult to discern in the field against the background noise that accompanies on-scene or in-transport assessment. Use of the stethoscope to auscultate the abdomen is of limited value in the field. The bowel sounds are difficult to appreciate, and proper assessment takes too much time, usually 4 to 5 minutes. Bowel sounds are a diagnostic evaluation best performed in the emergency department.

Heart sounds may also be evaluated through auscultation. Place the bell of the stethoscope over the heart valves at approximately the 3rd intercostal space, just left of the sternum. The bell is used to listen to the closing of the valves and to pick up any extraneous sounds of that process. The bell must be carefully placed over the heart. Too much pressure will cause the skin beneath it to stretch and act like the diaphragm. It will then transmit the higher-frequency sounds, not the low-frequency sounds of the valves closing. (See Figure 10-22.)

Warm the diaphragm of the stethoscope before applying it to the patient's chest or abdomen. A cold stethoscope can startle the patient, causing him or her to distrust further intervention. Apply the diaphragm of the stethoscope gently and explain to the patient what you're doing and why.

Percussion

Percussion is the evaluation of a surface and the tissue beneath by sending a vibration through it. It is accomplished by transmitting the thump of one index finger impacting against the knuckle of the other over the site. The resonance, or lack thereof, may tell whether the underlying region is filled with air, air under pressure, a fluid, or normal tissue. For example, the sound (or feel) of resonance may be hollow and vibrating, suggesting a tension pneumothorax. The dull response to percussion may indicate fluid or blood in the cavity. The results are most reliable when compared with the sounds produced on the uninjured or unaffected side. Percussion is a skill that requires regular practice. Infrequent use will limit its ability to discern various conditions. For this reason, percussion is not commonly used in the field. (See Figure 10-23.)

Head-to-Toe Evaluation

To keep the process of the secondary assessment uncomplicated and at reasonable length, the differential diagnoses and treatment modalities for traumatic and medical problems will be discussed in the chapters to follow. The order in which the physical assessment is performed is not important. What is important is that it be done completely. To that end, paramedics should identify a particular order and stick to it with each patient assessed. It may be easiest to evaluate head-to-toe, then assess the upper extremities. This is a simple approach that's easy to remember. It takes into consideration that more significant injury and life threat can occur with thigh and leg pathology than with arm and forearm.

Head.   For evaluation purposes, the head is divided into the cranium and the facial region. The cranium should be palpated with the fingers over its entire surface. (See Figure 10-24.) It should be swept from the occiput to the superior surface, as well as laterally. This should be accomplished without any significant displacement of the head forward to protect against spinal injury. Remember that in any patient with potential for spine injury the spine should be stabilized in the primary assessment and stabilization maintained throughout care.

Cranium.   The general contour of the cranium should be noted, as well as any deformities, such as depressions or protrusions. (See Figure 10-24.) The presence of any discoloration, unusual warmth, or lack of symmetry should be recorded. Blood can flow into the hair and go unnoticed if care is not taken during this assessment. Examine your gloved fingers periodically for blood or other body fluids. (See Figure 10-25.) Many of the overt signs of head pathology, such as "**Battle's Sign**" and **bilateral periorbital ecchymosis (Raccoon Eyes)**, are delayed because of late development of the associated discoloration. Battle's sign is an ecchymotic

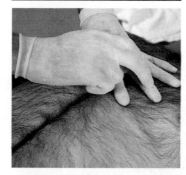

FIGURE 10-23   Percussion is the process of striking the body in order to evaluate the transmission of sounds and vibration. It is only used occasionally in prehospital care.

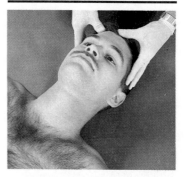

FIGURE 10-24   The first step in the head-to-toe examination is palpation of the head.

■ **Battle's sign** a black-and-blue discoloration over the mastoid process (just behind the ear), characteristic of a basilar skull fracture.

■ **bilateral periorbital ecchymosis** A black-and-blue discoloration of the area surrounding the eyes. It is normally associated with a basilar skull fracture.

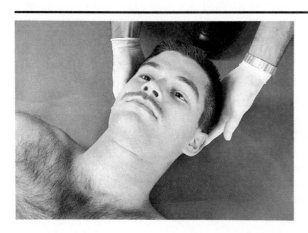

FIGURE 10-25   It is important to periodically inspect your fingers for the presence of blood. Wearing gloves, while necessary, can affect your sensation of touch and you may not notice the presence of anything on your hands.

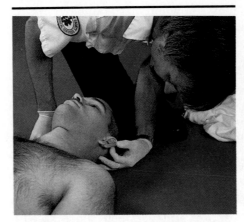

FIGURE 10-26 The ears should be externally inspected. The presence of blood or clear fluid draining from the ear should be documented.

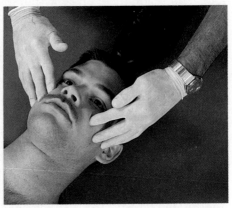

FIGURE 10-27 Gently palpate the bones of the face. Any crepitus, pain, or irregularity may indicate facial bone fracture.

■ **cerebrospinal fluid (CSF)** the clear, watery fluid that bathes the brain and spinal cord.

■ **crepitation** a grating or crackling sensation, felt or heard in such conditions as subcutaneous emphysema, or bone fracture.

(black-and-blue) discoloration over the mastoid process (the bony process just posterior to the ear). Raccoon eyes is a similar discoloration, surrounding and including the orbits (eye sockets). Either of these signs indicates possible basilar skull fracture. Their discovery in the early prehospital setting should direct you to consider the possibility of a previous injury.

Ears. The ears should be examined for soft-tissue injury and fluid drainage from the external auditory canal. Move your head to where you can visualize the external auditory canal with a flashlight. Blood coming from the canal may reflect a pressure injury or possible skull fracture. Clear fluid discharge may be secondary to fracture or infection. If blood and **cerebrospinal fluid** are mixed, and the fluid is allowed to drip on a sheet or pillow case, it will yield a characteristic halo or target sign (a darker red circle surrounded by a lighter one). (See Figure 10-26.)

Facial Region. The facial region is one of the more important areas of your assessment. Observation and palpation should begin the evaluation process, with pupillary exam and an in-depth assessment of the orifices to follow. Palpation is accomplished with the pads of the fingers over the entirety of the facial bones. The orbits are felt for stability, as should be the nasal bones and cartilage. Instability or asymmetry of these regions should lead to suspicion of facial fracture. Palpation of the upper jaw region may reveal deformity or instability, often due to maxillary fracture secondary to trauma. The mandible should demonstrate mobility, as evidenced by opening and closing the mouth, as well as some slight lateral movement. The motion should not elicit pain. **Crepitation,** limited motion, or mandibular fixation would indicate fracture or dislocation. (See Figure 10-27.)

Eyes. While it is not recommended that pressure be applied to the globes of the eye, palpation of the area may reveal softness. This condition may be associated with severe dehydration or possible diabetic hyperglycemia and ketoacidosis.

The pupils should be examined very closely. (See Figure 10-28.) They represent a window into the brain. They are controlled by some of the higher cranial nerves and their blood supply is closely related to that

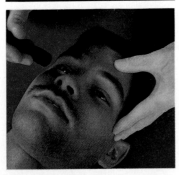

FIGURE 10-28 The pupils should be closely examined with a pen light.

of the brain itself. The rate at which the pupil of the eye reacts to light is a good indicator of cerebral perfusion. Under normal circumstances, the pupils will react briskly to changes in light intensity, constricting to increases in light and dilating to decreases. In intense indoor lighting or normal daylight, it may be appropriate to shade both eyes to check pupil reactivity, rather than to direct a flashlight beam into the pupil. Additionally, the pupils should respond consensually. That is, when the light intensity change is directed at one pupil, both pupils will respond to it. Abnormal pupillary responses may reflect intracranial pathology. A sluggish pupil reaction to light changes may be a reflection of central nervous system depression, due to hypoxia, **hypercarbia,** injury, or the effects of drugs. The extreme of this condition is dilated and non-reactive (fixed) pupils.

On the other hand, very small or pinpoint pupils suggest intoxication from the opiate derivatives (narcotics). While pupil inequality (called **anisocoria**) is present in a small percentage of the population, it may imply head injury or stroke. This is especially true if the reactivity of the larger pupil is less brisk than that of the constricted one. The sign may reflect pathology on either the same side or the opposite side of the brain.

Pupillary movement should be carefully evaluated within the secondary assessment. If the pupils fail to move together, or seem to be looking in different directions (**dysconjugate gaze**), this may be an indication of a pre-existing problem, muscle entrapment, or optic nerve damage. If the eyes move with the head as it's turned, instead of remaining fixed in the original direction (known as the **doll's eye response**), severe head injury may have occurred. Don't attempt this maneuver on any patient with suspected spine injury.

Finally, if the eyes are unable to follow your finger as you draw an imaginary "X" in front of them, there may be nerve damage or orbital fracture that may be impinging the extra-ocular muscles. (See Figure 10-29.) Examination will also reflect the evidence of direct eye trauma. While the eyes are well-protected by the orbits, eye trauma can produce serious, sight-threatening injury. Any signs of discoloration, bleeding, or impaled object or particles, and any laceration to the eye's surface should be protected and reported to the Emergency Department personnel.

Close examination of the eye should reveal the presence of contact lenses. (See Figure 10-30.) They may be left in place unless the uncon-

■ **hypercarbia** an increased level of carbon dioxide in the body.

■ **anisocoria** pupils of unequal size.

■ **dysconjugate gaze** failure of the eyes to rotate simultaneously in the same direction.

■ **doll's eye reflex** the eyes turning as the head is turned. An unnatural response, indicative of head injury.

✱ The testing for doll's eye response is not, typically, a prehospital procedure. It should never be used in the trauma patient.

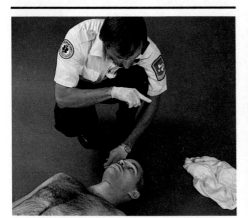

FIGURE 10-29 Briefly check extraocular eye movements by having the patient follow your finger as you draw an imaginary "X."

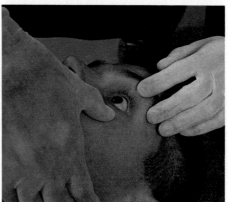

FIGURE 10-30 Inspect the cornea for the presence of a contact lens or obvious corneal lesion.

scious patient will be transported for more than 15 minutes. If there is a chance that toxic material has contaminated the eye, remove the lenses and irrigate the eye.

The evaluation of the eye may reveal many things. The surface of the normal eye should sparkle in the light. If the eye is dull or lacks its normal luster, a circulatory deficit should be suspected. If the sclera of the eye appears yellow, it may be the characteristic discoloration called icterus, caused by liver dysfunction.

Mouth. The mouth should be gently opened and examined for any signs of obstruction, potential obstruction, toxic inhalation, toxic ingestion, or trauma. (See Figure 10-31.) Should an unresponsive patient have loose false teeth, remove them. The examiner's fingers should be protected any time they enter the patient's mouth. It may be necessary to position the head to protect the airway. An endotracheal tube or an oral airway may have to be placed if the patient has no gag reflex. Any odor from the patient should be consciously evaluated. (See Figure 10-32.) The odor of alcohol is a common finding. It may mask other more significant odors, such as those of ketones from the diabetic, or the signs and symptoms of traumatic or acute medical disease. Any changes in the mental state of a patient who has been drinking should not be attributed to alcohol, unless all other causes have been ruled out (not likely in the field). Other problems may present with characteristic odors that should be kept in mind during the entire assessment process. Various poisonings may be determined by the smells they produce. Fecal odor emanating from the mouth may indicate lower-bowel obstruction; the smell of gastric contents may forewarn of emesis and possible aspiration.

Fluids in the oral cavity can provide clues to the underlying pathology. A coffee-grounds-like material can signal bleeding into the stomach, where the gastric contents begin to break down the blood. Fresh blood can reflect a recent hemorrhage within the upper gastrointestinal tract. Pink-tinged sputum may indicate congestive heart failure. A green or yellow phlegm may suggest respiratory infection. Vomitus may reflect gastrointestinal or brainstem problems, among many others. Because of the airway's importance, any indication of hazard or potential hazard should be cared for immediately.

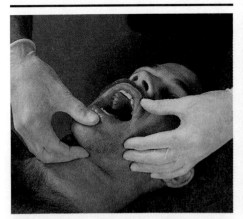

FIGURE 10-31 The mouth should be briefly inspected for any signs of obstruction, potential obstruction, or trauma.

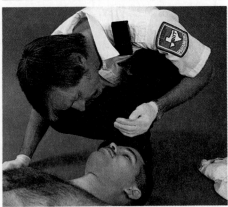

FIGURE 10-32 Any odors on the patient's breath should be noted and documented.

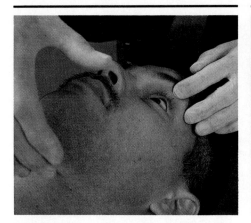

FIGURE 10-33 Quickly inspect the nose for any bleeding or for the presence of clear fluid drainage.

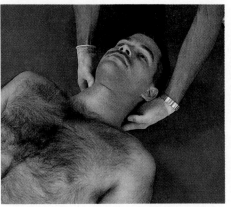

FIGURE 10-34 Re-examine the posterior aspect of the neck in much the same manner as in the primary survey. Note any tenderness, irregularity, or edema.

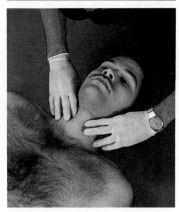

FIGURE 10-35 Examine the anterior aspect of the neck as well. Pay particular attention to tracheal deviation.

As another part of the airway, the **nares** are important areas to assess. They should be examined for flaring, a sign of airway distress. Pay special attention to infants less than 1 month old. They are obligatory nasal breathers, and need a clear and unobstructed nasal cavity for respiration. The presence of fluid may indicate internal trauma or infection. Blood and spinal fluid are signs of internal laceration, skull fracture, or both. Bleeding within the nasal cavity may be severe and very difficult to control. (See Figure 10-33.) It may also contribute to nausea and vomiting if the patient has swallowed much blood.

Neck. The neck has been examined carefully in the primary assessment, but should be reassessed with a focus on the less obvious pathology. The lateral surfaces should be palpated, as should the anterior and posterior ones. (See Figure 10-34.) Any apparent deformity, warmth, or discoloration should be noted and appraised further. Soft-tissue injury, edema, or laceration to the neck can be life-threatening. The arterial vessels located lateral to the trachea provide critical circulation to the brain. Penetrating injury to these large, high-pressure structures can result in massive blood loss. The venous vessels, which carry a high volume of blood, can allow the aspiration of air directly into the circulatory system. During inspiration, the neck veins may maintain intravascular pressures below that of atmospheric. If there is an open wound, air may be drawn in, resulting in massive air **emboli.** Any significant penetrating, soft-tissue injury in this area should be evaluated for bleeding and for the possibility of air emboli. (See Figure 10-35.)

Examine the jugular veins for distention. (See Figure 10-36.) In the supine, normotensive patient, they should be slightly distended. However, as the body is brought to a 45-degree angle, they should empty. Distention beyond 45 degrees is indicative of pathology: cardiac tamponade, tension pneumothorax, right heart failure, or cor pulmonale (right heart failure secondary to increased pulmonary vascular resistance). (See Figure 10-37.) If the veins are not distended in the supine position, hypovolemia is the probable cause.

The anterior neck should be palpated for tracheal location and movement. The trachea should be midline and stationary during breathing ef-

■ **nares** the openings of the nose that lead into the nasal cavity.

■ **emboli** a clot or other particle brought by the blood from another vessel, and forced into a smaller one.

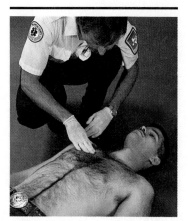

FIGURE 10-36 The jugular veins should be slightly distended when the patient is in the supine position.

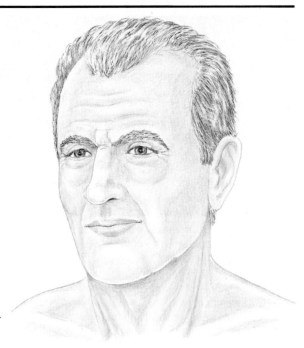

FIGURE 10-37 Jugular venous distention is often a sign of congestive heart failure or chronic obstructive pulmonary disease.

■ **contralateral** relating to the opposite side of the body

■ **ipsilateral** on, or referring to, the same side.

■ **subcutaneous emphysema** the presence of air within the subcutaneous tissues, often associated with pneumothorax.

forts. If it's displaced to one side, it may indicate a tension pneumothorax on the **contralateral** (opposite) side. If it tugs or moves toward one side with each inspiration, there might be an airway obstruction on that side (**ipsilateral**). The neck may also display **subcutaneous emphysema,** which may cause crepitation as the air moves about under your palpation. This may be due to a developing tension pneumothorax or a tracheal tear. If the patient coughs or exhales forcibly while a tracheal tear exists, the air will be forced into the neck tissue, enlarging the region.

Chest. The chest exam is best performed with the chest completely exposed. Care should be taken to protect the patient from embarrassment and the environment. The shoulders must be visualized and palpated for symmetry. (See Figure 10-38.) Asymmetry or deformity suggests fracture of one of the bones composing the joint, a dislocation or soft-tissue damage with resultant edema. The clavicles should be palpated over their entire length, bilaterally. (See Figure 10-39.) They remain the most fre-

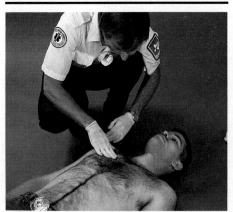

FIGURE 10-38 Visually inspect the chest for asymmetry.

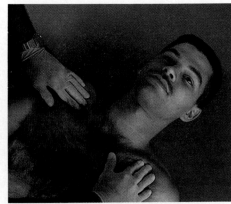

FIGURE 10-39 Palpate the clavicles.

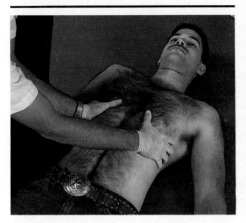

FIGURE 10-40 Palpate the chest noting AP diameter, symmetry, and air exchange.

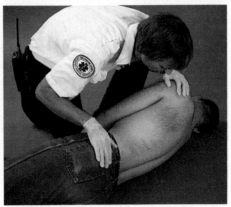

FIGURE 10-41 Palpate the posterior aspect of the chest. This maneuver should be deferred if a cervical spine injury is suspected.

quently fractured bones in the human body. Although their fracture is not of major significance, the tissue beneath them may be injured. The clavicles are located directly over the subclavian artery and the superior-most aspect of the lung. Fracture and displacement may disrupt the artery or lung tissue, leading to hemothorax, pneumothorax, or both. The region just above the clavicles (supraclavicular space), the intercostal spaces, as well as the suprasternal notch, may present with retraction during inspiration. This is a sign of partial or complete airway obstruction. It occurs when the atmospheric pressure significantly exceeds that of inspiration. It is a serious sign that demands clearing of the airway: pharmacologically, as in asthma; physically, as in removing an airway obstruction with the laryngoscope and **Magill forceps;** or mechanically, with an endotracheal tube.

The surface of the thorax is examined for bilateral excursion with respiration. This should be accomplished by placing one hand on each of the lower halves of the thorax, just below the nipple line or breast area. (See Figure 10-40.) Normal respiration should cause the hands to move very slightly in and out with each breath. Each breath should be smooth and regular, with symmetrical motion. Determine the general shape to the chest cavity. Is the anterior-posterior dimension normal, or is the chest large and barreled (a condition suggestive of chronic, obstructive lung disease)? Are there any deformities that appear congenital or traumatic? Palpate and observe the entirety of the thoracic surface. Are there any signs of trauma, discoloration, or edema? Once again, the classical soft-tissue injury signs may not be present in the field. Look for the erythema caused by impact to the ribs. There may be an outline of discoloration silhouetting the ribs and sternum. Visually inspect for any penetrating trauma. If found, assess for signs of air exchange (open pneumothorax) and a possible exit wound. Compress the lateral aspects of the chest medially. They should pose a moderate resistance, yet elicit no tenderness. The lateral and anterior surface of the chest should be palpated. In the case of a female, your palpation should work around the breast, not directly over it. You can assess the entirety of the breast during the chest evaluation, without assessing it as one unit. This will reduce the risk of the patient taking offense at your action. Finally, the posterior surface of the thorax should be evaluated. (See Figure 10-41.) Once spine injury is ruled out, the spine is stabilized, or, during a log roll or other movement

■ **Magill forceps** instrument used in airway management for reaching into the oropharynx to manipulate a foreign body, endotracheal tube, or similar item.

✽ If a penetrating chest wound is found, suspect and search for an exit wound.

technique, the region should be completely palpated. Gentle evaluation should reveal any deformity, warmth, fluid loss, or evidence of soft-tissue injury. If, during palpation of the chest, you notice a crackling sensation (much like crushing Rice Krispies), suspect tension pneumothorax. This sensation is called subcutaneous emphysema, which arises from an increase in intrathoracic pressure that causes air in the **pleural** space to be forced into the soft tissues. The subcutaneous air will normally flow from the upper chest to the neck and head. In some cases, the patient's facial features will change before your eyes.

The chest should be auscultated at the bases (the lower border of the rib cage), at the apices (just below the clavicles at their midpoint), and along the mid-axillary line (in the armpit at about the nipple line). (See Figures 10-42 and 10-43.) The respiratory sounds should be evaluated anteriorly and then posteriorly. The normal patient should present with normal breath sounds in all regions. Normal breath sounds are less distinct than abnormal sounds. The sounds heard at the locations mentioned above are called **vesicular.** Soft and low-pitched, they are often described as sighing in quality. You should notice that inspiratory sounds last longer then expiratory sounds. If you assess the lung sounds closer to the sternum, you will hear the sounds of bronchial and tracheal passageways. Louder and higher-pitched, these sounds display almost equal inspiratory and expiratory phases.

Abnormal breath sounds on auscultation include rales, rhonchi, wheezes, and stridor. **Rales** are fine crackling sounds, similar to the sound of hair being rolled between your fingers. They indicate fluid in the lungs and minor alveolar obstruction. **Rhonchi** are coarser sounds that suggest more significant fluid or mucous accumulation. **Wheezes** reflect airway narrowing, and are generally associated with bronchial constriction and asthma. They will present with a prolonged higher-pitched sound on expiration. The sound of stridor needs no stethoscope to be audible. It is high-pitched and occurs because of obstruction at the larynx from local swelling or spasm of the vocal folds (**laryngospasm**). Breath sounds are truly hard to determine unless you listen to them frequently. To keep an appreciation of the technique and the quality of the sounds listened for, periodically auscultate your own breath sounds and those of

■ **pleura** a membrane covering the lungs and the interior of the thoracic cage.

■ **vesicular** breath sound heard in the normal lung.

■ **rales** abnormal breath sound due to the presence of fluid in the smaller airways.

■ **rhonchi** abnormal breath sound due to the presence of fluid or mucous in the larger airways.

■ **laryngospasm** a spasm of the vocal folds that may occlude the airway. It is a protective mechanism to prevent the aspiration of foreign bodies into the airway.

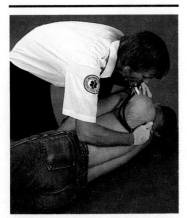

FIGURE 10-42 Auscultate the posterior chest, beginning at the bases.

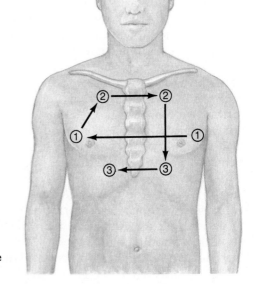

FIGURE 10-43 Method for auscultating the anterior chest.

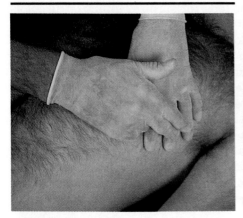

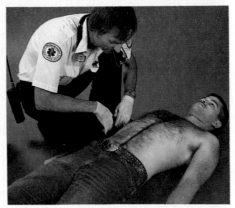

FIGURE 10-44 Percussion of the chest can help determine the presence of pneumothorax or hemothorax.

FIGURE 10-45 The examination of the abdomen should begin with inspection. Note any swelling, discoloration, or wounds.

fellow co-workers at the station. In the field, listening to your own lung sounds will give you a benchmark for evaluating those of your patient.

Auscultation can tell much beyond the sounds of respiration. If the respiratory sounds are not bilaterally equal, they may indicate a pneumothorax. If the respiratory or heart sounds are distant and muffled, the pathology may be hemothorax. If only the heart sounds are diminished, the patient may have a pericardial tamponade. (Be advised that these differentiations are impossible to make without several signs and symptoms that support a specific pathology.)

Percussion can provide evidence regarding chest pathology. (See Figure 10-44.) If the region is hyperresonant, the thorax may contain air under pressure (tension pneumothorax). If the region is dull to percussion, it may be filled with the blood of a hemothorax or other fluid (pleural **effusion**). Be sure to compare the sounds left-to-right and front-to-back to confirm your evaluation.

Examine the patient's respiratory function. Reassess the volume of air moved, as was done in the primary assessment. Determine the exact rate of respiration over at least 30 seconds. A good technique is to count both the inspirations and expirations over the 30 seconds. The result will give you the number of breaths per minute. Examine the respiratory pattern for pathology. A rapid deep pattern can be due to head injury (central neurogenic hyperventilation); metabolic problem, as in diabetic coma (**Kussmaul respirations**); extreme exertion; or hyperventilation syndrome. The respiratory pattern known as **Cheyne-Stokes** is a repeated series of increasing, then decreasing, breath volume with periods of apnea in-between. Another pattern, **Biot's respirations,** consists of agonal, gasping, breaths, irregular in rate and depth. Biot's and Cheyne-Stokes respirations are related to increasing intracranial pressure or severe brain-stem injury or both.

Abdomen. The abdomen should be inspected and, if indicated, gently palpated for signs or symptoms of disease or trauma. Observe for any overt motion or pulsation. (See Figure 10-45.) The abdomen in the thin supine patient will pulsate with the pulsing of the abdominal aorta. Aneurysm should be suspected if this pulsation is exaggerated or localized, especially if it is accompanied with "tearing" pain. Exaggerated abdominal-wall motion to assist respiration may be caused by spinal injury, or may reflect airway obstruction or failure of the muscles of respiration. The ex-

■ **effusion** the escape of fluid, normally from the vascular space, into a cavity (e.g., pleural effusion).

■ **Kussmaul respirations** a very deep gasping respiratory pattern, found in diabetic coma.

■ **Cheyne-Stokes respirations** breathing pattern characterized by progressive increase in the rate and volume of respirations that later gradually subsides. Usually associated with a disturbance in the respiratory center of the brain.

■ **Biot's respirations** breathing pattern characterized by irregular periods of apnea and hyperpnea associated with increased intracranial pressure.

amination of the abdomen should also look for signs of injury or discoloration, especially any abrasions, contusions, open wounds, or erythema. Two characteristic ecchymotic discolorations of the abdomen are **Cullen's Sign,** around the **umbilicus** (navel), and **Grey Turner's Sign,** along the flanks. Both are secondary to internal bleeding, of traumatic or acute medical origin. They also develop late and may point to an earlier injury.

Before palpation, you must determine whether any pain present is generalized, regional, or limited to a specific point. Be certain to evaluate the pain carefully in the field setting. As the pathology progresses (during your care and transport), the pain may become more general, while guarding and increased pain may prevent accurate palpation. This may mask the true location of the problem from the hospital staff and slow the diagnostic process unless you perform a comprehensive and accurate assessment in the field.

The four quadrants (LUQ, RUQ, LLQ & RLQ) of the abdomen should be evaluated for tenderness and **rebound tenderness.** Palpation should occur gently, assessing last any quadrant with pain. (See Figure 10-46.) To elicit rebound tenderness, the paramedic should release quickly the gentle pressure of palpation. Any pain that occurs with this release is probably related to inflammation of the **peritoneum** (the tissue that covers most of the abdominal organs and the interior of the abdominal cavity). Gentle palpation should not elicit any muscle spasm or contraction. Such a response is termed guarding and is reflective of disease. Any masses, specifically painful areas, or the location of guarding should be recorded in your documentation. If the abdomen appears to be distended or feels spongy during palpation, ascites should be suspected. **Ascites** is an accumulation of fluid within the abdominal cavity, caused by backed-up pressure in the systemic circulation (right heart failure) or in the **portal system** (cirrhosis of the liver).

Palpate the flank (lateral) region of the abdomen, while looking for the signs of trauma: deformity, swelling, laceration, or discoloration. Continue the palpation underneath the small of the back from each side and to the vertebral column. (See Figure 10-47.) This area may present with dependent edema, a fluid buildup in the lower parts of the body (the legs and lower back), due to chronic circulatory backup. The edema in the lumbar region is called **presacral** (above the sacrum) **edema.** It is reflective of a systemic problem, possibly due to heart failure. This sign is more commonly seen in the patient who is recumbent for prolonged periods.

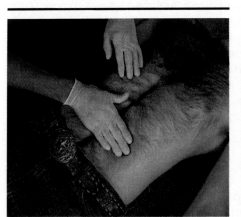

FIGURE 10-46 Palpation of the abdomen in the prehospital phase should be limited. Leave the quadrant where pain exists until the end.

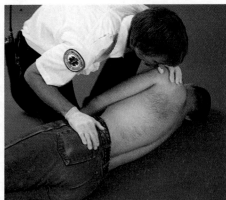

FIGURE 10-47 Be sure to inspect the back of the abdomen if not already accomplished during the chest exam. This should not be attempted if a cervical spine injury is suspected.

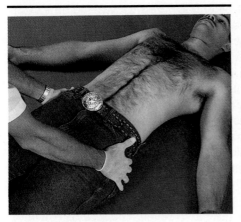

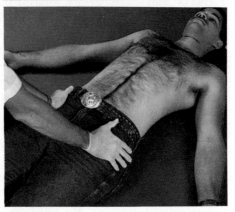

FIGURE 10-48 Assess the integrity of the pelvis by pressing medially on the pelvic ring.

FIGURE 10-49 Compress the pelvis posteriorly to complete the examination of the pelvis.

Because of how long it takes to auscultate, and the unreliability of what is heard, the assessment of bowel sounds is not a field procedure.

Pelvis. The bony pelvis is an extremely strong structure. Only very powerful forces can fracture it (except in the elderly or those with degenerative bone disease). With pelvic fracture, there is a potential for vascular injury. The vessels running through the pelvis are rather large and are near the bones. Because of this, these injuries commonly have associated severe internal bleeding.

Assessment of the pelvis must be comprehensive. The pelvic ring is evaluated for fracture by applying pressure to the iliac crests (the bony prominences, anterior and lateral, that support the belt). (See Figures 10-48 and 10-49.) The pressure is best directed medially, then posteriorly. Posterior pressure should also be applied to the symphysis pubis, the bone just above the genitalia. Be careful not to trap the genitalia of the male, nor rock the pelvis in either sex. The pressure applied in any of these areas may elicit pain, crepitation, or instability. If it does, suspect pelvic fracture and be prepared to care for what may be severe hypovolemic shock.

Genitalia. The genital region is another area that needs special attention during the assessment. Male and female patients may present with different mechanisms of injury, signs, and symptoms. The male genitalia, which are external and extremely vascular, can be subjected to traumatic injury and extreme blood loss. This can be overlooked in the assessment because clothing may contain the hemorrhage (especially the denim of blue jeans). Evaluation of the male genitalia can also reveal the presence of injury to the spinal cord. **Priapism,** a painful erection of the penis, is caused by unopposed parasympathetic stimulation, which comes with spinal cord interruption or certain types of brain problems. Such a finding should be followed by complete spinal immobilization and assessment.

The female genitalia, on the other hand, are internal and relatively well-protected from all but penetrating injury. They are moderately vascular, but not often injured in trauma because of their location. Traumatic injury can occur in sexual abuse and rape. If either is suspected, attempt to have the patient assessed and treated by a member of the same sex. This may relieve any hostilities and anxiety that could be directed toward a caregiver of the opposite gender. In cases of possible sexual

■ **priapism** a painful, prolonged erection of the male penis, due to spinal injury or disease process. (It may occur in sickle cell anemia).

✱ In cases of rape or sexual assault, have the patient treated by a care giver of the same gender, if possible.

abuse or rape, the patient should not be encouraged to bathe. The examination should be limited to what is essential to the patient's stabilization. Other assessment and care may destroy evidence needed to prosecute, and might increase the psychological trauma.

In the acute medical (gynecological) or obstetrical emergency, there may be discharge from the vaginal canal. Blood, amniotic fluid, or some other fluid may be involved. An estimation of the quantity and type of discharge should be made. It may be helpful for the woman to approximate the volume by indicating the number of pads or tampons needed to absorb the discharge. Since the etiology of this problem is internal and inaccessible, PASG may be the only method of hemorrhage control available. If the patient even begins to show the signs of developing shock, transport immediately.

Evaluation of the genital region may also reveal the loss of bowel or bladder control (incontinence). The reasons for this problem should be sought. Causes include deep coma, stroke, or spinal injury. The occurrence of either of these signs is indicative of deep central nervous system depression or interruption. The buttocks should be palpated to rule out hemorrhage, contusion, or other injury. Though predominantly soft tissue, this area is a large mass. It can account for considerable internal blood loss, often with no obvious signs.

Lower Extremities.   The lower extremities are the thigh, leg, and foot. In examining this area, the surfaces should be palpated anteriorly, posteriorly, laterally, and medially over the entire length of the extremity. (See Figure 10-50.) Examination is directed at evaluating for tenderness, crepitation, or deformity. Any abnormal motion, such as joint-like characteristics where a joint shouldn't exist, or resistance to normal motion, should be thoroughly evaluated. Evaluation of the distal pulse will ensure that no circulatory compromise has occurred. The pulse can be taken using either the dorsalis pedis or medial malleolar (posterior tibial) pulse. The dorsalis pedis pulse is located on the arch of the foot, along the anterior surface about 1/3 the distance from the medial to the lateral side. (See Figure 10-51.) This pulse is normally absent in about 10% of the population. The posterior tibial pulse can be felt medially, just posterior and inferior to the inside protrusion of the ankle (medial malleolus). The posterior tibial pulse may be more practical to use in the field because landmarks make it easier and faster to find. If no pulse can be found, the ade-

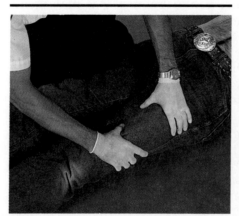

FIGURE 10-50   Palpate the thigh noting any deformity, swelling, or crepitus.

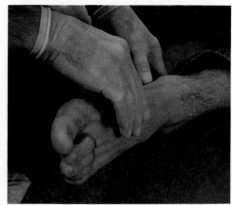

FIGURE 10-51   Palpate the dorsalis pedis pulse on each foot.

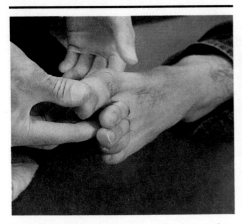

FIGURE 10-52 Briefly assess the status of sensation in the leg and foot.

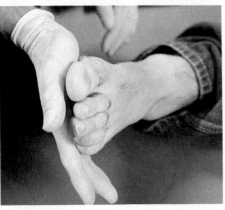

FIGURE 10-53 Test motor function, if a fracture is not suspected, by asking the patient to press his foot against your hand.

quacy of perfusion can be determined by capillary refill or by assessing the temperature, color, and moisture of the skin of the foot. If the pulse is absent, the limb is cool, capillary refill is slow or does not occur, and the skin is ashen or cyanotic, presume there is circulatory compromise to the distal limb.

Evaluation of the lower aspect of the extremity may reveal edema. If the extremity is swollen, the overlying skin may be depressed with the examiner's finger. Edema is present if the depression remains following removal of the finger. This phenomenon is called pitting edema, a sign of severe and chronic systemic fluid retention.

The extremity should also be evaluated for motor and sensory function. (See Figures 10-52, 10-53.) Ask the patient to tell you when he or she feels a firm (but gentle) touch with the blunted end of a bandage scissors or similar device. It is not recommended to ask "Do you feel this?" If the answer is "no," a patient will know there's a deficit and become anxious about it. You should also ask the patient to push firmly against your hand with his or her foot, provided the extremity has been assessed as uninjured. Repeat the procedure on the opposite side and compare the results. If the strength appears unequal, retry the procedure, switching hands. If the difference still remains, suspect nervous impairment or injury.

Upper Extremities. The assessment of the upper extremities is similar to that of the lower extremities. The only exceptions are the use of the radial pulse and asking the patient to squeeze your first and second finger, rather than push your hand. (See Figures 10-54, 10-55.) As with the lower extremities, compare the strength and pulse from one side to the other. You might also examine the fingers for clubbing. **Clubbing** is a widening of the distal portion of the finger, resulting from central cyanosis, a chronic hypoxic condition caused by cardiovascular or respiratory disease. The neck, ankle, wrist, and the wallet should be checked for medic alert identification. An orange, red, or blue star of life or other medical symbol will help identify these materials. They usually contain pertinent information about the patient's medical history, allergies, or special treatment considerations. Search for this information and use it to guide your care.

■ **clubbing** the enlargement of the distal fingers and toes, often due to chronic respiratory or cardiovascular disease.

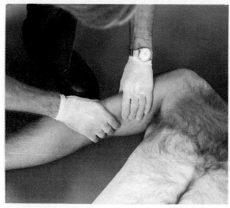

FIGURE 10-54 Palpate the upper extremity.

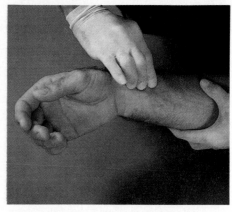

FIGURE 10-55 Palpate the radial pulse.

Neurological Assessment. CNS dysfunction can be evaluated objectively by looking at the patient's orientation and response to physical stimuli.

The level of orientation should be judged through patient questioning. As a patient moves away from a state of complete alertness, orientation to the environment diminishes in a specific order. Initially, the patient will be completely conscious and oriented to person, place, and time. As the level of consciousness drops, the first noticeable loss is orientation to time. The patient will often be unable to identify the day of the week, day of the month, year, and time of day. At the scene of a medical emergency, it is common for patients and bystanders to complain of long response times when arrival actually happens within minutes of the call. This finding is normally associated with excitement or stress. It is not very significant to the patient's overall condition. As the level of consciousness continues to slip, patients begin to lose orientation to place. They will not know where they are, and will not be able to recognize familiar surroundings, such as the interior of an ambulance. While this can be caused by stress and excitement, it may reflect a deeper decline in cerebral function. (See Figure 10-56.)

On the same plateau of orientation is the loss of recollection of what happened. The patient is unaware of how he or she was injured, and of the events leading up to the incident. This is termed orientation to the event. The next step in the downward progression of consciousness is the loss of orientation to person. The patient may fail to recognize close

✱ A patient's orientation will diminish in a specific order from orientation to time, to place (or event), to persons, and to one's own person, as he or she moves from alert and oriented to unresponsive.

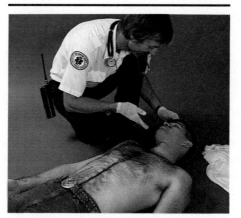

FIGURE 10-56 Determine the patient's mental status.

friends or relatives. He or she may also be unable to determine or remember who you are, even though you are in uniform and have introduced yourself several times. The last of the orientations to be lost is that of one's own person. The patient, while still responsive to verbal commands, will not be aware of his or her own name. He or she may recognize it once said, but will not be able to remember without hearing it. As the patient moves toward unconsciousness and coma, he or she can be further evaluated objectively by observing the physical responses to stimuli. Patients may respond by moving their extremities or opening their eyes, when the paramedic shouts the patient's name or issues a loud verbal command (verbal **stimuli**). They may speak, but the communication is incoherent, garbled, or unintelligible.

As the level of consciousness continues to diminish, the patient will no longer respond to verbal stimuli, but may respond to painful stimulation. A good location to elicit this pain is the fleshy region between the thumb and first finger (of an uninjured extremity). Watch the motion carefully. If the patient responds by moving away from the pain or by brushing your hand away, the response is called purposeful. If the hand and forearm move, but not effectively, the response is called purposeless. The patient who is completely unconscious and unresponsive will fail to move to any stimuli. This is identified as unresponsive and is reflective of deep coma. With these two scales, a continuum can be established from complete consciousness to deep and profound coma. A patient will progress from the orientations of time, place, person, and own person, to the levels of response—purposeful, purposeless, and unresponsive.

The results of an evaluation can be objectively compared to repeated serial evaluation. Any changes in state of consciousness will be apparent.

Glasgow Coma Scale. A system for evaluation of the neurologically disabled patient is the Glasgow Coma Scale. (See Figure 10-18.) It consists of three areas of assessment: eye-opening, motor response, and verbal response. The scale awards points for the best patient response achieved. The resulting value can give an indication of the patient's Central Nervous System deficit. A score of 15 is the maximum, and is the most common finding. A score of 9 or above is indicative of consciousness; anything below 7 is coma. Note that the lowest score obtainable is 3. Any system or approach used in the assessment of consciousness should be repeated serially.

The initial level is determined during the primary assessment. It should be re-evaluated every few minutes thereafter. The re-evaluation will identify any deterioration or improvement. In addition to the failure of the patient to move to stimuli, look for the general muscle tone. Even patients in coma will display some muscle tone. If the tone seems absent (flaccid), it may indicate severe central nervous system injury or cord damage. If the flaccidity is unequal, it may suggest a head injury or stroke and hemiplegia.

The patient, in cases of severe brain injury, may respond with either decorticate or decerebrate posturing. Decerebrate posturing is present when the arms and legs are extended with the back bowed under extreme muscle contracture. Decorticate posturing differs only in that the upper extremities are flexed rather than extended. Either posturing may be present continuously, or may occur with painful stimuli. An attempt should be made to determine if the patient has lost consciousness or orientation at any time since the accident. If unconsciousness has occurred, the index of suspicion toward serious internal head injury should be increased. The patient with this history should be watched very carefully for any change

■ **stimulus (pl. stimuli)** any factor or input into the sensory system that causes an action or response.

in his or her level of consciousness. The history should be communicated to the emergency department personnel. A change in the level of consciousness or any other physical indication of possible neurologic dysfunction demands immediate transport.

Summary of Head-to-Toe Assessment. As the head-to-toe assessment is completed, the results should be carefully and completely recorded. Analysis should determine if the signs support one problem or several problems occurring together. Any unusual or questionable findings must be reassessed to ensure validity and accuracy. Summarize the findings of the head-to-toe assessment and identify the apparent injuries. Place them in priority order, from the greatest to the least severity. Keep these findings in mind as you move to the assessment of the vital signs and patient history.

Vital Signs

There are four basic vital signs in medicine: pulse, blood pressure, respiration, and temperature. The first three are of prime importance in prehospital care, while the last, temperature, may be of limited use. Respiration was evaluated early in the primary assessment and has already been discussed in detail. Blood pressure and pulse, however, are important diagnostic signs that should be taken periodically during patient care.

Blood Pressure

Blood pressure determination is a basic but important skill to the paramedic. (See Figure 10-57.) It can give an indication of the state of the circulatory system and the effects of its compensatory mechanisms. Its greatest shortfall is that blood pressure drops late in the progression of shock, too late to be of much value in preventing shock. (See Chapter 12.) In shock, the blood pressure is well-maintained as the body becomes hypovolemic. The vasculature constricts, the cardiac output increases, and the circulation shunts to just those organs and systems that require continuous perfusion. The result is a blood pressure that remains normal until the compensatory mechanisms give way. At that point, the patient's blood pressure drops, and he or she moves to uncompensated shock, then very quickly into irreversible shock, then death.

However, blood pressure can be of significant value in the evaluation of other pathologic conditions. Head injury, stress, hypertensive crisis, and heat stroke are common causes of acute elevation of the blood pres-

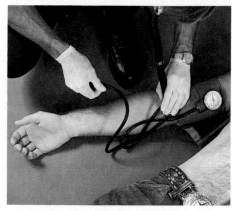

FIGURE 10-57 Following the head-to-toe examination, the vital signs should be obtained. The blood pressure should be recorded using a sphygmomanometer and stethoscope.

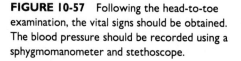

sure. Chronic **hypertension** may also be a contributing factor to cerebrovascular and cardiovascular emergencies. The ideal adult blood pressure, regardless of age, is 120 mm Hg systolic. Females are expected to have a slightly lower pressure, at least until menopause. However, a significant proportion of the female population has hypertension. It is necessary to recognize that a blood pressure of 120 mm/Hg in one patient may reflect hypotension, while in another, it may indicate hypertension.

Blood pressure must be used in concert with several factors to determine the overall state of the cardiovascular system and circulation. Blood pressure determination can be a difficult task in the field. The sounds normally produced by the arterial blood against the wall of the artery and the stethoscope can be difficult to distinguish, especially with extraneous noise at the scene. A helpful technique is to raise the patient's extremity (presuming it's uninjured), wait for a moment, then inflate the cuff rapidly. Bring the arm down to the normal position, and have the patient flex and extend the fingers a few times. Let the cuff down slowly, 3 mm to 4 mm of mercury per second, while you auscultate. The amplitude of the sound should increase markedly, making the values easier to hear.

Even under the best of circumstances, blood pressure may be an inaccurate measure. Reasons include the fact that the sphygmomanometer is only accurate to the closest even number. In addition, there is a large variation in pressure readings between cuffs, and hearing sensitivity differs between care providers. These factors make the value a rough estimate. Add the excitement, noise, and distraction of the field environment, and you see why blood pressure values are generally unreliable when considered alone. If the blood pressure is too difficult to hear, consider taking it by palpation. (Note that a blood pressure taken by palpation is about 10 mm Hg lower than the actual systolic pressure and no diastolic value will be found.) If it cannot be determined by either palpation or auscultation, report that you were unable to obtain a pressure. Some circumstances that are common in the field make it nearly impossible to determine blood pressure.

A technique that is becoming more prevalent in the field for determining blood pressure is the ultrasonic doppler. (See Figure 10-58). It is a device that uses high frequency sound waves to pick up the movement of blood through an artery. The device is able to pick up arterial pulses that are not otherwise audible. It is helpful in the evaluation of both pulse rate and blood pressure. However, only a systolic value can be determined. The doppler is an electronic stethoscope, which is placed over the artery. A small amount of conductive gel is used to help conduct the sound waves. The volume is adjusted until the "whooshing" of the artery is heard. Then the pulse is timed or the blood pressure is taken.

■ **hypertension** an arterial blood pressure that is elevated above normal. It may be either chronic or acute.

✱ The blood pressure must be used in concert with several factors to assess the overall state of the cardiovascular system and circulation.

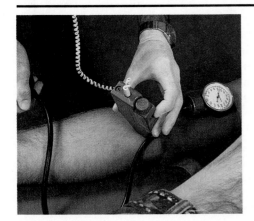

FIGURE 10-58 If the blood pressure is difficult to hear a doppler stethoscope may be employed.

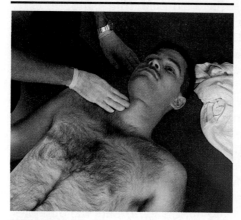

FIGURE 10-59 The pulse rate and character should be recorded.

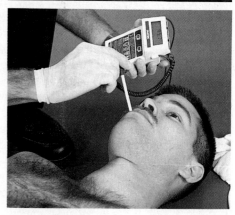

FIGURE 10-60 If indicated, the patient's temperature should be determined.

As you evaluate the blood pressure, also look to the difference between the systolic and diastolic readings. This value, called the pulse pressure, reflects the effectiveness of the cardiac output against the flexibility of the arterial system. The wider the pulse pressure, to a point, the better the state of the circulatory system. A narrow pulse pressure may indicate pericardial tamponade or tension pneumothorax, or may be an early finding in shock.

Pulse

The pulse is a valuable tool in the assessment of the patient's circulatory function. (See Figure 10-59.) It will begin the compensatory response to hypovolemia and may be the first indication that something is going wrong. A rise of more than 20 beats per minute when the patient moves from supine to a seated position suggests significant blood loss, generally more than 500 ml. As the hypovolemia becomes more significant, the pulse will become tachycardic in any position and the strength of the pulse will diminish. The pulse may support the diagnosis of conditions other than shock. A slow and bounding pulse may reflect head injury or heat stroke. A rapid and strong pulse may indicate excitement or other form of **sympathetic stimulation.** As with any tool in the evaluation of a patient, the pulse should be taken periodically to determine any trends in patient condition.

Temperature

The body works hard at maintaining a temperature of 37 degrees Centigrade (98.6 degrees Fahrenheit). This temperature reflects a balance between heat production and heat loss through the skin and respiratory system. Any variance, even a slight one, can mean that significant events are going on within the body. Temperature is taken to approximate the internal or core environment. In emergency medical service it is normally taken orally or occassionally, rectally. The battery-operated thermometer is preferred to glass because the danger of breakage is reduced and the speed and accuracy of the device is better. (See Figure 10-60.) An increase in body temperature indicates either the effects of environmental extremes or the body's desire to make the internal environment inhospitable to invading pathogens. Fever will present with a history of illness and

■ **sympathetic stimulation** a stimulous that triggers the sympathetic nervous system, increasing heart rate and blood pressure, as well as other actions of the sympathetic nervous system.

a high skin and internal temperature. The skin will be relatively dry until the fever breaks and the body's cooling mechanisms begin to take effect. In environmental extremes, the body will utilize its cooling mechanisms to maintain core temperature. The body's temperature will only rise when these mechanisms are no longer effective, as in extreme heat and humidity, or in cases like heat stroke, where the CNS control of the cooling mechanisms fail. As the body temperature rises, it will begin to threaten body processes and specifically the brain. A temperature of up to 102°F will increase metabolism markedly. As it rises above 103°F, the neurons begin to denature, and, much above 105°F, the brain cells will begin to die and the patient may have seizures. Extremes of cold will also affect body temperature. When peripheral vasoconstriction and shivering mechanisms can no longer reduce heat loss, the core temperature drops. At a body temperature of 34°C (93°F) the normal body warming mechanisms begin to fail. As the core temperature drops below 31°C (90°F), the heart sounds diminish and cardiac irritability increases. If the body temperature drops much below 22°C (70°F), the patient will present with a death-like appearance and, possibly, irreversible asystole. Most thermometers will not record below 96 degrees Fahrenheit and will not be of assistance in evaluating the hypothermic patient.

Determine the overall patient condition, which is suggested by the results of the vital-sign assessment. Compare it with the general patient condition that you would suspect from the injuries found during the head-to-toe evaluation. If the vital signs suggest a more serious problem than already found, look for the cause. If the apparent injuries should account for poorer vital signs, then consider re-evaluation of the vital signs. In either case, always look for the worst and treat in anticipation of it. Vital signs should be taken serially. In the patient who is suspected of serious pathology, the evaluation should be repeated every few minutes. If the patient appears stable, taking vital signs every ten or fifteen minutes will be acceptable. Compare the findings to ensure that the patient's condition is not deteriorating.

✱ To determine the patient's overall condition, compare the results of the mechanism of injury analysis, physical assessment, and the vital sign assessment.

Other Modalities

Cardiac Monitoring.   Cardiac monitoring should be an element of trauma and medical patient assessment. (See Figure 10-61.) While the analysis of an ECG is normally associated with cardiac problems, the skill is also of great value in assessing both the trauma and general medical patient. In addition to cardiogenic problems, head injury, chest trauma, stroke, drugs, and respiratory and metabolic problems can cause dysrhythmias.

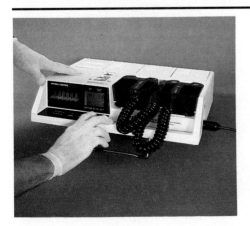

FIGURE 10-61   Cardiac monitoring should be routinely employed in prehospital care.

The elements of this portion of the assessment will be discussed in detail in Chapter 21.

■ **pulse oximetry** assessment modality that measures the oxygen saturation level of the blood through a noninvasive sensor placed on a finger or ear lobe.

Pulse Oximetry. If available, **pulse oximetry** should be used with all patients. (See Figure 10-62.) The pulse oximeter is a quick and accurate tool that can objectively determine the oxygenation status of the patient during the primary survey. The pulse oximeter provides immediate continuous evaluation of the delivery of oxygen to the body tissues. It quantifies the effect of interventions, including oxygen therapy, medication, suctioning, and ventilatory assistance. The pulse oximeter functions by measuring the transmission of red and infrared light through an arterial bed, such as those present in a finger, toe, or earlobe. The reliability and validity of the pulse oximeter is well-documented, and the device is widely used in a variety of critical care settings.

The pulse oximeter should give a reading of 96% to 99% oxygen saturation in the patient who has effective respiration. Should respiration be compromised, even slightly, oxygen saturation, as displayed on the digital display of the pulse oximeter, will fall. Any patient whose saturation is below 90% should receive aggressive oxygenation and possibly positive pressure ventilation.

The pulse oximeter is a valuable evaluation tool, useful in virtually any medical emergency. It does, however, have disadvantages. In low-flow states, such as hypothermia, the device may not sense accurately. The presence of carbon monoxide on the **hemoglobin** molecule tends to elevate the value displayed on the pulse oximeter above actual saturation level. In a chronic smoker, this may account for up to 10% of the saturation value. While the uncompromised patient has adjusted to this level, the smoker who is having respiratory problems may show a saturation higher than the actual value.

■ **hemoglobin** an iron-containing compound, found within the red blood cell, that is responsible for the transport and delivery of oxygen to the body cells.

In patients with anemia, and in some cases of hypovolemia, the paramedic must be careful in using the oximeter. The reading may be within the normal range, but, because of the decreased hemoglobin, the oxygen-carrying capacity of the blood is diminished. The vital signs should be monitored carefully, and high-flow oxygen administered.

Glucose Determination. Field glucose tests, through the use of a blood glucose test kit, may provide an indication of the blood-sugar level and possible hypoglycemia. Currently, the tests are dependent on proper and uniform technique and have had only limited success. The process in-

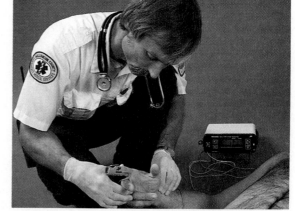

FIGURE 10-62 Pulse oximetry allows you to rapidly and accurately determine the oxygenation status of the patient.

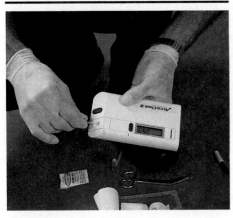

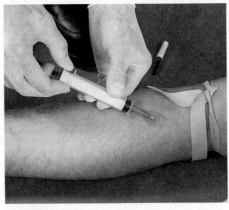

FIGURE 10-63 Determine the blood glucose with either a glucometer or Dextrostix®.

FIGURE 10-64 If performing a blood glucose, or starting an IV, collect a sample of blood if required by local protocols.

volves smearing a small amount of blood on a test strip and comparing the resultant color against a color scale that corresponds to blood-sugar level. Many EMS units carry glucose monitors, which give a relatively accurate, numeric blood-glucose reading. These are preferable to the standard reagent sticks. (See Figure 10-63.)

Certain drugs can assist in the patient evaluation. Naloxone, which is a narcotic antagonist, can reverse the effects of narcotic overdose, and glucose administration will bring a patient out of a hypoglycemic coma. Neither drug will generally cause harm and a dramatic reversal of the patient's condition gives good evidence to the nature of the problem.

Venipuncture. During the assessment process, several invasive diagnostic tests may be performed by drawing blood for analysis by the Emergency Department personnel. The blood draw will do little to help with the patient assessment for the prehospital care provider. It may, however, assist the medical control physician when it is analyzed at the hospital. It may reveal pre-care levels of alcohol, glucose, or narcotics, as well as the ratio of red blood cells to serum by volume (**hematocrit**). Some systems draw blood during prolonged extrication and have the sample transported to the hospital before the patient. The blood may be typed and cross-matched, so that, when the patient arrives at the emergency department, blood is ready and waiting. (See Figure 10-64.)

✳ Blood should be drawn, according to local protocol, to help determine the pre-care condition of the patient.

■ **hematocrit** the percentage of blood occupied by red blood cells.

HISTORY

Patient questioning is the evaluation of the patient to obtain information (generally symptoms) not gained in the physical assessment. (See Figure 10-65.) It is also a time when you begin to appreciate the patient's perspective toward the emergency. It can begin as part of the primary assessment, when you determine the level of consciousness, and will continue until the patient is delivered to emergency department personnel. Patient questioning should progress through several steps. The chief complaint should be obtained and a detailed explanation elicited regarding intensity, duration, and associated complaints. A pertinent medical history must be obtained, including pre-existing conditions, medications, and allergies. Finally, the significant information must be organized and com-

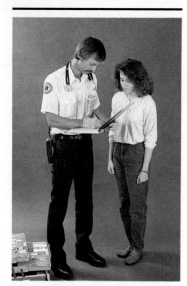

FIGURE 10-65 Obtain a brief, yet pertinent history from family members or the patient.

✱ At the completion of your assessment you should have an exact description of the chief complaint, including its location, quality, intensity, duration, onset, and aggravating and alleviating factors.

municated through radio, and both verbal and written reports. The medical control physician needs to know the patient's condition, to allow the emergency department to prepare for your arrival and to be able to provide permission and direction for medical care.

The arrival at the hospital should continue this exchange of information and culminate with written documentation of the significant circumstances and events of the call. Several elements are essential to the complete and appropriate patient assessment. They include the chief complaint, the history of the present illness, and a previous medical history.

Chief Complaint

The chief complaint is the pain, discomfort, or dysfunction that caused the patient to request your help. It may be a spouse calling for help when her husband cannot be aroused from sleep, a bystander calling for assistance to a "man down," or an auto accident with injuries radioed in by the police. As you arrive and begin to interview and assess the patient, the chief complaint becomes more and more specific. The chief complaint may be different from the primary problem. The chief complaint is a sign or symptom noticed by the patient. The primary problem is the principal medical problem present. For example, a patient may complain of left leg pain. This is his or her chief complaint. The primary problem, on the other hand, may be a left tibia fracture.

By the time you have finished your assessment, you should have an exact description, in terms of location, quality, intensity, duration, circumstances of onset, and alleviating or aggravating factors. The information gathered through patient questioning is guided by you. You have the choice to use open-ended questions, which allow the patient to explain in detail what he or she feels, or to use closed questions, which limit the patient's response and reduce the time taken for your verbal evaluation. The open-ended question is one that calls for an answer in a sentence or paragraph, such as "Describe the pain in your chest." The closed question asks for a one-word or short-phrase response. An example would be "Are you on any medications?" Select the type of question that provides you with the needed information, yet keeps questioning to a reasonable length. In either case, you should not use questions that suggest their answers (e.g., "Do you have a crushing pain in your chest?").

The questioning process should result in the patient feeling comfortable with you, confident in your care, and supportive of your control of the situation. Ensure that you are at the patient's eye level and that you focus your attention on him or her. Give patients' requests and concerns a high priority, even though they may not be medically significant. For example, if they mention they're cold, cover them with a blanket. It may not only make them feel warmer, it may give them confidence in your desire and ability to help. If a complaint cannot be cared for immediately, let them know you are concerned about it and will take care of it shortly. The patient should also be addressed with regard to his or her station in life. Ask for his or her name and use it frequently during the assessment. You should also ask how a patient wants to be addressed—Mr. Jones, James, or Jim—and respect his or her wishes.

During the patient assessment, the paramedic must carefully listen to what the patient says. All too often, we anticipate the problem, then suffer from tunnel vision. We fail to look for other signs, symptoms, or conditions that could account for what is wrong with our patient. If we carefully listen to all that the patient says, we can seldom go wrong. You must record what is said versus what you feel the patient meant to say.

Paramedics, because of their medical background, tend to use words that are very specific and ones that convey special meanings. The best method to record a symptom is to use the patient's "exact" words. Should the patient's description of a symptom change, it then means that the condition is changing, rather than that an error was made in assessment.

To make the patient questioning organized, efficient, and complete it is necessary to look at a few aspects of the chief complaint. Your questions should investigate the location, quality, intensity, duration, circumstances of onset, and **aggravating** and **alleviating** factors. Examining these components of the chief complaint will ensure that it is well-investigated and the "whole" picture is seen.

■ **aggravate** to worsen or increase in severity.

■ **alleviate** to reduce or eliminate. It usually refers to a problem or discomforting feeling.

Evaluation of Chief Complaint

Location. It is essential to identify the exact location of the pain, discomfort, or dysfunction. Does the patient complain of pain "here" while holding a clenched fist over the sternum, or does he or she grasp the entire abdomen with both hands and moan? Identify its specific location, or the boundary of the pain if it is regional. Also determine if the pain is truly pain or tenderness (pain on touch). Determine whether the pain moves or is radiating. Localized pain is found in one very specific area, while radiating pain travels outward and away from the source, in either one, many, or all directions. Moving pain should be evaluated as to initial location, progression, and any factors that affect its movement. Referred pain should also be noted. The two most common areas that produce referred pain are the heart and the diaphragm. The pain of the myocardial infarction or angina is most commonly referred to the left arm, with occasional referral to the neck, jaw and back. The pain associated with irritation of the diaphragm (most commonly blood in the abdomen of the supine patient) is generally referred to the clavicular region.

Quality. Investigate how the patient perceives the pain. Is it described as crushing, tearing, oppressive, gnawing, crampy, or otherwise? Use the patient's exact words to describe the pain in your oral and written reports. If the patient reports the pain feels as though "someone has put my chest in a vise," then report it to medical control in those exact words. We tend to put things into medical terms when, in fact, the patient's words are a more exact description.

Intensity. Intensity is the degree of pain that the patient feels. Any and all pain is uncomfortable. The difficulty with its assessment is that there is no standard of measurement. You may be able to get an idea of the patient's pain by asking about previous events that caused pain. An example might be asking a chest pain patient how severe his pain is compared with the pain of fractured ribs he had a few years ago. In addition to the way the patient describes pain, the paramedic must evaluate the amount of discomfort the patient displays. Sweating usually means that the pain is severe and the patient is concerned about it. A patient who is writhing about, or reluctant to move at all, is in significant pain. If, despite attempts to distract him or her through questioning, the patient keeps reverting back to concern about the pain, it must be severe.

Duration. How long has this symptom affected the patient? Is it something that started suddenly, or is it a problem that developed over time? Is this the first occurrence, or has it occurred before? If so, how often?

When did it first start? Was the course of its development slow and gradual, or mild then suddenly severe?

Onset. What if any actions or events seem to precede the onset of the symptom? Evaluate the activities immediately before, and at the time of, the experience. Evaluate the patient's environment. If it was trauma, look to the mechanism of injury. If it was medical, look to what he or she was doing at the time of the problem's development. In trauma, look beyond the mechanism of injury, as assessed in the scene survey. Compare the chief complaint to the mechanism of injury, and ask yourself, "How much damage is there to the vehicle interior where the knee impacted the dash?" The interior damage should be commensurate with the damage to the knee. The patient's narration of the accident should also confirm what appears to have happened. If there is any disagreement between the evidence of trauma, the assessed injuries, and the patient's narration or complaint, reassess each element.

If the problem was caused by a traumatic incident, was it precipitated by a medical problem? Was the patient driving an auto when he experienced a myocardial infarction and hit a tree? Was the patient hypoglycemic when she passed out and fell down a flight of stairs? A good investigation into the events leading up to the incident may reveal the precipitating, and possibly a more important, medical problem.

In the medical emergency, investigate what the patient was doing when or shortly before the symptoms or signs developed. Were they exercising or exerting themselves, or at rest or sleeping? Were they eating or drinking, and if so, what? Have they recently changed their lifestyle in any way that could account for this occurrence? A topic that may merit investigation in the medical circumstance is the possible relationship of emotional events. Situations such as divorce, a recent move, job loss, recent retirement, or the death of a close friend or family member may impact physiologically as well as psychologically. Attempt to correlate any event with the beginning or progression of the illness.

Look also to the environment where the patient is found. Examine not only for the physical elements, such as temperature, presence of odors, or airborne particles. Also check the general appearance of the home, any offending agents (e.g., medications, alcohol containers, drug paraphernalia), signs of neglect, etc. During this phase of the assessment, you may also notice the attitudes toward the disease or accident by the bystanders, family members, and patient. These attitudes may reflect how the patient is perceiving his or her infirmity. If the social environment is not supportive, the patient may feel uncomfortable about the problem and may not wish to discuss it in much detail.

Aggravating and Alleviating Factors. In many illnesses or injuries, certain factors either increase or decrease the pain, discomfort, or dysfunction. These include motion, pressure, jarring, ingestion of solids or fluids, and rest or sleep. In some cases, the position will be a factor. A patient may wish to lie on his or her side in the fetal position to reduce the abdominal pain. The congestive heart failure (CHF) patient will insist upon remaining in the seated position to ease the breathing effort and effectiveness. The CHF patient may also experience paroxysmal nocturnal dyspnea, a sleep-disturbing dyspnea caused by fluids building up in the lungs while the patient is supine. The patient will often sleep with several pillows under the head and chest, or sleep in a seated position to ease the discomfort. Ask your patient how breathing affects the discomfort. A patient with pleuritic pain or the pain of rib fractures will not breathe deeply, whereas breathing may not affect the pain of the angina patient. Deep breathing may also increase the pain of the acute abdomen patient. Any patient with pain during respiration will breathe with more frequent and shallow breaths.

If a medication is taken shortly before you arrive, its effect or lack of effect on the patient may help determine the pathology. Drugs such as bronchial dialators, hypoglycemic agents, and anti-convulsants are commonly prescribed and taken at home. Be sure to investigate any medications used to alleviate the problem and note their effectiveness. Many factors will affect various patients in various ways. Ask for and record any activity, position, medication, or other circumstance that either alleviates or aggravates the chief complaint.

In evaluating the patient, the paramedic should note pertinent negatives. For example, if a patient complains of shortness of breath, and denies chest pain and cardiac history, the run report and radio message should mention it. Any element of the history or physical assessment which does not support a suspected or possible diagnosis should be noted.

Previous Medical History

The determination of the previous medical history is essential to almost all medical and many traumatic injuries. The greatest difficulty in evaluating this component of the assessment is determining what is pertinent and what is not. While it is hard to know what histories are important, it may likewise be difficult for the patient to know what is worthwhile to mention. A helpful method is to divide the previous medical history into pre-existing medical problems, medications, allergies, and the patient's personal physician.

Pre-Existing Medical Problems. A pertinent medical history will tell much about the patient in either the medical or traumatic situation. It is often difficult to gain an appropriate history because the patient may not really know what is pertinent. During the assessment you might ask if he or she has been to a physician or been hospitalized recently. If this elicits information, that information can be questioned further. If no information is forthcoming, ask more open-ended questions. If a pre-existing medical problem is found, investigate what effects it has had on the patient, when the patient was last affected by the disease, and if the patient is on any prescribed medications or restricted in activity. Record any appropriate information for transferral to the receiving hospital.

Medications. Any medications the patient has had prescribed should be noted in the record and considered. (See Figure 10-66.) The medication may give a clue to the underlying medical problem. If not taken as prescribed, it may be responsible for the current medical problem—by not reaching therapeutic levels or by possible over-medication. The medication, if just recently prescribed and taken as ordered, may be causing an allergic or **untoward** (severe and unexpected) reaction. It may also be out of date and no longer able to provide the expected effect. The patient should be asked why he or she is on a particular medication. The response may be simplistic, but will usually be helpful to identify any pre-existing conditions. It may also provide you with an awareness of the patient's general understanding of medical terminology and ability to comprehend medical problems. Any medications found with the patient

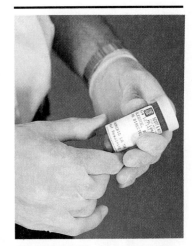

FIGURE 10-66 Note the names, dosages, and dates of any medications taken by the patient.

■ **untoward** an unexpected reaction, usually associated with the administration of a drug.

or at home should be communicated to medical control, taken with the patient to the hospital, and recorded in the ambulance report.

Allergies. Ask about any known allergies. This information may not be obtainable at the Emergency Department if the patient becomes unconscious or otherwise disoriented. Ask especially about allergy to penicillin, the "caine" family (local anesthetics), or tetanus toxoid. These agents are frequently given in the emergent situation and knowledge of the patient's allergy may prevent additional complications on the emergency department visit.

Personal Physician. Obtain the name of the patient's personal physician. He or she may be contacted by the Emergency Department personnel to gain further medical history. The personal physician will also be asked to follow up with the patient after the emergency has subsided.

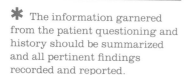

*The information garnered from the patient questioning and history should be summarized and all pertinent findings recorded and reported.

It may be helpful to use a system to remember the elements of the patient history. Many systems utilize the "AMPLE" pneumonic. The A reflects allergies, the M medications, the P past medical history, the L for last meal or oral intake, and the E for events leading up to the incident. (The last meal may be important if the patient will need surgery.) As with the head-to-toe assessment, the vital signs, and investigation of the chief complaint, the information gained from the medical history should be summarized. Summarizing will help identify the pertinent elements of the medical history and help prepare for the radio communication to medical command.

COMMUNICATION OF ASSESSMENT FINDINGS

The communication between you and the Emergency Department Medical Control physician is extremely important. The information passed to the physician about the patient must be concise, correct, and pertinent to his or her condition. The information should be presented in a consistent way to allow both the paramedic and physician to easily organize what is communicated. (See Figure 10-67.)

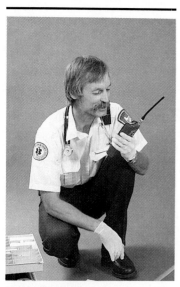

FIGURE 10-67 Relay the patient report to medical control.

Radio Communications. Many services, hospitals, and EMS systems have created pocket notebook forms to provide a format for the basic composition of the radio message. The most common format identifies: age, sex, patient's weight, chief complaint (mechanism of injury), short history, level of consciousness, vital signs (pulse rate and character, blood pressure, respiratory rate and volume), supporting signs and symptoms, medications, allergies, family physician, request for care procedures, and estimated time of arrival. The use of this or a similar form ensures that the needed information will be transmitted quickly and efficiently and will be anticipated and recorded at the medical command facility. The objective of radio communication between the field paramedic and medical control is the conveyance of just enough information to support the request for care and to allow the emergency department to prepare for the patient's arrival. Only the information that is essential to that purpose should be communicated. There is rarely a need to communicate all signs and symptoms or all patient information to medical command. The following is an example of a radio communication that might be expected for a moderately serious accident with a patient injured, yet stable.

"Unit 96 to United Hospital. We are at the scene of an auto/train accident with a 55-year-old male patient, weighing 100 kilograms. He is complaining of leg and cervical pain with numbness in his hands but not feet. The patient also has an apparent open fracture of the left femur. The patient is conscious and alert, with a blood pressure of 136 over 88, a pulse of 110, and respirations of 18 and regular. The patient denies any previous medical history other than an allergy to Xylocaine. He is currently on moderate-flow oxygen, cervical immobilization is in place, and we are awaiting extrication to apply a traction splint to the femur. We request permission to start an IV of lactated Ringer's solution, and Nitronox for pain. We expect a ten-minute extrication and a 15-minute transport to your facility."

Once the interventions have been instituted and the patient is ready for transport, the paramedic should update the medical control physician.

"Unit 96 to United Hospital. We have initiated an IV in the left anterior forearm, and have administered Nitronox. The patient remains alert, with a blood pressure of 132 over 86 and a pulse of 94. Respirations are 20 and regular. The patient's pain has diminished some. We have applied the traction splint, loaded him into the ambulance, and are enroute to your facility; estimating arrival within 15 minutes."

Communication of the results of your assessment is essential to a successful request for critical intervention. It is also very important to the continuity of care as you present your patient at the emergency department. If the medical control physician is accurately informed of the patient's condition, he or she, and the department staff, will be prepared physically and mentally for your arrival. They will have a picture of the condition of the patient long before the doors of your ambulance are opened.

> ✳ Communication of the results of your assessment is essential to a successful request for critical intervention from medical control.

Emergency Department Arrival. With arrival, you are responsible for updating the staff with any change in the patient's condition, as well as with any other pertinent information that was not communicated via radio. (See Figure 10-68.) This should include any patient interventions and the results of those interventions. As the emergency department physician begins the assessment and care, your communication will be compared with the physical findings. If your assessment (and the condensation of it in the radio report) was concise and accurate, the patient will continue to receive increasing and appropriate care. If the picture of the patient the physician received was not what he or she saw when you arrived, the continuity of care will be interrupted while the patient is re-evaluated, and your credibility as a field care provider will be questioned.

Documentation Reports. The final component of the patient assessment is the recording of the findings and events during the call. This information is recorded in detail on the ambulance report form. It must be complete, neat, and accurate, since it will serve several functions. It is part of the patient's medical record, a written report of the medical care the patient received, which began in the field and ended with discharge from the hospital. It is documentation of what occurred in the field, of what patient findings were noted, and of the care you offered at the scene and during transport. It may also be the documentation that comes to your defense (or incrimination) if the patient care you offered is questioned in a court of law or by medical command. The ambulance report form should provide space to record the dispatch information, what was found as you

> ✳ The ambulance report form must be complete, neat, and accurate, since it will become part of the patient's medical record and a legal document.

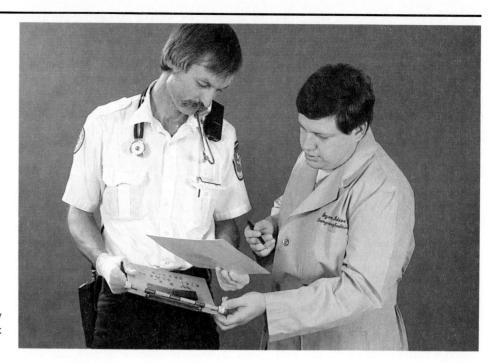

FIGURE 10-68 Relay any additional information to the emergency department physician upon arrival at the hospital.

reached the scene (including medical care given before you arrived), what signs, symptoms, and other patient information were obtained through your assessment, what care was instituted, and the impact that care had on vital signs and on the patient in general. The form should be well-organized, so that it allows you to record information in the order in which it was obtained, and allows anyone reviewing it to rapidly gain the information they need. A well-designed ambulance report form will facilitate complete and orderly documentation.

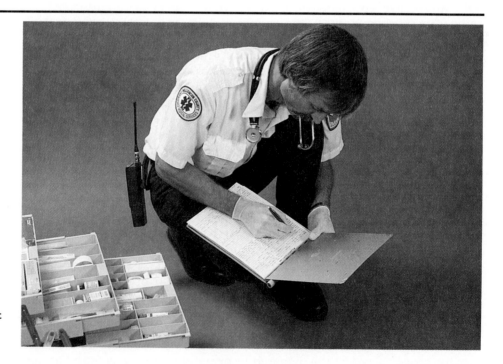

FIGURE 10-69 Document the response as soon as possible so that crucial details will not be overlooked.

The Patient Assessment Process
A Comparison of Trauma *vs.* Medical

The assessment process is identical for trauma and medical problems up to the application of the secondary assessment. It is understood that each emergency is unique and this template for assessment will vary depending on the exact circumstances presented to the paramedic.

Review of Dispatch

Determine the nature of the emergency, the number of patients involved, and the exact location; and identify any hazards which may exist at the scene.

↓

Scene Survey

Identify any immediate hazards to the patient or rescuers; determine the best access to the patient, the number of patients, any mechanism of injury or evidence to suggest the patient's problem, and the best route by which to remove the patient.

↓

Primary Assessment
Airway

Ensure the patient's airway is patent, and protect the cervical spine.

↓

Breathing

Ensure the patient is breathing adequately.

↓

Circulation

Evaluate distal pulses to ensure adequate circulation.

↓

Disability neurologic

Assess level of consciousness (AVPU).

↓

Expose for critical injuries

Quickly observe the head, neck, chest, abdomen, pelvis, and extremities for signs of severe hemorrhage or other life-threatening hemorrhage.

↓

At the conclusion of the primary assessment the paramedic should not only have addressed any life threatening problem encountered but should also determine the seriousness of the patient's problem.

FIGURE 10-70

Secondary Assessment

Trauma

Medical

Physical Assessment

The head-to-toe assessment examines for the signs and symptoms of tramua including pain, tenderness, deformity, discoloration, crepitus, skin temperature variation, and other indications of injury. The distal extremities are examined for circulation and feeling.

Special focus is directed to the areas of potential injury as suggested by the mechanism of injury, though the entire anatomy is assessed if the patient's condition and time permit. (The assessment may continue or be completed during transport.)

At the conclusion of the head-to-toe assessment all suspected injuries are identified and placed in priority for care.

The physical assessment for the medical patient may also progress from head to toe and involve the entire body, although it is most commonly directed to the areas (and signs and symptoms) which either support or disprove a suspected diagnosis.

The assessment looks for specific information such as systemic findings like pitting edema or hemiparalysis or local findings like pain, paresthesia, or tenderness. A strong emphasis is placed on the relationship between the signs found and the patient's description of the problem (specifically, the symptoms).

The physical assessment of the medical patient is more interactive with, and more directed by, the patient questioning than the trauma assessment.

Vital Signs

Vital signs are used with the mechanism of injury and the findings of the primary and physical assessment to determine the patient's general state. They are determined early during the patient evaluation process.

Vital signs are determined early in the assessment process to assist in determining the seriousness of the patient problem. They also form a baseline patient evaluation to help determine any trend in the patient's condition.

Patient History

Patient history is directed toward the events preceding the injury, the injury itself, and specifics of the patient's chief and secondary complaints. Medical history of allergies, medications, and past medical problems is important.

Patient history for the medical patient addresses the chief complaint with a focus on the nature of the complaint, its severity, and related symptoms. The history also examines past medical problems, allergies, last meal, personal physicians, and so on.

FIGURE 10-71

SUMMARY

Patient assessment is the orderly evaluation of all the information available to you as a paramedic, from the original dispatch to the passing of patient responsibilities to the emergency department staff. It uses the senses of sight, hearing, touch, and smell to determine what is most likely wrong with the patient. It is an organized and progressive evaluation of the entire patient, from the evaluation of dispatch information, to the complete head-to-toe assessment and medical history. The process must progress using information from the dispatch information, survey of the scene, primary assessment, secondary assessment, determination of vital signs, and patient history. This information is used to anticipate and prepare for what might happen during care and transport. It is used to ensure that the airway, breathing, and circulation are stable. It is used to decide whether to stabilize at the scene or immediately transport the patient. It is used to identify what is most probably wrong with the patient. It is used to support your request for advanced field interventions.

And finally, it is used to complete the ambulance report form and other documentation of the call. The execution of a proper patient assessment will guide you to the appropriate and timely care of the patient. If performed well, patient assessment will allow you to accomplish your objective—quality advanced patient care. If poorly performed, at the very best you will not be able to provide the needed care. Assessment is a primary and absolutely essential skill upon which any further care or intervention is predicated.

FURTHER READING

AMERICAN COLLEGE OF SURGEONS, COMMITTEE ON TRAUMA. *Advanced Trauma Life Support Course: Student Manual.* American College of Surgeons, 1989.

AMERICAN COLLEGE OF SURGEONS, COMMITTEE ON TRAUMA. *Advanced Trauma Life Support Course: Student Manual.* American College of Surgeons, 1989.

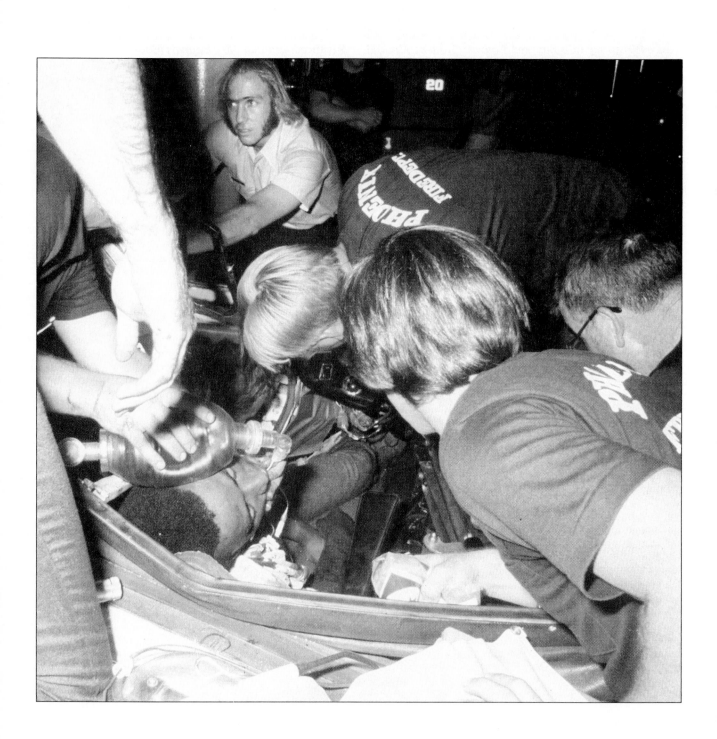

Advanced Airway Management and Ventilation

Objectives for Chapter 11

Upon completing this chapter, the student should be able to:

1. Describe the anatomy of the upper airway, including the mouth, nose, pharynx, epiglottis, and larynx.

2. Name the three regions of the pharynx.

3. Identify the relationship between the larynx and the tongue, pharynx, epiglottis, esophagus, and vocal cords.

4. Describe the procedures used to open the airway manually.

5. Discuss indications, contraindications, and methods for insertion and use of the oropharyngeal airway, nasopharyngeal airway, esophageal obturator airway, esophageal gastric tube airway, and pharyngeo-tracheal lumen airway.

6. List the equipment used to perform endotracheal intubation.

7. Recall the indications, contraindications, and alternatives of endotracheal intubation.

8. Explain the need for rapid placement of the endotracheal tube.

9. Describe the methods used to assure correct placement of the endotracheal tube.

10. List and demonstrate the steps in performing endotracheal intubation.

11. State the precautions that should be used when intubating a trauma patient.

12. Discuss indications, contraindications, and methods for using the pocket mask, bag-valve-mask device, and demand valve resuscitator.

13. Identify the indications, contraindications, and methods of performing percutaneous transtracheal catheter ventilation and a cricothyrotomy.

14. Discuss the indications, contraindications, and methods of performing suctioning.

Medic 1 is called to see a patient who has collapsed at home. Upon arrival, paramedics Al and Emma find a 58-year-old female supine on the floor next to her living room couch. After quickly moving a coffee table in order to reach the patient, they find her unresponsive. Al employs the head-tilt/chin-lift technique to open her airway. He then checks for breathing, only to find that she is not breathing. An oropharyngeal airway is inserted, and the paramedics provide ventilatory support with a bag-valve-mask device and 100 percent oxygen. As resuscitative efforts continue, Emma determines that the patient is pulseless and initiates chest compressions. Before Al can perform endotracheal intubation, though, the patient regurgitates. Still, the upper airway can be suctioned enough to place an endotracheal tube. During resuscitation efforts, it was noted that breath sounds on the right side of the patient's chest had disappeared. Immediately determining the problem, Al slowly pulls back the endotracheal tube until breath sounds can again be heard bilaterally.

Although the patient responded to initial treatment modalities, the crew is unable to convert her to an effective electromechanical rhythm. Resuscitative efforts continue until they reach the hospital, where the patient is pronounced dead on arrival.

INTRODUCTION

■ **aspiration** the act of taking foreign material into the lungs during inhalation.

■ **ventilation** breathing, moving air in and out of the lungs.

■ **hypoxia** a reduction of oxygen supply to the cells.

■ **patent** open.

As a result of medical and trauma-related emergencies, many patients in prehospital care settings may experience an obstructed airway, **aspiration,** inadequate **ventilation,** or **hypoxia.** These are all life-threatening conditions that require immediate intervention if the patient is to survive.

Paramedics need to be proficient in a wide range of skills, including securing a **patent** airway, maintaining appropriate ventilatory function, and oxygenating patients. Some procedures employed by the paramedic are manual and require no adjunctive equipment, while others demand sophisticated techniques and equipment. Unlike the hospital environment, where patient care is provided in a controlled setting, managing a patient in the field often involves too few hands, too little lighting, and an anxious crowd that expects the patient to be saved no matter how severe his or her condition. The paramedic must often deliver airway support while kneeling in blood or vomitus. All of these factors make the job difficult, to say the least. The quality of care cannot be reduced because a paramedic comes to the scene of an emergency ill prepared.

Airway management skills can be quickly forgotten, unless they are learned well initially and then continually reinforced. Among the aspects of a paramedic's education, learning airway management is one of the most important.

ANATOMY AND PHYSIOLOGY OF THE RESPIRATORY SYSTEM

The primary function of the respiratory system is to provide air flow into and out of the body. *Oxygen* is brought into the lungs, and *carbon dioxide*—a waste product of metabolism—is expelled. (Oxygen is required for the conversion of essential nutrients into energy.) In order for this process to continue, a patient must have a patent airway, intact muscles of respiration, unobstructed respiratory passageways, adequate pulmonary blood flow, and appropriate neurological stimulus.

The respiratory passageway is divided into two sections: an *upper airway* and a *lower airway*. The upper airway includes the nose, mouth, nasopharynx, oropharynx, hypopharynx, and larynx. (See Figure 11-1.)

The nose is one of two passageways into the respiratory tree. (The mouth is the second.) It is lined with a **mucous membrane,** which carries a rich blood supply. It is covered with **mucus** that is kept in motion by **ciliated** cells. This membrane filters air; warming, moistening, and cleaning it along the way. When inspired air finally reaches the distal air passageways (alveoli), it is at body temperature, 100 percent humidified, and free of airborne particles.

The external portion of the nose is made of cartilage and skin, and it is lined with mucous membrane. It has two openings, which are referred to as *nares,* or nostrils. The internal portion of the nose is separated into right and left cavities by the vascular midline **septum.** Each of the inner nasal cavities has three boney projections called the superior, middle, and

■ **mucous membrane** a membrane lining many of the body cavities that handle air transport; it usually contains small, mucous-secreting glands.

■ **mucus** a thick, slippery secretion that functions as a lubricant and protects various surfaces.

■ **ciliated** having hairlike processes projecting from the cells which propel mucus.

■ **septum** a wall that divides a chamber into two cavities.

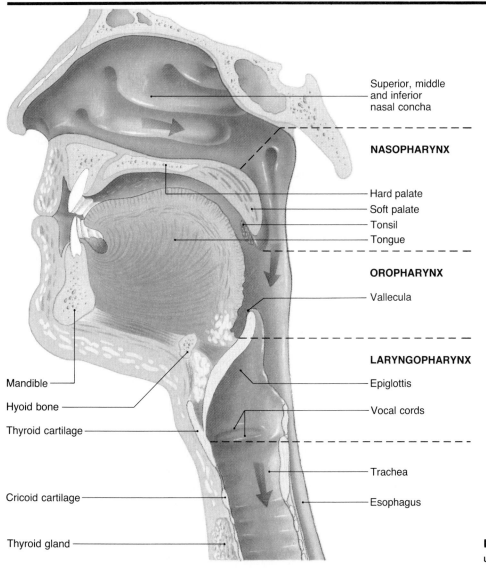

Superior, middle and inferior nasal concha

NASOPHARYNX

Hard palate
Soft palate
Tonsil
Tongue

OROPHARYNX

Vallecula

LARYNGOPHARYNX

Epiglottis

Vocal cords

Trachea

Esophagus

Mandible
Hyoid bone
Thyroid cartilage
Cricoid cartilage
Thyroid gland

FIGURE 11-1 Anatomy of the upper airway.

inferior turbinates (also referred to as conchae), which can be likened to shelves. Located on the lateral wall of each cavity, the turbinates cause eddies in the flowing air, forcing it to rebound in several directions during its passage through the nose. This action traps fine foreign particles, which the cilia then propel back to the pharynx to be swallowed. Introduction of an irritant can stimulate a sneeze necessary to expel it. At the posterior surface of the internal nose are two openings (called nares) that serve as passageways into the *nasopharynx.*

The mouth, or oral cavity, is bordered by the cheeks, the hard and soft *palates,* and the tongue. The lips are the fleshy folds surrounding the orifice of the mouth, with the gums and teeth located behind them. The top of the mouth is formed by the hard and soft palates, while the tongue—a large mass of muscle—is located on the bottom of the cavity. The tongue attaches anteriorly to the jaw (*mandible*), as well as to the hyoid bone, through a series of muscles and ligaments. The *hyoid bone,* shaped like a U, is located just beneath the chin. The hyoid is considered unique, as it is the only bone in the axial skeleton that's not jointed with any other bone. It is, instead, suspended by ligaments from the styloid process of the temporal bone of the skull.

The *pharynx,* or throat, is a muscular tube that extends vertically from the back of the soft palate to the upper end of the esophagus. It passes air into (and out of) the respiratory tract and foods and liquids into the digestive system. It contains several openings, including the **eustachian tube** (from the middle ear), the posterior nares, the mouth, the larynx, the esophagus, and tonsils. This pharynx is divided into three regions: the *nasopharynx,* the *oropharynx,* and the *laryngopharynx.* The nasopharynx is the uppermost part of the pharynx; it extends from the back of the nasal opening to the plane of the soft palate. The oropharynx is the section that extends from the soft palate in the back of the mouth to the hyoid bone below the lower jaw. The laryngopharynx extends from the

■ **eustachian tube** a tube connecting the pharynx and the middle ear.

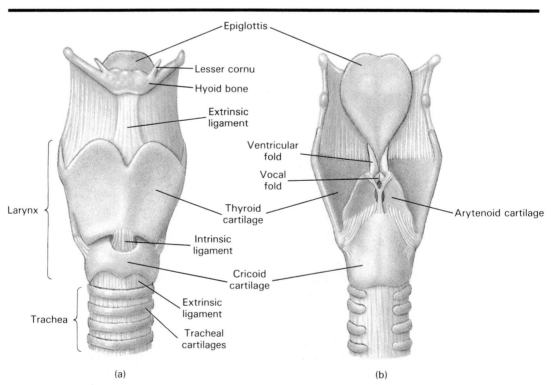

FIGURE 11-2 Internal anatomy of the upper airway. (a) Anterior view; (b) posterior view.

hyoid bone at the base of the tongue to the esophagus, posteriorly, and to the trachea, anteriorly. The laryngopharynx—also known as the *hypopharynx*—is important, relative to airway management techniques employed in field and hospital settings. Because the mouth and pharynx serve dual purposes, there are a number of mechanisms to prevent their accidental blockage and also to stop foreign objects from being aspirated into the lungs. Sensitive nerves activate the body's cough and swallowing mechanisms, as well as the **gag reflex,** and prevent foreign material from entering the **glottis,** and trachea.

Located anteriorly in the pharynx are the epiglottis, the laryngeal inlet, and the mucous membrane-covered arytenoid and cricoid cartilages of the larynx. (See Figure 11-2.) Just behind the hypopharynx are the fourth and fifth cervical vertebral bodies. The *epiglottis,* a leaf-shaped cartilage, prevents food from entering the respiratory tract during the act of swallowing. Just above this is the **vallecula.** On either side are recesses known as pyriform fossa. The epiglottis is connected to the hyoid bone and mandible by a series of ligaments and muscles.

The *larynx* is the tubular structure that joins the pharynx with the trachea. Lying midline in the neck, inferior to the hyoid bone and anterior to the esophagus, it consists of the *thyroid cartilage, cricoid cartilage,* the upper end of the *trachea, vocal cords,* and **arytenoid folds.** The walls of the larynx are supported by cartilages that prevent it from collapsing during inhalation.

The main laryngeal cartilage is the *thyroid cartilage,* or Adam's apple. In adults, the portion of the thyroid cartilage housing the vocal cords is the narrowest part of the upper airway. The thyroid cartilage consists of two large plates that form the anterior wall of the larynx and give it its V-shaped appearance. The posterior wall of the thyroid cartilage is open and consists of muscle. The upper end of the thyroid cartilage is attached to the hyoid bone by the thyrohyoid membrane. The thyroid cartilage is larger in males than in females.

Beneath the thyroid cartilage is the *cricoid cartilage.* It forms the inferior walls of the larynx and is attached to the larynx's first ring of cartilage. Unlike the thyroid and tracheal cartilages, which are open on their posterior surfaces, the cricoid cartilage forms a complete ring. Just behind this lies the esophagus. In children, the narrowest part of the laryngeal airway is the cricoid cartilage. Connecting the inferior border of the thyroid cartilage with the superior aspect of the cricoid membrane is the **cricothyroid membrane.**

Lying on the rear surface of the cricoid cartilage are two pyramid-shaped arytenoid cartilages. These attach to the vocal folds and pharyngeal walls, and can open and close the vocal cords. Within the laryngeal cavity lie the true and false vocal cords. True vocal cords regulate the passage of air through the larynx and control the production of sound. As the muscles in the larynx contract, these cords change shape and vibrate, thus producing sounds of different pitches. The vocal cords can also close together to prevent foreign bodies from entering the airway. The space between the vocal cords is referred to as the glottic opening. The passage of an endotracheal tube between the vocal cords interferes not only with the creation of sound, but also with coughing. The false vocal cords are located above the true vocal cords.

Most of the larynx is lined with a ciliated tissue that secretes mucus. This membrane, richly lined with nerve endings from the vagus nerve, is so sensitive that any irritation sparks a cough, or forceful exhalation of a large volume of air. To initiate a cough, air must first be drawn into the respiratory passageways. Next, the glottic opening shuts tightly, in or-

■ **gag reflex** the act of retching or striving to vomit; a normal reflex triggered by touching the soft palate or the throat.

■ **glottis** the slit-like opening between the vocal cords.

■ **vallecula** the depression between the epiglottis and the base of the tongue.

■ **arytenoid folds** cupped or ladle-shaped tissues found posterior to the vocal cords.

■ **cricothyroid membrane** the membrane located between the cricoid and thyroid cartilages of the larynx.

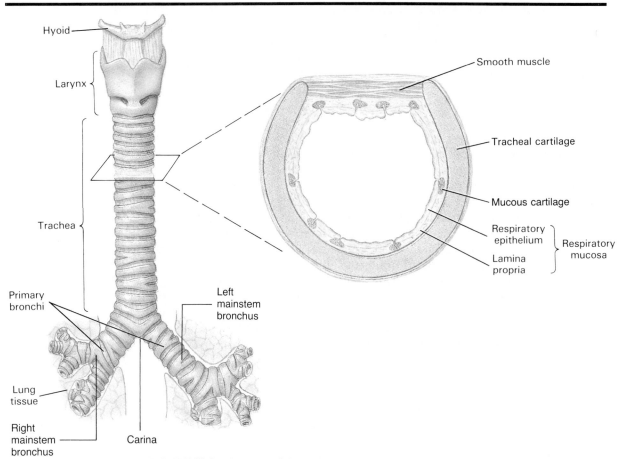

Hyoid

Larynx

Trachea

Primary
bronchi

Lung
tissue

Right
mainstem
bronchus

Carina

Left
mainstem
bronchus

Smooth muscle

Tracheal cartilage

Mucous cartilage

Respiratory
epithelium

Lamina
propria

Respiratory
mucosa

FIGURE 11-3 Anatomy of the lower airway.

■ **carina** the point at which the trachea bifurcates into the right and left mainstem bronchi.

der to trap the air within the lungs. Then the abdominal and thoracic muscles contract, pushing against the diaphragm and increasing intrathoracic pressure. The vocal cords suddenly open, and the sudden burst of air forces foreign particles out of the lungs. Due to the degree of vagal innervation, stimulation of the laryngeal mucous membrane (by a laryngoscope or endotracheal tube) can cause bradycardia, hypotension, and a decreased respiratory rate.

The lower airway consists of the trachea, right and left mainstem bronchi, the secondary bronchi, bronchioles, and the alveoli. (See Figure 11-3.) The *trachea* is the tube extending from the lower edge of the larynx to the **carina** at the level of the fifth or sixth thoracic vertebra. Its purpose is to conduct air between the larynx and the bronchi. It is approximately ten to 15 centimeters in length and is supported by C-shaped cartilaginous rings that are open posteriorly. The trachea is lined with respiratory epithelium, which contain cilia and mucus-producing cells. They warm and humidify air and also trap foreign materials. These foreign particles are propelled upward through the airway by the cilia. The smooth muscle of the trachea is innervated by the parasympathetic branch of the autonomic nervous system.

At the carina, the trachea divides into right and left *mainstem bronchi,* with the right bronchi—a more direct passageway from the trachea—being the wider and shorter of the two. Like the trachea, the bronchi are lined with ciliated mucous layers and reinforced with cartilaginous rings. Upon entering the lung, each bronchus divides to form smaller *bronchi.* This subdivision continues, forming progressively smaller tubes. The more distant branches are referred to as *bronchioles.* These bronchioles, in turn, branch still farther into even narrower tubes called *terminal bronchioles*. The continuous branching of the trachea into primary bronchi, secondary bronchi, bronchioles, and terminal bronchioles resembles a tree trunk with branches; thus it is commonly referred to as the bronchial tree. At the end of the terminal bronchioles are clusters of air sacs, or **alveoli.** These alveoli are hollow, with a shell only one to two cell layers thick. They are the most important functional units of the respiratory system, the places where oxygen and carbon dioxide are exchanged.

The process of moving air in and out of the lungs is known as the *respiratory cycle.* It includes inspiration (breathing in) and expiration (breathing out).

The brain initiates *inspiration* by signalling the muscles of respiration to increase the size of the chest cavity. The *diaphragm* and the *intercostal muscles* are stimulated to contract. The diaphragm, the major inspiratory muscle, accounts for 70 percent of air flow into and out of the lungs. It flattens downward against the abdominal structures in breathing, thus increasing the vertical dimensions of the thoracic cavity. Normal quiet breathing is accomplished almost entirely by this muscle. The intercostal muscles lift the rib cage upward and outward, increasing the horizontal and transverse dimensions of the thoracic cavity. These actions create a vacuum that draws air into the lungs. Airway resistance must be overcome if breathing is to continue smoothly. Changes in airway caliber will affect resistance.

Expiration occurs when respiratory muscles relax and the chest cavity decreases in size. The reduced thoracic volume increases the intrathoracic pressure, and air is forced from the lungs. This is generally a passive act, with its driving force provided by lung recoil.

Enough air must be moved into and out of the lungs to accommodate normal, as well as extraordinary, physiological requirements. The amount of air breathed in and out over the course of a minute is referred to as the respiratory **minute volume ($\dot{V}_{min}$).** It equals the respiratory rate multiplied by the volume. The normal respiratory rate in an adult is approximately 12 to 20 breaths per minute. In children, it is 24, while in infants the rate varies from 40 to 60. The *tidal volume ($\dot{V}_T$),* or the amount of air inhaled and exhaled in a single respiratory cycle, usually equals approximately 500 mL. Of that, *dead space air ($\dot{V}_D$),* or the amount of air remaining in the air passageways and unavailable for gas exchange, equals approximately 150 mL. *Alveolar air ($\dot{V}_A$),* that which reaches the alveoli for gas exchange, equals approximately 350 mL.

Oxygen enters the body through the respiratory system during the process of inspiration. Inspired air contains a higher oxygen concentration (21 percent) than expired air. Once it reaches the alveoli, it will interface with the venous blood stream. Oxygen diffuses across the *alveolar/ capillary membrane,* going from an area of higher concentration to an area of lesser concentration. (See Figure 11-4.)

In the bloodstream the majority of oxygen will bind with the hemoglobin of red blood cells. Some, however, is carried in the plasma. This oxygen-enriched blood is transported back to the heart via the pulmonary bloodstream. Once in the heart, it is circulated through the systemic circulation, where it is transported to the cellular level and diffuses. In the cells, oxygen assists with the production of energy.

The amount of carbon dioxide in the body also depends on ventilatory effectiveness. Under normal conditions, increasing ventilation will decrease the level of carbon dioxide. If ventilations are decreased, then the volume of carbon dioxide will rise. In other words, carbon dioxide levels vary inversely with ventilations. The amount of carbon dioxide in the

■ **alveoli** the microscopic air sacs where the oxygen–carbon dioxide exchange takes place.

■ **minute volume ($\dot{V}_{min}$)** the amount of air inhaled and exhaled in one minute; it equals the respiratory rate times the tidal volume.

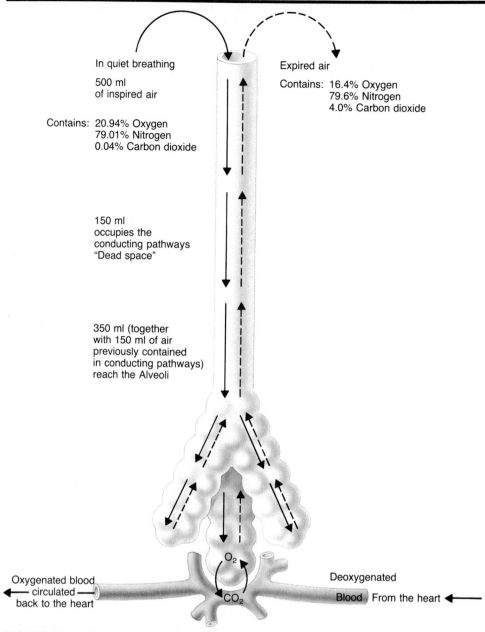

In quiet breathing

500 ml
of inspired air

Contains: 20.94% Oxygen
79.01% Nitrogen
0.04% Carbon dioxide

Expired air

Contains: 16.4% Oxygen
79.6% Nitrogen
4.0% Carbon dioxide

150 ml
occupies the
conducting pathways
"Dead space"

350 ml (together
with 150 ml of air
previously contained
in conducting pathways)
reach the Alveoli

O_2

CO_2

Oxygenated blood
circulated
back to the heart

Deoxygenated

Blood From the heart

FIGURE 11-4 Gas exchange in the alveoli.

body can have a significant impact, as carbon dioxide combines with water to form carbonic acid. Thus, if there is an acute increase in carbon dioxide, it will cause an increase in the body's concentration of carbonic acid. Just the opposite will happen with an acute decrease in carbon dioxide. As carbonic acid is a weak acid, the pH of the body will be affected. When there are increases in carbonic acid, the pH will drop toward more acidic levels. Acidosis, when profound, affects the body adversely by depressing the cells, and it eventually lead to cellular death.

CAUSES OF UPPER AIRWAY OBSTRUCTION

Upper airway obstruction may be defined as "an interference with air movement through the upper airway." This interference can come from the tongue, foreign bodies, vomitus, blood, teeth, or something else. Most often, upper airway obstruction in an unconscious patient can be blamed on the tongue. (See Figure 11-5.) Normally, the submandibular muscles provide direct support of the tongue and indirect support of the epiglottis. In the absence of sufficient muscle tone, though, the relaxed tongue falls back against the rear of the pharynx, thus occluding the airway. The epiglottis may also block the airway at the level of the larynx. If the tongue and epiglottis are in this position, airflow into the respiratory system is at least diminished, and breathing efforts may inadvertently suck the base of the tongue into an obstructing position. Airway blockage by the base of the tongue depends on the position of the head and jaw, and can occur regardless of whether the patient is in a lateral, supine, or prone position.

* Airway obstruction by the tongue can occur whether the patient is supine, lateral, or prone.

Large, poorly chewed pieces of food can also obstruct the upper airway by becoming lodged in the laryngopharynx. (Alcohol consumption and dentures are often involved in these cases.) This sort of emergency, often occurring in restaurants, is frequently mistaken for a heart attack, and is thus referred to commonly as a "cafe coronary." The patient may clutch his or her neck between the thumb and fingers, a universal distress signal. Children, especially toddlers, can easily aspirate foreign objects, as they have the tendency to put everything they can find into their mouths, including not only food, but also balloons, marbles, beads, and thumbtacks. In adults, dentures, teeth, and vomitus are likely to obstruct the airway. Vomitus is made up of food particles, protein-dissolving enzymes, and hydrochloric acid that have been regurgitated from the stomach into the oropharynx. This mixture, if allowed to enter the lungs, can result in increased interstitial fluid and pulmonary edema, and can severely damage the alveoli. Saliva, like vomitus, contains digestive enzymes for starches (primarily amylase) and can also fill the alveoli. Gas exchange can be seriously impaired by the marked increase in alveolar/capillary distance, thus causing **hypoxemia** and **hypercarbia.** These complications occur in 50 percent to 80 percent of patients who aspirate foreign matter, and can usually be avoided by proper airway management and suction.

■ **hypoxemia** a condition of reduced partial pressure of oxygen in the blood.

In trauma, particularly when the patient is unconscious, the airway may be obstructed by loose teeth, facial bones or tissue, and clotted blood. Blood contains many components, including proteins, fibrin, water, and electrolytes, which may clog the alveoli, bronchioles, and bronchi if al-

■ **hypercarbia** excessive partial pressure of carbon dioxide in the blood.

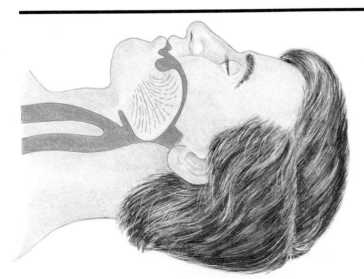

FIGURE 11-5 One of the most common causes of airway obstruction is the tongue. In the unconscious patient, it can fall into the back of the throat, effectively closing the airway.

lowed to enter the lungs in large amounts. Additionally, penetrating or blunt trauma may obstruct the airway by fracturing or displacing the larynx, and allowing the vocal cords to collapse into the tracheal lumen.

Laryngeal spasm is another form of upper airway obstruction. Since the glottis is the narrowest part of an adult's airway, edema or spasm of the vocal cords is a potentially lethal condition. Even moderate amounts of edema can severely obstruct airflow through the glottis, and result in asphyxia. Just beneath the mucous membrane that covers the vocal cords is a layer of loose tissue, where blood or other fluids can accumulate. This tissue may swell following injury. Swelling due to an accumulation of fluids in the vocal cords is slow in subsiding. Causes of laryngeal spasm include anaphylaxis, epiglottitis, and inhalation of super-heated air, smoke, or toxic substances.

CAUSES OF VENTILATORY INEFFECTIVENESS

As stated earlier, the intake of adequate oxygen and the removal of sufficient carbon dioxide depend greatly on a person's ability to maintain sufficient minute volume respirations. A reduction of either the rate or the volume of inhalation leads to a reduction in minute volumes. In some cases, the respiratory rate may be rapid, but the depth of breathing is so shallow that little air exchange takes place. This state of **hypoventilation** may be brought on by depressed respiratory function, fractured ribs, a drug overdose, spinal injury, or head injury, and can lead to hypercarbia or hypoxia.

■ **hypoventilation** a reduced rate or depth of breathing; it often results in an abnormal rise of carbon dioxide in the system.

CAUSES OF HYPOXIA

Hypoxia, or a reduction in oxygen supply to the cells, has a number of adverse consequences on the body. At the cellular level, it leads to anaerobic metabolism and the development of metabolic acidosis. In the heart, hypoxia causes cardiac **dysrhythmias,** and it also increases the myocardial and respiratory workloads as these systems are used to offset the hypoxia. Causes of hypoxia include:

■ **dysrhythmia** a disturbance in the normal rhythm of the heart.

Causes	Examples
Insufficient oxygen in the inspired air	smoke toxic gases high altitude
Failure of the ventilatory mechanism	pneumothorax fractured ribs muscular paralysis kyphoscoliosis
Upper airway compromise	foreign body obstruction epiglottitis croup edema of vocal cords
Lower airway compromise	chronic bronchitis acute asthma attack tumors pneumonia pulmonary edema emphysema fibrosis

Causes	Examples
Circulatory deficiency	pump failure
	congestive heart failure
	congenital defects
	blood loss (hemorrhage)
	shock
	anemia
	carbon monoxide poisoning
Cellular deficiency	cyanide poisoning
	toxic shock syndrome

ASSESSMENT OF THE PATIENT

As with any patient-care situation, paramedics who are assessing the breathing abilities of a patient can obtain a great deal of information:

❑ Is the patient breathing?
❑ Is the patient conscious?
❑ How well does the patient appear to be moving air in and out of his or her lungs?

All these questions can usually be answered by the time a paramedic reaches the patient's side. Airway blockage and ineffective breathing efforts require that the paramedic take immediate corrective steps. Once at the patient's side, and then throughout the time a paramedic provides care to that patient, assessment should proceed in a logical and systematic manner.

Indicators used to assess respiratory function include:

❑ rise and fall of the chest
❑ color of the skin
❑ breath sounds
❑ outward signs (flaring of the nares, retraction, noisy breathing)
❑ air movement at the nose and mouth
❑ compliance
❑ pulse rate

The rising and falling of the chest will tell a great deal about the adequacy of air exchange. (See Figure 11-6 and 11-7.) Normally, a person's chest will rise and fall with each respiratory cycle. In an adult patient, the respiratory rate generally ranges between 12 and 20 breaths per minute. Breathing should be spontaneous and regular. Irregular breathing suggests a significant problem and usually requires some ventilatory support. The chest wall should be observed for any area of asymmetrical movement. This condition, known as **paradoxical breathing**, suggests a **flail chest.** When assisting a patient's breathing with a ventilatory device (bag-valve-mask device or demand-valve resuscitator), or after placing an airway adjunct (nasopharyngeal airway, Esophogeal Obturator Airway, or endotracheal tube), monitor the rise and fall of the chest to determine correct usage and placement. Feel the chest wall to determine that the ribs are parting and the wall is rising and falling. Watch for symmetry of chest wall movement.

The color and texture of the patient's skin will also provide information regarding oxygenation. Early in respiratory compromise, the sympathetic nervous system will be stimulated to help offset the lack of oxygen.

✳ The assessment of the "A" and "B" of the primary survey will evaluate respiratory effectiveness.

■ **paradoxical breathing** an asymmetrical chest wall movement caused by a defect (flail chest) which lessens respiratory efficiency.

■ **flail chest** a defect in the chest wall that allows for free movement of a segment. Breathing will cause paradoxical chest wall motion.

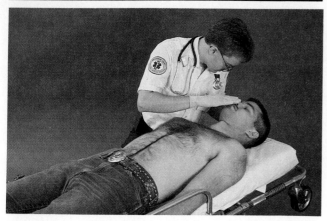

FIGURE 11-6 When assissing the airway, feel for the movement of air with your hand or cheek.

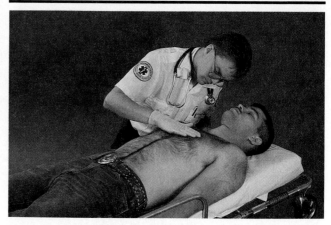

FIGURE 11-7 Assess rise and fall of the patient's chest.

When this happens, the skin will often appear pale and diaphoretic. Cyanosis is another sign of respiratory distress. When oxygen binds with the hemoglobin the blood appears "bright red." Deoxygenated hemoglobin is blue and will give the skin a bluish color (cyanosis). However, this is not a reliable sign, since severe tissue hypoxia is possible without cyanosis. In fact, cyanosis is considered a late sign of respiratory compromise. When it does appear, cyanosis will usually affect the lips, fingernails and skin.

Auscultation of the chest provides information regarding airflow into and out of the lungs. (See Figure 11-8.) In a prehospital-care setting, the sites to be auscultated include the right and left apex (just beneath the clavicle), the right and left base (eighth or ninth intercostal space, midclavicular line), and the right and left mid-axillary line (fourth or fifth intercostal space, on the lateral side of the chest). There are also six locations on the posterior chest that can be monitored. When the patient's condition permits, the posterior surface is actually preferred over the anterior one, as heart sounds there do not interfere with auscultation. However, since patients are usually supine during airway management, the anterior and lateral positions are most accessible.

When assessing the effectiveness of ventilatory support or the correct placement of an airway adjunct, realize that, in some cases, air movement into the epigastrium may mimic breath sounds. Thus, listening to the chest should be only one of several means used to assess air movement. Another method of checking correct placement of an airway adjunct is to auscultate over the epigastrium: it should be silent during ventilation. When providing ventilatory support, watch for signs of gastric distension. This will suggest inadequate hyperextension of the head, that too much pressure is being generated by the ventilatory device, or that airway adjuncts have been improperly placed. Listening over the sternal notch will also confirm the presence of airflow when an endotracheal tube is correctly placed in the trachea.

Other signs of respiratory compromise include nasal flaring (nostrils wide open during inspiration), **tracheal tugging,** retraction of the intercostal muscles, and use of the diaphragm and neck muscles to assist with breathing. Sounds can also point to airflow compromise.

✱ Air movement into the epigastrium may mimic breath sounds; hence auscultation is only one of several means used to confirm proper airway placement.

■ **tracheal tugging** when an Adam's apple appears to be pulled upward on inspiration; occurs in the presence of airway obstruction.

Sound:	Indicates Airway Obstruction Due To:
Snoring respirations	the tongue
Gurgling sounds	accumulation of blood, vomitus, or other secretions
Stridor (a harsh, high-pitched sound heard on inhalation)	laryngeal edema or constriction

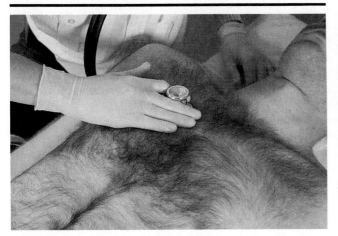

FIGURE 11-8 Auscultation of the chest provides a great deal of information regarding air movement through the lungs.

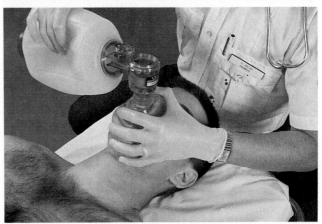

FIGURE 11-9 When providing ventilatory support with a bag-valve-mask, gauge the effectiveness of airflow into the lungs by noting lung compliance and how quickly the bag empties.

When assessing respiratory function, feel for air movement at the patient's nose and mouth. If an endotracheal tube is in place, the proximal end can be checked for this movement. The paramedic should use either the back of his or her hand or cheek to determine airflow.

When providing ventilatory support with the bag-valve-mask device, the paramedic can gauge airflow into the lungs by noting compliance. (See Figure 11-9.) *Compliance* refers to the stiffness or flexibility of the lung tissue, and it is determined by how easily air flows into the lungs. When compliance is good, airflow occurs with a minimum amount of resistance. Poor compliance means that ventilation is harder to achieve. Compliance is often poor in diseased lungs and in patients suffering from chest wall injuries or tension pneumothorax. It will decrease when the upper airway is obstructed by the tongue. If a patient shows poor compliance during ventilatory support, the paramedic should look for potential causes.

✳ If compliance is poor or changing, the paramedic should look for the cause.

- ❑ Is the airway open?
- ❑ Is the head properly extended?
- ❑ Is the patient developing tension pneumothorax?
- ❑ Is the endotracheal tube occluded?
- ❑ Has the endotracheal tube been inadvertently pushed into the right or left mainstem bronchus?

A bag that compresses too quickly or "collapses" should arouse suspicion. It may indicate incorrect placement of the endotracheal tube into the esophagus or a defect in the bag-valve-mask device.

Pulse rate abnormalities may also suggest respiratory compromise. Tachycardia usually accompanies hypoxemia in an adult, while bradycardia hints at anoxia with imminent cardiac arrest. (See Figure 11-10.)

The history of a patient experiencing airway obstruction or compromise may be evident, as was the case with the "cafe coronary." However, causes will usually not be so easily determined. When time and the patient's condition permit, ask appropriate questions to establish his or her medical history, the history of the present complication, or the mechanism of injury.

Airway obstruction is referred to as either "partial" or "complete." Partial airway obstruction allows for either adequate or poor air exchange.

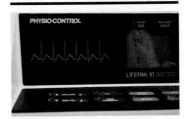

FIGURE 11-10 Tachycardia may indicate hypoxemia.

Adequate air exchange makes it possible for the patient to cough effectively. Patients suffering poor air exchange are no longer able to generate an effective cough, often give off a high-pitched noise while inhaling, and may experience increased breathing difficulty and cyanosis. Complete airway obstruction exists when the patient cannot speak, breathe, or cough; when airflow is not felt or heard from the nose and mouth; when efforts to breathe spontaneously result in retraction of the supraclavicular and intercostal areas; and when there is no chest expansion. A patient with complete airway obstruction will quickly become unconscious, and death will occur if the obstruction is not relieved. In the absence of spontaneous breathing, complete airway obstruction can be recognized by the difficulty encountered when trying to ventilate the patient.

MANAGING THE UPPER AIRWAY

On first encountering a patient, the paramedic must determine if an open airway is present. (If the possibility of spinal injury exists, this must be done in conjunction with appropriate cervical spine stabilization.) Whenever airway compromise is evident, it must be resolved. Once the airway is clear, respiratory effectiveness must be assessed. If the patient is not breathing enough to maintain adequate respiratory minute volumes, the paramedic must provide ventilatory support. Following that, circulatory effectiveness needs to be evaluated and measures taken to resolve any life-threatening deficiencies. In most cases, manual airway control, ventilation, and oxygenation should precede attempts to place an endotracheal tube. (This is particularly important when a patient has been "down" for several minutes before medical help arrived at the scene.) Manual efforts allow an initial correction of the hypoxic and hypercarbic states that are most likely present. However, due to the high pharyngeal pressures generated by most ventilatory support measures and devices, an endotracheal tube should be placed as soon as possible to prevent aspiration.

Whenever the paramedic must place his or her hands into a patient's mouth to perform airway management, protective latex gloves should be worn. Additionally, whenever there is a chance that bodily fluids will be splashed, the paramedic should don protective eyewear and, possibly, protective overalls. (See Figure 11-11.)

As stated earlier, the tongue is the most common cause of airway obstruction in an unconscious patient. Any of the following techniques may be attempted to open and maintain the airway. However, if cervical spine injury is suspected, the procedures should be applied as recommended in Chapter 15.

Head-Tilt/Chin-Lift

The preferred technique for opening an airway is the *head-tilt/chin-lift*. (See Figure 11-12.) This maneuver is considered superior to the head-tilt/neck-lift and other procedures, because direct manipulation of the jaw will lift the tongue and epiglottis up and out of their obstructing positions. Steps in performing the head-tilt/chin-lift are as follows:

1. With the patient supine, position yourself at the side.
2. Place one hand on the patient's forehead and tilt the head back by applying firm downward pressure with your palm.

* The endotracheal tube should be placed as soon as is practical in the nonbreathing patient.

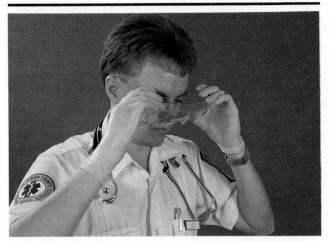

FIGURE 11-11 Protective equipment—gloves and goggles—should be worn when performing airway maneuvers.

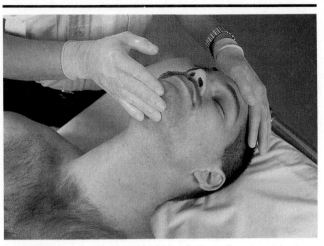

FIGURE 11-12 The head-tilt/chin-lift is an effective method to open the airway if cervical injury is not suspected.

3. Use your other hand to grasp the chin, placing your thumb on the anterior mandible and your index finger on the inferior mandible. This should be done without applying undue pressure on the jaw. Be particularly careful to keep your fingers on the bony part of the chin. This will avoid compressing the soft tissues underneath, an act that can lead to airway obstruction.

4. Lift the jaw anteriorly to open the airway. (See Figure 11-13.)

Jaw-Thrust

This is another useful technique for opening an airway. (See Figure 11-14.) When employed with the head-tilt and retraction of the lower lip, it is referred to as the triple airway maneuver. Steps in performing the

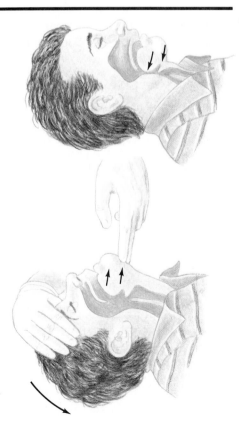

FIGURE 11-13 The head-tilt/chin-lift maneuver effectively elevates the tongue, opening the airway.

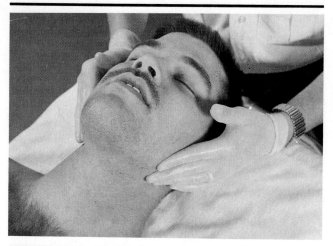

FIGURE 11-14 The jaw-thrust maneuver is also effective in opening the airway.

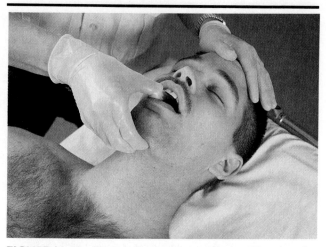

FIGURE 11-15 The jaw-lift maneuver is effective. However, the paramedic must use caution, as it requires that fingers be placed in the mouth.

jaw-thrust are as follows:

1. With the patient supine, kneel at the top of his or her head.
2. Place the fingertips of each hand on the angles of the patient's lower jaw.
3. Forcefully displace the jaw forward, while gently tilting your patient's head backward.
4. Retract the patient's lower lip with your thumbs.

Jaw-Lift

The *jaw-lift* may be used to open an airway. However, it should be employed carefully, as the paramedic must place his or her fingers in the patient's mouth. (See Figure 11-15.) Steps used in performing the jaw-lift are as follows:

1. With the patient supine, position yourself at his or her side.
2. Use one hand to grasp the jaw, placing your thumb on the lower incisor and positioning your index finger on the inferior mandible.
3. Pull the jaw anteriorly to open the airway.

Chin-Lift or Jaw-Thrust Without Head-Tilt

In trauma patients who may have spinal injuries, initial attempts to open the airway should be done while the head is in a neutral position. (See Figure 11-16.) Chin-lift or jaw-thrust techniques can often be successful without the head-tilt. If the airway remains obstructed, then the head-tilt should be added slowly and gently until the airway is open.

Any of these maneuvers should be tried before airway adjuncts are employed, and ideally there should be two rescuers involved. Airway adjuncts should be deferred, because activation of the gag, cough, or swallowing mechanisms (potential side effects of airway devices) may cause significant cardiovascular stimulation and increase intracranial pressure. In some situations, such as those involving a spontaneously breathing patient, opening the airway may be all that is required.

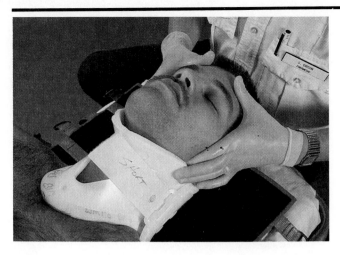

FIGURE 11-16 In cases of trauma, or if cervical spine injury is suspected, the chin-lift without head-tilt should be employed. This can be performed with rigid cervical collars in place.

When an airway adjunct is necessary, you have a variety to choose from, some offering more features and complications than others.

Oropharyngeal and Nasopharyngeal Airways

Both the oropharyngeal and nasopharyngeal airways are designed to lift the base of the tongue forward and away from the posterior oropharynx. An *oropharyngeal airway* is inserted into the mouth, while a *nasopharyngeal airway* fits into the nostril. With either airway in place, the proper head position is still important, as oropharyngeal and nasopharyngeal airways only assist with maintaining an open airway.

The oropharyngeal airway is a semicircular device, made of plastic or rubber and designed to conform to the curvature of the palate. It is used to hold the base of the tongue away from the posterior oropharynx. When properly positioned, it allows air to pass around and through the tube, countering obstruction by teeth and lips. The oropharyngeal airway is particularly useful in managing an unconscious patient who is breathing spontaneously or who needs to be ventilated by a bag-valve-mask device or other ventilatory apparatus. It makes suctioning of the pharynx easy, as a large suction catheter can pass on either side. It can be used as a block to prevent a patient from biting down on and closing an endotracheal tube.

There are, however, disadvantages to using an oropharyngeal airway:

- ❑ It does not isolate the trachea.
- ❑ It cannot be inserted when the teeth are clenched.
- ❑ It may obstruct the airway if it is not inserted properly.
- ❑ It can be dislodged easily.

Use of an oropharyngeal airway is inadvisable with conscious or semiconscious patients who have a gag reflex, as its insertion may stimulate vomiting (by stimulating the posterior tongue gag reflexes) or laryngospasm.

Oropharyngeal airways come in a number of sizes, ranging from #0 (for infants) to #6 (for large adults). Selecting the proper size for your task is important, because an airway that is too long can press the epiglottis against the entrance of the larynx, resulting in airway obstruc-

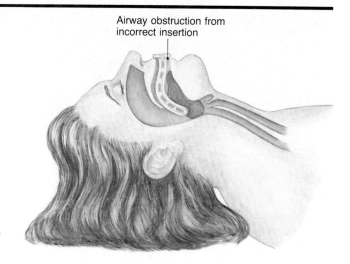

Airway obstruction from incorrect insertion

FIGURE 11-17 Improper placement of the oropharyngeal airway can cause airway obstruction.

tion. (See Figure 11-17.) An airway that is too small will not hold the tongue forward. Measure the airway by placing its flange beside the patient's cheek, parallel to the front teeth. A properly sized airway will extend from the patient's mouth to the angle of his or her jaw. To insert the oropharyngeal airway (See Figure 11-18):

1. Hyperextend the patient's head and neck.
2. Assure or maintain effective ventilatory function; if indicated, **hyperventilate** the patient with 100 percent oxygen.
3. Grasp the patient's tongue and jaw, and lift anteriorly.
4. With your other hand, hold the airway at its proximal end and insert it into the mouth. Make sure the curve is reversed, with the tip pointing toward the roof of the mouth.
5. Once the tip reaches the level of the uvula, the airway should be turned 180 degrees until it comes to rest over the tongue.
6. Verify appropriate position of the airway. (Clear breath sounds and chest rise indicate correct placement).
7. Hyperventilate the patient with 100 percent oxygen (if indicated).

Make sure the airway is correctly positioned. Improper placement can push the tongue back against the posterior oropharynx, thus obstructing the airway. (An indicator of improper placement is when the tube advances out of the mouth during ventilatory efforts.) An alternative method of inserting the device is to use a tongue blade to depress the tongue while pushing the airway past it.

The *nasopharyngeal airway* is an uncuffed tube that's made of soft rubber or plastic. (See Figure 11-19.) Ranging from 17 to 20 cm long, its diameter ranges from 20 to 36 french. At its proximal end is a funnel-shaped projection, which helps prevent the tube from slipping inside a patient's nose and becoming lost or aspirated. The distal end is bevel-shaped to facilitate passage. The nasopharyngeal airway is designed to follow the natural curvature of the nasopharynx, passing through the nose and extending from the nostril to the posterior pharynx just below the base of the tongue. (See Figure 11-20.) The nasopharyngeal airway is used to relieve soft-tissue upper airway obstruction in cases where use of an oropharyngeal airway is not advised.

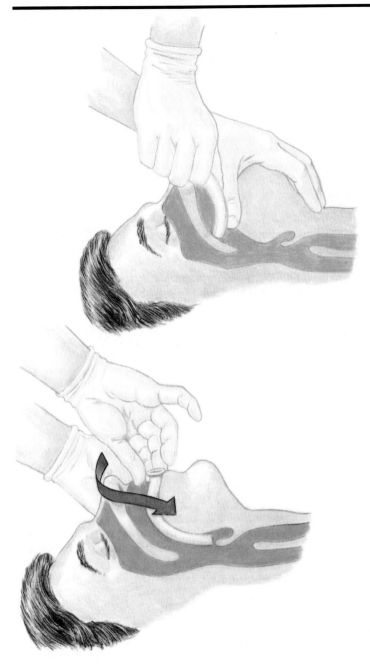

FIGURE 11-18 The oropharyngeal airway should be inserted in a twisting manner. It is an effective airway adjunct in the unresponsive patient.

Advantages of the nasopharyngeal airway:

- ❏ It can be rapidly inserted.
- ❏ It bypasses the tongue.
- ❏ It may be used in the presence of a gag reflex.
- ❏ It can be used when the patient has suffered injury to his or her oral cavity (anything from trauma to the mandible or maxilla, to significant soft tissue damage to the tongue or pharynx).
- ❏ It can be used when the patient's teeth are clenched.

Disadvantages of the nasopharyngeal airway:

- ❏ It is smaller than the oropharyngeal airway.
- ❏ It does not isolate the trachea.

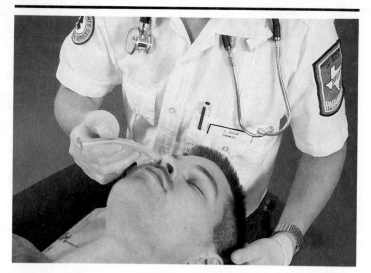

FIGURE 11-19 The nasopharyngeal airway is easy to insert and usually well-tolerated by the patient. It should not be used if basilar skill fracture is suspected.

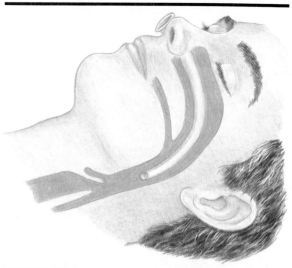

FIGURE 11-20 The nasopharyngeal airway rests between the tongue and the posterior pharyngeal wall, thus maintaining an open airway.

❑ It is difficult to suction through.
❑ It may cause severe nosebleeds if it's inserted too forcefully.
❑ It may cause pressure necrosis of the nasal mucosa.
❑ It may kink and clog, obstructing the airway.
❑ It is difficult to insert if nasal damage (old or new) is present.
❑ It cannot be used if there is a basilar skull fracture.

Cases when the use of a nasopharyngeal airway are not advisable include those involving patients who are predisposed to nosebleeds or who have a nasal obstruction. The nasopharyngeal airway should not be used in the presence of a basilar skull fracture, as the tube can inadvertently pass into the brain.

The proper-sized airway is slightly smaller in diameter than the patient's nostril; it is equal to or slightly longer than the distance from the patient's nose to his or her earlobe. Selecting the appropriate size is important, because too small a tube will not extend past the tongue, and one that is too long may pass into the esophagus and result in hypoventilation and gastric distension with artificial ventilation.

Steps in inserting a nasopharyngeal airway:

1. Hyperextend the patient's head and neck.
2. Assure or maintain effective ventilatory function. If indicated, hyperventilate the patient with 100 percent oxygen.
3. Lubricate the exterior of the tube with a water-soluble gel to prevent trauma during insertion. If possible, use a lidocaine gel in the conscious or semiconscious patient, because its anesthetic effect on the mucosa will make insertion more comfortable.
4. Push up on the tip of the nose and pass the tube into the right nostril. Avoid pushing against any resistance, as this may cause tissue trauma and airway kinking. In some cases, when the septum is deviated and insertion into the right nostril cannot be accomplished, the left nostril must be used.
5. Verify appropriate position of the airway. (Clear breath sounds and chest rise indicate correct placement; also feel for airflow at the proximal end of the device on expiration).
6. Hyperventilate the patient with 100 percent oxygen, if indicated.

While semiconscious patients tolerate use of a nasopharyngeal airway better than they do an oropharyngeal one, it may precipitate vomiting and laryngospasm. Insertion of the nasopharyngeal airway may injure the nasal mucosa, leading to bleeding, aspiration of clots into the trachea, and the need for suctioning to remove the secretions or blood. Forceful insertion of the airway may lacerate the adenoids, causing considerable bleeding.

Esophageal Obturator Airway

The *esophageal obturator airway (EOA)* is a large-bore, flexible tube, approximately 37 cm long. (See Figure 11-21.) Its proximal end is open, and it has a rounded and closed distal end. Upon its insertion into the esophagus, a distal cuff—inflated with 30 to 35 mL of air—will close the esophagus, preventing regurgitation. Ventilations are delivered through the open end, which is housed in a detachable clear-plastic mask. When a proper seal is maintained between the patient's face and the EOA mask, air exits the tube through 16 holes located at the level of the hypopharynx. Although endotracheal intubation is the preferred technique for managing the airway, the esophageal obturator airway is an alternative in cases where personnel are not trained or permitted to perform endotracheal intubation; where the equipment to perform endotracheal intubation is not available or not working; or where endotracheal intubation is not technically possible or desirable. Because insertion of the EOA will stimulate the gag reflex, this device should only be used to secure and maintain a patent airway in an unconscious patient. If the patient becomes responsive, the device must be removed. (See Figure 11-22.)

✱ The preferred technique for managing the airway of an unconscious patient is by endotracheal intubation.

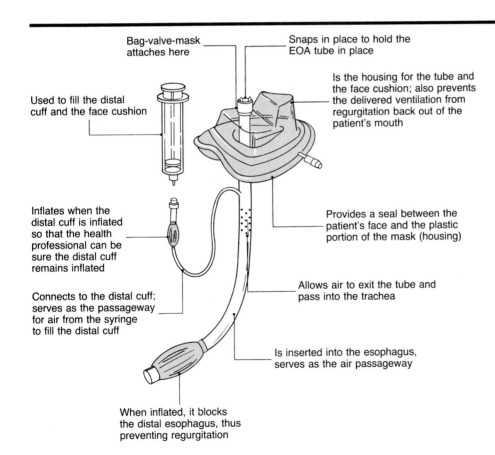

Bag-valve-mask attaches here

Snaps in place to hold the EOA tube in place

Is the housing for the tube and the face cushion; also prevents the delivered ventilation from regurgitation back out of the patient's mouth

Used to fill the distal cuff and the face cushion

Inflates when the distal cuff is inflated so that the health professional can be sure the distal cuff remains inflated

Provides a seal between the patient's face and the plastic portion of the mask (housing)

Connects to the distal cuff; serves as the passageway for air from the syringe to fill the distal cuff

Allows air to exit the tube and pass into the trachea

Is inserted into the esophagus, serves as the air passageway

When inflated, it blocks the distal esophagus, thus preventing regurgitation

FIGURE 11-21 The Esophageal Obturator Airway (EOA).

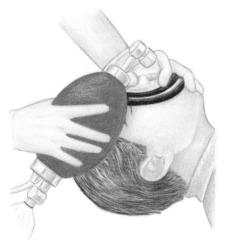

FIRST; Hyperventilate the patient with a bag-valve-mask and 100% oxygen

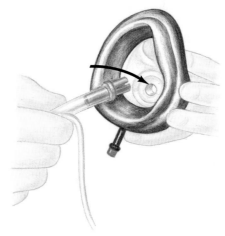

SECOND; Attach the EOA mask to the tube

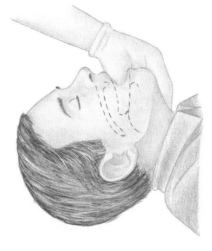

THIRD; Use the tongue-jaw lift to prepare for insertion

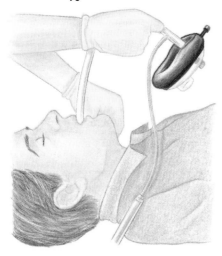

FOURTH; Insert the tube blindly into the mouth

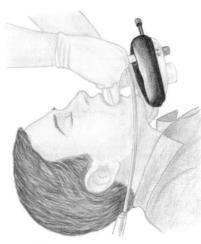

FIFTH; Insert the tube in the midline, following the natural curvature of the pharynx

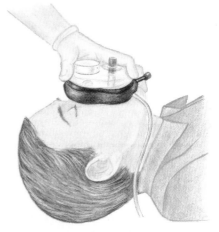

SIXTH; Pass the tube directly into the esophagus advance it until the mask rests on the patient's face

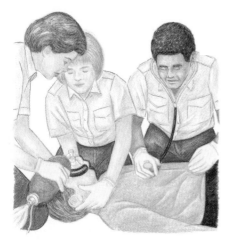

SEVENTH; check for proper placement of EOA mask

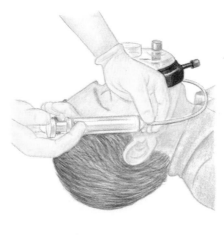

EIGHTH; Inflate the distal cuff with 30-35 ml of air

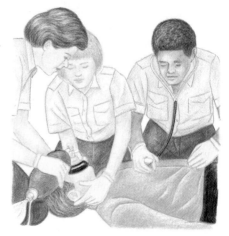

NINTH; Recheck the proper placement of EOA mask

FIGURE 11-22   Insertion of the EOA.

Advantages of the esophageal obturator airway:

- ❏ It is easy to insert and does not require that the paramedic see the larynx.
- ❏ It prevents gastric distension and regurgitation.
- ❏ It delivers ventilations at the level of the hypopharynx.
- ❏ It can be used on trauma victims who may have spinal injuries, as there is no need for hyperextension or flexion of the neck during insertion.
- ❏ It makes it easier to insert an endotracheal tube, as there is only one passageway remaining.
- ❏ A high oxygen concentration can be delivered through the device.

Two potential hazards associated with use of the EOA, however, are accidental endotracheal placement and pharyngeal or esophageal trauma. Since the tube is closed at its distal end, placement in the trachea will block airflow into the lungs. Ventilatory effectiveness, then, must be checked immediately after insertion of this device (even before inflation of the distal cuff). A rising chest and breath sounds will indicate that the tube has been placed properly in the esophagus. To prevent accidental insertion of the device into the trachea and esophageal laceration, a number of rules must be followed:

1. The patient's head and neck must be placed in a neutral position or flexed forward, because a hyperextended position may inadvertently direct the tip of the tube anteriorly into the trachea.
2. A tongue-jaw-lift should be used with one hand, while the device is inserted with the other.
3. When inserting the device, grasp it between the upper and middle thirds of the tube, in the same way that you would grasp a pencil. This facilitates gentle maneuvering of the tube posteriorly and reduces the risk of pharyngeal trauma.
4. The tube must be stored in a natural position. Small storage compartments may inadvertently curl the tube, thus increasing the likelihood that it will aim upward into the trachea during insertion.
5. Never use force during insertion of the tube. Whenever you meet resistance, withdraw the device slightly, improve the jaw-lift, and readvance the tube. This will avoid pharyngeal and esophageal trauma.
6. And finally, the amount of air used to inflate the distal cuff should be considered patient-dependent, with smaller patients needing less.

A third problem with using an EOA is that it's difficult to maintain an effective seal between the mask and the patient's face. The EOA may, therefore, fail to deliver adequate ventilatory volumes, a difficulty that may come up also when using the bag-valve-mask device.

Use of the esophageal obturator airway is contraindicated when treating:

- ❏ persons under the age of 16
- ❏ persons under 5 feet or over 6 feet, 7 inches tall
- ❏ persons who may have ingested caustic poisons
- ❏ persons who have a history of esophageal disease or alcoholism

The esophageal obturator airway should be used with caution in patients who may be suffering from drug overdose (which can be reversed by naloxone) or hypoglycemia (which can be treated with dextrose), because improvements in mental status may activate the gag reflex and lead to vomiting. Also, the EOA does nothing to protect a patient from aspirating foreign materials that are present in the mouth and pharynx. Appropriate suctioning techniques must be used to clear the airway.

Steps to inserting an esophageal obturator airway (See Procedure 11-1):

1. While maintaining ventilatory support, hyperventilate the patient with 100 percent oxygen.
2. Assemble and check the equipment.
3. Connect the tube to the mask. The tube is seated properly when its proximal end clicks into place on the mask.
4. Pull back on the plunger of the syringe and draw in 30 to 35 mL of air. Attach the syringe to the one-way valve of the inflation tube. (It is beneficial to tape the inflation tube to the EOA tube to prevent it from being accidentally severed). When inserting the tip of the syringe into the inflation valve, use a twisting action to seat it properly.
5. Place the patient's head in a neutral position.
6. With your left hand, grasp the patient's jaw in your fingers. Insert your thumb deep into the subject's mouth behind the base of the tongue.
7. Lift the jaw and tongue anteriorly away from the posterior pharynx.
8. With your right hand, grasp the esophageal obturator tube between its upper and middle thirds, holding it in a J-shaped position.
9. Insert the EOA over the patient's tongue, with the tube in the midline; follow the natural curvature of the pharynx.
10. Continue inserting the tube until the mask rests on the patient's face. If resistance is met, withdraw the tube and try again.
11. Attach a ventilatory device to the 15 mm connector, and deliver a breath. Look for chest rise and listen for breath sounds. If chest rise and breath sounds are absent with ventilation, suspect placement into the trachea, and withdraw the tube.
12. If the patient's chest rises and breath sounds are present, inflate the distal cuff with 30 to 35 mL of air. Check the pilot bulb to verify that air is inflating the distal cuff. (A filled pilot balloon indicates that the distal cuff is inflated).
13. Remove the syringe from the one-way valve, using a reverse twisting action to prevent accidental loss of air.
14. While hyperventilating the patient, recheck the EOA's placement, chest rise, and breath sounds, and auscultate over the stomach.

Keep in mind that when the esophageal obturator is fully inserted, its distal cuff typically lies below the level of the carina (where the trachea divides into right and left mainstem bronchi). However, in some cases the cuff will lie above the level of the carina. Inflation of the distal cuff in these cases may cause tracheal obstruction as the posterior membranous portion of the trachea is compressed. Check for this problem if breath sounds and chest rise, which were present prior to distal cuff inflation, disappear after 30 to 35 mL of air are introduced. To resolve the problem, withdraw air from the distal cuff until effective ventilations are restored. It may be necessary to remove the esophageal obturator airway if there is any indication that the obstruction remains.

When ventilating a patient with the EOA in place, the subject's head should still be tilted backward in order to maintain an open airway, unless trauma is suspected. Use of a lubricant is usually unnecessary in the field, as there are sufficient secretions to allow for easy passage of the device. If the patient's upper airway is dry, lubricate the distal end of the obturator with a water-soluble gel.

In some circumstances, it may be necessary to remove the EOA in the field setting. Note that patients may vomit when the device is removed, so place the patient on his or her side and have suction readily available.

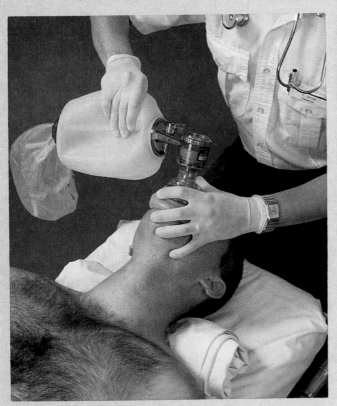

11-1A.   Hyperventilate the patient.

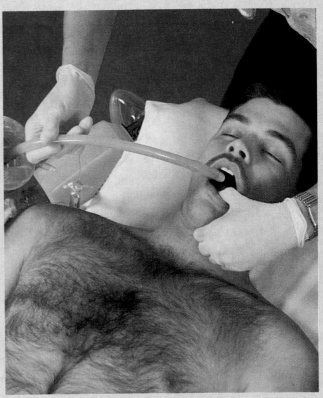

11-1B.   Flex the head slightly and insert the airway.

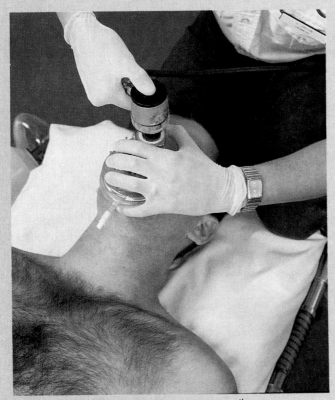

11-1C.   Seal the face mask and attempt to ventilate.

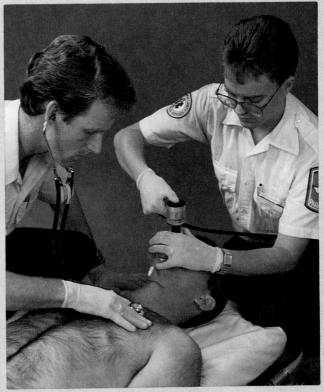

11-1D.   Assess the quality of ventilations.

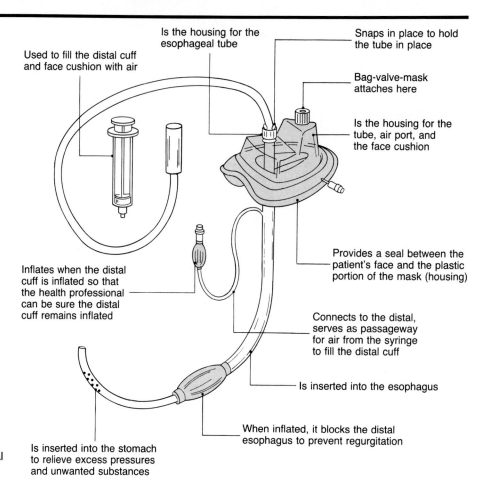

Used to fill the distal cuff and face cushion with air

Is the housing for the esophageal tube

Snaps in place to hold the tube in place

Bag-valve-mask attaches here

Is the housing for the tube, air port, and the face cushion

Inflates when the distal cuff is inflated so that the health professional can be sure the distal cuff remains inflated

Provides a seal between the patient's face and the plastic portion of the mask (housing)

Connects to the distal, serves as passageway for air from the syringe to fill the distal cuff

Is inserted into the esophagus

When inflated, it blocks the distal esophagus to prevent regurgitation

Is inserted into the stomach to relieve excess pressures and unwanted substances

FIGURE 11-23 The Esophageal Gastric Tube Airway (EGTA).

Ideally, an endotracheal tube will be in place to protect the airway from aspiration. To remove the EOA, deflate its distal cuff and withdraw the tube in a steady and gentle manner.

Esophageal Gastric Tube Airway

The *esophageal gastric tube airway (EGTA)* is an alternative to the EOA. (See Figure 11-23.) An EGTA's primary advantage is that it allows for suctioning of the patient's stomach contents, so gastric distension can be alleviated prior to removal of the device.

The EGTA consists of an inflatable face mask and a tube, which is open throughout its length to permit passage of a gastric (Levine) tube necessary for decompression of the stomach. The transparent face mask has two ports: one for attachment of the esophageal tube, and the other—a standard 15 mm connector—which serves as the ventilation port. During ventilation, air is blown into the upper port of the mask. With the esophagus blocked, air has nowhere to go but into the trachea and lungs. The technique for insertion and the complications in using an EGTA are the same as those presented by the EOA.

Pharyngeo-tracheal Lumen Airway (PtL)

Several new devices are available to assist in airway management. Among the more popular is the *pharyngeo-tracheal lumen airway (PtL)*. (See Figure 11-24.) This device can be described as a two-tube system. The first

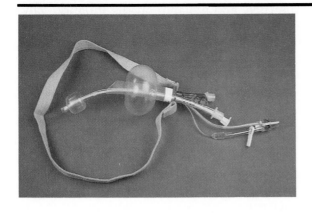

FIGURE 11-24 The Pharyngeo-tracheal Lumen (PtL) airway.

tube is short and wide (green in color at the proximal end), and has a balloon situated along its lower third. When inflated, this balloon seals the entire oropharynx. Air introduced through the tube at the proximal end will enter the pharynx. The second, clear tube travels through the first one, and extends approximately 10 cm past its distal end. This second tube may be inserted into either the trachea or the esophagus, and it has a distal cuff that is inflated to seal off whichever anatomical structure contains it. When the second tube is in the esophagus, the patient will be ventilated via the first tube. When the second tube is in the trachea, the patient will be ventilated through it. The PtL can be inserted blindly and placed when the patient's head is in a neutral position. (See Figure 11-25.) Thus, it is useful in cases that may involve spinal injury. Because of the oropharyngeal balloon, this device eliminates the need for a face mask, so it presents no problems in dealing with a patient who has sustained facial trauma or burns. Additionally, the pharyngeo-tracheal lumen airway may also protect the trachea from upper airway bleeding and secretions. Its other features include: a 15/22mm connector at the proximal end of each tube, which allows for the attachment of a standard ventilatory device; a semi-rigid plastic stylet housed in the clear plastic tube,

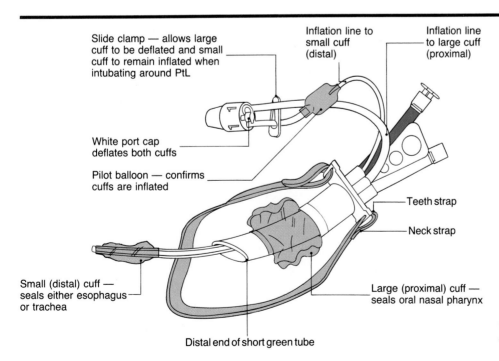

Slide clamp — allows large cuff to be deflated and small cuff to remain inflated when intubating around PtL

Inflation line to small cuff (distal)

Inflation line to large cuff (proximal)

White port cap deflates both cuffs

Pilot balloon — confirms cuffs are inflated

Teeth strap

Neck strap

Small (distal) cuff — seals either esophagus or trachea

Large (proximal) cuff — seals oral nasal pharynx

Distal end of short green tube

FIGURE 11-25 The PtL airway is designed for blind insertion.

allowing for redirection of the tube; and a clamp on the inflation valve that permits deflation of the oropharyngeal cuff while the other cuff remains inflated. When the long, clear tube is positioned in the esophagus, deflation of the cuff in the oropharynx allows the device to be moved to the left side of the patient's mouth. This permits endotracheal intubation while continuing esophageal occlusion. The device also has an adjustable, cloth neck strap that holds the tube in place.

Steps for inserting the pharyngeo-tracheal lumen airway are as follows:

1. While maintaining ventilatory support, hyperventilate the patient with 100 percent oxygen.
2. Assemble and check the equipment.
3. Place the patient's head into the appropriate position. Use a hyperextended position if there are no potential spinal injuries. In the presence of possible spinal injury, maintain the patient's head and neck in neutral position, while a fellow team member provides in-line stabilization.
4. Insert the device using a tongue-jaw lift.
5. Once it is in place, inflate the PtL's distal cuffs simultaneously with a sustained breath fed into the inflation valve (referred to as valve #1).
6. Deliver a breath into the green, or oropharyngeal, tube. If the patient's chest rises, the long clear tube is in the esophagus and ventilations should be continued via the green tube.
7. If the chest does not rise, it means the long, clear tube is in the trachea. In this case, remove the stylet from the clear tube and ventilate the patient through the tube.
8. Attach a ventilatory device to the 15 mm connector and continue delivering ventilatory support. Reassess for proper placement on an ongoing basis. (See Figure 11-26.)

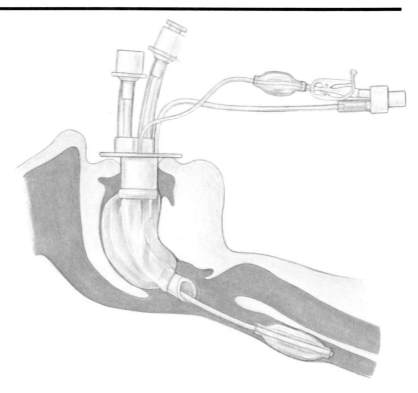

FIGURE 11-26 The PtL airway in place.

Sellick's Maneuver

Gastric regurgitation occurs all too often during ventilatory support and intubation efforts. As stated earlier, vomitus that enters the airway can be a severe complication. To prevent regurgitation, employ a simple procedure referred to as the *Sellick's maneuver*. (See Figure 11-27.) In this procedure, slight pressure—directed posteriorly—is applied over the cricoid cartilage. Since the esophagus lies just behind the cricoid, this exertion against the cartilage at the front will close off the esophagus to pressures as high as 100 cm/H_2O. (To locate the cricoid cartilage, palpate the depression just below the thyroid cartilage, or Adam's apple. This depression is the cricothyroid membrane. The prominence just below this membrane is the cricoid cartilage.)

Using the thumb and index finger of one hand, apply pressure to the anterior and lateral aspects of the cartilage just next to the midline. More pressure is required to prevent regurgitation than gastric distention.

This technique is valuable when you're providing ventilatory support (with a bag-valve-mask device or demand valve resuscitator), and during endotracheal intubation attempts.

Endotracheal Intubation

Endotracheal intubation means the placement of an open-ended tube directly into the trachea. This is the preferred technique for managing a patient's airway in the field setting. However, it is a sophisticated skill which should only be performed by persons trained and proficient in the procedure.

Endotracheal intubation is used to secure an open airway when a patient is experiencing, or is likely to experience, upper airway compromise. This includes patients who:

- ❑ are in respiratory or cardiac arrest
- ❑ are unconscious and without a gag reflex
- ❑ have a decreased tidal volume, due to decreased respiratory rate or volume
- ❑ may have an airway obstruction due to foreign bodies, trauma, or anaphylaxis

There is only one type of case in which endotracheal intubation is inadvisable: in the presence of epiglottitis, when attempts at endotracheal intubation may precipitate laryngospasm. Some local protocols, though, do

✳ Sellick's maneuver may be effective in preventing regurgitation during attempts at placing an endotracheal tube.

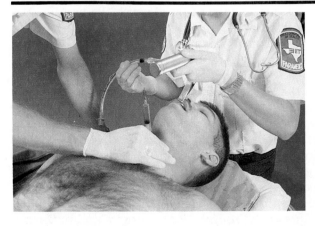

FIGURE 11-27 Sellick's maneuver (anterior cricoid pressure) is effective in preventing gastric regurgitation.

permit endotracheal intubation in patients who are experiencing epiglottitis and whose condition is worsening.

Endotracheal intubation offers a number of advantages:

❑ Complete control of the airway is achieved, since the trachea is isolated. Most other airway devices do nothing to prevent blood, vomitus, and other foreign materials from being aspirated into the trachea. When the endotracheal tube is in place and the cuff is inflated, the trachea is sealed against aspiration of these elements.

Since air is passed directly into the trachea, gastric distension is prevented.

❑ Most other procedures require that an effective seal be maintained between the patient's face and the mask of a ventilatory device. No such problem exists with endotracheal intubation, as the tube is placed directly into the trachea. Ventilating the patient in this manner is much easier and more efficient.

❑ With a direct route into the respiratory passageway, the trachea can be easily suctioned.

❑ Medications (such as epinephrine, atropine, lidocaine, and naloxone) can be administered via the endotracheal tube. This is particularly useful in the presence of peripheral vascular collapse, which often occurs with cardiac arrest.

Endotracheal intubation is accomplished either orotracheally or nasotracheally. Endotracheal intubation can also be accomplished digitally, via the orotracheal route. Equipment and supplies used to perform endotracheal intubation include: a laryngoscope (handle and blade); an appropriately sized endotracheal tube; a 10 mL syringe; a stylet; a bag-valve-mask device; a suction device; a bite block; Magill forceps; and tie-down tape or a commercial tube-holding device.

The *laryngoscope* is an instrument for lifting the tongue and epiglottis out of the way, so that the vocal cords can be seen. Typically, it is used in placing an endotracheal tube, but may also be used in conjunction with Magill forceps to retrieve a foreign body obstructing the upper airway.

A laryngoscope consists of a handle and blade. The handle is made of a reusable or a disposable material. It houses several batteries, which power a light that's located in the distal third of the laryngoscope blade. This light illuminates the airway, making it easier for the paramedic to see upper airway structures. The attachment point between the handle and blade is the "fitting." When connected, it locks the blade in place and provides electrical contact between the batteries and the bulb.

In preparing for intubation, the indentation of the laryngoscope's blade is attached to the bar of the handle. It will click into place when properly seated. (See Figure 11-28.) To determine if the laryngoscope is functional, the blade should be elevated to a right angle with the handle. (See Figure 11-29.) If properly positioned, the light should go on, bright white and steady. A yellow, flickering light will not sufficiently illuminate anatomical structures. If the light fails to go on, the problem may be with either the batteries (are they dead?) or the bulb (is it loose?). Infrequently, the failure is in the contact point(s) or the wire that travels through the blade to the bulb.

The laryngoscope blade is made of either a reusable or a disposable material. Two common types of blades are the *curved* (or MacIntosh) blade and the *straight blade* (often referred to as the Miller, Wisconsin, or Flagg blade). (See Figures 11-30, 11-31, 11-32.) Laryngoscope blades come in a variety of sizes, ranging from 0 (for the infant) to 4 (for the large adult patient). The curved blade is designed to fit into the *vallecula*. When the handle is lifted anteriorly, it elevates the tongue and indirectly

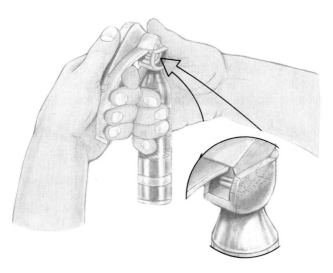

FIGURE 11-28 Engaging the laryngoscope blade.

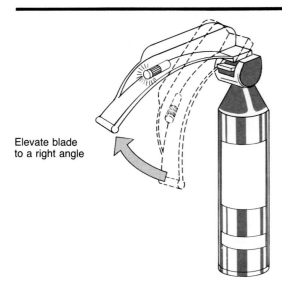

Elevate blade to a right angle

FIGURE 11-29 Elevating the laryngoscope blade to activate the light source.

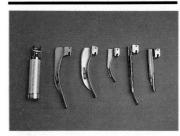

FIGURE 11-30 Laryngoscope blades.

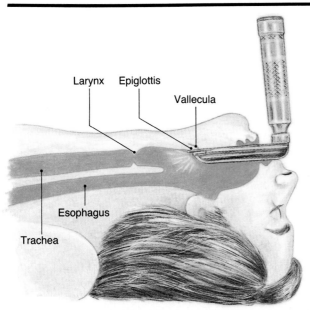

Larynx Epiglottis

Vallecula

Esophagus

Trachea

FIGURE 11-31 The straight blade should be used to elevate the epiglottis.

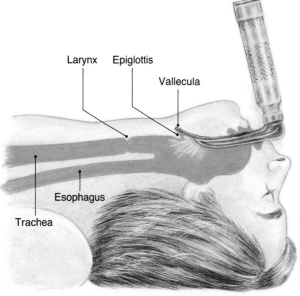

Larynx Epiglottis

Vallecula

Esophagus

Trachea

FIGURE 11-32 The curved blade should be gently guided into the vallecula so as to indirectly elevate the epiglottis.

elevates the epiglottis, allowing the medic to see the glottic opening. Because the curved blade does not touch the larynx itself, it should not traumatize or accidentally stimulate the very sensitive gag receptors located on the posterior surface of the epiglottis. The curved blade also permits more room for viewing and tube insertion. The straight blade, on the other hand, is designed to fit under the epiglottis. When its handle is lifted anteriorly, it directly lifts the epiglottis up and out of the way. A straight blade is preferred in treating infants, since it provides greater displacement of the tongue and better visualization of the glottis.

There are advantages and disadvantages to each type of blade, of course, and use of one over the other depends largely on individual preference. The paramedic should be skilled in the use of both blades, though, as patient peculiarities sometimes call for the specific use of one type.

The *endotracheal tube* is flexible, translucent, approximately 35 to 37 cm long, and open at both ends. (See Figure 11-33.) The proximal end features a standard 15/22 mm adapter, which attaches to a ventilatory device, while the distal end has an inflatable 5- to 10-mL cuff that's used to seal the trachea. Air from a syringe used to fill the distal cuff is pushed through a thin inflation tube, which runs the length of the main tube and empties into the distal cuff. At the proximal end of the inflation tube is a valve that permits air to enter the distal cuff without allowing it also to leak inadvertently. A pilot balloon, located between the one-way valve and the distal cuff, indicates whether the distal cuff has inflated. The distal cuff should always be checked for leaks prior to insertion.

An endotracheal tube is typically supplied prewrapped in a curved shape. The reason for this shape is that the trachea lies anteriorly in the neck; in most patients the tube must be directed upward if it's to pass through the glottic opening. Some endotracheal tubes are equipped with an O-shaped ring that connects to a plastic wire. This wire runs the length of the tube and terminates distally. When the ring is pulled, the distal end of the tube bends upward, helping to redirect the angle of the distal end of the tube and allowing for passage into the glottic opening.

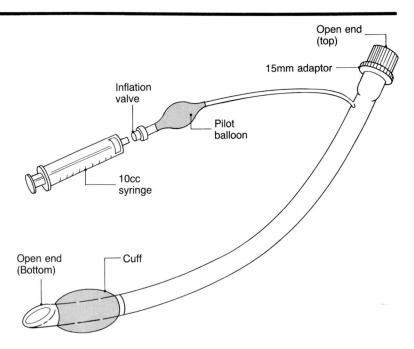

FIGURE 11-33 The endotracheal tube.

Endotracheal tubes come in a variety of sizes. Markings on the tube indicate the internal diameter (i.d.) in millimeters. The table below lists the typical tube sizes for average-sized patients:

✱ The endotracheal tube may be sized to approximate the diameter of the patient's little finger.

Newborn	2.5 to 3.5 i.d.
Infant	3.5 to 4.0 i.d.
Child	4.0 to 6.0 i.d.
Adult	7.0 to 9.0 i.d. (females 7.0 to 8.0 i.d.; males 7.5 to 8.5 i.d.)

In an emergency, a good standard-size endotracheal tube for both adult female and male patients is 7.5 i.d.

Noncuffed endotracheal tubes are usually used with infants and children under the age of 8, because the round narrowing of the cricoid cartilage will serve as a suitable cuff in those cases. Selection of the appropriate tube diameter for children is critical. Tube size can be correctly determined by measuring the outside diameter of the tube against the diameter of the child's smallest finger. A tube that is too large can cause tracheal edema and/or damage to the vocal cords, while too small a tube may not allow for delivery of adequate ventilatory volumes. A tube that is too small may also produce a negative pressure in the lungs, which can lead to pneumothorax and pulmonary edema.

The *malleable stylet* is a metal wire covered with plastic. (See Figure 11-34.) It is used to direct the endotracheal tube anteriorly when a patient's larynx and trachea lie pronouncedly forward and in cases where the patient has a short, fat neck that makes optimal positioning of the head difficult. The stylet allows the endotracheal tube to be pulled into a J or hockey stick shape. (See Figure 11-35.) Because it is a wire, the stylet may inadvertently cause tissue damage during intubation attempts if it is allowed to extend past the distal end of the endotracheal tube. So, when inserting the stylet into the endotracheal tube, the wire's distal end should be recessed at least one-half inch from the tip of the tube. A stylet is not employed in all cases, but it should be readily available in those where the tube needs to be directed anteriorly.

A tie-down or umbilical tape is used to secure the endotracheal tube in place once it has entered the trachea. The reasons for securing the endotracheal tube are twofold. First, during the process of resuscitation and transportation, when the patient is being moved about, the tube can be dislodged easily. Even when the tube isn't dislodged, movement can still cause injury to the tracheal mucosa, cardiovascular stimulation, and an elevation in intracranial pressure. Second, the person providing ventilatory support may accidently push down on the endotracheal tube, forcing it into the right or left mainstem bronchus. Tying the tube in place prevents this accidental movement or displacement. Tying is preferred over taping, as tape tends to loosen when either the patient's face or the tube is moist. A number of commercial tube-holding devices are also available.

The *Magill forceps* are scissor-style clamps with circle-shaped tips. (See Figure 11-36.) It is used to remove foreign materials or redirect the endotracheal tube during nasotracheal intubation.

Water-soluble lubricants help facilitate the tube's insertion.

A *suction unit* should be available, in order to remove secretions and foreign materials from the oropharynx during intubation attempts. (This is particularly important, since the patient in cardiac arrest often has large volumes of secretions.)

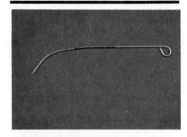

FIGURE 11-34 Stylet for use during endotracheal intubation. It should be formed into the desired shape to facilitate use.

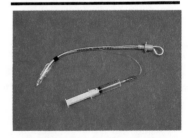

FIGURE 11-35 Cuffed endotracheal tube with the stylet in place.

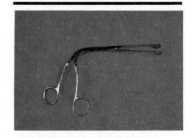

FIGURE 11-36 McGill forceps.

An oropharyngeal airway should also be on hand during an endotracheal intubation. It is used as a block to prevent the patient from biting down on and collapsing the endotracheal tube.

Orotracheal Route Using a Laryngoscope.   The most common route for performing endotracheal intubation is through the mouth. An orotracheal procedure allows the paramedic to see the upper airway and glottic opening, using a laryngoscope, and then gently and accurately pass the endotracheal tube through the vocal cords.

Steps for performing endotracheal intubation, using the orotracheal route and when no spinal injuries are suspected, are as follows (See Procedure 11-2):

1. While maintaining ventilatory support, hyperventilate the patient with 100 percent oxygen.

2. Assemble and check your equipment. Pull back on the plunger of the syringe and draw in 5 to 10 mL of air. Attach the syringe to the one-way inflation valve on the distal cuff, using a twisting action to properly seat the syringe. Tape the inflation tube to the endotracheal tube to prevent it from being accidentally severed.

3. Place the patient's head and neck in an appropriate position. To achieve direct visualization of the larynx, the three axes—those of the mouth, the pharynx, and the trachea—must be aligned. To establish this alignment, place the patient's head into a "sniffing position." This is accomplished by flexing the patient's neck forward and the head backward, and perhaps by also inserting a rolled towel under the patient's shoulders or the back of the head. Establishing this position is extremely difficult in patients with short, fat necks or whose motion is limited by such conditions as arthritis.

4. Hold the laryngoscope in your left hand. Most laryngoscopes are designed for right-handed persons; that is, the right-handed person must hold it in his or her left hand in order to use the right one for manipulating the endotracheal tube.

5. Insert the laryngoscope blade into the right side of the patient's mouth. With a sweeping action, displace the tongue to the left. This pushes the tongue out of your line of vision and allows more room to manipulate the endotracheal tube.

6. Move the blade slightly toward the midline, and advance it until the distal end is positioned at base of tongue. Simultaneously, move the patient's lower lip away from the blade using the index finger of your right hand.

7. Lift the laryngoscope handle slightly and move it forward to displace the jaw but not put pressure on the teeth. At this point vomitus, or secretions lying in the posterior pharynx can usually be seen, and suctioning is necessary to clear the airway. If suctioning fails to resolve the airway obstruction, placing the patient on his or her side will facilitate drainage of the secretions. It may be necessary to insert an esophageal obturator airway to prevent further regurgitation of stomach contents.

8. Look for the tip of the epiglottis, and place the laryngoscope blade into its proper position. If you're using a curved blade, direct its tip into the vallecula. With a straight blade, extend it behind the epiglottis and lift. Frequently, the blade tip will not be perfectly positioned when the lifting maneuver is first employed. The epiglottis should come into view, unless the blade has been inserted too deeply. If you suspect that this has happened, withdraw the blade until you can again see the epiglottis. On the other hand, the blade may need to be advanced. To do this, place your right thumb in the patient's mouth, grasp the chin, and lift the jaw while advancing the laryngoscope.

9. With your left wrist straight, use your shoulder and arm to continue lifting the mandible and tongue at a 45-degree angle to the ground until the glottis

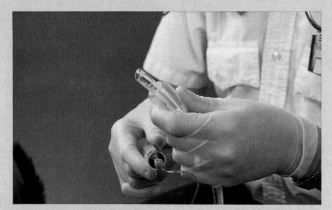

11-2A. Prepare equipment.

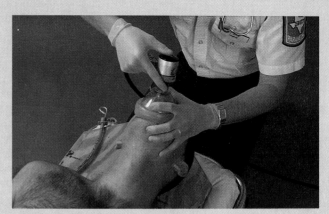

11-2B. Hyperventilate the patient.

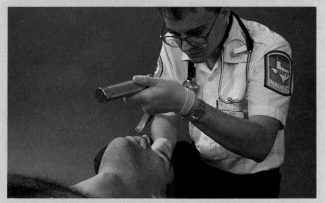

11-2C. Insert the laryngoscope.

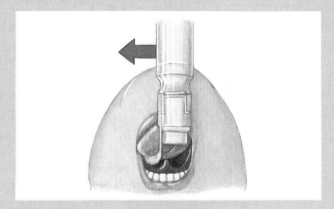

11-2D. Slide the tongue to the left.

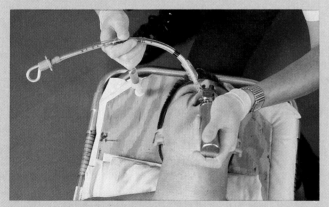

11-2E. Visualize the larynx.

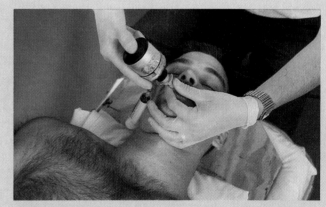

11-2F. Insert the tube, and ventilate.

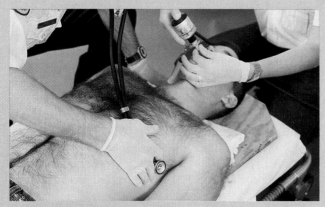

11-2G. Assess ventilations.

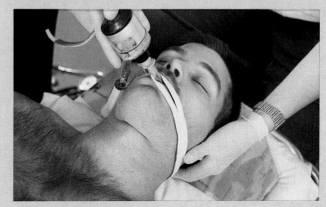

11-2H. Secure the tube.

is exposed. Often the glottis will not be seen in its entirety, but at least its posterior third or half should be visible. If the larynx lies anteriorly, you may want another member of your team to apply firm downward pressure on the patient's neck in the region of the cricoid cartilage (the Sellick's maneuver). This will push the larynx backward, allowing a better view. A stylet may prove useful in this situation, as the tube can be redirected anteriorly.

10. Grasp the endotracheal tube in your right hand, holding it as you would a pencil. This permits gentle maneuvering of the tube. It may also help you hold the tube so that the curve is in a horizontal plane (bevel sideways). Advance the tube through the right corner of the patient's mouth. Typically, you must direct the device's distal end up or down in order to pass it into the larynx.

11. Under direct observation, insert the endotracheal tube into the glottic opening and pass it through until the distal cuff disappears past the vocal cords. Then advance it another half-inch or full inch.

12. Hold the tube in place with your hand to prevent its accidental displacement. Attach a bag-valve device to the 15/22 mm adapter on the tube and deliver several breaths.

13. Check for proper tube placement. Watch to see that the chest rises and falls with each ventilation, and listen for equal, bilateral breath sounds in the chest. There should an absence of sounds over the epigastrium when ventilations are delivered.

14. Inflate the distal cuff with 5 to 10 mL of air. To avoid tracheal trauma due to excessive cuff pressure, use only enough air to fill the distal cuff. Determine the minimum amount of air needed by listening for air leakage around the tube prior to distal cuff inflation. The cuff should be filled only to the point where this leakage ceases. When removing the syringe, use a reverse twisting action to prevent any accidental leakage of air.

15. Recheck for proper tube placement. Observe the chest's rise and fall. Listen for breath sounds. Also check the proximal end of the tube for breath condensation during each exhalation. Condensation is simply the moisture present in exhaled air. It should disappear each time the patient breathes in or a ventilation is delivered. The absence of breath condensation during exhalation suggests improper placement of the tube. (Recheck tube placement any time the patient is moved.)

16. Hyperventilate the patient with 100 percent oxygen. Insert an oropharyngeal airway to serve as a bite block.

17. Secure the endotracheal tube with umbilical tape, while maintaining ventilatory support. Loop the tape around the tube at the level of the patient's teeth, attaching it tightly to the tube without kinking or pinching it. Then wrap the tape around the patient's head and tie it at the side of the neck.

18. Continue supporting the tube manually while maintaining ventilations. Check periodically to ensure proper tube positioning.

One problem that can occur while attempting to visualize the cords is bringing your face too close to the patient's. This makes it difficult to properly identify the anatomical structures and may make it difficult to insert the tube.

While endotracheal intubation is the preferred technique for managing the airway, there are a number of disadvantages associated with its use. Endotracheal intubation requires that the person performing the procedure be sufficiently trained and experienced in its application. It also demands specialized equipment, the retrieval of which can slow efforts to secure the airway. The time lost is increased when the equipment malfunctions—for instance, when a laryngoscope fails to light. Use of an airway kit or "intubation wrap" reduces time loss, as all of the necessary equipment and supplies are readily available. To eliminate surprise equipment failures, the kit and all its contents should be inspected at the begin-

✳ To ensure the equipment functions and is readily available it should be tested before each shift and kept together in one kit or airway wrap.

ning of every work shift. In volunteer settings, where specific coverage is not provided, the equipment should be checked at least once a week. These inspections are effective in reducing equipment malfunction.

Injury to the tissues or teeth can occur when the intubation equipment is not handled carefully. This hazard can be eliminated, however, using the laryngoscope as an instrument, not a tool. When inserting this device into the mouth and pharynx, be sure to guide it gently into place, avoiding accidental pressure on the teeth. When manipulating the jaw anteriorly, use upward traction rather than a rotation and flexing of your wrist, as that will cause the laryngoscope to function as a lever. As all levers require a fulcrum, and the only fulcrums available in this case will be the patient's upper incisors, a rotating/flexing action may break teeth. To avoid this hazard, lift the laryngoscope's handle (exposing the epiglottis) after the blade is applied to the base of the tongue. After this, the left wrist should remain straight, and any lifting should be done by the shoulder and arm.

Inadvertent delays in oxygenation prior to successful intubation result from lengthy intubation efforts or failure to provide ventilatory support between procedures. Hypoxia may occur during endotracheal intubation, due to the inexperience of the operator. The uniqueness of each patient's anatomy and unusual clinical situations can challenge even the most experienced paramedic. So follow one basic rule during intubation: Each attempt should be limited to 30 seconds. To gauge this time, some paramedics hold their breath from the point at which they stop ventilating a patient until ventilatory support is reinitiated. Note that it is seldom necessary to place the endotracheal tube on your first attempt. That initial effort should at least give the paramedic a "lay of the land," some orientation to the patient's anatomy. Placing the tube can be accomplished in some subsequent attempt (each of which is scheduled between hyperventilations, using a bag-valve-mask device and 100 percent oxygen).

A catastrophic complication associated with endotracheal intubation is unrecognized misplacement of the tube into the esophagus, the pyriform sinus, or one of the mainstem bronchi.

If the endotracheal tube is inserted too anteriorly, it may lodge in the vallecula; if it strays from the midline, it can get hung up on either side of the epiglottis, in the pyriform sinus. These errors will cause the skin to "tent up" on either side of the laryngeal prominence. Forceful efforts can perforate these tissues, leading potentially to serious bleeding and **subcutaneous emphysema.** In the case of misplacement in the pyriform sinus, the problem can be resolved by slightly withdrawing and rotating the tube to the midline.

Accidental misplacement of the tube into the esophagus will cut off the patient's ventilation or oxygenation. If not corrected, esophageal misplacement of the tube will lead to severe hypoxia and brain death.

Indications of esophageal intubation include:

❑ an absence of chest rise and breath sounds with ventilatory support
❑ gurgling sounds heard over the epigastrium with each breath delivered
❑ an absence of breath condensation in the endotracheal tube
❑ a persistent air leak, despite inflation of the tube's distal cuff
❑ cyanosis and a progressive worsening of the patient's condition
❑ **phonation** (any noise made by the vocal cords).

Correct placement of the endotracheal tube should be routinely and visually checked, using a laryngoscope. If there is any suspicion that the tube is in the esophagus, remove it immediately.

✱ Hyperventilate the patient before and after each attempt to place the endotracheal tube, and take no longer than 30 seconds for tube placement.

■ **subcutaneous emphysema** the presence of air beneath the skin (in the subcutaneous tissues), giving it a characteristic crackling sensation upon palpation.

■ **phonation** the process of generating speech and other sounds.

■ **intubation** to pass a tube into an opening of the body.

In some cases of esophageal intubation, vomitus will propel from the tube. This results from high gastric pressures brought on by resuscitation efforts, particularly by the several breaths that a paramedic may have delivered in order to check a patient for chest rise. When vomiting occurs, leave the tube in place; removing it may cause the vomitus to travel into the pharynx and be aspirated into the trachea. Instead, move the tube to one side of the mouth and ventilate your patient with a bag-valve-mask device until his or her trachea can be successfully intubated.

A number of commercially available devices also detect endotracheal placement of the tube. Some, attached to the proximal end of the tube, whistle with each expiration only when the tube is properly positioned. One new device, the End-Tidal CO_2 Detector, detects instead the presence of CO_2 in the expired air.

The End-Tidal CO_2 Detector, designed for single-patient use, contains a non-toxic chemical indicator that changes color in reaction to expired tracheal CO_2. The reversibility of this change allows a paramedic to determine when esophageal or tracheal intubation is finally successful. After six breaths from the patient, a yellow color on expiration indicates correct placement in the trachea, while purple shows that the device is misplaced in the esophagus.

✱ If breath sounds are absent or diminished on one side, suspect that the endotracheal tube is in too far.

Aside from misplacement of an endotracheal tube, there is also the problem of its being inserted too deeply. When it reaches the bifurcation of the trachea, it will pass into either the right or left mainstem bronchus. Endobronchial intubation results in one-lung ventilation and hypoxia. It is evidenced by breath sounds on one side of the chest but diminished or absent on the other. Poor compliance (felt when delivering ventilations with the bag-valve device), cyanosis, and other signs of hypoxia, such as cardiac dysrhythmias, may also indicate endobronchial intubation. To resolve the problem, withdraw the tube until breath sounds are again heard equally on both sides of the chest.

You can prevent the tube from being inserted too far if you follow a few guidelines:

1. Advance the distal cuff past the vocal cords no more than half an inch to one full inch
2. Once it is in this position, hold the tube in place with one hand, preventing it from being accidently pushed any further
3. Inflate the cuff and firmly secure the tube in place with umbilical tape or a commercial tube-holding device
4. Mark the side of the endotracheal tube at the level where it emerges from your patient's mouth. This will allow you to quickly identify any changes in tube placement.

Endotracheal Intubation with an EOA in Place. Given the prevalence of EOA use, there will be some situations in which the paramedic will have to place an endotracheal tube in a patient who has already been intubated with an EOA. While it's a somewhat cumbersome process, this is possible to do.

The steps for performing endotracheal intubation with an EOA in place are as follows:

1. While maintaining ventilatory support, hyperventilate the patient with 100 percent oxygen.
2. Assemble and check the equipment.
3. Place the patient's head and neck into their appropriate positions.
4. Hold the laryngoscope in your left hand.

5. Remove the EOA mask by pinching its obturator tube where it extends through the plastic housing, and then lifting the mask off. (See Figure 11-37.)

6. Insert your laryngoscope blade into the right side of the patient's mouth. With a sweeping action, displace the tongue and EOA tube to the left. Proceed with intubation in the usual manner. (See Figure 11-38.)

7. Under direct observation, insert the endotracheal tube into the glottic opening and pass it through until the distal cuff disappears past the vocal cords. Then advance the tube another half-inch to full inch. Appropriate precautions should be used to ensure that the tube is in the larynx, as the distensible esophagus can easily accommodate both the esophageal obturator and the endotracheal tube. (See Figure 11-39.)

8. Hold the endotracheal tube in place with one hand to prevent displacement. Then attach a bag-valve device to the 15/22 mm adapter of the tube and deliver several breaths.

9. Check for proper tube placement by observing breath sounds, chest rise, and the absence of sounds in the epigastrium when ventilations are delivered.

10. Inflate the distal cuff with 5 to 10 mL of air, and remove the syringe.

11. Recheck for proper placement of the tube.

12. Hyperventilate the patient with 100 percent oxygen.

13. Secure the endotracheal tube with umbilical tape while continuing to maintain ventilatory support.

14. With suction available, deflate the EOA's distal cuff. Then hold the endotracheal tube firmly in place while you steadily remove the EOA tube. The EOA tube must be extracted to prevent esophageal or tracheal damage, which may result from having two distal cuffs in place at the same time.

15. Maintain ventilatory support, checking periodically to ensure proper tube position.

Endotracheal Intubation in the Trauma Patient. Establishing and maintaining an open airway is a critical aspect of trauma care. It requires the use of special techniques, because the head and neck must be stabilized in a neutral, in-line position that will prevent spinal injuries. Endotracheal intubation is the preferred technique, as long as it can be accomplished without extension, rotation, or flexion of the neck. It must be emphasized that a cervical collar alone will not provide adequate stabilization of the cervical spine.

✳ The head and neck must be maintained in a neutral position during intubation if trauma and spine injury are suspected.

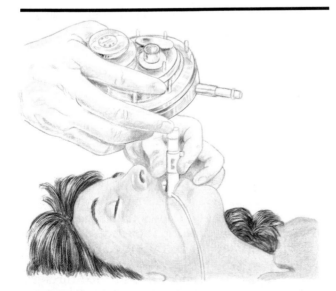

FIGURE 11-37 Remove the EOA mask.

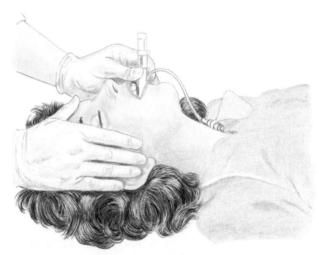

FIGURE 11-38 Move the EOA tube to the left side of the mouth.

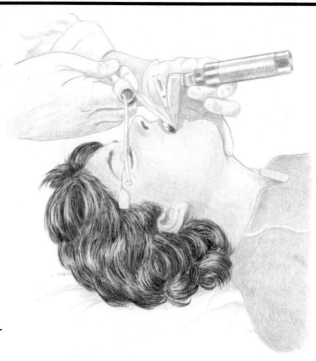

FIGURE 11-39 Perform endotracheal intubation.

There are several techniques for performing endotracheal intubation in the trauma victim, including: orotracheal intubation using in-line stabilization; nasotracheal intubation; digital intubation; and lighted stylet intubation.

Among the methods for performing orotracheal intubation using in-line stabilization, one has the paramedic assume a sitting position and then stabilize the patient's head between his or her thighs. This immobilizes the head and cervical spine while enabling the paramedic to see the glottic opening with a laryngoscope. Another calls for one team member to immobilize the head and spine while a second performs endotracheal intubation.

The steps involved in two people carrying out endotracheal intubation with in-line stabilization are as follows (See Procedure 11-3):

1. One team member assumes a position at the patient's side, facing the patient
2. He or she then places both hands over the patient's ears with the little, ring, and middle fingers under the occiput, the index finger over the tragus (the cartilaginous projection on the anterior ear), and the thumbs on the face over the maxillary sinuses

■ **caudally** of, at, or near the foot end of the body.

3. Slight pressure is applied **caudally** to support and immobilize the head
4. The paramedic charged with performing the intubation assumes a sitting position on the ground with each leg straddling one of the patient's shoulders
5. He or she then moves forward gently until the patient's head is secured between the thighs. At this point, firm pressure is applied with the thighs to the patient's head in order to prevent movement. The grip of both team members is extremely effective in preventing movement during intubation
6. The laryngoscope blade is inserted into the right side of the patient's mouth, and with a sweeping action, the tongue is displaced to the left. Intubation is continued in the manner described earlier.

Nasotracheal Intubation. The passing of an endotracheal tube through the nose and into the trachea is accomplished either "blindly" or by using

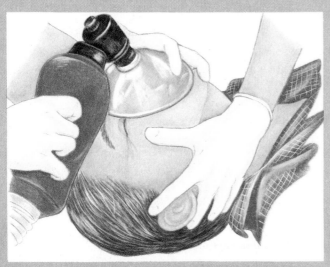

11-3A. Hyperventilate the patient with the cervical spine manually immobilized.

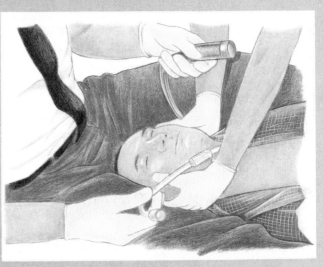

11-3B. Maintaining immobilization, prepare to visualize the airway.

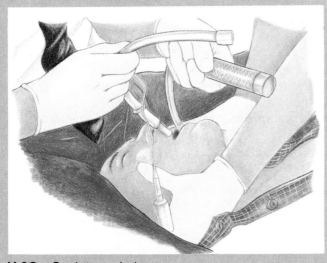

11-3C. Gently insert the laryngoscope.

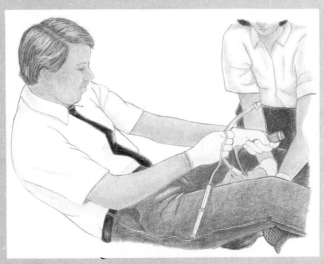

11-3D. Visualize the airway without moving the patient's neck.

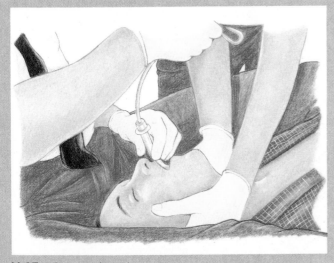

11-3E. Remove the stylet.

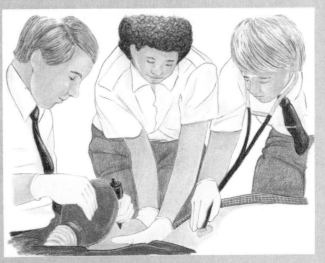

11-3F. Assess ventilations.

239

a laryngoscope. (See Figure 11-40.) Cases in which nasotracheal intubation is called for in the field include:

- those involving patients who may have spinal injuries
- those involving patients who are not in arrest or deeply comatose
- those in which the patient's mouth cannot be opened due to clenched teeth
- those involving a patient with a fractured jaw
- those involving oral or maxillofacial injuries
- those involving patients who have recently undergone oral surgery
- those that involve a severely obese patient or one whose neck arthritis prevents placing him or her into the sniffing position
- those involving a the patient who cannot be ventilated by another means

Nasotracheal intubation is not recommended in cases that involve nose fractures, basilar skull fractures, a deviated nasal septum, or nasal obstruction.

Advantages of nasotracheal intubation include:

- The tube can be placed while the patient's head and neck are immobilized.
- It is more comfortable for the patient than insertion of an oral endotracheal tube.
- The nasotracheal tube will not be bitten.
- The tube can be easily anchored.

Disadvantages of the procedure are that nasotracheal intubation is more difficult and time-consuming to perform than orotracheal intubation, and it is potentially more traumatic for patients. The tube may also kink or clog more easily than an oral endotracheal tube. Passage of the

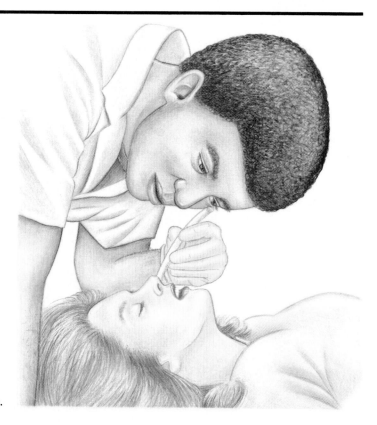

FIGURE 11-40 Blind nasotracheal intubation.

tube may lacerate the pharyngeal mucosa or larynx during insertion. It poses a greater risk of infection, because it introduces nasal bacteria into the trachea. It should not be attempted if a basilar skull fracture is suspected. Nasotracheal intubation is less predictable, as the tube cannot be seen as it passes through the glottic opening. And, finally, this method of intubation requires that the patient be breathing.

Blind Nasotracheal Intubation. Steps to performing blind nasotracheal intubation are as follows:

1. While maintaining ventilation, hyperventilate the patient with 100 percent oxygen.
2. Assemble and check your equipment, and lubricate the distal end of a proper-sized tube. If time permits, apply a local spray of 4 percent lidocaine (a topical anesthetic) mixed with 0.25 percent phenylephrine (a potent vasoconstrictor) to the nasal mucosa. This will make tube insertion more comfortable to the patient and reduce the amount of possible hemorrhage.
3. Place the patient's head and neck into a relaxed position. If spinal injury is suspected, maintain the head and neck in a neutral, in-line position.
4. Inspect the nose, and select the larger nostril as your passageway.
5. Insert your tube into the nostril, with the flanged end of the tube along the floor of the nostril or facing the nasal septum, in order to avoid damaging the turbinates. Then gently guide it in an anterior to posterior direction.
6. As the tube is felt to drop into retropharyngeal space, listen closely at its near end for the patient's respiratory sounds. These sounds are loudest when the tube is proximal to the epiglottis. Care must be taken when the tube tip reaches the posterior pharyngeal wall, because it must then be directed toward the glottic opening. At this point in the procedure, the tip of the tube may become "hung up" in the pyriform sinus. You can recognize this by the "tenting up" of skin on either side of the Adam's apple. Pyriform sinus placement is easily resolved by slightly withdrawing the tube and rotating it to the midline.
7. With the patient's next inhaled breath, advance the tube rapidly into the glottic opening, and then continue passing it until the distal cuff is just past the vocal cords. At this point, the patient may cough, buck, or strain. Gagging is a sign of esophageal placement, but bulging and anterior displacement of the larynx usually indicates correct placement of the tube. When correctly placed in the trachea, the patient's exhaled air will be felt coming from the proximal end of the tube. At the same time, breath condensation should intermittently fog the clear plastic tube.
8. Hold the tube in place with one hand to prevent displacement.
9. Inflate the distal cuff with 5 to 10 mL of air.
10. Recheck for proper placement of the tube by observing breath sounds, chest rise, and the absence of sounds over the epigastrium.
11. Hyperventilate the patient with 100 percent oxygen.
12. Secure the endotracheal tube with umbilical tape while continuing to maintain ventilatory support.

Even the most experienced paramedic will find patients in whom blind nasotracheal intubation is extremely difficult to perform. Either tube passage is stopped in the retropharynx, because the tube is angled away from the midline, or it passes posteriorly into the esophagus.

The route of a tube passing into the esophagus may be corrected if you extend the head further and then repeat the procedure. The tube can also be directed into the glottic opening using a laryngoscope and Magill forceps. (See Figure 11-41.) The procedure for this laryngoscopy is identical to that described for orotracheal intubation. With the glottic opening exposed, redirect the laterally malpositioned tube tip by rotating its proxi-

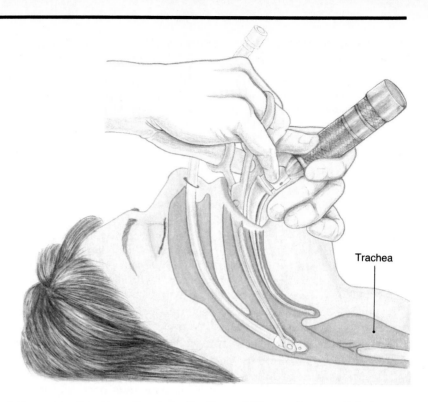

FIGURE 11-41 The McGill forceps are useful in performing nasotracheal intubation.

Trachea

mal end. After repositioning the tube in the midline, advance it between the vocal cords. In the case of a posteriorly directed tube that fails to pass through the glottic opening with repositioning, use the Magill forceps to grasp it and direct it anteriorly. While the operator holds the tube and manipulates it anteriorly, another member of the team or an assistant should carefully advance the tube by applying pressure on its proximal end. In this way, the operator is free to guide the tube without having to pull it along with the forceps.

Digital Intubation. During the 18th century, intubations were performed without the benefit of a laryngoscope. The technique used at the time was known as "digital" (finger) or "tactile" (touch) intubation. Today this procedure is still useful for a number of situations in the prehospital-care setting. Digital intubation is suggested when a patient is deeply comatose or in cardiac arrest, and when proper positioning is difficult to achieve. The classic example involves a trauma patient with suspected cervical spine injury. Since the digital technique does not require manipulation of the head and neck, it is of great value here, as it may also be in extrication situations where a patient cannot be properly positioned. Additionally, because this technique does not require visualization, it may be useful when patients have facial injuries that distort the anatomy or when copious amounts of blood, vomitus, or other secretions cannot be suctioned out for a proper view of the airway. (See Figure 11-42.)

The steps used in performing digital intubation are as follows:

1. While maintaining ventilatory support, hyperventilate the patient with 100 percent oxygen.
2. Assemble and check your equipment. Needed in this procedure are an appropriately sized endotracheal tube, a malleable stylet, water-soluble lubricant, a 5- to 10-mL syringe, a bite block, and latex examining gloves. Insert the stylet into the endotracheal tube and bend the tube/stylet into a J shape.
3. While a fellow team member or your partner stabilizes the patient's head and neck in an in-line position, kneel at the patient's left shoulder. Be sure you

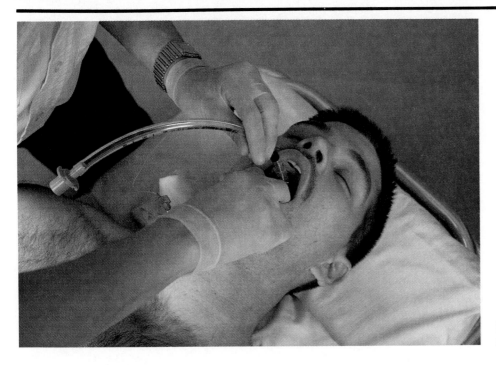

FIGURE 11-42 Blind Orotracheal intubation by the digital method.

are facing the patient. Place the bite block (or other such device) between the patient's molars to prevent injury to your fingers.

4. Insert the middle and index fingers of your left hand into the patient's mouth. (See Figure 11-43.) By alternating fingers, "walk" your hand down the midline, while simultaneously tugging forward on the tongue. This lifts the epiglottis up and away from the glottic opening, positioning it within reach of your probing fingers.

5. Palpate the epiglottis with your middle finger. (See Figure 11-44.)

6. Press the epiglottis forward and insert the endotracheal tube into the mouth anterior to your fingers. (See Figure 11-45.)

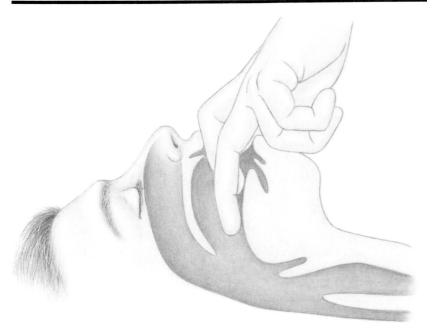

FIGURE 11-43 Insert the middle and index finger into the patient's mouth.

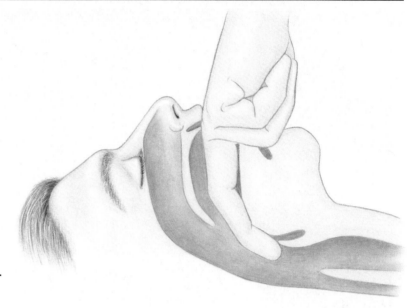

FIGURE 11-44 "Walk" the fingers down, and palpate the epiglottis with the middle finger.

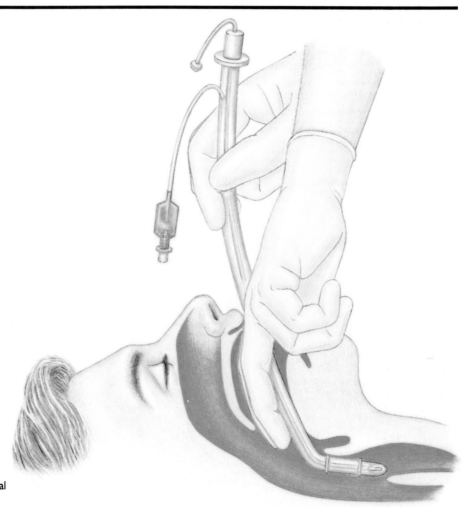

FIGURE 11-45 Insert the endotracheal tube while elevating the epiglottis.

7. Advance the tube, pushing it with your opposite hand. Then use your index finger to maintain the tip of the tube against the middle finger. This will direct the tip to the epiglottis.

8. Use your middle and index fingers to direct the tube tip between the epiglottis (in front) and the fingers (behind). Then, advance the tube through the cords, at the same time pressing the tube forward with the index and middle fingers to prevent it from slipping posteriorly into the esophagus.

9. Hold the tube in place with one hand. Attach a bag-valve device to the 15/22 mm adapter of the tube and deliver several breaths

10. Check for proper tube placement by observing breath sounds, chest rise, and the absence of sounds in the epigastrium when ventilations are delivered.

11. Inflate the distal cuff with 5 to 10 mL of air, and then remove the syringe.

12. Recheck for proper placement of the tube.

13. Hyperventilate the patient with 100 percent oxygen.

14. Secure the endotracheal tube with umbilical tape while you continue ventilatory support.

15. Maintain ventilation, periodically checking to ensure proper tube position.

Transillumination (Lighted Stylet) Intubation. Recently, another alternative concept in endotracheal intubation was introduced: the transillumination method. It is based on the assumption that a bright light, introduced into the larynx or trachea, can be seen shining through the soft tissues of a patient's neck. This allows the paramedic to pass an endotracheal tube through the glottic opening without having to directly visualize the structures. Endotracheal intubation can be performed in this way without manipulating the head and neck. The transillumination technique calls for a special device, known as a lighted stylet. (See Figure 11-46.) This stylet is a malleable, plastic-coated wire that features a small, high-intensity bulb at its distal end. Power for the device is supplied by a small battery housed at the proximal end, and is controlled by an on-off switch.

Several studies have shown the transillumination technique to be fast, dependable, and atraumatic. Because the head and neck do not have to be manipulated, it can be used in a trauma patient. The biggest problem associated with this method of intubation is that ambient illumination can make it difficult to see the stylet light. When attempting this procedure, then, ambient light should be reduced. The method works best in a dark-

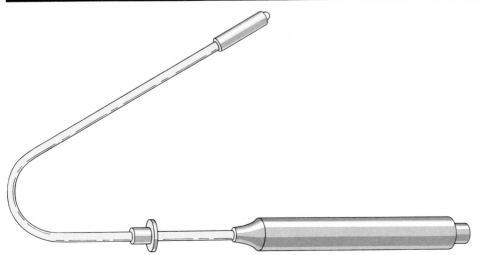

FIGURE 11-46 Lighted stylet for endotracheal intubation.

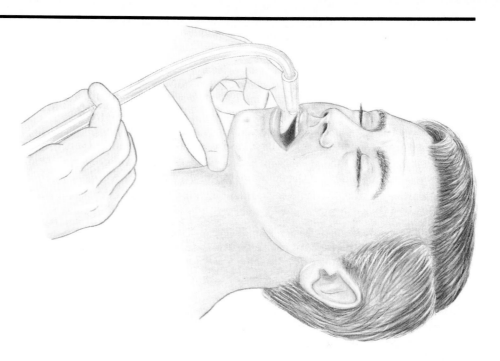

FIGURE 11-47 Insertion of the lighted stylet/endotracheal tube.

ened room and with thin patients. In direct sun or bright daylight, the patient's neck should be shielded.

Use the following steps to perform the transillumination technique (See Figure 11-47):

1. While maintaining ventilatory support, hyperventilate the patient with 100 percent oxygen.

2. Assemble and check your equipment. The endotracheal tube should be 7.5 to 8.5 i.d., and will need to be cut to 25–27 cm in order to accommodate the stylet. Place the stylet into the tube and bend it just proximal to the cuff.

3. Kneel on either side of the patient, facing his or her head.

4. Turn on the stylet light.

5. With your index and middle fingers inserted deeply into the patient's mouth and your thumb on the chin, lift the patient's tongue and jaw forward.

6. Insert the tube/stylet combination into the mouth and advance it through the oropharynx into the hypopharynx. (See Figure 11-48.)

7. Use a "hooking" action with the tube/stylet to lift the epiglottis out of the way.

8. When you see a circle of light at the level of the patient's Adam's apple, hold the stylet stationary. Advance the tube off the stylet into the larynx approximately one-half to one full inch. A diffuse, dim, or hard-to-see light indicates that the tube/stylet combination is in the esophagus. (See Figure 11-49.) A bright light that appears laterally to the upper aspect of the laryngeal prominence indicates that it has moved into the right or left pyriform fossa. Both of these situations can be corrected by withdrawing the tube and reattempting intubation after the patient has been ventilated with 100 percent oxygen for several minutes.

9. Hold the tube in place with one hand and then remove the stylet. Attach a bag-valve device to the 15/22 mm adapter of the endotracheal tube and deliver several breaths.

10. Check for proper tube placement by observing breath sounds, chest rise, and the absence of sounds in the epigastrium when ventilations are delivered.

11. Inflate the distal cuff with 5 to 10 mL of air.

12. Recheck for proper tube placement and continue delivering ventilations while securing the tube in place.

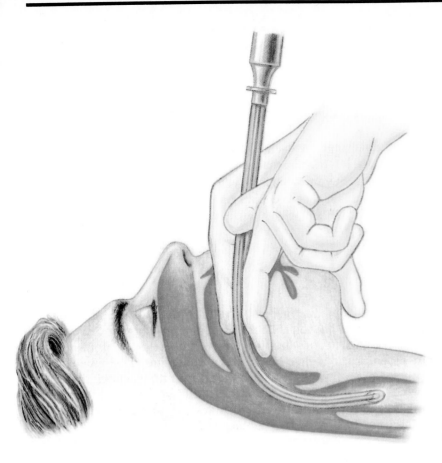

FIGURE 11-48 Lighted stylet/endotracheal tube in position.

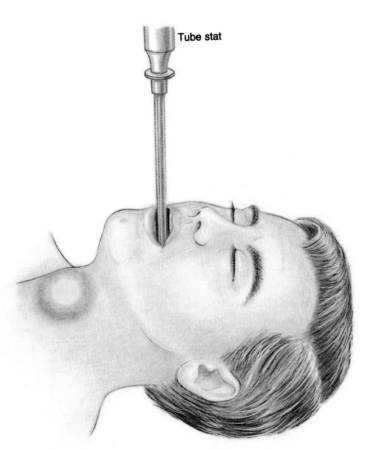

Tube stat

FIGURE 11-49 The light of the stylet, when in proper position, should be visible on the front of the patient's neck.

Endotracheal Intubation in Children. While the procedure for performing endotracheal intubation in children is similar to that used with adults, there are differences. These come as a result of differences in the anatomy of a child's airway. (See Figure 11-50.) Note that in the airway of a pediatric patient:

■ **cephalic** toward the head end of the body.

❏ the structures are proportionately smaller and more flexible than an adult's
❏ the tongue is larger in relation to the oropharynx
❏ the epiglottis is narrow and "floppy"
❏ the glottic opening is higher and more anterior in the neck
❏ the vocal cords slant upward, toward the back of the head (postero-**cephalic**) and they are closer to the base of the tongue
❏ the narrowest part of the upper airway is at the cricoid cartilage, not the glottic opening.

Also important to consider is that infants and small children are believed to have greater vagal tone. Therefore, laryngoscopy and passage of an endotracheal tube are more likely to precipitate a vaso-vagal response, dramatically slowing the child's heart rate and decreasing cardiac output and blood pressure. Heart rate must be monitored throughout the procedure to guard against this complication. If it falls below 60 beats per minute (or below 80 beats per minute in an infant), the procedure should be stopped and ventilations (with 100 percent oxygen) should be delivered.

The cases in which endotracheal intubation is called for in a pediatric patient are the same as those pertaining to adults: ventilatory support with a bag-valve-mask device seems inadequate; cardiac or respiratory arrest ensues; it is necessary to provide a route for drug administration or ready access to the airway for suctioning; or there is a need for pro-

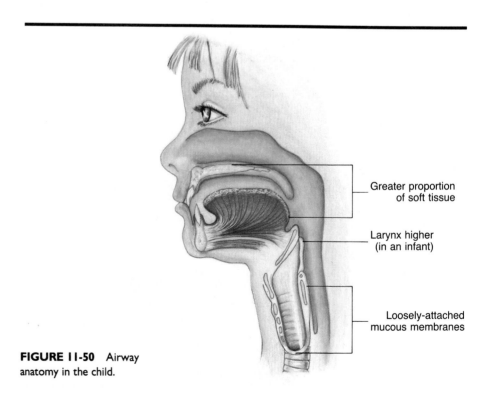

Greater proportion
of soft tissue

Larynx higher
(in an infant)

Loosely-attached
mucous membranes

FIGURE 11-50 Airway anatomy in the child.

longed artificial ventilation. Additionally, and if local protocols allow it, endotracheal intubation may be used in a child who's suffering from croup or epiglottitis and an increasingly compromised airway.

Steps used in performing endotracheal intubation on a pediatric patient are as follows (See Procedure 11-4):

1. While maintaining ventilatory support, hyperventilate the patient with 100 percent oxygen. If time allows, hyperventilate the patient for a full two minutes.

2. Assemble and check your equipment. As stated earlier, a straight blade laryngoscope is preferred with infants and small children, since it provides greater displacement of the tongue and better visualization of the relatively cephalad and anterior glottis. Also, with children younger than 8 years old, use a noncuffed endotracheal tube. Due to the distance between the mouth and the trachea, a stylet is rarely needed to properly position the tube.

3. Place the patient's head and neck into an appropriate position. With a pediatric patient, the head should be maintained in a "sniffing" position maintained by placing a towel under the head.

4. Hold the laryngoscope in your left hand.

5. Insert your laryngoscope blade into the right side of the patient's mouth. With a sweeping action, displace the tongue to the left.

6. Move the blade slightly toward the midline, and then advance it until the distal end is positioned at the base of the tongue.

7. Look for the tip of epiglottis and place the laryngoscope blade into its proper position. Keep in mind that in a child (and particularly an infant), the airway is shorter and the glottis sits higher than an adult's. Because of this, you'll see the cords much sooner than you expect.

8. With your left wrist straight, use your shoulder and arm to lift the mandible and tongue at a 45-degree angle to the floor until the glottis is exposed. Use the little finger of your left hand to apply gentle downward pressure to the cricoid cartilage. This will permit easier visualization of the cords.

9. Grasp the endotracheal tube in your right hand. To pass the tube into your patient's mouth it may be helpful to hold it so that its curve is in a horizontal plane (bevel sideways). Insert the tube through the right corner of the child's mouth.

10. Under direct observation, insert the endotracheal tube into the glottic opening and pass it through until its distal cuff disappears past the vocal cords—approximately 5 to 10 mm. As the tube is advanced, it should be rotated into the proper plane. It some cases, it will be difficult to advance an endotracheal tube at the level of the cricoid. Do not force the tube through this region, as it may cause laryngeal edema.

11. Hold the tube in place with your left hand. Attach an infant- or child-size bag-valve device to the 15/22 mm adapter of the tube and deliver several breaths.

12. Check for proper tube placement. Watch for the chest to rise and fall with each ventilation, and listen for equal, bilateral breath sounds. There should also be an absence of sounds over the epigastrium when ventilations are delivered.

13. If the tube used has a distal cuff, inflate the tube with the recommended amount of air.

14. Recheck for proper placement of the tube and hyperventilate the patient with 100 percent oxygen.

15. Secure the endotracheal tube with umbilical tape while maintaining ventilatory support.

16. Continue supporting the tube manually while maintaining ventilations. Check periodically to ensure proper tube position. As with adults, allow no more than 30 seconds to pass without ventilating your patient.

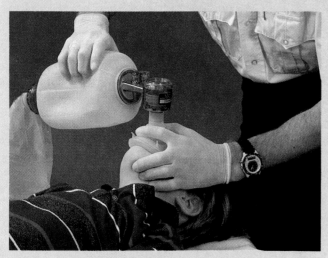

11-4A.   Hyperventilate the child.

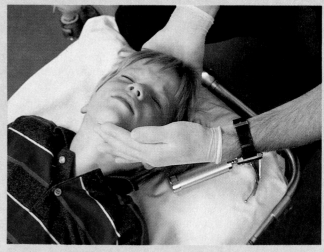

11-4B.   Position the head.

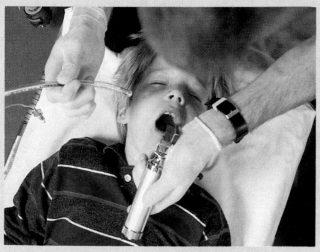

11-4C.   Insert the laryngoscope and visualize the airway.

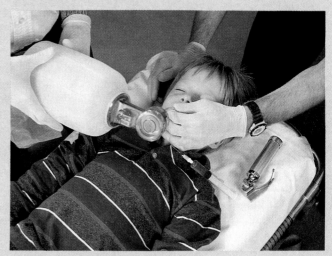

11-4D.   Insert the tube and ventilate the child.

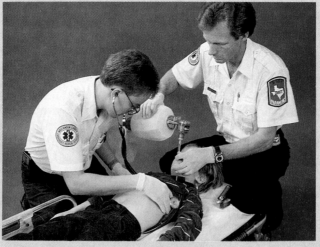

11-4E.   Confirm tube placement.

PERCUTANEOUS TRANSTRACHEAL CATHETER VENTILATION AND CRICOTHYROTOMY

As explained earlier, the larynx houses the vocal apparatus. The opening between the vocal cords, referred to as the glottic opening, or glottis, is the narrowest point along the upper airway. Foreign material, such as pieces of food, often become lodged here and obstruct the airway. Gag and other protective reflexes may restrict the airway, preventing the material from traveling deeper. Other conditions that cause laryngospasm or swelling of the vocal cords can also close the airway completely.

In cases where an upper airway obstruction cannot be relieved by conventional methods, it may be necessary to open a patent airway below the vocal cords to allow ventilation. Circumstances that make this appropriate may involve severe laryngeal edema, facial or upper laryngeal trauma, and an airway obstructed by a foreign body. Because the cricoid membrane does not have an extensive blood supply, it can be **cannulated** in a relatively bloodless manner, making it an excellent point of entry.

■ **cannulated** to have a tube inserted into a body duct or cavity.

The cricothyroid membrane can be located by palpating the patient's neck, starting at the top. (See Figure 11-51.) The first prominence felt will be the thyroid cartilage, while the second is the cricoid cartilage. The space between these two, noted by the small depression, is the cricoid membrane. (See Figure 11-52.)

Complications associated with penetrating the cricoid membrane to create an open airway include:

❑ It may produce hemorrhage at the insertion site, particularly if the thyroid is perforated.
❑ Faulty placement of the cannula into the subcutaneous tissues, rather than into the trachea may result in subcutaneous or mediastinal emphysema.

Percutaneous Transtracheal Catheter Ventilation

Percutaneous transtracheal catheter ventilation is the insertion of an over-the-needle catheter into the cricoid membrane, followed by intermittent jet ventilation. It is a temporary, last-resort procedure that provides oxygenation in cases where the patient is experiencing asphyxia due to

✱ Percutaneous transtracheal catheter ventilation is a temporary, last-resort procedure when all other methods of obtaining an airway have been unsuccessful.

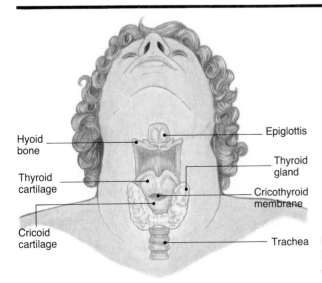

Hyoid bone
Thyroid cartilage
Cricoid cartilage
Epiglottis
Thyroid gland
Cricothyroid membrane
Trachea

FIGURE 11-51 Anatomical landmarks associated with the cricothyroid membrane.

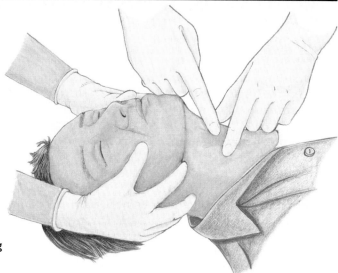

FIGURE 11-52 Locate the cricothyroid membrane by palpating inferior to the thyroid cartilage and superior to the cricoid cartilage.

some unresolved upper airway obstruction. Percutaneous transtracheal catheter ventilation takes only about 30 seconds to perform and can be done without interrupting resuscitative efforts. The equipment needed to carry out this procedure includes:

- ❏ a 14-gauge (or larger) over-the-needle catheter, preferably with side holes (See Figure 11-53.)
- ❏ a 5- or 10-mL syringe
- ❏ a manual jet ventilator device that is capable of delivering driving pressures of at least 50 psi
- ❏ a regulating valve attached to a high-pressure oxygen supply
- ❏ providone-iodine swabs
- ❏ adhesive tape or tie

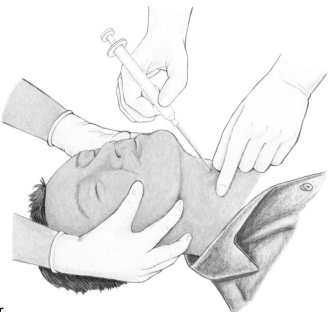

FIGURE 11-53 Perform the puncture with the 14-gauge catheter.

Steps in performing percutaneous transtracheal catheter ventilation are as follows:

1. While continuing efforts to ventilate and oxygenate your patient, place him or her into a supine position and hyperextend the head and neck. If spinal injury is suspected, the head and neck should be maintained in a neutral, in-line position. (See Figure 11-54.)

2. Locate the patient's cricothyroid membrane (See Figure 11-55.)

3. Prep the area quickly with povidone-iodine swabs.

4. Attach the 14-gauge (or larger) plastic catheter with a needle to the 5- or 10-mL syringe. The syringe can be can be filled with 1 to 2 cc of saline, in order to allow easy visualization of air entry after the trachea is penetrated.

5. Carefully insert the needle and catheter in the midline, through the patient's skin and membrane. Direct it downward and caudally at a 45-degree angle to the trachea. A pop can be felt as the needle penetrates the trachea.

6. Maintain negative pressure on the syringe as the needle and catheter are advanced. The needle has entered the patient's trachea when air readily fills the syringe.

7. Once in the trachea, advance the catheter over the full length of the needle until the catheter hub comes to rest against the skin.

8. Hold the hub of the catheter in place to prevent accidental displacement, and then remove both the needle and the syringe.

9. Reconfirm the position of the catheter by aspirating it again with the syringe.

10. Connect one end of the flexible tubing to the catheter hub, and the other to the oxygen source.

11. Open the release valve to introduce an oxygen jet into the trachea. Adjust the pressure to allow adequate lung expansion.

12. Watch the chest carefully, turning off the release valve as soon as the chest rises. Exhalation then occurs passively, due to the elastic recoil of the lungs and chest wall. A rate of at least 20 breaths per minute should be delivered. The inflation-deflation time ratio should approximate that of normal respiration, or 1:2.

13. Check for adequacy of ventilations. Look for chest rise with each ventilation, and listen for breath sounds in the chest.

14. Fasten the catheter hub securely to the skin and continue ventilatory support.

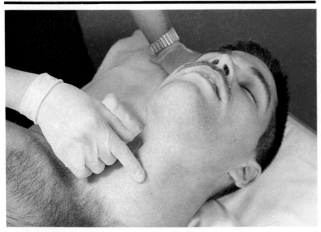

FIGURE 11-54 Palpate the cricothyroid membrane.

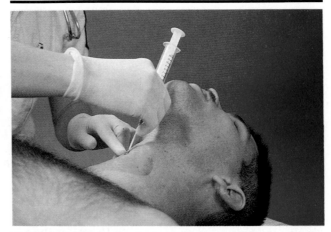

FIGURE 11-55 Position for performing a cricothyroid puncture.

Disadvantages of percutaneous transtracheal catheter ventilation:

❑ The high pressure generated during ventilation and air entrapment may rupture a patient's lungs.
❑ If the needle is inserted too far, it may perforate the esophagus.
❑ The procedure does not allow for direct suctioning of secretions.
❑ It may not allow for efficient elimination of carbon dioxide.

✱ For transtracheal ventilation via a large bore catheter to be successful, the airway must be partially open to allow for expiration.

Passive exhalation is achieved through the upper airway, so it must be at least partially open in order to avoid lung rupture during this procedure. In cases of complete upper airway obstruction, a second large-bore tracheal catheter needle should be inserted next to the first one. This will accommodate exhalations. It may also be necessary to provide intermittent suction to the catheter, promoting effective expiration. If the chest remains distended, a cricothyrotomy may be called for. When ventilating a patient via percutaneous transtracheal catheter ventilation, neither the bag-valve device nor the demand valve resuscitator should be used, as they cannot provide sufficient driving pressures. This makes clear another disadvantage to percutaneous transtracheal catheter ventilation: special equipment must be available in order to perform the procedure and maintain ventilations. Cricothyrotomy, then, may be preferred in some cases, as it can be done without restrictions.

Cricothyrotomy

Cricothyrotomy allows rapid entrance to a patient's airway for temporary ventilation and oxygenation. It is used in cases where airway control is not possible by other methods. *Cricothyrotomy* means making an incision in the cricoid membrane and placing an airway tube. Use the largest available cannula that does not cause injury to the larynx. A 6 mm (outside diameter) tracheostomy tube or similar-sized device can be used on adults, while a 3 mm (outside diameter) tube can be used on large children. The device should be equipped with a standard 15/22mm adapter for connecting a ventilatory device. A 12-gauge over-the-needle catheter may be employed with small children and infants.

The steps used to perform cricothyrotomy are as follows:

1. Place the patient on his or her back, and then hyperextend the head and neck.
2. Grasp the larynx with your thumb and middle finger. Locate the cricoid membrane with the index finger.
3. Prep the area quickly with providone-iodine swabs.
4. Make a horizontal incision—less than 1/2 inch long—with the scalpel, cutting through the patient's skin and the membrane. The incision should be made with the blade angled away from the head, lest there be injury to the vocal cords. (See Figure 11-56.)
5. Keeping your left hand on the larynx to stabilize it, insert the scalpel handle and rotate it 90 degrees to spread the cartilage.
6. Insert the small tube or cannula into the opening, making sure the tip points toward the patient's feet. (See Figure 11-57.) Use controlled force to advance it until the flange is flush with the skin.
7. Hold the catheter or tube to prevent accidental displacement.
8. Attach a bag-valve unit to the tube in order to provide oxygen and ventilations. (See Figure 11-58.)
9. Check for the adequacy of ventilations. Look for chest rise with each ventilation, and listen for breath sounds in the chest.

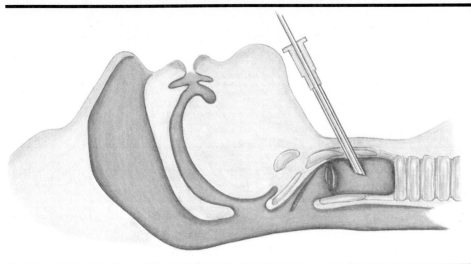

FIGURE 11-56 Cannula properly placed in the trachea.

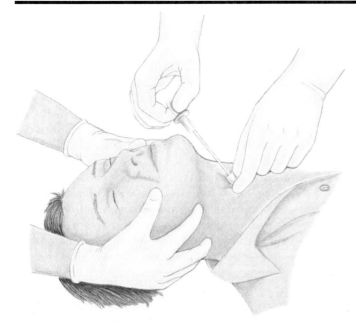

FIGURE 11-57 Advance the cannula.

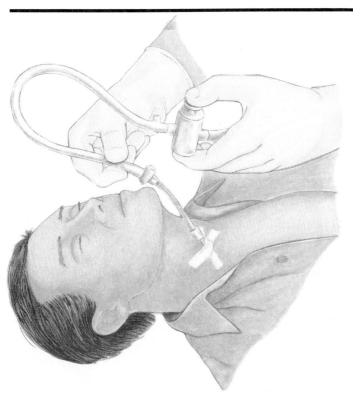

FIGURE 11-58 Ventilate the patient as shown.

10. When the catheter or tube is correctly positioned, secure it in place.

11. Continue providing ventilatory support.

One advantage in using cricothyrotomy is that it allows for suctioning.

SUCTIONING

In the field, an airway may be compromised by a number of elements. Suctioning will remove vomitus, blood, and other fluids and secretions from the airway.

A variety of devices are available for suctioning patients in the prehospital-care setting, including portable ones (hand-, foot-, oxygen-, and battery-powered) and stationary units (electrical or vacuum powered in connection with an engine manifold). The ones that are most effective in an emergency situation generate vacuum levels of at least 300 mmHg when the distal end is occluded and allow a flow rate of at least 30 liters per minute when the tube is open.

A pair of recently introduced units offer tremendous portability. One is hand operated, weighs only a pound or so, and is capable of generating excellent suctioning pressures. Because it is hand powered, this device can be used without concern for a power source, and its small size allows it to be stored easily in an airway kit. The other new portable suction device is powered by a rechargeable battery and offers excellent suctioning capabilities (550 mmHg with a flow rate in excess of 30 LPM).

The most common types of suction catheters used in prehospital-care settings are those with "tonsil tips" and "whistle tips." (See Figures 11-59 and 11-60.) The *tonsil tip,* or *Yankauer, suction* is a rigid tube with a large tip and multiple holes at its distal end. (A newer, large-bore version is open at the tip.) The tonsil tip catheter can remove larger particles and a greater quantity of secretions than the whistle tip variety. However, it can only be used to suction the upper airway, and its vigorous insertion can cause lacerations and other injuries. Tonsil tip devices are inserted along an oropharyngeal airway, or are used during laryngoscopy. On the other hand, the whistle tip suction catheter is a long, flexible tube that's easy to use, small, and can extend into the lower respiratory tract. Unfortunately, *whistle tip* catheters cannot remove large volumes of secretions rapidly, and are often unable to retrieve even small food particles. The whistle tip catheter can be inserted through the nares, into the orophar-

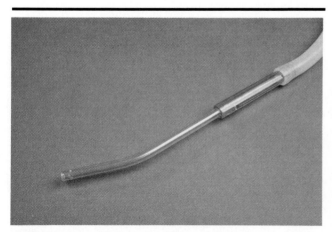

FIGURE 11-59 Yankauer "tonsil" suction device.

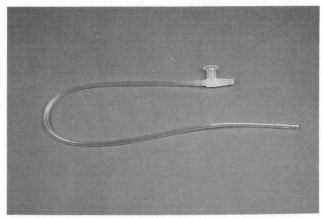

FIGURE 11-60 "Whistle tip" suction catheter.

ynx or nasopharynx, through a nasopharyngeal airway, along an oropharyngeal airway, or through an endotracheal tube.

Since suctioning reduces a patient's access to oxygen, each attempt
should be limited to ten seconds. If possible, hyperventilate the patient
with 100 percent oxygen prior to and following each suctioning effort.
Clear the airway first if there are fluids in the upper airway and assisted
breathing will cause aspiration. Do not apply suction during insertion of
the catheter. Only when the catheter is properly positioned should suction be applied and the catheter withdrawn.

✱ Suctioning of the airway
should be limited to ten seconds
with the patient hyperventilated
before and after the procedure.

Most suction catheters have an open port or orifice at their proximal
ends, which allows the paramedic to selectively initiate or stop the negative pressure being generated through the catheter. When the suction device is not equipped with this orifice, you can create one by making a
small slit in the catheter or suction tubing. You can also control the suction by turning the unit on and off as needed. When the fluid present in
the upper airway is so great or so thick that neither the tonsil tip nor
whistle tip catheter provides adequate suctioning, it may be beneficial to
replace the catheter with thick-walled, wide-bore suction tubing. It may
also be necessary to place your patient on his or her side and use your
fingers to clear substances from the mouth.

The principal hazards associated with these procedures relate to hypoxia brought on by lengthy suctioning attempts. Serious cardiac dysrhythmias can occur during suctioning, due to decreases in myocardial
oxygen supply. Suctioning can stimulate the vagus nerve, causing hypertension and tachycardia, or bradycardia and hypotension. Finally, suctioning may stimulate the airway's mucosa and start the patient coughing. This can increase intracranial pressure and reduce cerebral blood
flow.

The steps taken in suctioning a patient are as follows:

1. While maintaining ventilatory support, attempt to hyperventilate the patient.
2. Determine the depth of catheter insertion by measuring from the patient's
   earlobe to his or her lips.
3. Insert the catheter into your patient's pharynx to the predetermined depth
   (without the suction operating).
4. Turn on the suction unit or place your thumb over the suction control orifice, limiting suction to ten seconds.
5. Withdraw the catheter. When using a whistle tip catheter, rotate it between
   your fingertips.
6. While maintaining ventilatory support, hyperventilate the patient with 100
   percent oxygen.

In many cases you will be suctioning out extremely viscous or thick
secretions, which can obstruct fluid flow through the tubing. To reduce
this problem, suction water through the tubing between suctioning attempts. This dilutes the secretions and facilitates flow to the suction can-
ister. Most suction units are supplied with small water canisters that can
be used for this purpose.

OXYGENATION AND VENTILATION

Oxygen Administration

Oxygen administration is an important aspect of patient care. It's essential in cases that involve suspected hypoxia of any cause, chest pain due
to myocardial ischemia, and cardiorespiratory arrest. Administering sup-

plemental oxygen to a hypoxic patient raises his or her oxygen level by:

- ❏ increasing their inspired percentage of oxygen
- ❏ increasing oxygen concentration at the alveolar level
- ❏ increasing arterial oxygen levels
- ❏ increasing the amount of oxygen delivered to the patient's cells

Oxygen administration decreases hypoxia, reduces the volume of respiration necessary to oxygenate the blood, and reduces the myocardial work demanded to maintain a given arterial oxygen tension.

Oxygen therapy is provided through either a high-flow or low-flow system. A high-flow system uses a Venturi adapter to draw in relatively large amounts of room air for each liter of oxygen provided by the regulator. This allows for the delivery of a precise oxygen concentration, regardless of the patient's inspiratory efforts.

In a low-flow system, oxygen travels directly from the regulator to the patient. If the regulator is set at 6 liters per minute, for instance, that is precisely what the patient will receive. With a low-flow system, ambient air is drawn into the respiratory passageways with each breath. This dilutes the oxygen concentration from 100 percent (being delivered through the oxygen tubing). The concentration delivered to the patient depends on the flow rate and the type of oxygen-delivery device being used. With some oxygen-delivery devices, oxygen concentration can vary with increases and decreases in the respiratory minute volume (rate x depth of breathing). So a hyperventilating patient will receive less oxygen as he or she breathes in more room air. Conversely, the barbiturate overdose patient whose breathing is slow and shallow dilutes the delivered oxygen flow with less room air, so receives a higher concentration of oxygen. The devices most vulnerable to variations in the percentage of oxygen delivered to patients are the nasal cannula and simple masks. The least vulnerable are the partial and nonrebreather masks.

✱ There are no absolute contraindications to oxygen therapy, although it should be used with caution in premature infants and in patients with chronic respiratory problems.

There are no absolute contraindications to oxygen administration. However, it should be used with caution in premature infants and patients who are prone to carbon dioxide retention (hypoxic drive). It should be administered at lower flow rates with COPD patients—1 to 3 liters delivered via nasal cannula, or 24 percent to 28 percent delivered via Venturi mask. If your patient develops respiratory depression, breathing should be assisted with a bag-valve-mask device. When ventilating via a bag-valve-mask device, use 100 percent oxygen. When providing oxygen to a premature infant, hold the mask over the face, not directly on it.

Devices commonly used to administer oxygen in the field include the nasal cannula, the simple face mask, the nonrebreather mask, and the Venturi mask.

Nasal cannula. This is a comfortable and easily tolerated device that can deliver an oxygen concentrations of 24 percent to 44 percent. (See Figure 11-61.) Flow rates administered through the nasal cannula range from 1 to 6 liters per minute.

Liter flow	Oxygen concentration delivered
1	24
2	28
3	32
4	36
5	40
6	44

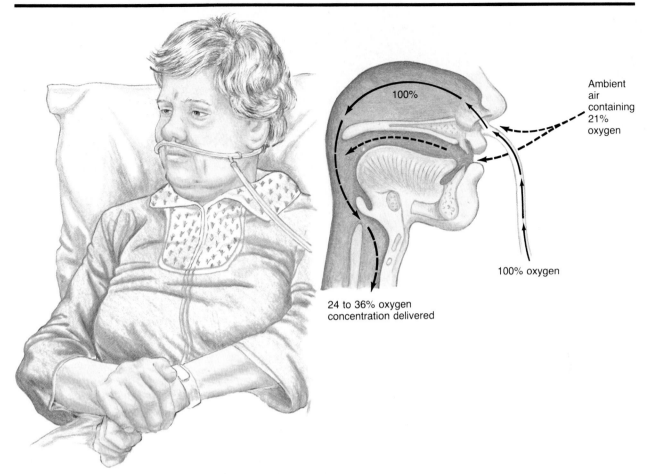

Ambient
air
containing
21%
oxygen

100%

100% oxygen

24 to 36% oxygen
concentration delivered

FIGURE 11-61   The nasal cannula is comfortable and convenient.

Flow rates of greater than 6 liters per minute do little to increase inspired oxygen concentrations, since the anatomical reserve (nasal cavity) is already filled. Higher flow rates will dry the mucous membrane and cause headaches.

The nasal cannula is used with patients who are experiencing minor to moderate hypoxia; who are prone to carbon dioxide retention; who are frightened or feeling suffocated by an oxygen mask; and who are experiencing nausea or vomiting. One benefit of the nasal cannula is that it doesn't stop the patient from talking, so the paramedic can continue gathering patient information during the procedure. The only contraindication for use of a nasal cannula is nasal obstruction.

Simple face mask.   This device includes oxygen tubing and a face mask. (See Figure 11-62.) On the outside of the mask are two inlet/outlet ports. Oxygen is delivered through the bottom of the mask via its oxygen inlet port. The simple face mask will deliver an oxygen concentration of 40 percent to 60 percent. Flow rates administered through the simple face mask range between 8 and 12 liters per minute. No fewer than 6 liters should be administered through this device, as expired carbon dioxide can otherwise accumulate in the mask. Flow rates in excess of 8 liters are needed to "wash out" any expired carbon dioxide.

The simple face mask provides oxygen to patients who are suffering from moderate hypoxia. Its disadvantages are that it may feel confining to the patient, it is difficult to hear the patient speaking when the device is in place, and the mask requires a tight face seal. Because the mask

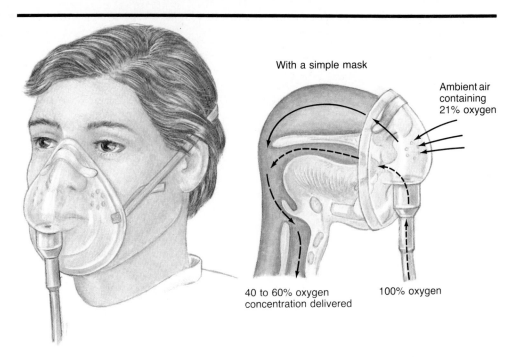

With a simple mask

Ambient air containing 21% oxygen

40 to 60% oxygen concentration delivered

100% oxygen

FIGURE 11-62 Simple mask.

covers the patient's face, it should be used with caution in cases that involve nausea or vomiting. With the pediatric patient, a flow rate of 6 to 8 liters per minute is generally considered acceptable.

Nonrebreather mask.   This device consists of oxygen tubing and a face mask with an attached reservoir bag. (See Figure 11-63.) On the outside of the mask are two air inlet/outlet ports, one covered with a thin rubber flap. Oxygen delivered through the oxygen tubing fills the reservoir. When the patient inhales, the 100 percent oxygen contained in the reservoir is drawn into the mask and the patient's respiratory passageways. Ambient air is prevented from entering the mask by the rubber flap that closes over the inlet/outlet ports during inspiration. When the patient exhales, the flapper valve is forced open to allow the expired air an exit. Preventing the expired air from entering the reservoir bag is a one-way valve situated between the mask and the reservoir.

Among oxygen administration devices, the nonrebreather mask delivers the highest concentration of oxygen. When supplied with 10 to 15 liters per minute, it can deliver an 80 percent to 100 percent oxygen concentration. No fewer than 8 liters of oxygen per minute should be admininstered through this device. Because it is a relatively closed system, restricting the inspiration of ambient air, its reservoir bag should not be allowed to deflate totally, for that might allow the patient to suffocate. The nonrebreather mask is similar to the simple face mask in that it requires a tight seal. This may be difficult to obtain with some patients, and they may find the mask confining. This device should be employed with caution in nauseated patients, but should be used in the treatment of severely hypoxic patients—those suffering respiratory compromise, shock, acute myocardial infarction, trauma, or carbon monoxide poisoning.

Venturi mask.   This high-flow device includes oxygen tubing, a face mask, and a Venturi system. As oxygen passes through a jet orifice in the base of the mask, it entrains room air, and the resulting mixture is deliv-

✱ When using the nonrebreather mask, oxygen should be run at no less than 8 L per minute, and the reservoir bag should not be allowed to collapse.

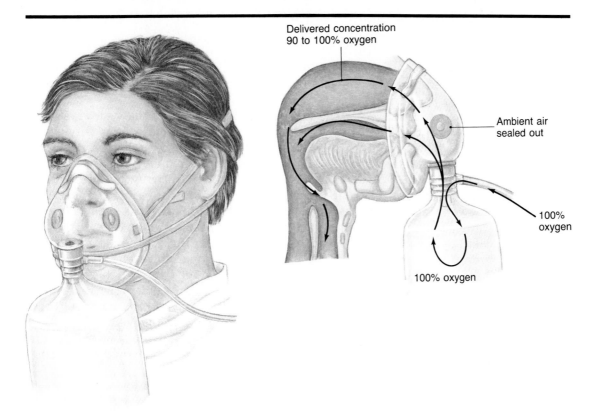

Delivered concentration
90 to 100% oxygen

Ambient air
sealed out

100%
oxygen

100% oxygen

FIGURE 11-63   Non-rebreather mask.

ered to the patient. The same amount of ambient air is always entrained, regardless of the respiratory rate or depth. With this device, relatively precise concentrations of oxygen can be provided. The Venturi mask is particularly useful in cases that involve COPD patients, where careful control of inspired oxygen concentration is desirable. To control the amount of ambient air a patient takes in, some Venturi masks are supplied with dial selection, while others come with interchangeable caps. These devices deliver oxygen concentrations of 24 percent, 28 percent, 35 percent, or 40 percent. The liter flow depends on the oxygen concentration desired.

Ventilation

In the field, paramedics will be called upon in many cases to provide ventilatory support, from those that involve apneic patients to less obvious situations in which patients are experiencing depressed respiratory function. Remember that when a patient is unconscious, his or her respiratory center may not function at a satisfactory level. A significant decrease in the patient's rate or depth of breathing will lead, in turn, to decreased respiratory minute volume, hypercarbia, hypoxia, and a lowered pH. If not corrected, respiratory or cardiac arrest may occur.

With this in mind, paramedics must remain on guard for situations that require ventilatory assistance. Procedures and devices used to provide ventilatory support include:

❑ mouth-to-mouth and mouth-to-nose ventilation
❑ mouth-to-mask ventilation
❑ the bag-valve-mask device

- ❏ the demand valve resuscitator
- ❏ the automatic ventilator

To achieve effective ventilatory support, an adequate rate and volume of oxygen must be delivered: at least 800 mL of O_2 at a rate of 12 to 20 breaths per minute.

One problem associated with ventilatory support is that you must generate enough force to overcome the elastic resistance of the lungs and chest wall as well as frictional resistance in the respiratory passageways. This can be likened to blowing up a balloon: resistance must be overcome in order to inflate the rubber. Keep in mind that air will travel the path of least resistance. In other words, if a tight seal is not maintained between the ventilation mask and your patient's face, air will leak from the gaps rather than travel through the respiratory passageways. Effectively ventilating a patient, then, requires that his or her airway be in an open position; that a closed system be established and maintained between the patient and the rescuer's ventilation mask or mouth; and that adequate ventilatory volumes be delivered. However, be careful because generating the pressure necessary to ventilate the lungs may lead to patient regurgitation. So use caution in selecting devices for use in the field.

Because carbon dioxide is removed during the process of expiration, the patient should always be allowed to exhale between delivered breaths.

Mouth to Mouth/Mouth to Nose. Mouth-to-mouth and mouth-to-nose breathing can provide effective ventilatory support to a patient. They require no adjunctive equipment, it is easy to maintain an effective mouth (or nose) seal, and, when applied properly, both procedures deliver sufficient ventilatory volumes. The only limitations on mouth-to-mouth and mouth-to-nose breathing have to do with the capacity of the person delivering the ventilations and the fact that both methods provide only limited oxygen (expired air from the rescuer, after all, will contain only 17 percent oxygen).

What makes them less-than-attractive techniques, though, is the fact that patients often have copious secretions, bleeding, and gastric regurgitation, and that they may be suffering from transmittable diseases.

✻ When possible, the pocket mask should be used to ventilate a patient when other adjuncts are not available.

Pocket Mask. The *pocket mask* is a clear plastic device that sits over a patient's face, covering both the mouth and nose. This mask prevents contact between the rescuer and the patient's mouth, thus reducing the risk of contamination and subsequent infection during resuscitation.

There are a variety of pocket masks available. Some are reusable, while others are disposed of after a single use. Most offer the versatility of being small and compact, so that they can be carried with the paramedic at all times or stored in a pocket or purse. The device is usually designed with a one-way valve that prevents the patient's expired air from coming into contact with the rescuer. It may also provide an inlet for the administration of supplemental oxygen. With an oxygen flow rate of 10 liters per minute, combined with mouth-to-mask breathing, an inspired oxygen concentration of approximately 50 percent can be delivered through the device.

Steps for using the pocket mask are as follows:

1. Kneel just above your patient's head.
2. Use the head-tilt/chin-lift to properly position the patient's head (except in trauma).
3. If needed, insert an oropharyngeal airway.

Bag-valve-mask devices should not feature a pop-off valve. When you are providing ventilatory assistance to a patient with high airway resistance and poor lung compliance, a pop-off valve will prevent effective ventilation.

There are a number of reasons for recommending use of the bag-valve-mask device. It provides an immediate means of ventilatory support. It can give an oxygen-enriched mixture to the patient. It conveys a sense of compliance from the patient's lungs. And, it can be used to assist a patient's breathing or to administer high oxygen concentrations to one who is already breathing spontaneously.

However, the bag-valve-mask device is not without its problems. To begin with, it is difficult to maintain a tight seal between the patient's face and the mask. Mask leakage is a serious problem, decreasing air volume delivered to the oropharynx by as much as 40 percent. The medical literature describes a number of ways to hold the mask, of which probably the easiest and most effective is the clamp technique:

1. Take the hand that you'll be using to hold the mask and form it into the shape of a "C."
2. Place your thumb across the apex of the mask and your first and second fingers over the base of the mask.
3. Fit the apex of the mask over the bridge of your patient's nose and seat its base into the groove between his or her lower lip and chin.
4. Once that is done, apply firm downward pressure to the patient's face with the mask.
5. While providing ventilatory support to the patient, listen continuously for air leaks around the mask. An air leak indicates that a better seal needs to be established and maintained.

Another problem with the bag-valve-mask device is that it is difficult to use it and also sustain hyperextension of the patient's head and neck, particularly when you're applying downward pressure on the mask to maintain a seal. In order to achieve good hyperextension, the paramedic must assume a position behind the patient; trying to ventilate a patient from the side is difficult and unproductive. While applying firm downward pressure on the mask, hook your ring and little fingers under the chin. Next, pull the chin upward and backward while tilting the head with your free hand. This hyperextension of the head and neck can then be maintained by applying continuous backward pressure on the jaw.

Finally, forcing enough air from the bag to adequately expand your patient's lungs is most challenging. Current teaching suggests that at least 800 mL of air should be delivered with each breath. Depending on the manufacturer, bag-valve-mask units have capacities of between 1,000 and 1,600 mL. But just because a device has a certain capacity doesn't mean it will deliver that much air to the patient's lungs. Small bags are easier to handle, but have less capacity than larger ones. The larger the bag, though, the more difficult it will be to compress, especially for paramedics who have small hands. To achieve optimal compression of the bag, hold it parallel to the ground or floor (it is difficult to effectively empty a bag which is all "scrunched up"). When compressing the bag, squeeze it like a loaf of bread, with your thumb under the bag and your four other fingers of your hand over the top. Compress the bag as completely as possible, using a smooth and steady action. Between each compression, allow the bag to refill completely. The paramedic may choose alternately to compress the bag against his or her thigh or knee.

Once an endotracheal tube is placed, ventilatory support can be accom-

* The bag-valve-mask can provide the patient with an oxygen-enriched mixture and can allow the paramedic to feel the compliance of the lungs.

plished without regard to mask leakage. Steps used to ventilate a patient with a bag-valve-mask device are as follows:

1. Connect the bag-valve-mask to an oxygen supply.
2. Select a properly sized mask for the patient.
3. Open the airway by employing the head-tilt/chin-lift.
4. Position yourself behind the head of the patient.
5. Insert an oropharyngeal airway.
6. Position the mask over your patient's face, with the apex of the mask positioned over the bridge of the nose and the base resting between the lower lip and the projection of the chin.
7. With one hand, firmly hold the mask to your patient's face, making a good seal.
8. Squeeze the bag as completely as possible to force air into the patient's lungs.
9. Watch for chest rise and auscultate the lung fields to assure proper ventilation.

Because this device presents problems, it should be used only by trained and experienced personnel. What's more, application of a bag-valve-mask device should be practiced periodically on a CPR mannequin, as the skills necessary for its efficient use tend to deteriorate rapidly.

Ventilation with a bag-valve-mask device may be best delivered by two people, rather than one: While the first person holds the mask in place and maintains an open airway, the second can squeeze the bag with two hands. The trouble is that, in a field setting, where there are not enough persons or space available, double-teaming may not be possible.

Demand Valve.   The *demand valve resuscitator,* also called the "manually triggered oxygen-powered breathing device," will deliver 100 percent oxygen to a patient at its highest flow rates (40 to 60 liters per minute). (See Figure 11-66.) The device is compact, easy to handle, rugged, and has an

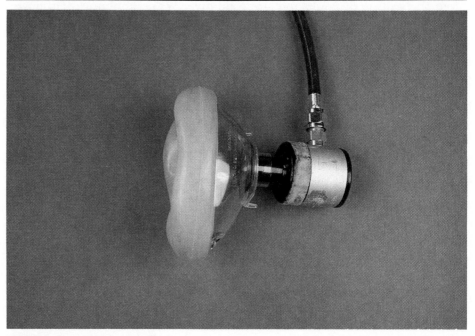

FIGURE 11-66   Demand valve.

easily located manual control button. It can be attached to a face mask or an EOA. The complete system consists of high-pressure tubing, which connects to an oxygen supply, and a valve that is activated by a push button or lever. When the valve is opened, oxygen flows to the patient. Most of these units also contain an inspiratory release valve that makes them useful in treating spontaneously breathing patients who need high oxygen concentrations. The slight negative pressure created by inhalation opens the valve. The greater the inspiratory effort, the higher the flow. When inhalation ceases, so does the oxygen flow.

Positive attributes of the demand valve resuscitator are that it's easy to use and provides high oxygen concentrations. However, there are also negative aspects. During ventilation, the device does not provide the paramedic with a sense of chest compliance; thus, you must take care not to overinflate the lungs. Due to the high pressures generated by the device, lungs may experience pressure-related injury, which can lead to pneumothorax and subcutaneous emphysema. The demand valve resuscitator may open the esophagus, causing gastric distension in patients who have not been intubated. Since the oxygen flow rate is so high, the demand valve resuscitator will quickly drain the contents of a portable oxygen cylinder. Another means of ventilatory support will need to be employed if the cylinder requires changing during patient management. The demand valve resuscitator is not recommended for use with patients under the age of 16. And, finally, because of the sudden high pressures that this device can supply, it should be used with extreme caution, if at all, in intubated patients.

Steps used to ventilate a patient with a demand valve resuscitator are as follows:

1. Open the regulator valve to the oxygen supply.
2. Select a properly sized mask for the patient.
3. Open the airway by employing the head-tilt/chin-lift.
4. Position yourself behind the head of the patient.
5. Insert an oropharyngeal airway.
6. Position the mask over your patient's face, with the apex of the mask positioned over the bridge of the nose and its base resting between the lower lip and the projection of the patient's chin.
7. With both your hands, hold the mask firmly against the patient's face to make a seal, while at the same time maintaining head and neck hyperextension.
8. Deliver a ventilation by pushing the device's control button.
9. Watch for chest rise and auscultate the lung fields to assure proper ventilation.
10. As soon as the patient's chest rises, release pressure on the button to allow for passive expiration. The flow of oxygen then ceases, and the expired air is released through a one-way valve.

Automatic Ventilators. Up to this point, all of the devices listed have been operator dependent. But a new device—the time-cycled, constant-flow, gas-powered ventilator—has recently been introduced to the prehospital-care setting. Designed for convenience and easy use during patient care and transport, this lightweight, compact ventilator is typically equipped with two controls: one for the ventilatory rate, the other for tidal volume. The automatic ventilator is dependable even in temperature extremes (from -30 F to 125 F). In order that it can be attached to a variety of airway devices, it is equipped with a standard 15mm ID/22 mm OD adapter. Some of these automatic units deliver controlled ventilation only, while

* The demand valve should be used with extreme caution in the intubated patient.

others function as intermittent mandatory ventilators, reverting to controlled mechanical ventilation in patients who are not breathing. Most units provide an adjustable tidal volume, while the ventilatory rate is either fixed or adjustable. The inspired oxygen concentration is usually fixed at 100 percent but it may be adjustable.

Many of these ventilators sport a "pop-off" valve that prevents pressure-related injury. This valve vents away some of the tidal volume when its preset level of airway pressure is exceeded. However, the pop-off feature can be detrimental in the presence of cardiogenic pulmonary edema, Adult Respiratory Distress Syndrome, pulmonary contusion, bronchospasm, and other disorders that demand that high airway pressures be overcome.

When providing ventilatory support to an intubated patient, use of the ventilator will allow a paramedic to perform other vital tasks.

Gastric Distention.   If your patient's airway is obstructed by inadequate positioning, or if excessive pressures are used during ventilation, he or she may experience gastric distention. This occurs when air takes the path of least resistance and enters the stomach instead of the lungs. Gastric distention can have severe consequences. It may cause the patient to regurgitate and possibly aspirate his or her stomach contents, and it can decrease vital capacity, due to elevation of the diaphragm and gastric rupture that comes as a result of overdistention.

When gastric distention occurs in the field and interferes with ventilatory efforts, it may be necessary to relieve it. Do this by turning the patient onto his or her side and then using one of your hands to exert moderate pressure over the patient's epigastrium, between the umbilicus and the rib cage. (See Figure 11-67.) A suction unit should be available to clear the upper airway in case of regurgitation. As easy as it sounds, note that gastric distention should be relieved only with extreme caution and when absolutely necessary.

✱ Gastric distention may reduce vital capacity, may cause the patient to vomit, and may cause gastric rupture.

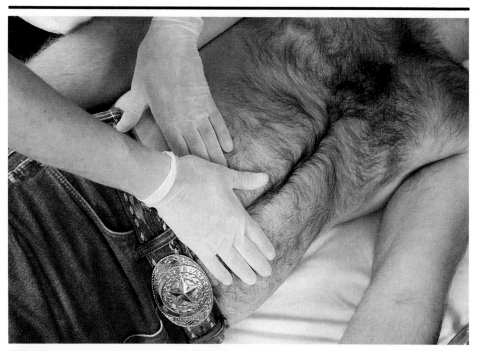

FIGURE 11-67   To relieve gastric distention, turn the patient to the side (if cervical spine injury is not suspected, and compress the stomach gently.

SUMMARY

As stated many times in this chapter, airway management is one of the most important aspects of prehospital care. It is not always easy to accomplish. Effective airway management depends on paramedics continually reinforcing their skills, so that they can perform procedures automatically.

Of foremost importance in airway management is that the patient's respiratory system be able to perform its primary function of moving air in and out of the body, thereby supplying the bloodstream with adequate oxygen. This requires that the patient have a patent airway, that there be adequate supplies of oxygen in the inspired air, and that the patient's respiratory minute volumes must be sufficient to remove appropriate levels of carbon dioxide.

The paramedic is armed with training in a number of procedures that can help sustain a critically ill or injured patient. All of them, however, require first that the airway be secured. Basic manipulations, such as the head-tilt/chin-lift, can then be used to move the tongue and epiglottis away from obstructing positions. In the presence of possible cervical spine injuries, the chin-lift should be employed without the head tilt. Endotracheal intubation is the preferred technique for securing an airway, as it prevents aspiration of foreign materials and allows for efficient delivery of ventilatory support. It presents hazards, though, as inadvertent misplacement of the tube can have severe consequences. Great care must be taken when performing endotracheal intubation, so as to prevent injury to the teeth and tissues. While traditional orotracheal intubation is the most commonly used procedure, others are useful when head and neck manipulation are inadvisable. These include: orotracheal intubation with in-line stabilization using two persons; nasotracheal intubation; digital intubation; and the transillumination method. Breathing efforts can be supported with a variety of devices. Among these, the bag-valve-mask device probably offers the most advantages, but it is difficult to use when you're trying to ventilate a nonintubated patient. Only frequent practice in using the bag-valve-mask device will ensure proficiency during emergency situations. Inspired oxygen concentrations can be increased with a number of different delivery devices, each of which has specific criteria for use. (Of the options, the nonrebreather mask delivers close to 100 percent oxygen.) Finally, recent introductions in the area of suctioning afford even greater portability of devices and ease of use.

FURTHER READING

American College of Surgeons, Committee on Trauma, *Advanced Trauma Life Support Course: Student Manual.* American College of Surgeons, 1984.

American Heart Association, *Textbook of Advanced Cardiac Life Support,* 2nd ed. Dallas, TX: American Heart Association, 1987.

APPLEBAUM, EDWARD L., and BRUCE, DAVID L. *Tracheal Intubation.* Saint Louis, MO: W.B. Saunders Company, 1976.

BLEDSOE, BRYAN E. *Atlas of Paramedic Skills.* Englewood Cliffs, NJ: Prentice-Hall, Inc., 1987.

CAMPBELL, JOHN E. *Basic Trauma Life Support,* 2nd ed. Englewood Cliffs, NJ: Prentice-Hall, Inc., 1988.

SHADE, BRUCE, et. al. *Advanced Cardiac Life Support: Certification, Preparation, and Review.* Englewood Cliffs, NJ: Brady Communications, Inc., 1988.

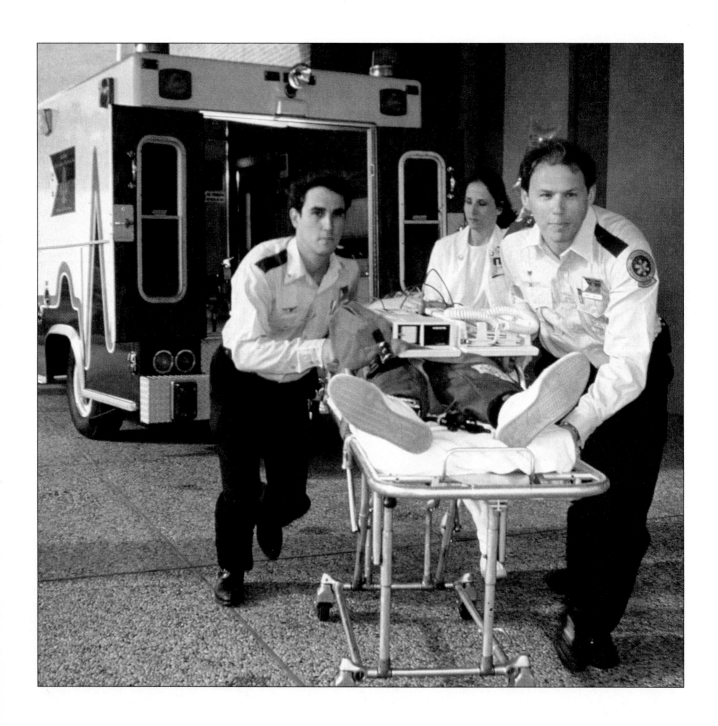

12

Pathophysiology of Shock

Objectives for Chapter 12

Upon completing this chapter, the student should be able to:

1. Identify the body's major fluid compartments and the proportion of total body water they contain.

2. Describe the abnormal states of hydration and their common causes and effects on the human system.

3. List the major electrolytes and the role they play in maintaining a fluid balance within the human body.

4. Define diffusion, osmosis, active transport, and facilitated diffusion and explain the roles they play in human fluid dynamics.

5. Identify the major elements of the blood and describe their purpose.

6. Explain the ABO blood typing system and its significance to emergency medical care.

7. List the various fluid replacement products and describe the advantages and disadvantages of field use.

8. Describe the acid-base balance system and its impact on the human body as it applies to shock and fluid therapy.

9. Illustrate the structure and function of the cardiovascular system.

10. Define shock and explain the shock process and the body's compensatory mechanisms.

11. Describe the pathophysiology of hypovolemic, cardiogenic, and neurogenic shock.

12. Describe and demonstrate the assessment of the shock patient.

13. Describe and demonstrate the management of the shock patient.

14. Identify the indications, contraindications, and application process for the PASG.

15. Explain the indications for, and the initiation of, intravenous therapy.

16. List the equipment commonly used for intravenous therapy and explain its purpose and use.

17. Identify the common complications of intravenous therapy and the process of preventing or correcting those complications.

CASE STUDY

City Ambulance 1 is dispatched to assist a basic life support ambulance in another city that is working with a 39-year-old male who is trapped under an overturned bulldozer. Upon arrival, the paramedics find the patient to be alert. His pelvis and lower extremities are pinned by the side of the overturned bulldozer.

Rescue personnel do not have the equipment immediately available to lift the dozer. Bob, the senior paramedic, quickly performs the primary assessment and no problem is detected. The EMTs already have oxygen flowing using a non-rebreather mask.

Bob begins the secondary assessment. The patient has good breath sounds. He is not able to feel his feet. A pelvic fracture is highly suspected. Vital signs are: blood pressure 110/68, pulse 100, respirations 24, oxygen saturation 99 percent. Two IVs of lactated Ringer's are established, one infusing wide open. The PASG and a backboard are prepared. The paramedics converse with the patient while rescue equipment is readied. Vital signs are measured every four minutes or so and they remain stable. Finally, the bulldozer is slowly lifted and the patient is removed to the waiting backboard. The PASG is applied and inflated. After removal, it is apparent that fractures of the pelvis, bilateral femur, and left tibia are present. Both IVs are opened wide.

After the equipment is elevated the patient reports an increase in pain. He then becomes restless and attempts to get up. Shortly, he becomes somewhat lethargic. The oximetry reveals the saturation has dropped to 94 percent and the pulse rate is up to 130 beats per minute. With time, the patient's level of consciousness improves. The pulse rate remains elevated. Both IVs are placed in pressure bags and the patient transported to the ambulance before any splinting is completed. Upon arrival at the hospital the patient remains stable, yet tachycardic. Type O-negative blood is started and a third IV established. Within 20 minutes the patient is transported to surgery with the PASG in place. The patient survives the incident. His rehabilitation will continue for more than a year due to the multiple fractures.

INTRODUCTION

The paramedic differs from the EMT in several ways. The paramedic can perform advanced patient assessment, and possesses knowledge of specialized skills and procedures, medication administration, and IV fluid therapy. However, the paramedic's performance is dependent upon a thorough understanding of the body's normal physiology as well as common pathophysiology.

■ **shock** a state of inadequate tissue perfusion.

This chapter will address the topics of fluid and electrolyte therapy, acid-base balance and **shock**. First, normal physiology will be presented. This will be followed by pertinent pathophysiology and prehospital management.

FLUID AND ELECTROLYTES

Water

Water is the most abundant substance in the human body. In fact, approximately 60 percent of the total body weight is due to water. The total amount of water in the body at any given time is referred to as the *total body water* (TBW). In a person weighing 70 kilograms (154 pounds) the amount of total body water would be approximately 42 liters (11 gallons).

Water is usually distributed into various compartments of the body. These compartments are separated by cell membranes. The largest compartment is the **intracellular fluid (ICF)** and includes all of the fluid found inside body cells. Approximately 75 percent of all body water is found within this compartment. The fluid found outside of the cells is called the **extracellular fluid (ECF).** The remaining 25 percent of all body water is in the extracellular compartment.

There are two divisions of the extracellular fluid compartment. The first includes fluid found outside of cells and within the circulatory system and is called **intravascular fluid.** It is essentially the same as the blood plasma. The remaining compartment includes all fluid found outside of cell membranes, yet not within the circulatory system. It is called the **interstitial fluid.** The following represents the body fluid compartments (see Figure 12-1):

■ **water** the universal solvent. Approximately 60 percent of the weight of the human body is due to water.

■ **intracellular fluid** portion of the body fluid inside the body's cells.

■ **extracellular fluid** portion of the body fluid outside the body's cells.

■ **intravascular fluid** portion of the body's fluid outside the body's cells and within the circulatory system.

■ **interstitial fluid** portion of the body fluid found outside the body's cells, yet not within the circulatory system. Interstitial fluid is that fluid found within the interstitial space between the cells.

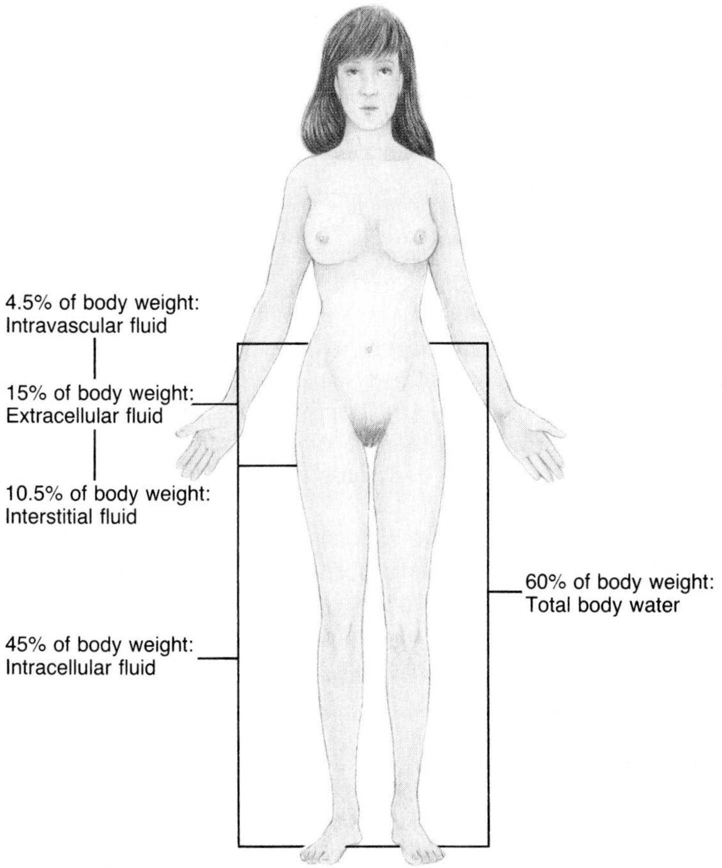

4.5% of body weight: Intravascular fluid

15% of body weight: Extracellular fluid

10.5% of body weight: Interstitial fluid

60% of body weight: Total body water

45% of body weight: Intracellular fluid

FIGURE 12-1   Percentage of total body weight due to water as distributed in the various fluid compartments.

Compartment	Percentage of Total Body Water	Volume in 70 kg Adult
Intracellular Fluid	75%	31.50 L
Extracellular Fluid	25%	10.50 L
Interstitial Fluid	17.5%	7.35 L
Intravascular Fluid	7.5%	3.15 L

Abnormal States of Hydration

■ **homeostasis** the body's natural tendency to keep the internal environment constant.

Water is the universal solvent and is necessary for many of the biochemical reactions that occur. Normally, the total volume of water in the body as well as the distribution of fluid in the three body compartments remains relatively constant. This occurs despite wide fluctuations in the amount of water that enters and is excreted from the body on a daily basis. The water coming into the body is referred to as *intake*. The water that is excreted from the body is referred to as *output*. To maintain relative **homeostasis,** or balance, the intake must equal the output.

Intake

digestive system:	1,000 mL
• liquids	
• food (solid)	1,200 mL
metabolic sources:	300 mL
	————
TOTAL:	2,500 mL

Output

lungs:	400 mL
kidneys:	1,500 mL
skin:	400 mL
intestines (feces):	200 mL
	————
TOTAL:	2,500 mL

Several mechanisms work to maintain a relative balance between input and output. As an example, when the fluid volume drops, the pituitary gland at the base of the brain secretes the hormone, ADH (anti-diuretic hormone). ADH causes the kidney tubules to reabsorb more water back into the blood and excrete less urine. This helps in building the fluid volume back up.

Thirst also regulates fluid intake. The sensation of thirst normally occurs when body fluids decrease, stimulating the person to take in more fluids orally. On the other hand, when too many fluids enter the body, the kidneys are activated and more urine is excreted, thus eliminating excess fluid. The body also maintains fluid balance by shifting water from one body space to another.

■ **dehydration** an abnormal decrease in total body water.

Dehydration. **Dehydration** is an abnormal decrease in the total body water and can result from several factors. These include such things as:

❑ *gastrointestinal losses:* Gastrointestinal losses result from prolonged vomiting, diarrhea, or malabsorption disorders.

❑ *increased insensible loss:* Loss of water through normal mechanisms can be increased in fever states, during hyperventilation, or with high environmental temperatures.

❑ *increased sweating:* A significant amount of fluid can be lost through sweating, or diaphoresis. This can occur with many medical conditions or in areas of high environmental temperature.

❑ *internal losses:* Fluid can be lost into various body fluid compartments, commonly called "*third space*" losses. This can occur with peritonitis, pancreatitis, or bowel obstruction. It can also occur in poor nutritional states where there is not enough protein in the vascular system to retain water.

❑ *plasma losses:* Plasma losses occur from burns, surgical drains and fistulas, and open wounds.

Dehydration may involve only the loss of water. However, more commonly, there is also a loss of **electrolytes.** Hospital-based fluid replacement will be based on both fluid and electrolyte deficits.

■ **electrolytes** chemical substances that dissociate into charged particles when placed in water.

Clinically, the dehydrated patient will exhibit dry mucous membranes and poor skin turgor. There often is excessive thirst. As it becomes more severe, dehydration will be accompanied by an increased pulse rate, decreased blood pressure, and orthostatic hypotension. In infants, the anterior fontanelle may be sunken and the diaper may be dry or reveal the presence of highly concentrated urine.

The treatment for dehydration is replacement of fluid. Since electrolyte deficits cannot be determined in the field, an isotonic fluid such as normal saline or lactated Ringer's should be used. This should be infused at 100–200 mL per hour.

Overhydration. **Overhydration** can occur as well. The major sign of overhydration is *edema.* Patients with heart disease may manifest overhydration much earlier than patients without heart disease. In severe cases of overhydration, overt heart failure may be present.

■ **overhydration** an excess of total body water.

Treatment is directed at removing the excessive fluid. An IV of D5W should be infused at a TKO ("to keep open") rate. The medical control physician may request the administration of a **diuretic.** In severe cases, phlebotomy may be indicated.

■ **diuretic** a medication that stimulates the kidneys to excrete water.

Electrolytes

The various chemical substances present throughout the body can be classified either as electrolytes or non-electrolytes. Electrolytes are substances that dissociate into charged particles when placed into water. The charged particles are referred to as **ions.** Ions with a positive charge are called **cations** while ions with a negative charge are called **anions.**

■ **ion** a charged particle.

An example of this would be the dissociation of the drug sodium bicarbonate when placed into water. Sodium bicarbonate is a neutral salt. When placed into water it dissociates into two charged particles as illustrated:

$$NaHCO_3 \longrightarrow Na^+ + HCO_3^-$$

Neutral Salt $\longrightarrow$ *Cation* + *Anion*

■ **cation** a positively charged ion. It is attracted to the negative pole of an electrode (cathode), hence the name.

Sodium bicarbonate is an example of a medication. However, there are many naturally-occurring electrolytes present in the body.

The most frequently occurring *cations* are:

■ **anion** a negatively charged ion. It is attracted to the positive pole of an electrode (anode), hence the name.

1. **sodium (Na⁺):** Sodium is the most prevalent cation in the extracellular fluid. It plays a major role in regulating the distribution of water. In fact, it is often said that water "follows sodium." Sodium also is important in the

✱ Water follows sodium.

transmission of nervous impulses. An increase in the relative amount of sodium in the body is called *hypernatremia* while a decrease is referred to as *hyponatremia.*

2. **potassium (K$^+$):** Potassium is the most prevalent cation in the intracellular fluid. It is also important in the transmission of electrical impulses. An abnormally low potassium level is called *hypokalemia* while a high potassium level is referred to as *hyperkalemia.*

3. **calcium (Ca^{++}):** Calcium has many physiological functions. It plays a major role in muscle contraction as well as nervous impulse transmission.

4. **magnesium (Mg^{++}):** Magnesium is necessary for several biochemical processes that occur in the body, and is closely associated with phosphate in many processes.

The most frequently occurring *anions* are:

1. **chloride (Cl$^-$):** Chloride is an important anion. Its negative charge balances the positive charge associated with the cations. It also plays a major role in fluid balance and renal function. Chloride has a close association with sodium.

2. **bicarbonate (HCO$_3^-$):** Bicarbonate is the principle **buffer** of the body. It neutralizes the highly acidic hydrogen ion (H$^+$) and other organic acids.

3. **phosphate (HPO$_3^-$):** Phosphate is important in body energy stores. It is closely associated with magnesium in renal function. It also acts as a buffer, primarily in the intracellular space, in much the same manner as bicarbonate.

Many other compounds carry negative charges. Among these are some of the proteins, certain organic acids, and other compounds. Electrolytes are usually measured in **milliequivalents** per liter (mEq/L).

Non-electrolytes are molecules that have no electrical charge. These include glucose, urea, and similar substances.

Osmosis and Diffusion

The various fluid compartments, previously discussed, are separated by cell membranes. These membranes are unique and said to be **semipermeable membranes.** That is, they allow the passage of certain materials and restrict the passage of others. Compounds with small molecules, such as water (H$_2$O), pass readily through the membrane while larger compounds, such as proteins, are restricted. This is accomplished by the presence of pores within the membrane. Only compounds small enough to pass through the pores can enter or exit the cell. Electrolytes do not pass as readily as water through the membrane. This is not due so much to their size as to their electrical charge.

The natural tendency of the body is to keep the balance of electrolytes and water equal on each side of the cell membrane. This is an example of homeostasis. If one side of a cell membrane has an increased quantity of a given electrolyte, there will be a shift of water and the electrolyte to resume the balanced state.

When solutions on opposite sides of a semi-permeable membrane are equal in concentration, the relationship is said to be **isotonic.** When the concentration of a given solute on one side of the membrane is greater than the other, it is said to be **hypertonic.** When the concentration is less on one side of the cell membrane, as compared to the other, it is referred to as **hypotonic.** (See Figure 12-2.) This difference in concentration is often referred to as the *osmotic gradient.* When there is an unequal relationship, the solute will diffuse across the cell membrane from the area of

■ **buffer** substance that neutralizes or weakens a strong acid or base.

■ **milliequivalent** weight of a substance contained in one milliliter of a normal solution.

■ **semipermeable membrane** specialized biological membrane, such as that which encloses the body's cells, which allows the passage of certain substances and restricts the passage of others.

■ **isotonic** a state where solutions on opposite sides of a semipermeable membrane are in equal concentration.

■ **hypertonic** a state where a solution has a higher solute concentration on one side of a semipermeable membrane compared to the other side.

■ **hypotonic** a state where a solution has a lower solute concentration on one side of a semipermeable membrane compared to the other side.

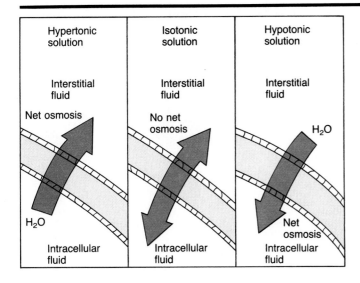

FIGURE 12-2   Fluid shifts across a semi-permeable membrane.

higher concentration to the area of lower concentration. (See Figure 12-3.) This process is referred to as **diffusion** and does not require energy. It will continue until the natural balance is again attained.

Water also moves across the cell membrane so as to dilute the area of increased electrolyte concentration. The movement of water is more rapid than the movement of electrolytes and is referred to as **osmosis.** (See Figure 12-4.) It occurs in the opposite direction of solute movement. For example, if a semi-permeable membrane separates a solution of water and sodium, and the concentration of sodium is two times higher on one side of the membrane as on the other, then two things will occur. Sodium will diffuse from the area of higher concentration (the hypertonic side) to the area of lesser concentration (the hypotonic side). Concurrently, water will diffuse in the opposite direction. That is, water will leave the hypotonic

■ **diffusion** the movement of solutes (substances dissolved in a solution) from an area of greater concentration to an area of lesser concentration.

■ **osmosis** the movement of a solvent (water) across a semi-permeable membrane from an area of lesser (solute) concentration to an area of greater (solute) concentration. Osmosis is a form of diffusion.

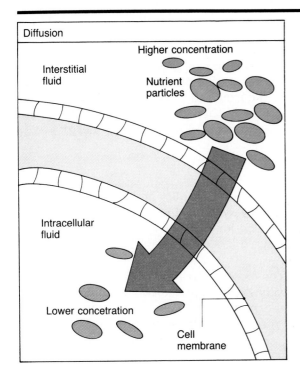

FIGURE 12-3   Diffusion is the movement of a substance from an area of greater concentration to an area of lesser concentration.

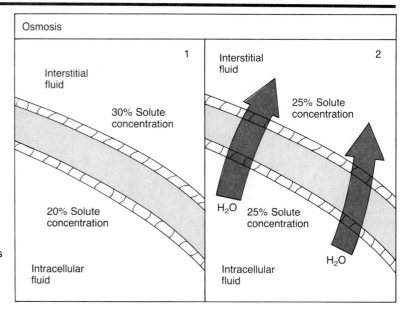

FIGURE 12-4 Osmosis is the movement of water from an area of higher WATER contentration to an area of lower WATER concentration. Because water is a solvent, it moves from an area of lower SOLUTE concentration, to an area of higher SOLUTE concentration.

■ **active transport** biochemical process where a substance is moved across a cell membrane, often against a gradient, using energy.

■ **facilitated diffusion** biochemical process where a substance is selectively transported across a membrane, using "helper proteins" and energy.

side and diffuse across the membrane to the hypertonic side. This will continue until both components, water and sodium, have equalized.

In addition to diffusion, other substances can be transported across cell membranes by one of two different mechanisms. **Active transport** is the movement of a substance across the cell membrane against the osmotic gradient. For example, the body requires cells of the myocardium (heart muscle) to be negatively charged on the inside of the cell as compared to the outside. Sodium, however, tends to passively diffuse back into the cell. This would destroy the negative charge inside the cell. In order to maintain the desired gradient, sodium is actively pumped out of the cell by a mechanism known as the sodium-potassium pump. Active transport is faster than diffusion and requires expenditure of energy. Proteins are moved across the cell membrane in a similar fashion.

Certain molecules can move across the cell membrane by a process known as **facilitated diffusion.** Glucose is an example of such a molecule. Facilitated diffusion requires the assistance of "helper proteins" on the surface of the cell membrane. These proteins, once activated, bind to the glucose molecule. Following binding, the protein changes its configuration and transports the glucose molecule to the inside of the cell where it is released. The transport protein is then ready for another glucose molecule. This process, like active transport, often requires energy.

Fluid Replacement Therapy

Intravenous therapy is the introduction of fluids and other substances into the venous side of the circulatory system. It is used for fluid replacement, for electrolyte replacement, and for introduction of medications directly into the vascular system.

Blood and Blood Components. The *blood* is the fluid of the cardiovascular system. An adequate amount of blood is required for perfusion and for transport of nutrients, oxygen, hormones, and heat. Blood consists of the liquid portion, or *plasma,* and the formed elements, or blood cells. (See Figure 12-5.)

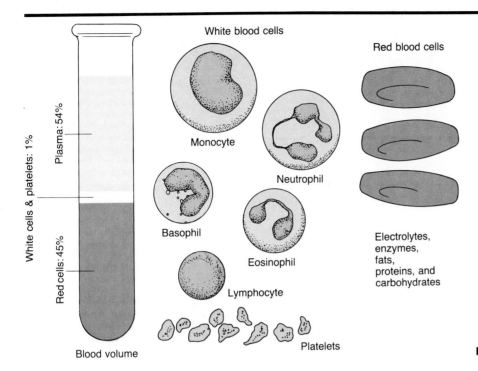

White blood cells

Monocyte

Neutrophil

Basophil

Eosinophil

Lymphocyte

Platelets

Red blood cells

Electrolytes, enzymes, fats, proteins, and carbohydrates

Plasma: 54%

White cells & platelets: 1%

Red cells: 45%

Blood volume

FIGURE 12-5 Blood components.

Plasma is made up of approximately 92 percent water, 6 to 7 percent proteins, and a small portion consisting of electrolytes, lipids, enzymes, clotting factors, glucose, and other dissolved substances.

The formed elements include the red blood cells, or *erythrocytes;* the white blood cells, or *leukocytes;* and the platelets, or *thrombocytes.*

More than 99 percent of the cells are red blood cells. Red blood cells contain hemoglobin and are responsible for transporting oxygen to the peripheral cells. **Hemoglobin** is an iron-based compound that binds with oxygen in the pulmonary capillaries and transports it to the peripheral tissues where it can be unloaded. Factors such as pH and oxygen concentration affect the amount of oxygen transported by hemoglobin.

The white cells are responsible for immunity and fighting infection. The platelets play a major role in blood clotting. The *viscosity* (thickness) of the blood is determined by the ratio of plasma to formed elements. The lesser the ratio of plasma to formed elements, the greater the viscosity.

The plasma can be separated from the formed elements by centrifugation. That is, blood can be placed in a test tube inside a centrifuge and spun at high speed. The heavier cells, the erythrocytes, will be forced to the bottom of the tube, leaving the plasma portion at the top. Usually, the red blood cells will account for approximately 45 percent of the blood volume. The percentage of blood occupied by red blood cells is referred to as the **hematocrit.** (See Figure 12-6.)

Blood is a type of tissue and varies from patient to patient. Blood can be categorized into various "types" as determined by the presence of proteins known as antigens on the erythrocytes. The major system of blood classification is the **ABO system.** (See Table 12-1.) This system is based on the type of antigen present on the cell.

There are two major antigen types, A and B. A patient can have either the A antigen, the B antigen, both antigens, or neither antigen. The blood type of a patient is genetically pre-determined. Persons, with a few exceptions, can only receive blood that is of the same type as their own. Persons

■ **hemoglobin** the iron-containing substance in blood responsible for transport of oxygen

■ **hematocrit** the percentage of the blood consisting of the red blood cells, or erythrocytes (usually 35–45 percent).

■ **ABO system** system of blood typing based on the presence of proteins on the surface of the red blood cells.

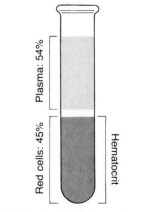

Plasma: 54%

Red cells: 45%

Hematocrit

FIGURE 12-6 The percentage of the blood occupied by the red blood cells is termed the hematocrit.

TABLE 12-1   Blood Typing—ABO System

Blood Type	Antigen Present on RBC	Antibody Present in Serum
O	None	Anti-A, Anti-B
AB	A and B	None
B	B	Anti-A
A	A	Anti-B

with type A blood have the A antigen on the erythrocyte. Since they do not have the B antigen, they have antibody to B. If they were to receive type B blood, the immune system would determine that the blood was foreign and a reaction would occur.

There are two exceptions to this. Persons with type AB blood do not have antibody to either A or B since they carry both antigens. Therefore, in an emergency, they can receive blood of any type. Because of this, persons with type AB blood are referred to as **universal recipients.** Type O blood does not contain either the A or B antigen. Therefore, in emergencies, it can be administered to a patient of any blood type. Because of this it is referred to as the **universal donor** blood type. (See Table 12-2.) In addition to the ABO types, there are many additional minor blood types. In routine medical practice blood is matched as closely as possible, considering both major and minor blood types.

One additional blood type worthy of mentioning is the *Rh factor.* Rh factor is present in approximately 85 percent of the population. Persons who are Rh negative usually do not have anti-Rh antibodies. However, if exposed to Rh positive blood through transfusion, these persons become "sensitized." Sensitization means that the patient has developed antibodies to Rh factor. If the patient were to receive an additional transfusion of Rh positive blood, then a severe or even fatal reaction could occur.

Fluid Replacement.   The most desirable fluid for replacement is whole blood. There are several reasons for this. First, blood contains hemoglobin, which can transport oxygen. In addition, it is the most natural replacement. However, even in the hospital setting, the routine use of whole blood is not practical. (See Table 12-3.)

Blood is a precious commodity and it must be conserved so that it can benefit the most people. Because of this, blood is often fractionated, or separated into parts. The red cells are packaged separately as *packed red blood cells.* The white cells are used for other purposes. Plasma is packaged as *fresh frozen plasma* for use when plasma or clotting factors are needed. Thus, with the exception of true hemorrhagic shock, where

TABLE 12-2   Compatibility Among ABO Blood Groups

Cells of Donor	Reaction with Serum of Recipient			
	AB	B	A	O
AB	−	+	+	+
B	−	−	+	+
A	−	+	−	+
O	−	−	−	−

− = Nonagglutination
+ = Agglutination

TABLE 12-3   Resuscitation Fluids

Diagnosis	Resuscitation Fluid Used			
	1st Choice	**2nd Choice**	**3rd Choice**	**4th Choice**
Hemorrhagic Shock	Whole Blood	Packed RBCs	Plasma or Plasma Substitute	Lactated Ringer's or Normal Saline
Shock due to plasma loss (burns)	Plasma	Plasma Substitute	Lactated Ringer's or Normal Saline	
Dehydration	Lactated Ringer's or Normal Saline			

whole blood is the fluid of first choice, packed red blood cells are now more frequently used than whole blood.

Before blood, or blood products, can be administered to a patient, they must typed and cross-matched to prevent a severe allergic reaction. The exception to this is fresh frozen plasma, which does not require cross-matching. If there is not adequate time for typing and cross-matching, O-negative blood can be administered, since it is the universal donor type.

Transfusion Reaction.   For obvious reasons, blood and blood products are not used in the field. However, on occasion, the paramedic may be called upon to transport a patient with blood infusing. Because of this, the paramedic must be able to recognize the signs and symptoms of a *transfusion reaction*. Common signs and symptoms of a transfusion reaction include fever, chills, hives, hypotension, palpitations, tachycardia, flushing of the skin, headaches, loss of consciousness, nausea, vomiting or shortness of breath.

If a transfusion reaction is suspected, IMMEDIATELY stop the transfusion and save the substance being transfused. The blood should be replaced by an electrolyte solution to keep the vein open. Quickly complete an adequate assessment of the patient's mental status. Oxygen should be administered and the medical control physician should be contacted. The medical control physician may request the administration of mannitol, diphenhydramine, or furosemide. These drugs are used to maintain renal function, which is often severely compromised during a transfusion reaction.

In addition to overt reaction, the paramedic must always be alert for signs of fluid overload and congestive heart failure secondary to transfusion. This is evidenced by increased dyspnea, pulmonary congestion, edema, and altered mental state. If this is suspected, the infusion should be stopped and a crystalloid solution should be started at a TKO ("to keep open") rate. The patient should receive oxygen and the medical control physician should be contacted for additional orders.

Intravenous Fluids.   Intravenous fluids are the most common products used in prehospital care for fluid and electrolyte therapy. (See Table 12-4.) Intravenous fluids occur in two general forms; colloids and crystalloids.

Colloids contain proteins, or other high molecular weight molecules, which tend to remain in the intravascular space an extended period of time. In addition, colloids have **colloid osmotic pressure,** which means

■ **colloid osmotic pressure** pressure generated by the presence of colloids in the vascular system or interstitial space.

TABLE 12-4 Crystalloid Intravenous Fluids: Approximate Ionic Concentrations (mEq/l) and Calories Per Liter

	Ionic Concentrations (mEq/l)					Calories per liter	Osmolarity * (mOsm/l)	pH Range **
	Sodium	Potassium	Calcium	Chloride	Lactate			
5% Dextrose Injection, USP	0	0	0	0	0	170	252	3.5–6.5
10% Dextrose Injection, USP	0	0	0	0	0	340	505	3.5–6.5
0.9% Sodium Chloride Injection, USP	154	0	0	154	0	0	308	4.5–7.0
Sodium Lactate Injection, USP (M/6 Sodium Lactate)	167	0	0	0	167	54	334	6.0–7.3
2.5% Dextrose & 0.45% Sodium Chloride Injection, USP	77	0	0	77	0	85	280	3.5–6.0
5% Dextrose % 0.2% Sodium Chloride Injection, USP	34	0	0	34	0	170	321	3.5–6.0
5% Dextrose & 0.33% Sodium Chloride Injection, USP	56	0	0	56	0	170	365	3.5–6.0
5% Dextrose & 0.45% Sodium Chloride Injection, USP	77	0	0	77	0	170	406	3.5–6.0
5% Dextrose & 0.9% Sodium Chloride Injection, USP	154	0	0	104	0	170	560	3.5–6.0
10% Dextrose & 0.9% Sodium Chloride Injection, USP	154	0	0	154	0	340	813	3.5–6.0
Ringer's Injection, USP	147.5	4	4.5	156	0	0	309	5.0–7.5
Lactated Ringer's Injection, USP	130	4	3	100	28	9	273	6.0–7.5
5% Dextrose in Ringer's Injection	147.5	4	4.5	150	0	170	561	3.5–6.5
Lactated Ringer's with 5% Dextrose	130	4	3	109	28	180	525	4.0–6.5

* Normal physiologic isotonicity range is approximately 280–310 mOsm/liter. Administration of substantially hypotonic solutions may cause hemolysis and administration of substantially hypertonic solutions may cause vein damage.
** pH ranges are USP for applicable solution, corporate specifications for non-USP solutions.
(Adapted with permission from Travenol Laboratories, Inc., Deerfield, Illinois)

they tend to attract water into the intravascular space. Thus, a small amount of a colloid can be administered to a patient with a greater than expected increase in intravascular volume. This is because the colloid will draw water from the interstitial space and the intracellular compartment in order to increase the intravascular volume. Common examples of colloids include:

- **plasma protein fraction (Plasmanate®):** Plasmanate is a protein-containing colloid. The principle protein present is **albumin,** which is suspended, along with other proteins, in a saline solvent.
- **salt-poor albumin:** Salt-poor albumin contains only human albumin. Each gram of albumin holds approximately 18 milliliters of water in the blood stream.
- **Dextran®:** Dextran is not a protein but a large sugar molecule with osmotic properties similar to albumin. It comes in two molecular weights (40,000 and 70,000 Daltons). Dextran 40 has two to two and one-half times the colloid osmotic pressure of albumin.
- **hetastarch (Hespan®):** Hetastarch, like Dextran, is a sugar molecule with osmotic properties similar to protein. It does not appear to share many of Dextran's side-effects.

■ **albumin** protein found in almost all animal tissues that constitutes one of the major proteins in human blood.

Colloid replacement therapy does not have a role in prehospital care except under rare circumstances. The colloid products are expensive and have a short shelf-life.

Crystalloids are the primary compounds used in prehospital intravenous fluid therapy. There are multiple fluid preparations. It is often helpful to classify them according to the **tonicity** related to plasma:

■ **tonicity** the number of particles present per unit volume.

- **isotonic solutions:** Isotonic solutions have electrolyte composition similar to the blood plasma. When placed into a normally hydrated patient they will not cause a significant fluid or electrolyte shift.
- **hypertonic solutions:** Hypertonic solutions have a higher solute concentration than the cells. These fluids will tend to cause a fluid shift out of the intracellular compartment into the extracellular compartment when administered to a normally hydrated patient. Later, there will be a diffusion of solute in the opposite direction.
- **hypotonic solutions:** Hypotonic solutions have less of a solute concentration when compared to the cells. When administered to a normally hydrated patient they will cause a movement of fluid from the extracellular compartment into the intracellular compartment. Later, solutes will move in an opposite direction.

Replacement fluids should be chosen based on the needs of the patient and the patient's underlying problem. As a rule, hemorrhage occurs so fast that there has not been time for a significant fluid shift between the extracellular and intracellular space. Because of this, the replacement fluid should be isotonic. It is for this reason that lactated Ringer's and normal saline are often used. If the patient is dehydrated due to fluid loss from diarrhea or fever, then there is a greater deficit of water than sodium. In these cases, hypotonic fluids such as half-normal saline are chosen.

Some replacement fluids contain a single element, such as sodium chloride or dextrose, while others contain multiple elements. Solutions, such as lactated Ringer's, are designed so that the concentration of electrolytes is very similar to that of the plasma. It is because of this that these are referred to as *balanced salt solutions.*

Three of the most commonly used solutions in pre-hospital care include: lactated Ringer's solution, 0.9% sodium chloride (normal saline), and 5% dextrose in water (D5W).

- ❑ **lactated Ringer's:** Lactated Ringer's solution is an isotonic, electrolyte solution. It contains sodium chloride, potassium chloride, calcium chloride and sodium lactate in water.
- ❑ **normal saline:** Normal saline is an electrolyte solution containing sodium chloride in water which is isotonic with the extracellular fluid.
- ❑ **5% dextrose in water:** D5W is a hypotonic, glucose solution used to keep a vein open and to supply calories necessary for cell metabolism. While it will have an initial effect of increasing the circulatory volume, glucose molecules rapidly diffuse across the vascular membrane with a resultant free water increase.

Both lactated Ringer's solution and normal saline are used to replace fluid volume because their administration causes an immediate expansion of the circulatory volume. However, as was noted earlier, due to the movement of the electrolytes and water, two thirds of either of these solutions is lost to the interstitial space within one hour.

ACID–BASE BALANCE

Acid-base balance is a dynamic relationship which reflects the relative concentration of hydrogen ions (H^+) in the body. Hydrogen ions are acidic and the concentration of these within the body must be maintained within fairly strict limits. Any deviation in the hydrogen ion concentration adversely affects all of the biochemical events that occur in the body. The hydrogen ion concentration is dynamic, changing from second to second.

The total number of hydrogen ions present in the body at any given time is very high. Because of this the **pH** system of measurement is utilized. The pH scale is a **logarithmic** value, inversely related to hydrogen ion concentration. That is, the greater the hydrogen ion concentration, the lower the pH. The lower the hydrogen ion concentration, the higher the pH. The following formula represents pH:

$$pH = \log \frac{1}{[H^+]}$$

The pH scale ranges from 1 to 14. A pH of 1 means that only hydrogen ions are present. A pH of 14 means that there are no hydrogen ions present. The pH of water is 7.0, which is a neutral pH. The pH of the body is normally 7.35 to 7.45. A pH above 7.45 is referred to as **alkalosis** while a pH below 7.35 is called **acidosis.** A variation of only 0.4 of a pH unit in either direction (6.9 or 7.8) can be fatal.

The body is constantly producing acids through metabolism and other biochemical processes. Therefore, these acids must be constantly eliminated from the body. There are three major mechanisms to remove acids (hydrogen ions) from the body. The fastest mechanism is often referred to as the buffer system or the bicarbonate buffer system.

The two components of the bicarbonate buffer system are bicarbonate ion (HCO_3^-) and carbonic acid (H_2CO_3). These two compounds are in equilibrium with hydrogen ion (H^+):

$$H^+ + HCO_3^- \leftrightarrow H_2CO_3$$

For every molecule of carbonic acid, there are 20 molecules of bicarbonate ion. Any change in this 20:1 ratio is immediately corrected without significant change in the total pH. Thus, an increase in hydrogen ion causes

■ **pH** scientific method of expressing the acidity or alkalinity of a solution. It is the logarithm of the hydrogen ion concentration divided by one. The higher the pH, the more alkaline the solution. The lower the pH, the more acidic the solution.

■ **logarithm** mathematical concept that eases calculation of large numbers. The log of a number is the exponent of the power to which a given base must be raised to equal that number. For example, the log of 100 is 2 ($100 = 10^2$), and the log of 1,000 is 3 ($1,000 = 10^3$).

■ **alkalosis** a state where the pH is higher than normal due to a decreased hydrogen ion concentration.

■ **acidosis** a state where the pH is lower than normal due to an increased hydrogen ion concentration.

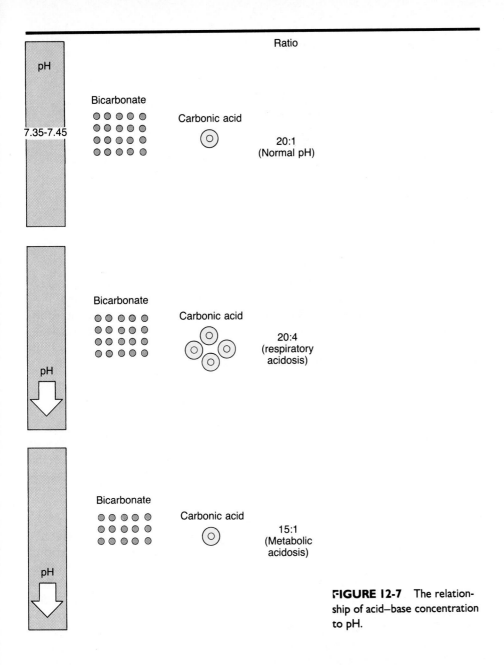

FIGURE 12-7 The relationship of acid–base concentration to pH.

an increase in carbonic acid. A decrease in hydrogen ion concentration causes a decrease in carbonic acid. (See Figure 12-7.) For example:

Increased Acid

$$\uparrow H^+ + HCO_3^- \rightarrow \ \uparrow H_2CO_3$$

Decreased Acid

$$\downarrow H^+ + HCO_3^- \rightarrow \ \downarrow H_2CO_3$$

The above process occurs very rapidly. Carbonic acid is a weak, volatile acid and better tolerated by the body than pure hydrogen ion. However, the body carries this reaction further. Carbonic acid must also be eliminated.

Normally, over time, carbonic acid will eventually dissociate into carbon dioxide and water. This process is slow and ineffective. The erythrocytes contain an enzyme called *carbonic anhydrase.* Most buffering of acid in the body occurs in the erythrocytes. Carbonic anhydrase causes carbonic acid to be very rapidly converted to carbon dioxide and water.

✳ The lower the patient's pH, the more acidic the patient.

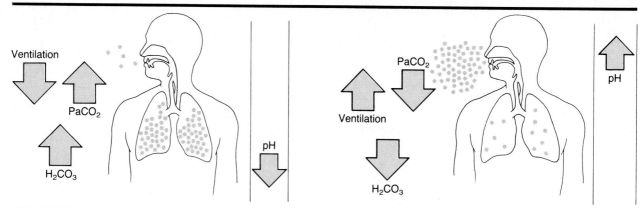

FIGURE 12-8 The respiratory component of acid-base balance.

This reaction occurs so quickly that carbonic acid only exists for a fraction of a second before it is converted into carbon dioxide and water.

The enzyme also works in a reverse fashion, which allows carbon dioxide and water to be quickly converted into carbonic acid. Thus, with the aid of carbonic anhydrase, there is an equilibrium between hydrogen ion and carbon dioxide. The following equation illustrates this relationship.

$$\text{H}^+ \quad + \quad \text{HCO}_3^- \quad \longleftrightarrow \quad \text{H}_2\text{CO}_3 \longleftrightarrow \text{H}_2\text{O} \quad + \quad \text{CO}_2$$
hydrogen ion   bicarbonate ion   carbonic acid   water   carbon dioxide

Thus an increase in acid (hydrogen ion) would result in an increase in carbonic acid. With the aid of carbonic anhydrase, carbonic acid would quickly dissociate into water and carbon dioxide. Therefore, an increase in CO_2 causes an increase in hydrogen ion concentration and a decrease in pH. Thus:

$$\uparrow \text{H}^+ \longleftrightarrow \uparrow \text{CO}_2$$

In addition, the body regulates acid-base balance by two other mechanisms. The CO_2 level can be altered by the lungs. Increased respirations cause increased elimination of CO_2, which results in a decrease in hydrogen ions and an increase in pH. Conversely, decreased respirations cause CO_2 to be retained. This causes an increase in hydrogen ions and a decrease in pH. (See Figure 12-8.)

The kidneys also can regulate the pH by altering the concentration of bicarbonate ion in the blood. Increased elimination of HCO_3^- results in a lowered pH while retention of HCO_3^- causes an increase in pH. In addition, the kidneys affect the acid-base balance by removing or retaining various chemicals. Normally, the kidneys remove larger metabolic acids, excreting them in the urine.

Acid–Base Derangements

An increase in hydrogen ion drives the equilibrium described above to the right. Hydrogen ion is immediately combined with bicarbonate ion. This combination results in the formation of carbonic acid, which subsequently dissociates into carbon dioxide and water with the assistance of carbonic anhydrase. Carbon dioxide is eliminated by the lungs and water is eliminated through the kidneys. Any change in a component of this equation affects the other components. For example, if the amount of hydrogen ion in the body is increased, as occurs in cardiac arrest, the equation is altered. For example:

$$\uparrow H^+ + HCO_3^- \rightarrow \uparrow H_2CO_3 \rightarrow H_2O + \uparrow CO_2$$

Conversely, if the amount of carbon dioxide is increased the equation is driven the other direction resulting in the formation of acid.

$$\uparrow CO_2 + H_2O \rightarrow \uparrow H_2CO_3 \rightarrow \uparrow H^+ + HCO_3^-$$

Both types of acid-base derangements, alkalosis and acidosis, can be divided into two categories based on the underlying causes. Changes in the concentration of CO_2 result from changes in the respiratory system. Thus, an acidosis caused by retained CO_2 is referred to as respiratory acidosis. An alkalosis caused by the excess removal of CO_2 is called respiratory alkalosis. However, if acidosis results from the production of metabolic acids, such as lactic acid, then metabolic acidosis is said to exist. If an alkalosis is caused by the excess elimination of hydrogen ion, then it is termed metabolic alkalosis.

Respiratory Acidosis. Respiratory acidosis is caused by the retention of CO_2. This can result from impaired ventilation due to problems occurring either in the lungs or in the respiratory center of the brain. The pH is decreased and the CO_2 level is increased. Treatment is directed at improving ventilation.

* The primary treatment for any patient where acidosis is suspected is to increase ventilations.

$$\downarrow \text{RESPIRATION} = \uparrow CO_2 + H_2O \rightarrow \uparrow H_2CO_3 \rightarrow \uparrow H^+ + HCO_3^-$$

Respiratory Alkalosis. Respiratory alkalosis results from the excessive elimination of CO_2. This can occur with anxiety or following ascent to a high altitude. The pH is increased and the CO_2 level is decreased. Treatment, if required, consists of increasing the CO_2 level by having the patient rebreathe CO_2.

$$\uparrow \text{RESPIRATION} = \downarrow CO_2 + H_2O \rightarrow \downarrow H_2CO_3 \rightarrow \downarrow H^+ + HCO_3^-$$

Metabolic Acidosis. Metabolic acidosis results from the production of metabolic acids such as lactic acid. In addition, it can result from diarrhea, vomiting, diabetes, and medication usage. The pH is decreased and the CO_2 level is normal. Treatment primarily consists of ventilation, which causes the elimination of CO_2 and, subsequently, hydrogen ion. (See Figure 12-9.) On rare occasions, additional bicarbonate, usually in the form of sodium bicarbonate ($NaHCO_3$), may be required.

$$\uparrow H^+ + HCO_3^- \rightarrow \uparrow H_2CO_3 \rightarrow H_2O + \uparrow CO_2$$

Metabolic Alkalosis. Metabolic alkalosis occurs much less frequently than metabolic acidosis. It is usually caused by the administration of diuretics, loss of chloride ions associated with prolonged vomiting, or the overzealous administration of sodium bicarbonate. The pH is increased and the CO_2 level is normal. Treatment consists of correcting the underlying cause.

$$\downarrow H^+ + HCO_3^- \rightarrow \downarrow H_2CO_3 \rightarrow H_2O + \downarrow CO_2$$

Usually, both a respiratory and a metabolic component is present. The type of acid-base derangement present can only be determined by arterial blood gas studies. These, of course, are only available in the hospital setting. Arterial blood gasses report the pH, the $PaCO_2$, PaO_2, bicarbonate concentration, and oxygen saturation. Pulse oximetry is now available for field use and is quite accurate in determining oxygen saturation levels.

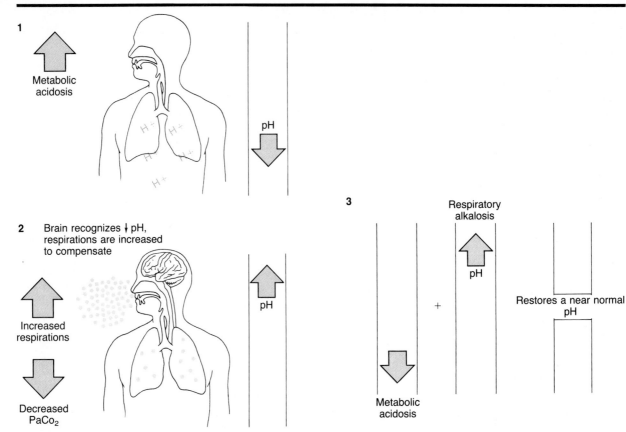

FIGURE 12-9 Compensation for metabolic acidosis begins with an increase in respirations.

SHOCK

■ **shock** a state of inadequate tissue perfusion.

Shock, from a medical standpoint, is defined as inadequate tissue perfusion. It can occur for many reasons such as trauma, fluid loss, heart attack, infection, spinal cord injury, and other causes. Although the causes are different, all forms of shock have the same underlying pathophysiology at the tissue level.

Physiology of Perfusion

■ **perfusion** fluid passing through an organ or a part of the body.

As mentioned above, the common factor in all types of shock is inadequate **perfusion** of the various body tissues. Shock occurs first at a cellular level. If allowed to progress, organ failure, organ system failure, and ultimately, death will occur.

The cells of the body require a constant supply of oxygen and other essential nutrients. These are provided by the circulatory system, in conjunction with the respiratory and gastrointestinal systems. In addition, cells require the elimination of waste products such as carbon dioxide and metabolic acids.

Perfusion is dependent on a functioning and intact circulatory system. The three components of the circulatory system are:

❑ the pump (heart)
❑ the volume (blood)
❑ the container (blood vessels)

A derangement in any one of these components can adversely affect perfusion. (See Figure 12-10.)

The Pump. The *heart* is the pump of the cardiovascular system. It receives blood from the venous system, pumps it to the lungs where it is oxygenated, and subsequently pumps it to the peripheral tissues. The amount of blood ejected by the heart in one contraction is referred to as the *stroke volume*. Several factors affect stroke volume. These are:

- ❏ preload
- ❏ contractile force
- ❏ afterload

Preload is the amount of blood delivered to the heart during diastole and is dependent on venous return. The venous system is a capacitance, or storage, system. That is, it can be contracted or expanded as needed to meet the physiological demands of the body. When additional oxygenated blood is required, the venous capacitance is reduced, thus increasing the amount of blood delivered to the heart. The greater the preload, the greater the stroke volume.

■ **preload** the pressure within the ventricles at the end of the diastole.

Preload also affects **cardiac contractile force.** The greater the volume of preload, the more the ventricles are stretched. The greater the stretch, up to a certain point, the greater will be the subsequent cardiac contraction. This is referred to as the *Frank-Starling mechanism* and can be illustrated by a rubber band—the more it is stretched, the greater will be its velocity when released.

■ **cardiac contractile force** the force generated by the heart during each contraction.

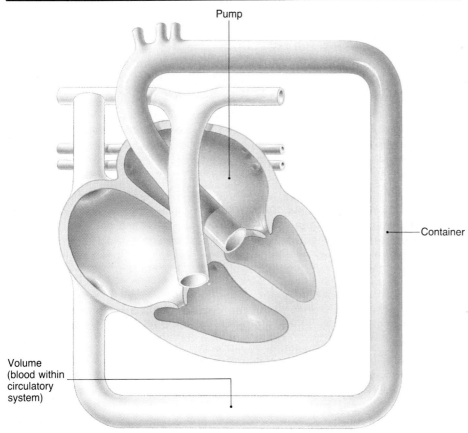

Pump

Container

Volume (blood within circulatory system)

FIGURE 12-10 Components of the circulatory system.

■ **catecholamine** class of hormones which act upon the autonomic nervous system. They include epinephrine, norepinephrine, and similar compounds.

■ **afterload** the resistance against which the heart must pump.

■ **cardiac output** the amount of blood pumped by the heart in one minute.

■ **peripheral vascular resistance** the resistance to blood flow due to the peripheral blood vessels. This pressure must be overcome for the heart to pump blood effectively.

In addition, cardiac contractile strength is affected by circulating **catecholamines** (epinephrine and norepinephrine), and sympathetic nervous system tone. Catecholamines enhance cardiac contractile strength by action on the beta-adrenergic receptors.

Finally, stroke volume is affected by **afterload.** The *afterload* is the resistance against which the ventricle must contract. This resistance must be overcome before ventricular contraction can result in ejection of blood. Afterload is determined by the degree of peripheral resistance; this in effect, is due to the amount of vasoconstriction present. The arterial system can be expanded and contracted as required to meet the metabolic demands of the body. The greater the resistance offered by the arterial system, the less the stroke volume.

The amount of blood pumped by the heart in one minute is referred to as the **cardiac output** and is a function of heart rate and stroke volume. It is usually expressed in liters per minute. It can be defined as:

Stroke Volume × Heart Rate = Cardiac Output

The equation illustrates the factors that can affect cardiac output. An increase in stroke volume or an increase in heart rate can increase cardiac output. Conversely, a decrease in stroke volume or a decrease in heart rate can decrease cardiac output. The *blood pressure* is representative of cardiac output. In fact:

Cardiac Output × Peripheral Vascular Resistance = Blood Pressure

Peripheral vascular resistance is the pressure against which the heart must pump. Since the circulatory system is a closed system, increasing either cardiac output or peripheral vascular resistance will increase blood pressure. Likewise, a decrease in cardiac output or a decrease in peripheral vascular resistance will decrease blood pressure.

The body strives to keep the blood pressure relatively constant through feedback mechanisms. Sensory fibers, commonly referred to as *baroreceptors,* are present in the carotid bodies—small structures that contain nerve tissue at the branch of the carotid arteries—and the arch of the aorta. These baroreceptor centers closely monitor blood pressure.

If blood pressure increases, the baroreceptors send signals to the brain that cause the blood pressure to be returned to its normal values. This is accomplished by decreasing the heart rate, decreasing the preload, or decreasing peripheral vascular resistance. If the blood pressure falls, the baroreceptors are stimulated. This results in activation of the sympathetic nervous system. The heart rate is increased, as is the strength of the cardiac contractions. In addition, the peripheral blood vessels are also affected. There is arteriolar constriction, venous constriction (which results in decreased container size), and overall increased peripheral vascular resistance. Finally, the adrenal medulla is stimulated. This results in the secretion of epinephrine and norepinephrine, which further enhance the response.

The Fluid. Blood is the fluid of the cardiovascular system. A viscous fluid, blood is thicker and more adhesive than water, and because of this it flows more slowly than water.

An adequate amount of blood is required for perfusion. The cardiovascular system is a closed system, with no major movement of fluid into or out of the system. Because of this, the volume of blood present must be adequate to fill the container. Blood, which consists of the plasma and the formed elements, transports oxygen, carbon dioxide, nutrients, hormones, metabolic waste products, and heat.

The Container. Blood vessels serve as the container of the cardiovascular system. The blood vessels can be thought of as a continuous, closed, and pressurized pipeline that moves blood throughout the body. Comprised of arteries, arterioles, capillaries, venules, and veins, the blood vessels play a significant role in maintaining blood flow. Although the heart is considered to be the pump of the circulatory system, the blood vessels—under the control of the autonomic nervous system—can regulate blood flow to different areas of the body by adjusting their size as well as by selectively rerouting blood through the large microcirculation.

While the arteries and veins, like the heart, are subject to direct stimulation from sympathetic portions of the autonomic nervous system, the microcirculation is primarily responsive to local tissue needs. The capability of some vessels in the capillary network to adjust their diameter permits the microcirculation to selectively supply undernourished tissue while temporarily bypassing tissues with no immediate need. Capillaries have a sphincter at the origin of the capillary, called the *pre-capillary sphincter,* and another at the end of the capillary, called the *post-capillary sphincter.* The pre-capillary sphincter responds to local tissue demands, such as acidosis, and opens as more arterial blood is needed. The post-capillary sphincter opens when blood is to be emptied into the venous system.

Blood flow through the vessels occurs because of two characteristics: peripheral resistance and pressure within the system. *Peripheral resistance* is defined as the resistance to blood flow. Vessels with larger inside diameters create less resistance, while vessels with smaller inside diameters create greater resistance. Peripheral resistance is dependent on three factors: the length of the vessel, the diameter of the vessel, and blood viscosity.

There is very little resistance to blood flow through the aorta and arteries. A significant change in peripheral resistance occurs at the arteriole level. This is because the inside diameter of the arteriole is much smaller, as compared to the aorta and arteries. Additionally, the arteriole has the pronounced ability to change its diameter as much as fivefold. It tends to do this in response to local tissue needs and autonomic nervous signals.

Contraction of the venous side of the vascular system results in decreased capacitance and increased cardiac preload. The arterial system, on the other hand, provides systemic vascular resistance. An increase in arterial tone increases resistance, which increases blood pressure.

Oxygen Transport

In addition to perfusion, oxygenation of the peripheral tissues is also essential. Oxygen is brought into the body via the respiratory system. During inspiration, approximately 500 to 800 mL of atmospheric air is taken into the lungs. Of this atmospheric air, 21 percent is oxygen. This air passes through the upper and lower airways, coming to rest in the *alveoli* of the lungs.

Surrounding the alveoli are capillaries, which are perfused by the arterial side of the pulmonary circulation. The arterial blood, which has been pumped through the pulmonary circulation by the right side of the heart, is low in oxygen, approximately a 16-percent concentration. The partial pressure of oxygen in the alveoli is greater than the deoxygenated blood within the pulmonary circulation. Thus, oxygen diffuses across the *alveolar-capillary* membrane and into the bloodstream. The red blood cells "pick-up" this oxygen while passing through the microcirculation of the pulmonary capillary bed. Oxygen binds to the hemoglobin molecule of the red blood cells, which serve as the primary carriers of oxygen within the bloodstream.

Under normal situations, between 97 percent and 100 percent of the hemoglobin is saturated with oxygen. The oxygen-enriched blood then circulates back to the heart via the venous side of the pulmonary circulation. Passing through the left atrium and into the left ventricle, the oxygen-enriched blood is pumped throughout the body via the systemic circulation.

Upon reaching the capillary circulation, the blood interfaces with the tissues. The tissues contain cells that are oxygen-deficient due to normal metabolic activity. Since the concentration of oxygen is greater in the bloodstream than the tissues, oxygen will diffuse from the red blood cells, into the tissues and cells. Overall, the movement and utilization of oxygen in the body is dependent upon:

1. adequate concentration of inspired oxygen,
2. appropriate movement of oxygen across the alveolar/capillary membrane into the arterial bloodstream,
3. adequate number of red blood cells to carry the oxygen,
4. proper tissue perfusion,
5. efficient off-loading of oxygen at the tissue level.

These elements are collectively known as the "*Fick Principle.*"

Tissue Perfusion

Tissue perfusion is dependent upon each component of the circulatory system. In addition, in terms of tissue oxygenation, it is dependent upon the respiratory system. If tissue perfusion is compromised, several things begin to occur.

Factors that can cause decreased perfusion include:

1. inadequate pump
    • inadequate preload
    • inadequate cardiac contractile strength
    • excessive afterload
    • inadequate heart rate
2. inadequate fluid
    • hypovolemia (abnormally low circulating blood volume)
3. inadequate container
    • dilated container without change in fluid volume
    • inadequate systemic vascular resistance

Usually, the body is able to compensate for any of the changes described above. However, when the compensatory mechanisms fail, shock develops.

Shock at the Cellular Level

Shock affects the entire organism. The cell is the ultimate target of inadequate tissue perfusion. Following an interruption of oxygen supply to the cell, metabolism will switch from an *aerobic* (with oxygen) to an *anaerobic* (without oxygen) mode.

The primary energy source for the cells is glucose, taken into the cell with the aid of insulin. There, in anaerobic metabolism, it is broken down

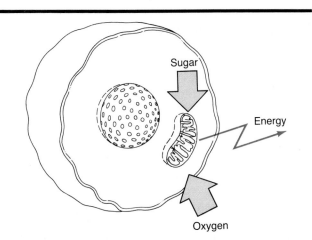

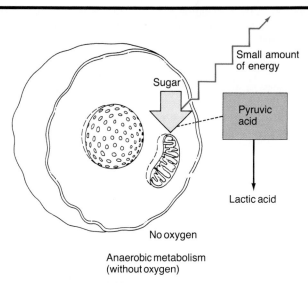

FIGURE 12-11 Aerobic metabolism requires oxygen and is most efficient.

FIGURE 12-12 Anaerobic metabolism yields much less energy and toxic by-products such as lactic acid.

into a compound called pyruvic acid in a process termed *glycolysis.* Glycolysis does not require oxygen, yet only yields a small amount of energy. Glycolysis alone is an inefficient utilization of glucose. Because of this, in the normal state, pyruvic acid is further degraded into carbon dioxide, water, and energy, in a process termed the *Krebs* or *citric acid cycle.* This aerobic process yields considerably more energy than glycolysis, and it requires oxygen. (See Figures 12-11, 12-12.)

In poor perfusion states, and in hypoxia, an inadequate amount of oxygen is presented to the cells. Thus, glucose can only complete glycolysis and cannot enter into the citric acid cycle. This causes an accumulation of pyruvic acid. In these cases, pyruvic acid is quickly degraded to lactic acid. If time elapses, and lactic acid and other metabolic acids accumulate, cellular death will occur. If this is allowed to continue, cell death will ultimately lead to tissue death. Tissue death will lead to organ failure. Organ failure will ultimately lead to death of the individual.

Stages of Shock

Shock can be divided into three distinct stages. These are:

- ❏ compensated shock
- ❏ decompensated shock
- ❏ irreversible shock.

Compensated Shock. Shock can be hidden by compensatory mechanisms such as generalized vasoconstriction and increases in the heart rate. Initially, these mechanisms are aimed at preserving cardiac output. These compensatory mechanisms serve to maintain an adequate blood pressure and to perfuse the vital organs.

Initially, following the onset of inadequate tissue perfusion, the various compensatory mechanisms of the body will be stimulated. The heart rate and strength of cardiac contractions will increase. There will be an increase in systemic vascular resistance that will assist in maintaining the blood pressure. These compensatory changes will continue until the

✱ Compensated shock is the most difficult stage of shock to detect. However, prompt recognition and treatment are essential.

body is unable to maintain blood pressure. Additionally, certain medications that the patient may be taking can contribute to the problem. Medications, such as propranolol, that act to block the beta receptor sites are just one example. They can initially hide the signs and symptoms of shock by hindering the compensatory increase in the heart rate and the ability of myocardial tissue to contract.

Decompensated Shock. In the later stages of shock blood pressure begins to fall. Prior to the fall in blood pressure, blood supply to essential organs diminishes. In addition to falling cardiac output, changes occur in the microcirculation that further interfere with oxygen delivery to the cells. The pre-capillary sphincters relax and the post-capillary sphincters remain closed. The result is the slowing of blood flow and sludging. Ultimately, the pressure driving the erythrocytes is diminished. This renders the erythrocytes unable to bend. Under routine capillary pressures, the erythrocytes can bend to facilitate movement through the capillary. However, when inadequate capillary pressure is present, the erythrocytes do not bend and simply stack, like a roll of coins, in a formation called a *rouleaux*. This causes further stagnation of capillary blood flow.

Irreversible Shock. Ultimately, after failure of the compensatory mechanisms, cellular death will begin. At some point, when enough cells in vital organs are disrupted, shock becomes irreversible and death is inevitable, even if vital signs are restored.

The heart is an amazing organ, so much so that even in a patient with no palpable blood pressure or pulse, adequate cardiac output (at least within normal values) can be restored with appropriate definitive care. While many patients recuperate from shock, others are not so fortunate.

As the initial insult of shock progresses, it becomes more deadly. Cells begin to die and so do organs. Vital organs such as the kidneys, liver, lungs and even the heart begin to falter and eventually become ineffective. A patient may be revived, only to die several days later as a result of end-organ failure—defined as the deleterious deterioration of the vital organs as a result of inadequate perfusion. Conditions that may occur during this phase include adult respiratory distress syndrome (ARDS), renal failure, liver failure, and sepsis.

Types of Shock

Hypovolemic Shock. Shock due to a loss of intravascular fluid volume is referred to as *hypovolemic shock*. Possible causes of hypovolemic shock include:

❏ internal or external hemorrhage
❏ traumatic injury
❏ long bone or open fractures
❏ severe dehydration from vomiting or diarrhea
❏ plasma loss from burns
❏ diabetic ketoacidosis from osmotic diuresis
❏ excessive sweating

Hypovolemic shock can also be due to internal third-space loss such as that which occurs with bowel obstruction, peritonitis, pancreatitis, or liver failure which results in ascites (accumulation of fluid within the abdominal cavity).

Cardiogenic Shock. An inability of the heart to pump enough blood to supply all body parts is referred to as *cardiogenic shock*. Cardiogenic shock is usually the result of severe left ventricular depression, secondary to acute myocardial infarction or congestive heart failure. The hypotension that accompanies this form of shock aggravates the situation by decreasing coronary perfusion. With decreased coronary perfusion the heart muscle becomes even more damaged, thus establishing a vicious cycle that ultimately results in complete pump failure.

During cardiogenic shock the activation of compensatory mechanisms can actually worsen the situation. When the peripheral resistance increases in an attempt to maintain blood pressure, the myocardial workload increases. This, in turn, increases the myocardial oxygen demand, further aggravating myocardial ischemia and infarction. Cardiac output is further depressed.

While the most common cause of cardiogenic shock is severe left ventricular depression, a number of other factors can have the same clinical manifestations. These include chronic progressive heart disease, such as cardiomyopathy, rupture of the papillary heart muscles or interventricular septum, and end-stage valvular disease (mitral or aortic stenosis). Most patients who experience cardiogenic shock will have normal blood volume. However, some patients will be hypovolemic from an excessive use of prescribed diuretics or the severe diaphoresis that accompanies some acute cardiac events. Patients may also experience relative hypovolemia (neurogenic shock) from the vasodilatory (blood vessel dilation) effects of such drugs as nitroglycerin.

Neurogenic Shock. *Neurogenic shock* may be described as inadequate peripheral resistance due to widespread vasodilation. With this inappropriate vasodilation a disproportionate amount of blood collects in the capillary bed. This reduces venous return, cardiac output, and arterial blood pressure. Neurogenic shock is most commonly due to an injury that results in severe spinal cord injury or total transection of the cord. Other causes of neurogenic shock include: central nervous system injury, septicemia from bacterial infection, anaphylactic reaction, insulin overdose, and Addisonian crisis (a disorder of the adrenal glands). With neurogenic shock there is an absence of the "sympathetic response."

Evaluation of the Shock Victim

Shock will present itself in a variety of ways. Depending on the degree of compensation, some patients will display few signs while others will be "classically symptomatic." Your initial approach can often yield a great deal of information. Before reaching the patient's side you can observe mental status, respiratory effort, and skin color. In situations where the patient is obviously in shock you must be aggressive with your assessment and treatment.

As with any patient care situation, assessment should begin with the "ABC's." (See Figure 12-13.) First, check the airway. The conscious patient who is able to speak usually has a patent (open) airway, whereas the unconscious patient is often subject to airway obstruction—particularly by the tongue—which tends to fall back against the posterior oropharynx. In trauma-related shock, bleeding in the oropharynx is often present, which can further compromise the airway. Once an open airway has been ensured, the adequacy of air exchange should be checked. While compensatory hyperventilation tends to occur in early shock, the unconscious shock patient will often hypoventilate. Hypoventilation occurs

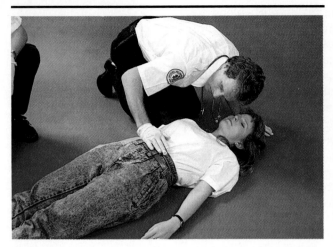

FIGURE 12-13 As with any emergency patient, assess the ABC's first.

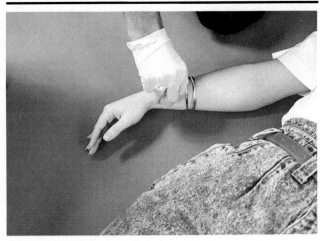

FIGURE 12-14 The presence and character of the pulse is a good indicator of the status of the patient's circulatory system.

when the respiratory center of the brain becomes depressed due to hypoperfusion.

When evaluating the ventilatory status, be sure to check both the rate and depth of respirations. Watch for patients who exhibit rapid, shallow breathing. This type of breathing is just as ineffective as slow or irregular respirations. Rapid, shallow breathing results in severely reduced minute volumes since an inadequate amount of air is being exchanged.

After patency of the airway and ventilatory effectiveness have been assured, turn your attention to evaluating circulation. First, evaluate the pulse for rate and character. Then examine the patient for obvious external bleeding. Because of compensatory mechanisms, a normal pulse rate may be seen even in the presence of a 10-percent to 15-percent volume deficit. A fast, weak, or thready pulse suggests decreased circulatory volume.

The location of the palpable pulse can also be an important indicator of circulatory status. Although these are rough estimates, they can be quite helpful. The presence of a radial pulse indicates that the patient has a systolic blood pressure of at least 80 mm Hg. If the radial pulse cannot be palpated, the femoral pulse or carotid pulse should be checked next. A palpable femoral pulse indicates a systolic blood pressure of 70 mm Hg. while a palpable carotid pulse indicates a systolic blood pressure of 60 mm Hg. (See Figure 12-14.)

In the case of profound shock where severe vasoconstriction is present, you might not be able to a palpate a pulse at all. Based on your findings of reduced perfusion, it would be appropriate to take immediate measures to restore circulation. In cases of obvious hypotension, as determined by using the above "rule" for checking the location of a palpable pulse, you don't need to take the time to auscultate a blood pressure before applying the anti-shock trousers or placing intravenous lines. The color, appearance and temperature of the skin can also serve as a useful indicator of circulatory effectiveness. As discussed earlier, the skin may appear normal in the initial stages of shock. Then as compensatory mechanisms such as vasoconstriction are activated and the blood is routed to the central circulation, the skin becomes pale (decreased perfusion), cyanotic (stagnant pooling of blood with inadequate oxygenation), mottled (combination of both; a late sign of shock), and cool to the touch and diaphoretic.

Often, the appearance of the skin will indicate shock even before there are any noticeable changes in the blood pressure.

Another method of assessing the circulation is to check the capillary refill. Capillary refill testing is performed by applying pressure to the nail bed of one of the patient's fingers. This pressure should cause a blanching of the nail bed. When the pressure is released, the nail should return to its normal pink color within two seconds. (See Figure 12-15.) You can approximate this time period by saying "capillary refill." If the normal pink color does not return to the nail bed, it can be assumed that there is decreased perfusion to this area. Since the nail bed is the most distal part of the circulation, poor capillary refill is an early indicator of decreased perfusion to the whole body. However, use of the capillary refill test has limited value in the field setting due to poor lighting conditions and other environmental factors.

The level of consciousness or mentation should also be assessed throughout the initial survey. In fact, the level of consciousness is probably a better indicator of decreased tissue perfusion than most other signs. Because of the high energy requirements of the brain, any reduction in cerebral blood flow will be manifested by:

❑ agitation
❑ disorientation
❑ confusion
❑ an inability to respond to questions or commands appropriately
❑ unconsciousness

Any significant alteration in the level of consciousness must be viewed as a indication of critical hypoperfusion or hypoxia. Additionally, with an increased secretion of catecholamines, the patient often becomes anxious or apprehensive.

Another factor that clouds the picture in trauma-related shock is that mind-altering substances are often involved. When alcohol and/or drugs interfere with the patient's normal thought processes, it is extremely difficult to gain an accurate view of the mental status. Your job as a health care provider can also be taxed by the fact that the intoxicated or "high" patient often behaves in a less than social manner. Keep in mind, however, that just because the patient has been drinking or taking drugs, doesn't mean that there may not be a serious underlying problem. Whenever the likelihood of a serious trauma or medical emergency exists, it is

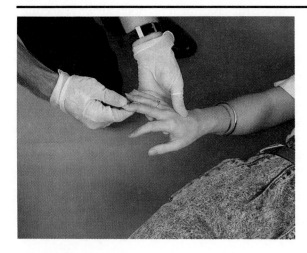

FIGURE 12-15 Normal capillary refill takes two seconds or less.

probably best to assume that any altered mental status is due to decreased cerebral perfusion.

After completion of the primary survey and initiation of the necessary treatment, a secondary survey should be performed. The thoroughness of the secondary survey is dependant upon the severity of the patient's condition. Obvious life-threatening problems that cannot be corrected in the pre-hospital care setting warrant rapid transportation of the patient to an appropriate definitive care facility. Ideally, when assessing the seriously injured patient, you should expose and inspect the head, neck, chest, and abdomen. Throughout the secondary survey, and while providing treatment and transporting the patient to the hospital, you must continually reassess the temperature and moisture of the skin, blood pressure, pulse rate, and respiratory rate.

In shock—due to the presence of hypoxia, acidosis and increased secretion of catecholamines—cardiac dysrhythmias must be considered a potential complication. Because of this, you should include the continual monitoring of the patient's ECG rhythm in your assessment. Look for rapid or slow heart rates as well as irregular rhythms, as these indicate potential life-threatening problems. Additional information can be obtained by asking your patient the appropriate questions. Find out how he feels. Is the patient thirsty, weak, nauseous, dizzy, etc.? Does he have a history of significant medical conditions or take any medications? This will give you additional information upon which you can base your treatment.

Evaluation of the trauma victim for shock, then, is begun in the primary survey, where the most obvious signs of decreased tissue perfusion may be present. It is continued during the secondary survey, where more subtle clues may be found. The patient is then continually assessed for signs of developing shock until he is placed in the hands of receiving medical personnel.

General Management

Providing aggressive care to the patient who is experiencing shock begins during the resuscitation phase of the primary survey and continues until appropriate tissue perfusion and cellular oxygenation has been restored. The primary aspects of patient management include maintaining a patent airway; ensuring an adequate ventilatory rate and volume; providing supplemental oxygen; supporting circulation; and stabilizing suspected fractures or injuries.

Although it is taught in the classroom that patient care should always progress in a systematic fashion—first, maintain an open airway; second, ensure adequate breathing; and third, deal with circulation—the reality of the field setting is that many times there is a need to provide all primary treatments at essentially the same time. To accomplish this, you and your partner (or members of your crew) must work as a team. Ideally, while one person is maintaining a patent airway, assuring adequate ventilations, and providing supplemental oxygen, the other paramedics should control any significant bleeding, position the patient appropriately, apply the PASG and establish one or more intravenous lines. As part of applying the anti-shock trousers, the patient should be log-rolled onto a full backboard. This way, many tasks are being performed at relatively the same time.

Maintaining a Patent Airway. As indicated earlier, the presentation of the patient in shock can range from alert to unresponsive and apneic. Usu-

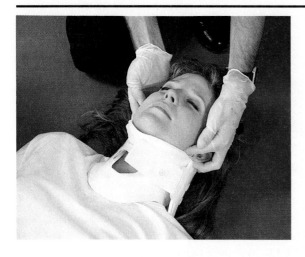

FIGURE 12-16 The airway in the shock patient should be assessed and maintained. If cervical spine injury is suspected, use the jaw-thrust maneuver.

ally, the appearance of the patient falls somewhere in-between. If the patient is unable to maintain his own airway, adjuncts should be utilized to prevent the tongue from falling back against the posterior oropharynx and obstructing the airway. Additionally, fluids and other foreign objects should be removed to prevent aspiration into the trachea.

Whenever the potential exists for the patient to have sustained head or spinal injury, you must employ the appropriate cervical spine support in all aspects of airway management and ventilatory support. (See Figure 12-16.) Options that can be used to prevent obstruction of airflow through the upper airway include placement of an oropharyngeal airway, nasopharyngeal airway, esophageal obturator airway (EOA) or endotracheal tube (ET). When dealing with the shock patient who is unresponsive, particularly in the presence of bleeding into the pharynx (as commonly occurs secondary to trauma-related shock), endotracheal intubation is the preferred airway technique. The reason: The trachea can be effectively sealed off to prevent aspiration. Endotracheal intubation is also better tolerated than adjuncts such as an EOA in a case where the patient starts to awaken after application of the pneumatic anti-shock garment, or ventilation and oxygenation efforts improve cerebral blood flow and oxygenation.

Blood or fluids should be cleared with appropriate suctioning techniques, taking care not to stimulate the gag reflex or create inadvertent hypoxia. Larger foreign objects, such as teeth, should be removed utilizing the finger sweep technique. In the presence of ongoing fluid accumulation in the pharynx, it may be necessary to place the patient onto his side. Although this is an effective alternative, as fluids will seek the lowest point and drain out, it is cumbersome to maintain cervical spine support and assist ventilations while the patient is in this position.

Maintaining Adequate Respiratory Function. Remember, an effective ventilatory volume is dependent upon two variables: adequate rate and sufficient depth of respirations. In shock, both of these may be less than normal. To complicate matters more, the patient may appear to be breathing at a sufficient rate or even display tachypnea. But in reality, the patient may be exchanging very little air with each breath. The unconscious patient should be closely monitored to be sure that he is maintaining adequate respiratory minute volumes. (See Figure 12-17.) If there is any indication of hypoventilation, you must assist the patient's breathing with a bag-valve-mask device or other ventilatory assistance adjunct. Another

* Your first action when caring for any shock patient should be the primary assessment.

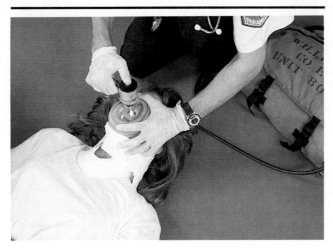

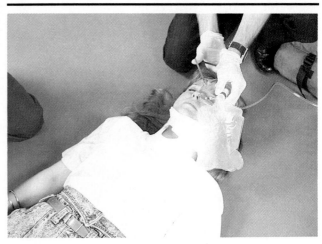

FIGURE 12-17 If necessary, assist or provide respirations and oxygenation.

FIGURE 12-18 Provide high-flow oxygen.

variable to consider is that application of the anti-shock trousers can decrease thoracic capacity by forcing the abdominal organs up against the diaphragm, thus creating a situation where the patient is moving an inadequate amount of air. Again, any indication of hypoventilation should prompt you to consider employing ventilatory assistance. Other conditions occurring with shock that result in respiratory compromise must be dealt with. These include administration of diuretics, bronchodilators, and emergency chest decompression.

Oxygenation of the Patient. Once the airway has been secured, the patient should receive as high a concentration of supplemental oxygen as possible. If the patient is breathing sufficiently, a non-rebreather mask with a liter flow of 10 to 15 liters per minute should be applied. Pay attention to the amount of oxygen that remains in the reservoir of the device at the end of each inspiration. Patients experiencing compensatory hyperventilation can deplete the reservoir, in which case a simple face mask should be employed to prevent suffocation. If the patient becomes nauseous or is frightened by the mask, a nasal cannula with a liter flow of 6 to 8 liters per minute can be employed. When there is a need to assist ventilations, as occurs in the presence of hypoventilation or when an endotracheal tube has been placed, 100 percent oxygen should be delivered via a bag-valve device, manually triggered demand-valve device, or automatic ventilator device. (See Figure 12-18.)

Control of Major Bleeding. Next, attention is directed to the control of any major bleeding. Usually, direct pressure to sites of rapid external bleeding will be sufficient to contain blood loss. (See Figure 12-19.) In cases where peripheral hemorrhage cannot be controlled by direct pressure, other measures must be employed, including application of a tourniquet. Application of the pneumatic anti-shock trousers may be useful in controlling intra-abdominal (aorta, liver, spleen, retroperitoneal, pelvic) and lower extremity hemorrhage.

Managing Hypotension. Hypotension can be managed in a variety of ways including elevation of the patient's legs, applying and inflating the anti-shock trousers, establishing intravenous lifelines and administering vasopressor (vasoconstrictor) agents.

Positioning of the Patient. In shock, the preferred position for the patient is generally supine, with the legs elevated 10 to 12 inches. This position promotes increased venous return to the heart and increased cerebral perfusion. In some situations, elevation of the legs alone will be sufficient to raise the blood pressure. However, this position is directly opposite of that which is best suited for easing respirations. In cases where the patient is experiencing respiratory compromise, e.g. acute pulmonary edema secondary to cardiogenic shock, an upright, sitting position is preferred. In addition, elevating the legs in patients with concomitant head injury can increase intracranial pressure and worsen an already bad situation. (See Figure 12-20.)

When attempting to determine the appropriate position for the patient experiencing shock accompanied by respiratory compromise, you must weigh the benefits of easier breathing against the disadvantages of reduced cerebral perfusion. If the respiratory compromised patient is placed in a supine position you must take the necessary precautions to assure appropriate air exchange. It may be necessary to use a bag-valve-mask device or demand valve to assist the patient's breathing.

Pneumatic Anti-shock Garment. If the patient is hypotensive, the *pneumatic anti-shock garment (PASG)* should be applied and inflated until an adequate blood pressure is obtained. The pneumatic anti-shock garment is a three-chambered unit that is wrapped around both lower extremities and the abdomen. When inflated by use of an external pump, it applies circumferential pneumatic counter pressure to the structures beneath it. While quite a bit of controversy surrounds use of the pneumatic anti-shock garment, there does seem to be benefit to its application in the field setting. The positive effects obtained include:

❏ an increase in the blood pressure
❏ increased blood flow to the heart, brain and lungs
❏ control of bleeding
❏ stabilization of fractures of the lower limbs and pelvis.

Currently, there are two main theories regarding how application of the pneumatic anti-shock garment works to increase blood pressure and blood flow to the heart, brain, and lungs. The first theory suggests that inflation of the garment produces pneumatic counter pressure, which

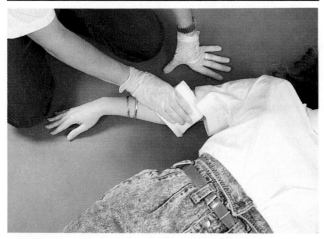

FIGURE 12-19 Control any obvious bleeding.

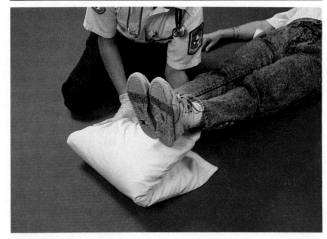

FIGURE 12-20 Elevate the feet if a head injury is not suspected.

acts to reduce the container size of the venous circulation. This redistributes as much as two units of blood from the lower half of the body to the central circulation. This "autotransfusion" produces a reversible increase in preload. More recent studies, however, suggest that only a minimal amount of blood is autotransfused—as little as 300 mL in a 150-pound man.

The second theory suggests that application of the pneumatic anti-shock garment affects the blood pressure by increasing arterial impedance. When circumferential pneumatic counter pressure is applied to the lower half of the body, blood vessels under the suit constrict. This decreases blood flow to the lower half of the body and increases peripheral vascular resistance. An elevated blood pressure and increased blood flow to the central portion of the body (heart, brain, and lungs) then occurs. Review of recent literature seems to indicate that neither the "autotransfusion theory" or "increased systemic vascular resistance theory" can be ruled out. In fact, it is likely that the reversal of hypotension is dependent on the clinical situation as well as the potential that several mechanisms may, in fact, work together.

Regardless of how it works, application of the garment can produce impressive changes in the patient's condition. Because of the improved cerebral blood flow, it is not uncommon for the unconscious patient to wake up. Usually, this is not a problem. But when the patient is intubated, or there are mind altering substances or psychiatric problems involved, it may be necessary to use restraints to prevent injury to the patient or yourself.

PASG indications. Indications for application of the PASG include:

- ❑ **Control of bleeding:** The pneumatic anti-shock garment acts to control bleeding by applying direct pressure to the injury site. This pneumatic counter pressure creates circumferential tension, which improves hemostasis and decreases blood flow to torn vessels beneath the garment. It is also believed to exert a tamponade effect on bleeding within the abdomen.
- ❑ **Stabilization of fractures:** By enclosing both the lower extremities and pelvis, and producing effects similar to a large air splint, the garment prevents movement. Application of the pneumatic anti-shock garment is indicated in cases where the hypotensive patient has sustained fractures to the lower extremities. Use of the device allows you to treat both problems at essentially the same time, thus permitting rapid packaging and transportation of the patient. Because inflation of the device can raise the patient's blood pressure, it should only be used for fracture stabilization in cases where the patient is hypotensive. Other splinting devices (traction, vacuum, and/or board splints) should be used to immobilize fractures when the patient is normotensive or hypertensive.
- ❑ **Blood pressure:** Since use of the pneumatic anti-shock garment may make cannula placement easier, application of the garment should precede the placement of these lines in the severely hypotensive patient.

Contraindications and Complications. Use of the pneumatic anti-shock garment is contraindicated in the presence of pulmonary edema occurring secondary to heart failure. This is because adding fluid volume to the central circulation may further compromise an already failing heart. Relative contraindications for inflation of the abdominal section include pregnancy beyond the second trimester, evisceration, and an impaled object in the abdomen. However, these precautions should not deter use of this device in the treatment of the severely hypotensive patient.

Potential complications associated with use of the pneumatic anti-shock garment include lower extremity compartment syndromes, metabolic acidosis after prolonged use due to decreased lower extremity tissue perfusion, decreased renal function, and decreased respiratory vital capacity resulting from compression of the abdominal organs against the diaphragm. Because of the potential for decreased diaphragmatic excursion—with resultant decreased vital capacity—caution should be exercised when using the device in the presence of any dyspnea.

Application of the PASG. Techniques for applying the pneumatic anti-shock garment are shown in Procedure 12-1. While some teach that the patient's clothing should be removed prior to application of the pneumatic anti-shock garment, there is little evidence to support that there is any real benefit to this practice. Additionally, in the field setting, many factors make this practice virtually impossible: environmental conditions (weather, temperature, presence of onlookers), severity of the patient's injuries, and the patient's unwillingness to be disrobed.

Due to the environmental conditions (broken glass, splintered wood, spilled gasoline, etc.) and urgency of the situation under which these devices are typically applied, the inflation pressure should be frequently checked as the possibility for damage to the garment and subsequent leaks is always present. Additionally, changes in temperature or altitude may cause significant fluctuation in pressure within the device. This is especially true when the patient is taken from a cold environment to a warm one, or when there is an increase in altitude such as that which occurs when the patient is transported by air. Both of these situations can cause pressure in the suit to increase dramatically.

Once inflated, the pneumatic anti-shock garment should not be deflated without specific direction from a physician. The reason for this is that the device, by increasing the preload and/or the systemic vascular resistance, only acts to provide a temporary, interim elevation of the blood pressure. Deflation of the garment prior to restoration of adequate circulating blood volume can have life-threatening consequences as the cardiac output and blood pressure often drop precipitously.

Restoration of adequate circulating blood volume is unlikely in the field setting. Once the patient has received stabilizing care at a definitive care facility you may be instructed to remove the pneumatic anti-shock garment. The release of air from the compartments should take place over several minutes, beginning with the abdominal section and then moving to each leg. At no time should the entire garment be deflated at once. Throughout the deflation of each compartment, the patient's blood pressure and appearance should be constantly monitored. In cases where the patient becomes hypotensive and/or symptomatic, it may be necessary to reinflate the garment.

Intravenous Fluid Therapy. Intravenous cannulation is a procedure used to directly access the venous circulation. The primary reasons for intravenous cannulation in the field setting include establishing a route for:

1. administration of drugs
2. replacement of fluid
3. obtaining specimens of venous blood for laboratory determinations

While many drugs can be administered subcutaneously or intramuscularly, absorption of the drug into the circulatory system is severely hampered during states of decreased cardiac output (e.g. shock). Intravenous

* The PASG should not be removed in the field setting.

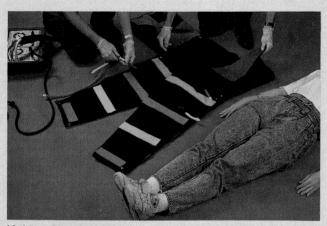

12-1A.   Prepare the PASG.

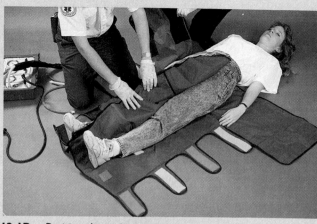

12-1B.   Position the patient.

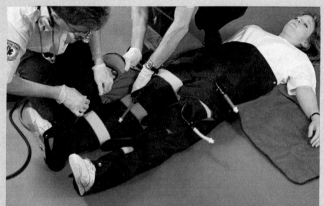

12-1C.   Wrap the legs following manufacturer's recommendations.

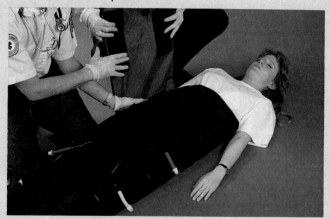

12-1D.   Wrap the abdomen last.

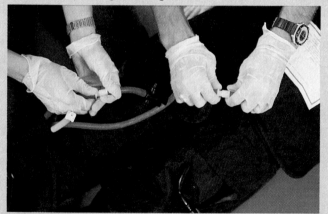

12-1E.   Connect the tubing.

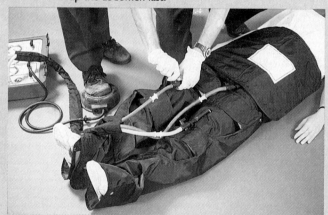

12-1F.   Inflate the PASG, both legs first.

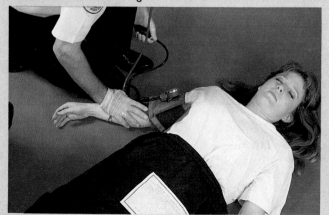

12-1G.   Monitor the patient.

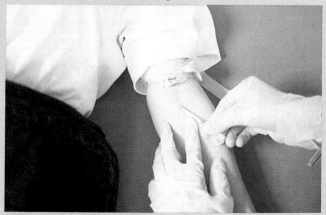

12-1H.   Establish an IV.

administration of drugs usually ensures that they will reach the circulation.

Necessary supplies. Typical supplies needed for intravenous cannulation include: protective latex gloves, intravenous solution, administration tubing, extension set, cannulas (assorted sizes), venous constricting band, tape, antibiotic swabs, antibiotic ointment, tape and gauze dressings (2×2's, 4×4's), 35 mL syringe, and a padded armboard. (See Figure 12-21.)

Intravenous solutions. Intravenous solutions, as discussed earlier in the chapter, are divided into two groups: colloids (whole blood, packed red blood cells, plasma, plasma substitutes) and crystalloids. Colloid solutions contain molecules that are too large to easily pass through the capillary membranes. Thus, these solutions tend to remain in the vascular space for a considerable period of time.

On the other hand, crystalloid solutions contain electrolytes and water but no proteins or larger molecules. Therefore, without larger molecules to keep the fluid in the vascular space, crystalloid solutions easily move across the capillary walls into the tissues. Because crystalloid solutions often have a transitory effect, there is a need to administer two to three times the amount of blood lost when treating patients who have experienced hemorrhagic shock.

Although colloids are particularly useful in maintaining the vascular volume, their use is prohibitive in the field setting due to the cost and special requirements for storage. However, because you may be asked to assist with their administration in the emergency department or in the case of a lengthy entrapment or disaster scene, where medical personnel are brought in to assist, you should be familiar with the more common types.

Administration set. Intravenous solutions are almost always administered through clear, plastic tubing. This allows for easy viewing in the case of air bubbles or precipitation of certain medications administered through the tubing. There are two primary types of intravenous administration sets: the *microdrip* (pediatric) and the *macrodrip* (standard). (See

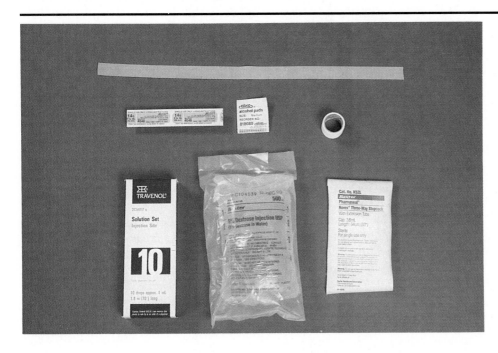

FIGURE 12-21 Supplies for initiating IV therapy.

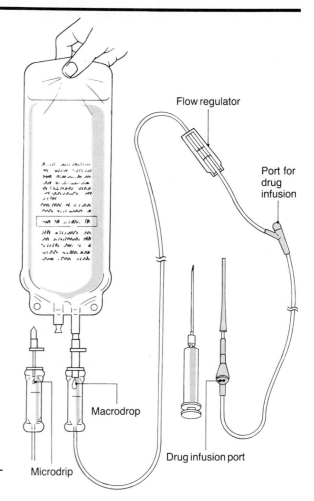

FIGURE 12-22 Comparison of macrodrip and microdrip IV administration sets.

Flow regulator

Port for drug infusion

Macrodrop

Drug infusion port

Microdrip

Figure 12-22.) The microdrip is typically used in situations where it is necessary to restrict the amount of fluids administered, e.g. cardiac, medical, and pediatric emergencies. When administering solutions through the microdrip administration set, 60 drops is equal to 1 milliliter. The macrodrip is used in situations where large amounts of fluid are to be administered, e.g. shock, fluid replacement. With the macrodrip administration set, 10 drops is equal to 1 milliliter. However, it is important to note that, depending on the manufacturer, the drop size may vary. Be sure to read the box that the administration set comes in.

Cannulas. There are three types of cannulas:

1. hollow needles, e.g., butterfly, or winged, needles;
2. plastic catheters inserted over a hollow needle, e.g. Angiocath®
3. plastic catheters inserted through a hollow needle, e.g. Intracath®

In the field setting, the over-the-needle catheter is generally preferred, since it can be anchored better and permits freer movement of the patient. Additionally, the puncture in the vein is exactly the same size as the plastic catheter. Thus, there is less chance for bleeding around the venipuncture site. The outside diameter of the needle is called a gauge. The larger the gauge number, the smaller the diameter of the shaft. For example, a 22 gauge cannula is small, whereas a 14 gauge cannula is

✱ The shorter the length of an IV catheter, and the greater the diameter, the greater will be the volume that can be delivered through it.

large. A large diameter catheter (14 gauge) provides a much greater fluid flow than does a small diameter catheter (22 gauge). Cannulas used for pre-hospital care come in a variety of sizes:

- ❑ 24 gauge
- ❑ 22 gauge (used for fragile and/or small veins, pediatric patients)
- ❑ 20 gauge (used for average sized adult patients)
- ❑ 18 gauge, 16 gauge, and 14 gauge (used for volume replacement or where viscous medications such as glucose are to be administered)

The other variable that should be considered when selecting an intravenous cannula is its length. The longer the cannula, the less the flow rate will be. The flow rate through a 14 gauge, 5 cm catheter (approximately 125 mL/minute), is twice the flow rate through a longer, 16 gauge, 20 cm catheter. For cannulation of a peripheral vein, a needle and catheter length of 5 cm is adequate while the cannulation of a central line requires a needle length of 6–7 cm and catheter length of at least 15–20 cm.

Venous access.   As discussed earlier, in the field setting, use of peripheral veins is preferred over central vein cannulation. The technique is relatively easy to master, it provides an effective route for administration of fluids and medications, and it does not interfere with other life-sustaining measures such as cardiopulmonary resuscitation and airway management. Cannulation of central veins often takes longer, requires the use of sterile procedures (gloves, drapes, prep, solution.), has a higher complication rate (pneumothorax, arterial injury, abnormal placement) and usually necessitates that a chest X-ray be taken immediately after placement to ensure correct positioning. However, central veins are useful in situations where peripheral veins have collapsed.

For peripheral cannulation, the veins of the dorsal aspect of the hand, forearm, and antecubital fossa are the most convenient. The veins on the back of the hand offer the advantage of permitting the patient to freely move his arm. Additionally, if a problem develops with these more distal veins, another site higher up on the arm can be selected. The disadvantage of the more distal veins is that they are sometimes fragile and difficult to cannulate. In addition, in states of decreased cardiac output, medications administered through these vessels take longer to reach the central circulation.

The veins of the forearm and antecubital fossa offer the advantage of being larger and easier to cannulate. Additionally, because they are closer, medications will reach the central circulation quicker. In cardiac arrest and other states of decreased perfusion, the forearm, or antecubital fossa, is the preferred site for cannulation. In the presence of hypovolemia, application of the pneumatic anti-shock garment should precede venous cannulation, as the garment makes it easier to find and cannulate the vein.

An alternative to central line placement is the external jugular vein. This vein is easily accessed and relatively free of complication. (See Figure 12-23.)

In children, several veins are available. In addition to the veins of the arm and leg, the external jugular vein is available as well as several scalp veins.

While repeated practice makes starting IVs easier, there are some patients in whom cannulating a vein is particularly difficult. Among them: obese patients, patients experiencing shock and cardiac arrest, chronic

✳ Central line placement is not indicated in prehospital care.

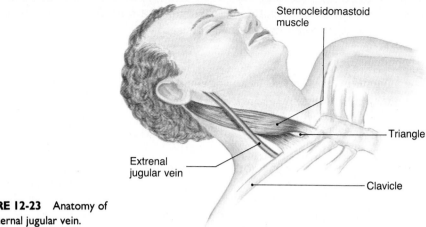

FIGURE 12-23 Anatomy of the external jugular vein.

"main line" IV drug users, elderly patients with "fragile" or "rolling veins," and small children. (See Procedure 12-2.)

When the IV does not flow. In some cases the IV will not flow as it should. The following should be considered:

1. Has the venous constricting band been removed? This is probably the most common mistake made in both the hospital and field settings. Additionally, check to make sure that the patient is not wearing restrictive clothing that may be interfering with venous flow.
2. Is there swelling at the cannulation site? This indicates infiltration into the tissues.
3. Are the tubing control valves open? Be sure to check both the primary control valve and any control valves that are part of the extension set.
4. Is the cannula up against a valve or wall of the vein? This can be checked by slightly repositioning the cannula. It may be necessary to untape the cannula and retape it after a good flow rate has been achieved by repositioning. It may be necessary to use a padded armboard to keep the patient's hand or arm in the appropriate position.
5. Is the IV bag high enough? Sometimes when moving the patient the cannulation site is raised higher than the bag; subsequently it interferes with gravity, which is required to move the fluid.
6. Is the drip chamber completely filled with solution? This can be easily corrected by simply inverting the bag and squeezing the drip chamber to return some of the fluid to the bag. If the flow is still slow or absent, lower the IV bag below the level of the insertion site. If blood return is seen in the IV tubing, the site is patent. If problems still persist, the IV should be removed and reestablished on another extremity.

Complications of intravenous therapy. Complications that can occur with intravenous therapy include:

Pain. Pain at the puncture site may be due to penetration of the skin with the needle or **extravasation.** Pain can lead to increased anxiety, which can predispose the patient to cardiac dysrhythmias. Pain can be minimized by using a smaller gauge catheter, anesthetizing the overlying skin using 1 percent lidocaine (without epinephrine) prior to penetration, or by using the sharp tip of a smaller needle to make an incision in the skin through which a larger cannula can pass more easily.

Hematoma or infiltration. Hematoma or infiltration at the puncture site results from injury to the blood vessel, or the catheter becoming dislodged from the vein. Fluid then accumulates in the interstitial space. In

■ **extravasation** the leakage of fluid or medication outside a blood vessel.

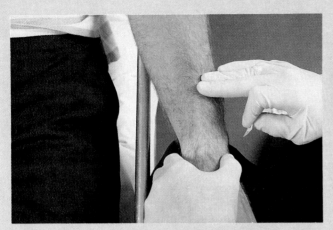

12-2A. Apply the tourniquet and select a suitable vein.

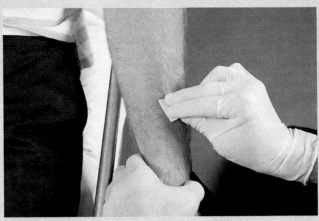

12-2B. Prep the site with an anti-bacterial solution.

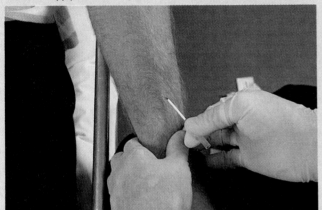

12-2C. Insert the needle into the vein.

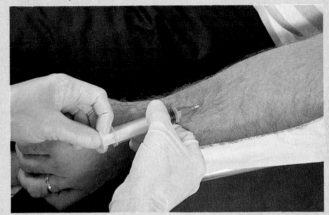

12-2D. Withdraw any blood samples needed.

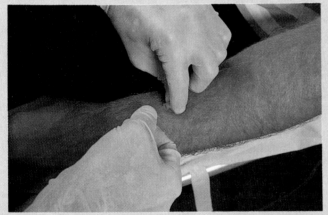

12-2E. Connect the IV tubing.

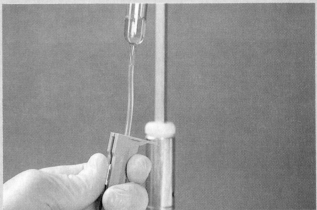

12-2F. Turn on the IV and check the flow.

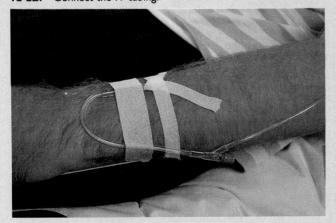

12-2G. Secure the site.

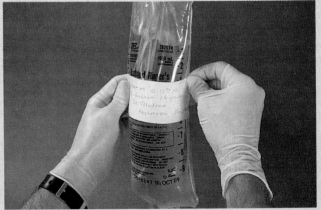

12-2H. Label the bag.

the presence of a hematoma or infiltration at the puncture site, the catheter should be removed and the IV reestablished at another site.

Local infection. Local infection occurs when appropriate cleansing techniques are not utilized and bacteria are introduced into the puncture site.

Pyrogenic reaction. A pyrogenic reaction occurs when **pyrogens** (foreign proteins capable of producing fever) are present in the administration set or intravenous solution. It is characterized by the abrupt onset of fever (100–106° F), chills, backache, headache, nausea, and vomiting. Cardiovascular collapse may also result. Reaction usually occurs within one-half to one hour following initiation of IV therapy. If a pyrogenic reaction is suspected the IV should be immediately terminated and established in the other arm using a new administration set and solution. The potential for this complication to occur emphasizes the need to discard any IV bag that shows leakage or cloudiness.

Catheter shear. A catheter shear occurs when the catheter is pulled back through (Intracath) or over (Angiocath) the needle after it has been advanced forward. Since the catheter is plastic it easily snags on the sharp edge of the needle and is sheared off, becoming a plastic emboli. For this reason the catheter should never be drawn back over or through the needle. Always withdraw the needle first and then withdraw the catheter.

Inadvertent arterial puncture. Because of its sometimes close proximity to veins, an artery may be inadvertently punctured. Arterial puncture is recognized by the appearance of spurting, bright red blood. When arterial puncture occurs, immediately withdraw the catheter and apply direct pressure to the site, for at least 5 minutes, and until the bleeding has stopped.

Circulatory overload. Circulatory overload occurs when too much intravenous solution is administered for a given patient's condition. This emphasizes the need to closely monitor the IV flow rate, particularly in patients prone to heart failure. Constantly watch the patient for signs of developing congestive heart failure—rales, tachypnea, external jugular vein distension—in which case the IV flow rate should be significantly reduced or terminated.

Thrombophlebitis. Inflammation of the vein is particularly common when intravenous therapy is long-term. Thrombophlebitis is manifested by redness and edema at the puncture site, and pain along the course of the vein, which is sometimes accompanied by inflammation and tenderness. Typically, thrombophlebitis does not occur immediately, but is more common after several hours of intravenous therapy. When thrombophlebitis is suspected the IV should be terminated and warm compresses should be applied to the site.

Air embolism. Air embolism occurs when air is allowed to enter the vein. It is more likely to occur during central vein cannulation or when air has not be cleared from the IV administration set appropriately.

Flow rates. In the field setting, there are typically two rates for administering intravenous solutions. In medical emergencies, where intravenous lines are placed prophylactically or for the purpose of administering medications, the flow is usually maintained at a "keep open" rate. In trauma or other situations, where intravenous fluids are being used to replace circulatory volume, the flow rate should be based on the patient's response (improvements in pulse, blood pressure, capillary refill, and cerebral function). In the severely hypovolemic patient, the solution should be administered at a rapid flow rate. The maximum amount of intrave-

■ **pyrogen** any substance capable of causing fever.

nous fluids that should be administered to an adult in the field setting is about 2 to 3 liters. When treating the patient with severe blood loss, the flow rate can be increased three to four times normal by wrapping a blood pressure cuff around the IV bag and inflating it to 300 mm Hg or using a commercial pressure infuser.

Maintaining Body Temperature. In the course of treating the patient for shock the body temperature should be maintained as close to normal as possible. (See Figure 12-24.) Pay attention to factors that affect body temperature including environmental/weather conditions, temperature of the oxygen and intravenous fluids, and the location where the patient is found, to name a few. Persons lying on the ground, particularly during inclement weather, are prone to hypothermia. Body temperature can be maintained by protecting the patient from the elements and by removing any wet clothing. Cover the patient to avoid heat loss, but be careful not to overbundle. Too much heat produces vasodilation, which counteracts the body's compensatory mechanism of vasoconstriction and increases fluid loss by perspiration.

Use of Medications in the Treatment of Shock. Medications that may be used in the treatment of some forms of shock include alpha- and beta-stimulating catecholamines, vasodilators, corticosteroids, diuretics, antidysrhythmics and naloxone.

Hypovolemic shock. In the field setting, medications are rarely used in the treatment of hypovolemic shock. The primary effort is directed toward replacing circulatory volume and improving cellular oxygenation.

Cardiogenic shock. When cardiogenic shock is caused by severe myocardial depression, sympathetic stimulating agents such as dopamine, dobutamine and norepinephrine may be used to improve the pumping action of the heart and cardiac output. The exact doses of these medications are based on patient response and must be administered with great care.

✳ Medications are never used in the treatment of hypovolemic shock unless fluid replacement has been carried out. Thus, they are very rarely used in the prehospital management of hypovolemic shock.

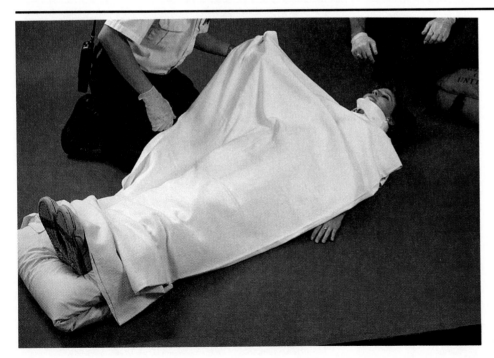

FIGURE 12-24 Always maintain the patient's body temperature.

Typically, when dopamine is used it should be titrated to maintain a systolic blood pressure of 80 to 100 mm Hg. The lowest dose consistent with the desired result should be used. When cardiac dysrhythmias result in depressed cardiac output, antidysrhythmic agents such as lidocaine, bretylium, procainamide (ventricular origin), atropine, isoproterenol (bradycardia) and verapamil, propranolol (supraventricular tachycardia) may be used to restore normal cardiac output.

Neurogenic shock. Vasopressors such as dopamine or norepinephrine may be used to treat some forms of inappropriate systemic vascular resistance seen with neurogenic, septic or anaphylactic shock. Definitive therapy is directed toward correction of the underlying cause.

Rapid packaging and transport of the patient. The patient should then be transported to the hospital as rapidly as possible, under constant monitoring. Packaging is a skill that should be repeatedly practiced. (See Figure 12-25.)

Shock resuscitation in the severely injured patient. The severely injured patient requires definitive, often surgical, in-hospital care. Field stabilization should be rapid, with many procedures initiated enroute. The steps in field management of the severely injured patient include:

Extrication. The patient should be removed as rapidly as possible utilizing standard techniques and methods of stabilization.

PASG. The PASG should be readily available. Even if the patient appears stable, the PASG should be in place. Should the patient deteriorate, it can be inflated enroute.

Stabilization. Brief stabilization of the airway, breathing, and circulation should be completed. In addition, any major sources of hemorrhage should be controlled.

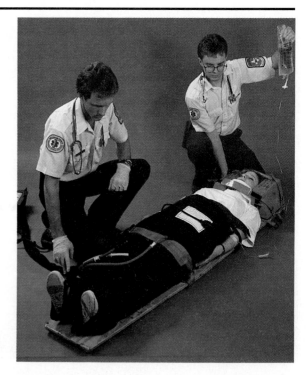

FIGURE 12-25 The packaged patient.

Load for transportation. The patient should be placed in the ambulance and prepared for transport.

IV therapy. While the IV is being prepared, transport should be initiated. While en route the venous constricting band should be applied, the vein identified, the tape prepared, the IV prepared, and the skin prepped. Then, the driver should pull to the side of the road for cannula placement. As soon as the cannula is in place, transport should resume. The cannula is subsequently stabilized and the flow rate adjusted.

SUMMARY

This chapter has presented fundamental physiology, pathophysiology and management of fluid and electrolyte disorders, acid-base balance, and shock. Shock is the final, common denominator of a large variety of disease processes and represents a life-threatening decompensation of vital functions. It demands immediate recognition and treatment.

FURTHER READING

American College of Surgeons, Committee on Trauma. *Advanced Trauma Life Support Course: Student Manual.* American College of Surgeons, 1989.

BLEDSOE, BRYAN E. *Atlas of Paramedic Skills.* Englewood Cliffs, NJ: Prentice Hall, Inc., 1987.

BLEDSOE, BRYAN E., BOSKER, GIDEON, and PAPA, FRANK J. *Pre-hospital Emergency Pharmacology,* 2nd ed. Englewood Cliffs, NJ: Prentice Hall, Inc., 1988.

BUTMAN, ALEXANDER M., and PATURAS, JAMES L. *Pre-Hospital Trauma Life Support.* Akron, OH: Emergency Training, 1986.

CAMPBELL, JOHN E. *Basic Trauma Life Support,* 2nd ed. Englewood Cliffs, NJ: Prentice Hall, Inc., 1988.

SHADE, BRUCE, et al, *Advanced Cardiac Life Support: Certification, Preparation, and Review.* Englewood Cliffs, NJ: Brady Communications, Inc., 1988.

TINTINALLI, JUDITH E., KROME, RONALD L., and RUIZ, ERNEST. *Emergency Medicine: A Comprehensive Study Guide,* 2nd ed. New York, NY: McGraw-Hill Book Company, 1988.

13

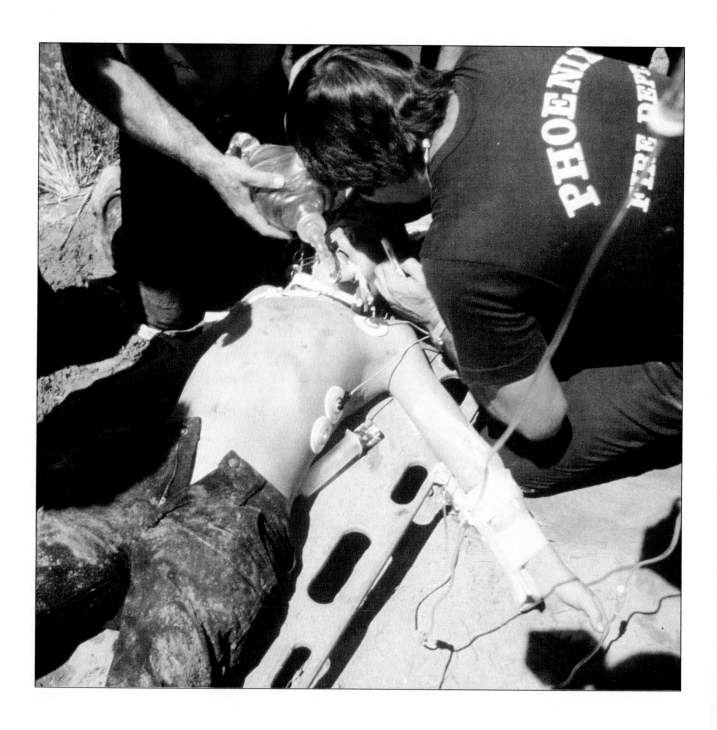

Emergency Pharmacology

Objectives For Chapter 13

Upon completing this chapter, the student should be able to:

1. Define:
   - pharmacology
   - drug
   - pharmacodynamics
   - pharmacokinetics
2. List four drug sources and give an example of a drug derived from each source.
3. Name three federal legislative acts that regulate drugs.
4. List the five drug schedules and give an example of a medication from each.
5. List the four names for a drug.
6. Describe three common drug references. Be able to readily find an assigned medication in one of these references.
7. List several examples of both liquid and solid drugs.
8. Define "parenteral medication."
9. Define:
   - ampule
   - vial
   - prefilled syringe
10. Define important pharmacological terms presented in this chapter.
11. Define a drug's mechanism of action.
12. List four factors that influence the quantity of drug present in the body.
13. List two factors that slow drug absorption and two factors that enhance it.

14. Define "blood brain barrier."
15. Describe the theory of drug receptors and give an example of one.
16. Define:
   - agonist
   - antagonist
   - sympathomimetic
   - sympatholytic
   - parasympathomimetic
   - parasympatholytic
17. Describe the principles of "therapeutic threshold," "therapeutic index," and "minimum effective concentration."
18. Describe, in detail, the autonomic nervous system and its role in pharmacology.
19. Describe the location and action of α and β adrenergic receptors.
20. Define the metric system.
21. Be able to make routine calculations and conversions using the metric system.
22. Be able to calculate any given drug dose for all medications used in your EMS system.
23. List six routes of medication administration and give the advantages and disadvantages of each.

Engine and EMS 28 are dispatched to 4817 West Fuller on a "chest pain" call. As the ambulance pulls up, a sheriff's deputy runs to the vehicle, stating, "This guy looks bad."

The paramedics grab the drug kit, airway bag, monitor/defibrillator, and the stretcher and enter the residence. Seated in a recliner is a male in his late 50s. He is pale, slightly diaphoretic, and short of breath. When asked what is wrong he states, "I'm having chest pain. I've never had anything like this in my life. I think I'm gonna die."

The senior paramedic quickly completes the primary assessment while his partner places a non-rebreather mask to administer oxygen. The airway is patent, the patient is moving air, and the pulse is present, yet weak. The patient's mental status is alert. One of the EMTs from Engine 28 begins to take the vital signs while the secondary assessment is carried out. The second paramedic places the ECG electrodes and sets up the monitor. The patient's wife reports he was watching baseball on television when the pain started. He has a history of diabetes but controls it with oral medication. He is hypertensive and has an appointment with his family doctor next week for a stress test. He is not allergic to any medications.

The EMT reports the blood pressure is 150/90, the pulse rate 100, and the respiratory rate 20. The ECG reveals a sinus rhythm with frequent premature ventricular contractions. An IV of D5W is started at a "to keep open" rate in the left arm. The senior paramedic contacts medical control and presents the patient report. The medical control physician requests the administration of 1 milligram per kilogram of lidocaine. In addition, he orders the administration of morphine in 2 milligram increments until the pain is improved. The paramedics recall that lidocaine can be effective in suppressing PVCs while the morphine helps to alleviate pain and decrease anxiety.

The paramedics administer the lidocaine bolus as ordered and 2 milligrams of morphine. Shortly thereafter the patient has a short epi-

INTRODUCTION

■ **pharmacology** Pharmacology is the study of drugs and how they affect the body.

■ **drug** A drug is a chemical agent used in diagnosis, treatment, and prevention of disease.

This chapter presents the fundamentals of pharmacology. **Pharmacology** is the study of drugs and how they affect the body. **Drugs** are defined as chemical agents used in diagnosis, treatment, and prevention of disease. The many medications used in the prehospital phase of emergency care will also be covered in this chapter. Additional clinical correlation will be presented in the clinical chapters.

The use of medications is an area of prehospital care that separates paramedics from EMTs and First Responders. Most of the drugs used in prehospital care are for cardiovascular emergencies. The medications used in an EMS system will vary by system. It is the paramedic's responsibility to be familiar with all medications used in his or her system.

DRUG SOURCES

Drugs are derived from four primary sources: plant, animal, mineral, and synthetic. Among the emergency medications derived from plants are atropine, morphine, and digitalis. Insulin and pitocin are examples of

sode of seizure activity and becomes unresponsive. The paramedics check the pulse and find it absent. The ECG shows ventricular fibrillation. The paramedics move the patient to the floor, a precordial thump is administered, and the pulse is rechecked. The pulse is still absent. The defibrillator is readied and a 200 joule countershock is delivered. The patient remains in ventricular fibrillation. A second countershock, this time at 300 joules, is applied. The patient remains in ventricular fibrillation and pulseless. Another countershock, this time at 360 joules, is applied. The patient remains unresponsive, pulseless, and in ventricular fibrillation. CPR is started, the patient ventilated with a bag-valve-mask unit, and a 1 milligram dose of epinephrine is administered intravenously.

The paramedics remember that epinephrine makes ventricular fibrillation more susceptible to direct current countershock. An endotracheal tube is placed without problem. Approximately 1 minute after the epinephrine dose another 360 joule countershock is delivered. The patient converts to a idioventricular rhythm with a faint pulse. The heart rate quickly increases, the pulse becomes strong, and the ECG resumes a sinus pattern. The blood pressure is 100/60 and the pulse is 120. The medical control physician is again contacted and an order for 0.5 milligrams per kilogram body weight of lidocaine is received. In addition, the medical control physician requests a lidocaine drip at 2 milligrams per minute. The drugs are administered and the patient prepared for transport.

The transport to the hospital goes without problem. Upon arrival the patient is alert and calm with good respiratory effort. In the emergency room a 12 lead ECG shows the presence of an anterior wall myocardial infarction. Tissue plasminogen activator (TPA) is started. The patient's chest pain resolves completely within the hour. He is transferred to the CCU where he remains stable.

medications derived from animals. Two medications derived from minerals are calcium chloride and sodium bicarbonate. By far, the majority of emergency medications are man-made, or synthetic. Bretylium tosylate, lidocaine, and procainamide are examples of synthetic medications.

DRUG LAWS

Governmental agencies strictly control medications used in the United States. Most of these agencies resulted from several landmark pieces of drug legislation. The most sweeping revision was the *Federal Food, Drug, and Cosmetic Act, of 1938.* This act required the names of all ingredients of foods and medications to be placed on the product label. It also required that the label state whether any of the ingredients are habit-forming and cite the percentages of those drugs present.

Narcotics, because of their addictive nature, have always been a problem. In 1915, the federal government enacted the *Harrison Narcotic Act.* This act regulated the sale, importation, and manufacture of the opium plant and its derivatives. Opium is a primary source of narcotic products. In 1970, the government further regulated addictive medications through the *Controlled Substances Act.* This act classified addictive medications into five schedules, summarized below:

1. *Schedule I:* These drugs have a high potential for abuse and no accepted medical indications. Examples are heroin, LSD, and marijuana.
2. *Schedule II:* These drugs have a high potential for abuse, yet also have accepted medical indications. Emergency medications in this class include morphine, meperidine, and Dilaudid.
3. *Schedule III:* Drugs classified here have a lesser degree of abuse potential and accepted medical indications. An example is the fixed combination acetaminophen with codeine (Tylenol #4).
4. *Schedule IV:* This group of drugs has a low potential for abuse, but may cause physical or psychological dependence. An example is the anticonvulsant, diazepam (Valium).
5. *Schedule V:* Schedule V drugs have a low potential for abuse, yet contain small quantities of narcotic preparations. Several cough preparations and anti-diarrheal agents fall under this classification.

In addition to establishing drug classifications, the Controlled Substances Act prohibits the refilling of prescriptions for Schedule II drugs and requires that the original prescription be filled within 72 hours. Enforcement of the Controlled Substances Act rests with the Drug Enforcement Administration (DEA).

DRUG NAMES

Drugs can be identified by four names. The most elemental is the *chemical name,* which identifies the drug's chemical structure. The *generic name* is usually an abbreviated version of the chemical name and is frequently used. The *trade name* is the name given a drug by its manufacturer. A medication may appear under several trade names if it is made by a number of manufacturers. Finally, the *official name* is the name that's published in the United States Pharmacopeia. The official name is followed by the letters U.S.P. As an example, here are the four names of the analgesic preparation meperidine:

Chemical Name:	*ethyl-1-methyl-4-phenylisonipecotate hydrochloride*
Generic Name:	meperidine hydrochloride
Trade Name:	Demerol Hydrochloride
Official Name:	meperidine hydrochloride, U.S.P.

DRUG REFERENCES

Valuable sources of information concerning medications include:

AMA Drug Evaluations. This manual, published by the American Medical Association, provides information on all drug groups. It covers dosages, side-effects, indications, and contraindications.

Physicians' Desk Reference (PDR). The Physicians' Desk Reference is a standard that should be on board every paramedic unit. It contains a very useful Product Identification Guide, with photographs of various medications showing actual size and color, as well as information on most drugs currently on the market. The PDR is published yearly by the Medical Economics Company.

Drug Inserts. The written literature packaged with most drugs is a good source of information. These inserts can be collected in a notebook for personal use.

DRUG FORMS

Drugs come in many forms. Each form has advantages and disadvantages. Here are some common drug preparations.

Liquids

Liquid drugs usually consist of a powder dissolved in a liquid. The drug is referred to as the *solute*. The liquid part is called the *solvent*. In liquid drug preparations, it is primarily the solvent that distinguishes one from another.

Solutions. Solutions are preparations in which the drugs are dissolved in a solvent, usually water (for example, 5% dextrose in water).

Tinctures. Tinctures are drug preparations in which the drug was extracted chemically with alcohol. They will usually contain some dilute alcohol (for example, tincture of iodine).

Suspensions. Suspensions are liquid drug preparations that do not remain dissolved. After sitting for even a short time, these preparations will tend to separate. They must always be shaken well before use (for example, amoxicillin preparations).

Spirits. Spirit solutions contain volatile chemicals (chemicals that quickly vaporize) dissolved in alcohol (for example, spirit of ammonia).

Emulsions. Emulsions are preparations in which an oily substance is mixed with a solvent that will not dissolve it. After mixing, globules of fat form and float in the solvent. These preparations are similar to what occurs in a mixture of oil and vinegar.

Elixirs. Elixirs are preparations that contain the drug in an alcohol solvent. Flavoring, frequently cherry, is added to improve the taste (for example, Tylenol Elixir).

Syrups. Often drugs are suspended in sugar and water to improve the taste. These are referred to as syrups (for example, cough syrup).

Liquid drugs administered into the body through intramuscular, subcutaneous, or intravenous routes are called **parenteral drugs.** These drugs are introduced through routes outside of the digestive tract (also called the enteral system). Most drugs used in emergencies are parenteral. These preparations must be sterile because they are introduced into the body.

Parenteral Drug Containers. Parenteral medications are packaged in several types of container. *Ampules* are sterile parenteral containers designed to carry a single patient dose. (See Figure 13-1.) Generally, ampules are broken, and the drug is drawn into a syringe for administration.

■ **parenteral drugs** drugs administered into the body without going through the digestive tract are referred to as parenteral drugs.

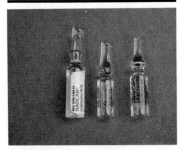

FIGURE 13-1 Ampules

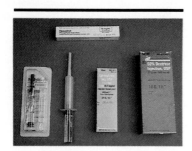

FIGURE 13-2 Prefilled syringes.

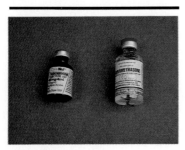

FIGURE 13-3 Vials.

In emergency medicine, most of the drugs are provided in *prefilled syringes* to save time. (See Figure 13-2.) Containers of parenteral medications that contain more than one dose are called *vials*. (See Figure 13-3.) A few of the drugs used at emergencies are provided in vials. Today, single-dose vials are available that do not require breakage in order to withdraw the drug.

Solid Drugs

Solid drugs are usually administered orally, but can be administered rectally or vaginally. They include:

Pills. Pills are drugs that are shaped into a form that's easy to swallow. They are often coated to improve taste.

Powders. Powders are drugs in powdered form. They are not as popular as pills, yet some are still in use (for example, B.C. Powder).

Capsules. Capsules are gelatin containers into which a powder has been placed. The gelatin dissolves, liberating the powder into the gastrointestinal tract (for example, Dalmane capsules).

Tablets. Tablets are similar to pills. They are composed of a powder that has been compressed into an easily swallowed form.

Suppositories. Suppositories are mixed into a base that is solid at room temperature (approximately 70 degrees F). When placed into the body, rectally or vaginally, they dissolve and are absorbed into the surrounding tissue.

PHARMACOLOGICAL TERMINOLOGY

There are several important pharmacological terms that prehospital personnel should be familiar with. They include:

❑ *Antagonism.* Antagonism signifies the opposition between two or more medications (for example, between naloxone and morphine).

   Bolus. A bolus is a single, often large dose of medication (for example, lidocaine bolus, which is often followed by a lidocaine infusion).

❑ *Contraindications.* Contraindications are the medical or physiological conditions present in a patient that would make it harmful to administer an otherwise appropriate medication.

❑ *Cumulative Action.* A cumulative action occurs when a drug is administered in several doses, causing an increased effect. This is usually due to a buildup of the drug in the blood.

❑ *Depressant.* A depressant is a medication that decreases a bodily function or activity.

❑ *Habituation* Habituation is physical or psychological dependence on a drug.

❑ *Hypersensitivity.* Hypersensitivity is a state of altered reactivity to a foreign substance (including medications), with an exaggerated immune response.

❑ *Idiosyncrasy.* An idiosyncrasy is an individual reaction to a drug that is unusually different from that normally seen.

❑ *Indication.* An indication refers to the medical condition or conditions in which a drug has proven to be of therapeutic value.

❑ *Potentiation.* Potentiation is the enhancement of one drug's effects by another (for example, barbiturates and alcohol).

❏ *Refractory*. Patients who do not respond to a drug are said to be refractory to the drug (for example, a patient with premature ventricular contractions who does not respond to lidocaine).

❏ *Side Effects*. Side effects are the unavoidable, undesired effects that a drug often causes, even in therapeutic dosages.

❏ *Stimulant*. A stimulant is a drug that increases a bodily function or activity (for example, caffeine in coffee).

❏ *Synergism*. Synergism is the combined action of two drugs. It is much stronger than the effects of either one.

❏ *Therapeutic Action*. A therapeutic action is the intended action of a drug given in the appropriate medical condition.

❏ *Tolerance*. When a patient has been on a drug for a long time, he or she may require larger dosages to achieve a therapeutic effect. This increased requirement is termed tolerance.

❏ *Untoward Effect*. An untoward effect is a side effect harmful to the patient.

ACTIONS OF DRUGS

For a drug to exert its desired effects upon the body, it must reach its targeted tissue in suitable form and in sufficient concentration. The study of how drugs enter the body and reach their site of action, and how they are eventually eliminated is called **pharmacokinetics.** Once drugs reach their targeted tissue, they begin a chain of biochemical events that ultimately lead to the physiological changes desired. These biochemical and physiological events are called the drug's *mechanism of action.* The study of a drug's action upon the body is called **pharmacodynamics.** The following section covers the fundamentals of pharmacokinetics and pharmacodynamics as they apply to prehospital emergency care.

■ **pharmacokinetics** the study of how drugs enter the body and reach their site of action, and how they are eventually eliminated.

■ **pharmacodynamics** the study of a drug's action upon the body.

Pharmacokinetics

Several factors influence the concentration of a drug at its site of action. These factors include *absorption* of the drug into the circulatory system; *distribution* of the drug throughout the body; *biotransformation* of the drug into its active form; and, finally, *elimination* of the drug from the body. It is important to understand that not all of these factors are involved in every medication used in prehospital care. However, a fundamental understanding of each factor is essential.

Drug Absorption. Most medications used in prehospital care are given by the intravenous, intramuscular, or subcutaneous route. A drug administered into a muscle or into subcutaneous tissue must be absorbed, through the walls of the capillaries, into the circulation. It can then be transported to its sites of action. Several factors may affect the rate of absorption. Factors that delay absorption from parenteral sites include shock, acidosis, and peripheral vasoconstriction due to hypothermia. Factors that can increase the rate of absorption include peripheral vasodilation, which can occur in hyperthermia and fever. Muscles, as a rule, are more richly supplied with blood vessels than subcutaneous tissue. Therefore, a drug should be absorbed more rapidly from muscle than from subcutaneous tissue. Other factors that can affect drug absorption include the size, age, and general medical condition of the patient.

Drug absorption delays may be avoided by injecting the medication directly into the circulatory system through the veins. (See Figure 13-4.) The desired effects are seen much sooner and the eventual blood levels of

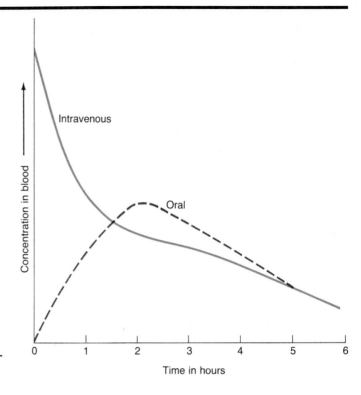

FIGURE 13-4 Comparison of intravenous and oral administration of the same drug.

the medication are much more predictable. Because of this, most critical care medications are administered intravenously.

Distribution. Once in the circulatory system, a drug is distributed throughout the body tissues. Most medications pass easily from the intravascular compartment, through the interstitial spaces, to the target cells. These drugs tend to have a rapid onset of action and short duration of effect. Some drugs, on the other hand, are immediately bound to serum proteins after entering the circulation. These drugs tend to have a delayed onset of action and remain in the circulatory system for a prolonged time.

Generally, drugs will concentrate in tissues with good blood supplies, such as the heart, brain, liver, and kidneys. It is important to remember that in critical situations, such as shock, the tissues receiving the most blood are the heart and brain. Delivery of blood to the brain is limited by a protective mechanism called the **blood brain barrier.** It selectively allows the entry of only a limited number of compounds into the brain. Drugs that are protein-bound, or drugs in an ionized form, are weak penetrators of the blood brain barrier.

■ **blood brain barrier** a protective mechanism that selectively allows the entry of only a limited number of compounds into the brain.

Biotransformation. Many drugs are inactive when administered. Once absorbed, they are converted into an active form, either in the blood or by the target tissue. The process of changing a drug to another form, either active or inactive, is called *biotransformation*. It results in chemical variations of the drugs, which are called metabolites.

Several drugs used in prehospital care must be converted into an active form to take effect. Diazepam, for example, is relatively inactive as administered. Once in the body, it is biotransformed into an active metabolite. Other drugs are active as administered, but are biotransformed into an inactive metabolite before elimination. Epinephrine is an example of a medication that is quickly biotransformed to an inactive metabolite.

Because of this rapid biotransformation, epinephrine must be readministered approximately every five minutes.

Elimination. Drugs are eventually eliminated from the body in either their original form or as metabolites. Drugs may be excreted by the kidneys into the urine, by the liver into the bile, by the intestines into the feces, or by the lungs into the expired air. The rate of elimination varies with the medication and the condition of the body. During shock states, the kidneys are poorly perfused, and drugs may remain in the body longer. The slower the rate of elimination, the longer the drug stays in the body.

Pharmocodynamics

Once a drug has reached its target tissue, it must induce the desired biochemical or physiological response. To do that, most drugs must bind to drug receptors. (See Figure 13-5.) *Drug receptors* are proteins present on the surface of cell membranes; they are often compared to locks. Drugs are the keys for these locks. Once the drug has bound to the receptor—i.e., the key is in the lock—biochemical actions begin that lead to the desired biochemical response. Drugs that bind to a receptor and cause a response are referred to as *agonists.* Certain drugs, however, may bind to a receptor and block a biochemical response. Their presence on the receptor may prevent other drugs from binding. These drugs are known as *antagonists.* (See Figure 13-6.) Classic illustrations of these principles are the drugs epinephrine and propranolol (Inderal). Epinephrine is transported to the target tissues—namely the heart, lungs, and peripheral blood vessels. Once there, it binds to its receptors, alpha (α) and beta (β) adrenergic receptors. If the drug binds to these receptors, the desired physiological response will be seen. However, there are several drugs, which are themselves inactive, that can bind to the β receptors in much the same manner as epinephrine. These medications are referred to as beta blockers. The prototype of this group is propranolol. If the beta blocker is already bound to the receptor, then epinephrine cannot bind and its β effects are effectively inhibited.

To be effective, a medication must reach a certain concentration in

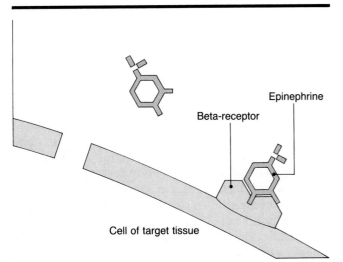

FIGURE 13-5 Example of drug (epinephrine) interacting with a drug receptor (β receptor).

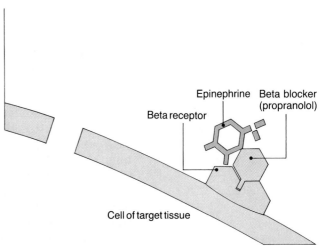

FIGURE 13-6 Drug receptor blocked by antagonist (β blocker).

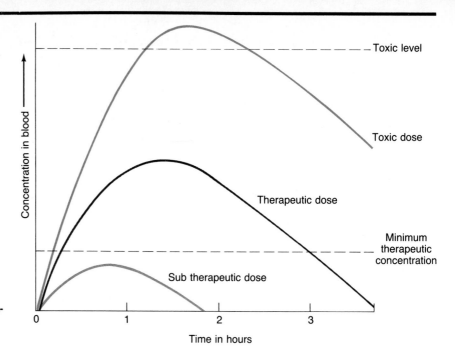

FIGURE 13-7 Comparison of sub-therapeutic, therapeutic, and toxic doses of the same drug.

the target tissues. The minimal concentration of a drug necessary to cause the desired response is referred to as the *therapeutic threshold* or *minimum effective concentration*. A concentration below this threshold will not induce a clinical response. Conversely, there is a point at which the drug concentration can get high enough to be toxic or even fatal. The general goal of pharmacological therapy is to give the minimum concentration of a drug necessary to obtain the desired response.

The difference between the minimum effective concentration and the toxic level varies widely between drugs. The difference between effective and toxic concentrations is called the *therapeutic index*. (See Figure 13-7.) It is usually determined in the laboratory. With certain drugs, digitalis (Lanoxin) among them, there is little difference between effective and toxic doses. These drugs are said to have a *low therapeutic index*. Drugs such as naloxone (Narcan), the narcotic antagonist, have a significant margin between effective and toxic doses. Drugs of this kind are said to have a *high therapeutic index*. Paramedics must be familiar with the therapeutic indices of medications used in their system.

THE AUTONOMIC NERVOUS SYSTEM

■ **autonomic nervous system**
the part of the nervous system responsible for control of involuntary actions.

The **autonomic nervous system** is the part of the nervous system responsible for control of involuntary actions. Many medications used in prehospital care directly affect the autonomic nervous system. It is essential that prehospital personnel have a good understanding of this aspect of the nervous system and how emergency medications affect it.

The two functional divisions of the autonomic nervous system are the *sympathetic nervous* system and the *parasympathetic nervous system*. The sympathetic nervous system allows the body to function under stress. It is often referred to as the "fight or flight" aspect of the nervous system. When stimulated, the sympathetic nervous system causes pupillary dilation, an increase in heart rate, increased force of cardiac contractions, peripheral vasoconstriction, and increased metabolic rate. The sympathetic nervous system, when stimulated, releases norepinephrine, which acts on specialized chemical receptors. These receptors are located throughout the body. Once stimulated by the appropriate hormone, in this case norepinephrine, they cause a response in the organ or organs they control.

The two known types of receptors are the adrenergic receptors and the dopaminergic receptors. The *adrenergic receptors* are generally divided into four types. These four receptors are designated *alpha 1* (α_1), *alpha 2* (α_2), *beta 1* (β_1), and *beta 2* (β_2). The α_1 receptors cause peripheral vasoconstriction and, on occasion, mild bronchoconstriction. Discussion of the α_2 receptors is complex and not within the scope of this text. The β_1 receptors cause an increase in heart rate, cardiac contractile force, and an increase in cardiac automaticity and conduction. The β_2 receptors will cause vasodilation and bronchodilation. *Dopaminergic receptors,* although not fully understood, are believed to cause dilation of the renal, coronary, and cerebral arteries. Medications that stimulate the sympathetic nervous system are referred to as **sympathomimetics.** Medications that inhibit the sympathetic nervous system are called **sympatholytics.** Some medications are pure α **agonists,** while others are pure α **antagonists.** Some medications are pure β agonists, while others are pure β antagonists. Medications such as epinephrine stimulate both alpha and beta receptors. Other medications, such as the bronchodilators, are termed β selective, since they act more on β_2 receptors than upon β_1.

The parasympathetic nervous system is in constant opposition with the sympathetic nervous system. It primarily controls vegetative functions, such as digestion of food, and decreases heart rate. It is often referred to as the "feed or breed" aspect of the autonomic nervous system. (See Table 13-1.) The parasympathetic nervous system exerts control pri-

■ **sympathomimetic** a drug or other substance which causes effects like those of the sympathetic nervous system (also called adrenergic).

■ **sympatholytic** a drug or other substance which blocks the actions of the sympathetic nervous system (also called antiadrenergic)

■ **agonist** a drug or other substance that causes a physiological response.

■ **antagonist** a drug or other substance which blocks a physiological response or that blocks the action of another drug or substance.

TABLE 13-1 Comparison of the Physiological Effects of the Sympathetic and Parasympathetic Components of the Autonomic Nervous System

Structure	Sympathetic	Parasympathetic
Eye: Pupil	Dilatation	Contraction
Ciliary muscle	Relaxation and distance vision accommodation	Contraction and close-up vision accommodation
Glands: nasal, lacrimal, gastric, pancreatic, parotid, submaxillary	Vasoconstriction thus altering secretion	Increases thin, copious secretions
sweat glands	Profuse sweating	No effect
Heart: Muscle	Increased rate and strength of contraction	Slows rate of contraction
Coronary arteries	Dilatation	Constriction
Lungs: Bronchi	Dilatation	Constriction
Blood vessels	Mild constriction	No effect
Intestine: Muscle	Decreased peristalsis	Increased peristalsis
Sphincter	Increased tone	Decreased tone
Liver	Glycogenolysis stimulated	No effect
Kidney	Output decreased	No effect
Penis	Ejaculation	Erection
Blood vessels: Abdominal	Constriction	No effect
External genitalia	Constriction	Dilatation
Skeletal muscle	Increased strength and glycogenolysis	No effect
Mental activity	Accelerated	No effect
Blood: Glucose	Increased	No effect
Coagulation	Increased	No effect

parasympatholytic a drug or other substance that blocks or inhibits the actions of the parasympathetic nervous system (also called anticholinergic).

parasympathomimetic a drug or other substance which causes effects like those of the parasympathetic nervous system (also called cholinergic).

marily through the vagus nerve, and, to a lesser degree, through some other cranial nerves. It uses the neurotransmitter acetylcholine. When released, acetylcholine tends to decrease the heart rate, promote increased salivation, and cause pupillary constriction.

The emergency medication atropine is an antagonist to the parasympathetic nervous system and is used to increase heart rate. Atropine binds with acetylcholine receptors thus preventing acetylcholine from exerting its effect. Medications like atropine, which block the actions of the parasympathetic nervous system, are referred to as **parasympatholytics.** Medications that stimulate the parasympathetic nervous system are referred to as **parasympathomimetics.**

MEDICATIONS

When studying a medication, you must determine and understand the following:

- ❑ What is the usual dose of the medication?
- ❑ What, if any, is the required dilution?
- ❑ What is the drug's action?
- ❑ What are the prehospital indications and uses?
- ❑ What precautions should you take when administering the medication?
- ❑ What are the contraindications to administering the medication?
- ❑ What are the compatibilities and incompatibilities with other medications?
- ❑ What are the common side effects?
- ❑ What, if any, are the antidotes to the medication?

You should learn all these elements about every medication used in your system. Many paramedics choose to keep this information on cards for ready reference.

WEIGHTS AND MEASURES

metric system The metric system is a system of weights and measures widely used in science and medicine. It is based on a unit of 10.

apothecary's system The Apothecary's system is an antiquated system of weights and measures used widely in early medicine.

The **metric system** is used worldwide as the standard system of weights and measures in science and medicine. It is the principal system of weights and measures used in pharmacology. However, because of tradition, the mostly antiquated **Apothecary's system** of weights and measures remains in occasional use.

The metric system was devised by the French and is based on the unit 10. All units are 10 times larger than, or 1/10 as large as, the next unit. Because the metric system is based on the unit 10, conversion from one unit to another is simple. The change from one set of units to another requires moving only a decimal point.

Making physical descriptions involves three measurements: mass, length, and volume. *Mass* is the quantity of matter in a substance. *Length* is the distance between two points. *Volume* is the space occupied by a substance. The metric system has three fundamental units for these measurements. The fundamental unit for measuring mass is the gram (G). The fundamental unit for measuring length is the meter (M). The fundamental unit for measuring volume is the liter (L). All other metric units used to describe mass, length, and volume are derivatives of these three fundamental, or base, units. Instead of using a lot of zeros in metric conversions, simply change the prefix. Common metric system prefixes are:

kilo = 1000 (k)
hecto = 100 (h)
deka = 10 (D)
Fundamental Unit = 1 (gram, liter, or meter)
deci = 1/10 or 0.1 (d)
centi = 1/100 or 0.01 (c)
milli = 1/1000 or 0.001 (m)
micro = 1/1,000,000 or 0.000001 (μ)

The most common prefixes in prehospital care are: kilo-, centi-, milli-, and micro-.

Metric Conversions

To change a prefix, move the decimal point the indicated number of decimals left or right. Common examples of metric conversions are:

1,000 liters = 1 kiloliter
1,000 grams = 1 kilogram
1/1000 gram = 1 milligram (0.001 gram = 1 milligram)
1/100 meter = 1 centimeter (0.01 meter = 1 centimeter)

Multiplication of decimals is easily accomplished by moving the decimal point. For example, when multiplying a decimal by 10, move the decimal one place to the right:

10 milliliters × 10 = 100 milliliters
0.1 centimeter × 10 = 1 centimeter

When multiplying a decimal by 100, simply move the decimal point two places to the right:

10 liters × 100 = 1,000 liters
0.01 milliliter × 100 = 1 milliliter

To divide a decimal, simply move the decimal point the indicated number of places to the left. For example, to divide a decimal by 10, simply move the decimal point one place to the left:

1 liter ÷ 10 = 0.1 liter
100 centimeters ÷ 10 = 1 centimeter

To divide by 100, simply move the decimal point two places to the left. For example:

1000 milligrams ÷ 100 = 10 milligrams
10 milliliters ÷ 100 = 0.1 milliliter

Conversion between cubic centimeters and milliliters is often used in medicine. One milliliter of water occupies 1 cubic centimeter of space. Thus:

1 cubic centimeter (cm^3) = 1 milliliter (mL)

Milliliter (mL) is replacing "cubic centimeter" (cc) as the preferred term.

Occasionally, orders will be received for certain drugs in the old apothecary's system. The most common apothecary measure likely to be seen is the grain. Some physicians still prescribe certain medications, such as analgesics, in grains. The conversion is:

1 grain = 60 milligrams

thus

1/4 grain = 15 milligrams

The English system of weights and measures is generally used by the lay public. To bring the metric system into perspective, here are some common conversions:

$$1 \text{ centimeter} = 0.39 \text{ inches}$$
$$1 \text{ meter} = 39.37 \text{ inches}$$
$$1 \text{ liter} = 1.05 \text{ quarts}$$
$$1 \text{ kilogram} = 2.2 \text{ pounds}$$
$$2.54 \text{ centimeters} = 1 \text{ inch}$$

Drug Dosage Calculations

Most medications are provided in stock solutions. Paramedics, as well as other health care workers, must calculate the quantity of medication to be administered. There are several methods for accomplishing this. This text will present a simple method that works for all prehospital applications.

When preparing to administer a medication to a patient, the paramedic will usually have certain information available:

1. *The Desired Dose.* The desired dose is the quantity of medication or fluid the medical control physician wants administered to the patient. This is usually expressed in milligrams, grams, or grains.
2. *The Concentration of the Drug on Hand.* The concentration of the drug on hand is the amount of the drug present in the ampule or vial. This is usually expressed in milligrams, grams, or grains, and is found on the label.
3. *The Volume of the Drug on Hand.* The volume of the drug on hand is the amount of fluid within the ampule or vial in which the drug is dissolved. This is usually represented in milliliters and found on the label.

Based on these three pieces of information, you can calculate the volume of the drug to be administered. The following formula represents this relationship:

$$\text{Volume administered } (X) = \frac{(\text{Volume on hand})(\text{Desired dose})}{\text{Concentration on hand}}$$

Example 1. A physician wants 5 milligrams of a medication administered to a patient. The ampule contains 10 milligrams of the drug in 2 milliliters of solvent. The following calculation can then be made:

$$\text{Volume administered } (X) = \frac{\text{Volume on hand (2 mL)} \times \text{Desired dose (5 mg)}}{\text{Concentration on hand (10 mg)}}$$

To solve, multiply:

$$X = \frac{(2 \text{ mL})(5 \text{ mg})}{(10 \text{ mg})}$$

Thus:

$$X = \frac{10}{10}$$

Then:

$$X = 1 \text{ mL}$$

Example 2. A physician wants a patient to receive 75 milligrams of lidocaine administered in a bolus. The drug is supplied in prefilled syringes that contain 100 milligrams of the drug in 5 milliliters of solvent. To calculate the number of milliliters to be administered:

$$X = \frac{(5 \text{ mL})(75 \text{ mg})}{100 \text{ mg}}$$

Thus:
$$X = \frac{375}{100}$$

Then:
$$X = 3.75 \text{ mL}$$

This formula works for all drug calculations routinely used in emergency medicine, but it only works if all measurements are in the same units.

Variations On A Theme. The formula presented above is useful for calculating the infusion rate of IV drips. All that is required is to multiply X, the volume to be administered, by the drops per milliliter delivered by the set you are using. The result will be the number of drops per minute that must be delivered.

Example 3. A physician wants 2 milligrams per minute of lidocaine administered to a patient. She orders 2 grams of lidocaine to be placed in 500 milliliters of 5% dextrose in water. A minidrip administration set that delivers 60 drops per minute is being used. The problem can be solved as follows:

$$\frac{(500 \text{ mL})(2 \text{ mg/minute})}{2000 \text{ mg}} \times 60 \text{ drops/mL} = X \text{ drops/minute}$$

Then:

$$\frac{1000}{2000} = 0.5 \times 60 \text{ drops/mL} = 30 \text{ drops/minute}$$

Other Calculations. Occasionally, an order will be received to administer a drug to a patient based on the patient's weight. The drug dosage must be calculated based on the patient's weight and can then be plugged into the formula.

Example 4. A physician wants a patient to receive 5 milligrams per kilogram of a medication. The patient weighs 220 pounds. The medication is supplied in an ampule containing 500 milligrams of the drug in 10 milliliters of solvent. How many milliliters of the drug should be administered?

In order to solve this problem, you must make two preliminary calculations. First, convert the patient's weight to kilograms. Second, multiply the patient's weight, in kilograms, by the number of milligrams per kilogram to be administered. The calculation is:

1. *Convert the patient's weight to kilograms:*

   220 pounds ÷ 2.2 pounds/kilogram = 100 kilograms

2. *Calculate the desired dose:*

   100 kilograms × 5 milligrams/kilogram = 500 milligrams

3. *Calculate the volume to be administered:*

$$X = \frac{(10\ \text{mL})(500\ \text{mg})}{500\ \text{mg}}$$

Then:

$$X = \frac{5000}{500}$$

Thus:

$$X = 10\ \text{mL}$$

Frequent practice is essential to mastering drug dosage calculations. This should be practiced routinely during paramedic training and after graduation. There are sample problems in the accompanying workbook. Review them periodically.

MEDICATION ADMINISTRATION ROUTES

In emergency medical services, medications must be administered promptly, in the correct dose, and by the correct route. If given by an inappropriate route, many drugs can be fatal. This section will detail the common methods of medication administration used in prehospital care.

General Administration Routes

The two primary channels for getting medications into the body are through the digestive tract and by parenteral routes. Most critical-care medications are administered parenterally because the onset of action is much quicker and more predictable.

Parenteral Routes. Any method of drug administration that does not involve passage through the digestive tract is termed parenteral. Parenteral routes include:

- ❑ *Intradermal.* Drugs can be injected into the dermal layer of the skin. The amount of medication that can be administered by this route is limited and systemic absorption is very slow. Generally, this route is reserved for diagnostic skin testing, such as allergy testing or tuberculin skin tests.
- ❑ *Transdermal.* Several medications are now available that can be placed on the skin and absorbed, through the skin, into the circulatory system. Medications available in this form include nitroglycerin, blood pressure medications, and hormone preparations.
- ❑ *Subcutaneous.* With subcutaneous administration, medications are injected directly into the fatty, subcutaneous tissue under the skin that overlies the muscle. Absorption from this route is slow, resulting in a delayed onset of action and prolonged effect. (See Procedure 13-1.)
- ❑ *Intramuscular.* The most commonly used route of parenteral medication administration is the intramuscular route. The drug is injected into the muscle tissue, from which it is absorbed into the bloodstream. (See Figure 13-8.) This method of administration has a predictable rate of absorption, but has an onset of action considerably slower than intravenous administration. (See Procedure 13-2.)
- ❑ *Intravenous.* The majority of medications used in prehospital care are administered by the intravenous route. This can be in the form of an intrave-

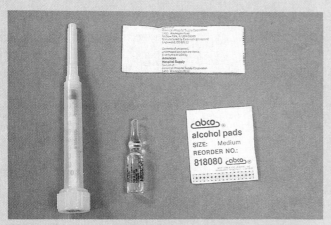

13-1A. Prepare the equipment.

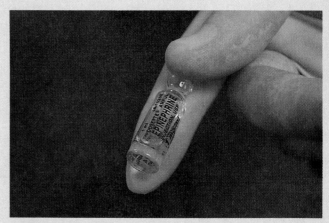

13-1B. Check the medication.

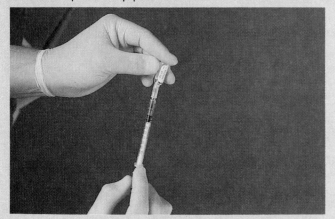

13-1C. Draw up the medication.

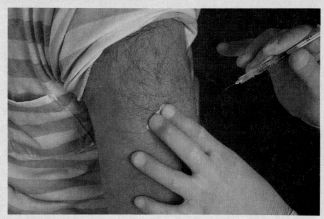

13-1D. Prep the site.

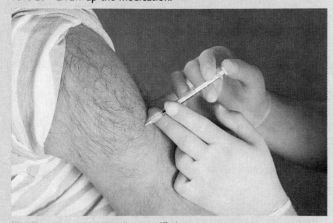

13-1E. Insert the needle at a 45-degree angle.

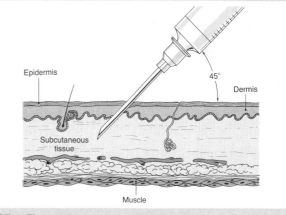

13-1F. The needle should enter the subcutaneous tissue.

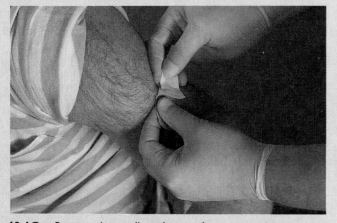

13-1G. Remove the needle and cover the puncture site.

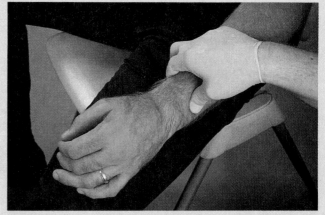

13-1H. Monitor the patient.

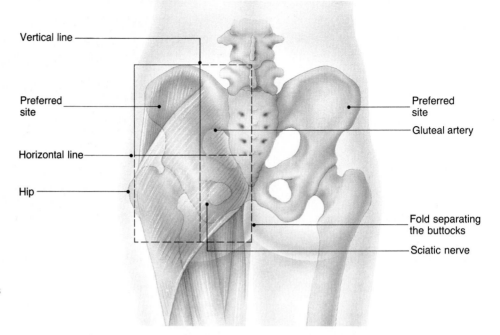

Vertical line

Preferred site

Horizontal line

Hip

Preferred site

Gluteal artery

Fold separating the buttocks

Sciatic nerve

FIGURE 13-8 Desired placement for intramuscular medications in the prehospital setting.

nous bolus (see Procedure 13-3), or as a slow, intravenous infusion, sometimes referred to as a "piggyback" infusion (see Procedure 13-4). The rate of absorption is rapid and predictable. However, of the routes frequently employed, intravenous administration of drugs has the most potential for causing adverse reactions.

❑ *Endotracheal.* When an IV cannot be started, it is often possible to administer emergency medications down an endotracheal tube, which permits absorption into the pulmonary capillaries of the lungs. It has been documented that this route of medication administration has a rate of absorption as fast as the intravenous route for certain drugs. Drugs that can be administered endotracheally include naloxone, atropine, epinephrine, and lidocaine. (See Procedure 13-5.)

❑ *Sublingual Injection.* In the rare instance when neither an IV nor an endotracheal tube can be used, certain drugs can be injected into the vast capillary network immediately under the tongue. Lidocaine and epinephrine are the most common.

❑ *Intracardiac.* Injection of medication directly into the ventricle of the heart is referred to as intracardiac injection. Once quite popular, it is seldom used today because of its inherent complications, such as pericardial tamponade and laceration of the coronary vessels, as well as its lack of documented effectiveness.

✱ Remember the five "R"s of correct medication administration:
• the Right drug
• the Right dose
• the Right route
• the Right patient
• the Right time

Enteral Routes. Very few medications used in prehospital care are administered into the digestive tract. Common methods of enteral medication administration include:

❑ *Sublingual.* Certain emergency medications, such as nitroglycerin and nifedipine (Procardia), can be placed under the tongue for rapid absorption into the capillary bed. The sublingual route is better for these medications because intravenous nitrates are difficult to administer and nifedipine is not available in parenteral form.

❑ *Oral.* The most convenient way of administering medication is by mouth. Medications used in prehospital care which are administered orally include syrup of Ipecac and activated charcoal.

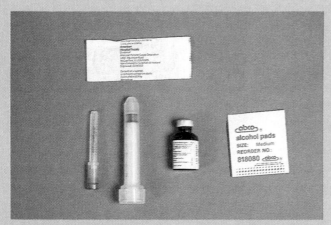

13-2A. Prepare the equipment.

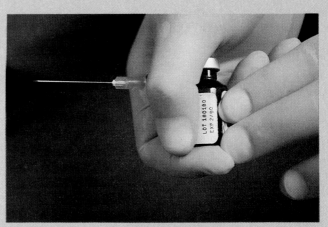

13-2B. Check the medication.

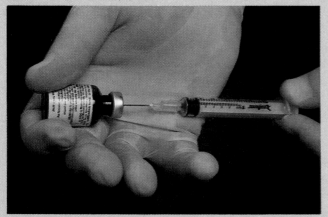

13-2C. Draw up the medication.

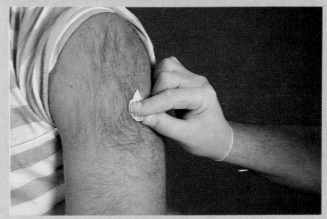

13-2D. Prep the site.

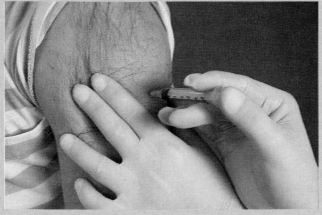

13-2E. Insert the needle at a 90-degree angle.

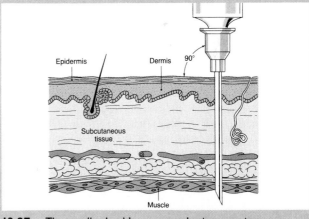

13-2F. The needle should enter muscle tissue; aspirate to ensure that a blood vessel has not been entered; inject medication.

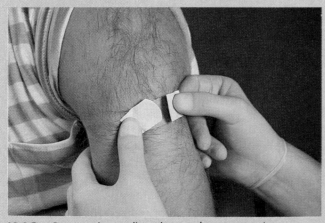

13-2G. Remove the needle and cover the puncture site.

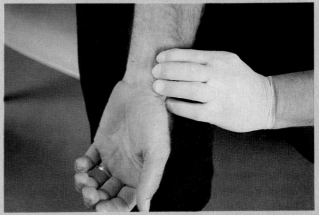

13-2H. Monitor the patient.

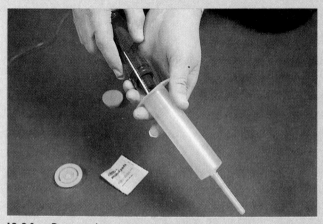

13-3A. Prepare the equipment.

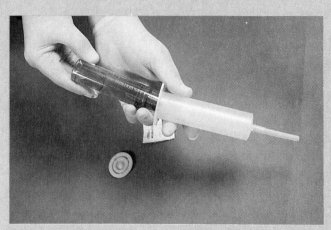

13-3B. Prepare the medication.

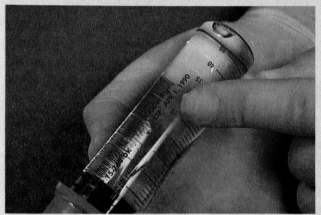

13-3C. Check the label.

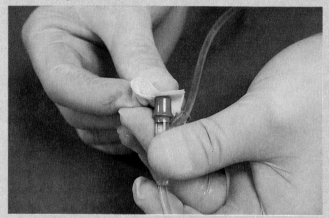

13-3D. Select and clean an administration port.

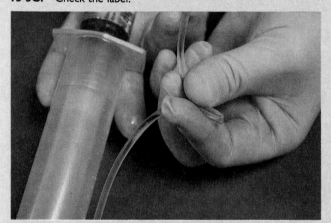

13-3E. Pinch the line.

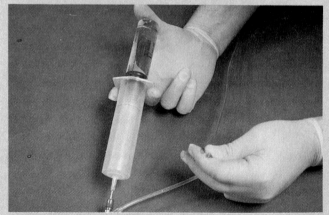

13-3F. Administer the medication.

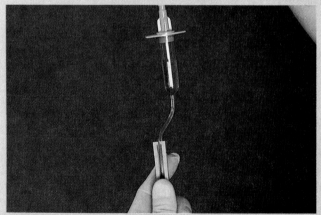

13-3G. Adjust the IV flow rate.

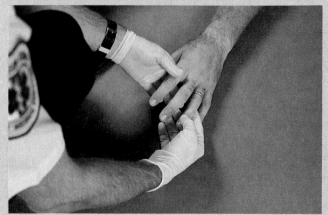

13-3H. Monitor the patient.

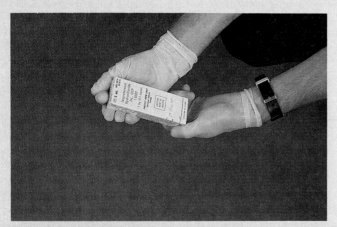

13-4A. Select the drug.

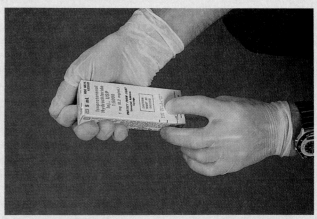

13-4B. Check the label.

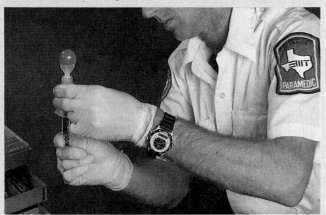

13-4C. Draw up the drug.

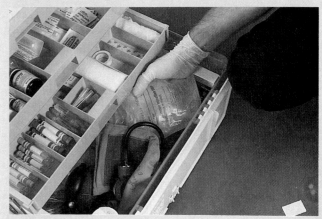

13-4D. Select IV fluid for dilution.

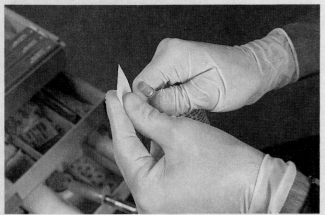

13-4E. Clean the medication addition port.

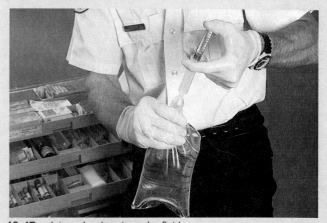

13-4F. Inject the drug into the fluid.

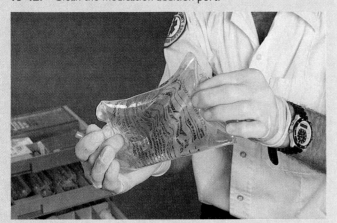

13-4G. Mix the solution.

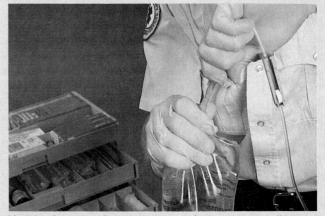

13-4H. Insert an administration set and connect to main IV line with needle.

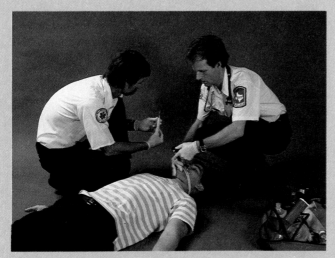

13-5A. Hyperventilate patient.

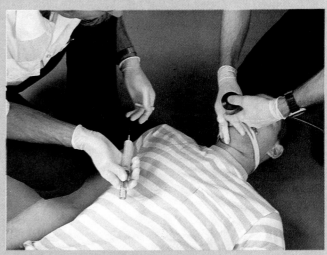

13-5B. Remove the ventilation device.

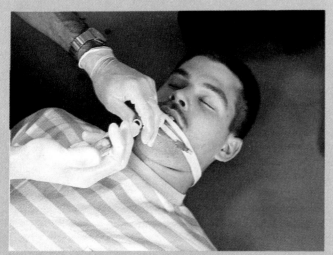

13-5C. Inject the drug.

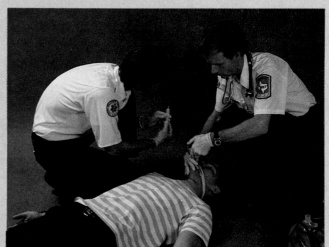

13-5D. Reconnect the bag and ventilate.

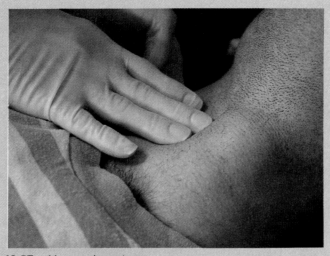

13-5E. Monitor the patient.

When preparing medications for administration, the paramedic must remember to:

- Concentrate on the task.
- Assure that the medical control physician understands the situation.
- Assure that the medical control physician's orders are clearly understood.
- Repeat orders back to the medical control physician to confirm them before administering the medication.
- Read drug labels carefully.
- Check the expiration date of the medication.
- Double-check all calculations before administration.
- Use correct, properly-operating equipment.
- Use aseptic technique.
- Check for incompatibility problems.
- Monitor the patient for the desired effects, as well as any unexpected side effects.

DRUGS USED IN PREHOSPITAL CARE

Drugs Used In Cardiovascular Emergencies

Oxygen

Description. Oxygen is one of the most important emergency drugs and is required by the body to facilitate the breakdown of glucose into a usable energy form. It is an odorless, tasteless, colorless gas necessary for life. It passes into the body through the respiratory system. Oxygen is transported to body cells by hemoglobin, a substance found in the red blood cells.

Indications. Oxygen should be administered to the hypoxic patient. It should also be administered if it appears hypoxia might soon develop or if oxygen demands may be increased. It should be routinely used in the management of cardiac arrest. Oxygen should also be administered to any patient with chest pain that may be due to cardiac ischemia.

✱ Never withhold oxygen from a hypoxic patient.

Contraindications. High-flow oxygen should not be used in patients with chronic CO_2 retention, who have a hypoxic drive to breathing, unless respiratory failure is imminent. Instead, low flow devices, such as nasal cannulas, should be used.

Precautions. Caution should be used when administering oxygen to patients with chronic obstructive pulmonary disease. These patients have ceased depending on the level of carbon dioxide in the blood to regulate their respiratory pattern. Their disease makes them dependent on the amount of oxygen in the blood. Administration of large quantities of oxygen to such patients can result in apnea.

The prolonged administration of high quantities of oxygen to newborn infants can result in eye damage. Prehospital personnel should confirm desired oxygen concentrations with the attending physician prior to prolonged oxygen therapy. This is especially important in long-distance neonatal transport, whether by ambulance or aircraft.

Dosage

- ❏ *Cardiac Arrest:* 100% or as close to that as possible
- ❏ *Hypoxia:* 10–15 liters per minute
- ❏ *Chest Pain:* 6–8 liters per minute
- ❏ *COPD:* 0–2 liters per minute

The Sympathomimetics. The term *sympathomimetic* means to mimic the actions of the sympathetic nervous system. Drugs in this group will either act directly on receptors of the sympathetic nervous system, or act indirectly by stimulating the release of endogenous catecholamines. *Catecholamine* is the name used to describe several chemically similar drugs that act on the sympathetic nervous system.

Epinephrine 1:10,000

✱ Epinephrine increases the rate and force of the cardiac contraction and causes peripheral vasoconstriction.

Description. Epinephrine is a potent α and β stimulant. The 1:10,000 dilution, frequently used in the treatment of cardiac emergencies, contains 1 milligram of epinephrine in 10 milliliters of isotonic sodium chloride. When administered, it has an effect on both α and β adrenergic receptors. However, its effect on β receptors is much more profound. In asystole, it is used to initiate electrical activity in the myocardium. Once that activity is initiated, electrical defibrillation may be attempted.

■ **inotrope** a drug or other substance which affects the contractile force of the heart.

Because of its strong **inotropic** and **chronotropic** properties, epinephrine increases myocardial oxygen demand. When administering epinephrine in the emergency setting, keep these effects in mind. Like most other drugs in emergency medicine, epinephrine is only effective when the myocardium is adequately oxygenated.

■ **chronotrope** a drug or other substance which affects the heart rate.

Epinephrine effects appear within 90 seconds of administration, and they are usually of short duration. Therefore, the drug must be administered every five minutes to maintain therapeutic levels.

Indications

- ❏ Fine ventricular fibrillation
- ❏ Asystole
- ❏ Electromechanical dissociation (EMD)
- ❏ Anaphylactic shock

Contraindications. Epinephrine 1:10,000 is contraindicated in patients who do not require extensive cardiopulmonary resuscitative efforts. With asthma, or acute anaphylaxis, the 1:1000 dilution is administered subcutaneously.

Precautions. Epinephrine, like all catecholamines, should be protected from light. It can be deactivated by alkaline solutions such as sodium bicarbonate. Because of this, it is essential that the IV line is adequately flushed between the administration of epinephrine and sodium bicarbonate.

Dosage. Epinephrine is administered in doses of 0.5 to 1.0 milligram. The dose should be repeated every 5 minutes until the patient is resuscitated.

Route. The most common route of administration used in emergency medicine is intravenous (IV). However, if an IV line cannot be established, the drug may be given via the endotracheal route. Because of the inherent complications, intracardiac injection should be avoided.

Norepinephrine (Levophed)

Description. Norepinephrine acts predominantly on α receptors. Thus, it is a potent peripheral vasoconstrictor. This vasoconstriction increases blood pressure in cardiogenic shock and other hypotensive emergencies. Because norepinephrine also tends to constrict the renal and mesenteric blood vessels, an undesirable action, it has fallen into relative disuse. Dopamine, which maintains renal and mesenteric perfusion when used in appropriate dosage, is preferred.

> ✱ Norepinephrine is primarily a vasoconstrictor with minimal cardiac effects.

Indications

- ❏ Cardiogenic shock
- ❏ Neurogenic shock

Contraindications. Norepinephrine should not be given to patients who are hypotensive from hypovolemia.

Precautions. Because of the powerful effects of norepinephrine, it is essential to measure the blood pressure every 5 to 10 minutes to prevent dangerously high levels. Norepinephrine should be given through the largest vein readily available, because it may cause local tissue necrosis if infiltrated. In addition, it can be deactivated by alkaline solutions, such as sodium bicarbonate.

Dosage. The current dosage recommended by the American Heart Association for norepinephrine is 2 to 12 micrograms per minute for adults. The best dilution comes from placing 8 milligrams in 500 milliliters of 5% dextrose in water. This will give a concentration of 16 micrograms per milliliter. The infusion should be started at 2 micrograms per minute (7.5 drops per minute using a 60-drop-per-milliliter set). This can be increased as required. The same concentration can be obtained by placing 4 milligrams in 250 milliliters of 5% dextrose in water. (See Figure 13-9.)

Routes. Because of its potency, norepinephrine is given only in extremely diluted intravenous infusions. To control its administration, the

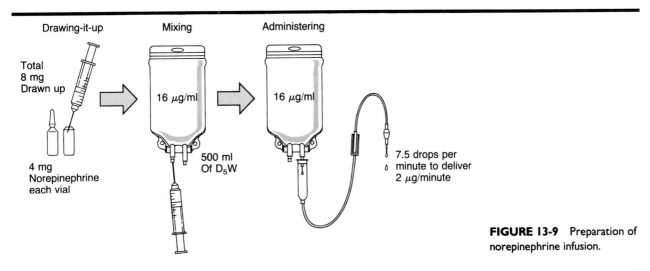

FIGURE 13-9 Preparation of norepinephrine infusion.

drug should be "piggybacked" into an already established line of 5% dextrose in water.

Isoproterenol (Isuprel)

Description. Isoproterenol is a potent, synthetic catecholamine that acts exclusively on β receptors. Because it has virtually no α receptor-stimulating capabilities, its actions are primarily on the heart and lungs. In cardiac emergencies it is used to increase heart rate in bradycardias that are refractory to atropine. Moreover, it causes an increase in cardiac output, owing to its positive inotropic and chronotropic actions. It is important to be careful when administering isoproterenol. Like epinephrine, it significantly increases myocardial oxygen demand. The increase in myocardial oxygen consumption may increase myocardial infarction size. In patients who have not suffered a myocardial infarction, isoproterenol may cause myocardial ischemia. The emergency physician must weigh the benefits of isoproterenol against its risks. (See Figure 13-10.)

Indications

■ **refractory** a disorder or condition that resists treatment.

❑ Bradycardias **refractory** to atropine
❑ Bradycardias due to high-degree heart blocks (that is, Second Degree Mobitz II and Third Degree Blocks)

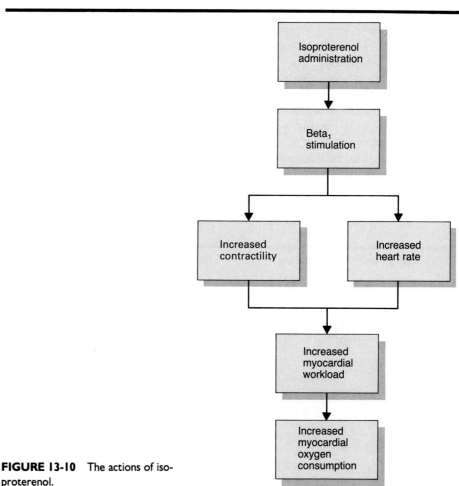

FIGURE 13-10 The actions of isoproterenol.

Contraindications. Isoproterenol is not used to increase blood pressure in cardiogenic shock. It should only be used in shock due to bradycardias. Other sympathomimetics, such as dopamine and norepinephrine, should be used in cases of cardiogenic shock.

Precautions. When administering isoproterenol, you must monitor the patient for signs of ventricular irritability. These may take the form of premature ventricular contractions, ventricular tachycardia, or even ventricular fibrillation. Lidocaine should be readily available whenever you administer isoproterenol.

Because isoproterenol causes significant increases in myocardial oxygen demand, it should be avoided in cases of acute myocardial infarction.

Isoproterenol can be deactivated by alkaline solutions such as sodium bicarbonate.

Dosage. One milligram of isoproterenol should be diluted in 500 milliliters of 5% dextrose in water. This will give a concentration of 2 micrograms per milliliter. It should be **titrated** until the desired heart rate is attained, or until signs of ventricular irritability, such as premature ventricular contractions, occur. The recommended infusion rate is 2 to 10 mcg/minute. Doses of greater than 10 mcg/minute are rarely necessary. (See Figure 13-11.)

■ **titration** estimation of the appropriate dosage by slowly changing the rate of administration.

Route. Because of its potency, isoproterenol should only be given by intravenous infusion. An established line of 5% dextrose in water, into which the isoproterenol is piggybacked, should be maintained.

Dopamine (Intropin)

Description. Dopamine is one of the most commonly used agents in the treatment of hypotension associated with cardiogenic shock. It is chemically related to both epinephrine and norepinephrine. Dopamine acts primarily on β_1 receptors, exerting a positive inotropic effect on the heart. The drug does not cause an increase in myocardial oxygen demand to the degree that isoproterenol does; nor does it have the same powerful chronotropic effects. Unlike norepinephrine, dopamine maintains renal and mesenteric blood flow when it's used in therapeutic dosages. For these reasons, dopamine is the most commonly used vasopressor. Table

✱ Dopamine increases cardiac contractile force and thus cardiac output and is the drug of choice for the management of cardiogenic shock.

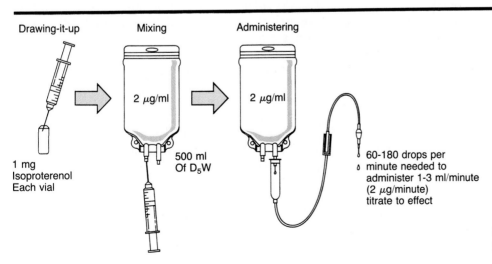

Drawing-it-up   Mixing   Administering

2 µg/ml   2 µg/ml

1 mg   500 ml   60-180 drops per
Isoproterenol   Of D₅W   minute needed to
Each vial   administer 1-3 ml/minute
                                   (2 µg/minute)
                                   titrate to effect

FIGURE 13-11 Preparation of isoproterenol infusion.

TABLE 13-2 Intropin® (Dopamine HCl) Dosage Phenomena

The Effects of Intropin® at Three Dose Ranges	2–5 mcg/kg/min	5–20 mcg/kg/min	Over 20 mcg/kg/min
Cardiac output	no change	increase	increase
Stroke Volume	no change	increase	increase
Heart Rate	no change	there is an initial increase followed by a decrease toward normal rates as infusion continues	
Myocardial Contractility	no change	increase	increase
Potential for Excessive Myocardial Oxygen Demands	low* coronary blood flow increased	low* coronary blood flow increased	data unavailable
Potential for Tachyarrhythmias	low*	low*	moderate
Total Systemic Vascular Resistance	slight decrease to no change	no change to slight increase	increase
Renal Blood Flow	increase	increase	decrease**
Urine Output	increase	increase	decrease**

* Low but needs monitoring
** Relative to peak values achieved at lower dosages.
© 1981 American Critical Care Division of American Hospital Supply Corporation
(Courtesy of American Critical Care, Division of American Hospital Supply Corporation, McGaw Park, Illinois, 1983)

13-2 illustrates the dosage phenomena of dopamine. Dopamine will increase the systolic blood pressure and the pulse pressure (the difference between the systolic and diastolic blood pressures). However, as a rule, there is usually less effect on the diastolic pressure.

Indications

❑ Cardiogenic shock
❑ Hypovolemic shock (only after complete fluid resuscitation)

Contraindications. Dopamine should not be used as the sole agent in the management of hypovolemic shock, unless fluid resuscitation is well under way.

Precautions. Dopamine should not be administered in the presence of tachydysrhythmias or ventricular fibrillation. Like all of the sympathomimetic vasopressors, it can be deactivated by alkaline solutions, such as sodium bicarbonate. If the patient is taking monoamine oxidase inhibitors (a type of antidepressant), the dose should then be reduced to prevent possible hypertensive crisis.

Dosage. The standard preparation for a dopamine infusion is to place 800 milligrams in 500 milliliters of 5% dextrose in water. You can also get this dilution by adding 400 milligrams to 250 milliliters of 5% dextrose in water. This gives a concentration of 1600 micrograms per milliliter. The effects of dopamine are dose-dependent. The infusion should be started at a dosage of 2–5 micrograms per kilogram per minute. Table 13-3 illustrates the dosage of dopamine based on body weight. (See Figure 13-12.)

Route. Dopamine is administered only by intravenous infusion, which should be piggybacked into an already established infusion of 5% dextrose in water.

TABLE 13-3 Intropin® (Dopamine HCl) Dosage Chart

For A Concentration of 1600 mcg Dopamine HCl/ml (800 mg Intropin Per 500 ml—Or—400 mg Intropin Per 250 ml)

Body Wt lbs	**77**	**88**	**99**	**110**	**121**	**132**	**143**	**154**	**165**	**176**	**187**	**198**	**209**	**220**	**231**	**242**
kgs	**35**	**40**	**45**	**50**	**55**	**60**	**65**	**70**	**75**	**80**	**85**	**90**	**95**	**100**	**105**	**110**
Flow Rate in Drops* Per Minute																
5	3.8	3.4	2.9	2.6	2.4	2.2	2.0	1.9	1.8	1.6	1.55	1.5	1.4	1.3	1.25	1.2
10	7.6	6.7	5.9	5.3	4.9	4.5	4.1	3.8	3.6	3.3	3.1	3.0	2.8	2.7	2.5	2.4
15	11	10	8.9	8.0	7.3	6.6	6.1	5.7	5.3	5.0	4.7	4.4	4.2	4.0	3.8	3.6
20	15	13	12	11	9.7	8.9	8.2	7.6	7.1	6.7	6.3	5.9	5.6	5.3	5.1	4.9
25	19	17	15	13	12	11	10	9.5	8.9	8.4	7.8	7.4	7.0	6.6	6.3	6.0
30	23	20	18	16	15	13	12	11	11	10	9.4	8.9	8.4	8.0	7.6	7.3
35	27	23	21	19	17	16	14	13	12	12	11	10	9.8	9.3	8.9	8.5
40	31	27	24	21	19	18	16	15	14	13	13	12	11	11	10	9.7
45	34	30	27	24	22	20	18	17	16	15	14	13	13	12	11	11
50	38	33	30	27	24	22	21	19	18	17	16	15	14	13	13	12
55	42	37	33	29	27	24	23	21	20	18	17	16	15	15	14	13
60	46	40	36	32	29	27	25	25	21	20	19	18	17	16	15	15
70	53	47	42	37	34	31	29	27	25	23	22	21	20	19	18	17
80	61	53	47	43	39	36	33	31	28	27	25	24	23	21	20	19
90	69	60	53	48	44	40	37	34	32	30	28	27	25	24	23	22
100	76	67	59	53	49	45	41	38	36	33	31	30	28	27	25	24

Dosage = mcg Dopamine HCl/kg/min

* Based on a microdrip calibration of 60 drops equal to 1.0 milliliter
Note: All dosages of 10 mcg/kg/min and above have been rounded off to the nearest mcg/kg/min.
(Courtesy of American Critical Care, Division of American Hospital Supply Corporation, McGaw Park, Illinois, 1983)

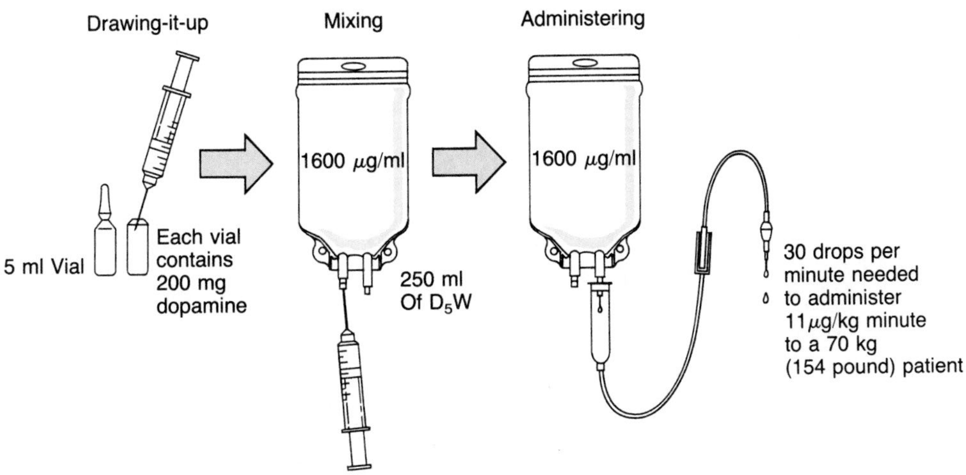

Drawing-it-up
Mixing
Administering
5 ml Vial
Each vial contains 200 mg dopamine
1600 μg/ml
250 ml Of D5W
1600 μg/ml
30 drops per minute needed to administer 11μg/kg minute to a 70 kg (154 pound) patient

FIGURE 13-12 Preparation of dopamine infusion.

Dobutamine (Dobutrex)

Description. Dobutamine, like isoproterenol, is a synthetic catecholamine. It acts primarily on β receptors but is less of a β agonist than isoproterenol. Dobutamine increases the force of the systolic contraction (positive inotropic effect), with little chronotropic activity. For these reasons, it is useful in the management of congestive heart failure when an increase in heart rate is not desired.

Indications. Short-term management of congestive heart failure when an increased cardiac output is desired, without an increase in cardiac rate.

Contraindications. Dobutamine should not be used as the sole agent in hypovolemic shock, unless fluid resuscitation is well under way. To increase cardiac output in severe emergencies, like cardiogenic shock, dopamine is the preferred agent.

Precautions. Tachycardia and an increase in the systolic blood pressure are common following the administration of dobutamine. Increases in heart rate of more than 10 percent may induce or exacerbate myocardial ischemia. PVCs can occur in conjunction with dobutamine administration. Lidocaine should be readily available. As with any sympathomimetic, blood pressure should be monitored frequently.

Dosage. The desired dosage range for dobutamine is between 2.5 and 20 micrograms per kilogram per minute. Dobutamine should be administered according to the patient's response.

Route. Dobutamine should be diluted in either 500 milliliters, or 1 liter, of 5% dextrose in water, and administered via IV infusion. (See Figure 13-13.)

The Sympathetic Blockers. Sympathetic blockers are a unique class of drugs that antagonize (block) adrenergic receptor sites. Certain drugs will block only α receptors, while others block only β receptors. Some of the β blockers are so selective that they block only β_1 or β_2 receptors. The drugs that block the β receptors are used the most.

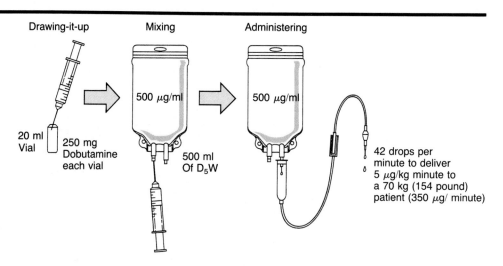

Drawing-it-up   Mixing   Administering

500 µg/ml   500 µg/ml

20 ml Vial   250 mg Dobutamine each vial   500 ml Of D₅W   42 drops per minute to deliver 5 µg/kg minute to a 70 kg (154 pound) patient (350 µg/ minute)

FIGURE 13-13 Preparation of dobutamine infusion.

Labetalol (Trandate) (Normodyne)

Description. Labetalol acts very differently from the other β blockers. Like propranolol (the prototype β blocker), labetalol is a nonselective β adrenergic antagonist showing no preference for either β_1 or β_2 receptors. However, unlike the other β blockers, labetalol also blocks α_1 adrenergic receptors. Blockage of α_1 receptors inhibits peripheral vasoconstriction, thus causing peripheral vasodilatation. Because of these properties, labetalol is a potent agent for lowering blood pressure in cases of hypertensive crisis. It does this by decreasing cardiac output through its β_1 blocking properties and by causing peripheral vasodilatation through its α_1 blocking properties.

Indications. Labetalol is indicated for the acute management of hypertensive crisis.

Contraindications. Labetalol is contraindicated in patients with bronchial asthma, congestive heart failure, heart block, bradycardia, or cardiogenic shock.

Precautions. With all β blockers, you should continuously monitor the blood pressure, pulse rate, ECG, and respiratory status. Prehospital personnel should be alert for signs and symptoms of congestive heart failure, bradycardia, shock, heart block, or bronchospasm when administering labetalol. The appearance of any of these is an indication for discontinuing the drug.

Because of the effects of labetalol on β_1 receptors, postural hypotension might occur and should be anticipated. The patient should be supine at all times during drug administration.

Dosage. There are two accepted methods of administering labetalol in the treatment of hypertensive crisis:

1. Twenty milligrams of labetalol can be administered by slow intravenous injection over 2 minutes. Immediately before the injection, and at 5 minutes and 10 minutes after the injection, record the supine blood pressure. Additional injections of 40 milligrams can be given every 10 minutes until a desired supine blood pressure is achieved, or 300 milligrams of the drug has been given.

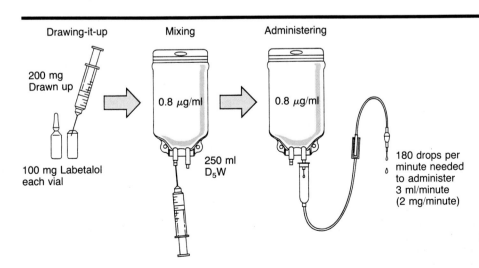

Drawing-it-up   Mixing   Administering

200 mg
Drawn up

0.8 μg/ml

0.8 μg/ml

100 mg Labetalol
each vial

250 ml
D$_5$W

180 drops per
minute needed
to administer
3 ml/minute
(2 mg/minute)

FIGURE 13-14 Preparation of labetalol infusion.

2. Two ampules (200 milligrams) of labetalol can be added to 250 milliliters of 5% dextrose in water (D5W). This gives a concentration of 0.8 milligram per milliliter. This solution should be administered at a rate of 2 milligrams per minute (2.5 milliliters per minute). The blood pressure should be continuously monitored. (See Figure 13-14.)

The Antidysrhythmics. Many drugs are useful in the treatment and prevention of cardiac dysrhythmias. Some are useful in the treatment of atrial dysrhythmias, while others are useful in the treatment of ventricular dysrhythmias. It is essential to distinguish between ventricular and atrial dysrhythmias.

Lidocaine (Xylocaine)

✱ Lidocaine suppresses ventricular ectopic activity and is thus useful in the treatment of many ventricular dysrhythmias.

Description. Lidocaine is probably the most frequently used antidysrhythmic agent in the treatment of life-threatening cardiac emergencies. Moreover, it has been proven effective in suppressing premature ventricular contractions, and in treating ventricular tachycardia and some cases of ventricular fibrillation. It has also been found to increase the fibrillation threshold in acute myocardial infarction.

In prehospital care, the most common cause of life-threatening ventricular dysrhythmias is acute myocardial infarction. Lidocaine suppresses ventricular ectopy in the setting of myocardial infarction and increases the ventricular fibrillation threshold. This aids in the prevention of PVCs, which can induce ventricular fibrillation. After acute myocardial infarction, the ventricular fibrillation threshold is often significantly reduced. Moreover, because electrical defibrillation tends to cause ventricular irritability, patients who have been successfully defibrillated should be treated with lidocaine.

Lidocaine seems to be successful in suppressing ventricular dysrhythmias only when the level of the drug in the blood is between 1.5 and 6.0 micrograms per milliliter of blood. A 1 mg/kg bolus of lidocaine will maintain adequate blood levels for only 20 minutes. (See Figure 13-15.) Therefore, a lidocaine bolus should be followed by a 2 to 4 mg/minute infusion to assure therapeutic blood levels. (See Figure 13-16.)

It is important to recognize patterns of premature ventricular contractions that are likely to lead to serious dysrhythmias. Premature ventricular contractions (PVCs) that may lead to life-threatening dysrhythmias are called *malignant premature ventricular contractions.* These include:

❑ More than 6 unifocal PVCs per minute
❑ PVCs that appear to be coming from more than one ectopic focus (for example, multifocal PVCs)

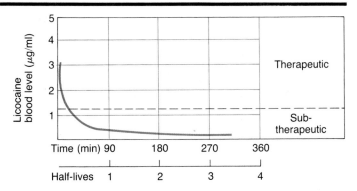

FIGURE 13-15 Blood levels of lidocaine following bolus alone.

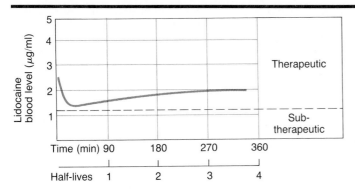

FIGURE 13-16 Blood levels of lidocaine following bolus and continuous infusion.

❑ PVCs that occur in couplets (two PVCs together without a normal QRS complex in between)

❑ Runs of more than 2 PVCs, or ventricular tachycardia

❑ PVCs falling in the vulnerable period of the preceding normal complex (R on T phenomena).

Premature ventricular contractions, as well as ventricular tachycardia and ventricular fibrillation, must be treated aggressively with lidocaine.

Indications

❑ Malignant premature ventricular contractions

❑ Ventricular tachycardia

❑ Ventricular fibrillation (after the initial series of resuscitative procedures, including electrical defibrillation)

❑ Dysrhythmia prophylaxis in patients suffering acute myocardial infarction

Contraindications. Lidocaine is generally contraindicated in second-degree Mobitz II and third-degree blocks, since it may further slow conduction of the electrical impulse from the atria to the ventricles. Decreased ventricular rates may accompany high-grade heart block, resulting in escape beats that are premature ventricular contractions. Whenever premature ventricular contractions occur in conjunction with bradycardia (heart rate less than 60), the bradycardia should be treated first. The drug of choice is atropine sulfate, followed by isoproterenol if atropine is not effective. If PVCs are still present after increasing the rate, lidocaine should be administered.

Precautions. Central nervous system depression may occur when the dosage exceeds 300 milligrams per hour. Symptoms of central nervous system depression include a decreased level of consciousness, irritability, confusion, muscle-twitching, and, eventually, seizures. Excessive doses can result in coma and death.

Dosage. The initial bolus is 1 milligram per kilogram body weight (generally 50 to 75 milligrams), followed by subsequent boluses of 0.5 milligram per kilogram every 8–10 minutes until the dysrhythmia resolves, or a maximum loading dose of 3 milligrams per kilogram is reached. The initial loading dose should be decreased by 50% in patients 70 years of age or older. This is followed by a maintenance infusion of 2 to 4 milligrams per minute. For the infusion, 2 grams of lidocaine are diluted in 500 milliliters of 5% dextrose in water. (See Figure 13-17.)

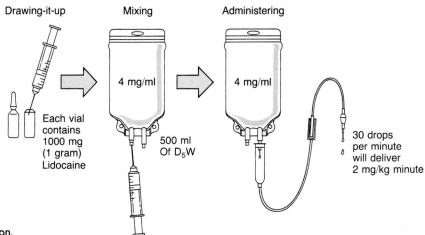

Drawing-it-up   Mixing   Administering

Each vial contains 1000 mg (1 gram) Lidocaine

4 mg/ml

500 ml Of D₅W

4 mg/ml

30 drops per minute will deliver 2 mg/kg minute

FIGURE 13-17 Preparation of lidocaine infusion.

Routes. Lidocaine is generally given in an IV bolus, followed by an infusion. However, it can also be given endotracheally if an IV line cannot be established. A preparation of lidocaine is also available that can be given intramuscularly for ventricular dysrhythmias. This should be reserved for times when an IV cannot be established and the patient is not intubated.

> ### Bretylium Tosylate (Bretylol)

✱ The pharmacological effects of bretylium are often delayed 3–5 minutes or more following administration. Other resuscitative measures should be carried out in the interim.

Description. Bretylium tosylate was approved for use in emergency care in 1978 and has proven effective in the treatment of ventricular fibrillation, ventricular tachycardia, and certain ventricular ectopic rhythms. Its use, however, is reserved for those cases that fail to respond to lidocaine. It has been demonstrated that, like lidocaine, bretylium increases the ventricular fibrillation threshold. Bretylium seems to raise the ventricular fibrillation threshold through postganglionic adrenergic blockade. A side effect of this blockade is bradycardia and postural hypotension, which is commonly seen within 24 hours. Bretylium will sometimes convert ventricular fibrillation or ventricular tachycardia to a supraventricular rhythm. Because of this action, bretylium is sometimes referred to as a "chemical defibrillator." (See Figure 13-18.)

Bretylium's effects are often not evident until 3 to 5 minutes after administration. Cardiopulmonary resuscitative procedures should be continued in the interim.

Indications

❑ Ventricular fibrillation refractory to lidocaine
❑ Ventricular tachycardia refractory to lidocaine
❑ Malignant premature ventricular contractions refractory to first-line agents

Contraindications. There are no contraindications to bretylium when used in the management of life-threatening ventricular dysrhythmias.

Precautions. Postural hypotension occurs in approximately 50 percent of patients receiving bretylium. This side effect should be anticipated and the patient maintained in a supine position.

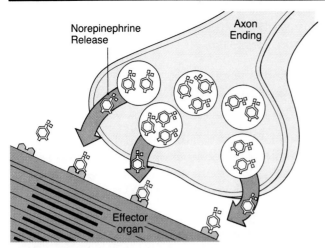

A. Bretylium provokes the release of norepinephrine from the axon ending

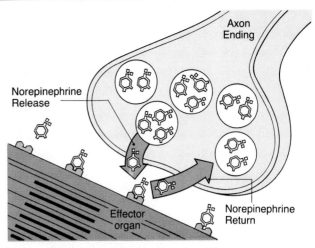

B. Normally norepinephrine is released and then taken back up to the axon ending

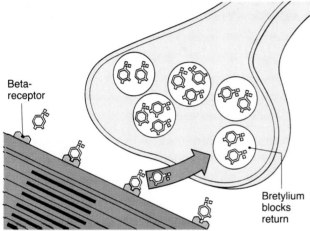

C. Bretylium blocks the return of norepinephrine to the axon ending

FIGURE 13-18 Pharmacological actions of bretylium.

Dosage. Bretylium should be administered at a dose of 5 milligrams per kilogram of body weight. If the dysrhythmia persists, a second dose can be repeated at a dosage of 10 milligrams per kilogram body weight. Additional doses may be repeated at 15–30 minute intervals, to a maximum dose of 30 milligrams per kilogram of body weight.

Route. Bretylium should be administered by IV bolus. On rare occasions, an intravenous infusion may be ordered.

Procainamide (Pronestyl)

Description. Procainamide is used in the treatment of ventricular dysrhythmias. Because lidocaine is the drug of choice, procainamide should be withheld until at least 3 milligrams per kilogram of lidocaine have been administered and found to be unsuccessful in treating ventricular ectopy.

❑ Premature ventricular contractions refractory to lidocaine
❑ Ventricular tachycardia refractory to lidocaine

Procainamide is used to treat ventricular ectopic activity refractory to lidocaine.

Contraindications. Procainamide should not be administered to patients with severe conductive system disturbances, especially second- and third-degree heart blocks.

Precautions. Procainamide should not be administered to patients with premature ventricular contractions in conjunction with profound brady-cardia (escape beats). The heart rate should be first increased with atro-pine. Only after increasing the heart rate can the PVCs be treated with lidocaine or procainamide.

Hypotension is common with intravenous infusion. The constant monitoring of blood pressure is essential.

Dosage. In treating premature ventricular contractions or ventricular tachycardia, 100 milligrams should be administered every 5 minutes at a rate of 20 milligrams per minute. This should be discontinued if any of the following occurs:

❑ The dysrhythmia is suppressed
❑ Hypotension ensues
❑ The QRS is widened by 50 percent or more of its original width
❑ A total of 1 gram of the medication has been administered

The maintenance infusion of procainamide is 1–4 milligrams per minute. The duration of procainamide's effect is shorter than that of lido-caine.

Route. Procainamide should only be administered intravenously.

Verapamil (Isoptin) (Calan)

Vererapamil slows AV conduction and is effective in treating supraventricular tachydysrhythmias.

Description. Verapamil is a calcium-ion antagonist that slows conduc-tion through the AV node. The advantages of this are twofold. First, vera-pamil will inhibit dysrhythmias caused by a reentry mechanism, such as paroxysmal supraventricular tachycardia. Second, it will decrease the rapid ventricular response seen with atrial tachydysrhythmias, such as atrial flutter and atrial fibrillation. Verapamil also decreases myocardial oxygen demand because of its negative inotropic effects and causes coro-nary and peripheral vasodilation.

Indications

❑ Paroxysmal supraventricular tachycardia
❑ Atrial flutter with rapid ventricular response
❑ Atrial fibrillation with rapid ventricular response

Contraindications. Verapamil should not be administered to any pa-tient with severe hypotension or cardiogenic shock. In addition, vera-pamil should not be administered in the prehospital setting to patients with ventricular tachycardia.

Before treating a patient suffering atrial flutter or atrial fibrillation, the paramedic must be sure that the patient does not suffer from **Wolff-Parkinson-White** syndrome.

■ **Wolff-Parkinson-White** a dis-order of the heart characterized by early contraction of the heart muscle.

NOTE: Verapamil should not be administered to patients receiving intravenous beta blockers.

Precautions.   Verapamil can cause systemic hypotension. Constant monitoring of the blood pressure is essential.

Dosage.   In the treatment of paroxysmal supraventricular tachycardia, a 3–5 milligram intravenous dose should be given initially over a 2- to 3-minute period. A second dose of 5 to 10 milligrams can be given after 10–15 minutes if PSVT persists and there has been no adverse reaction. The total dose of verapamil should not exceed 15 milligrams in 30 minutes.

Route.   Verapamil should be administered intravenously.

The Parasympatholytics.   Drugs that inhibit the actions of the parasympathetic nervous system are referred to as parasympatholytics. Sometimes they are referred to as anticholinergics. The parasympathetic nervous system plays a major role in the maintenance of homeostasis. The primary nerve of the parasympathetic nervous system is the vagus nerve, also called the tenth cranial nerve. When stimulated, it causes acetylcholine to be released from the presynaptic nerve endings. Acetylcholine then activates acetylcholine receptors, on either the post-synaptic membrane or the target organ, such as the heart. This results in slowing of the heart rate and other activities. However, a second compound—*acetylcholinesterase*—is released almost immediately, which deactivates acetylcholine, terminating its effect.

   Several medications affect this mechanism. Atropine binds to acetylcholine receptors, blocking the action of acetylcholine. Organophosphates, a common class of insecticides, bind irreversibly to acetylcholinesterase, prolonging the effect of acetylcholine. Pralidoxime (2-PAM), an antidote for organophosphate poisoning, reactivates acetylcholinesterase.

Atropine Sulfate

Description.   Atropine sulfate is a potent parasympatholytic. It blocks acetylcholine receptors, thus inhibiting parasympathetic effects. In emergency medicine it is used primarily to increase the heart rate in life-threatening bradycardia. Although it has positive chronotropic properties, it has little or no inotropic effect. Atropine also plays a role in the management of organophosphate poisonings.

✳ Atropine blocks the action of the parasympathetic nervous system and the vagus nerve. It is effective in the treatment of symptomatic bradycardias.

Indications.

❑ Bradycardias accompanied by hemodynamically significant hypotension or frequent ectopic escape beats. It is of some use in the treatment of second-degree Mobitz type II and third-degree heart block in the setting of myocardial infarction.
❑ Asystole
❑ Organophosphate poisonings

Contraindications.   None in the emergency setting.

Precautions.   A maximum dose of 2.0 milligrams should only be exceeded in the case of organophosphate poisonings. If the heart rate fails to increase after a total of 2.0 milligrams, then isoproterenol or cardiac pacing is indicated.

Dosage. The initial dose in the treatment of bradycardias is 0.5 milligram. This can be administered every 5 minutes up to a total of 2.0 milligrams. For treating asystole, the initial dose is 1.0 milligram.

In cases of organophosphate poisoning, a test dose of 1.0 milligram should be administered to determine whether the patient is tolerant to atropine. If the patient responds to the initial dose, he or she is probably not severely poisoned. If there is no improvement following the test dose, a second dose of 2.0–5.0 milligrams may be indicated for an adult.

Route. Atropine should be administered by intravenous bolus. If an IV cannot be established, administer the drug down an endotracheal tube.

The Alkalinizing Agents. Alkalinizing drugs, such as sodium bicarbonate, are used to buffer the acids present in the body during and after severe hypoxia. Normal body pH is 7.4 (7.35–7.45). During hypoxia, serum pH may fall quickly. Sodium bicarbonate will help correct metabolic (usually lactic acid) acidosis until hypoxia is corrected. The following reaction illustrates the role of sodium bicarbonate in acid-base balance:

$$H^+ \quad + \quad HCO_3^- \quad \longleftrightarrow \quad H_2CO_3 \quad \longleftrightarrow \quad H_2 \quad + \quad CO_2$$

| Hydrogen ion | Bicarbonate ion | Carbonic acid | Water | Carbon Dioxide |

Bicarbonate combines with strong acids, such as lactic acid, and forms a weak, volatile acid. This acid is subsequently degraded to carbon dioxide and water. The end-products are removed via the kidneys or lungs.

Excessive administration of sodium bicarbonate can cause metabolic alkalosis, which can be worse than the metabolic acidosis being treated. Sodium bicarbonate delivers 50 mEq of sodium with each prefilled syringe, which can cause additional problems.

The primary treatment of metabolic acidosis in the setting of hypoxia or cardiac arrest is adequate oxygenation and blood-pressure support.

Sodium Bicarbonate (NaHCO₃)

Description. Sodium bicarbonate was the cornerstone of advanced cardiac life support for many years. However, recent studies have questioned its role. Sodium bicarbonate is now reserved for use late in cardiac arrest, after ventilation has been adequately addressed.

Sodium bicarbonate provides bicarbonate ion to buffer strong acids.

Indications

- ❏ Severe acidosis
- ❏ Cardiac arrest after ventilation and other problems have been corrected
- ❏ Tricyclic antidepressant overdosage

Contraindications. When used in the treatment of severe hypoxia, late in cardiac arrest, there are no contraindications.

Precautions. Sodium bicarbonate can cause metabolic alkalosis following overzealous administration. In addition, most vasopressors, such as dopamine, can be deactivated by the alkaline environment provided by so-

✱ The role of sodium bicarbonate in advanced cardiac life support is questionable due to the absence of proven effectiveness and numerous adverse reactions.

dium bicarbonate. Also, sodium bicarbonate should not be administered concurrently with calcium chloride because a precipitate can develop.

Dosage. The initial dose of sodium bicarbonate is 1 mEq per kilogram of body weight. This can be repeated, if required, at 0.5 mEq per kilogram of body weight.

Route. Sodium bicarbonate should be administered intravenously.

The Analgesics. Drugs that have proven effective in alleviating pain are referred to as analgesics. Although they may be administered in many types of emergencies, they are usually reserved for the treatment of emergencies involving the cardiovascular system, especially myocardial infarction.

Morphine Sulfate

Description. Although morphine sulfate is one of the most potent analgesics, it also has hemodynamic properties that make it extremely useful in emergency medicine. It increases peripheral venous capacitance and decreases venous return. This effect is sometimes called a "chemical phlebotomy." Morphine also decreases myocardial oxygen demand. This action is due to the decreased systemic vascular resistance and the sedative effects of the drug. Patient apprehension and fear can significantly increase myocardial oxygen demand; in some cases, it may even increase the size of myocardial infarction. Its hemodynamic properties make morphine one of the most important drugs used in treating pulmonary edema. Morphine is frequently administered to patients with signs and symptoms of pulmonary edema who are not having chest pain.

Morphine is a narcotic derivative of opium. With a high tendency for addiction and abuse, it is covered under the Controlled Substances Act of 1970. It is classified as a Schedule II drug. Many EMS systems have opted to use the synthetic analgesics, like nalbuphine (Nubain) and pentazocine (Talwin), to avoid the legal complications involved in using morphine and meperidine (Demerol).

In higher dosages, morphine causes severe respiratory depression. This is especially true in patients who already have some respiratory impairment. The narcotic antagonist naloxone (Narcan) should be readily available whenever the drug is administered.

Indications

❑ Severe pain associated with myocardial infarction, kidney stones, etc.
❑ Pulmonary edema, with or without associated pain

Contraindications. Morphine should not be used with patients who are volume-depleted or severely hypotensive because of the hemodynamic effects. Morphine should not be administered to any patient with a history of hypersensitivity to the drug or to patients with apparent head injury or abdominal pain.

Precautions. Morphine can cause respiratory depression. The paramedic should always have naloxone available to reverse the effects of the drug if respiratory depression ensues. Patients who are extremely ill, or who may have pre-existing respiratory depression, may be extremely sensitive to the depressive effects of morphine.

* A common method of dosing morphine in the prehospital phase is in 2 milligram increments until pain is relieved ("2 + 2").

Dosage. There are many approaches to the administration of morphine. An initial dose of 2 to 5 milligrams IV is standard. This can be augmented with additional doses of 2 milligrams every few minutes, and can be continued until the pain is relieved, or until signs of respiratory depression occur. Intramuscular injection, as a rule, requires 5 to 15 milligrams, based on the patient's weight.

Routes. Morphine is routinely given intravenously in emergency medicine. However, it can also be given intramuscularly.

Nitronox

Description. Nitronox is a blended mixture of 50% nitrous oxide and 50% oxygen. When inhaled, it has potent analgesic effects. These effects quickly dissipate, however—within 2 to 5 minutes after administration.

The Nitronox unit consists of one oxygen and one nitrous oxide cylinder. The gases are fed into a blender that combines them at the appropriate 50%/50% concentration. It is then delivered to a modified demand valve for administration to the patient.

Nitronox is self-administered. It is effective in treating most varieties of pain encountered in emergency medicine, including pain from trauma. The high concentration of oxygen delivered with the nitrous oxide will increase the oxygen tension in the blood, thus reducing hypoxia.

Indications

❑ Musculoskeletal pain
❑ Burns
❑ Suspected ischemic chest pain
❑ States of severe anxiety

Contraindications. Nitronox should not be administered to patients who:

❑ cannot comprehend verbal instructions
❑ are intoxicated with alcohol or other drugs
❑ have a head injury sufficient to impair their mental status
❑ have thoracic injury suspicious of pneumothorax
❑ have abdominal pain and distention suggestive of a bowel obstruction
❑ who have COPD where the high oxygen concentration may depress respirations

Precautions. It is essential that Nitronox be self-administered, if possible. Also, nitrous oxide may cause nausea and vomiting in susceptible individuals. This reaction should be anticipated. The duration of administration should be documented.

* Nitronox should only be self-administered by the patient.

Dosage. Nitronox should be self-administered until the patient drops the mask, or the pain is significantly relieved.

The Diuretics. One of the more common cardiovascular emergencies is congestive heart failure. Congestive heart failure occurs when the heart loses its ability to pump blood effectively. In congestive heart failure, the veins leading to the heart become engorged. Failure of the left side of the heart causes a buildup of blood in the pulmonary circulation. Failure of the right side of the heart results in congestion of the peripheral circulation, which often manifests as peripheral edema. Common signs of right-heart failure include jugular venous distention, ascites, and pedal (ankle or pretibial) edema.

Drugs that cause the elimination of fluid from the body, via the kidneys, are referred to as diuretics. Furosemide is the most commonly used diuretic in prehospital care.

Furosemide (Lasix)

Description. Furosemide is a potent diuretic that inhibits sodium and chloride reabsorption in the kidney. It also causes venous dilation. It is extremely useful in the treatment of congestive heart failure and pulmonary edema. Its effects are usually evident within five minutes of administration.

Indications

- ❑ Congestive heart failure
- ❑ Pulmonary edema

Contraindications. Usage in pregnancy should be limited to life-threatening situations. Furosemide has been known to cause fetal abnormalities.

Precautions. Dehydration and electrolyte depletion can result from excessive doses of potent diuretics. Furosemide should be protected from light.

Dosage. The standard dosage of furosemide is 40 milligrams, given by slow IV push in patients already on chronic oral furosemide therapy; and 20 milligrams IV in patients who are not regularly taking the drug orally. Dosages as high as 80 milligrams IV may be indicated in severe cases.

Route. Furosemide should be given intravenously in emergency situations.

The Antianginal Agents. A common manifestation of advanced cardiovascular disease is *angina pectoris*. It results from a narrowing of the coronary arteries, due to the buildup of atherosclerotic plaques, or coronary artery vasospasm. In exercise, and other stressful situations, the amount of blood that can be carried by the coronary arteries may not be sufficient to meet the oxygen demands of the myocardium. This results in myocardial hypoxia, causing the classic pain syndrome called angina pectoris. Sublingual nitroglycerin usually gives immediate relief by causing a decrease in cardiac work, and, to a lesser degree, dilatation of the coronary arteries.

In recent years, nitroglycerin has been tried with patients suffering myocardial infarction in the hope of decreasing the extent of myocardial damage. Nitroglycerin is often administered to patients complaining of chest pain to rule out angina as the cause. When cardiac pain is not relieved by nitroglycerin, morphine and other potent analgesics are administered.

Nitroglycerin is generally administered sublingually. Recently, however, it has been given intravenously in some cases of unstable angina and acute myocardial infarction.

Calcium ion antagonists, such as diltiazem (Cardizem) and nifedip-

✱ Furosemide promotes venous pooling and stimulates the kidneys to excrete water and is thus a mainstay in the treatment of congestive heart failure.

ine (Procardia), have proven effective in the management of angina, especially if it's due to coronary artery vasospasm. In certain areas, these two agents may be on prehospital drug lists.

Nitroglycerin (Nitro Stat)

Description. Nitroglycerin is a rapid smooth-muscle relaxant that causes decreased cardiac work. To a lesser degree, it also causes vasodilatation of coronary arteries, thus increasing perfusion of ischemic myocardium. Pain relief occurs within two minutes, and therapeutic effects can be observed up to 30 minutes later.

Indications

- Chest pain associated with angina pectoris
- Chest pain associated with acute myocardial infarction
- Acute pulmonary edema

Contraindications. Nitroglycerin is contraindicated in patients with increased intracranial pressure.

Precautions. Patients taking nitroglycerin may develop a tolerance for the drug, which requires increasing the dosage. Headache is a common side effect of nitroglycerin, resulting from vasodilation of cerebral vessels. Nitroglycerin deteriorates rapidly once the bottle is opened. When a bottle of nitroglycerin is opened, it should be dated. Nitroglycerin should also be protected from light.

Dosage. One tablet (0.4 milligram) sublingually for routine angina pectoris. The dose may be repeated as required.

Routes. Nitroglycerin should be administered sublingually, making sure the patient doesn't swallow it. Intravenous nitroglycerin is sometimes used in emergency departments and ICU units, but the sublingual route works in most prehospital situations. Nitroglycerin is also available in patches and in ointment.

Nitroglycerin Spray (Nitrolingual Spray)

✳ Nitroglycerin deteriorates quickly following exposure to air. Thus, paramedics should always be sure that the nitroglycerin in stock is current and fresh.

Description. Nitroglycerin spray is an aerosol preparation of nitroglycerin that delivers precisely 0.4 milligram of nitroglycerin per spray. Peak effects occur within four minutes.

Indications

- Chest pain associated with angina pectoris
- Chest pain associated with acute myocardial infarction

Contraindications. Nitroglycerin is contraindicated in patient with increased intracranial pressure.

Precautions. Patients taking nitroglycerin routinely may develop a tolerance for the drug. Headache is a common side effect, which results from dilation of cerebral blood vessels. This should be anticipated.

Dosage. One spray (0.4 milligram) should be sprayed under the tongue at the onset of an angina attack. Do not exceed three sprays in a 25-minute period. *The spray should not be inhaled.*

Route. Nitroglycerin spray should be applied to the sublingual mucous membranes.

The Anti-hypertensives

Nifedipine (Procardia)

Description. Nifedipine is a calcium-channel blocker in widespread emergency usage. It is effective in reducing coronary artery spasm in angina. The drug causes decreased peripheral vascular resistance, as evidenced by a decrease in both systolic and diastolic blood pressures.

* Nifedipine causes relaxation of the smooth muscle which encircles the blood vessels, causing vasodilation, thus decreasing blood pressure.

Indications

- Severe hypertension
- Angina pectoris

Contraindications. Nifedipine is contraindicated in patients with known hypersensitivity to the drug. It is also contraindicated in a patient with hypotension.

Precautions. Nifedipine can cause a significant drop in blood pressure. Thus, the blood pressure should be frequently measured. Nifedipine should be used with caution in patients with heart failure.

NOTE: Nifedipine should not be administered to patients receiving intravenous beta blockers.

Dosage. One 10-milligram capsule should have several small puncture holes placed in the capsule and placed under the tongue, where it can be absorbed. Alternatively, the capsule can be bitten by the patient and swallowed with about the same rate of onset.

Route. Nifedipine should only be administered orally or sublingully.

Diazoxide (Hyperstat)

Description. Diazoxide is effective in the treatment of hypertensive crisis. It decreases both systolic and diastolic pressures by causing vasodilatation of the peripheral arterioles.

* Diazoxide is rarely used in prehospital care due to the introduction of safer drugs such as nifedepine and labetalol.

Indication. Malignant hypertension, if a prompt decrease in diastolic blood pressure is indicated.

Contraindications. None of consequence in the field.

Precautions. Hypotension may occur. If severe, it should be treated with sympathomimetics. Because of the rapid onset of action of diazoxide, blood pressure must be monitored every minute.

Dosage. The standard dose of diazoxide is 1 to 3 milligrams per kilogram of body weight, up to 150 milligrams in a single rapid injection. This may be repeated at intervals of 5 to 15 minutes until a satisfactory reduction in blood pressure is seen.

Route. Diazoxide is administered intravenously and only in a peripheral vein.

Other Cardiovascular Agents

Calcium Chloride

Description. Calcium chloride causes a significant increase in the myocardial contractile force and seems to increase ventricular automaticity.

Although used for many years in the management of cardiac arrest, especially if due to asystole and electromechanical dissociation (EMD), recent studies raise serious questions about calcium chloride's role, even in these cases.

Indications

✱ Calcium chloride is rarely indicated in prehospital care.

❏ Hyperkalemia (dangeroulsy high potassium level)
❏ Hypocalcemia (dangerously low calcium level)
❏ Calcium channel blocker toxicity

Contraindications. Caution is warranted when calcium chloride is administered to patients receiving digitalis, because it may precipitate digitalis toxicity.

Precautions. It is extremely important to flush the IV line between administrations of calcium chloride and sodium bicarbonate to avoid precipitation.

Dosage. The standard dose for calcium chloride is 250 to 500 milligrams intravenously. This may be repeated every 10 minutes or so as requested by medical control.

Route. Calcium chloride should only be given intravenously.

Drugs Used In The Treatment Of Respiratory Emergencies

Introduction. Oxygen is the most commonly used drug in the management of respiratory emergencies. In addition to oxygen, however, several pharmacologic agents have proven effective in the prehospital phase of emergency medical care.

Another agent frequently used in the management of respiratory emergencies is aminophylline. Aminophylline, chemically unrelated to the catecholamines, belongs to a class of drugs called *xanthines*. A commonly encountered drug in the xanthines class is caffeine. Aminophylline causes relaxation of the bronchiole smooth musculature, thus relieving bronchospasm.

In addition to oxygen and aminophylline, the β agonists play a major role in the treatment of respiratory emergencies. Drugs are now available that act predominantly on β_2 receptors. These agents are preferred to non-selective agents because of the decreased incidence of side effects, such as rapid heart rate.

Oxygen

Description. Oxygen is an odorless, tasteless, colorless gas necessary for life. Supplemental oxygen added to inspired air increases the amount of oxygen in the blood, thus increasing the amount of oxygen delivered to the tissues.

Indications. Oxygen is indicated in these situations:

❏ suspected hypoxemia or respiratory distress from any cause
❏ acute chest pain if myocardial infarction is suspected
❏ shock from any cause
❏ major trauma
❏ carbon monoxide poisoning

Precautions. Oxygen alone should not be used in patients who are not breathing adequately. These patients should be ventilated as well. A nasal cannula on an apneic patient is a waste of oxygen. Oxygen should be used cautiously in patients with COPD, because significant increases in PaO_2 may cause suppression of hypoxic drive.

If possible, all oxygen should be humidified, since non-humidified oxygen tends to dry mucous membranes. Oxygen supports combustion and should not be used around an open flame. Smoking should not be permitted when oxygen is in use.

Dosage

- Low Flow: 1–2 liters/minute
- Moderate Flow: 4–6 liters/minute
- High Flow: 10–15 liters/minute

Epinephrine 1:1,000

Description. Epinephrine is a potent catecholamine, with both alpha (α) and beta (β) properties; the effect on β receptors is the more profound. It is used in the treatment of respiratory emergencies because of its significant effects on β_2 adrenergic receptors.

Indications. In respiratory emergencies, epinephrine is indicated in these situations:

- severe, systemic allergic reactions
- asthma in persons under 40 years of age
- exacerbation of COPD

Precautions. Epinephrine, like the other catecholamines, should not be added to solutions that contain sodium bicarbonate, such as bicarbonate infusions, since the drug can be inactivated by the alkaline solution. When using epinephrine for allergic reactions, you should remember that the increased cardiac work caused by the drug can precipitate angina or myocardial infarction in susceptible patients. Because of its peripheral vasoconstrictive effects, epinephrine should be used cautiously in patients with peripheral vascular insufficiency.

Wheezing in an elderly person may be due to such causes as pulmonary edema or pulmonary embolism; epinephrine may not be indicated.

Anxiety, tremors, palpitations, tachycardia, and headache are common and expected side effects. The drug should be used cautiously, if at all, in patients with hypertension, hyperthyroidism, ischemic heart disease, or cerebrovascular insufficiency.

Dosage. The initial adult dose of epinephrine 1:1,000 should be 0.3–0.5 milligrams. In children, the dose is 0.01 mg/kg body weight.

Route. Epinephrine 1:1,000 should only be administered subcutaneously.

* Epinephrine 1:1,000 is for subcutaneous administration only.

Aminophylline

Description. Aminophylline is a bronchodilator used occasionally in emergency care. It sometimes proves effective in cases in which sympathomimetics have not been effective. Aminophylline achieves its bronchodilation effects via a different mechanism from that of the sympathomimetics. In addition to bronchodilation, aminophylline has mild diuretic properties, increases the heart rate and the cardiac output, and may precipitate dysrhythmias.

Owing to its mild diuretic and inotropic effects, aminophylline is also used in the management of congestive heart failure and pulmonary edema.

In prehospital emergency care, aminophylline is given by slow intravenous infusion. However, the use of aminophylline is on the decline with the β selective agonists (albuterol, isoetharine, etc.) being preferred.

Indications

- ❑ Bronchial asthma
- ❑ Reversible bronchospasm associated with chronic bronchitis and emphysema
- ❑ Congestive heart failure
- ❑ Pulmonary edema

Contraindications. Aminophylline should not be administered to any patient with a history of hypersensitivity to the drug.

Precautions. Extreme caution should be used when administering aminophylline to any patient with a history of cardiovascular disease or hypertension. Any patient receiving aminophylline should be placed on a cardiac monitor. You should be alert for any signs of cardiac irritability, especially PVCs and tachycardia. Hypotension can follow rapid administration.

Many patients are chronically on theophylline preparations. Often, the initial prehospital dosage of aminophylline should be reduced for such patients.

Dosage. Two major regimens are used in administering aminophylline.

The first is for patients in whom fluid overload or edema does not appear to be present (that is, acute bronchial asthma):

1. Place 250 to 500 milligrams in 90 or 80 milliliters of 5% dextrose, respectively. This can be done with a 100 milliliter IV bag or with a Buretrol- or Volutrol-type administration set. This is then infused over 20 to 30 minutes. This slow infusion tends to reduce the chances of dysrhythmias.

For patients with congestive heart failure, or for patients in whom any additional fluid might be dangerous, a more concentrated infusion is prepared:

2. Place 250 or 500 milligrams (2 to 5 mg/kg) in 20 milliliters of 5% dextrose in water. This is then infused over 20 to 30 minutes using a Buretrol- or Volutrol-type administration set.

Route. Parenteral aminophylline should only be given by slow intravenous infusion by one of the regimens discussed above.

Racemic Epinephrine (microNEFRIN) (Vaponefrin)

Description. Racemic epinephrine is slightly different chemically from the epinephrine compounds already discussed. Compounds that differ only in chemical arrangement are called *isomers*. This form is occasionally used to treat croup in children.

Racemic epinephrine should only be administered by inhalation.

Indication. Croup (laryngotracheobronchitis).

Contraindications. Racemic epinephrine should not be used in the management of epiglottitis.

Precautions. Racemic epinephrine can result in tachycardia and possibly dysrhythmias.

Dosage. 0.5 milliliters of a 2.5% solution should be mixed with 4 milliliters of normal saline and placed in a small-volume nebulizer. It should only be used initially and not repeated.

Route. Racemic epinephrine should be given only by inhalation, usually through a small-volume updraft nebulizer.

Terbutaline (Brethine)

Description. Terbutaline is a synthetic sympathomimetic that is selective for β_2 adrenergic receptors. It causes bronchodilation with less cardiac effect than epinephrine. Its onset of action is similar to that of epinephrine.

Indications

- ❑ Bronchial asthma
- ❑ Reversible bronchospasm associated with chronic bronchitis and emphysema

Contraindications. Terbutaline should not be administered to any patient with a history of hypersensitivity to the drug.

Precautions. Palpitations, anxiety, nausea, and dizziness may be seen with terbutaline. As with any sympathomimetic, the patient's vital signs must be monitored. Use caution when administering terbutaline to patients with cardiovascular disease or hypertension.

Dosage. The standard dose of terbutaline is 0.25 milligrams injected subcutaneously. If therapeutic effects are not seen within 15 minutes, a second dose may be administered.

Route. Terbutaline should only be administered subcutaneously.

Albuterol (Proventil) (Ventolin)

Description. Like the agents metaproterenol and terbutaline, albuterol is a sympathomimetic that is selective for β_2 adrenergic receptors. Once administered, it causes bronchodilation with minimal side effects. Albuterol's duration of action is approximately five hours.

✱ The aerosolized β agonists are rapidly becoming the drug of choice in the management of asthma.

Indications

- ❑ Bronchial asthma
- ❑ Reversible bronchospasm associated with chronic bronchitis and emphysema

Contraindications. Albuterol should not be administered to any patient with a known history of hypersensitivity to the drug.

Precautions. Palpitations, anxiety, nausea, and dizziness may be seen with albuterol. As with any sympathomimetic, the patient's vital signs must be monitored. Use caution when administering albuterol to patients with a history of cardiovascular disease or hypertension.

Dosage. The usual adult dosage is 2 inhalations repeated every four to six hours. In addition, 2.5 milligrams of the drug can be placed in 2–3 milliliters of normal saline and administered by hand-held updraft nebulizer.

Route. In prehospital emergency care, albuterol should only be administered by inhalation.

Drugs Used In The Treatment Of Endocrine And Metabolic Emergencies

Introduction. Glands that secrete hormones directly into the blood, without the aid of ducts, are called *endocrine glands.* With the exception of the pancreas, they rarely cause emergency disorders. Occasionally the thyroid, the endocrine gland that controls metabolic rate, will begin secreting excess thyroid hormones. This disorder, called "thyroid storm," is characterized by increased heart rate, loss of body weight, and congestive heart failure. Fortunately, it is rare and probably would not be diagnosed in prehospital emergency medical care.

50% Dextrose In Water

Description. "Dextrose" is used to describe the six-carbon sugar *d-glucose,* which is the principal form of carbohydrate used by the body. In hypoglycemia, the rapid administration of glucose is essential. When the hypoglycemic patient is comatose, glucose cannot be given by mouth and should be given intravenously.

Indications

- ❑ Acute alcoholism with coma
- ❑ Hypoglycemia
- ❑ Altered level of consciousness

Contraindications. There are no major contraindications to the intravenous administration of 50% dextrose in water to a patient with suspected hypoglycemia. Even if a patient was suffering from ketoacidosis, the amount of glucose present in 50 milliliters of 50% dextrose would have no adverse effects.

Precautions. If possible, determine the glucose level and draw a sample of blood before initiating an IV infusion and giving 50% dextrose. Localized venous irritation may occur when smaller veins are used.

Dosage. The standard dosage of 50% dextrose in hypoglycemia is 25 grams (50 milliliters of a 50% solution) intravenously. If an initial dose is ineffective, a second dose of 25 grams can be given.

Route. Fifty percent dextrose is only given intravenously. Concentrated glucose solutions can cause venous irritation if administered for an extended period.

Thiamine

✳ In coma of unknown cause, always consider the administration of Thiamine, D50W, and Naloxone.

Description. Thiamine is an important vitamin commonly referred to as vitamin B1. A *vitamin* is a substance that the body cannot manufacture but requires for metabolism. The body gets most of the vitamins it needs through food. Thiamine is required for the conversion of glucose into energy. Without thiamine, a significant amount of the energy available in glucose is unavailable. The brain is extremely sensitive to thiamine deficiency.

Chronic alcohol intake interferes with the absorption, intake, and utilization of thiamine. A significant percentage of alcoholics have thiamine deficiency. During extended periods of fasting, neurological symptoms may occur from thiamine deficiency. Any comatose patients, especially suspected alcoholics, should receive intravenous thiamine prior to the administration of 50% dextrose or Narcan.

Indications

❑ Coma of unknown origin, especially if alcohol may be involved
❑ Delirium tremens

Contraindications. There are no contraindications to the administration of thiamine in the emergency setting.

Precautions. A few cases of hypersensitivity to thiamine have been reported.

Dosage. The emergency dose of thiamine is 100 milligrams intravenously or intramuscularly.

Route. Thiamine can be given either intravenously or intramuscularly. The intravenous route is preferred in emergency medicine.

Drugs Used In The Treatment Of Neurological Emergencies

Introduction. Emergencies involving the nervous system can be devastating. In addition, they are notoriously difficult to manage. Signs and symptoms of neurological disorders can range from slight headache to coma. Prompt recognition and treatment of neurological emergencies is essential.

Dexamethasone (Decadron) (Hexadrol)

Description. The role of steroids in the management of cerebral edema remains controversial. The mechanism by which and extent to which dexamethasone decreases cerebral edema, if it does, is unclear.

The role of steroids in the prehospital setting is controversial. Always follow local protocols regarding their usage.

Dexamethasone is a synthetic steroid chemically related to the natural hormones secreted by the adrenal cortex. Dexamethasone is classified as a long-acting steroid with a plasma half-life of about five hours. In general medical practice steroids have many uses. Effective as anti-inflammatory agents, they are used in the management of allergic reactions and occasionally in the management of shock.

It is generally agreed that a large single dose of steroids has little harmful effect. Consequently, dexamethasone is used frequently in patients with cerebral edema, both in the emergency department and in the prehospital setting.

Indications

❑ Cerebral edema
❑ Asthma
❑ Anaphylactic reactions
❑ Possibly effective as an adjunctive agent in the management of shock

Contraindications. There are no major contraindications to the use of dexamethasone in the acute management of cerebral edema.

Precautions. A single dose of dexamethasone is all that should be given in prehospital care. Long-term steroid therapy can cause GI bleeding, prolonged wound healing, and suppression of adrenocortical steroids.

Dosage. The dose of dexamethasone varies considerably. The usual range is 4 to 24 milligrams, with 12 milligrams IV being a commonly used dose. However, high-dose Decadron therapy, using up to 100 milligrams of the drug, is sometimes given.

Route. Dexamethasone is administered intravenously for treatment of acute cerebral edema.

Diazepam (Valium)

Description. Diazepam is one of the most frequently prescribed medications in the United States. It is used in the management of anxiety and stress. Diazepam is effective in treating the tremors and anxiety associated with alcohol withdrawal. It is also an effective skeletal-muscle relaxant, which makes it an effective adjunct in orthopedic injuries. It is a good premedication for minor operative procedures and cardioversion because it induces amnesia, which diminishes the patient's recall.

In emergency medicine diazepam is principally used for its anticonvulsant properties. It suppresses the spread of seizure activity through the motor cortex of the brain.

Indications

❑ Major motor seizures
❑ Status epilepticus
❑ Premedication prior to cardioversion
❑ Skeletal-muscle relaxant
❑ Acute anxiety states

Contraindications. Diazepam should not be administered to any patient with a history of hypersensitivity to the drug.

Precautions. Because diazepam is a relatively short-acting drug when administered intravenously as an anti-convulsant, seizure activity may recur. In such cases, an additional dose may be required.

Dosage. The typical dosage of diazepam in status epilepticus is 2–5 milligrams intravenously. On occasion, doses of up to 15 milligrams may be required.

Route. In the emergency setting, the intravenous route is preferred.

Drugs Used In The Treatment Of Obstetrical And Gynecological Emergencies

Introduction. Prehospital care for most obstetric and gynecologic emergencies is supportive. However, there are two complications that necessitate intervention with pharmacological agents. These are toxemia of pregnancy and severe post-partum vaginal bleeding. Magnesium sulfate has proven effective in controlling the convulsions associated with toxemia of pregnancy. Pitocin, a drug chemically identical to the hormone oxytocin, is effective in causing uterine contraction and will slow many cases of postpartum vaginal bleeding.

✱ Valium may effectively suppress the source of seizure activity in the brain, making it an effective medication in the acute management of seizures.

Oxytocin (Pitocin)

Description. Oxytocin is a naturally occurring hormone that is secreted by the posterior pituitary. It causes contraction of uterine smooth muscle and plays a role in lactation.

Oxytocin is used to induce labor in selected cases and is also effective in inducing uterine contractions following delivery, thereby controlling postpartum hemorrhage.

When a baby is placed on the breast, the sucking action causes the posterior pituitary to release oxytocin. It is important to remember this inherent mechanism whenever confronted with a patient suffering moderate to severe postpartum bleeding.

Indications. Postpartum hemorrhage.

Contraindications. In the prehospital setting, oxytocin should be administered only to patients suffering severe postpartum bleeding. Before administration, it is essential to verify that the baby has been delivered and that there is not an additional fetus in the uterus.

Precautions. Excess oxytocin can cause overstimulation of the uterus and possible rupture. Hypertension, cardiac dysrhythmias, and anaphylaxis have been reported in conjunction with oxytocin. Vital signs and uterine tone should be monitored.

Dosage. There are two regimens for the administration of oxytocin in the management of patients with postpartum hemorrhage.

- ❑ 3 to 10 units can be administered IM following delivery of the placenta.
- ❑ 10 to 20 units can be placed in either 500 or 1000 milliliters of normal saline or lactated Ringer's. This should be titrated according to the severity of the bleeding and the uterine response.

Route. Oxytocin should only be administered intramuscularly or by slow intravenous infusion.

Magnesium Sulfate

Description. Magnesium sulfate is a central nervous system depressant effective in the management of seizures associated with toxemia of pregnancy (eclampsia). It is used for the initial therapy of convulsions. After cessation of seizure activity, other anticonvulsant agents may be administered.

Indications. Eclampsia (seizures associated with toxemia of pregnancy).

Contraindications. Magnesium sulfate should not be administered to any patient with heart block or recent myocardial infarction.

Precautions. Magnesium sulfate, like other CNS depressants, can cause hypotension, circulatory collapse, and depression of cardiac and respiratory function. The most immediate danger is respiratory depression. Calcium chloride should be readily available for IV administration as an antidote to respiratory depression.

Dosage. The standard dosage for the management of convulsions associated with toxemia of pregnancy is 1 gram intravenously.

Route. In the setting of eclampsia, magnesium sulfate should only be administered intravenously.

Drugs Used In The Management Of Toxicological Emergencies

Diphenhydramine (Benadryl)

Description. When released into the circulation following an allergic reaction, histamine acts on two different histamine receptors. The first type of receptor, called H^1, when stimulated, causes bronchoconstriction and contraction of the gut. The second type of receptor is called H^2. When stimulated, it causes peripheral vasodilation and secretion of gastric acids.

Antihistamines are administered after epinephrine in the treatment of anaphylaxis. Epinephrine causes immediate bronchodilaton by activating β_2 adrenergic receptors, while diphenhydramine inhibits histamine release.

Indications

- ❏ Anaphylaxis
- ❏ Allergic reactions
- ❏ Urticaria (hives)

Contraindications. Diphenhydramine should not be used in the management of lower-respiratory diseases such as asthma.

Precautions. Hypotension, headache, palpitations, and tachycardia have been known to occur following administration of diphenhydramine. Sedation, drowsiness, and disturbed coordination are common.

Dosage. The standard dosage of diphenhydramine is 25 to 50 milligrams, either intravenously or intramuscularly.

Routes. Diphenhydramine should be administered intravenously or intramuscularly.

Syrup Of Ipecac

Description. Syrup of ipecac is a potent and effective emetic. It acts as a local irritant on the enteric tract and on emetic centers within the brain, thus causing emesis. To assure complete evacuation of the stomach, the administration of ipecac is followed by several glasses of warm water. Some recent studies have advocated the use of carbonated beverages, instead of warm water, as they may cause emesis sooner. Emesis, following administration, usually occurs within 5 to 10 minutes.

Indications

- ❏ Poisoning
- ❏ Overdose

Contraindications. Vomiting should not be induced in any patient with impaired consciousness. It should also not be induced when the ingested substance is a strong acid base or petroleum distillate.

In addition, administration of syrup of ipecac is not indicated when the ingested agent was an antiemetic, especially of the phenothiazine type.

Precautions. It is important to monitor constantly the patient's airway during and following emesis. Activated charcoal should only be administered after vomiting.

Dosage. The standard dose of syrup of ipecac is 15 to 30 milliliters orally, followed by several glasses of warm water or carbonated soda.

Route. Syrup of ipecac should only be administered orally.

Activated Charcoal

Description. Activated charcoal is a fine black powder with a large surface area. It binds and absorbs ingested toxins still present in the gastrointestinal tract following emesis. Once bound to the activated charcoal, the combined complex is excreted.

Indication. Poisoning (following emesis, or in cases where emesis may be contraindicated).

Contraindications. There are no major contraindications to the use of activated charcoal in severe poisoning, unless the airway cannot be adequately controlled.

Precautious. Activated charcoal should only be administered after emesis has been induced with syrup of ipecac, or in those cases in which emesis is not contraindicated.

Dosage. The standard dosage in the management of poisoning is 2 tablespoons (50 grams) mixed with a glass of water. This is then administered orally or through a nasogastric tube.

Route. Activated charcoal should only be administered orally in a slurry solution made with water, as described above. Premixed solutions, such as ACTIDOSE with SORBITOL, are preferred in the prehospital setting.

Naloxone (Narcan)

Description. Naloxone is an effective narcotic antagonist and has proven effective in the management and reversal of overdoses caused by narcotics or synthetic narcotic agents. Recent studies have shown that naloxone may also be effective in reversal of coma associated with alcohol ingestion.

Indications

- For the complete or partial reversal of depression caused by narcotics, including the following agents:

  morphine   Demerol   heroin   Percodan   methadone
  paregoric   Dilaudid   codeine   Fentanyl

- For the complete or partial reversal of depression caused by synthetic narcotic analgesic agents, including the following drugs:

  Nubain   Stadol
  Talwin   Darvon

- Alcoholic coma
- Treatment of coma of unknown origin

Contraindications. Naloxone should not be administered to a patient with a history of hypersensitivity to the drug.

Precautions. Naloxone should be administered cautiously to patients who are known or suspected to be physically dependent on narcotics. Abrupt and complete reversal by naloxone can cause withdrawal-type effects. This includes newborn infants of mothers with known or suspected narcotic dependence.

Dosage. The standard dosage for suspected or confirmed narcotic or synthetic narcotic overdoses is 1 to 2 milligrams IV. If unsuccessful, then a second dose may be administered 5 minutes later. Failure to obtain reversal after 2 to 3 doses indicates another disease process or overdosage on non-opioid drugs.

Larger than average doses (2 to 5 milligrams) have been used in the management of Darvon overdoses and alcoholic coma.

An intravenous infusion can be prepared by placing 2 milligrams of Naloxone in 500 milliliters of 5% dextrose in water. This gives a concentration of 4 micrograms per milliliter. One-hundred milliliters per hour should be infused, thus delivering 0.4 milligrams per hour.

Route. In the emergency setting, Naloxone should be administered intravenously only. When an IV cannot be established, IM, subcutaneous, or endotracheal administration can be performed.

Drugs Used In The Management Of Behavioral Emergencies

Haloperidol (Haldol)

Description. Haloperidol is a frequently used major tranquilizer. It has proven effective in the management of acute psychotic episodes. It has pharmacological properties similar to other medications of the phenothiazine class of drugs, including sedation and dry mouth. Haloperidol is believed to block dopamine receptors in the brain associated with mood and behavior.

Indications. Acute psychotic episodes.

Contraindications. Haloperidol should not be administered if other drugs, especially sedatives, may be present. Haloperidol should not be used in the management of dysphoria caused by Talwin, because it may promote sedation and anesthesia.

Precautions. Haloperidol may impair mental and physical abilities. Hypotension, occassionally orthostatic, may be seen. Caution should be used when administering haloperidol to patients on anticoagulants or those known to be hypertensive. The dosage should be reduced for the elderly.

Extrapyramidal, or Parkinson-like reactions, have been known to occur following the administration of haloperidol, especially in children.

Dosage. A dose of 2 to 5 milligrams intramuscularly is standard in the management of an acute psychotic episode with severe symptoms.

Route. Haloperidol should be given intramuscularly only.

Other Medications

Promethazine (Phenergan)

Description. Promethazine is a phenothiazine with potent antihistamine effects. It also has considerable anticholinergic activity and is an effective and commonly used antiemetic. Unlike hydroxyzine (Vistaril), it can be given intravenously. It is often administered with analgesics, particularly narcotics, to enhance their effect.

Indications

❑ Nausea and vomiting
❑ Motion sickness
❑ To enhance the effects of analgesics

Contraindications. Promethazine is contraindicated in comatose patients and in patients who have received a large amount of depressants. Also, it should not be administered to any patient with a history of hypersensitivity to the drug.

Precautions. Promethazine may impair mental and physical ability. Care must be taken to avoid accidental intra-arterial injection. It should never be administered subcutaneously.

Dosage. The standard dosage of promethazine in the management of nausea and vomiting is 12.5 to 25 milligrams, either intravenously or intramuscularly.

The standard dosage for adjunctive use with analgesics is 25 milligrams.

Route. Promethazine should be given by intravenous or deep intramuscular injection only. Care must be taken to avoid accidental intra-arterial injection.

SUMMARY

This chapter has presented the fundamental aspects of pharmacological therapy as it applies to prehospital care. The medications used in prehospital care vary among EMS systems. It is your responsibility, as a paramedic, to be familiar with all medications in your EMS system. Infrequently used medications should be periodically reviewed. Overall, it is important to appreciate the inherent dangers of emergency medications and to use them properly. The rule to remember is "When in doubt, do no harm."

✳ "When in doubt, do no harm."

FURTHER READING

AMERICAN HEART ASSOCIATION. *Textbook of Advanced Cardiac Life Support.* 2nd ed. Dallas: American Heart Association, 1987.

AMERICAN HEART ASSOCIATION AND AMERICAN ACADEMY OF PEDIATRICS. *Textbook of Pediatric Advanced Life Support.* Dallas: American Heart Association, 1988.

BLEDSOE, BRYAN E., GIDEON BOSKER, AND FRANK J. PAPA. *Prehospital Emergency Pharmacology.* 2nd ed. Englewood Cliffs, NJ: Prentice Hall, 1988.

GOODMAN, L.S., AND A. GILMAN. *The Pharmacological Basis of Therapeutics.* 7th ed. New York: MacMillan, 1985.

SHADE, BRUCE, ET AL. *Advanced Cardiac Life Support: Certification, Preparation, and Review.* Englewood Cliffs, NJ: Brady Communications, 1988.

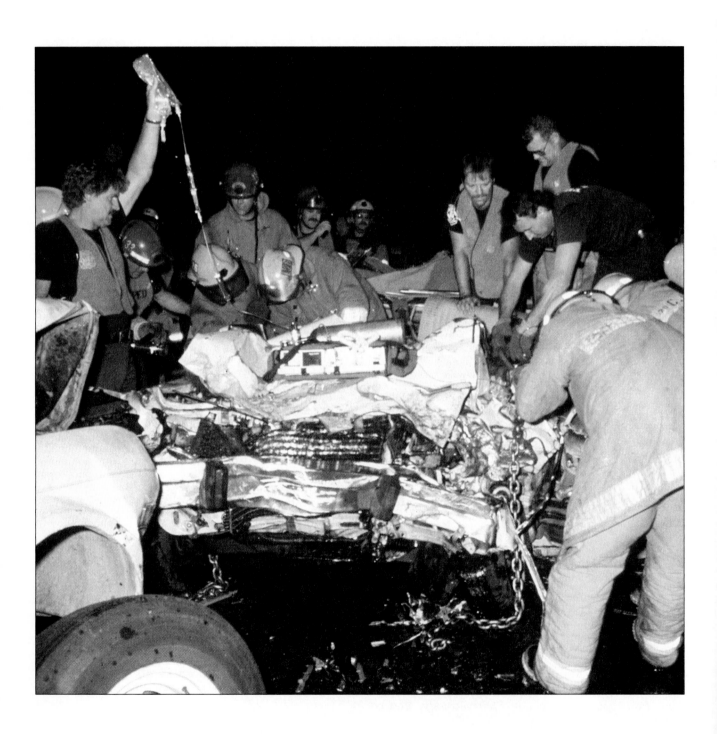

14

The Kinetics of Trauma

Objectives for Chapter 14

Upon completing this chapter, the student should be able to:

1. Describe the prevalence and significance of traumatic injury.

2. Explain the "Golden Hour" concept and the component of it that emergency medical service utilizes.

3. Identify, and explain by example, Newton's Laws of Inertia and Conservation of Energy.

4. Apply the principles of the kinetic energy and force formulas to the various types of trauma.

5. Compare and contrast the types of impact associated with auto and motorcycle accidents.

6. Predict the injuries expected from the various types of auto impacts and other blunt and penetrating trauma.

7. Relate the benefits and disadvantages of auto restraints and motorcycle helmets.

8. Associate the various types of penetrating injuries with the extent of injury they can involve.

9. Describe the significance and meaning of the terms velocity, cavitation, and profile as they relate to penetrating trauma.

10. Describe how the environment and mechanism of injury can alert the paramedic to specific types of injury.

City Ambulance is called to the scene of a multivehicle accident at the freeway interchange. Two cars are involved and multiple persons are reported injured. Traffic is backed up, so the ambulance is directed to enter the exit ramp.

Police have just arrived at the scene. Police update the en route ambulance, indicating that a stalled auto was hit by another traveling at freeway speed. There are three injured parties, one in the red car, which was stopped, and two in the green vehicle.

As the ambulance arrives at the scene the two cars are found separated by about 100 yards. The green car has severe front-end damage with two "spider webs" in the windshield. The steering column is deformed. The officer in charge reports that neither of the two people in the car wore seat belts.

The second car has sustained severe rear-end damage. The windshield is intact. The driver was wearing a seatbelt and the head rest is in the up position. The paramedics call for another unit to back them up and secure the scene. They head to the green car, expecting the worst injuries to be found there.

They assess the two victims quickly and find the driver to have chest trauma where she impacted with the steering wheel. She is experiencing difficult and painful breathing, although the airway is clear. Her pulses are strong, regular, and at a moderate rate. Physical exam reveals a forehead contusion, a reddened anterior chest with crepitation, and clear breath sounds bilaterally.

The passenger is unconscious and cannot be aroused. She has a rapid, barely palpable pulse and is breathing with shallow rapid breaths. Her forehead is badly contused and is bleeding moderately. Her thighs appear noticeably shortened and physical assessment displays instability of the pelvis and both femurs.

A first-responder-trained police officer indicates that the driver of the other car is conscious, alert, and appears only shaken up. He has a blood pressure of 126/84, a pulse of 86, and is breathing normally at a

INTRODUCTION

■ **trauma** a physical injury or wound caused by external force or violence.

The three most frequent causes of death in the United States are cardiovascular disease, cancer, and **trauma.** Trauma is the leading cause of death for persons under the age of 44 and is responsible for more than 140,000 lives lost each year. Approximately 50,000 of those deaths occur on the nation's highways. These statistics clearly define the significance of trauma as it relates to prehospital emergency care.

Trauma is a serious life threat, though the nature of its presentation can distract from the true immediacy of the patient's condition. Extremity injuries, for example, rarely cause a threat to life yet are frequently obvious and grotesque. Life-endangering problems, such as internal bleeding and shock, almost always occur with very subtle signs and symptoms. In trauma, assessment must look beyond the obvious injuries to those injuries and syndromes that threaten life.

As emergency medical service evolved in the middle and late 1960s,

rate of 20. The paramedic in charge asks the officer to stay with the driver of the other car.

She also asks the driver of this car not to move and prepares to remove the passenger rapidly, using spinal precautions. The board is prepared with the PASG, and the patient receives a cervical collar and is moved rapidly onto the board. There the spine is immobilized with a cervical immobilization device.

The second unit arrives, and the crew is given a quick briefing and assigned to the other two patients. The patient with the pelvic instability is loaded into the ambulance, a police officer is assigned to drive, and transportation begins. The vitals are taken quickly, revealing a blood pressure of 82 by palpation, a very weak carotid pulse of 130, and absent peripheral pulses. Capillary refill time is over 3 seconds. Medical command is contacted and given a brief report, and orders are received.

The PASG is inflated, two large-bore IVs are started, and fluids are run under pressure infusers. Oxygen is administered by non-rebreathing mask, the patient is hyperventilated, and the intubation equipment is readied.

The ambulance is stopped to allow intubation, and the head is immobilized while nasotracheal intubation is attempted. It is unsuccessful. The tube is withdrawn, the patient is hyperventilated, and digital intubation is tried. Lung sounds are clear, chest excursion is good, and oximetry readings begin to rise.

The patient arrives at the Trauma Center with just under 2,000 mL of fluid infused, the PASG fully inflated, and the operating room prepared. The C-spine is cleared by X-ray. The vascular injuries associated with the pelvic fracture are repaired, six units of typed and cross-matched whole blood are infused, the broken femurs are pinned, and the pelvis is stabilized. The patient recovers after a few weeks of hospitalization and will walk again with only slight reminders of the injuries and care she received.

emphasis was on providing definitive care at the scene of auto accidents, where care had not been given before. Later, however, it was found that many seriously injured trauma patients were receiving care at the scene for injuries that were not life-threatening while they bled internally. They would often reach the emergency department and surgery too late to have their internal problems corrected and would die. The approach for treating the trauma patient has since been modified to ensure that the seriously injured patient is promptly recognized and immediately transported to a trauma center.

Assessment of the trauma patient must take into consideration two things:

1. the mechanism of injury
2. the index of suspicion

These criteria are important for deciding whether to stabilize the patient at the scene or provide rapid transport to the hospital.

MECHANISM OF INJURY

✱ The mechanism of injury is the exchange of forces that results in injury to the victim.

In the case of an auto accident, the *mechanism of injury* is the process by which forces are exchanged between the auto and what it struck, the patient and the interior of the auto, and the various tissues and organs within the patient as they collide with one another. Close inspection of the auto and these forces can lead to formulation of an index of suspicion for possible injuries.

INDEX OF SUSPICION

✱ The index of suspicion is the anticipation of the nature and severity of injury to the patient gained by analysis of the mechanism of injury.

The *index of suspicion* is the anticipation of the nature and severity of patient injury. It is arrived at by analysis of the mechanism of injury. A pedestrian struck by a car moving 30 miles per hour has a much higher chance of being injured than does a pedestrian struck by a car moving 5 miles per hour. Thus, the index of suspicion for injury would be higher in the first pedestrian than the second. Since the paramedic usually attends to the patient shortly after the accident, the signs and symptoms of shock—or the discoloration of a contusion—are not frequently seen. This makes it even more important to try and establish the mechanism of injury and an index of suspicion regarding the seriousness of the patient's injuries. It is very easy to detect fractures and lacerations. However, it is also very easy to be distracted by these less threatening injuries and ignore the subtle signs of impending shock. Many serious injuries will be missed if the index of suspicion is not high enough.

THE GOLDEN HOUR

■ **Golden Hour** the 1-hour period following a severe injury. Based on research, it has been demonstrated that severe trauma patients who reach surgery within this period have a higher survival rate.

The last consideration in the overall approach to the trauma patient is a focus on the time spent at the scene. The **Golden Hour** has been greatly publicized by the Maryland Institute for Emergency Medical Services of Baltimore and is well accepted as the standard for emergency intervention. (See Figure 14-1.) The institute's research has shown that if the severely injured patient can be in surgery within 1 hour after the accident, his or her chances of survival are greatly enhanced.

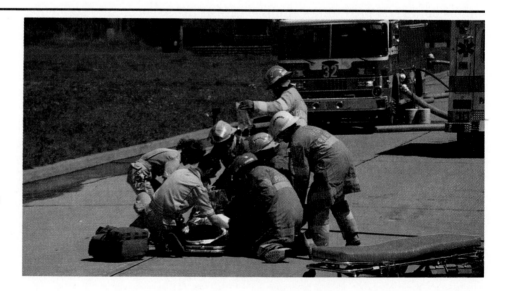

FIGURE 14-1 Victims of severe trauma have enhanced chances of survival if they can be delivered to the operating room within 1 hour after their accident (the "Golden Hour").

Of that hour, prehospital care is given about 10 minutes of on-scene time for paramedics to assess, stabilize (in an emergent sense), package, extricate, and begin transporting the critical or potentially critical patient. Scene time is short, and the paramedic's responsibilities are great.

The care provided can be extremely effective if responding paramedics focus on recognizing which patients need stabilization at the scene and which ones need rapid transport for surgical intervention. The paramedic must be able to evaluate the accident scene and trauma patient rapidly and accurately to make the best decision.

TRANSPORT VERSUS ON-SCENE STABILIZATION

The decision to either transport a patient immediately or attempt stabilization at the scene is among the most difficult decisions paramedics must make. As a rule, the following types of emergencies should be immediately transported with intravenous access and other procedures attempted en route. (See Figure 14-2.) They include:

- ❏ Cardiopulmonary arrest
- ❏ Uncorrectable airway problems
- ❏ Any embarrassment of the respiratory system
- ❏ Any wounds that deform or penetrate the chest, head, or abdomen
- ❏ Significant external, or suspected internal, blood loss
- ❏ Signs and symptoms of compensatory shock
- ❏ Multiple fractures, especially pelvic ring or bilateral femur fractures
- ❏ Lowered or changing level of consciousness
- ❏ Mechanism of injury suggestive of severe trauma

This list is not all-inclusive but can serve as a general guideline in decision-making regarding immediate transport.

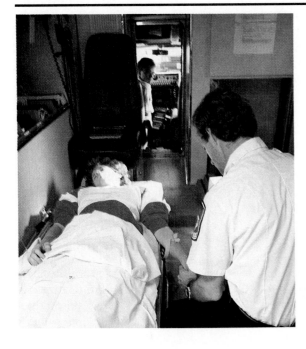

FIGURE 14-2 Victims of major trauma should be immediately transported with stabilization procedures, such as IV therapy, attempted enroute.

Kinetics is the study of **motion** as caused by external forces. The mechanics of trauma are related to physics—specifically, the laws of motion. The two laws of physics important to the emergency care provider are the Law of **Inertia** and the Law of the Conservation of **Energy.** An appreciation of these laws and the principles of physics can help emergency personnel in assessing the severity of patient injuries. In addition, these laws can aid in providing an understanding of the causes and effects that occur during the auto accident or other traumatic event.

Newton's First Law

The laws of motion, as described by Sir Isaac Newton, can help explain what happens during the traumatic insult. His first law states, "A body in motion will remain in motion unless acted upon by an outside force." Two examples of this are identical autos slowing down from 55 miles per hour, one braking for a red light and the other stopping abruptly as it collides with the abutment of a bridge. In both cases the auto is slowed by an "outside force," either the brakes or the bridge, yet the results are very different.

The first law of motion continues, "A body at rest will remain at rest unless acted upon by an outside force." Examples of this include an auto accelerating from a stop sign, or a vehicle being struck from behind by another and then accelerating forward. The resulting effects on passengers of both autos will be an **acceleration** forward. In the second case, however, the danger of injury to the occupants is increased.

Conservation of Energy

The Law of the Conservation of Energy states that energy can neither be created nor destroyed. It can only be changed from one form to another. In the auto crash, as in other trauma, this change is important for understanding what energy forces are involved and where the energy of **impact** goes. **Kinetic energy,** the energy a car and its passengers possess, is transformed into other forms of energy during the crash. The eventual result is the auto, and those inside it, coming to rest. The resulting transformations of energy might include the deformity of the front of the car, the sound of the impact, the heat generated in the structural steel as it bends and is compressed, and damage to the interior of the vehicle as passengers collide with the steering wheel or other objects inside the automobile.

Kinetic Energy

Kinetic energy is the total amount of energy possessed by an object in motion. It is a function of the mass of the item and the **velocity** at which it is moving. The total kinetic energy any object has while in motion can be defined by the following formula:

$$\text{Kinetic Energy} = \frac{\text{Mass (weight)} \times \text{Velocity}^2}{2}$$

This formula illustrates that as the weight of an object is doubled, the energy of its motion is also doubled. It would be twice as damaging to be hit by a 2-pound baseball as to be hit by a 1-pound ball. It would be three times as damaging to be hit by a 3-pound ball, and so on.

■ **kinetics** the branch of dynamics that deals with motion, taking into consideration mass and force.

■ **motion** the process of changing place; movement.

■ **inertia** the tendency of an object to remain at rest or to remain in motion unless acted upon by an external force.

■ **energy** the capacity to do work in the strict physical sense.

■ **acceleration** the rate at which speed or velocity increases.

■ **impact** forceful contact or collision. It is the forceful exchange of energy that results frequently in trauma.

■ **kinetic energy** the energy an object has while it is in motion. It is related to the object's velocity and mass.

■ **velocity** a rate of motion in a particular direction in relation to time.

Mass and weight are not truly identical. However, for this discussion they can be considered equal. The same is true for velocity and speed. As the speed (velocity) is increased, there will be a larger increase (squared) in the net energy. Being hit with a 1-pound baseball traveling at 20 miles per hour would cause four times the trauma as being hit with it at 10 miles per hour. If the speed were increased to 30 miles per hour, the trauma expected would be nine times worse. This concept plays an important role in understanding the devastating effects of a gunshot wound.

It is important to understand that kinetic energy is the measure of how much energy an object in motion has, not necessarily how much injury will occur. Two autos traveling at 55 miles per hour have about the same amount of kinetic energy. The same two autos would have equal kinetic energy once they have stopped, even if one came to rest by hitting a bridge abutment, and the other stopped by braking. The difference between the two events is the rate of slowing, or **deceleration.** Deceleration (or acceleration) is the rate of speed change and is related to the force of the accident.

■ **deceleration** the rate at which speed decreases.

Force

The second of Newton's formulas which plays a role in understanding the forces at work in the accident is identified below:

$$\text{Force} = \text{Mass} \times \text{Acceleration (or Deceleration)}$$

This formula brings into focus the importance of the rate at which an object changes speed, either increasing (acceleration) or decreasing (deceleration). Slow deceleration is rather uneventful. Normal stopping, as for a stop sign, covers about 120 feet (from 55 miles per hour to 0 miles per hour at a braking rate of 22 feet/10 miles per hour) and usually does not result in injury. On the other hand, colliding with a bridge and slowing from 55 miles per hour to 0 miles per hour in a matter of inches produces tremendous force and devastating injuries.

TRAUMA

When the energies explained by Newton's laws are directed at the human anatomy, the result is *trauma*. Trauma is defined as a wound or injury that is externally or violently produced.

Trauma can be classified as being either blunt or penetrating in nature. *Blunt trauma* results from deceleration and compression, which most often fails to break the skin yet causes injury beneath it. In blunt trauma the injury is caused by the compression or the stretching of tissue in the area that is affected. The injury generally extends into the tissues beneath the impact site through a chain reaction process, trapping consecutive layers of tissue between others that are either accelerating or decelerating. This is very much like hitting your thumb with a hammer while driving a nail. The tissue is trapped between the hammer (which pushes the tissue) and the board (which resists the motion).

✱ Trauma can be classified as either blunt or penetrating.

Significant internal injury can occur within the thorax or abdomen through this mechanism. Traumatic compression may cause hollow organs to rupture, spilling their contents, causing blood loss and, later on, inflammation. Solid organs, such as the spleen, may be contused or lacerated, leading to blood loss, swelling, or both.

Further trauma may occur secondary to organ attachment and rapid deceleration or acceleration. The liver, for example, is suspended by the *ligamentum teres.* During severe deceleration the liver may be sliced by the ligament similar to the way cheese is cut by a wire cheese cutter. The aorta may be injured as the chest slows and the heart, suspended by the great vessels, twists on impact. The aorta is often disrupted as the various layers of vascular tissue rip apart, leading to a tearing chest pain, circulatory compromise, and possible immediate or delayed exsanguination (blood loss).

Penetrating trauma is defined as an injury where the skin is broken and the trauma extends beneath the open wound. The injury is caused by direct contact with the energy source as it progresses into the body. Energy may also be transmitted to surrounding body tissue, further extending the area of injury. This is seen with bullet wounds.

Various sources of penetrating and blunt trauma can be identified and placed into categories. Motor vehicle trauma (generally blunt) can include automobile, motorcycle, recreational vehicle, and pedestrian accidents. Other blunt trauma can include sports injuries, falls, and blast injuries.

Penetrating trauma is associated with many different mechanisms, the most common being stabbing and gunshot. Stabbing is generally considered low-velocity, while the gunshot is considered high-velocity. The gunshot injury is further subdivided into medium-energy (the handgun) and high-energy (the rifle).

MOTOR VEHICLE TRAUMA

Automobile fatalities account for over one-third of the yearly death toll attributed to accidents. While more than 50,000 people die secondary to vehicular trauma, many more are severely injured, and some disabled for life. Since the auto accident accounts for a large proportion of paramedic responses, it is essential that care for the victim is timely and appropriate. To this end, the paramedic must look carefully at the various auto accident mechanisms so as to improve the accuracy of the index of suspicion for life-threatening injury. These injuries result from various types of impacts, each possibly producing a different scenario of injuries. The types of impacts include:

- ❏ frontal
- ❏ rear end
- ❏ lateral
- ❏ rotational
- ❏ rollover

Each collision type has secondary impacts associated with it. The typical chain of events includes the following:

1. *Vehicle collision.* The vehicle collision occurs when the vehicle strikes an object, resulting in the transfer of energy from the vehicle to the stationary object. The energy of motion is transformed into damage to the vehicle. The motion of the car is stopped by bending of the frame. (See Figure 14-3.)

2. *Body collision.* Body collision occurs when the body strikes the interior of the vehicle, transferring energy between the body and the vehicle. Motion of the occupant continues until energy is absorbed by bending of the occupant or bending of the restraining device. (See Figure 14-4.)

3. *Organ collision.* Organ collision results when the organs are propelled against other organs or the wall of the body cavity, resulting in trauma to the organ. Damage can result from compression or deceleration. (See Figure 14-5.)

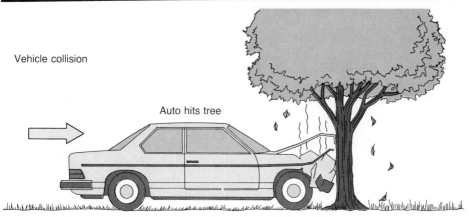

Vehicle collision

Auto hits tree

FIGURE 14-3 Step 1—Vehicle collision. The vehicle strikes an object.

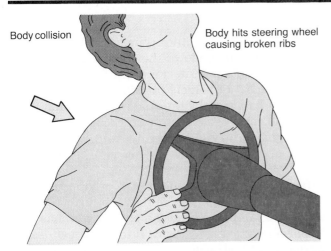

Body collision

Body hits steering wheel
causing broken ribs

FIGURE 14-4 Step 2—Body collision. The occupant continues forward and strikes the inside of the automobile.

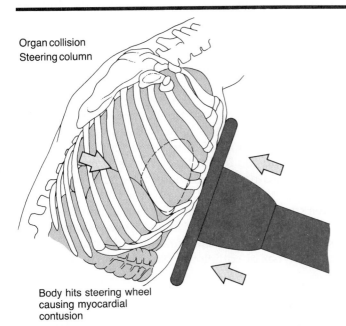

Organ collision
Steering column

Body hits steering wheel
causing myocardial
contusion

FIGURE 14-5 Step 3—Organ collision. The organs continue to move forward and strike the inside of the chest or other organs.

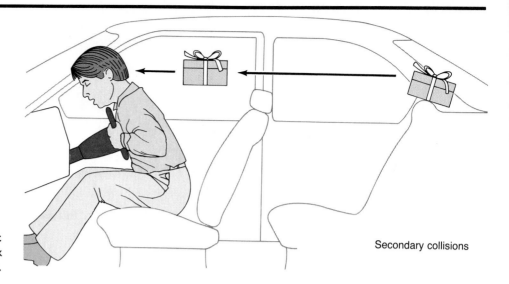

FIGURE 14-6 Secondary impact results when the occupant is struck by loose objects within the vehicle.

Secondary collisions

In the typical automobile accident, the initial impact is between the vehicle and the object struck. The impact slows the vehicle, and as a result the unrestrained occupant impacts the interior of the slowed car. The skin comes in contact with an aspect of vehicle interior and slows while the tissue behind collides with it, causing the internal injury. In addition, loose objects within the vehicle may become projectiles, impacting the passenger and causing additional injury. (See Figure 14-6.) Finally, rebounding of the vehicle and patient may cause additional impacts and consequent injury.

✱ When evaluating the effect of the auto accident or other traumatic event, the paramedic must realize the significance of secondary impact to a patient.

In evaluating the effect of the auto accident and other traumatic mechanisms of injury, the paramedic must realize the significance of secondary impact to a patient. For example, consider a patient who has sustained a fracture of his or her femur in an accident. It took a great deal of energy to cause the fracture initially. However, the energy now needed to displace the already fractured bone-ends and cause further, possibly more severe, injury might be relatively small. It is important to consider what effect a second impact would have on the injury site and the patient's overall condition. (For example, the car hits a culvert after colliding with another car).

✱ The visual examination of the auto accident can begin to tell a good deal about what happened to the patient and what injuries should be expected.

The visual examination of the auto accident can begin to tell a good deal about what happened to the patient and what injuries might be expected. The direction of the forces expressed upon the auto represent the direction of forces expressed upon the patient. By looking carefully at the vehicle and analyzing the damage it received, the nature and severity of the injuries can be anticipated. The angle of impact will propose a set of potential injuries to suspect. The extent of auto deformity will give an idea of the strength of impact and the strength of forces experienced by the patient. These elements of evaluation will help determine what may have happened.

The following is a breakdown of motor vehicle trauma and the types of vehicular impacts. The figures are given for an urban setting; in a more rural area, anticipate an increase in the incidence of frontal impact with a reduction in the other types of collisions. (See Figure 14-7.) These include:

Frontal:	32 percent
Lateral:	15 percent
Rotational:	38 percent
Rear End:	9 percent

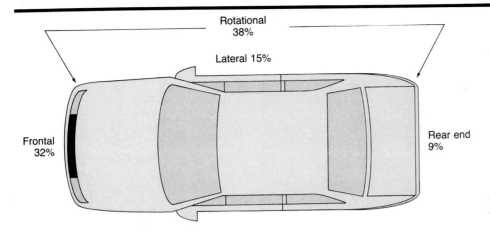

Rotational
38%

Lateral 15%

Frontal
32%

Rear end
9%

FIGURE 14-7 Motor vehicle trauma based upon the type of impact.

(See Figure 14-7. Rotational impact actually includes four categories of impacts: left front, right front, left rear, and right rear).

Frontal Impact. Frontal impact is the most common. (See Figure 14-8.) Frontal impact generally involves one of three pathways of injury for the patient. These are down and under, up and over, or ejection. A comprehensive understanding of these pathways can lead to a greater anticipation of the injuries likely to result from the frontal impact. This will help assure the patient receives the needed care.

The down-and-under pathway involves the driver or passenger who slides downward as the vehicle comes to a stop. The knee contacts the fire wall (under the dash) causing possible knee, femur, and hip dislocations or fractures. As the lower body slows due to the impact, the upper body is brought forward, pivoting at the hip, and crashes against the steering wheel. This action may cause such chest injuries as flail chest, myocardial trauma, or aortic trauma. It may also cause what is referred to as the "paper bag syndrome." (See Figure 14-10.) In this case the occupant takes a deep breath and holds it in anticipation of the collision. The lung tissue bursts, as a paper bag would, as the chest impacts the steering wheel or dash. The impact and bursting tissue leads to possible pneumothorax and pulmonary contusion. There is also a chance of tracheal trauma if the patient's anatomy is small or the contact with the steering wheel is anatomically high.

The up-and-over pathway involves the upper half of the occupant

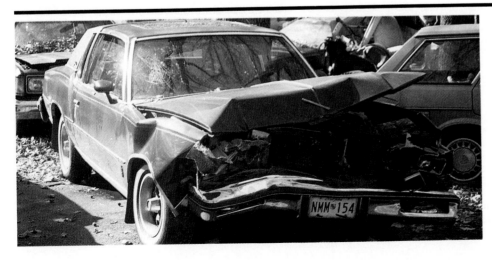

FIGURE 14-8 Frontal impact.

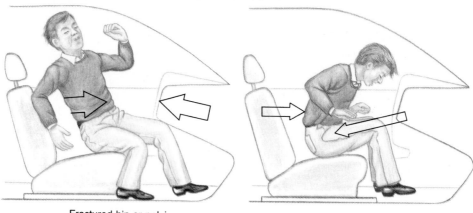

Fractured hip or pelvis   Dislocated hip or knee

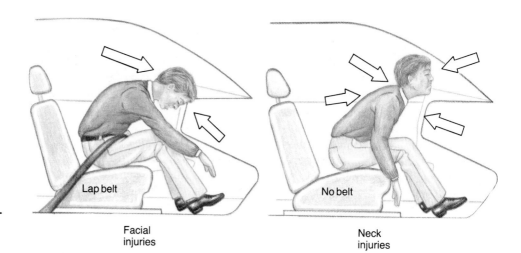

FIGURE 14-9 Examples of injury mechanisms associated with frontal impact.

Facial injuries   Neck injuries

moving forward and upward first, either due to the nature of the impact or the tensing of the occupant's lower extremities. The steering wheel impinges the femurs, causing bilateral fractures. In addition, the steering wheel tends to compress or decelerate the abdominal contents, causing hollow-organ rupture and liver laceration. Impact of the chest and steering wheel may also be responsible for some of the same thoracic injuries seen with the down-and-under pathway. (See Figure 14-11.)

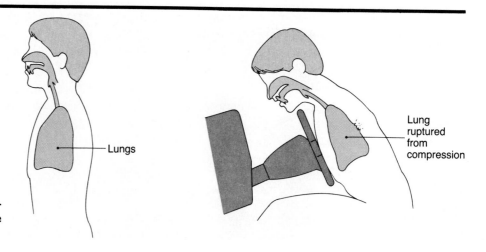

FIGURE 14-10 The "paper bag" syndrome results from compresssion of the chest against the steering column.

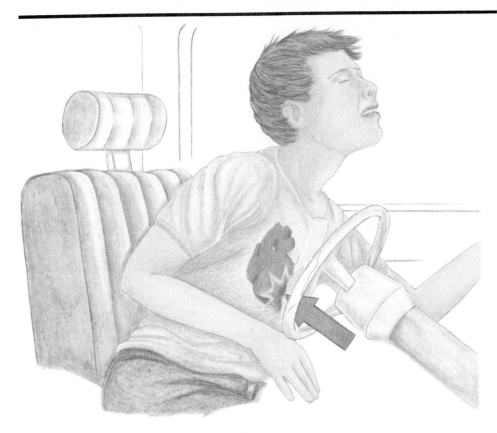

FIGURE 14-11 Myocardial contusion can result from impact with the steering wheel.

The contact of the head with the windshield can cause skull fracture or internal injury, while neck injury can be caused by the compressional forces of windshield impact as well as hyperextension, or **axial loading.** It should be noted that over half of all vehicular deaths can be attributed to the injuries caused by the up-and-over pathway.

An additional component of the up-and-over pathway is ejection. The victim of this type of motion experiences two impacts: the initial accident with the windshield and the impact with the ground, tree, or other secondary object. This mechanism of injury is responsible for about 27 percent of vehicular fatalities. While ejection may occur from other types of impact, the most common cause is the frontal impact.

Rear Impact. In the rear impact, the auto is pushed forward by the forces of the collision. (See Figure 14-12.) The passenger or driver is propelled forward by the vehicle seat. The head, however, is relatively unsupported and remains stationary. The neck extends severely and will then snap forward quickly. This rapid and extreme hyperextension followed by hyperflexion may result in soft tissue and skeletal neck injuries. (See Figure 14-13.) There is also the risk of secondary collisions in the auto with objects that are thrown about.

Lateral Impact. The kinetics of the lateral impact are relatively the same as for the frontal impact with two exceptions. (See Figure 14-14.) The passenger within the vehicle presents a different profile (turned 90 degrees) to the forces of the collision, and the amount of structural steel between the impact site and the interior of the vehicle is greatly reduced. It is important to note that the lateral impact is responsible for about 22 percent of vehicular fatalities, yet is the mechanism of impact for only 15 percent of auto accidents. The lateral impact accident, for these reasons, should carry a high index of suspicion for serious injury.

■ **axial loading** places the forces of trauma along the axis of the spine and may result in compression fractures.

✱ The lateral impact accident is associated with a high index of suspicion for serious injury.

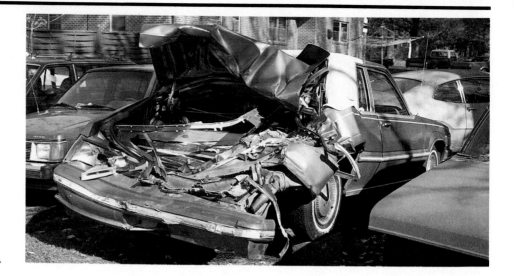

FIGURE 14-12 Rear impact.

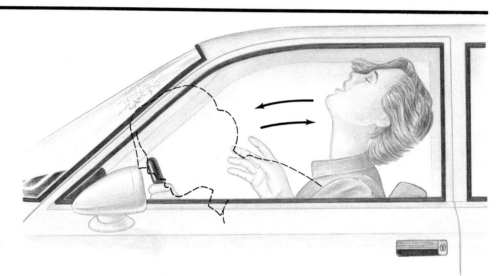

FIGURE 14-13 Movement in rear-impact collision.

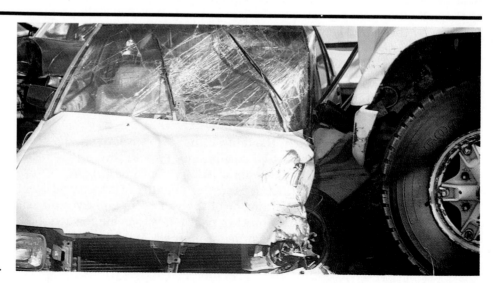

FIGURE 14-14 Lateral impact.

The injuries expected from this type collision are different from the scenario presented with the frontal. There is an increase in upper extremity injuries and a reduction in the incidence of rib fractures (although they may still occur). The clavicle may fracture as may the pelvis and femur on the impacted side. Cervical spine injury is common, as are skull fractures and internal head injuries.

The lateral compressional forces on the body cavity may give rise to diaphragm rupture, pulmonary contusion, aortic tear, and much more. The complete accident evaluation should take into consideration the effects of an unrestrained passenger opposite the impact site. If the driver's side is struck and the passenger is not belted, he or she will become an object striking and injuring the driver shortly after the initial impact.

Rotational Impact. In rotational impact the auto is struck at an **oblique** angle causing it to turn as the forces of the collision are expended. (See Figure 14-15.) The forces of acceleration (or deceleration) are greatest further from the center of mass of the auto and closest to the point of impact. The ensuing rotation and forces can cause scenarios with injuries much like the frontal and lateral impacts. While the injuries sustained in the rotational impact can be severe, they are often less than expected from other types of collisions. The autos involved are deflected from their paths rather than being stopped abruptly. The "stopping distance" for the occupant inside is much greater, and therefore the injury expected is less.

Rollover. The rollover of an automobile is normally caused by a change in elevation and/or a high vehicle center of gravity. (See Figure 14-16.) The occupant is subjected to various impacts with each vehicle impact. The type of injuries expected would be related to the specific impacts involved. Remember that any injury occurring during the first collision can be severely compounded with subsequent impacts because many of the normal protective mechanisms are compromised. A common result of this type of collision is ejection or partial ejection with a limb or head being trapped and injured.

Restraints. Statistics demonstrate that restraints greatly reduce injury and death in the auto accident. In the severe accident, the seat belt and shoulder strap may cause some injury as they prevent some of the more

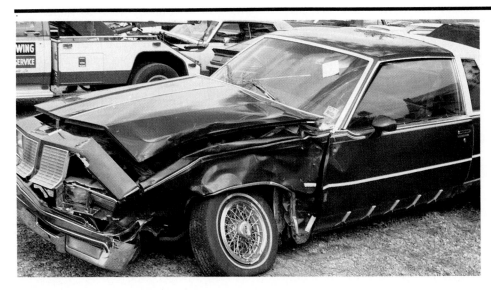

FIGURE 14-15 Rotational impact.

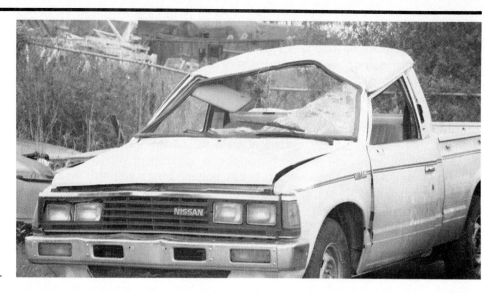

FIGURE 14-16 Roll over.

severe trauma that would normally occur. The value of seat belt use is demonstrated frequently. The use of seat belts should be required of all EMS personnel, especially while driving the vehicle. The seat belt provides positive positioning of the driver so that he or she is not so affected by the gravitational forces ("G" forces) sometimes associated with emergency driving.

If the lap belt is worn alone, head and cervical spine injury can occur. If it is worn too high, it may cause abdominal compression and possibly spinal (T12 to L2) fractures. If the lap belt is worn too low, it may cause hip dislocations. The shoulder strap, if worn alone, may cause severe neck injury or decapitation in the violent accident. If worn, as intended, with the lap belt, the shoulder strap may account for contusions, rib fractures and compressional injuries. With the exception of the shoulder alone, the injuries secondary to seatbelt use are much less than those expected without their use. The air bag passive restraint system is effective for the frontal impact only. It is not effective for any lateral or secondary collisions. It is, however, a highly effective restraint for the most common (frontal) impact.

Intoxication. Alcohol is an important consideration when examining vehicular accidents, as it is a contributing factor in many auto accidents. In states where alcohol-level testing is mandatory following a fatal accident, it has been found that one or more of the drivers are over the legal intoxication level in 50 percent of the incidents. It is also a contributing factor in recreational-vehicle accidents, boating accidents, and accidental drownings.

In addition to its contributing effects in the auto accident, alcohol intoxication can interfere with the recognition of symptoms and assessment of the level of consciousness. It can mimic the signs of head injury, lower the level of orientation, and anesthetize the patient to the pain of traumatic injury. The intoxicated patient handicaps the patient assessment process. This makes assessment of the mechanism of injury and index of suspicion even more important. Otherwise, significant injuries may be overlooked.

Vehicular Mortality. Examination of the overall effect of motor vehicle trauma on the body shows that certain areas are more prone to produce

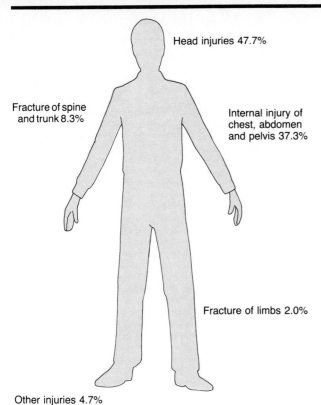

Head injuries 47.7%

Fracture of spine and trunk 8.3%

Internal injury of chest, abdomen and pelvis 37.3%

Fracture of limbs 2.0%

Other injuries 4.7%

FIGURE 14-17 Types of injuries resulting in death in motor vehicle collisions.

life-threatening trauma than others. A study of the incidence of mortality and the associated location of the trauma which caused it is identified in Figure 14-17.

The figures associated with Figure 14-17 clearly demonstrate head and body cavity injury account for a substantial 85 percent of vehicular mortality. It is easy to conclude that assessment of the auto accident patient should be directed to a rapid and thorough evaluation of these areas.

✳ Head and body cavity injuries account for 85 percent of auto fatalities.

Motorcycle Accidents.   Motorcycle accidents are very significant from the standpoint of injury because the rider is not provided the protection of the automobile. (See Figure 14-18.) Injury can be extreme, with an especially high incidence of head trauma. The impacts of the motorcycle accident are somewhat different than those of the auto and include: frontal, angular, ejection, and sliding.

In a frontal or head-on impact, the bike dips downward, causing the rider to be propelled upward and forward. This can lead to either the lower abdomen or pelvis being caught by the handle bars and resulting in abdominal injury and/or pelvic fracture. In some cases the rider is propelled through a higher trajectory, with the femurs being trapped by the handle bars, resulting in bilateral femur fractures.

Angular impacts are caused when the bike strikes an object at an oblique angle. The rider's lower extremity is frequently trapped between the bike and the object struck. This may cause fractures and crushing injuries to the foot, ankle, knee, and femur. Often the wounds are open.

Ejection during the accident involving a motorcycle is common and usually severe. It may occur with either of the mechanisms previously described. The ejection may cause several impacts:

❑ the initial bike/object collision
❑ the rider/object impact
❑ the rider/ground impact

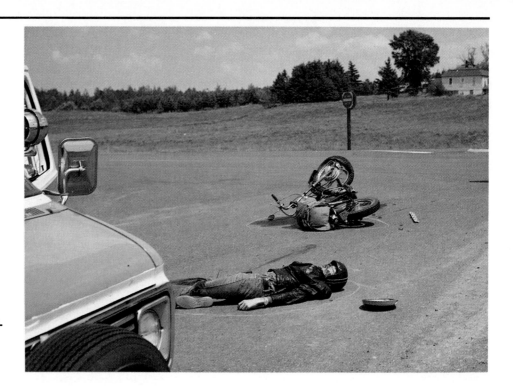

FIGURE 14-18 Motorcycle accidents can result in many types of trauma due to lack of protection for the rider.

Injuries that are likely to occur include skull fracture and/or internal head injury, spinal fractures and paralysis, and, frequently, extremity fractures.

Sliding impact occurs when an experienced rider, faced with an imminent crash, often "lays the bike down." The rider slides the bike sideways into the other vehicle or object, thereby reducing the chances of ejection and allowing the bike to "run interference" for him or her. The result is an increase in lacerations, abrasions, and minor fractures, with a decrease in some of the more serious injuries.

Whether or not a rider was wearing a helmet or leather clothing during an accident affects the severity of injury. Wearing a helmet considerably reduces the incidence of head injury, but it neither increases nor decreases the incidence of spinal trauma. Leather clothing will protect the wearer against open soft tissue injury but may hide an underlying contusion or fracture from the assessing paramedic.

Pedestrian Accidents. Pedestrian accidents differ between the adult and child, not only because of the anatomical differences but because of the way the victim responds to the impending trauma. (See Figure 14-19.) Paramedics can use this information to anticipate injuries and guide treatment.

The adult will generally turn away from the source of impact and present a rather lateral surface to the approaching vehicle. Anatomically, the impact is low with the bumper striking the lower leg first and causing fractures of the tibia and fibula. The transmitted impact can lead to ligament injury in the opposing knee.

As the lower extremity is propelled forward with the car, the upper and lateral body crashes into the hood causing fractures to either the femur, lateral chest, or upper extremity. The next impact sees the victim contacting the windshield, leading to the possibility of shoulder, neck, and head trauma.

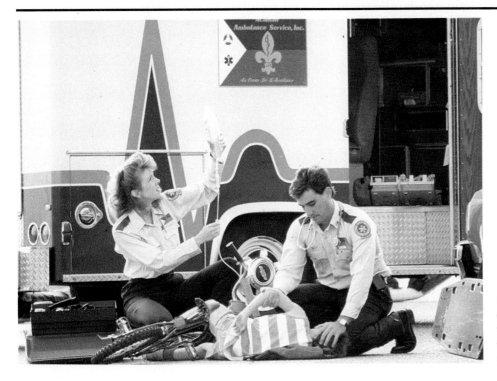

FIGURE 14-19 The injuries associated with pedestrian accidents will vary based on the size of the patient, the velocity of the vehicle, and the part of the body struck.

In contrast to the adult, the child will turn into the oncoming vehicle, presenting a slightly different list of problems to suspect. Also, because of the child's smaller anatomy, injury tends to be located anatomically higher than in the adult. The bumper will impact the femur, causing fracture. The secondary contact from the hood may lead to chest as well as upper-extremity and head injury. The windshield may produce head and neck injury. Both the child and the adult may be further injured when they are thrown and contact the ground. This traumatic collision may cause additional injury or compound those that occurred earlier in the accident. The child is frequently thrown in front of the vehicle because of the child's smaller size and lower center of gravity. (See Figure 14-20.)

Recreational Vehicle Accidents. Over the past few years the use of recreational vehicles has increased, and with it, the incidence of related trauma. (See Figure 14-21.) Recreational vehicles often present similar types of injuries. In addition, there is often difficulty detecting, reaching, and retrieving the victim.

Two of the major types of recreational vehicles commonly involved in accidents are the snowmobile and the all-terrain vehicle (ATV). Common to the snowmobile are crush injuries secondary to rollover and glancing blows against obstructions in the snow. Snowmobiles are also prone to cause severe head and neck damage due to collisions with other vehicles, including autos and other snowmobiles, or with stationary objects, such as trees. Snowmobile-related trauma may include severe neck injury occurring when the vehicle and rider run into an unseen wire fence. The anterior neck may be deeply lacerated yielding airway compromise, severe bleeding, and quite possibly complete severance of the head.

There are two types of ATVs: the three-wheel and the four-wheel versions. The three-wheeled version is notoriously unstable, especially when ridden by children, young adults, persons of lower body weight,

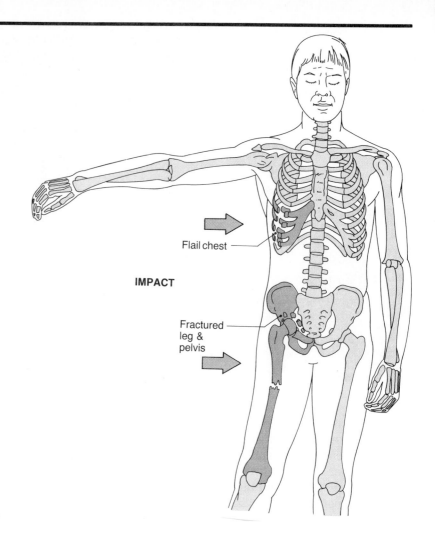

Flail chest

IMPACT

Fractured
leg &
pelvis

FIGURE 14-20 Typical auto-pedestrian injuries.

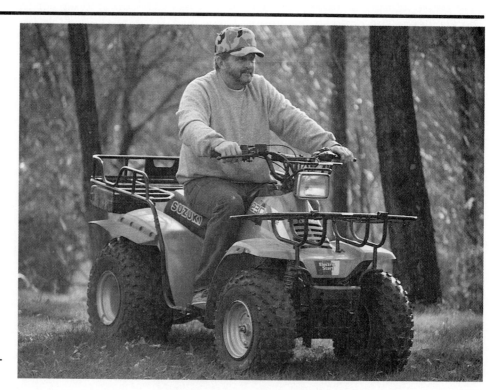

FIGURE 14-21 All-terrain vehicles (ATV) can cause a multitude of injuries due to their speed and instability.

and those with limited vehicle experience. The center of gravity is relatively high, contributing to frequent rollover during quick turns. As with the snowmobile, there is also a significant incidence of frontal collision. The injuries expected might include upper and lower extremity fracture, and head and spine injury.

A problem that may compound the ATV and snowmobile accident is the distance from the accident to the closest passable road. This distance can be long and may lead to significant delay in discovery of the accident, calls for help, and the arrival of paramedics. Once at the patient's side, the paramedic must consider transport to the ambulance, possibly over rough terrain, and possibly over a long distance.

Other Blunt Trauma

Falls. In terms of physics, the fall is nothing more than the release of stored gravitational energy. The greater the height, the greater the energy of impact, and the greater the trauma. As with the auto accident, stopping distance is possibly of more importance than the height of a fall. A person may dive pleasurably from a 12-foot-high platform into deep water, but the fall from a second-story window to the concrete below would be quite a different matter. Another of Newton's Laws, Force = Mass times Acceleration (or Deceleration), comes into play once more. The resulting trauma is dependent on the area of contact. If the victim lands feet first, the energy of the fall is transmitted up the skeletal structure leading to possible fractures of the calcaneus, femur, or lumbar spine. (See Figure 14-22.) The lumbar spine is especially prone to trauma because of its support of the entire upper body. The forces of deceleration are transmitted through this region, causing compression injury and possible displacement.

As the body continues the collision, the individual will either fall forward or backward. In the forward displacement, attempts will be made to break the fall with the outstretched arm, resulting in shoulder, clavicle (the most commonly fractured bone in the human body), and wrist fractures.

A posterior pathway may lead to pelvic and head injury. Should the victim impact with other body areas initially, the trauma will be transmitted from that area and cause problems such as pelvic, spinal, and/or upper extremity fractures, as well as chest, shoulder, head, and neck injury. In the severe fall, one in which a person falls more than 15 feet to an unyielding surface, attention should be turned to internal injury. The rapid deceleration of impact with the ground causes many of the internal organs to be compressed and twisted. The heart, for example, may be twisted with such force that it tears the aorta, leading to almost immediate exsanguination.

Sports Injuries. The field of sports medicine is growing very rapidly. It is an extensive field, which certainly could not be covered in detail in this chapter. For the purpose of understanding, some basic principles are important to address.

The sports injury is most commonly produced by extreme exertion, fatigue, or by the direct forces of trauma. The injury can be secondary to acceleration, deceleration, compressional forces, rotational forces, and hyperextension or hyperflexion. The forces can leave behind soft-tissue damage to the skin and muscle, connective tissue injury to the tendons and ligaments, skeletal trauma to the long bones or spinal column, as well as internal damage to either hollow or solid organs.

✳ The potential injury from a fall depends on the height and the stopping distance.

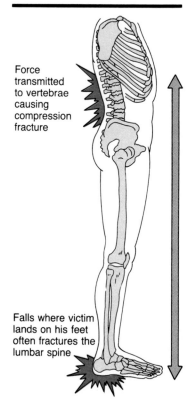

Force transmitted to vertebrae causing compression fracture

Falls where victim lands on his feet often fractures the lumbar spine

FIGURE 14-22 In falls, the energy is transmitted up the skeletal system.

Protective gear can afford effective protection. But once the destruction has occurred, such equipment may hinder assessment and patient stabilization. In the major contact sports, especially football, shoes are designed to give maximum traction. The soles have cleats to lock the foot firmly in position. When the player is struck and the body is forcibly turned, it twists on an immobile foot. This can cause severe and debilitating leg injury, frequently tearing the ligaments of the knee.

Contact sports also are responsible for some severe and sudden impact to an unknowing participant. If the trauma leads to head injury and/or any loss of consciousness, the individual should be seen by emergency department personnel. There is often a strong desire by coaches and players alike to return to the game. However, until a head or cervical spine injury can be ruled out, such action must be discouraged.

Blast Injuries. Blast injuries are not uncommon in prehospital emergency care. Natural gas, gasoline, fireworks, and even the dust within a grain elevator can give rise to a violent explosion and the specific scenario of injuries that accompany this mechanism of injury. Insult to the patient results from three specific phases of the explosion:

Primary. The primary event is the initial air blast. Injuries are primarily due to compression of air-containing organs and include:

- ❏ auditory injuries (usually involve ruptured tympanic membranes)
- ❏ sinus injuries
- ❏ lung injuries (may include pneumothorax, **parenchymal** hemorrhage, and alveolar rupture)
- ❏ stomach injuries
- ❏ intestinal injuries

Secondary. Secondarily, the victim is struck by debris propelled by the force of the blast.

Tertiary. Finally, there is the trauma caused when the victim is thrown away from the source of the blast. Injuries are much the same as would be expected from ejection from a vehicle. (See Figure 14-23.)

Penetrating Trauma

The knife, arrow, bullet, and other mechanisms of injury can be responsible for penetrating trauma. The extent of damage depends on Newton's Laws of Motion, most notably the formula for kinetic energy. As you recall, kinetic energy is equal to the mass of an object times the square of its velocity.

$$KE = \frac{Mass \times Velocity^2}{2}$$

This is then divided by two. The importance of this relationship is that as the mass of an object is doubled, its energy is doubled. However, if the speed is doubled, the energy is quadrupled. Hence a very small and light bullet traveling at a very high speed can do tremendous damage within the human body.

The law of conservation of energy states, "Energy can neither be created nor destroyed, only changed." It shows that the kinetic energy of the projectile will be transferred to the object it strikes. If the bullet remains within the object struck, then all the energy has been expended. If it

■ **parenchymal** referring to the essential parts of an organ, concerned with its function and not its framework.

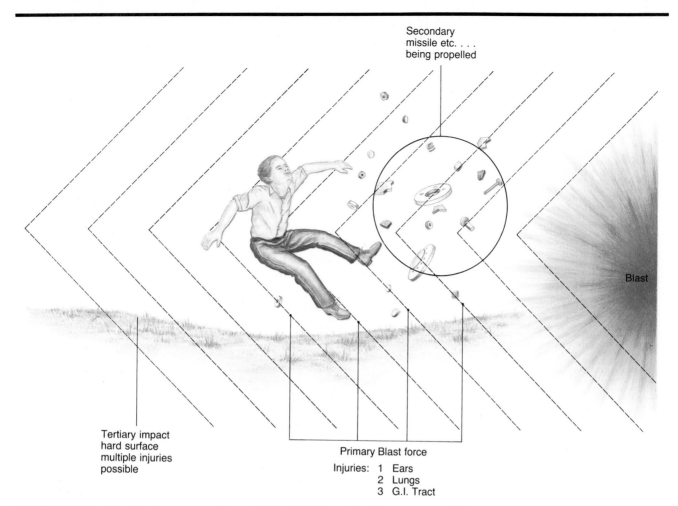

Secondary
missile etc. . . .
being propelled

Blast

Tertiary impact
hard surface
multiple injuries
possible

Primary Blast force
Injuries: 1 Ears
2 Lungs
3 G.I. Tract

FIGURE 14-23 Blast injuries can cause injury with the initial blast, when the victim is struck by debris, or by the victim being blown away from the site of the blast.

passes through, then the energy expended is equal to the energy just prior to entering the body minus the energy remaining as the projectile leaves the body.

Ballistics. Ballistics is the study of the properties and characteristics of projectiles. The major aspects of this study are trajectory and those factors that affect the dissipation of energy. These include drag, expansion, **profile,** and **cavitation.** The trajectory is the curved path that a bullet follows once fired from a gun. As it travels through the air it is constantly pulled downward by gravity at an acceleration of 32 ft/s^2. The faster the bullet, the flatter the curve of its travel (the straighter its trajectory).

The second and more significant aspect of the study of projectile travel is the dissipation of energy. As the bullet travels through the air, it experiences wind resistance, or drag. The faster it travels, the more drag it experiences and the greater the slowing effect. Since this represents a reduction in the bullet's speed, it also means that, if all else is equal, the damage caused by a bullet fired at close range will be more severe than that caused by a bullet fired from a great distance.

The damage done by the bullet as it enters the victim is dependent upon a number of elements. The first element is the bullet's profile. The larger the diameter of the projectile, the greater the area of tissue it con-

■ **ballistics** the study of projectile motion and its effects upon any object it impacts.

■ **profile** the size and shape of a projectile as it contacts a target.

■ **cavitation** formation of a partial vacuum, and subsequent cavity, within a liquid. This describes the action of a high-velocity projectile on the human body which is 60 percent water.

tacts, and the more rapid the exchange of energy. The small .22 caliber bullet (about 1/4 inch in diameter) would be expected to lose less energy as it traveled through the body than the .45 caliber bullet (about 1/2 inch in diameter). As the diameter doubles from 1/4 inch to 1/2 inch, the increase in the surface area that transmits the energy of impact increases by four. (See Figures 14-24, 14-25, and 14-26.)

To increase the dissipation of energy, some bullets are designed to expand on entry. An example of this is the soft-point, hollow-tipped bullet (dum-dum or wad cutter), which will mushroom and/or fragment on impact. A bullet that rotates or tumbles will also present a wider profile and increase the rate of energy transfer. (See Figure 14-27.) As the bullet travels into and through fluid or human flesh, it creates a wave of pressure. This pressure wave, called cavitation, extends the damage beyond the initial pathway of the object. (See Figure 14-28.)

The size of the cavitational wave is very dependent on the rate of energy being expended. With a knife or arrow, the speed is relatively low and the damage is limited to the actual path of the projectile. However, with a high energy projectile, such as a rifle bullet, the damage is many times larger than the actual pathway.

Pathway expansion is an important concept in understanding the pathology of bullet wounds. As the bullet contacts the patient's semi-fluid body, the cavitation wave is generated. The organs and tissue are com-

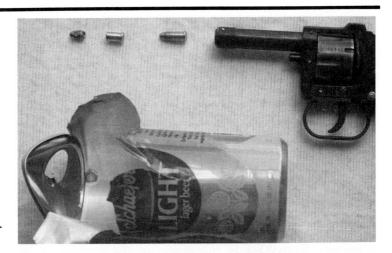

FIGURE 14-24 Destructive effect of .22 caliber hand gun.

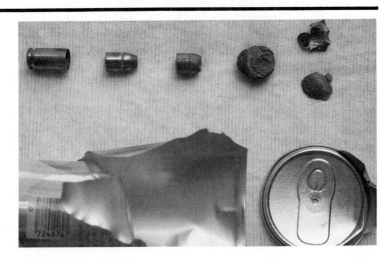

FIGURE 14-25 Destructive effect of .32 caliber hand gun.

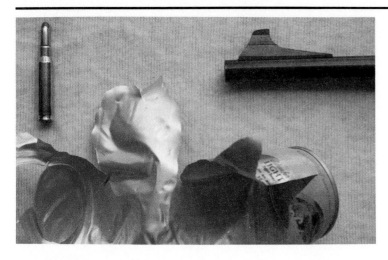

FIGURE 14-26 Destructive effect of .308 caliber rifle.

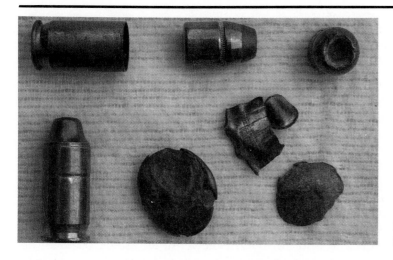

FIGURE 14-27 The profile of a bullet will vary based on its design.

pressed drastically, causing contusion, rupture, and fracture. The faster the bullet travels, and the greater profile it presents to the body tissue, the greater will be the rate of energy transfer, the larger the cavitation wave, and the larger the resultant damage.

There are three categories of projectile injury. These are:

❑ low-velocity
❑ high-velocity/medium-energy
❑ high-velocity/high-energy

Low Velocity. The low-velocity injury is the trauma caused by a knife, ice pick, or arrow. The kinetic energy involved is limited by the relatively slow speed of the object as it enters the body. The most common of these would probably be a stabbing where an individual, weighing about 150 pounds, strikes another at 50 mph. The speed is noticeably less than that of a bullet, yet the weight behind the penetration is much more. The expected trauma would be limited to the pathway of the knife alone.

An important consideration of low-velocity penetrating wounds is that the entrance wound may not be reflective of the total extent of injury.

✱ The faster the bullet travels, and the greater the profile it presents, the greater will be the rate of energy transfer, and the larger the cavitational wave and the resultant damage.

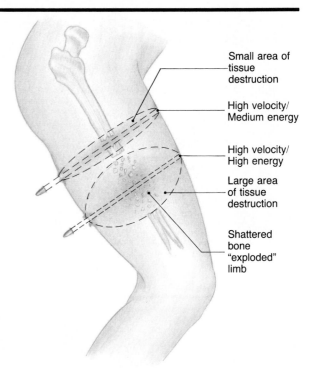

Small area of tissue destruction

High velocity/ Medium energy

High velocity/ High energy

Large area of tissue destruction

Shattered bone "exploded" limb

FIGURE 14-28 The severity of injury associated with penetrating trauma is, in many ways, related to the velocity of the penetrating object.

The knife, for example, may have been twisted, moved about, or inserted at an oblique angle. If the entrance wound is in an area close to the rib margin, the structures involved may be either abdominal, thoracic, or both. It is important to remember that the border between the abdominal and thoracic cavities moves up and down with respiration.

There are also some characteristics of the attack to be considered. Gender makes a difference in the expected injuries. The male will most often strike with an outward or crosswise stroke, while the female will strike with an overhand and downward blow. As an attack occurs, the victim attempts to protect him or herself by using the upper extremities. Deep lacerations of the upper extremities (commonly called "defense wounds") will probably occur. If the attack is "successful," the injuries are generally directed to the chest, abdomen, or back.

High Velocity. The high-velocity injury, most commonly caused by a bullet, is subdivided into medium- and high-energy wounds. The medium-energy wound often results from shotgun pellets or handgun bullets. High-energy trauma is usually caused by the high-power, high-speed rifle bullet.

The energy delivered to the victim can be immense. A bullet with a muzzle velocity of 1,000 feet per second is traveling about 720 miles per hour. Newton's Laws state that kinetic energy is equal to weight times the speed squared. Thus it is easy to see that even a very small object, such as a bullet, at this speed has tremendous energy. The trauma caused by the high-velocity projectile is normally much greater than would be expected by just noting the entrance and exit wounds (if an exit wound exists).

The energy is transmitted beyond the bullet pathway. The resulting cavitation wave is smaller with the medium-energy projectile than with the high-energy event.

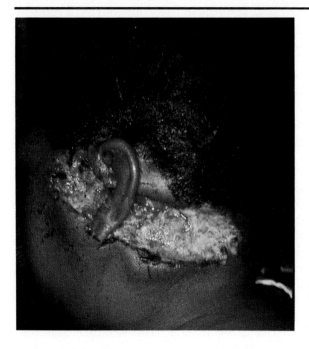

FIGURE 14-29 Wound resulting from close-range shotgun blast. Note the tattooing of the skin from the gun powder.

The entrance wound may appear abraded around its margin and may show some signs of powder burns (tattooing) if the gunshot was delivered at close range. (See Figure 14-29.) The exit wound will be larger and probably more severe since the cavitational wave extends to all sides of the bullet as it passes through the tissues. Should all the energy be expended within the victim, no exit wound would exist and the projectile would remain lodged inside the patient.

Pathologies of Penetrating Trauma. The stabbing, gunshot blast, and other penetrating trauma can cause numerous injuries. Several specific areas where trauma can occur need to be investigated and emphasized. These include the head, neck, thorax, abdomen, and extremities.

The head can be divided into two regions for the discussion of penetrating trauma. The facial area is often severely damaged in the attempted suicide. When a rifle or shotgun is used, the victim places the barrel under the chin, or in the mouth, and reaches for the trigger. As the trigger is squeezed, the head is tilted back and the blast impacts the mandible, maxilla, and nasal bones. Occasionally, this fails to kill the individual. In these cases, the resultant injuries are a true threat to the airway and are very difficult to manage.

The second area of the head is the cranium. Because the cranium is a container of fixed volume and inflexible shape, the impact of the bullet and the cavitation it causes is increased. Ricochet or deflection which follows the curve of the skull's interior may further increase the damage within the skull and pose a serious threat to life. Most gunshot injuries in which the projectile enters the cranium are fatal.

The neck area is a location where the concern for airway and breathing are first priority. The trachea is at the anterior surface of the neck and is thus exposed to any frontal or penetrating injury. There should be concern for hemorrhage from the large arterial and venous vessels that traverse this area. It should be noted that the venous system, at times,

✳ Most gunshot injuries in which the projectile enters the cranium are fatal.

does carry a pressure less than that present in the atmosphere (a relative negative pressure). A large open wound may allow air to be taken into a large vein, leading to air emboli.

Finally, some concern should be afforded the cervical spine. Although very well protected skeletally, its importance to survival and bodily function make it an extremely important structure. Any injury in this region must be treated as a spinal injury until ruled out by X-ray and in-hospital evaluation. Care for these injuries should be directed at spinal stabilization, control of severe bleeding, airway protection, and prevention of air embolization from a venous injury.

The thorax is a large and relatively common target of both the low- and high-velocity penetrating injuries. The lung is rather tolerant to injury. The spongy structure of the lung, with its air-filled alveoli, is better able to withstand the cavitation wave than most other tissue. However, the structures of the mediastinum (heart, great vessels, trachea, esophagus, etc.) are not so tolerant. Pulmonary contusions or pneumothorax may occur as well as pericardial tamponade, esophageal injury, rupture of the great vessels, and rapid exsanguination.

Open pneumothorax is of concern in almost any penetrating injury to the chest. However, it does not routinely occur with knife or gunshot injury unless the wound is rather large in size. The shotgun blast, at close range, may very well cause a sucking chest wound, but most other gunshot injuries do not. (See Chapter 16.)

If the ribs are subjected to high energy impact they may fracture, allowing for greater dissipation of energy, possible bullet deflection, and fragmentation of the projectile. This will increase the size of the damage pathway and possibly the significance of the injury.

The abdomen carries with it the danger of injury secondary to the damage caused by the passage of the object through the viscera. The contents of the large bowel may be spilled into the peritoneal cavity, giving rise to massive infection. Another example is damage to the pancreas. This may affect the metabolism of glucose and digestion as well as allowing strong digestive enzymes to leak into the abdominal cavity. Almost any combination of internal problems can occur with the abdominal-penetrating wound.

The extremities are rarely of life-threatening concern when subjected to penetrating trauma. However, injuries can be very extensive since the long bones are large and strong, and their impact can provide for a quick exchange of energy. The lack of involvement of critical structures reduces concern, except where significant bleeding occurs.

SUMMARY

Decisions regarding patient care should be based on an understanding of the mechanism of injury and a comparable index of suspicion, not just the grotesqueness of the wound or wounds. Understanding the kinetics of trauma can give paramedics the basis for making the right decisions at the right time.

By analyzing what happened to the patient, specifically the nature and severity of the forces of trauma, the paramedic may anticipate the nature and severity of the victim's wounds and overall condition. With this information, the paramedic is better able to assign priorities of patient care and determine if the patient is best served by care on-scene or during rapid transport.

FURTHER READING

American College of Surgeons, Committee on Trauma. *Advanced Trauma Life Support Course: Student Manual.* American College of Surgeons, 1984.

Butman, Alexander M., and Paturas, James L. *Pre-Hospital Trauma Life Support.* Akron, OH: Emergency Training, 1986.

Campbell, John E. *Basic Trauma Life Support,* 2nd ed. Englewood Cliffs, NJ: Prentice-Hall, Inc., 1988.

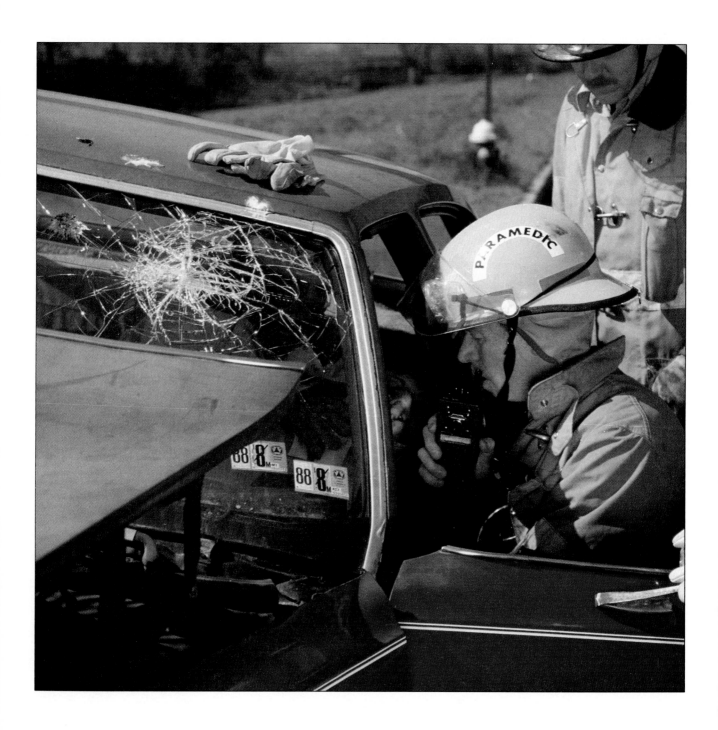

15

Head, Neck, and Spine Trauma

Objectives for Chapter 15

Upon completing this chapter, the student should be able to:

1. Identify the incidence, mortality, and morbidity for head, neck, and spine injuries respectively.

2. List the structures which protect the central nervous system from trauma and describe how they accomplish this function.

3. List the components of the central nervous system and explain how they help control the human body.

4. Identify the various head, neck, and spine injuries and explain the progression of their respective injuries.

5. List the signs and symptoms for each of the following: soft tissue injury (to the scalp, face, and neck), skull frac-

ture, central nervous system injury, and increased intracranial pressure.

6. List and explain the significance of the elements of the primary assessment as they relate to CNS injury.

7. Demonstrate the assessment of a head, neck, or spinal injury patient, while listing the care steps required for each finding.

8. Identify and demonstrate the proper care steps for: soft tissue injury (to the face, scalp, and neck), skull fracture, special sense organ injury, and central nervous system injury.

Unit 765 is responding to a one-car accident with reports of one patient injured. Upon arrival at the scene, the paramedics observe an auto against a tree. No wires are down and there does not appear to be leaking gas or any ignition source. The police have controlled traffic.

The vehicle is greatly deformed due to a frontal impact; the frame is obviously bent. On the driver's side, the windshield is broken in a spiderweb configuration. The driver's door is ajar, with only one patient visible. The police officer explains that the patient was initially unconscious but woke up a few minutes ago.

Assessment of the patient finds a 31-year-old male who is conscious and alert, though disoriented to time and event. He cannot remember what happened nor what day it is. His head is manually stabilized and a cervical collar is applied. He has a contusion to the left forehead and some moderate chest pain. The pain seems to vary with respiration and he denies any pain prior to the accident or any history of heart problems. Palpation of the chest region elicits pain and some crepitus. Lung sounds are clear and the monitor shows a normal sinus rhythm. Vital signs are: blood pressure of 130/88, pulse of 70 and strong both central and distal, rapid capillary refill, and deep respirations at a rate of 20. The patient denies any previous medical history, prescribed medications, or allergies.

As the assessment continues, the patient becomes agitated and then combative. Oxygen is applied but his condition worsens until he becomes unresponsive. His left pupil is noticeably dilated. The patient only responds to deep pain, and then with ineffective motion. He is rapidly moved to a long spineboard and transported. An IV line is started enroute and normal saline hung run at a rate to keep the vein open. Medical command is contacted and the patient report is given. The on-call physician diverts the ambulance to the regional neurocenter. The patient is intubated orally, while the head is firmly immobilized. He is hyperventilated, pulse oximetry is applied, and oxygen saturation reads 97%.

The receiving hospital is awaiting the patient's arrival. A quick assessment is made and he is evaluated by X-ray and CAT scan. No cervical spine injury is found, but a epidural hematoma is noted. The patient is taken to surgery and the blood is evacuated. He is conscious, alert, and doing well when the crew does their 24-hour follow-up.

INTRODUCTION

The head, neck, and spine are commonly-injured parts of the body. Injury to the head is the most frequent cause of vehicular death, while spinal injury accounts for a high incidence of serious debilitation. Because there is such a high frequency of trauma to these areas of the body, and because the consequences of head and spinal injury are so debilitating, it is important to ensure that care is proper and appropriate. Even though these injuries are frequent and dangerous, they are often difficult to assess and care for in the prehospital setting. The most overt and obvious signs and symptoms do not generally reflect life-threatening injuries. It is the subtle and unforeseen problems that quietly allow the patient to deteriorate while attention is directed toward more gruesome and visually apparent injuries. Even if a life-threatening problem is found, there is little definitive care that can be provided in the field. There are no heroic measures of care for these injuries, as in the cardiac arrest or tension pneumothorax. However, failure to recognize potential injury, and failure to provide proper stabilization and rapid transportation can also lead to death.

THE CENTRAL NERVOUS SYSTEM

Anatomy and Physiology

In order to adequately understand the pathology, assessment, and care of head, neck, and spine injury, it is necessary to understand the anatomy of the central nervous system.

The *central nervous system (CNS)*, which consists of the brain and spinal cord, is responsible for the regulation of all body functions. It maintains consciousness and permits awareness of the environment. Additionally, it controls voluntary movement. The CNS is made up of highly specialized cells, called neurons, which may extend up to 3 feet in length. They differ in design from the peripheral nerve cells as they have no protective sheath. If the CNS neuron is injured, repair and regeneration is unlikely. Consequently, such injuries have, at best, a poor prognosis.

Several protective layers prevent injury to the CNS in all but the most extreme circumstances. The scalp and hair fend off the effects of external temperature and traumatic stress. The hard plate of the skull and the rigid support of the vertebral column withstand rigorous kinetic force. And the final layer of protection, the **meninges** and the **cerebrospinal fluid,** surrounds and actually floats the brain and cord to further absorb shock and suppress injury.

During trauma, the head and neck are frequently injured. The head may be the initial point of impact in auto accidents or falls, because it protrudes from the body. It is in fact often the target of blunt or penetrating injury of an accidental or intentional nature. The neck, because of its support of the head, also experiences kinetic forces. Extension, flexion, compression, or lateral movement may lead to fracture, instability, and subsequent risk of spinal cord injury.

Central Nervous System Protection.   Important protective structures include:

Scalp.   The scalp protects the brain from both the effects of trauma and the extremes of weather. It is a strong and flexible mass of skin and fascia (bands of connective and muscular tissue) able to withstand and absorb tremendous kinetic energy. The scalp is also extremely vascular to ensure that the brain is always maintained at the proper core temperature.

Skull.   Under the soft tissue of the scalp are the bones making up the skull. (See Figure 15-1.) These include the facial bones and the cranium. The facial bones provide support and form for the nose, mouth, orbits,

■ **meninges** three membranes that surround and protect the brain and spinal cord. They are: the dura matter, the arachnoid membrane, and the pia matter.

■ **cerebrospinal fluid** fluid surrounding and bathing the brain and spinal cord (the central nervous system).

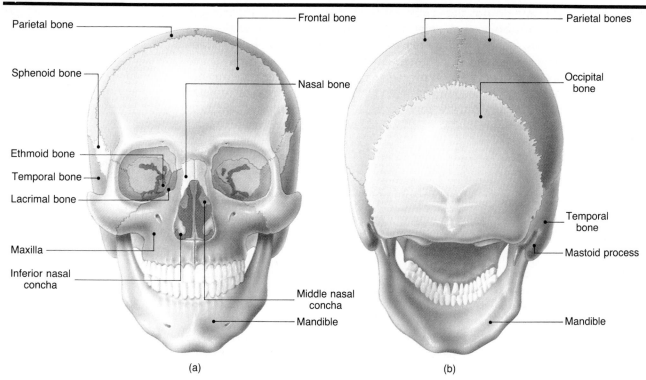

Parietal bone

Sphenoid bone

Ethmoid bone

Temporal bone

Lacrimal bone

Maxilla

Inferior nasal concha

Frontal bone

Nasal bone

Middle nasal concha

Mandible

Parietal bones

Occipital bone

Temporal bone

Mastoid process

Mandible

(a)　　　　　　　　　　　　(b)

FIGURE 15-1　The human skull.

■ **cranium** vaultlike portion of the skull encasing the brain.

and jaw. The **cranium** is the container for the brain. A knowledge of each of these bones is important in understanding the effects of trauma.

　The facial bones make up the anterior and inferior structures of the head and include the zygoma, maxilla, mandible and nasal bones. The *zygoma*, the prominent bone of the cheek, protects the eyes and the muscles controlling eye and jaw movement. The *maxilla* comprises the upper jaw and supports the *nasal bones.* These bones form the base for the nasal cartilage and the shape of the nose. The last of the facial bones is the *mandible,* or jawbone. It resembles two horizontal "L's" joined anteriorly and hinged underneath the posterior zygomatic arch. Besides forming the beginning of the airway and the alimentary canal, these bones are the protective and support structures for several sense organs including the tongue, eyes, and olfactory nerve. Injury to these bones can threaten the function of any of the organs of perception.

　The second component of the skull is the *cranium,* or cranial vault, which contains the brain. The skull is quite strong and consists of several bones fused together at pseudojoints called **sutures.** The bony plates forming the cranium consist of the *frontal, sphenoid, occipital, parietal,* and *temporal* bones. Under each lie regions of the brain called *lobes.* Each of these lobes bears the same name as the bone overlying it. Also, each of the cranial bones is actually composed of two plates of compact bone separated by a layer of spongy or **cancellous** bone in between. Such a configuration makes the skull strong yet light. The skull is, therefore, quite effective in protecting its contents from the direct effects of trauma. However swelling or bleeding occurring within the cranial vault has nowhere to expand. The result is increased internal pressure which can severely damage the brain.

■ **sutures** pseudo-joints that join the various bones of the skull to form the cranium.

■ **cancellous** having a lattice-work structure as in the spongy tissue of the bone.

Vertebral Column.　At its base, the skull is connected to the *vertebral column.* (See Figure 15-2.) This vertebral column is designed to protect the spinal cord and to allow for the mobility of the head, the upper body, and the thorax. A column composed of 32 to 34 separate and irregular bones, it is divided into the five spinal regions. These are the *cervical, thoracic, lumbar, sacral,* and *coccygeal* regions. Potential injury to the cervical spine is one of the key patient assessment considerations in prehospital care because of the spinal cord within. It is also a region which receives a high incidence of trauma due to the weight of the head it supports.

The cervical spine consists of 7 vertebrae numbered 1 through 7. The first, which is also called the *Atlas,* supports the skull and allows for the large range of motion as the head turns from left to right. The second cervical vertebra, the *Axis,* has a small fingerlike upward projection which acts as the pivot point for this motion. This protrusion, the **odontoid process** (or dens), is the primary structure keeping the upper reaches of the spinal column in line while the head turns. Because of its

■ **odontoid process** fingerlike projection of the second cervical vertebra, around which the first cervical vertebra rotates.

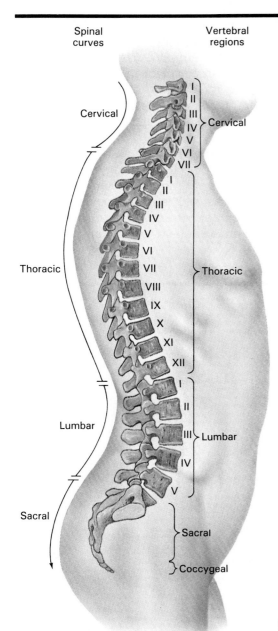

Spinal curves | Vertebral regions

Cervical

I
II
III
IV   Cervical
V
VI
VII

Thoracic

I
II
III
IV
V
VI
VII   Thoracic
VIII
IX
X
XI
XII

Lumbar

I
II
III   Lumbar
IV
V

Sacral

Sacral

Coccygeal

FIGURE 15-2   The human spine.

small size and fragile nature, minor kinetic forces can cause fracture of the odontoid. Movement of the neck following fracture of the odontoid can lead to injury or severance of the spinal cord. The cervical spine ends with the seventh cervical body. This vertebra can be palpated at the level of the shoulders. It is the first bony prominence noticed as you work your fingers down the posterior surface of the neck.

The next 12 vertebrae are *thoracic,* with one connected to each rib. This relationship, as well as the overlying scapulae, serve to protect the thoracic spinal column from injury.

The *lumbar spine* is made up of 5 of the largest vertebral bodies. This area is responsible for the support of the entire upper torso, neck, head, and upper extremities. It is prone to compressional fracture. Trauma to this region can also result in injury to the intervertebral discs.

The *sacrum* is the posterior aspect of the pelvis and is composed of fused vertebra. Five bodies are joined into one very strong plate forming the posterior component of the pelvic ring. The pseudojoint between the pelvis and the sacrum (called the sacroiliac joint) is an area of possible fracture, which, if it occurs, not only causes pain but instability.

The last region of the vertebral column is the *coccyx.* It is a series of 3, 4, or 5 small vertebrae that, early in development, fuse into two to four bones. Although the coccyx provides little support or function, it can be fractured in trauma secondary to falls and posterior impact. The share of weight each vertebra bears varies with its location. Moving from the top of the vertebral column to the bottom, the size of the bones increase. This occurs because the weight supported by the spine increases as you move down the column to the pelvis.

Each vertebra is made up of several components. (See Figure 15-3.) The major weight-bearing aspect is the *body.* It is a round cylinder that supports the structures above and allows rotational movement. Between the vertebral bodies are cartilaginous *discs.* The discs provide articular and weight-bearing surfaces for the spinal column. Their resilient outer capsule and inner semiliquid center enables them to cushion the column

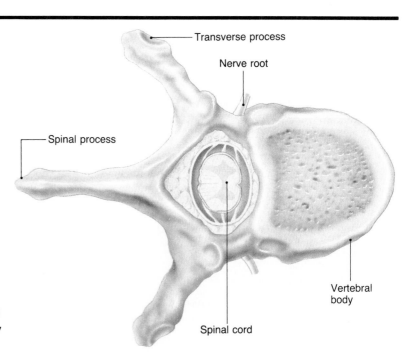

Transverse process

Nerve root

Spinal process

Vertebral body

Spinal cord

FIGURE 15-3 Although relatively well protected in the spinal canal, the spinal cord is subject to injury during accidents.

and the upper body from the jarring effects of walking. Similarly, they cushion the body when a person lands on his or her heels from a fall. They also give the column its flexibility in lateral motion as well as allowing flexion and extension. Posterior to the vertebral body are three processes—two lateral and one directly posterior. They provide for muscular and ligamentous attachment and afford some protection for the spinal cord. The distal end of the posterior process (called the spinous process) can be palpated from the seventh cervical vertebra to the sacrum. Central to the body and spinal processes is the opening for the spinal cord, called the **spinal foramen,** or canal. This hole provides a tube through which the spinal cord travels from the skull to the second lumbar vertebra where the cord ends. This tube must remain in alignment, as the spine supports the upper body.

The Meninges. The final protective mechanism for the brain and the spinal cord is the meninges. (See Figure 15-4.) They are a series of three tissues between the skull and the surface of the brain as well as between the spinal column and the cord. The outermost layer is called the **dura mater.** It is tough and a major source of central nervous system protection. The dura mater lies directly beneath the skull and lines the interior of the cranium and the vertebral column. It is actually the inner **periosteum** of the skull and is attached to the interior surface of the cranium as well as to the spinal column. The layer of the meninges closest to the brain and spinal cord is the **pia mater.** It is a delicate covering of all the convolutions of the brain and the cord. Weaker than the dura, the pia is much more substantial than brain and spinal cord tissue. Separating the two layers of mater is the **arachnoid membrane,** a strata of connective tissue suspending the brain in the cranial cavity and the cord in the spinal foramen. The arachnoid membrane is named for its weblike appearance. Beneath the **arachnoid** membrane is the subarachnoid space which

■ **spinal foramen** the opening in the vertebrae through which the spinal cord passes.

■ **dura mater** tough layer of the meninges firmly attached to the interior of the skull.

■ **periosteum** the exterior covering of a bone.

■ **pia mater** inner and most delicate layer of the meninges. It covers the convolutions of the brain and spinal cord.

■ **arachnoid membrane** middle layer of the meninges.

■ **arachnoid** weblike in appearance.

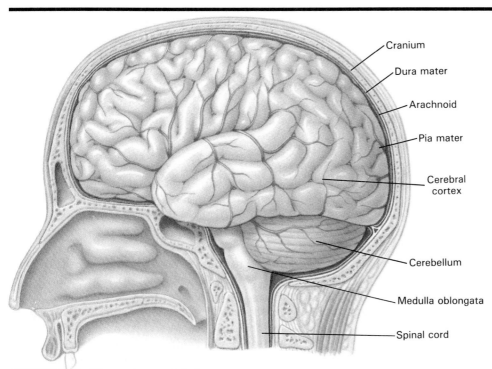

FIGURE 15-4 The meninges and skull.

is filled with cerebrospinal fluid. Cerebrospinal fluid is the medium which surrounds the central nervous system and acts to absorb shocks of minor deceleration.

Central Nervous System.   The functional unit of the central nervous system is the *neuron*. Neurons in the CNS are slightly different in appearance than those of the peripheral nervous system. CNS neurons do not have the protective protein sheath (called **neurilemma**) along their long arm, or *axon*. While this difference is subtle, it becomes important when considering the significance of injury and regenerative repair. In trauma to the peripheral nervous system, the nerve may regenerate along the pathway provided by the nerve sheath. Injury to the central nervous system which either interrupts the axon or kills the cell is, in contrast, generally permanent.

Brain.   The brain is composed of several structures, all essential to human function. They are the cerebrum, cerebellum, pons, and medulla oblongata. The *cerebrum* is the largest portion of the CNS, occupying most of the cranial cavity. The cerebrum is the center of conscious thought, personality, sensory and motor perception, and is also responsible for visual, auditory, and tactile (touch) perception. The cerebrum is regionalized into lobes generally lying beneath the bones of the skull. Its frontal region is anterior and controls the personality. The parietal region, which is superior and posterior, directs the motor and sensory activities. The occipital region, which is posterior and inferior, is responsible for sight. Laterally, the temporal region controls hearing and speech.

The cerebrum is divided into hemispheres by a structure called the *falx cerebri*. A ligamentous partition, the falx cerebri is suspended into the cranial cavity from the superior and interior surface of the skull. Corresponding to the falx cerebri is a fissure in the brain called the *central sulcus*. The fissure physically divides the cerebrum into the left and right hemispheres, each of which controls (for the most part) the activities of the opposite side of the body. The **tentorium** is a similar fibrous sheet within the occipital region and running at right angles to the falx cerebri. It separates the cerebrum from the cerebellum. The third cranial nerve, which controls pupil size, travels through this area. It may be compressed as **intracranial pressure** rises or the brain is displaced due to swelling or hemorrhage. This will cause pupillary disturbances which may manifest on either the same or the opposite side as the pathology. If the pressure is great enough, both pupils may dilate and fix.

Other anatomic points of interest within the skull are the cribriform plate and the foramen magnum. The **cribriform plate** is an irregular and sharp bony plane at the base of the skull. It has surfaces against which the brain may abrade, lacerate or contuse in severe deceleration. The *foramen magnum* is the largest opening in the skull. It is located at the base of the skull where it meets the spinal column and marks the point at which the spinal cord exits the cranium.

Located posterior and inferior to the cerebrum, the *cerebellum* is directly under the tentorium. It "fine tunes" motor control and allows the body to move smoothly from one position to another. Additionally, the cerebellum is responsible for maintaining muscle tone. The structure responsible for linking the cerebellum, the cerebrum, and the upper reaches of the spinal cord together is the *pons*. A bulb-shaped structure it is directly above the medulla oblongata. The pons acts as a communication interchange between the various components of the central nervous system and the spinal cord.

■ **neurilemma** thin, fibrous sheath surrounding the peripheral nerve fiber.

■ **tentorium** extension of the dura mater separating the cerebrum from the cerebellum.

■ **intracranial pressure** pressure exerted on the brain by the blood and cerebrospinal fluid.

■ **cribriform plate** thin, sharp plate in the central cranium.

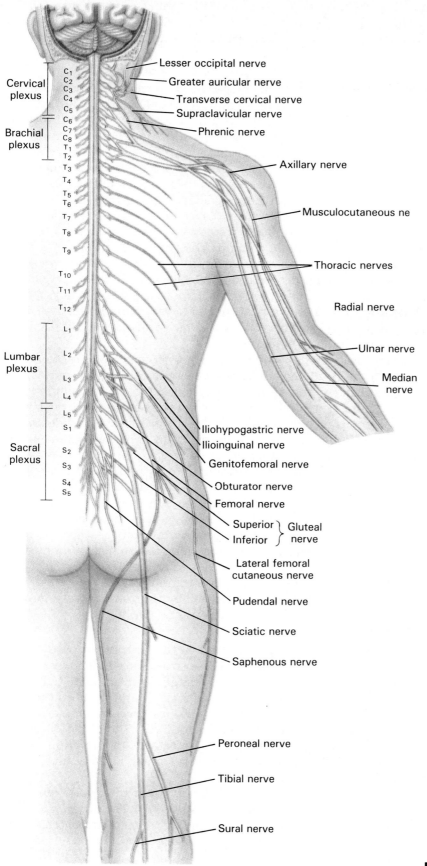

Cervical plexus

Brachial plexus

Lumbar plexus

Sacral plexus

C_1
C_2
C_3
C_4
C_5
C_6
C_7
C_8
T_1
T_2
T_3
T_4
T_5
T_6
T_7
T_8
T_9
T_{10}
T_{11}
T_{12}
L_1
L_2
L_3
L_4
L_5
S_1
S_2
S_3
S_4
S_5

Lesser occipital nerve
Greater auricular nerve
Transverse cervical nerve
Supraclavicular nerve
Phrenic nerve
Axillary nerve
Musculocutaneous ne
Thoracic nerves
Radial nerve
Ulnar nerve
Median nerve
Iliohypogastric nerve
Ilioinguinal nerve
Genitofemoral nerve
Obturator nerve
Femoral nerve
Superior } Gluteal
Inferior } nerve
Lateral femoral cutaneous nerve
Pudendal nerve
Sciatic nerve
Saphenous nerve
Peroneal nerve
Tibial nerve
Sural nerve

FIGURE 15-5   The spinal cord and its branches.

The last nervous system structure still within the cranial vault is the *medulla oblongata*. It is recognizable as a bulge in the very top of the spinal cord, and controls three vital signs: pulse rate, respiration, and blood pressure.

Spinal Cord. Nervous system messages leave the medulla via the spinal cord. The *spinal cord* is the body's main communication conduit. It carries the commands to and from the brain, collecting or dispersing them through the peripheral nervous system. (See Figure 15-5.) The cord virtually fills the spinal canal of the vertebral column, and is at great risk for injury if any swelling, displacement, or constriction should affect the lumen of the canal. The cord extends down the spinal column to the upper lumbar region. Early in fetal development, the cord runs the entire length of the column. Since the skeletal system grows much faster than the specialized cells of the nervous system, by full maturity, the cord is effectively pulled up the spinal column. The end of the spinal cord then lies at about the 2nd-lumbar level by adulthood. With skeletal growth, the spinal nerve roots are drawn into the lower spinal foramen with the cord. Because the lower spinal region looks like the tail of a horse, it is termed **cauda equina** (Latin for tail of the horse). This is the area into which a needle can be introduced to withdraw cerebrospinal fluid for diagnostic purposes (called a spinal tap).

The peripheral nervous system branches from the central nervous system between the skull and the atlas and between each of the vertebrae. These peripheral nerve roots divide into somatic and autonomic tracts which innervate the body. The **autonomic nervous system** provides nervous control over the body organs while the *somatic* tracts provide innervation of, among other things, the dermatomes. The **dermatomes** are topographical areas of the body's surface corresponding to various nerve roots. (See Figure 15-6.) As the peripheral roots branch off the spine, they perceive sensation lower and lower on the body. The lower cervical and first thoracic branches control sensation and skeletal movement in the upper extremity. The thoracic branches govern sensation over the chest and the back, while the lumbar and sacral branches provide sensation for the lower extremities. Four locations are of special interest to prehospital personnel because they are easy to locate. They are the collar region, sensed by the third cervical nerve, the nipple line, sensed by the fourth thoracic nerve, the umbilicus, sensed by the tenth thoracic nerve, and the soles of the feet, sensed by the first sacral nerve.

CNS Circulation. Blood flow to the brain is through two separate systems. The first is the *carotid arteries*. These two vessels ascend along the anterior surface of the neck. The other source of blood supply to the brain is the *vertebral arteries*. These vessels ascend along and through the vertebral column. Both the carotid and vertebral systems are connected by the *circle of Willis* in the base of the brain. From the circle of Willis branch various arteries which supply the substance of the brain itself. Venous drainage is initially through the dural sinuses. These ultimately drain into the internal jugular veins.

The spinal cord receives its blood supply from the *spinal arteries*. These vessels are derived from the vertebral artery. The *anterior spinal artery* supplies the anterior two-thirds of the spinal cord. In contrast, the *posterior spinal artery* supplies the posterior one-third. Venous drainage is through the spinal veins which follow a path similar to that of the spinal arteries.

■ **cauda equina** terminal portion of the spinal cord which is shaped much like the tail of a horse (Cauda Equina is Latin for tail of a horse).

■ **autonomic nervous system** portion of the nervous system responsible for the involuntary control of body functions.

■ **dermatome** topographical region of the body surface innervated by one specific nerve root.

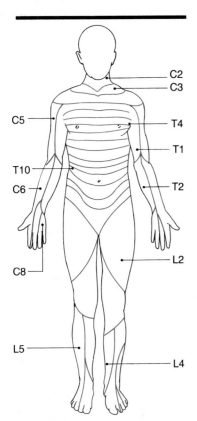

FIGURE 15-6 The dermatomes. Each dermatome corresponds to a spinal nerve.

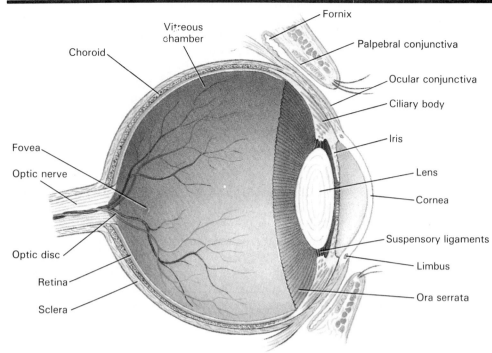

Labels on figure:

Choroid
Vitreous chamber
Fovea
Optic nerve
Optic disc
Retina
Sclera
Fornix
Palpebral conjunctiva
Ocular conjunctiva
Ciliary body
Iris
Lens
Cornea
Suspensory ligaments
Limbus
Ora serrata

FIGURE 15-7   The human eye.

Special Organs of Sense

The Eye.   The eyes are one of the most important special sense organs. They provide much of the sensory input we use to interact with the environment. They are placed in a position to scan the surroundings and yet are very well protected from injury. The frontal bones project above the globe of the eye, while the nasal bone protects medially. The zygoma rounds out the physical protection both laterally and inferiorly. These bones collectively form the orbits or eye sockets. Soft tissue of the eyelids and the eyelashes give the critical ocular surface additional protection.

The eye is a spherical globe, filled with fluid. (See Figure 15-7.) Its major compartment is the body of the eye which contains a gelatinous fluid called **vitreous humor.** The eye is lined with the actual light and color-sensing tissue, called the retina. The *retina* sends impulses through the optic nerve, which exits from the back of the globe. It enters the brain almost immediately. The structure separating the posterior from the anterior cavity is the *lens.* It is responsible for focusing light and images on the retina. The lens provides this service by thinning or thickening as controlled by small muscles. Regulating the amount of light penetrating the eye are structures located in front of the lens and within the anterior cavity. They include the iris and the aqueous humor, a fluid similar to that of the posterior cavity. The **iris** is the colored or pigmented diaphragm which controls the diameter of the opening (the pupil) that light travels through.

Several elements can be identified when the eye is examined from the front. The central black opening is the *pupil.* Surrounding it is the iris. Bordering the iris is the *sclera,* the white and vascular area which forms the remaining and underlying surface of the exposed eye. Both the pupil and the iris are covered by a very thin, clear, and delicate layer, called the *cornea.* Continuous with the cornea and extending out to the interior surface of the eyelid is the *conjunctiva.* It is also a delicate and smooth layer

■ **vitreous humor** clear watery fluid filling the posterior chamber of the eye. It is responsible for giving the eye its spherical shape.

■ **iris** pigmented portion of the eye. It is the muscular area that constricts or dilates to change the size of the pupil.

■ **lacrimal ducts** passageways carrying the lacrimal fluid (tears) from the lacrimal glands to the eye.

which, in the interior lid, slides over itself and the cornea. The eye is bathed by a fluid produced by the lacrimal glands. This fluid is transported by the **lacrimal ducts.** It is crucial to the cornea (which does not have blood vessels) because it is the source of lubrication, oxygen, and nutrients. If this important flow of fluid is prevented from traveling across the cornea, as for example, by a contact lens left in the unconscious patient, the surface of the eye may become damaged.

The motion of the eye is controlled by various small muscles located in the orbit (the eye socket) which in turn are controlled by cranial nerves. These muscles allow the eye to rotate through a wide degree of motion.

The Ear. The ear is also an essential sensory structure. Its functional structures are interior and exceptionally well protected from nearly all trauma. Only those involving great pressure differentials (i.e., blast and diving injuries), or basilar skull fracture, are likely to damage this area. The ear provides us with two very useful functions, hearing and positional sense. Hearing occurs when sound waves set the tympanic membrane (eardrum) to vibrating. The eardrum transmits the vibrations through three very small bones (the ossicles) to the **cochlea,** the organ of hearing. These vibrations stimulate the auditory nerve which transmits the signal to the brain.

■ **cochlea** snail-shaped structure within the inner ear containing the receptors for hearing.

The center responsible for the sense of position and motion is found in the **semicircular canals.** They are three hollow, fluid filled rings set at different angles. As the head moves, the fluid in the rings shifts and small, hairlike bodies sense the motion. These bodies send signals to the brain to maintain balance. They even tell how the head or body is moving when the eyes are closed. If this center is disturbed, and an excess of signals are sent to the brain, **vertigo** is experienced; that is, the person feels as though the head is spinning.

■ **semicircular canals** the three rings of the inner ear. They sense the motion of the head and provide positional sense for the body.

■ **vertigo** loss of positional sensation and the perception that the horizon and all points of reference are moving.

Neck. The neck region is a predominantly soft-tissue area containing several significant structures which are susceptible to trauma. The spinal column is, of course, midline and posterior. Lateral to the spine are large muscle masses which serve to strengthen and support the spine and neck. Anterior to the spinal column is the *trachea,* the hollow tube supported by C-shaped cartilage. The gasses of respiration travel through the trachea. Its posterior surface, shared with the *esophagus,* is purely soft tissue. Superior to the trachea is the *larynx,* a cartilaginous structure, consisting of the thyroid and cricoid cartilages. Like the trachea, it is hollow. The larynx houses the vocal cords and their supporting structures. Lateral to the trachea and the larynx are the carotid arteries and the jugular veins. Both have internal and external divisions and carry large volumes of blood to and from the head and brain. The carotid arteries are high pressure vessels that bleed profusely if opened. The jugular veins will also bleed profusely, although they generally carry low pressures.

PATHOPHYSIOLOGY OF HEAD, NECK, AND SPINAL TRAUMA

In considering trauma to the head, neck, and spine, it is best to focus on the following four areas: superficial, internal (CNS), sensory organ, and neck injuries. Superficial injuries include the scalp, underlying fascia, and the skeletal structures. Internal injury includes brain and spinal cord trauma. Sense organ injury involves the eye and inner ear, while neck trauma may involve only soft tissue.

Superficial Injury

The Scalp. The scalp can be the location of various types of soft tissue injuries expected from trauma. Contusions, lacerations, avulsions, and significant hemorrhage will often be obvious. Soft tissue injuries may manifest differently here than elsewhere on the body because the scalp covers the unyielding bony tissue of the skull. Minor swelling or internal bleeding has only one way to go, outward. It will be quite noticeable to palpation or close inspection. Sometimes, however, the assessment may be confounded by this arrangement. In blunt trauma the underlying fascia may be torn, while the overlying skin is still intact. Palpation may perceive a depression suggestive of depressed skull fracture where one does not exist. If a fracture does occur, the depression may be hidden due to internal bleeding and hematoma which either fills the depression or results in a spongy or firm bump. The scalp is not firmly attached to the skull from the frontal region to the occiput nor is it firmly attached laterally. If trauma is directed at a glancing angle, it may cause tearing and folding back of the scalp (an avulsion). The skull beneath may be exposed. Although the injury may be grotesque in appearance, it will generally heal well unless accompanied by gross contamination. Bleeding from the scalp and facial areas can be profuse because the blood supply in this region is great in order to protect the cranium and brain from heat loss in cold weather. The natural mechanisms that control hemorrhage are not as effective here as elsewhere in the body since the vessels are larger and not quite as muscular. Because blood loss can be severe and persistent, it can therefore contribute to shock.

Skull Fractures. Fractures of the skull underneath the scalp and soft tissue can range from very simple and minor breaks to those that are severe enough to cause life-endangering instability. Fractures of the cranium, facial region, and vertebral column are rarely of life-threatening proportions by themselves. It is the potential for central nervous system injury which is the deep and over riding concern. Therefore, any suspected fracture should receive the utmost consideration.

Because of its spherical shape, the skull will not fracture, unless trauma is extreme. Such fractures may present as linear, depressed, comminuted, or basilar in nature. (See Figure 15-8.) The linear fracture is a crack in the skull. In contrast, the depressed fracture is an actual displacement of its surface inward. In the comminuted fracture, fragments of the skull may penetrate the dura and cause physical harm to the cerebrum or cerebellum underneath. The basilar skull fracture affects the base of the skull. This area is permeated with *foramina* (openings) for the various cranial nerves and blood vessels. It also has hollow or open structures such as the sinuses, the orbits of the eye, the nasal cavity, the external auditory canal, and the inner ear. These spaces weaken the skull and make the basilar area prone to fracture. Signs and symptoms for this type of fracture vary, depending upon the areas involved. In the process of this fracture, blood vessels and other tissues are torn. The tearing of vasculature may cause internal bleeding which, in turn, may eventually cause classical discolorations. If the fracture affects the posterior region and the auditory canal, the blood may migrate to the mastoid (just posterior and slightly inferior to the ear). This discoloration is called **Battle's sign.** Another sign associated with basilar skull fracture, involving the orbits,

■ **Battle's sign** black and blue discoloration over the mastoid process (just behind the ear) which is characteristic of a basilar skull fracture.

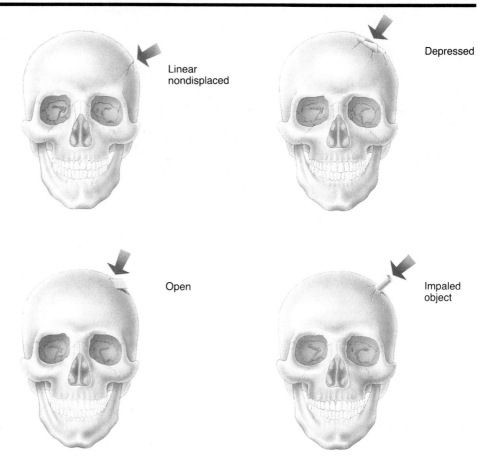

Linear
nondisplaced

Depressed

Open

Impaled
object

FIGURE 15-8 Types of skull fractures.

is called raccoon eyes. A discoloration around the eyes, it is more technically known as **bilateral periorbital ecchymosis.** (See Figure 15-9.) The ecchymotic (black and blue) discoloration and swelling will take time to develop and may not be visible during the prehospital phase of care. Basilar fracture can also cause an open wound between the subarachnoid space and either the nasal cavity or the external auditory canal. Such a

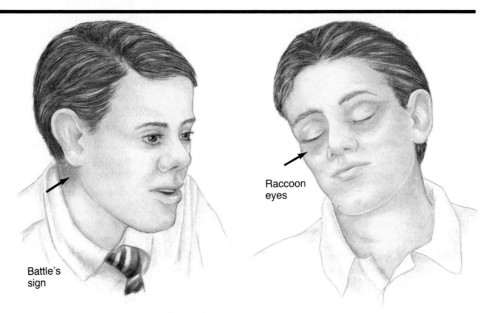

FIGURE 15-9 Battle's sign and racoon eyes may indicate a basilar skull fracture.

Battle's
sign

Raccoon
eyes

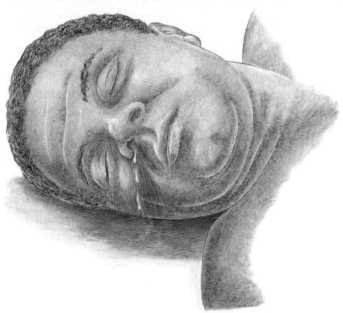

FIGURE 15-10 Drainage of blood or other fluid from the nose or ear may indicate a basilar skull fracture.

wound may allow for the leakage of cerebrospinal fluid. (See Figure 15-10.) While an open wound between the brain and the body's surface and the leakage of cerebrospinal fluid is of concern, it also may be beneficial. If intracranial pressure is increasing, the loss of CSF may help slow the rise in pressure. The fluid can be regenerated at a later time by the central nervous system.

Under some extreme traumatic circumstances, the skull can literally be destroyed. Because of its shape, it will resist trauma extremely well. However if sufficient trauma is experienced, it may shatter like an eggshell. Once again, the fracture of the skull is of minor concern when compared to injury to the contents it protects. Generally this type of skull fracture results in patient mortality due to severe physical injury to the cerebrum, cerebellum, or brainstem.

The Spinal Column. Spinal fracture may occur secondary to many mechanisms. Direct trauma may cause injury as may the compressional forces of head impact during a diving or auto accident. Compressional injury may also occur as the patient lands on his or her feet after a fall. Motion beyond the normal range, including hyperextension, hyperflexion, or extreme lateral or rotational motion, may contribute to injury. The spinal column may be subjected to direct trauma from blunt or penetrating sources. Blunt trauma may occur with falls against irregular surfaces or by contact with moving objects such as a baseball bat or industrial machinery. Penetrating injury may be initiated by a knife or gunshot wound to the neck or back. The wound pathway may enter anteriorly but may involve the spinal column without an exit wound. Remember that the spinal column is the only skeletal structure in the cervical and abdominal regions. Therefore, it may stop the projectile and absorb its energy without external signs. Compressional injury can also occur. Consider the forces involved as a diver impacts the bottom of a shallow pool, headfirst. Such an incident causes an extreme compressional force along the axis of the spinal column called **axial loading.** The resultant injury may be compressional fracture, intervertebral disc rupture, or both. The lumbar and the cervical spine is more frequently damaged than either the thoracic or sacral. The cervical region has a high incidence of injury because of the

■ **axial loading** extreme compressional forces applied to the axis of the vertebral spine.

support it provides for the head and the high range of motion it allows. Its relationship with the head is like that of a column of dominoes balancing a 20-pound bowling ball. While the vertebral "dominoes" are held together with strong ligaments, extreme acceleration or deceleration can cause injury.

The lumbar region is frequently injured by either axial loading (as in a fall) or by tangential forces (as in a seatbelt injury). The thoracic region is well protected by the support of the ribs, the overlying musculature, and by the **scapula.** Protection for the sacrum is provided by the ring structure of the pelvis and the musculature of the buttocks and the lower back. The ability of the column to protect the spinal cord is lost once a vertebral fracture has occurred. Any motion, direct (as in trying to move the head) or indirect (as in trying to lift the shoulders), may result in displacement of the cervical vertebra and damage to the cord. Since the space between the exterior of the cord and the interior of the spinal foramen is very small, especially in the cervical region, the slightest displacement can cause pressure, contusion, or laceration.

The Facial Region. Fractures of the facial bones are usually less dangerous than those of the vertebrae, yet they do represent significant trauma and potentially serious complications. Facial fractures may involve the zygoma, maxilla (upper jaw), and mandible. Most fractures will be stable with minor complications. The zygomatic fracture may entrap the muscles of the eye and limit motion. The **maxillary** fracture may present with little more than pain, crepitation, moderate deformity, and limited instability of the upper-jaw area. The mandible fracture may present with deformity, false motion, or limitation of the normal range of motion. Severe trauma and crushing fracture may require airway support. For example, in the attempted suicide using the shotgun placed under the jaw, the blast is often deflected away from the skull. Thus it injures the mandible, hard palate, maxilla, and zygoma. The resultant damage destroys the rigid support of the nasal and oral cavities, thereby possibly posing a serious threat to the airway which is difficult to manage.

Internal (CNS) Injury

Internal injuries of the central nervous system can be identified as originating from two distinct pathologies. The first are those that will generally improve with time: the concussion and the contusion. The second category are those which get worse as the injury progresses after the event. They include the intracranial, subdural, and epidural hemorrhage. Similar to most traumatic injury, brain and spinal cord injury may occur from blunt or penetrating trauma. Penetrating injury will usually be serious and life-threatening, and the signs of the injury mechanism will be obvious.

The Brain. Blunt trauma to the head is quite different from the fracture or soft tissue injury. Not only can the signs and symptoms be masked, but the existence of injury to the brain may be hard to discern. The brain is well protected from the effects of acceleration and deceleration by the scalp, skull, meninges, and the cerebrospinal fluid (CSF). To some degree, the brain floats in the CSF as you might do sitting in a bath tub. When deceleration occurs, the brain "sloshes" forward, pushing the CSF out of the way and gradually decelerating rather than stopping abruptly. Except for the most serious of decelerations, this mechanism protects the contents of the skull very well. If the trauma is too great, however, the

■ **scapula** large, flat and irregular bone located in the posterior shoulder which articulates with the humerus.

■ **maxillary** having to do with, or related to, the maxilla, the bone of the upper jaw.

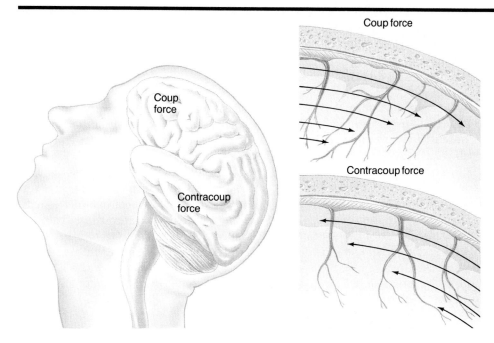

Coup force

Contracoup force

FIGURE 15-11 Coup and contrecoup movement of the brain.

brain will impact with the interior of the skull, causing the soft-tissue injuries one might expect: contusion, laceration, and hemorrhage. Such trauma also may cause the brain to "slosh" forward and then rebound, causing injury to the opposite surface of the brain. This phenomenon is called **contrecoup** (pronounced kontra koo) injury. (See Figure 15-11.) It is also important to note that the brainstem is the only location where the contents of the cranium are tethered. In the forceful acceleration or deceleration, the brain may tear or twist at this attachment. This causes a wide range of problems, ranging from the disruption of normal function, to tissue damage, to actual hemorrhage.

Physical impact may cause injury at various locations, dependent on the internal motions. The head may be impacted at the forehead, with associated frontal lobe injury. The cerebrum may then "slosh" back against the occipital region, causing a contrecoup injury. Concurrently, the cerebrum's motion may twist the brain stem, causing injury there. If we look at what happens to the brain during injury, we find it may be contused, lacerated, or it may hemorrhage either superficially or internally. The brain may also be jarred in such a way that it temporarily dysfunctions (a concussion).

Contusion/Concussion. The **concussion** is a transient loss of consciousness. It occurs when the brain has been violently shaken and its internal electrochemical function is disturbed. Dysfunction is brief, abating in under three to five minutes, or possibly extending to as much as one hour. Since the brain is not physically injured, complete recovery is expected. Concussion can occur simultaneously with other internal central nervous system injury.

The *contusion* is a more significant jarring with resultant cellular damage. Those tissues affected may dysfunction and swell, beginning an increase in the intracranial pressure and a decrease in the cerebral perfusion. There may also be some localized injury to a region of the brain manifested by a characteristic dysfunction or change in signs or symptoms. An example might be a change in patient personality noticed by relatives after trauma to the forehead, related to contusion of the frontal

■ **contrecoup** occurring on the opposite side; an injury to the brain opposite the site of impact.

■ **concussion** a transient period of unconsciousness. In most cases, the unconsciousness will be followed by a complete return of function.

lobe. Characteristic of both the contusion and the concussion is the improvement of the patient's level of consciousness and other physical signs after the insult. Only in cases where the pathology is progressive, as in intracranial hemorrhage, should the patient be expected to deteriorate after EMS arrival and intervention.

Intracranial Hemorrhage. Hemorrhage can occur at several locations within the cranium, each presenting with a different pathologic process. These injuries, from the deepest to the most superficial, are intracerebral, subdural and epidural.

The **intracerebral hemorrhage** is a rupture of a blood vessel within the substance of the brain with some limited bleeding into the nervous tissue. This particular injury is damaging, not only because of the area affected by the hemorrhage, but also the tissue edema resulting from the irritating effect of blood. The intracerebral hemorrhage will often present like a stroke with the manifestations of the insult occurring immediately. The presentation will be related to the function provided by the area involved in the injury. There will normally be some progression of the signs and symptoms with time.

Bleeding may also occur within the meninges, specifically beneath the dura and within the subarachnoid space. This is referred to as a **subdural hematoma.** (See Figure 15-12.) This hemorrhage is less dramatic in its growth and presentation than the epidural hematoma because blood loss is usually related to venous injury with smaller vessels involved. The subdural hemorrhage is also outside the brain, above the pia mater, and, therefore, does not cause cerebral irritation as the intracerebral hematoma does. The patient with a subdural hematoma will usually not present with overt signs and symptoms for hours or even days after the insult. This delayed presentation may allow the subdural hematoma to go undetected by the field and emergency department personnel. A week after the accident you may respond to a "Medical Call" only to find a patient with neurologic signs and symptoms. A careful assessment may uncover a history of an earlier injury which has caused the current presentation through this mechanism. This may especially occur in the elderly and chronic alcoholics. They are much more prone to subdural hematoma because the aging process and chronic alchoholism cause the brain to shrink. If paramedics are called to treat a patient suspected of chronic

■ **intracerebral hemorrhage** bleeding directly into the tissue of the brain.

■ **subdural hematoma** collection of blood directly beneath the dura matter.

✱ The subdural hematoma may not present with signs or symptoms for hours or even days after the injury.

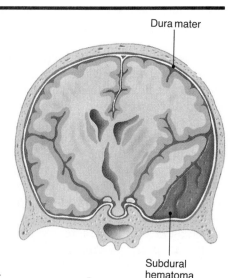

Dura mater

Subdural hematoma

FIGURE 15-12 Subdural hematoma.

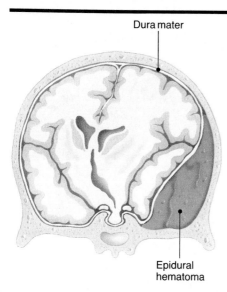

Dura mater

Epidural
hematoma

FIGURE 15-13   Epidural hematoma.

alcohol use, they should investigate for recent head trauma and be alert for any sign suggestive of internal CNS injury, even if the injury appears to be minor.

Bleeding between the dura mater and the interior surface of the skull is called **epidural hematoma.** (See Figure 15-13.) It usually involves arterial vessels (often the middle meningeal artery) and progresses rapidly toward unconsciousness. Since the bleeding is from a relatively high-pressure vessel, the intracranial pressure builds rapidly, compressing the cerebrum and increasing the pressure within the skull. The hemorrhage-induced intracranial pressure reduces oxygenated circulation to the nerve cells. Bleeding may be so extensive that the brain is displaced away from the injury site and pushed toward the foramen magnum. While the progression of this problem is rapid and quickly life threatening, immediate surgery can frequently reverse it.

The concussion, contusion, intracerebral hemorrhage, subdural hematoma, and epidural hematoma may occur in combination with each other. Occasionally the traumatic incident will cause the patient to sustain a concussion and epidural hematoma simultaneously. The concussion will result in immediate unconsciousness which lasts only minutes. The hematoma, over a period of 30 to 40 minutes, will begin to cause a decrease in the level of consciousness. Called a *lucid interval,* the interim period of consciousness is characteristic of the epidural hematoma.

Intracranial Pressure.   The circulation of blood through the brain tissue is a critical component in understanding the pathophysiology and significance of internal head injury. Since the cranium is a rigid container for the brain, cerebrospinal fluid, and the vasculature within, any expansion of one must be met by an equal reduction in another. The most mobile volume within the skull is the vascular space. Should any swelling, bleeding, or fluid accumulation occur, the circulating blood volume is reduced first. Then, as the pathology of the internal hemorrhage, cerebral edema, or both progress, the intracranial pressure increases. Such an increase initially causes the blood vessels to be compressed, limiting cerebral blood flow. As the cerebral blood flow is reduced, the brain becomes hypoxic and carbon dioxide concentrations rise. Hypercarbia causes the cerebral blood vessels to dilate and the systemic blood pressure to rise in an attempt to increase the cerebral circulation. This reflex also

■ **epidural hematoma** accumulation of blood between the dura mater and the cranium.

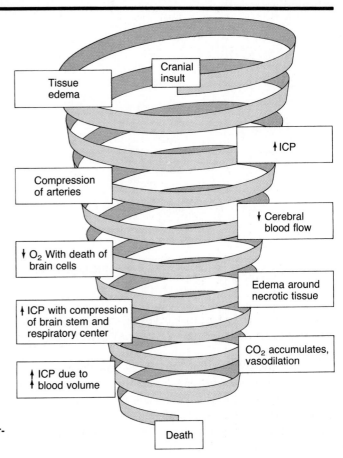

FIGURE 15-14 Pathway of deterioration following central nervous system insult.

Labels within figure:
- Cranial insult
- Tissue edema
- ↑ICP
- Compression of arteries
- ↓ Cerebral blood flow
- ↓ O₂ With death of brain cells
- Edema around necrotic tissue
- ↑ ICP with compression of brain stem and respiratory center
- CO₂ accumulates, vasodilation
- ↑ ICP due to ↑ blood volume
- Death

increases the rate at which the intracranial pressure rises. As the cycle of hypercarbia, increased blood pressure, and increased intracranial pressure continues, the pressure upon the brain causes it to displace away from the site of hematoma, hemorrhage, or edema and toward the foramen magnum. (See Figure 15-14.) This movement causes the third cranial nerve to become compressed (resulting in pupillary dilation) and the medulla oblongata to be compressed and displaced. The displacement will begin to push the medulla oblongata through the foramen magnum. Since the medulla controls respiratory rate and volume, as well as pulse rate and blood pressure, we see changes in these vital signs. Pulse rate will slow, the respirations will become rapid and deep or erratic, and blood pressure will rise. This collection of vital sign changes, called *Cushing's reflex,* is associated with increasing intracranial pressure. (See Figure 15-15.) The pressure on the medulla oblongata also causes other neurologic signs and symptoms. The patient may vomit without nausea, another sign that the medulla is being affected. Since the system responsible for consciousness, the **reticular activating system,** may be affected, the patient's level of consciousness will deteriorate.

The Spinal Cord.   Any cause to suspect head injury is also cause to suspect and treat the patient as though spinal fracture has occurred. Spinal injury may involve the vertebral structures, attaching ligaments, and/or the spinal cord. The greatest concern is directed at the injury or potential injury to the cord. Spinal column injury may occur with any movement beyond the normal range of motion for the patient. Extremes of energy are not necessary to induce injury, yet the results of injury can be devastating. Whenever the mechanism of injury includes events that could

✱ Increasing intracranial pressure may cause slowing pulse rate, deep or erratic respirations, and an increasing blood pressure (Cushing's Reflex).

■ **reticular activating system** the system responsible for consciousness. A series of nervous tissues keeping the human system in a state of consciousness.

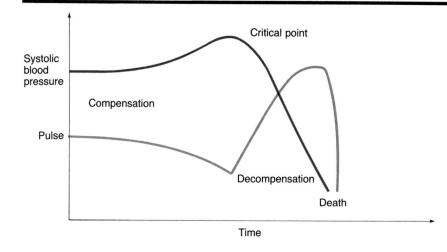

FIGURE 15-15 The response of systolic blood pressure and pulse during Cushing's Reflex.

Labels in figure: Systolic blood pressure, Pulse, Compensation, Critical point, Decompensation, Death, Time

have caused trauma to the spinal cord, the patient should be so treated until proven otherwise. That proof can only be gained in the emergency department with x-ray and other diagnostic tests.

Once significant forces have been directed at the spinal column, the danger of instability exists. Any motion, however slight, may cause the injury to compound. This may occur either by displacing the vertebral bodies to reduce the spinal foramen or apply pressure on the cord. The displacement may also compromise the vascular supply to the cord. Again, it is important to remember that the cells of the central nervous system are unable to repair themselves to any significant degree and thus any injury may be permanent.

Kinetic forces may also cause herniation of the intervertebral disc. If the herniation is directed toward the spinal foramen, it may place pressure on the cord causing dysfunction, physical damage, or both. The presentation of injury may vary with the degree of damage and the general condition of the patient. The signs and symptoms range from pain without motion, pain with motion, tenderness, point tenderness (tenderness at a specific location), to the complete absence of pain. More systemic signs may include bilateral paresthesia (a tingling or prickly sensation), anesthesia (absence of sensation), weakness, or paralysis. If injury to the cord has occurred, and disruption of its function exists, then a certain presentation would be expected. The patient should experience normal sensation and muscle control down to the dermatome corresponding to the affected vertebral area. Below that point he or she should experience bilateral sensory and motor loss. The absence of this severe presentation does not rule out the chance of vertebral fracture, instability of the column, nor the potential for catastrophic injury should the spine be mishandled.

The central nervous system injury will also affect activities under autonomic control. The blood vessels below the cord injury will be without innervation and will relax (dilate). In the shock patient, this will prevent the affected area from assisting with the normal response to shock, thereby contributing to the internal loss of blood volume. The skin of the affected area may be warm and dry when you would expect it to be cool and clammy. In the absence of shock, it may be cooler or warmer and drier than skin which still has autonomic control.

Cervical injury may compromise the sympathetic (thoraco-lumbar) nervous system so that it will no longer counter parasympathetic stimulation in the male. In this circumstance the patient will experience a prolonged penile erection, called *priapism*. Low-cervical injury may cause the patient to passively move the upper extremities to the so called "hold-up" position. The muscles pulling the arms down are paralyzed while those lifting them are intact. Any attempt by the patient to move the extremities will result in arms moving upward and into this position.

Although vertebral injury may not damage the spinal cord, it may injure the blood vessels, peripheral nerve roots, or connective tissue surrounding the vertebral body. Signs and symptoms may vary from localized pain to pain with attempted motion, to the signs of individual peripheral nerve root damage, generally involving one or more discrete dermatomes.

The forces injuring the spinal column are mostly transmitted. That is, initial impact occurred somewhere else and was transmitted to or through the spinal column. This transfer of the forces may leave more apparent injury elsewhere. The wound to the head and the patient's complaint of headache may distract you from cervical compression fracture. It is important to ensure that the potential for spinal injury is recognized even if the patient presents with frank signs and symptoms elsewhere.

Sense Organ Injury

The Eye. Although injury to the eye is not as frequent nor as life-endangering as spinal fracture, it is a serious injury which threatens one of the body's most important organs of perception. Since the eye is so well protected by the orbit around it, trauma is infrequent. Any insult must penetrate the eye socket to cause either blunt or penetrating injury. A serious threat to sight is laceration of the eye. The anterior structures are extremely delicate and the fluid within the chambers may not regenerate if lost. If significant penetrating injury occurs, especially if accompanied by aqueous or vitreous humor loss, it will result in loss of sight. Any object penetrating the eye will probably disturb the integrity of the anterior and/or posterior chambers. Its removal may allow the fluids to leak from the chambers and further threaten the patient's future vision.

Blunt trauma may result in several ocular presentations. *Hyphema* is a collection of blood in the anterior chamber and will present with a level of blood in front of the iris and pupil. It is secondary to bleeding within the anterior chamber. Hyphema requires evaluation by an opthalmologist. A less serious eye injury is *conjunctival hemorrhage*. Its presentation is dramatic in presentation yet will often clear without significant intervention or permanent vision loss. Two other, more serious ocular problems are central retinal artery occlusion and retinal detachment. *Acute retinal artery occlusion* is a vascular emergency in which the blood supply to the eye has been disrupted. It is a true emergency and a threat to future sight. The patient will complain of sudden and painless loss of vision in one eye. In *retinal detachment* the retina becomes separated from the posterior wall of the eye. The patient will complain of a dark curtain, obstructing part of the field of view.

Small foreign particles which land on the surface of the eye can cause ocular emergencies. The object may become embedded in the interior of the lid and then dragged across the cornea as the eye blinks. These corneal abrasions or lacerations will cause intense pain, even after the object has cleared.

Direct blows to the compressible globe can result in *blowout fractures*. A blowout fracture is a fracture of the thin bones comprising the orbit of the eye. The most common blowout fracture is of the inferior shelf of the orbit. Patients will often present with significant swelling. There may be pain in the maxillary sinus region. Some of the extraocular muscle can become entrapped, resulting in inability of the eye to look in a certain direction. These injuries are not life threatening but warrant evaluation in the emergency department.

The Ear. The middle and inner ear are infrequently injured due to their location and the skeletal integrity surrounding them. In cases of pressure or blast injury, rapid pressure differentials may injure the tympanum (the ear drum). The ear may also be affected in the basilar skull fracture which involves the auditory canal or the middle ear. The tympanum may be torn or the interior structures disrupted. Damage to the internal ear may result in hearing loss or vertigo.

Neck Injury

The neck is the last area of the head, neck, and spine to be examined regarding trauma. It is a critical area for concern because it contains structures which, if injured, can seriously endanger the patient's life. These include the trachea, larynx, esophagus, internal and external carotid arteries, and jugular veins.

The trachea and larynx are the most anterior structures of the neck. They are protected to some degree because the neck and chest protrude in front of them. Yet, they still are frequently injured. Injury may cause fracture and/or swelling which will compromise the lumen of these passageways or the function of the vocal cords. If the injury is sufficiently severe, the ability of the cartilaginous rings to maintain the tracheal opening may be lost. Consequently, the airway will close on inspiration. If penetrating injury is sustained by the trachea, it may cause subcutaneous emphysema. As the patient coughs or exhales forcefully, the resulting intratracheal pressure may push air into the soft tissue of the neck. Through palpation, the paramedic will feel the crackling of subcutaneous emphysema. Close observation will also detect a gradual increase in the diameter of the neck.

It is easy to overlook the importance of injury possibly involving the vasculature. The carotid and jugular vessels are major components of the circulatory system. If any of these vessels is damaged, the result can be severe blood loss, reduction in the cerebral circulation, and pulmonary emboli. Carotid artery bleeding will be severe, difficult to control, and may quickly lead to shock. The jugular veins, although rather low-pressure vessels, still carry large volumes of fluid. While blood loss may be extreme, there is a real concern for the aspiration of air. If a relatively large wound exists, the subatmospheric pressure of a strong inspiration may cause air to be drawn into the wound and the vein. The result may be massive and rapidly life threatening air emboli.

✱ If a large neck wound exists, it may allow for aspiration of air into the venous system.

ASSESSMENT AND CARE

Assessment of the trauma patient must be an orderly and comprehensive evaluation of the total patient, not simply a directed look for expected injuries. As described in Chapter 10, Advanced Patient Assessment, the paramedic must employ organized and well-practiced procedures to ensure proper priorities are observed and assessment is complete. The paramedic must review the dispatch information, survey the scene, and provide the primary and secondary assessment. He or she must also evaluate the vital signs and procure a patient history. These elements of the assessment are as important for the head, neck and spine injury patient as for any other trauma or medical emergency. The paramedic needs to remember that intervention and possible transport may precede the complete assessment should problems occur involving the ABC's, diminishing level of consciousness, or the development of shock.

The first element of the assessment following arrival at the accident scene is a rapid scene survey. The paramedic must rule out hazards present that may threaten both the patient and the rescuers. The number and location of patients must be identified as should the need for any additional assistance. Most importantly, and especially for the potential head and spine patient, the mechanism of injury must be determined and evaluated. The paramedic should examine the vehicle accident or other kinetic event. Ask yourself, "Were the forces involved great enough to cause any significant injury to the brain and/or spinal cord?" Look specifically for evidence of the strength of impact and the kinetic energy involved. Is the windshield broken? Are there deformities to the vehicle interior? Was the fall from a height over 15 feet? Was the trauma transmitted through or to the head or spinal column? If any of the questions are answered in the affirmative, then treatment must address possible head and spine injury.

* Both head and spine injury may occur without recognizable signs and symptoms; therefore the paramedic must maintain a high level of suspicion for these injuries.

Both head and spine injury may be present without recognizable signs or symptoms. It is essential that a high level of suspicion be kept whenever trauma is involved. If either of the conditions is suspected, rapid transport must be either under way or being arranged before the secondary assessment begins. If any possibility of spinal injury exists, the spine must be immobilized. The head should be manually and gently brought to the neutral position (unless resistance is felt) and maintained there while the primary assessment is performed. As soon as the patient's condition allows, the head should be mechanically stabilized through one of the techniques identified in this chapter. Assessment of the patient with central nervous system injury must look for associated injuries as well as establish a baseline to be followed by serial assessments. This will help identify whether the patient is improving, stable, or deteriorating. Careful attention must be given to detail so the slightest change in level of consciousness or other neurologic sign will be noticed.

Primary Assessment

The primary assessment, and the interventions called for by its findings, should be performed for any trauma victim, especially the suspected head, neck, or spine injury patient. CNS injury can easily account for problems with the ABC's. Therefore, their assessment and protection is of utmost significance. The D and E of this assessment also evaluates signs and symptoms possibly caused by injury of this nature. A well-performed primary assessment will quickly determine the extent of on-scene treatment required. (See Figure 15-16.) It will also determine if the patient would be better served by on-scene care, as in the suspected cervical spine injury.

The cervical spine must be immobilized immediately after injury is suspected. Initial stabilization should be manual. (See Figure 15-17.) The head should be gently brought to the neutral position, unless pain or resistance is felt. It is manually maintained in position with sufficient force to take the weight of the head off the spine and prevent its motion. This support is held by one of the team members. It will remain his or her responsibility until the head and torso are secured to the short spine board, long spine board or vest type device (e.g., K.E.D.). The head should be stabilized either from the front or from behind the patient. The head must

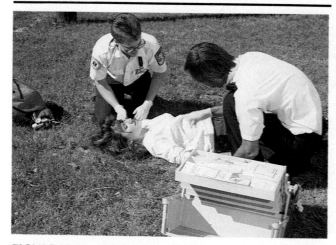

FIGURE 15-16 When treating a patient with a possible head injury, quickly assess the ABCs.

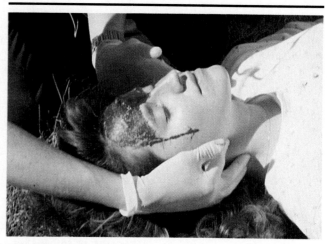

FIGURE 15-17 Maintain manual immobilization of the cervical spine while applying a rigid cervical collar.

be supported by grasping the mastoid and the angle of the mandible with the medial part of the palm of the hand. This support prevents movement posteriorly, anteriorly, or laterally. It is crucial to maintain the spine in a neutral position, a task not as easy as it first seems. The spine must be stabilized without displacement to the left or the right and in its normal curvature, anterior to posterior. The spine changes the direction of curvature from concave to convex, with each of the vertebral regions. The curvature of the cervical spine usually positions the patient's head about one to two inches above the surface of the spine board.

A cervical collar will help to limit any cervical motion and is essential in the spinal immobilization procedure. (See Figure 15-18.) It should be rigid and the proper size for the patient. The collar should fit snugly, limiting the motion of the cervical spine, but not causing hyperextension. Application of it should occur without any displacement of the spine or discomfort to the patient. Its sole purpose is to aid immobilization. Thus, it should never be counted on for any stabilization of the injured area. Manual immobilization should continue uninterrupted, until replaced by mechanical immobilization.

Airway should be assessed with a special watch for the loss of airway control and the potential for vomiting. Unresponsive patients who have

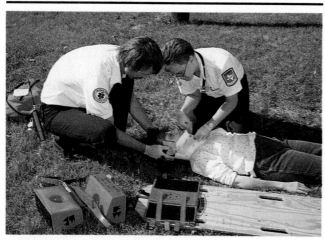

FIGURE 15-18 Apply a rigid cervical collar.

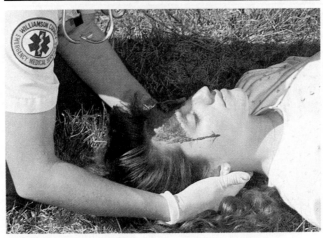

FIGURE 15-19 Manually immobilize the cervical spine. Use the modified jaw thrust maneuver to open the airway if necessary.

CNS injury may be without a gag reflex and the normal mechanisms of airway protection. They may also be prone to vomiting, sometimes without preceding nausea. The airway should be secured early in the assessment process if head injury is suspected. (See Figure 15-19.) Facial trauma may also endanger the airway. If there is indication of facial trauma, paramedics should assess the nasal and oral passages carefully, alert for any potential threat to the airway. That threat may be from fluids, edema, or possibly the loss of support for the airway due to massive facial fracture. If the airway is threatened, protect it with nasopharyngeal airway, oropharyngeal airway, endotracheal tube, or EOA/EGTA insertion, observing cervical spine precautions. (See Chapter 11.) Advanced airway care procedures should be employed if the patient has a lowered level of consciousness or reduced or absent gag reflex. (See Figure 15-20.)

Care should be observed to safeguard the cervical spine during the intubation. The head position should be maintained by one rescuer while the paramedic attempts oral, nasal, or digital intubation. Although oral intubation is discussed elsewhere in the text, it needs special modification

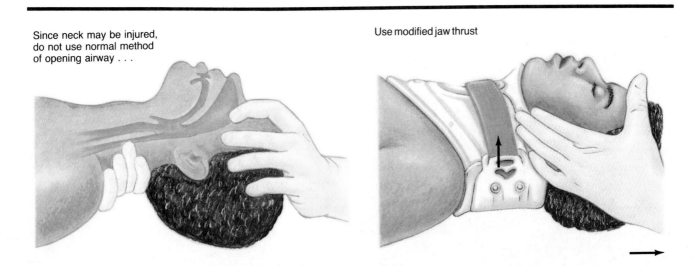

Since neck may be injured, do not use normal method of opening airway . . .

Use modified jaw thrust

FIGURE 15-20 The modified jaw-thrust maneuver should be used in patients suspected of having a spinal injury.

for the spinal trauma patient. Because of the potential for spinal injury in the unconscious patient, oral intubation must be accomplished without the normal flexion of the neck and extension of the head (the sniffing position). One care provider must rigidly immobilize the head by holding stabilization while another introduces the laryngoscope. Downward pressure may be applied to the thyroid cartilage to aid visualization of the vocal cords. Oral intubation under these circumstances is at best difficult, especially in the patient who is incompletely anesthetized, found supine on the floor or ground, and has an airway filled with vomitus.

Two other possibly useful techniques for these special patients are nasal and digital intubation. Nasal intubation, a blind procedure used in a breathing patient, allows the cervical spine to remain in the neutral position. The endotracheal tube is inserted into the largest naris. It is then directed posteriorly, curving toward the floor of the nasal cavity. The tube is advanced to the length of an oral airway (the distance between the earlobe and the corner of the mouth). At this point the insertion continues, but slowly, while the paramedic listens for the sounds of respiration. The tube is gently manipulated until the respiratory sounds are loudest and then is advanced during the inspiration. With luck, the tube will enter the trachea and the airway will be secure. There are specially designed endotracheal tubes (the Endotrol) that have tips which can be directed. Such a tube will assist in proper placement. This technique is difficult and determining proper placement is essential.

In digital intubation, the other technique, the paramedic "walks" his or her index and second finger along the patient's tongue until the epiglottis is felt and lifted. Stiffened with a stylet, the tube is inserted along the fingers and the epiglottis. During this procedure, it may be helpful for an assisting EMT or paramedic to place pressure on the thyroid cartilage to displace it slightly downward. This motion will bring the opening of the trachea more in line with the tube path and increase the probability of proper tube placement. The paramedic should gently advance the tube beyond his or her fingers and a few centimeters into the patient's trachea. The mouth must be kept open. Also the paramedic needs to protect his or her fingers should the patient decide to bite down during the procedure.

Once placement of the tube appears to be correct, it should be checked with auscultation of the axillary areas bilaterally. The paramedic should watch for bilaterally equal chest wall excursion. He or she should also listen to the epigastric area for sounds of esophageal intubation. If the tube is properly placed, the cuff should then be inflated and hyperventilation of the patient continued. This technique is quite effective, although it is essential to confirm placement by listening for breath sounds and the signs of adequate respirations. Attempts at endotracheal intubation can increase the parasympathetic (vagal) tone. This, in turn, may increase intracranial pressure and the bradycardia or other dysrhythmias already present from head injury. Thus, the intubation attempts should be rapidly executed. They should also be preceded and followed by hyperventilation with 100% oxygen.

The second step in the primary assessment, the evaluation of breathing, can reveal diagnostic signs suggestive of head injury. The particular pattern of respiration should be determined early in the assessment. If the patient displays any erratic, abnormally deep, or unusual respiratory pattern, it should be identified. Central neurogenic hyperventilation (very deep and rapid), Cheyne-Stokes (cyclic increasing, decreasing then apneic), Biot's (erratic and gasping), ataxic (irregular, forced and gasping), or agonal (infrequent gasping) respirations may reflect brain stem injury and the need for rapid transport. If, at this point, there is an indication that the patient might have sustained a head injury and is developing one of the CNS injuries discussed earlier in this chapter, he or she should be hyperventilated with high-flow oxygen. (Caution should be used if the patient is being ventilated by mask, as gastric distention and emesis may occur secondary to gastric insufflation.) Hyperventilation and high-flow oxygen will reduce the circulating carbon dioxide level and cerebral hypercarbia. It will also elevate the oxygen saturation of the blood and increase oxygen delivery to the brain. Both will help to reduce the development of the cerebral edema, decreasing the progression of intracranial pressure and the extent of the injury.

Within the standard primary assessment, the Circulatory status should be checked. The results may also support the possibility of head injury. If the pulse is slow and bounding, it may be a part of Cushing's reflex, especially if accompanied by a rapid and deep respiratory effort.

The Disability component of the primary assessment is important to the paramedic, especially when central nervous injury is present. Critical elements of a rapid central nervous system assessment occur during the primary patient evaluation. The level of consciousness should be established by assessing the patient's level of orientation or response to stimuli. To establish a CNS baseline, quickly check to see if the patient is oriented to time, place (or event), person, and one's own person or, if the patient does not respond to questioning, look for a response to verbal or painful stimuli. This will allow you to identify any deterioration or improvement during subsequent evaluations. If the evaluation reveals any response lower than orientation to place (or the event), CNS injury should be suspected. The patient should be carefully monitored for further deterioration and prepared for rapid transport to the emergency department.

If the patient appears fully oriented and there are no other reasons to suspect head or spine injury, the secondary assessment and care should continue at the scene. The level of consciousness determined here should act as a baseline for further CNS assessment during care and transport. To assist the paramedic and the medical control physician in determining the patient's condition, the Glasgow Coma Scale may be used. (See Table 15-1.) Determine the patient's best eye opening, motor response, and verbal response. If the score is below 12, immediate transport should be considered. At this time the patient may also be checked for other signs of serious CNS Deficit. If there is any loss in the normal muscle tone or any part of the extremities feels abnormally cool or warm, it should be carefully analyzed. A loss of muscle tone or unilateral temperature variation may reflect insult to the opposite hemisphere of the brain. If the lower parts of the body have lost tone or present with temperature difference bilaterally, the injury may be spinal. While the primary assessment must concentrate upon the overall assessment, findings may require these areas to be reassessed more carefully during the secondary assessment.

Additional findings of head, neck, and spine injury may be Exposed by the final component of primary assessment. The exam will look to the head, neck, chest and abdomen for early visible signs of developing life threat. Thus, the head may present with any of the soft tissue or skeletal injuries discussed earlier in the chapter. At this time the focus is on indications of central nervous system injury, whether internal head injury or cervical spine trauma. The neck area should be inspected for soft-tissue injury. Any sign of trauma, penetrating or blunt, should be investigated. The paramedic should especially watch for an open wound to the carotid arteries, jugular veins, the trachea, or esophagus.

TABLE 15-1 Glasgow Coma Scale

	Test	Patient's Response	Score
Eye Opening	Spontaneous	Opens eyes on own	4
	speech	Opens eyes when asked to in a loud voice	3
	Pain	Opens eyes when pinched	2
	Pain	Does not open eyes	1
Best Motor Response	Commands	Follows simple commands	6
	Pain	Pulls hand away when pinched	5
	Pain	Pulls a part of body away when examiner pinches him	4
	Pain	Flexes body inappropriately to pain (decorticate posturing)	3
	Pain	Body becomes rigid in an extended position when examiner pinches victim (decerebrate posturing)	2
	Pain	No motor response to pain	1
Verbal Response (Talking)	Speech	Carries on a conversation correctly and tells examiner where he is, who he is, month, and year	5
	Speech	Confused and disoriented	4
	Speech	Speech is clear but makes no sense	3
	Speech	Makes garbled sounds that examiner can not understand	2
	Speech	Makes no sounds	1

• Assess the patient's score in each category, and total the scores of the three categories. A total score of 7 or less indicates coma.
• Assess the patient's score in each category frequently, and record each observation and the time it was made. Keep a parallel record of vital signs.

Any severe bleeding from the head, neck or facial area should be controlled by direct pressure. (See Figure 15-21.) The paramedic should be careful to rule out an unstable skull fracture before applying pressure. If hemorrhage originates from the neck or there is an open wound to this area, it must be sealed with an occlusive dressing. The body must also be kept at a 15-degree angle, with the head down (unless otherwise contraindicated). This position will ensure that the venous pressure in the jugular veins remains positive and that the chance for air emboli is reduced.

Spinal injury may cause compromise of vascular control below the lesion. At best, this will keep the area from assisting with the compensatory mechanisms of shock (vasoconstriction) and at worse will contribute to hypovolemia. The PASG may provide needed support for the vascular system. It should be used cautiously if the patient is "belly breathing." Abdominal pressure may further compromise the efforts of the diaphragm to exchange the total respiratory volume. Should the patient be displaying the signs of compensated shock: rapid weak pulse, rapid shallow respirations, lowered sensorium, and so on; several steps should be taken. The PASG should be applied, and inflated. Then, once the primary assessment has been completed, two large bore IVs should be started with trauma tubing, running normal saline or lactated Ringer's solution, with

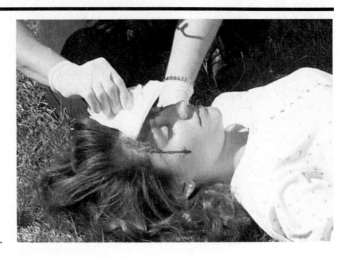

FIGURE 15-21 Control any bleeding.

pressure infusers ready. Respiration must be observed carefully for any signs of compromise from pulmonary edema or from the PASG impinging on respiratory excursion.

Assessment of the abdomen may provide the evaluator with signs of CNS problems. Should the belly be moving with exaggerated motion and the chest with little or opposing motion, then diaphragmatic breathing and high cervical injury should be suspected. Remember that the clear cut signs of head and spine injury may not appear until late in the assessment, during care, or patient transport. Just because there are no signs or symptoms of acute internal head injury at the end of the primary assessment does not rule out an underlying and progressing problem. If any part of the mechanism of injury or the primary assessment even suggests the possibility of head or spine injury, care must be instituted immediately. For the spine injury patient, that means immediate and continued spinal immobilization. For the head injury patient that includes high flow oxygen, hyperventilation at 25 full breaths per minute and immediate transport. The head injury patient must also be considered as having a spine injury and complete cervical immobilization should, therefore, be carried out.

The primary assessment should continue as should the care for any immediately life-threatening problems that are discovered. At its conclusion the decision should be made to either immediately transport or to care for the patient at the scene. Should the decision for immediate transport be made for a patient suspected of spine injury, the paramedic is confronted with one of the most difficult movement problems encountered in prehospital care. The patient must be rapidly extricated, yet any uncontrolled motion may permanently damage the spinal cord. Extreme care must be instituted to keep the spine in alignment, while the patient is moved to the waiting long spine board and stretcher. Teamwork must be used to keep the patient's nose, navel, and toes on the same plane without any flexion, extension, lateral motion, or rotation. (See Figure 15-22.) If the patient is seated, as in a car, then he or she must be rotated 90 degrees and carefully lowered to the board. The patient should be quickly secured, moved to the ambulance, and transported with further care enroute. If the need for movement is not so emergent, and the patient is found in the seated position, the more involved but safer procedure of short spine board or vest-type immobilization must be used. These movement devices provide a platform to which the shoulders, sacrum and oc-

✱ When rapid extrication of the spine-injured patient is required, it must be accomplished with extreme care to keep the spine aligned.

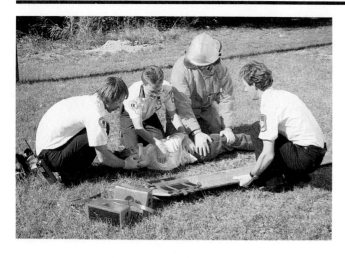

FIGURE 15-22 The patient should be moved as a unit keeping the entire spine in alignment.

ciput can be affixed and the spine immobilized. After the patient is placed in the supine position, the value of the movement device is diminished. The patient, device, and long board are then secured together.

The Secondary Assessment

The elements of the secondary assessment should progress in relatively the same way for the various types of trauma patients. The secondary assessment should include the head to toe assessment, evaluation of vital signs, and a complete patient history. Any findings should support the "whole picture" of the incident or they should be reevaluated to determine their significance. Any finding of injury, dysfunction, or patient complaint should be periodically reevaluated to determine what progression, if any, is occurring.

Head-to-Toe Assessment. The secondary assessment begins with the head. The cranium should be palpated and inspected over its entirety. Any deformity, wound (whether open or closed), or fluid loss should be carefully observed. While the characteristic discoloration of Battle's sign is a late sign, the region behind the ear should be visualized. The external auditory canal and nasal cavity should equally be assessed for the presence of cerebrospinal fluid, blood, or both. All visualization and palpation must be performed without displacing the head, neck or spine. The facial region should first be checked for soft tissue injury or fracture. The frontal, zygomatic, nasal and maxillary bones as well as the mandible should be palpated. Any swelling, crepitus, or instability will establish injury. The orbital ridge and nasal region should be carefully palpated since they are commonly involved in trauma. Any early signs of orbital swelling may suggest the presence of a basilar skull fracture or blowout fracture.

Paramedics should be careful in their estimation of the quantity and significance of blood loss when it involves the head. The tendency is to overestimate the hemorrhage from this area because it is very apparent and associated with the area related to personal identity. Blood loss from the head alone infrequently accounts for hypovolemic shock. If the signs and symptoms of shock exist, paramedics should look elsewhere for a possible cause. An exception to this rule, however, occurs with children, where blood loss can be both significant in relative volume and a threat to life.

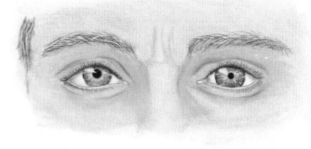

FIGURE 15-23 Anisocoria (unequal pupils) may indicate underlying CNS injury.

✳ The pupils are a direct window into the brain, and can quickly and accurately tell the general condition of the central nervous system.

Special attention should be given to the pupils. (See Figure 15-23.) They are a direct window into the brain and can quickly and accurately tell the general condition of the central nervous system. The eye will reflect the level of cerebral function as well as indicate some specific problems. If the pupil responds briskly to light-intensity changes, it can be generally presumed that the brain (and eye) are well perfused. If the pupil is slow to respond, CNS depression is present, either due to the effects of drugs or circulatory insufficiency. If the pupil is dilated and fixed, severe CNS injury or hypoxia may exist. If the pupillary signs are bilateral, the paramedic can presume the problem includes both hemispheres, while unilateral response reflects a problem on one side which may progress to involve the other. (See Figure 15-24.) The pupils should be examined for signs of trauma, impaled objects, and the presence of contact lenses. Specifically look for loss of aqueous or vitreous humor, foreign objects, or hyphema.

Reexamination of the nasal and oral cavities will ensure that they remain unobstructed from tissue swelling or deformity. It may also reveal hemorrhage, possibly containing cerebrospinal fluid. Fluid from the nose or ear that drops on a towel or sheet may show the target sign, or "halo sign" (a dark circle surrounded by a lighter one). While not absolute proof, this sign is suggestive of CSF in the blood and basilar skull fracture. (See Figure 15-25.)

The neck should be palpated over its entire surface; laterally, anteriorly, and posteriorly. Any tenderness, point tenderness, local warmth or

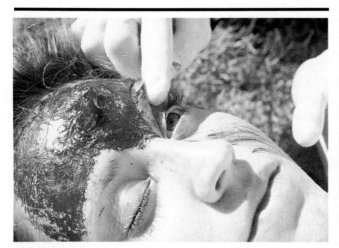

FIGURE 15-24 During the secondary assessment be sure to inspect both eyes.

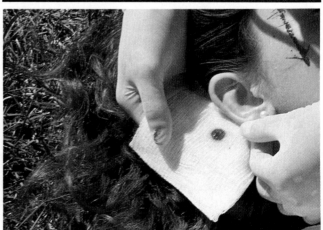

FIGURE 15-25 "Halo Test" to detect the presence of cerebrospinal fluid. If CSF is present, it will diffuse faster across a paper towel or sponge because it is thinner than blood.

outright pain along the vertebral column should call for immediate spinal immobilization. Blunt soft tissue injury of the neck, as determined by swelling, tenderness, or subcutaneous emphysema laterally or anteriorly, should direct concern to the vasculature and trachea traversing this region. The existence of an open wound should call for bleeding control and protection against vascular aspiration of air. The neck assessment should include palpation of the trachea to ensure its integrity has not been lost. Any deformity, swelling, crepitus or development of subcutaneous emphysema suggests injury.

During the head-to-toe assessment the entirety of the vertebral column should be palpated. Specific signs and symptoms examined for include pain, tenderness, deformity, and any signs of local warmth (suggesting early development of edema and injury).

The remainder of the physical assessment should look for the signs and symptoms of CNS injury. Any **flaccid** area, reduced sensation, weakness or outright paralysis should direct attention to head or spinal injury. Temperature variation affecting a specific body region, making it either cooler or warmer than the rest of the body, should be suspected of being of CNS origin. The paramedic should determine whether flaccidity or temperature variation is unilateral or bilateral and at what anatomic level the dysfunction begins. Blood pressure evaluation may support the probability of head injury. Elevated blood pressure may reflect an increase in intracranial pressure. It is the third of the signs of Cushing's reflex to be gathered during patient assessment. If serial blood pressure evaluation demonstrates an upward trend, this further indicates the presence of increasing intracranial pressure. The patient who is experiencing the effects of a head injury, or for that matter, any unconscious patient, should be monitored for dysrhythmias. CNS injury can present with bradycardia due to brain stem pressure, tachycardia due to vagus nerve interruption, and general irritability secondary to hypoxia, hypercarbia, or other metabolic disturbance.

MANAGEMENT

The management of the head, spine, and neck injury is a crucial part of total trauma care. Paramedics must ensure that the patient is not further harmed by rescuer actions (or the lack thereof). Thus, the patient must not remain at the scene after transport should have occurred, nor can the paramedic fail to provide stabilization and care as called for by the patient assessment. While spinal immobilization is predominantly a skill of the basic EMT, the paramedic is held to a higher standard of care in its application.

Prior to applying a movement device such as the vest or short spine board, the patient should be evaluated distally for motor and sensory function. It is essential to ensure the level of function before mechanical immobilization is applied. Serial assessment should continue during the application and patient transport to the hospital. The neutral position must be maintained during the immobilization and movement. Firm padding should be placed between the patient's occiput and the spine board or vest while the patient is seated. If the patient is found supine, or moved to this position through rapid extrication, the padding may be approximated. Ensure that it does not cause extension of the neck. Be careful not to place the padding behind the neck as it may cause pressure on the injured cervical spine or induce extension. (See Figures 15-26 and 15-27.) The head should be prevented from any lateral or turning motion by a

* Any sizeable open neck wound should be sealed against the possibility of vascular aspiration of air.

■ **flaccid** relaxed, flabby, or without muscle tone.

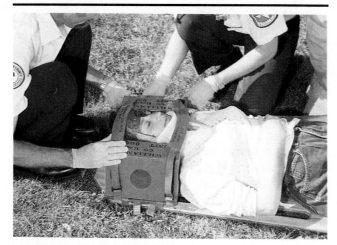

FIGURE 15-26   Stabilize the neck prior to transport.

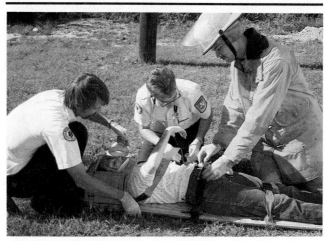

FIGURE 15-27   Secure the arms and legs.

cervical immobilization device (CID). The device may be commercial or fabricated from a blanket. It should place gentle but stabilizing pressure on the lateral sides of the head and trap the head firmly. This device should then be firmly affixed to the spine board. The head is further held in position with dressing materials or tape crossing the forehead and the chin flange of the cervical collar. Ensure that the collar flange does not restrict breathing or flex the neck.

If the patient who is found standing presents with a mechanism of injury suggesting that a spine injury could have occurred, he or she should be immobilized as found. (See Figures 15-29 through 15-31.) The long spine board should be placed behind the patient. Then he or she should be secured to it. The operation should not manipulate but immobilize the patient carefully to the device. Once the head, shoulders, pelvis and extremities are secured, the patient can be lowered to the supine position and transported. One of the paramedics should initiate an IV line to

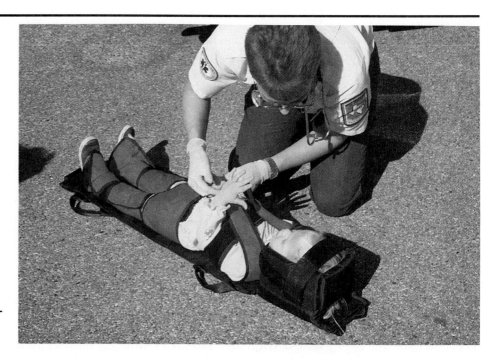

FIGURE 15-28   Pediatric immobilization devices are effective in immobilizing the spine of a child.

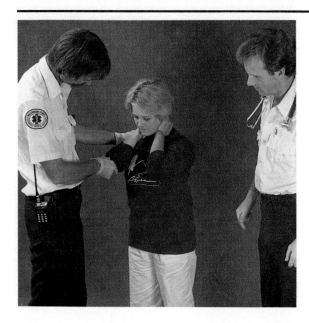

FIGURE 15-29 The standing patient complaining of neck pain following an injury should also receive spinal immobilization.

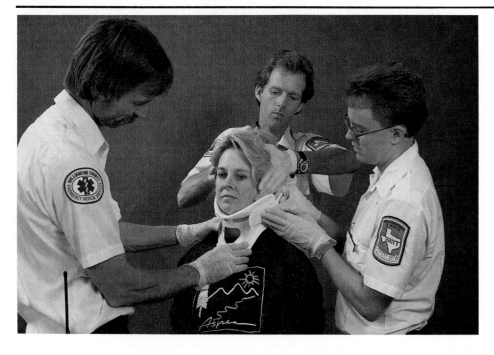

FIGURE 15-30 The cervical spine should be manually immobilized and a rigid cervical collar placed.

ensure rapid venous access. This should be accomplished enroute if the patient has been identified for immediate transport. It can be accomplished at the scene if the patient is receiving on-scene stabilization. The access should be accomplished with a large bore cannula and normal saline run slowly unless hypovolemia is suspected.

The patient suspected of central nervous system injury should be watched for hypothermia. Loss of nervous control over the peripheral capillary beds reduces the body's ability to control and maintain heat loss. The patient should be kept warm, with any heat loss reduced, except when the environment is extremely warm. In that circumstance, the paramedic should be careful to ensure that the patient does not overheat.

✳ Watch for and prevent hypothermia in the patient with central nervous system injury.

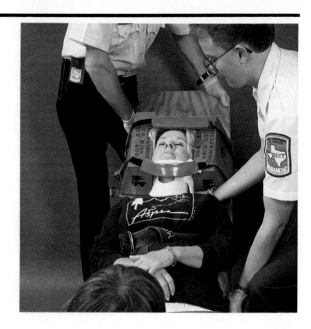

FIGURE 15-31 The long spine board can be applied while the patient remains standing.

Specific wounds to the head and neck can be cared for once the general concerns for central nervous system injury have been addressed. The paramedic should apply the basics of bleeding control and wound dressing. However, there are many special concerns for care of soft-tissue injuries to the head, neck, and special sense organs. Impaled objects, whether penetrating the skull, the neck, or the facial region, should be left in place. They should be protected, so further motion does not occur either from the object being bumped or from the forces of inertia during patient movement. The only exception to this rule is the object impaled in the cheek, threatening the airway. Since the cheek contains no critical structures and bleeding can be controlled, the object can be safely removed.

The nasal cavity can be a source of extensive hemorrhage which may be difficult to control. Nasal packing at the emergency department may be required in the posterior bleed to protect the airway both from blood loss and vomiting secondary to swallowing large volumes of blood. Anterior bleeding can be often slowed or stopped by compressing the nasal cartilage between the fingers. The paramedic needs to remember that it takes about 10 minutes for normal blood to clot. Nasal pressure must be held for at least that long.

Eye injuries must be protected and the patient transported. Any impaled object should be kept from jostling by a cup style dressing. Both eyes should be covered to reduce the sympathetic motion of the injured eye. These injuries cause a great deal of anxiety in the patient. If the patient's eyes are covered, the paramedic should warn the patient of any movement, such as transport to the ambulance, before it occurs. In the case of an unconscious or semiconscious patient, the hands may need to be tied to protect the wound from the urge to touch. Such a patient should be left supine if possible.

Patient History

Patient questioning is one of the key aspects of assessment of the head or spine injury victim. The elements of the chief complaint and past medical history can contribute greatly to the overall picture of what happened or may be happening. Questioning will allow close monitoring of the level of consciousness and simultaneously determine the mechanism of injury and symptoms of any injury. Evaluate the chief complaint for any indication of CNS problem. Any regionalized tingling sensations, numbness, weakness, or paralysis may indicate CNS injury. Complaint of headache should be investigated in detail to determine exactly where and how the pain presents to the patient. Although this information may not be specifically used to guide care, it may be invaluable to the emergency department staff.

The history should continue with an investigation looking into any unusual symptoms noticed by the patient. In the developing head injury, the patient may be aware of changes in vision, hearing, sensation, and motor control which could shed light on the location of the initial injury. As the problem progresses the level of consciousness may decline, and the patient may become unable to relate this information to the paramedic or emergency department staff. The paramedic should ensure that the complete results of the neurologic assessment are remembered and recorded. CNS changes may also be noticed by relatives and bystanders. They may possess a history that precedes your arrival and may see a progression before its recognizable to you. While casual observers may be unreliable, police or fire personnel are usually well practiced in objectively noting the circumstances of an emergency scene. Relatives may also be aware of otherwise unnoticeable changes from the preaccident personality. Paramedics should be especially aware of personality changes (including bizarre behavior) and changing level of consciousness. They must attempt to elicit the immediate history of the event, to determine what led up to the accident and what happened immediately afterwards. The patient may be unaware of these circumstances. Loss of memory preceding an event is called *retrograde amnesia*, while loss after it is called *antegrade amnesia*. Both are commonly found and may reflect effects of emotional rather than physiologic trauma. If central nervous system problems are suspected, the patient must be serially evaluated so any change in the level of orientation, or consciousness, or the presenting signs and symptoms will be rapidly apparent.

Drug Therapy

Once the immediate needs of the patient are cared for, certain pharmacological interventions may be ordered by medical control. These may include mannitol, furosemide (Lasix), dexamethasone (Decadron), and anticonvulsant medications (Valium).

Mannitol is one of the first-line drugs used in the care of cerebral edema. It is a potent diuretic which dehydrates the central nervous system, reducing cerebral edema, especially during the first 12 hours post-injury. It is a modified glucose molecule found naturally in fruits and vegetables. A relatively large molecule, mannitol remains in the extracellular space. There it draws out the cellular fluid, causing its elimination by the kidneys. Mannitol's major drawback is that by reducing brain mass and intracranial pressure, it may allow the rate of intracranial hemorrhage to increase. The drug should be used cautiously, if at all, in patients with chest trauma or signs of pulmonary edema, because transient increase in intravascular volume may exacerbate chest congestion. If any signs of pulmonary edema appear during therapy, the drip should be discontinued. Mannitol may also cause dehydration and electrolyte imbalance, although these problems usually develop after prolonged therapy. It should be given by IV drip only in doses of 0.5 to 2.0 g/kg of body weight and bolused slowly. Mannitol is normally supplied in 500 mL premixed IV bags of 15% or 20% solution or in 25 mL vials of a 20% solution. Use of the 20% mannitol solution in the 25 mL vial is recommended for field administration. The infusion must be filtered because mannitol may crystallize. This especially occurs if the higher concentrations are used and temperatures drop below 45 degrees. The crystals will dissolve if the solution is gently heated and agitated.

A second diuretic which may be ordered for the head injury patient is furosemide (Lasix). It is a potent diuretic frequently used during congestive heart failure and pulmonary edema. It may also be of benefit for treating the syndrome of increasing intracranial pressure. Lasix causes some vasodilation as well as rapid diuresis. These two effects reduce the cardiovascular volume and blood pressure, hence reducing the progression of cerebral edema. The drop in systemic blood pressure may cause the cerebral blood flow to slow, increasing hypoxia and hypercarbia. Lasix often comes in a preloaded syringe and is given in an IV bolus of 20 to 80 mg. The medication should be administrated very slowly, over 1 to 2 minutes. It is generally contraindicated for the pregnant female as it may cause some fetal abnormalities.

Probably the other most commonly used medication in head injury is dexamethasone (Decadron), a steroid similar to those produced and secreted by the adrenal cortex. Decadron has significant anti-inflammatory properties. In patients with cerebral edema, it may reduce the irritation and resultant swelling. Although steroids generally have a wide range of serious side effects, short-term high doses are relatively safe. Recent research, however, has shown that their use post-trauma may not be as effective as first thought. Decadron is supplied in vials and preloads of varying concentrations. Most common are 4, 10, and 24 milligrams per milliliter. It is normally administered in doses from 10 to 24 milligrams, with a maximum dosage as high as 100 mg. Administration should take between 1 and 2 minutes.

Dilantin is an anti-seizure drug which acts on the brain in a manner similar to lidocaine on the heart; it suppresses irritability. It will effectively reduce seizure activity. In the patient with increasing intracranial pressure, seizing is very likely. The intracranial pressure generally rises during seizure activity, worsening the injury and increasing patient mortality. Dilantin is given IV bolus or drip only. Since it may precipitate, dilantin should be administered in a line other than one established with D5W. Dosages of 150 to 250 mg are usual for an adult, administered from an ampule or a preloaded syringe.

Diazepam (Valium), another anticonvulsant, antianxiety agent may be useful in treating the head injury patient. It is the first-line drug in the control of major motor seizures. Valium should not be mixed with other drugs and is relatively short acting. The standard dosage is between 2 and 15 mg IV bolus. It should be administered very slowly, no more than 5 mg per minute. Large veins should be used to reduce venous irritation. The drug may need to be administered intramuscularly if the patient is seizing. Administration should be titrated to effect. The patient should be carefully watched and a follow-up dose of Valium given if its effects begin to subside. It is essential that the paramedic consult with the system medical director regarding the indications, dosage, and protocols for use of any drug mentioned within this text.

SUMMARY

Head, neck, and spine injuries are severe and significant injuries encountered in the field setting. They often present with signs and symptoms unreflective of their real significance. These injuries may progress quietly and rapidly, resulting in patient demise. The paramedic must ensure that assessment and care of the patient with a head, neck, or spine injury anticipates problems rather than awaits the signs and symptoms. He or she must ensure that the possible head injury patient is well ventilated at 20 to 25 breaths per minute with high flow oxygen. The airway needs to be protected with endotracheal intubation if the gag reflex is absent or diminished. The patient needs to be transported rapidly to definitive care. The spine injury patient needs immediate and continued immobilization from scene arrival until patient responsibility is assumed by the Emergency Department staff. Neck injuries also need to receive a high priority of care. Penetrating injury should increase suspicion for vascular or respiratory injury including airway compromise or air emboli. The neck should be sealed with an occlusive dressing, while any significant blood loss is controlled. The result of this aggressive focus on the head, neck, and spine injury will be better patient care and reduced morbidity and mortality.

FURTHER READING

AMERICAN COLLEGE OF SURGEONS, Committee on Trauma, *Advanced Trauma Life Support Course: Student Manual.* American College of Surgeons, 1984.

BUTMAN, A. M., AND PATURAS, J. L., *Pre-Hospital Trauma Life Support.* Akron, OH: Emergency Training, 1990.

CAMPBELL, J. E., *Basic Trauma Life Support,* 2nd ed. Englewood Cliffs, NJ: Prentice-Hall, Inc., 1988.

16

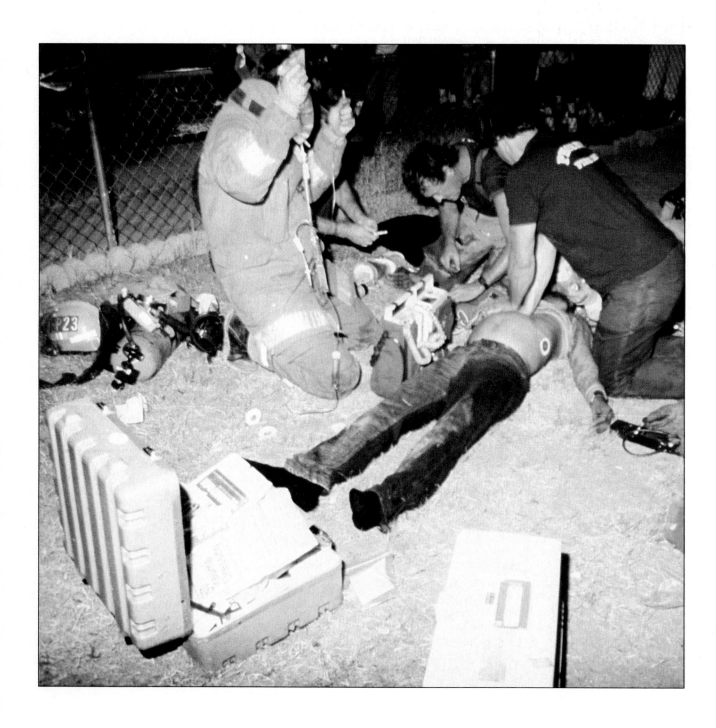

Body Cavity Trauma

Objectives for Chapter 16

Upon completing this chapter, the student should be able to:

1. Identify the incidence, mortality and morbidity of body cavity injury in the trauma patient.

2. Locate and explain the function of each of the organs and major structures found within the thorax and abdomen.

3. Explain the process of respiration, including the function of the bellows system, the pleura, and the airway.

4. Identify the various injuries associated with chest and abdominal trauma and explain the cause and effect relationship between the injury and its signs and symptoms.

5. Highlight the elements of primary assessment for chest and abdominal injury and explain how each element relates to the various injuries.

6. Demonstrate a complete assessment of the chest and abdomen, identifying the major signs and symptoms palpated, listened for, auscultated, and observed for during the assessment.

7. Identify the signs and symptoms expected for the various chest and abdominal injuries.

8. Identify, order, and demonstrate the care steps for chest and abdominal penetrating and blunt trauma.

CASE STUDY

Medic Rescue 3 is asked to respond to a small tavern downtown. A patient has been shot during an argument. The police have the suspect in custody. Upon arrival the paramedics find the scene secured by several police officers, one of whom directs them into the bar. The officer says that the victim was shot with a .357 magnum once in the chest. The patient is found to be sitting on the floor, propped up against the wall. He is a 24-year-old male who has some minor bleeding from the left upper chest, under a blood stained towel he's holding in place. The patient is conscious, alert, and somewhat agitated. He seems to have some trouble speaking in complete sentences and is slightly ashen in color. The airway is clear and his breathing is labored, at a rate of 36 per minute and shallow. Pulses (both central and distal) are strong but rapid. The chest has one small entrance wound, with a spray of burnt gunpowder around it. It is seeping a small stream of blood with no visible gurgling or bubbles. The posterior chest is evaluated to find a larger, more jagged wound with limited blood loss and no signs of air exchange. The rest of the primary assessment reveals no other signs of injury.

The wounds are sealed with occlusive dressings and high-flow oxygen is applied. The patient's color improves, although he seems to have more difficulty in moving air. Pulse oximetry is applied and oxygen saturation is 92%. The blood pressure is 100 by palpation (environmental noise is too loud to get a good reading). Lung sounds are difficult to hear with the background noise but appear diminished on the left. The patient begins to return to the earlier ashen color, and his jugular veins are becoming more prominent. The trachea looks to be midline. The patient's respirations continue to become more strained and his level of consciousness diminishes.

The patient is quickly loaded to the stretcher and transferred to the ambulance. Enroute to the hospital the report is given to medical command. Orders are received to start an IV of lactated Ringer's solution to be infused rapidly and repeat the breath sounds. The breath sounds are now severely diminished on the left and the trachea seems displaced to the right. Medical control orders decompression of the left chest. The occlusive dressing is removed and a gush of air exits the wound. The dressing is reapplied and taped on three sides. The patient's respirations improve as does his level of consciousness and oxygen saturation.

At the emergency department a chest tube is placed and put under suction. The patient is fully evaluated and taken to the ICU to be observed for a few days. He recovers completely.

INTRODUCTION

The body cavity, comprised of the thorax and abdomen, is an area commonly subjected to trauma. Body cavity injury is the second most frequent cause of vehicular death and is a common cause of mortality from other forms of traumatic insult. Injury can directly involve the respiratory, circulatory, digestive, or urinary system; or it can simultaneously affect multiple systems. These injuries account for a high percentage of mortality. However, if paramedics can rapidly recognize injury and correctly intervene, patient outcome will significantly improve. To accomplish this goal, paramedics must understand the underlying anatomy, physiology, and pathophysiology of chest and abdominal trauma. With this understanding they will be able to provide efficient and appropriate assessment and management for any injury to the body cavity.

The location of each organ is important to the overall assessment of traumatic injury. Forces directed to a specific location within the body cavity will most likely affect organs within that area. By assessing where, in which direction, and how much force was expressed, you can anticipate the specific organ or organs involved and the degree of injury. Knowledge of the purpose served by each abdominal and thoracic structure can provide further information about the potential harm an injury can cause. If a particular organ is injured, the effects of its dysfunction can be predicted locally and systemically. For example, if the structures that assist with the movement of air are damaged, dyspnea would be expected. The degree of dyspnea would depend on the specific structure involved and the degree of damage. It could be expected that hypoxia and hypercardia might also occur. Chest and abdominal trauma is usually not an isolated injury. Injury to one structure or organ may affect the function of other organs or structures. Kinetic forces directed to the chest wall may cause soft tissue injury and rib fracture. The injury may diminish the respiratory system's ability to move air. It may also compromise the seal that holds the lung tightly to the chest wall. The wound may act as a valve and allow pressure to build within the chest. This reduces the venous return to the heart, resulting in cardiovascular embarrassment. Associated blood loss into the thoracic cavity may contribute to hypovolemia.

A good understanding of body cavity injury is of little use unless the injury is quickly recognized. Assessment of the patient with body cavity trauma must be well performed. It is essential to identify the early signs of injury rather than wait until the injury has led to major dysfunction. For example, the developing tension pneumothorax must be recognized well before it results in cardiorespiratory arrest. The paramedic must assess the body cavity thoroughly and completely. At the same time he or she observes the overall trauma patient priorities. You must immediately stabilize the spine of patients with significant chest or abdominal trauma. You must secure the A-B-C-D-E's, and in most cases, you must complete the normal head to toe evaluation, take vital signs, and determine medical history. The assessment of the body cavity must be an integral part of this process to ensure that all important injuries are found and properly prioritized. Recognition of injury will help you determine whether the patient needs rapid transport or on-scene stabilization and care. The primary assessment must be thorough and specific concerning emergent injuries. The complete head to toe assessment must be sufficiently in-depth to ensure that even the most minute signs of internal injury to the body cavity are recognized. The on-scene assessment may be the only opportunity to evaluate signs and symptoms that will be masked later by the patient's diminished level of consciousness, or other injuries.

Unlike the head, neck and spine, the body cavity comprises a region where aggressive field care can significantly affect patient outcome. For chest and abdominal trauma the paramedic can utilize such procedures as positive pressure ventilation, high-concentration oxygenation, needle decompression of the chest, intubation, application of the PASG, rapid infusion of crystalloids, stabilization of the respiratory system, and rapid transport. With permission from medical control and in the appropriate

✱ Always suspect chest or abdominal cavity injury in the patient with multiple injuries.

✱ Assume a spinal injury also exists in any patient with body cavity trauma.

setting, these procedures can significantly affect the patient's chances for survival. To better understand injuries to these regions, and their effects on human survival, paramedics should look carefully at the anatomy and physiology of the cavities and the organs found within. Understanding the relationship between organ location and injury site, and organ function and the effects of organ injury, can prepare you to better recognize and manage the body cavity injury patient.

ANATOMY AND PHYSIOLOGY

The body cavity is really one large space extending from above the clavicles downward into the pelvis. It is divided into two smaller cavities by the *diaphragm,* a strong sheet of muscle and an active component in respiration. The upper cavity is the *thorax,* which contains the lungs on either side of the *mediastinum,* a central region housing the heart, trachea, esophagus, major blood vessels and several nerve pathways. The *abdominal cavity* is subdivided into three cavities: the abdomen, the retroperitoneal space, and the pelvic cavity.

The Thorax

The thorax is both a container and a dynamic functional part of the respiratory system. (See Figure 16-1.) It houses the major components of the respiratory and circulatory systems. It also changes volume very dramatically to accommodate respiration through the bellows system. The thorax is composed of skeletal and soft tissue. It is made up of twelve

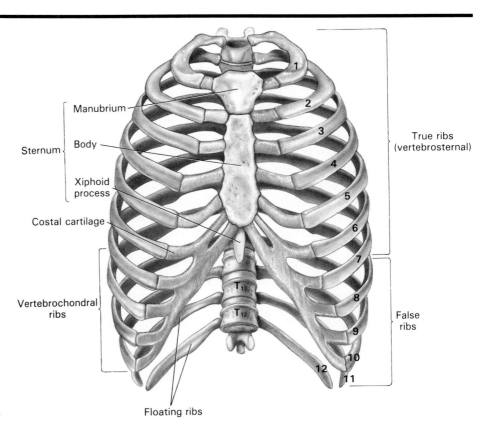

FIGURE 16-1 The thorax.

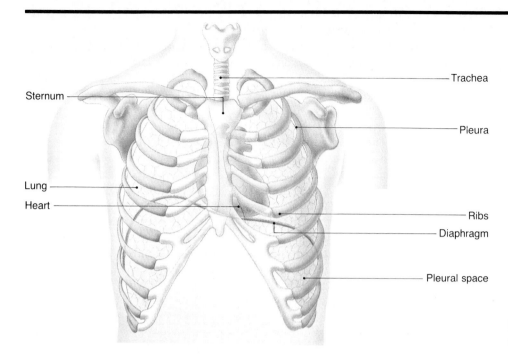

Sternum

Lung

Heart

Trachea

Pleura

Ribs

Diaphragm

Pleural space

FIGURE 16-2 The organs of the thorax.

C-shaped rib pairs, articulating directly with the vertebral column posteriorly. Through cartilage attachments, the upper six ribs are directly joined with the sternum anteriorly while the next four are indirectly attached. The last two ribs are not attached anteriorly and are, therefore, free to move through a modest range of motion.

The upper thorax is covered by the framework of the shoulder. (See Figure 16-2.) Sitting over the upper rib anteriorly, the clavicle articulates with the sternum medially and the humerus and scapula distally. The scapula overrides the upper four ribs posteriorly. Both musculature and structure of the shoulder girdle protect the upper thorax from the effects of trauma extremely well.

Central to the interior of the thoracic cage is an area called the **mediastinum** which houses several structures, essential to human function. The *trachea, vena cava, aorta,* and *esophagus* are major conduits for the respiratory, venous, arterial, and digestive systems respectively. The heart is a hollow muscular organ suspended within the mediastinum and is the pump of the circulatory system. (See Chapter 21.) It is divided by the septum into right and left sides and further subdivided into upper and lower chambers by the tricuspid and mitral valves. The heart walls are made up of very special muscle tissue providing the constant and rhythmic pumping function. The heart is supplied with oxygenated circulation through the coronary arteries found on the exterior surface of the heart muscle. A thin but strong sac called the **pericardium** surrounds it. Like the pleura, the pericardium provides a rather frictionless surface against which the heart can freely move as it pumps blood. In the acute setting the pericardium does not stretch and may, if filled with fluid, inhibit cardiac filling. The heart is secured centrally in the chest by the arch of the *aorta* and the *ligamentum arteriosum*. The aorta is attached to the base of the heart and is firmly stabilized against the thorax posteriorly. To some degree the aorta is immobilized by the innominate and subclavian arteries as they branch from the arch. The *ligamentum arteriosum* is all that remains of the fetal right heart-aortic circulation. After

■ **mediastinum** central cavity within the thorax containing the heart, great vessels, trachea, and esophagus.

■ **pericardium** two layered sac surrounding the heart.

birth it maintains the curve of the aorta. In lateral trauma it may contribute to damage to the vessel.

The lungs fill the chest cavity lateral to the mediastinum. Each lung is divided into regions called *lobes*—the right lung has three and the left lung has two. The lungs occupy between 6 and 8 liters of space, with the right lung slightly larger than the left. The left lung is smaller because of the heart's position in the mediastinum. The size of the thorax changes with inspiration and expiration.

The ribs lie at a downward orientation from posterior to anterior. They are lifted to a more horizontal position by the **sternocleidomastoid** and **intercostal muscles.** The sternocleidomastoid muscles raise the sternum and the anterior ribs, while the intercostal muscles bring the ribs closer together and help lift the lower ribs. The result is an increase in the anterior-posterior dimension. Simultaneously, the diaphragm contracts, displacing the abdominal contents downward and increasing the superior-inferior dimension of the thorax. This movement increases the total volume of the chest to allow respiration. As the volume of a container such as the thorax increases, the pressure within it falls. This causes air from the outside to rush in to equalize the pressure as *inspiration* occurs. When the muscles of respiration relax, the ribs settle, the diaphragm rises, and the volume of the chest decreases. This decrease causes the pressure within to rise and the air to rush out, a process called *expiration.*

The structure that ensures the lungs will expand within the thorax is the *pleura.* It is a double layer of smooth and delicate tissue lining the interior of the thorax (**parietal pleura**) and the exterior of the lungs (**visceral pleura**). Between the two layers is a potential space containing a small amount of pleural fluid to lubricate and hold the two layers together. The force securing the lung to the thorax resembles that which holds two pieces of glass together when water gets between them. Unless air is allowed to enter, the panes (or the lungs and thorax) will remain firmly together.

The **alveolus** is a hollow grape-shaped chamber where oxygen and carbon dioxide exchange takes place. There are about 300 million of these hollow spaces in the respiratory system, with a combined surface area half that of a basketball court. This surface area allows for an efficient and effective exchange of carbon dioxide and oxygen. It is the alveoli which give the lungs their spongy compliance, volume, and light weight. The thorax is a sealed and airtight container. As it changes volume, interior pressure changes and air moves in and out. The exterior of the lung is firmly held to the interior of the thorax by the pleura and hence expands and contracts with respiration. Because the alveoli are flexible and elastic, they are capable of expanding and contracting in volume. With each breath, they vary their diameter and change their volume to accommodate the chest motion. Under normal circumstances, air will, therefore, enter the airway and travel into the alveoli during inspiration.

The changing **intrathoracic** pressure is also responsible for some hemodynamic effects. The reduction of this pressure during inspiration assists venous return to the heart, while the increased pressure during expiration helps circulate arterial blood. The volume of blood pumped by the heart with each stroke is equal, left side versus right. Also, the volume of blood circulated through the pulmonary system is equal to that circulated through the systemic tissue. The pulmonary tissue is very vascular, and can result in severe swelling or hemorrhage if it is injured.

■ **sternocleidomastoid** muscle of the lateral neck and anterior thorax attaching at the mastoid, clavicle and sternum. It serves as an accessory muscle of respiration and lifts the sternum and anterior chest during deep respiration.

■ **intercostal muscles** muscles between the ribs that serve to expand the chest.

■ **parietal pleura** fine fibrous sheath covering the interior of the thorax.

■ **visceral pleura** fine lining covering the lungs. With the parietal pleura, it forms the seal holding the lungs to the interior of the thoracic cage.

■ **alveolus** one of the millions of microscopic chambers within the lung. It is the location where the gasses of respiration are exchanged. (pl. alveoli)

■ **intrathoracic** within the thoracic cage.

The Abdomen

The diaphragm, a dynamic organ, separates the thoracic and abdominal cavities. A dome-shaped muscle, the diaphragm is attached to the lower border of the rib cage. With each breath it moves a few inches superior, then inferior to the xiphoid process. The uppermost point of travel during a deep expiration is somewhere just below the nipple line. Thus, any penetrating or blunt trauma to the region may involve organs of the abdomen, thorax, or both. The abdomen is bordered posteriorly by the lower ribs and lumbar spine as well as the muscles of the lower back. It is bordered laterally by the flank muscles and anteriorly by the abdominal muscles. Its inferior border is the pelvis. The abdomen can be subdivided into three regions: the abdominal space, the retroperitoneal space, and the pelvic cavity. The **retroperitoneal** space contains the kidneys, aorta, vena cava, and part of the duodenum and pancreas. Its organs lack the protective covering of the peritoneum; hence the name. The *pelvic cavity* contains the organs within the pelvis: the bladder, rectum, and in the female, the **genitalia.** The last cavity, the *abdominal* space, houses the remaining organs.

The abdomen is divided into four quadrants by drawing an imaginary set of lines through the umbilicus, one superior to inferior and the other left to right. The *right-upper quadrant* contains the liver, right kidney, gall bladder, duodenum, and part of the pancreas. The *left-upper quadrant* includes the stomach, left kidney, spleen, and most of the pancreas. The *left-lower quadrant* houses the sigmoid colon, while the *right-lower quadrant* contains the appendix. All quadrants hold some of the small bowel, although the lower two have the largest portion. The large bowel begins in the right lower quadrant and travels upward, across and downward through all the remaining quadrants.

Beginning at the stomach, the alimentary canal travels through the abdomen. The esophagus empties into the stomach, where hydrochloric acid and **enzymes** are mixed and churned with the food to be digested. When the food reaches a semiliquid consistency, the lower end of the stomach allows it to travel into the **duodenum.** Here pancreatic juices and bile assist with the digestive breakdown. The food continues its motion through the canal via **peristalsis,** a wavelike muscular motion of the bowel. It moves through the **jejunum** and the **ileum** where most, if not all, nutrients are absorbed. Next, the food enters the large bowel at the *ileocecal valve,* a one-way structure in the right-lower quadrant. The large bowel contains bacteria which serve to break down the remaining material and release the water within it. The large bowel absorbs the water and other fluids, which are returned to the liver and then the circulatory system. As the digested and relatively dehydrated material leaves the alimentary canal, it passes the *rectum,* a holding area. Then it continues on to the anus, the sphincter muscle responsible for controlling the release of the large bowel contents.

Besides the hollow tube, which is the *alimentary canal,* there are accessory organs to digestion. These include the liver, gall bladder, and pancreas. The *liver* occupies the area below and under the rib cage in the right-upper quadrant and to a smaller extent, the left-upper quadrant. A large and vascular organ, it detoxifies the blood coming from the digestive field, stores body energy reserves, produces plasma proteins, and performs many other functions. Beneath and behind the liver is the *gall bladder,* a storehouse for **bile.** A product of the liver, bile helps in the

■ **retroperitoneal** behind the layers of the peritoneum. The organs within this space include the kidneys, spleen, and part of the pancreas.

■ **genitalia** reproductive organs of either the male or the female.

■ **enzyme** biochemical catalyst which speeds chemical reactions. The enzyme itself does not normally change during the process.

■ **duodenum** first part of the small bowel. About 10 inches in length, it receives the secretions of the liver and the pancreas.

■ **peristalsis** wavelike muscular motion of the esophagus and bowel which moves food through it.

■ **jejunum** second portion of the small bowel. It is approximately 8 feet in length and is located between the duodenum and ileum.

■ **ileum** third and longest portion of the small bowel. It is approximately 12 feet in length and extends from the jejunum to the ileo-cecal valve.

■ **bile** a yellow to green viscous fluid secreted by the liver and stored in the gall bladder. It is secreted into the small bowel, aids in digestion of fats, and gives the stool its normal coloration.

insulin pancreatic hormone needed to transport simple sugars from the interstitial spaces into the cells.

digestion of fats. The gall bladder will constrict in response to digestive material passing from the stomach (especially fats) and excrete bile, through the bile duct, into the duodenum. Through the common bile duct the *pancreas* also excretes digestive juices into the duodenum. Because it is very caustic, the pancreatic juice efficiently assists with the breakdown of food in the small bowel. The pancreas is also responsible for the body's production of **insulin,** the hormone necessary to move glucose across the cell membrane for use in metabolism. The pancreas is located in both of the upper quadrants, with most of its mass in the left. Another occupant of the left-upper abdominal quadrant is the *spleen.* Also a large vascular organ, it assists the body's mechanisms of protection against invasion of foreign organisms. Not only does the spleen help produce white blood cells it also houses the system which gives us immunity from diseases. Behind and beneath the spleen on the left and behind the liver on the right, lie the kidneys. They filter blood and draw from it water and waste products. The kidneys concentrate the waste and preserve the water/salt balance of the human system. Their product empties into the ureters, traveling to the urinary bladder.

peritoneum fine fibrous tissue surrounding the interior of most of the abdominal cavity and covering most of the small bowel and some of the abdominal organs.

The **peritoneum** is a tissue covering most of the abdominal organs. Similar to the pleura of the lungs, to some degree it performs the same function. The peritoneum is a delicate tissue covering both the organs (excepting those in the retroperitoneal space) and the interior of the abdominal cavity. Fluid within the peritoneum allows smooth motion between the various internal organs.

The abdomen also contains the abdominal aorta and vena cava. They are large vessels traveling along the posterior wall, next to the spinal column. Major branches off both vessels supply or receive blood to or from the major organs of the abdomen. They continue inferiorly to provide circulation to the pelvis and lower extremities.

mesentery double fold of peritoneum that supports the major portion of the small bowel, suspending it from the posterior abdominal wall.

Two specialized and important structures of the abdominal cavity are the **mesentery** and the **omentum.** The mesentery is a double fold of peritoneum extending from the posterior wall of the abdomen to the small bowel and providing it with circulation and innervation. It also keeps the bowel from becoming entangled during the process of digestion. Like the mesentery, the omentum is a double layer of peritoneum. It is suspended downward from the duodenum and the stomach in front of the abdominal organs. After a person's youth, it becomes covered with fatty tissue and insulates the anterior abdomen from trauma and temperature extremes. The peritoneum covers the anterior abdominal organs but not the kidneys, aorta, vena cave, nor parts of the duodenum and pancreas. These organs are identified as retroperitoneal and are well fixed by the peritoneum in their location.

omentum sheet of peritoneum and fat tissue, covering and protecting the anterior surface of the interior abdomen.

The Pelvic Cavity

The bladder, rectum and, in the female, the reproductive organs are contained within the pelvic cavity. This cavity also includes the iliac artery and vein, supplying and returning blood from the lower extremities. The pelvic cavity is generally considered to consist of the space from the opening of the pelvis (the pelvic inlet) to the pelvic floor and is well-protected from trauma.

PATHOPHYSIOLOGY

Injuries of the chest, abdomen, and pelvic cavity pose a serious threat to life due to blood loss, respiratory embarrassment, and compromise of critical organ function. Thus, they deserve serious evaluation and immediate consideration in traumatic insult. The paramedic needs to understand what internal injuries can occur, how they endanger human function, and the consequences which may follow.

Chest injuries can be divided into those that compromise the bellows system and the movement of air and those that injure the internal structures. The bellows system can be affected by restricted function due to pain, a breakdown of the bellows itself, or the failure of the lung to move in conjunction with the thoracic cage. Internal injuries can contuse or lacerate lung or mediastinal tissue, including the great vessels, trachea, esophagus, or the heart. Injury may be produced through a blunt or penetrating mechanism. The bellows may function inefficiently because of the pain of rib fracture. If the tidal volume drops much below the normal 500 ml, the minute volume and efficiency of respiration diminish. The dead space air remains the same while the volume of air exchanged is reduced. The result is more breaths, with a total reduced air exchange and more energy (and oxygen) required to support respiration. Since rib fractures are quite common and extremely painful, this is a frequent post-chest trauma problem. The respiratory restriction caused by rib fracture and the natural splinting due to pain, may result in other respiratory problems. Pain associated with deep breathing will limit chest excursion and lead to collapse of the alveoli, called **atelectasis.** The problem may be compounded by the patient suppressing the *sigh reflex.* This reflex causes periodic hyperinflation of the chest to expand those alveoli which have collapsed. Atelectasis may contribute to the development of pneumonia or other respiratory infection. It may also increase the effort needed to expand the chest during respiration.

During trauma, compression of the chest may contuse the lungs as it would any other body tissue. The pulmonary tissue will swell and develop edema, a typical sign of any contusion. Edema reduces lung compliance, making respiratory effort more difficult and less efficient. It also interferes with the diffusion of carbon dioxide, increasing $PaCO_2$ and decreasing the blood's pH. Trauma may be severe enough to fracture several ribs. If three or more ribs are fractured in multiple locations, the segment involved may become unstable, an injury called *flail chest.* (See Figure 16-3.) The segment may move due to intrathoracic pressures rather than by muscular control. As the patient attempts to inspire, the intact chest wall moves outward, and the intrathoracic pressure falls. The unstable, or flail segment, will be drawn in during inspiration. As the chest relaxes and moves inward during expiration, the increased intrathoracic pressure causes the flail segment to move outward. The motion of the flail segment, which is opposite to that of the rest of the chest, is called *paradoxical.* (See Figure 16-4.) It results in severe respiratory compromise because the air from beneath the segment travels to and from the good lung tissue instead of in and out of the airway. Not only does flail chest limit the useful air exchange from beneath the area of injury, it reduces the efficiency of the remaining bellows system.

Another extreme condition often associated with severe rib injury is **traumatic asphyxia.** In this injury the chest wall is pushed in and held, either by the nature of the rib fractures or by a compressional force such as the patient trapped between the auto seat and steering wheel. The compression severely limits chest **excursion** and results in hypoventilation. It also may tamponade the resultant intrathoracic hemorrhage and cause a backflow and back up of venous blood, especially within the neck and the head. The classical presentation of traumatic asphyxia includes bloodshot eyes, bulging blue tongue, distended neck veins, and a cyanotic

✱ Chest injuries account for one out of four trauma deaths in this country.

■ **atelectasis** collapse of the alveoli of the lung.

✱ Hypoxia is the most important concern in chest trauma.

■ **traumatic asphyxia** compression of the chest due to a crush injury. It limits chest excursion yet tamponades hemorrhage.

■ **excursion** extent of movement of a body part such as the chest during respiration.

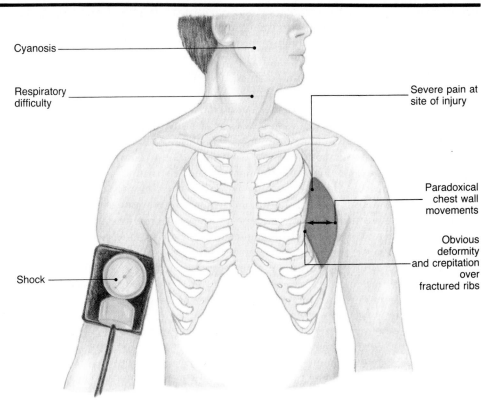

Cyanosis

Respiratory
difficulty

Severe pain at
site of injury

Paradoxical
chest wall
movements

Obvious
deformity
and crepitation
over
fractured ribs

Shock

FIGURE 16-3   Flail chest.

upper body. The prognosis is grave. The patient is suffering from severe hypoxia, yet relief of the chest compression may cause rapid deterioration. The removal of the compressing force may relieve the pressure which had been controlling the internal thoracic blood loss, as the PASG controls intraabdominal bleeding. When the chest is freed, the bleeding may induce rapid hypovolemia, shock, and death.

The bellows system may also fail because of loss of pleural seal integrity. If an internal or external wound allows air, blood, or fluid to enter the area between the pleural tissues, the potential space becomes an ac-

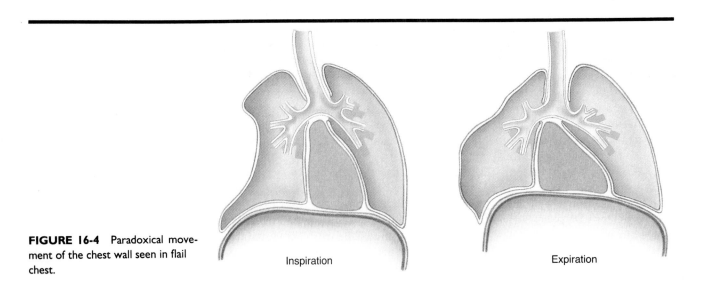

FIGURE 16-4   Paradoxical movement of the chest wall seen in flail
chest.

Inspiration

Expiration

tual space. The expansion of the pleural space reduces the effective expansion of the lung fields and compromises respiration. If the pleural space is expanded by air from an interior wound, it is called a *closed pneumothorax.* If the wound is external it is called an *open pneumothorax.* The opening may be the result of a torn bronchus, bronchiole, or alveolus, and can be caused by penetrating or blunt trauma, COPD, or congenital defect. The larger the tear and the structure involved, the more rapid the progression of the pneumothorax. In small tears, pneumothorax may self-seal and air will gradually be reabsorbed. If the tear involves the larger airways, the pneumothorax may be progressive. Trauma of the penetrating kind (open pneumothorax) will usually require a rather large hole to allow exchange or passage of air. Such trauma will result in gurgling or frothy blood.

A specific mechanism of injury that may precipitate the pneumothorax is compression of a hyperinflated chest during an auto accident. As passengers or driver sees the impending impact they tend to take a deep breath and to hold it. During the crash the chest impacts the steering wheel or dashboard, thereby compressing the hyperinflated thorax against the closed glottis. The alveoli and bronchioles rupture like a sealed paper bag between two hands clapping. This phenomenon, called the *paper bag syndrome,* results in a closed pneumothorax.

It should be noted that intermittent positive pressure ventilation (IPPV) may cause or worsen the pneumothorax in the trauma patient. If chest trauma has occurred, pulmonary tissue probably has been injured. The increased intrathoracic pressure which accompanies use of the bag-valve mask—or, to a greater degree, the demand valve—may rupture an already weak structure or blow air by an otherwise closed wound. The result is to induce or increase the size and rate of pneumothorax development. Exercise caution when using IPPV for the chest trauma patient.

If the external or internal wound acts as a one-way valve, **tension pneumothorax** may occur. Tension pneumothorax is a progressive pneumothorax that enlarges, builds in pressure, and begins to infringe upon the function of the opposite lung and the circulatory system. (See Figure 16-5.) The valve allows air to enter the pleural space during inspiration. As the patient expires, the valve closes and air cannot exit. The problem progresses and pressure within the thorax grows. This increases the effort needed to draw air in for respiration, pushes the mediastinum against the unaffected lung, retards venous return to the heart, reduces the heart's ability to fill, and possibly kinks the vena cava where it travels through the diaphragm. The overall effect upon the patient is extreme dyspnea and acute circulatory compromise.

Shifting of the trachea may occur with tension pneumothorax. It is a late sign, present only after there has been a significant shifting of the mediastinum. The degree of tension pneumothorax needed to displace the trachea, at least noticeably, is great. Tracheal deviation is not, therefore, a good sign to guide care. Instead, the paramedic should look at severe dyspnea, unilateral absent or severely diminished breath sounds, and the presentation of shock with no other apparent cause as an indication that this injury is occurring.

The pleural space may also be filled with fluid, most commonly blood. The accumulation will normally be slow. If the vessel involved is large enough, the blood loss may be severe and will significantly displace the pulmonary tissue. Remember that each lung occupies about 3 to 4 liters of space. Any rapid blood loss causing respiratory compromise will

■ **tension pneumothorax** buildup of air under pressure within the thorax. By compressing the lung, it severely reduces the effectiveness of respiration.

✳ Tension pneumothorax requires immediate decompression if permitted.

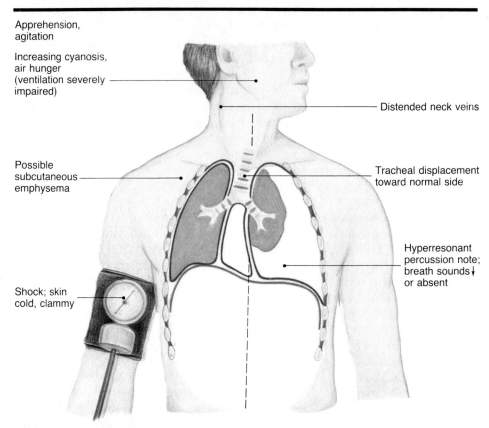

Apprehension, agitation

Increasing cyanosis, air hunger (ventilation severely impaired)

Possible subcutaneous emphysema

Shock; skin cold, clammy

Distended neck veins

Tracheal displacement toward normal side

Hyperresonant percussion note; breath sounds↓ or absent

FIGURE 16-5 Physical findings of tension pneumothorax.

thus result in hypovolemic shock. A mixed presentation, that is, pneumothorax and hemothorax together is also common. (See Figure 16-6.)

Decelerating trauma can affect the structures within the mediastinum, including the heart and great vessels. The heart can be contused, injuring the myocardium. While this injury often has a better prognosis than myocardial infarction, it presents similarly. The myocardial contusion may be acute in presentation and display life threatening dysrhythmias while the patient is within the prehospital setting. (Dysrhythmia recognition and care will be discussed in Chapter 21.)

Pericardial tamponade can occur secondary to either blunt or penetrating trauma. The coronary circulation may be torn, allowing blood to enter the pericardial space. As the sac fills with blood, it progressively restricts the passive filling of the heart. Cardiac output then drops quickly and without warning. In this injury the compensatory mechanisms for shock cause systemic vasoconstriction in order to maintain blood pressure. The patient's systolic pressure will remain relatively normal while the diastolic pressure rises. This narrowing of the pulse pressure is characteristic of tamponade, as are distended jugular veins and distant heart sounds. (See Figure 16-7.) If the syndrome continues, pericardial tamponade will eventually stop all blood flow through the heart, resulting in cardiopulmonary arrest.

The great vessels are subject to trauma in the severe deceleration accident. The aorta is one of the structures which supports the heart in its position within the chest. If sudden deceleration occurs, especially if it is

■ **pericardial tamponade**
filling of the pericardial sac with fluid which limits the filling of the heart.

✱ Cardiac tamponade most commonly results from penetrating injuries.

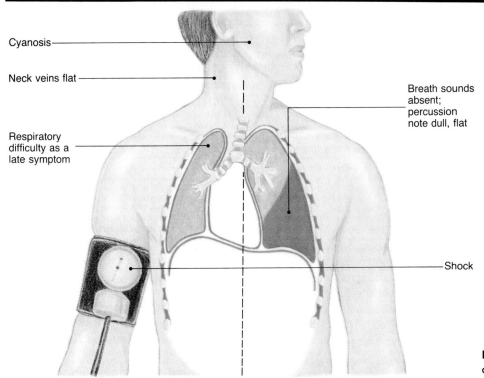

Cyanosis

Neck veins flat

Respiratory
difficulty as a
late symptom

Breath sounds
absent;
percussion
note dull, flat

Shock

FIGURE 16-6 Physical findings
of massive hemothorax.

lateral, the heart will twist on the aorta. This movement may cause the
layers of the aorta to break apart, causing an aneurysm, or weakness in
the vessel wall. Blood flows into and expands the aneurysm. It often impinges the left subclavian artery and diminishes circulation to the left
upper extremity. The patient may complain of a tearing sensation in the
central chest or back and numbness or tingling in the left extremity.

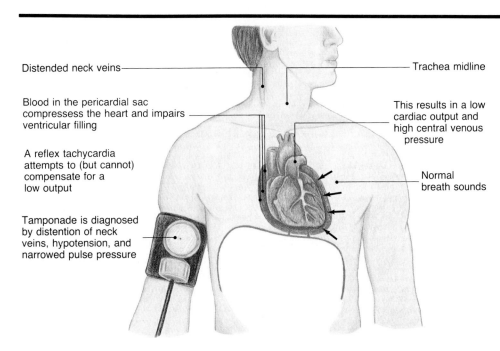

Distended neck veins

Blood in the pericardial sac
compressess the heart and impairs
ventricular filling

A reflex tachycardia
attempts to (but cannot)
compensate for a
low output

Tamponade is diagnosed
by distention of neck
veins, hypotension, and
narrowed pulse pressure

Trachea midline

This results in a low
cardiac output and
high central venous
pressure

Normal
breath sounds

FIGURE 16-7 Physical findings
of cardiac tamponade.

These may be accompanied by a diminished or absent pulse. If degeneration continues, the defect may rupture, with rapid exsanguination into the mediastinum. A very high percentage of patient's suffering from traumatic aortic aneurysm do not survive.

Other injuries of the mediastinal contents include rupture of the esophagus or trachea, or laceration to the inferior or superior vena cava. The tracheal tear may allow free air into the mediastinum, especially if the patient coughs or is placed on IPPV. Esophageal injury may allow gastric or other foreign materials into the mediastinum. While these may cause only minor problems in the field setting, they may eventually result in patient demise from infection. Vena cava damage, whether superior or inferior, may account for rapid, extensive and shock-inducing hemorrhage. Any of these injuries may be caused by blunt trauma, although penetrating trauma is a more likely cause.

Remember that the border between the abdomen and the thorax is dynamic. The abdominal or thoracic contents can be found two inches either above or below the xiphoid process due to the excursion of the diaphragm during respiration. Injury within this region may involve organs of the abdominal cavity, thoracic cavity, or both. Severe blunt abdominal trauma has been known to rupture the diaphragm, permitting abdominal contents to enter the thoracic cavity. This injury reduces the dynamics of the respiratory system and frequently makes the abdomen appear hollow or empty.

The Abdomen

The abdomen has less obvious signs and symptoms to indicate life threatening trauma. Assessment of this area is more difficult because of the pliability of the abdominal container and the delayed effects of hemorrhage or abdominal organ dysfunction. Thus, it is nearly impossible to predict the nature and the extent of injury. Therefore it is very important to recognize the potential for injury and to look for the most subtle indications that something might be amiss within this cavity. Abdominal injuries can also be divided into blunt and penetrating. Both have classical presentations and specific concerns. Penetrating injuries may be caused by rifle, handgun, knife, or other similar mechanisms. The faster the offending agent penetrates and the more rapid the exchange of energy, the greater will be the damage beyond the wound pathway. For example, a knife will ordinarily affect only those structures it actually contacts. A bullet's effects are more extensive.

The pathway of a penetrating abdominal injury is difficult to determine simply from the entrance wound. As weapon energy increases, damage extends increasingly further from the projectile's path. Cavitation of the hand gun bullet will involve a narrow cylinder around the path, while rifle injury may cause injury to organs quite distant from the path of the energy source. If the caliber of the weapon or even the designation—for example, rifle versus handgun—can be determined, it will aid in the degree of injury potential. For many reasons the expected pathway may not be the same as the real one. The bullet may tumble or deflect from a straight path and injure tissues outside the expected injury zone. Or it may fragment, causing injury along more than one pathway. The damage to body cavity organs can vary according to the particular tissue involved. The air filled lung is relatively tolerant to gunshot wounds. The cylinder of damage would be less than expected as air within the alveoli will compress when the cavitational wave pressurizes the tissue. The kidney, liver, spleen, and to a lesser degree, the pancreas are exactly the opposite. Solid, dense, and inelastic, they are damaged with much less force than the lung.

Evisceration, another type of penetrating injury which may occur in the abdominal region, is a rupture or laceration of the abdominal wall, allowing abdominal contents to escape through the opening. The small bowel is the most common viscera that protrudes. The danger from this form of injury is loss of circulation, tissue drying, bowel obstruction, and contamination.

Several types of injuries occur secondary to blunt abdominal trauma. Solid organs are contused, lacerated or fractured. Hollow organs rupture or the abdominal vasculature is torn. These injuries may be associated with hemorrhage, organ dysfunction, irritation, or destruction of the abdominal lining and organs.

Solid organs may be trapped between the posterior wall of the abdomen and the anterior surface during deceleration or acceleration. The tissue is contused, resulting in swelling, hemorrhage, and organ failure. The forces of injury may be severe enough to cause the solid organs to fracture. The hemorrhage will frequently be somewhat contained within the organ's peritoneal envelope or capsule. This may cause tamponade, which may cause rupture later and lead to rapid exsanguination.

The hollow organs can also be compressed during deceleration. If kinetic forces are great enough, the organ may rupture, spilling its contents into the abdominal cavity. The large bowel contains bacteria and other pathogens which, if spilled, cause severe infection. The gall bladder, stomach, and small bowel contain caustic fluids that chemically damage the abdominal contents if released into the peritoneal space.

The traumatic jarring or deceleration of abdominal contents may induce organs to tear at their attachment sites. Blood vessels are often torn where they branch from the abdominal aorta or vena cava or at the organ they supply. Injury involving the blood supply to any of the abdominal organs can result in rapid and extensive blood loss and organ dysfunction.

Ligamentous detachment can also lead to abdominal organ trauma. When the various organs within the cavity decelerate, ligaments and other connective tissue may restrain them. As was mentioned in Chapter 14, the liver is suspended by the *ligamentum teres.* As it moves forward while the lower boundary of the chest is decelerated, the liver may be sliced, as cheese is by a wire cutter. The laceration is severe, resulting in rapid hemorrhage.

The structures located within the pelvic cavity are extremely well protected by the design of the pelvis. The full bladder may be ruptured in rapid deceleration when the seat belt slows the body and expresses great force along the top of the pelvic ring. A similar injury may occur to a full sigmoid colon or to the rectum. The spilling of abdominal contents or blood into the peritoneal space will generally present in one of two ways. Blood, gastric or small bowel contents, or the digestive fluids (bile or pancreatic juices) are very irritating and will inflame the peritoneum within 12 hours. The highly infectious contents of the large bowel on the other hand, will develop peritoneal inflammation much more slowly, over 12 to 24 hours. The first indication of evolving injury may be rebound tenderness.

The female genitalia are most commonly injured from trauma directed specifically at that area. Child molestation and rape are the most prevalent causes of this injury. (See Chapter 31.) The mechanism of injury normally involves the forceful placement of objects into the vaginal canal. Tearing of the internal genitalia presents with moderate to severe internal and/or external bleeding. Because the male genitalia are external, they are more frequently injured and may present with profuse blood loss. The region is supplied with significant circulation and innervation. Laceration can cause large blood losses, while blunt trauma may lead to severe hematoma.

There is an obvious difference in the presentation of chest and abdominal injuries. While injuries in both locations can be life threatening, those of the chest tend to be more frequent and more immediately critical. The signs of chest injury are easily recognized by the soft-tissue injury to the chest wall, the pain of the rib fracture, and the dyspnea secondary to respiratory dysfunction. Moderate to severe pneumothorax, hemothorax, or flail chest contribute significantly to shock. Tension pneumothorax, traumatic asphyxia, pericardial tamponade, and aortic aneurysm may separately induce shock or in extreme cases cause cardiopulmonary arrest. On the other hand, abdominal injury may be much less obvious. The rupture of an internal, hollow organ may go relatively unnoticed, while the organ's contents spill into the cavity and begin the inflammatory process. Internal bleeding may also be unnoticed until shock develops, and the actual site of internal hemorrhage may be impossible to determine in the field. Trauma to the internal solid organs may only be evidenced by the mechanism of injury and non-specific signs and symptoms. These may offer few clues to the nature and severity of the injury inside. For patients with chest and abdominal trauma, the paramedic should exhibit a high degree of suspicion and must anticipate ongoing injury. It is better to anticipate serious consequences than to play catch-up once the grave signs of decompensatory shock evolve.

ASSESSMENT

During assessment of the trauma patient, you will direct your attention to the chest and abdomen several times. (See Figure 16-8.) Careful evaluation of the mechanism of injury and the signs and symptoms found during assessment will either suggest or rule out the probability of body cavity injury. This region houses important structures including the vital parts of the cardiovascular system, the respiratory system, and other essential organs. Assessment must be complete and thorough enough to identify any injury and specific enough to suggest proper care. If you overlook any evidence, further injury or mistreatment may result.

The mechanism of injury may suggest possible chest and abdominal injury. The gross nature of the incident may reveal the direction, strength, and point of contact of the insult. Examine the auto damage and, in your mind, relive what occurred in the passenger compartment. Try to picture the patient's impact against the auto interior. Observe any steering wheel or dash deformity. Determine whether the patient was restrained, and if so, approximate the deceleration against the seat belt.

Apply the same approach to the analysis of all types of injuries. Identify the impact direction, its strength and the point at which patient con-

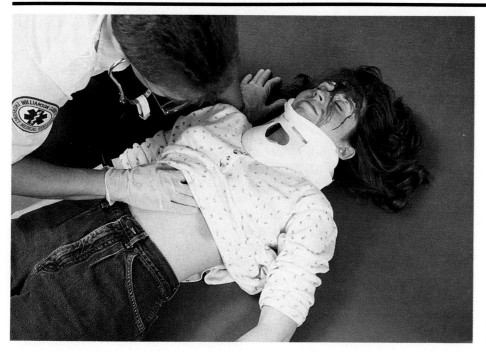

FIGURE 16-8 The chest and abdomen must be inspected for injury.

tact was made. Mentally record the possibilities of injury suggested by the mechanism of injury. They, however, should not affect application of the primary assessment.

Trauma assessment—especially, relating to the chest and abdomen—must be a complete procedure, one not specific nor focused. The paramedic must observe and evaluate completely for the A-B-C-D-E of the primary assessment. An assessment directed toward a suspected injury or patient complaint may lead the paramedic to miss the unexpected, less obvious, and possibly more serious problem. After you complete the primary assessment, the secondary assessment will allow you to evaluate anticipated injuries and patient complaints intensively.

Primary Assessment

With any suspected thoracic or abdominal trauma, the paramedic should be thinking of cervical-spine injury. Only after you immobilize the head and neck should you assess the A-B-C-D-E's. This early assessment will begin to identify the potential for and the effects of body cavity trauma. Evaluation of the *Airway* may begin to suggest chest injury, but the real evaluation of respiratory system function begins with the assessment of *Breathing*. The look, listen, and feel will really initiate the evaluation of respiratory effectiveness and the search for signs of chest trauma. The chest should be observed for equal, smooth, and symmetrical excursion. It should rise and settle gently in a rhythmic manner. Inspiration should be slightly shorter in duration than expiration. If respiratory effort varies from normal patterns, suspect chest injury. The "listen," or auditory assessment, may identify problems deep within the chest as well as the more common sounds of upper airway restriction. Wheezes or gurgling may reflect pulmonary edema, blood in the respiratory tract, or lower-airway narrowing. While the "feel" of air through the airway may not reflect the nature and the extent of chest or abdominal trauma, it may at least show that the patient is breathing. Remember that normal respiration is extremely quiet and unobtrusive. At the trauma scene it can be hard to distinguish from apnea unless the paramedic looks, listens, and feels very carefully. Chest wall movement may occur despite a complete airway obstruction. It is essential to confirm air movement even when the chest is moving.

The *Circulation* check during the primary assessment plays a key role in body cavity evaluation. Indications of hypovolemic shock, such as rapid and weak pulse, cool, clammy skin, poor capillary refill, and diminishing level of consciousness may mean that there is an internal source of blood loss within the chest or abdominal cavity. When these signs and symptoms are present and no site of hemorrhage can be located, the paramedic should suspect bleeding within the body cavity.

Assessment for *Disability* (including level of consciousness) may also heighten the suspicion of chest or abdominal injury. If the patient displays restlessness, anxiety, or central nervous system depression, suspect respiratory or circulatory compromise of body cavity origin.

As the assessment continues, the head, neck and chest are *Exposed*. Evidence of chest injury, then, may become more evident. The neck examination may reveal jugular venous distention (JVD), secondary to either increasing intrathoracic pressure caused by a tension pneumothorax or to venous backflow resulting from pericardial tamponade, traumatic asphyxia, or heart failure (myocardial contusion). Remember that JVD will be found in the normotensive supine patient. It is a significant finding only in a patient who is otherwise hypovolemic or whose upper torso is elevated higher than 45 degrees. The neck exam may also present displacement of the trachea. Displacement to the contralateral side may suggest tension pneumothorax, or to the ipsilateral side, an obstruction. Should the trachea be tugging toward one side with each inspiration, it may suggest **hemothorax** or simple (nontension) pneumothorax. Finally, the neck exam may identify subcutaneous emphysema. This finding is often associated with tension pneumothorax. Increased pressure within the thorax "pushes" air into the soft tissues, causing a crackling sensation in the area during palpation. The air will frequently migrate upward to the neck and head. Assessment of the chest should be performed with the chest exposed. The paramedic should be careful to protect the patient from the environment and the embarrassment of being viewed by bystanders. It is often best to cover the patient with a sheet or blanket to limit the vision of onlookers, maintain body temperature, and protect the patient from any adverse weather.

The paramedic should look for the signs of external trauma. Note any contusions, abrasions, lacerations or any penetrating wounds. Recognizing some of these signs may be difficult, if not impossible, since assessment occurs so quickly after the injury. View the action of the chest to determine if it is moving normally. Note if there is any paradoxical movement, any area which is moving less than the rest of the chest, or any retraction between the ribs, at the sternal notch or above the clavicles. Note any deformity in the thoracic cage, even if it appears to be stable and supporting normal respiration.

Quick auscultation will determine the relative effectiveness of the respiratory effort. Place the diaphragm of the stethoscope in each axilla,

■ **hemothorax** blood within the pleural cavity.

just above the nipple line. This location contains the least soft tissue between the disc and the lung tissue. It also provides auscultation of the sounds of the distal lung fields. If respiratory sounds heard here are normal, it can be presumed that good air exchange is occurring. The sounds should be equal bilaterally. If not, suspect an injury.

Observe and palpate the abdomen for signs of injury. Evaluate any discoloration, abrasion, laceration, evisceration, penetrating wound, or impaled object for the internal injury it may represent. If the abdomen or any quadrant is rigid, tender, exhibits rebound tenderness or contains an unusual or pulsing mass, note it. You should then suspect internal hemorrhage and perform further assessment later. Observe the abdomen for any signs of abnormal movement. Any pulsation may reflect abdominal aortic aneurysm, while exaggerated abdominal wall movement with respiration may indicate lower cervical spine injury.

At the conclusion of the primary assessment, treat injuries that threaten patient stability prior to initiating the secondary assessment. The patient should receive high flow oxygen by nonrebreathing mask. If he or she is unable to protect the airway, secure it with an endotracheal tube. Support inadequate respirations by intermittent positive pressure ventilation via the endotracheal tube. Limit any paradoxical motion by gentle immobilization. If an open pneumothorax is suspected, seal it immediately and carefully monitor respirations to observe for development of a tension pneumothorax. If primary assessment suggests a tension pneumothorax, confirm it by further assessment. Then decompress it (if allowed within protocol). Remember that internal bleeding—as may occur within the thorax or abdomen—presents with limited signs and symptoms until a great deal of blood is lost.

The paramedic should, with any significant trauma, always suspect hemorrhagic body cavity injury. Therefore, assess carefully for any sign or symptom forewarning of hypovolemia. After the primary assessment is completed, decide whether to transport immediately or remain at the scene. If the patient has or had a reduced level of consciousness or signs of respiratory or circulatory embarrassment, transport without delay. When in doubt, paramedics should transport.

Secondary Assessment

Secondary assessment gives the paramedic the opportunity to examine in detail any injury suspected from either the mechanism of injury or the results of the primary assessment. Even when a serious injury might call for immediate transport, evaluate the chest and abdomen completely during this period. If an immediate transport is unnecessary, continue the head-to-toe assessment, with special emphasis on the body cavity. Reassess the head and neck and then observe, palpate, and auscultate the entirety of the chest. Assessment should be complete and all-inclusive. No single sign, but several in combination, should be used to confirm the existence of a certain injury. Perform the entire chest assessment and use all the results to identify what may be going on within. A frequent shortfall of many field care providers is to find one or two signs of a particular injury and then focus on the suspected problem. But the various chest injuries, as well as many abdominal ones, present with similar symptoms. *If assessment is not comprehensive, you may miss the true injury.*

Assess both the chest and abdomen completely and comprehensively. Observe the excursion and rhythmic motion of the chest. Determine the rate of respiration and the approximate tidal volume. Multiply the two values to determine the minute volume and the relative effectiveness of the respiratory effort. Use of pulse oximetry is extremely helpful in determining if respirations are effective. (See Figure 16-9.) Oxygen saturation (SaO$_2$) should be maintained above 97% when possible. If the saturation drops much below 90%, give aggressive respiratory care. Paramedics should also consider the altitude of the patient above sea level, for this affects the overall SaO$_2$. Evaluate the chest carefully for discoloration or local swelling. Any developing erythema, ecchymosis, or deformity will become progressively more visible with time. Periodic assessment ensures that the effects of this delayed development do not go unnoticed. Direct special attention at the ribs and sternum, since the forces of trauma would trap the soft tissues between the offending object and these bony structures. If there is a penetrating wound, look for an exit wound, especially if a rifle, shotgun, or handgun was used. Examine the wound or wounds closely for air movement or frothy blood, both indicative of an open pneumothorax (sucking chest wound).

Note any other signs of respiratory distress outside the thoracic region. Any use of accessory muscles to assist the respiratory effort, such as the sternocleidomastoid or abdominal muscles, suggest respiratory problems. Anxiety, restlessness (especially in the presence of shock), or reduced level of consciousness hint of a possible respiratory problem. Systemic discoloration (cyanotic or ashen skin) may be due to respiratory insufficiency.

Palpate the entirety of the chest. Gently localize any crepitation, subcutaneous emphysema, or deformity and note it for the record. Place your hands on the lower borders of the patient's chest to evaluate the motion associated with each breath. This will allow you to easily count respirations, to determine rate, regularity, and symmetry of chest excursion.

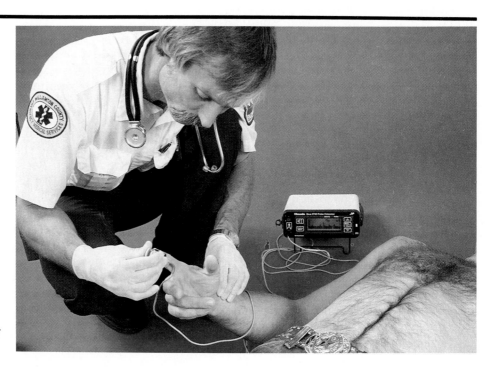

FIGURE 16-9 Pulse oximetry is effective in determining the status of oxygenation.

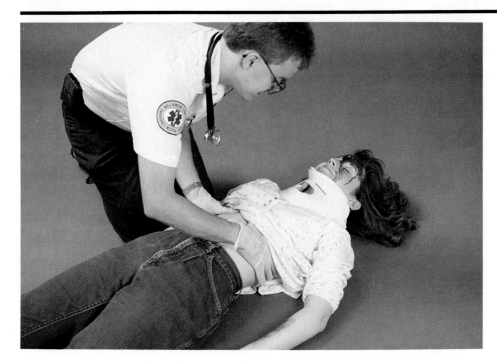

FIGURE 16-10 Paramedics should palpate the chest, noting any crepitus or subcutaneous emphysema.

If a rib fracture exists in a responsive patient, gentle compression of the lateral chest inward should elicit pain or crepitus. (See Figure 16-10.)

Auscultation should involve the complete thorax. Auscultate the anterior and posterior chest at the lung bases, apices, axillae and at the suprasternal notch. The lung sounds should be faint but without rales or rhonchi and equal in all regions. Be especially alert to the development of fine rales in the lower fields. These may be an early sign of pulmonary edema, which is frequently associated with lung contusion. Should lung sounds be unequal, search for the cause. Identify the presence of pneumothorax, tension pneumothorax, hemothorax, localized pulmonary edema, or bronchial obstruction.

Listen also to the heart sounds. If they are displaced from the normal position, which is just left of the sternum, a tension pneumothorax may be developing. If the heart sounds are distant and/or muffled, pericardial tamponade may be the cause. If a gallop (S_3) is heard, it may signal congestive heart failure secondary to myocardial contusion. Percuss the chest to assist in the confirmation of a particular injury. If the chest is dull to percussion, it may reflect the accumulation of fluid, most likely blood, in the thorax. If the vibration is hyperresonant, there may be air under pressure within, a sign of tension pneumothorax. Check one side against the other, anterior against posterior, and superior against inferior to determine the existence of inequality. Localize the absence or reduced resonance and determine if it is bilateral or regional.

The abdominal assessment should also include careful and complete observation and palpation. Carefully remove the patient's remaining clothing so the abdomen can be visualized in its entirety. Look for any signs of discoloration or deformity as well as any sites of pulsation. (See Figure 16-11.) Remember that these signs develop over time and serial assessment may be the only way to ensure that you do not miss them. The

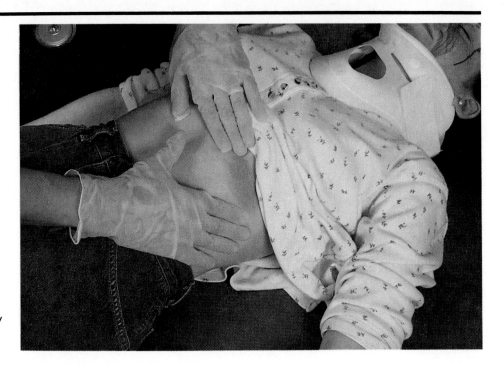

FIGURE 16-11 Paramedics should note any contusions possibly indicative of serious, underlying injury.

abdominal area lacks the bony protection of the chest. Therefore, patients with traumatic injury may not present with overt signs and symptoms.

The mechanism of injury, as well as any associated signs and symptoms, help determine the potential for injury. It is also important to remember that the signs and symptoms of underlying problems in the abdomen progress more slowly and inconspicuously than those of the chest. Spilling of bowel contents or blood into the peritoneal space may not manifest with pain until hours after the injury. Gently palpate the abdomen for symptoms of tenderness and rebound tenderness. Next, evaluate each quadrant by pushing lightly with fingers of one hand over those of the other hand. Feel for guarding, tenderness, pulsation or masses. Release the pressure quickly and note any discomfort (rebound tenderness). Relate any findings to the organs which lie beneath. Evaluate any other signs and symptoms in search of potential injury. Continue the palpation to the flanks and lower back. Ensure that no pain is felt on touch and that no deformities, swelling, or local warmth or coolness exist.

Often the determination that an injury has occurred within the abdomen is made more on the basis of ruling out injury and blood loss elsewhere than on finding frank abdominal signs. Careful evaluation of the rest of the patient and the vital signs are essential to assessment of abdominal injury.

Vital Signs. Vital signs are essential for complete assessment of the body cavity injury patient. Pulse, respirations, and blood pressure must be determined and carefully monitored during care and transport.

During the primary assessment, you evaluate the pulse briefly. Carefully reassess it for the development of shock. The rapid thready pulse in an anxious or CNS-depressed patient may be the only early indication of chest or abdominal hemorrhage.

Blood pressure can be an important tool in the evaluation of the patient with chest or abdominal injury. The hypotension associated with shock, although a late sign, should direct attention to the source of blood loss; possibly into the body cavity. Narrowing of the difference between the systolic and diastolic pressure may be a sign of pericardial tamponade. It may be even more specific of tamponade if the pulse is stronger during inspiration (*pulsus paradoxus*), in contrast to the normal pulse strength, which increases with expiration.

Patient History

Evaluate the patient for the normal symptoms of injury during the initial and secondary assessment of the chest and abdomen. Any complaint of pain, tenderness or abnormal feeling should be noted. Palpate carefully and inquire completely. Often, the patient will be distracted by more painful but less significant injury elsewhere. Explain to the patient that the major complaint will be addressed later. Now, however, a thorough exam is needed. Ask specifically if the respiratory effort is getting easier or harder. In traumatic chest compression, the alveoli may become collapsed (atelectasis) and the patient may complain that "I had the wind knocked out of me." The patient will find it difficult to move air at first. As the alveoli are reexpanded, respiration will become less and less difficult. On the other hand, the patient may complain of more and more effort needed to breathe. The lungs become stiff and edematous after a pulmonary contusion. Thus, the effort needed to move air becomes greater. Increased respiratory effort may also reflect an increasing pneumothorax, hemothorax, tension pneumothorax, or other progressing chest injury.

Abdominal symptoms can be very useful in determining the nature of any internal injury. Identify the exact location and type of pain the patient is experiencing. Record the description carefully in the patient's own words. Determine specifically if the pain is sharp, dull, tearing, constant, periodic, or throbbing. Identify the onset and progression of any abdominal pain. Did the pain begin immediately after the injury or was it delayed, and if so for how long? Has the pain grown worse, remained the same or gotten better since onset? Is there any position, movement or activity which makes it either better or worse? Document any findings. Then attempt to determine whether they reflect a specific or multiple-organ injury. Summarize and prioritize these findings. Decide what structures within the thorax, abdomen, and pelvis may be injured. Then place the injuries in order of significance for the patient's overall condition and identify priorities for care.

MANAGEMENT

As patient management begins, stabilize the spine, secure the airway, and support breathing as identified by the results of the primary assessment. Any significant trauma to the chest signifies vertebral injury until proven otherwise. Any patient who is unable to protect the airway should be intubated with an endotracheal tube. All trauma patients, and especially patients with body cavity injury, should receive high-flow oxygen.

If necessary, provide positive pressure ventilation. Begin PASG application and fluid resuscitation if the patient exhibits any early signs of shock. Initiate two large-bore IVs peripherally while the trousers are applied and prepared for inflation. The infusion may be assisted by the use of pressure infusion bags (or BP cuffs). If the abdomen shows signs of internal hemorrhage, consider inflating the abdominal compartment of the PASG, not only for its hemodynamic effect, but also for potential hemorrhage control. (The abdominal compartment may *only* be inflated with or after the inflation of the leg compartments.)

Should the patient present with any uncorrectable breathing or airway problem, or any signs or symptoms of central nervous system depression or of the early development of shock, transport immediately. Additionally, if the mechanism of injury suggest a threat to life, transport and provide care enroute. Once the primary care priorities have been addressed, the specific steps of body cavity injury care can begin.

Thoracic Trauma Care

If any internal chest injury is suspected, place the patient on the injured side unless contraindicated. Take serial vital signs, evaluate respiratory effectiveness, and auscultate breath sounds frequently. Record the results. Even if general care steps seem to alleviate a problem, continued and serial assessment is needed to ensure the injury doesn't redevelop or progress.

Soft-tissue injuries of the chest are important because of the potential injury beneath. Contusions, abrasions, and minor lacerations are superficial and can be cared for after the patient is completely stable. The only exception is the open pneumothorax. If a wound penetrates the thorax (see Figure 16-12) it should be sealed as if it were a sucking chest wound (open pneumothorax). Cover the wound with an occlusive dressing such as petroleum gauze, a defibrillator pad, or the inside of a trauma dressing wrapper. Seal three sides of the dressing so that any pressure build-up will escape and prevent the development of the tension pneumothorax. (See Figure 16-13.)

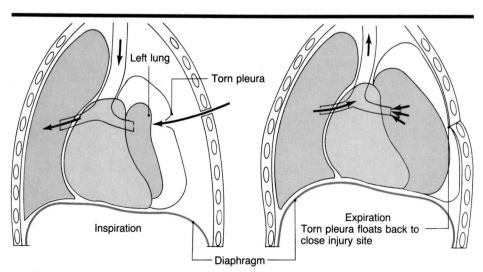

FIGURE 16-12 Sucking chest wound.

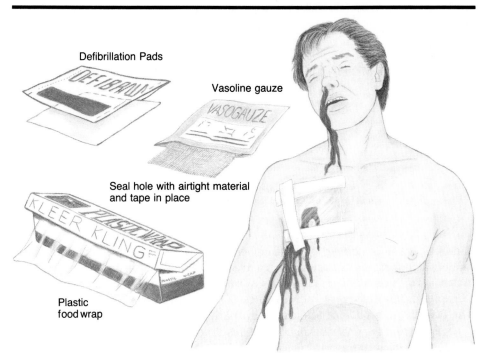

Defibrillation Pads

Vasoline gauze

Seal hole with airtight material
and tape in place

Plastic
food wrap

FIGURE 16-13 Prehospital treatment of a sucking chest wound should include the placement of an occlusive dressing secured on three sides.

Again, the patient is best placed on the injured side. There he or she should be monitored closely for the development of tension pneumothorax or other dyspnea-inducing problems. Placing the patient on the injured side allows gravity to assist the inflation of the unaffected lung. The weight of the injured or affected lung and the mediastinum will pull downward. This ensures that the unaffected lung is fully inflated with each breath.

Carefully monitor the patient's breath sounds to determine if, in fact, a pneumothorax does exist. Monitoring also ensures that the injury does not progress. Administer high-flow oxygen via a non-rebreathing mask and monitor oxygen saturation with pulse oximetry. If the saturation level drops much below 97%, attempt rigorous airway and respiratory support. If the saturation drops below 94%, use a bag-valve-mask device and endotracheal intubation with 100% oxygen.

If the patient assessment discovers any apparent rib fracture, monitor the respiratory effort. There will often be associated pulmonary contusions beneath the site which may cause pulmonary edema. The pain of the fracture will cause the patient to limit respiratory excursion, leading to poorer air exchange and possible atelectasis. Encourage the patient to breathe as deeply as tolerable.

Within some EMS systems the use of Nitronox may be suggested by protocol. Nitronox is an analgesic which may help manage the patient's limited respirations due to pain. It is a mixture of 50% oxygen and 50% nitrous oxide, self-administered by the patient through a mask arrangement. This prevents the patient from receiving too much drug and suffering central nervous system depression. Nitronox is a short-acting drug whose effects will subside within 2 to 5 minutes following administration. Nitrous oxide has proven safe in the field setting and should be con-

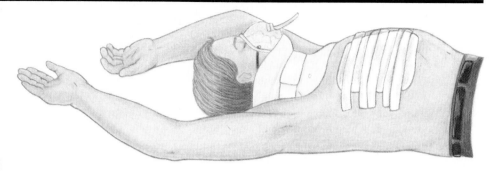

FIGURE 16-14 Flail chest should be treated with oxygen and gentle splinting of the flail segment with a pillow or a pad.

Tape pad in place, extending tape to both sides of chest

✳ Nitronox should not be used in cases of pneumothorax or in instances where bowel obstruction is possible.

sidered if it is approved by medical control. It does have a few side effects which affect its administration in trauma. Some patients will experience nausea and possibly emesis. This should be anticipated and prepared for. Nitrous oxide also may increase intracranial pressure. Thus its use with the head injury patient should be limited.

Special care may be needed if rib fractures are extensive and paradoxical chest wall motion is noted. Flail chest severely compromises respiration and the paradoxical motion must be stopped. Gentle pressure, as applied with a pad or pillow, will inhibit the outward excursion of the segment and decrease the negative effect of the flail segment. (See Figure 16-14.) In flail chest, positive pressure ventilation may reverse respiratory embarrassment. The conscious patient with spontaneous breathing may resist assisted respirations. Resistance usually abates once the effective exchange of air is accomplished, and the pain associated with respiration is diminished. It is helpful if the patient is allowed to signal when he or she feels the need for a breath. The use of positive pressure ventilation in any significant chest trauma may exacerbate injury to the pulmonary tissue, possibly beneath the flail segment. The bag-valve-mask may increase the incidence of associated pneumothorax and tension pneumothorax. In any case, the demand valve should rarely be used to assist the chest trauma patient. Its high-pressure inspiration significantly increases the incidence of simple and tension pneumothorax.

The final trauma-induced chest wall defect to be discussed is *traumatic asphyxia*. The patient with traumatic asphyxia should be rapidly transported to the hospital. Aggressive care should be administered during extrication and while enroute. The paramedic should anticipate the rapid development of hypovolemia as the chest compression is released. Initiate two IV access lines with large-bore catheters and trauma tubing. Prepare to run two 1000 mL bags of either normal saline or lactated Ringer's solution with pressure infusion. Apply and inflate the PASG as needed. Provide 100% oxygen by non-rebreather or bag-valve-mask and be ready to intubate the patient if unconsciousness ensues. Be prepared for this patient to rapidly deteriorate to trauma arrest.

Sodium bicarbonate for potential acidosis caused by traumatic asphyxia may be ordered by the medical control physician. Prolonged hypoxia followed by the release of chest compression may cause acidotic blood to return to the central circulation. Bicarbonate will counteract this problem by buffering the shift of the blood's pH. It will bind to the free hydrogen ions, forming water and carbon dioxide, and thus bring the acidity of the blood more toward normal. It should only be used when the hypoxia has been present for more than 10 minutes. It should be administered via IV bolus at a dosage of 1 mEq per kilogram of body weight during or shortly after the decompression of the patient's chest. Great care should be used in deciding to administer this drug. Its administration will place a high concentration of sodium ions in the vascular space which may contribute to systemic and pulmonary edema. (Edema is more of a concern in the overhydrated or CHF patient than in one suffering from hypovolemia; this precaution, then, may not apply to the traumatic asphyxia patient.) The alkalizing effects of bicarbonate may also reduce the effectiveness of the catecholamines used in cardiac arrest or protracted hypotension. Any administration of sodium bicarbonate should be guided by protocol and medical control.

If a closed pneumothorax is suspected or an open pneumothorax was sealed, the patient should be frequently evaluated for the development of tension pneumothorax. Continually check for the signs and symptoms of this injury. The pertinent negatives should be noted in the record, including tracheal displacement, breath sounds, jugular vein condition, and response to percussion. Tension pneumothorax is a serious, life-threatening insult to the respiratory and cardiovascular system. If it is present, the paramedic must relieve the pressure quickly by needle decompression, unless otherwise defined by your protocol. Carefully evaluate the patient's signs and symptoms and request permission to attempt the procedure from the on-line medical control physician. If permission is granted, one of two locations must be used. The midclavicular approach approximates the second or third intercostal space at the midclavicular line. This is found by locating the middle of the clavicle on the affected side and moving the fingers down to the first or second intercostal space. An alternate site is the midaxillary line at or around the fifth intercostal space. The intersection of the midaxillary and nipple line is used with the nearest intercostal groove palpated. A large bore (10–14 gauge) over-the-needle catheter is inserted just above the lower rib at a 90 degree angle until the sound of escaping air is heard. (See Figure 16-15.) At that point the catheter is advanced and the needle removed. Secure the hub of the catheter with tape and cover it with the finger of a rubber glove. Tie or tape it in place. Cut the tip to allow air to escape and not re-enter. (See Figure 16-16.) Once tension pneumothorax is relieved, monitor the patient frequently for the redevelopment of the injury. The catheter may become blocked or kinked, allowing the chest to repressurize. It may be necessary to decompress the chest with another needle inserted close to the original site.

The patient with cardiac contusion must be treated as aggressively as the patient with myocardial infarction. The implementation of the cardiac protocols (to be discussed later) should be considered, including oxygen, lidocaine, bretylium, procainamide, atropine, and isoproterenol.

It is necessary to ensure that the airway and respiration are optimally cared for. Any development of the signs and symptoms of shock should be supported with equally aggressive care. Pericardial tamponade is a dire emergency which is rarely correctable in the field setting. The procedure to relieve the pressure within the pericardial sac (pericardiocentesis) is extremely difficult under the best of conditions. (See Figure 16-17.) A large bore spinal needle must be inserted into the sac and the fluid withdrawn. It is difficult to ensure that the needle is in the sac and not the ventricle. By penetrating the myocardium, the needle may permit

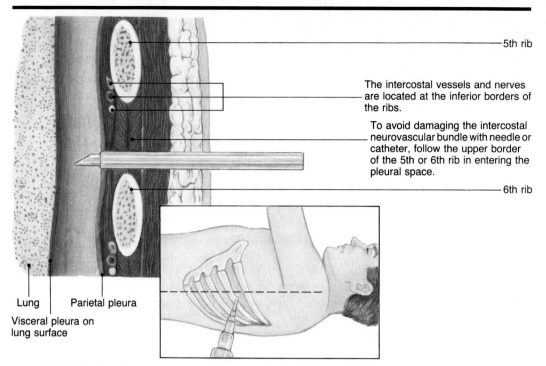

5th rib

The intercostal vessels and nerves are located at the inferior borders of the ribs.

To avoid damaging the intercostal neurovascular bundle with needle or catheter, follow the upper border of the 5th or 6th rib in entering the pleural space.

6th rib

Lung   Parietal pleura

Visceral pleura on lung surface

FIGURE 16-15   Needle decompression of a tension pneumothorax.

a more rapid redevelopment of the injury. Unless the paramedic is specifically trained and permitted by medical control to attempt this procedure, the patient should be packaged and transported immediately. Any patient suspected of suffering traumatic aortic aneurysm should receive rapid and gentle transport to definitive care. Bouncing, sudden movement, or increase in blood pressure, such as that caused by anxiety, may cause the

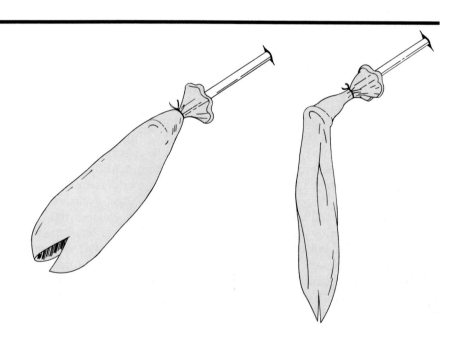

FIGURE 16-16   One-way valve constructed out of the finger of a latex glove.

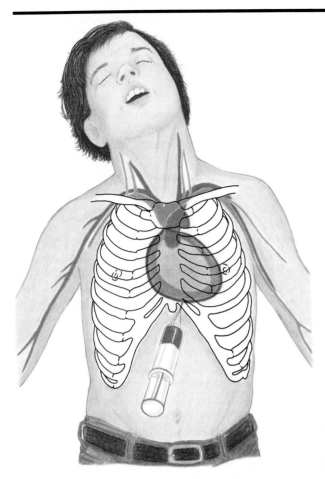

FIGURE 16-17   Technique for pericardiocentesis.

injury to progress. Shock should be treated conservatively, though good perfusion must be maintained. If blood pressure measurement must be obtained, the paramedic should use the right, upper extremity or one of the lower extremities. Using the left, upper extremity may cause additional back pressure on the aneurysm and increase the likelihood of its rupture.

If an object is found to be impaled in the chest, immobilize it in the same position as found. Cover the entry wound with an occlusive dressing and a bulky dressing. Completely stabilize the object so patient transport will not cause motion or dislodgment. If the object is very large or unwieldy, attempt to cut it. Fully immobilize the object prior to and during the efforts to shorten it. Remove the object only if it interferes with attempts to perform CPR in the cardiopulmonary arrest patient. Its removal may increase internal bleeding and further contribute to hypovolemia.

Abdominal Trauma Care

The care of the patient with suspected abdominal trauma should be directed at anticipation of internal hemorrhage and the need for rapid surgery. The patient with any significant signs, symptoms or mechanism of injury that suggest the potential for internal bleeding should be rapidly transported to the Emergency Department. Enroute, insert two large bore catheters and start IV fluids. The PASG should be applied and readied for inflation. Evaluate vital signs frequently, along with other signs possibly indicating the early development of shock. These include capillary refill, blood pressure, skin color, patient anxiety or restlessness, and pulse rate and strength.

In the presence of any significant sign or symptom of shock, it is imperative to provide aggressive fluid replacement to the abdominal trauma patient. Rapid blood loss can result from various sources and leave the patient with irreversible shock if not treated early. The crystalloid solutions used in the field will only remain in the vascular space for a short period. Thus, for every milliliter of blood lost, three milliliters of IV fluid must be infused. If the patient has lost 500 mL of blood preceding the paramedic's arrival, he or she needs 1,500 mL of fluids immediately and three times the blood volume lost during each minute thereafter. If care is delayed until the signs and symptoms of shock are obviously apparent, it may be necessary to infuse more fluid than possible in the field setting. The patient should receive aggressive fluid resuscitation enroute to the hospital and blood replacement once there. These should not be delayed. Following emergency measures aimed at preventing or treating shock, care for the specific abdominal injuries can begin.

Penetrating wounds of the abdominal cavity should be covered, as with any open wound. If it appears that bowel is protruding, cover the wound with a wet dressing and an occlusive dressing. This approach ensures that the tissues will not dry out. If an object remains impaled in the abdomen, carefully immobilize it in place. Patients with either an evisceration or an impaled object should have their hands restrained to prevent them from manipulating the wound.

If a rifle or handgun is suspected as the offending agent, examine the patient for an exit wound. If found, dress it as well. If the projectile expended all its energy within the patient, it may not emerge. Care for the blunt abdominal injury is basically supportive. Unless otherwise required, the patient should be placed in the most comfortable position, usually on the side, with the legs flexed. The transport to a trauma center should be rapid and as smooth as can be reasonably expected. Jarring may increase the patient's discomfort.

*The primary consideration in the management of the abdominal trauma patient is not to try and determine the exact injury, but to determine that an abdominal injury exists.

SUMMARY

Injury to the body cavity and the structures within is a frequent cause of serious injury and patient death. The evaluation of the mechanism of injury, signs and symptoms, as well as general patient presentation should result in a heightened suspicion of injury. It should also ensure that the focus still remains on total patient care. If there is any reason to suspect serious internal injury, perform a quick primary assessment and transport the patient immediately. The cervical spine, Airway, Breathing, and Circulation must be protected as should any immediately life-threatening head, neck, chest or abdominal injury. Additional care at the scene or enroute should include endotracheal intubation, high flow oxygenation, assisted respirations, hemorrhage control, and aggressive fluid replacement. If the patient appears stable, and there is no reason to suspect severe body cavity injury, he or she should be monitored carefully and continuously. In this way the development of internal problems will not go unnoticed. Provide oxygen, carry out the complete assessment, and provide general care steps provided for body cavity trauma.

Injury to the chest and abdomen account for a very high percentage of traumatic deaths. Therefore, the paramedic should have a high index of suspicion for injury to this region and be prepared for aggressive intervention. Such an approach will give emergency medical services its best opportunity to reduce patient mortality and morbidity.

FURTHER READING

AMERICAN COLLEGE OF SURGEONS, Committee on Trauma, *Advanced Trauma Life Support Course: Student Manual.* American College of Surgeons, 1989.

BLEDSOE, B. E., *Atlas of Paramedic Skills.* Englewood Cliffs, NJ: Prentice-Hall, Inc., 1987.

BUTMAN, A. M., AND PATURAS, J. L., *Pre-Hospital Trauma Life Support.* Akron, OH: Emergency Training, 1986.

CAMPBELL, J. E., *Basic Trauma Life Support.* 2d. ed. Englewood Cliffs, NJ: Prentice-Hall, Inc., 1988.

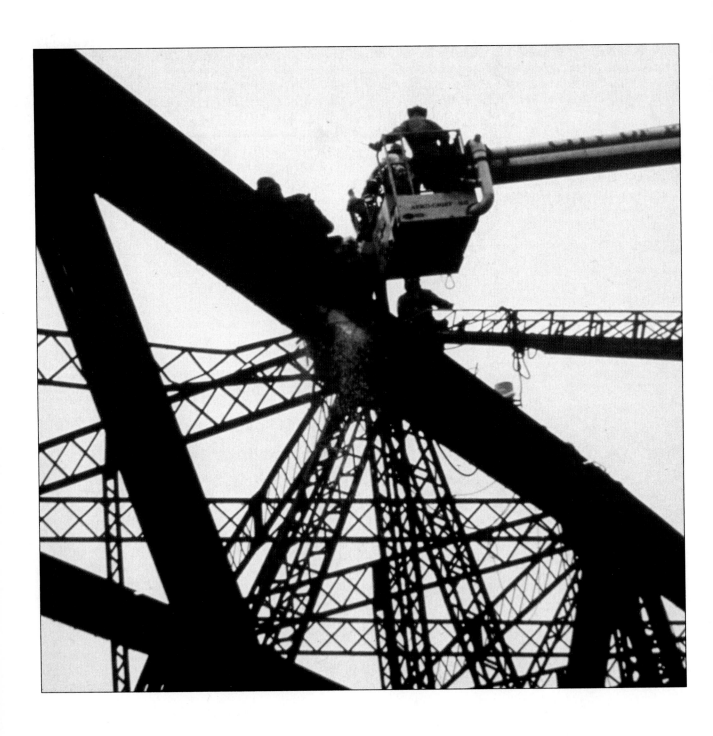

17

Musculoskeletal Injuries

Objectives for Chapter 17

Upon completing this chapter, the student should be able to:

1. Identify the long bones of the extremities and describe their general structure.

2. Describe the structure, attachment, and general action of the muscles of the extremities.

3. Compare and contrast the pathologies of sprain, strain, subluxation, dislocation and fracture.

4. List the signs and symptoms normally associated with musculoskeletal injury and their relative importance to the overall assessment process.

5. Order and demonstrate the steps of assessment for the trauma patient as they apply to extremity injury.

6. Identify the signs and symptoms of circulatory or nervous loss to a distal extremity and the steps to take to correct this deficit.

7. Explain fracture or dislocation immobilization techniques for the following locations: pelvis, hip, femur, knee, tibia and fibula, ankle, foot, shoulder, humerus, elbow, radius and ulna, wrist, hand, and finger.

CASE STUDY

Unit 93 is dispatched to a local nursing home to pick up a patient who fell out of bed. Upon arrival, the patient is found to be lying on a hallway floor. An 85-year-old female resident of the home, she explains that she fell while walking to the recreation hall. The patient denies any vertigo or any other symptoms either now or previous to the fall. She has limited pain in the thigh area and explains that she felt a snap as her hip gave way and she fell. Physical assessment reveals an angulated left thigh, crepitation, and instability beyond the hip joint. The attending nurse states that Mrs. Jones rarely complains and has had few medical problems. She is on oral hypoglycemic agents and a diuretic.

Vital signs reveal a blood pressure of 110/90, a pulse of 90, and respirations of normal depth and at a rate of 22. Her hands and unaffected leg are moist and cool, while her injured extremity is cold. The distal pulse is slightly diminished in the left leg, although present in the right. She is placed on moderate-flow oxygen; oximetry shows a saturation of 96%. She is gently moved to a spineboard via an orthopedic stretcher. One intravenous line is initiated, normal saline is hung and set to run at a to-keep-open rate. A dextrose stick indicates her glucose to be 120 mg/dl. She is transported to the ambulance and travels uneventfully to the Emergency Department where a hip fracture is confirmed by X-ray. Due to her age, the patient spends several weeks in the hospital and then several months ambulating in the nursing home.

INTRODUCTION

Musculoskeletal injuries are second in occurrence only to soft-tissue injuries. They usually are the result of direct or transmitted kinetic forces, but, occasionally, may be caused by penetrating insult. While most musculoskeletal injuries do not require more than basic care, these skills must be well applied to ensure that no harm occurs during care and transport.

The assessment and care of musculoskeletal injuries will be quite different for the unstable and for the stable patient. Unstable patients need immediate transport and will receive care directed at immediate support and rapid movement. They will be managed without the detailed and time-consuming splinting process. However, you still must consider possible musculoskeletal injuries when choosing movement and packaging techniques for these patients.

The patient who is found with an isolated long bone injury, or who is moderately injured and stable, should receive complete assessment and immobilization of any musculoskeletal areas. Any injury must be assessed carefully to ensure that circulation, motor control, and sensation remain intact during immobilization and transport. The injury site must be fixed in a physiologic position to allow the greatest comfort, adequate circulation, and efficient immobilization. Adjacent joints must be stabilized to prevent motion from being transmitted to, or through, the site. These objectives, if met, will ensure that patients receive optimal stabilization of their suspected injuries.

To properly respond to musculoskeletal emergencies the paramedic must maintain and build upon the knowledge and skills of the Basic EMT. These basic skills should be accompanied by a deeper understanding of the structure and function of the body elements, the process and progression of injury, and the assessment and care modalities the injuries require.

ANATOMY & PHYSIOLOGY

The musculoskeletal system is a complex system of levers and fulcrums that provide motion and support for the body. It consists of two distinct subsystems, the *skeleton* and the *muscles.* The skeleton is the superstructure of the human body, while the muscles supply the power of motion to the superstructure and various organs.

The Skeleton

Besides acting as the body's structural form, the skeleton serves several important functions. It is an exceptional protector of the vital organs. It allows us to move about efficiently against the forces of gravity. It is responsible for the storage of many needed salts and other materials for metabolism. And, it is responsible for the production of red blood cells used in the transport of oxygen. (See Figure 17-1.)

Although the skeleton is not often thought of as alive, it is exactly that. Its cells are alive, living in a matrix of protein fibers and salt deposits. These living cells are constantly changing the structure and dynamics of the human frame.

Bones are provided with a continuous supply of blood which brings in oxygen and nutrients and removes carbon dioxide and waste products. As with any body tissue, if the blood supply is damaged or lost, bone tissue will become ischemic and die. The bone will not show evidence of this degeneration during emergency care. However, the effects may be devastating afterwards. Numerous bones make up the framework of the body. They are divided into two major subdivisions: the axial and the appendicular skeletons. The *axial skeleton* consists of the skull, the vertebral column, and the thorax. The components of this subdivision have been discussed in Chapters 15 and 16. The *appendicular skeleton* is composed of the shoulder girdle and bones of the upper extremity, as well as the pelvis and bones of the lower extremity.

The extremity long bones are similar in design and structure. They consist of three regions, differing in construction and purpose. (See Figure 17-2.) The **diaphysis** is the long narrow cylinder or shaft of the bone. The articular and widened end is the **epiphysis.** Between the two is the **metaphysis,** which transitions from the hollow support member to the articular end.

The diaphysis is the central portion of the long bone comprised of very dense, compact bone. The actual weight-bearing portion of the shaft is a very thin and light hollow tube. Its interior is filled with *yellow bone marrow* which stores fat in a semiliquid form. The fat is a readily available energy source that the body can quickly and easily use.

The exterior of the diaphysis is covered with a tough membrane, the **periosteum.** Vascular and innervated, it initiates the repair cycle when the bone is fractured. The periosteum and compact bone are penetrated by blood vessels and nerves traveling through small passages called **haversian canals.** These canals allow the essential blood to pass into the interior and circulate to the bone ends.

■ **diaphysis** hollow shaft of the longbones.

■ **epiphysis** ends of the longbone, including the epiphyseal, or growth plate, and support structures underlying the joint.

■ **metaphysis** growth zone of the bone, active during the developmental stages of youth. It is located between the epiphysis and the diaphysis.

■ **periosteum** tough, hard covering of bone.

■ **haversian canals** small perforations of the longbones through which the blood vessels and nerves travel into the bone itself.

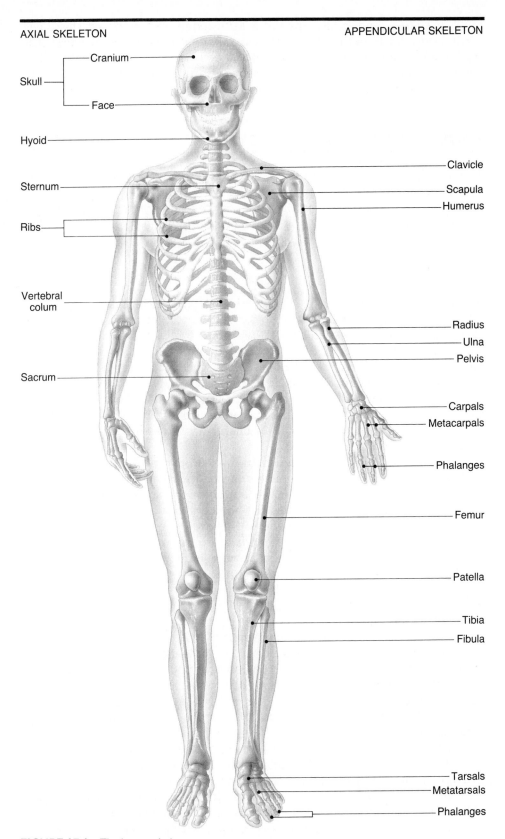

FIGURE 17-1 The human skeleton.

Toward the epiphysis, the bone structure changes dramatically. The hard, compact bone of the shaft changes into a network of fibers and strands. This network serves to spread the stress and pressure of support over a larger surface. The tissue in cross-section resembles a rigid bony sponge (**cancellous bone**). Covering this network of fibers is a thin layer of compact bone supporting the articular surface. The cancellous bone of the larger long bones is filled with *red marrow* which is responsible for the manufacture of erythrocytes. (See Figure 17-2.)

The **metaphysis** is an intermediate region between the epiphysis and diaphysis. It expands the dense, thin, and solid hollow tube of the diaphysis into the cancellous honeycomb of the epiphysis.

The epiphyseal surface is covered by a layer of connective tissue called **cartilage.** It is a smooth, strong, and flexible material which functions as the actual surface of articulation between bones. The cartilage allows for very easy movement between the ends of adjacent bones such as the femur and tibia. This tissue also absorbs some of the impact associated with walking, running, or any jarring activity.

The long bones are held together by a relatively sophisticated structure, the *joint*. It is banded together with strands of connective tissue called **ligaments.** They stretch and permit joint motion while holding the bone ends firmly in place. The flat band of the ligament is attached to the

■ **cancellous bone** spongy bone tissue found at the distal and proximal ends of the long-bones.

■ **cartilage** connective tissue providing the articular surfaces of the skeletal system.

■ **ligament** connective tissue connecting bone to bone and holding the joints together. The ligaments will stretch to allow joint movement.

STRUCTURE OF LONG BONE

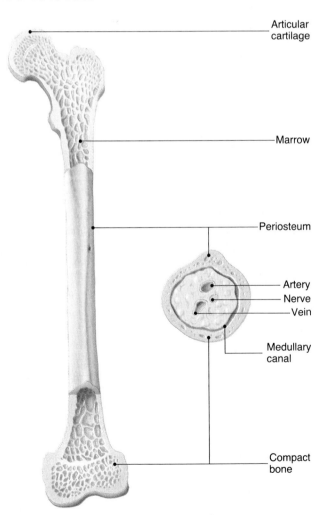

Articular cartilage

Marrow

Periosteum

Artery

Nerve

Vein

Medullary canal

Compact bone

FIGURE 17-2 The internal anatomy of a long bone.

joint end of each of the joint bones. Ligaments surround the articular region and cross it at many oblique angles. This arrangement ensures that the joint is held strongly together yet is flexible enough to move through the designed range of motion.

Contained by these ligamentous bands is the **synovial** capsule. It is a chamber that holds a small amount of fluid to lubricate the articular surfaces. This oily, viscous fluid assists joint motion by further reducing friction.

The structural design of the upper and lower extremities is similar. Both **articulate** with a joint supported by several bones and are affixed to the axial skeleton. Each has a single long bone proximally and paired bones distally. The terminal member, the hand or foot, consist of numerous bones with differing purposes yet parallel design.

Upper Extremity

The shoulder is composed of the clavicle and scapula, which sit high on the thoracic cage. The scapula is an irregularly-shaped bone located posteriorly and buried within the musculature of the upper back. It provides the glenoid depression, or fossa, which is the shallow socket in which the humerus sits. The scapula moves freely over the posterior thorax, providing some of the shoulder's large range of motion. The upper-back musculature effectively protects the scapula from fracture in all but the most direct and severe trauma.

The clavicle is anterior to the scapula and is not as well protected. It holds the scapula and shoulder joint at a fixed distance from the sternum. The clavicle is frequently fractured. It is, in fact, the most commonly fractured bone of the human body.

The humerus is the single bone of the proximal upper extremity. (This region is properly referred to as the arm.) It is secured against the shallow glenoid fossa of the shoulder joint proximally. The humerus articulates with the radius and ulna at the elbow.

The radius and ulna form the forearm. They move in conjunction with the humerus, and with each other. This articulation provides the ability to rotate the distal forearm to the palm up (**supination**) or palm down (**pronation**) position. It simultaneously allows for folding of the elbow.

The radius and ulna articulate with the carpal bones of the wrist. They, in turn, articulate with the metacarpals of the palm of the hand. The metacarpals articulate with the phalanges of the fingers. Each finger consists of three phalanges: the proximal, the middle, and the distal. The thumb has only two: the proximal and distal. The radius is on the thumb side of the forearm.

Lower Extremity

The lower extremity is supported, and allowed much of its motion, by the pelvis. A pair of fused bones and the sacrum compose the pelvis. The pubis, ilium, and iliac are joined collectively, making up the innominates. The two innominates together with the sacrum form the pelvic ring. This ring is very rigid and strong. It provides the basis for movement of the lower extremities and support when standing. The actual articular surface for the femur is the acetabulum. It is a hollow depression in the lateral pelvis into which the head of the femur fits.

The femur is the largest and strongest of the long bones. During the normal stress of walking, it often withstands pressures up to 1,200 pounds per square inch along its diaphysis. With such strength, a fracture of the femur must involve tremendous forces. Therefore, it probably will cause other related soft tissue, vascular, or nervous injury.

The femur is not a completely straight long bone. At its superior end, where the head meets the acetabulum, the femur makes an almost 90 degree turn. The head is supported by the neck, a narrow shaft, at almost a right angle to the uppermost aspect of the widened femoral shaft. This configuration permits the wide range of motion found in the joint and its great strength.

Meeting the femur distally is the tibia. It is matched with the fibula, a smaller, much more delicate bone. The tibia is the only bone of the lower leg that articulates with the femur. Since the fibula does not, its only function is to add control to the placement and motion of the foot during walking or other ambulation.

Both the tibia and fibula join the talus and calcaneus to form the ankle. The tibia forms the medial malleolus (protuberance of the ankle) while the fibula forms the lateral malleolus. In turn, the talus articulates with the tarsals. The tarsals, in turn, articulate with the metatarsals. Both articulate with the phalanges of the foot, in a parallel configuration to the bones of the wrist and hand.

The Muscular System

The muscles of the body can be divided into three types. Of these, the most specialized is the *myocardium,* a very specific and unique tissue. The myocardium is the muscle of the heart. It contracts rhythmically on its own, emitting an electrical impulse in the process. In this way it provides the lifelong rhythmic contraction and pumping function of the heart. (The particular properties of the myocardium are discussed in Chapter 21.)

The second muscle type is that of *smooth muscle.* These muscles are not under conscious control. They are found within the vascular system, the bronchioles, the bowel, and in many other organs. The autonomic nervous system controls them. Smooth muscle will contract to reduce (or relax to expand) the diameter of the lumen of the blood vessels, the bronchioles, or the digestive tract.

The remaining muscle tissue is that of the *skeletal muscles.* They are muscles over which we have conscious control. The skeletal muscles are associated with mobility of the extremities and the body in general. The largest component of the muscular system, they are the most commonly traumatized.

The skeletal muscles lie beneath the protective layer of the skin and subcutaneous fat. They are innervated and supplied with blood like any other tissues. The individual muscle fibers are layered together to form a muscle body, such as the triceps.

The skeletal muscles are attached to the skeletal system at a minimum of two locations. These attachments are called the origin and the insertion, depending on how the related bones move with contraction. The point of attachment that remains stationary is the **origin,** while the point that moves is the **insertion.** Specialized connective tissue bands called **tendons** accomplish the insertion, and in some cases the origin. These very fibrous ribbons, actually a part of the muscle, are extremely strong and will not stretch. They are so strong that in some instances they will break an area of bone loose rather than tear. The Achilles tendon

■ **origin** attachment of a muscle to the bone that does not move (or experiences the least movement) when the muscle contracts.

■ **insertion** attachment of a muscle to the bone that moves when the muscle contracts.

■ **tendon** band of connective tissue that attaches muscle to bone.

demonstrates the strength of this particular tissue. It can be felt as the band posterior to the malleoli of the ankle. This tendon is the muscle-controlled cord that allows us to lift the entire body weight and stand on our toes.

Muscles are usually paired, one on each side of a joint. This configuration is essential because the muscle is only able to contract with force. One muscle mass will move the extremity in one direction by contraction, while the opposing mass is stretched. The opposing mass can then contract, stretching the original muscle and moving the extremity in the opposite direction. This arrangement affords the opportunity to straighten the limb, called *extension*, and then bend at the joint, called *flexion*. By adding more muscle bodies with different origins and insertions, a wide variety of motion can be controlled. This relationship is nicely demonstrated in the shoulder. The shoulder muscles permit the humerus various degrees of motion. These include moving the extremity away from the body (**abduction**) or toward the body (**adduction**), as well as rotating the humerus at the elbow through about 60 degrees or circling the entire extremity through a 180-degree arch.

The sophistication of the muscle-tendon relationship is well demonstrated in the forearm. As the anterior muscles controlling the fingers contract, they can be felt tensing while the fingers flex. The movement of the tendons can also be visualized and palpated in the distal forearm and wrist as the fingers flex and extend. It is easy to appreciate the damage a deep transverse laceration can cause to the underlying connective tissue and muscle control of distal skeletal structures.

The muscle tissue is responsible not only for the body's ability to move about, but also for the production of heat energy. Through a chemical reaction between oxygen and simple sugars, energy of motion is produced. Heat, water and carbon dioxide are created as by-products of this reaction and must be excreted (as water in urine), expired (as carbon dioxide through respiration) and dissipated (as heat through radiation or convection). The requirements of muscle tissue for oxygen, nutrients and elimination of their waste products must constantly be met.

The blood vessels and major nerve pathways travel deep within the muscle masses and along the long bones. This orientation minimizes the effects of most trauma. If, however, the bone is fractured or dislocated, there is a good chance that these structures will be injured.

PATHOPHYSIOLOGY

The various injury processes that may occur to the muscular and skeletal systems are easy to identify. Muscles can be contused by blunt trauma or strained when excessive force or fatigue overexerts the fibers. The various joints may become injured because of extreme stress, as in a sprain. Or they become partially or completely displaced, as in subluxation or dislocation. The long bones themselves can be disrupted through the various types of fractures.

Muscular Injury

Muscular injury is common and may present painfully. Injuries may include contusion, strain, sprain, cramp, and spasm. None of the muscular injuries should contribute significantly to hypovolemia, with the exception of a severe contusion accompanied by internal hemorrhage.

■ **abduction** movement of a body part or extremity away from the midline.

■ **adduction** movement of a body part or extremity toward the midline.

✱ Muscular injuries rarely contribute significantly to hypovolemia, with the exception of a severe contusion accompanied by internal hemorrhage.

Muscular contusion is caused by blunt trauma. As with all contusions, small blood vessels rupture, causing dull pain, leakage of blood into the interstitial spaces, and the classical discoloration. The injury may allow pooling of blood beneath tissue layers and a resultant hematoma. Infrequently, large volumes of blood may accumulate and contribute to hypovolemia. This may especially occur when large vessels are involved in the major muscle masses of the thigh, buttocks, calf or arm.

The strain is an overstretching of the muscle and presents as pain. It is caused by extreme force on the muscle mass beyond the normal limits of exertion. The result is damage to fibers without internal bleeding or discoloration. Patients normally report pain when attempting to use the specific muscle affected.

Muscle cramping is not really an injury, but an "angina" of the tissue. The circulation does not supply the muscle mass with oxygen, or it fails to remove the waste products of metabolism, and muscle pain results. The pain begins during or immediately after vigorous exercise, or after the limb has been left in an unusual position for a period of time. Change of position may reduce or eliminate the pain. Once rest allows circulation to restore the metabolic balance, the pain usually subsides.

Spasm causes pain similar to that of muscle cramp and causes the muscle mass to contract firmly. A spasm may feel much like the deformity of a fracture to palpation. The problem, as with the cramp, will subside uneventfully with restored circulation.

Muscle injury may also occur with open wounds. Deep lacerations may penetrate the skin and subcutaneous tissues and affect the muscle mass, the tendons and the ligaments. Massive wounds affecting a large percentage of a muscle, or ones involving the tendons, may reduce the strength of the distal limb or render muscular control of it completely ineffective. As the tendons are cut, the muscle will retract them into the soft tissue. The opposing muscle will contract, moving the limb and also pulling the distal tendon away from the injury. Such injuries often call for surgical intervention to identify and rejoin the damaged connective bands.

Joint Injury

Joint injuries include the sprain, the subluxation, and the dislocation. The sprain is a tearing of the connective tissue of the joint capsule, specifically a ligament or ligaments. This injury causes exquisite pain at the site followed shortly by inflammation and swelling. Ecchymotic discoloration will occur over time, but not during the prehospital period. The ligaments have torn under tremendous tension, the joint is weakened, and continued use may cause complete joint failure.

A **subluxation** (partial dislocation) occurs when the joint is stressfully separated, stretching the ligaments. It differs from the sprain in that the joint integrity is more significantly reduced. In a subluxation, the articular surfaces are not held together tightly since more ligament damage has occurred. The site will be painful; the range of motion, limited; and the joint, unstable. The etiology of this injury is associated with hyperflexion, hyperextension, or lateral rotation beyond the normal range of motion. The injury may also be caused by extreme force pulling along the axis of the limb. Swelling and pain will normally accompany the injury.

Dislocation is a frank displacement of the bone ends from the joint. The joint is fixed in an abnormal position, with the joint area noticeably deformed. It will be painful and swollen. There is danger that blood ves-

■ **subluxation** incomplete dislocation of a joint. The surfaces remain in contact while the joint is somewhat deformed.

■ **dislocation** displacement of a longbone or other structure from its normal anatomical location.

sels and nerves have been entrapped, compressed, or torn. Dislocation occurs when the joint is moved beyond its normal range of motion with great force. The very nature of the injury means that it is associated with ligament damage and may also involve injury to the capsule and trauma to the articular cartilage.

Fractures

■ **fracture** disruption of the bone tissue. Types of fractures include: comminuted, greenstick, impacted, linear, oblique, spiral, and transverse.

The most dramatic of skeletal injuries is the **fracture.** A break in the continuity of the bone, it may involve not only skeletal tissue but blood vessels, nerves and other tissues within and surrounding the bone. If the fracture damages internal vasculature or nerves, it may limit the degree of repair possible and the post-accident use of the limb.

Paramedics deal with many types of fractures. These include impacted, hairline, and greenstick fractures. (See Figure 17-3.)

An *open fracture* is any fracture with an associated open wound. The wound communicates with the fracture site and provides a route for infectious materials to enter. Injury may occur when a penetrating object, such as a bullet, enters the body and then fractures the bone or when the bone breaks and is pushed through the skin. (See Figure 17-4.)

The *closed fracture* does not have an associated open wound. The prognosis for a closed fracture is generally better than for the open.

Two types of fractures which remain in-line and relatively stable are the hairline and the impacted fractures. The *hairline fracture* is a small crack in the bone with no actual displacement. The *impacted fracture* oc-

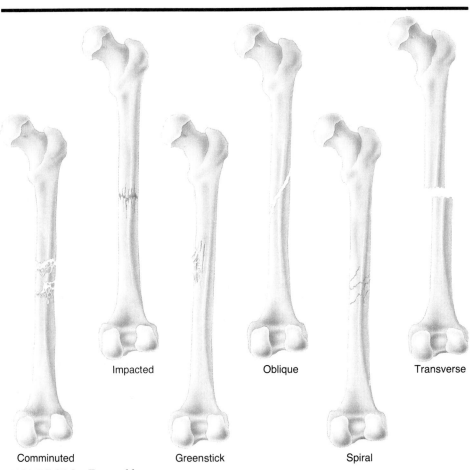

Impacted   Oblique   Transverse

Comminuted   Greenstick   Spiral

FIGURE 17-3 Types of fractures.

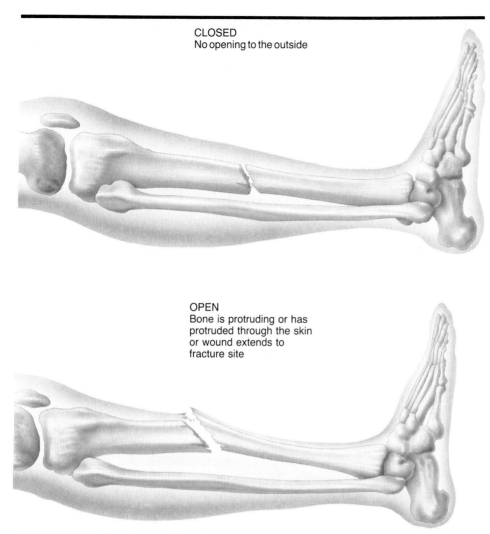

CLOSED
No opening to the outside

OPEN
Bone is protruding or has
protruded through the skin
or wound extends to
fracture site

FIGURE 17-4   Classification of fractures.

curs when the broken bone ends are compressed together providing the
fracture with some stability. In either fracture, the only evidence of a
problem may be the mechanism of injury and pain. The patient may use
the limb normally. But it is noticeably weakened and may, with stress,
collapse post-accident. The only way to rule out such an injury is with an
X-ray in the emergency department.

The *greenstick fracture* is a partial break, disrupting only one side
of the long bone. It most frequently affects pediatric patients because
their bone structure is less mature and more flexible than that of adults.
While incomplete as a fracture, it is significant because of the partial nature of the break. During the natural repair, the injured side will experience growth, while the other will not. The probable result will be a bone
which increases angulation as it heals. Often, the emergency department
staff will break the bone completely to ensure proper repair.

Skeletal injuries for the other end of the age spectrum, the geriatric
patient, are quite different. The skeletal system does not maintain its
strength late in life. Long bones may degenerate to a point where they
fracture easily or spontaneously. The patient will frequently describe
"feeling a snap" before falling. The injury process is relatively atraumatic. Thus, the patient feels less uncomfortable than someone who has
suffered an equivalent break because of trauma.

GENERAL CONSIDERATIONS

If we examine the skeletal structure and the musculature together, we can better anticipate the potential effects of trauma. It is important to note that long bones are smallest through the diaphysis and largest at the epiphyseal area, the joint. On the other hand, the diameter of the extremity is greatest surrounding the midshaft due to the placement of the skeletal muscles. This anatomical relationship is significant when looking at the potential for nervous or vascular injury.

Since the amount of soft tissue surrounding a joint is limited, joint fractures, dislocations, and, to a lesser degree, subluxations and sprains, may cause severe problems beyond the direct injury. Any swelling, deformity, or displacement may compromise the nerve and vascular supply to the distal extremity. Fractures near a joint may actually sever blood vessels or nerves. Dislocation may trap and compress these structures between the two displaced bone ends. The chance of blood vessel and nerve damage is much greater for injuries of the joint than for fractures of the longbone shaft.

The circulation supplying the epiphyseal areas of the long bones enters the bone through the diaphysis. If a fracture close to the epiphysis displaces the bone ends, it may compromise this circulatory supply, with devastating results. The distal end of the bone may die without the needed circulation. Thus the joint and its function are destroyed. Once the injury has occurred, the stability of the extremity is reduced. Any further movement can increase pain, soft-tissue damage, and the possibility of vascular or nerve involvement. Manipulation of the injury site may also increase the likelihood of bone fragments or fat emboli being introduced into the venous system. Even slight manipulation can cause internal trauma. The fractured ends of the femur are about the size of a broken broom handle. If, during extrication, splinting, and patient movement, it is allowed to flail within the soft tissue, the damage can be more severe than that which occurred with the initial fracture.

Another complication associated with long bone fracture is muscle spasm induced by the pain of injury. In the fractured long bone, especially the femur, pain causes the opposing muscles to contract. This forces the broken bone ends to override the fracture site. The result is two broom handle sized bones being driven into the muscles of the thigh. It is easy to recognize the damage and pain caused by an unstabilized fracture.

SPECIFIC CONSIDERATIONS

Certain longbone injuries are deserving of special attention. They may present management problems or necessitate immediate care and transport due to significant blood loss or threat to the affected limb.

Lower Extremeties

The pelvis is a large skeletal structure which most commonly fractures across the iliac crests or through the pelvic ring. Either fracture requires a great deal of force, although the pelvic ring fracture is generally much more severe. The injury usually affects two sites because of the circular anatomy of the pelvis. The ring fracture commonly involves the vasculature which runs along its interior and from there to the lower extremities. Pelvic fractures are frequently associated with severe hemorrhage, often in excess of 2 liters. They may also result in the loss of distal circulation.

The hip joint may be dislocated in two ways. The anterior dislocation displaces the femoral head anteriorly. The patient presents with the foot and knee rotated laterally. There may be a noticeable prominence in the inguinal area, reflecting the displaced femur head. The posterior dislocation moves the head of the femur into the buttocks. The patient presents with the knee flexed and the knee and foot internally rotated.

Fractures of the femur in the proximity of the hip may be difficult to differentiate from the anterior dislocation. While the broken leg is expected to be slightly shorter than the unbroken one, the difference may be slight and unnoticeable if the legs are not straight and parallel. Fractures involving the femur, either midshaft or otherwise, may affect the surrounding vasculature or significant soft tissue. The bleeding that follows can be extensive. Fractures to the femur, the pelvis and, to a limited degree, the humerus, can involve significant blood loss, possibly contributing to or inducing hypovolemia.

Knee dislocations will normally present with the knee at an angle and firmly fixed in position. The dislocation carries a high incidence of vascular and nervous injury because of the proximity of these structures to the injury site. Dislocation may also occur in combination with fracture since the energy needed to cause one is commonly sufficient to cause the other. Any fracture within 3 inches of a joint, especially the knee, the elbow, or the ankle should be treated similarly to a dislocation and immobilized as found. Dislocations of the patella are more common than those of the knee. But, to the untrained examiner, it may be difficult to distinguish between the two. Patellar dislocations, however, do not carry the increased incidence of vascular injury that knee dislocations do.

Fractures of the lower leg bones, the tibia and the fibula, can occur separately or together. The fractures are generally caused by direct trauma during auto or athletic accidents. The tibia will most commonly fracture, since it is the anterior bone and is responsible for weight bearing. If the fibula is intact the extremity may not angulate, but it will remain unstable. If only the fibula is broken, the limb may be rather stable.

Upper Extremeties

Shoulder dislocation may occur anteriorly, posteriorly, or inferiorly. The posterior dislocation will present with the shoulder hollow, the limb angled forward, the elbow internally rotated, and the arm away from the chest. The anterior displacement will present with a prominent shoulder and with the arm close to the chest as well as forward of the anterior axillary line. The inferior displacement locks the patient's extremity above the head.

Fracture may occur along the entire length of the humerus. Here the injury is particularly hard to stabilize because of the structure and mobility of the shoulder joint. The axillary artery runs through the axilla, making it difficult to apply any mechanical traction to the limb and providing the potential hazard of circulatory compromise.

Fractures in and around the elbow are particularly dangerous, especially in children. The soft-tissue depth is minimal and the skeletal diameter is large. Any fracture has a good probability of vessel or nerve involvement. Such damage may result in the eventual loss of function distal to the injury.

The forearm may fracture anywhere along its length. Commonly fracture will occur at the distal end of the radius, breaking it just above the articular surface. Known as *Colle's fracture,* it may present with the wrist turned up at an unusual angle. As with most joint fractures, the major concern is for distal circulation and innervation.

Fractures and dislocations affect living tissue which requires a constant and rich supply of oxygenated circulation. While the central nervous system, the heart and the kidneys will dysfunction more rapidly and more acutely than the skeletal system, the long bones may degenerate over time and leave the limb unable to carry out its intended function. Musculoskeletal injuries are of relatively low priority in the seriously injured patient. Yet their proper care is important to the patient's overall well being and recovery.

ASSESSMENT

Evaluation of the fracture, the dislocation or the muscular injury occurs late in the assessment process. These injuries infrequently threaten life or seriously contribute to the development of shock. On the other hand, they occur often in patients who present without other serious traumatic injury. In most circumstances, the fracture and dislocation will receive complete assessment and stabilization.

Primary Assessment

It is imperative that trauma assessment begin with the A-B-C-D-E's, followed by the head-to-toe, vital sign, and patient history evaluation. Musculoskeletal injury assessment and care must be deferred until the potential for life threat is ruled out. The risk for cervical-spine injury must be considered and evaluated. This may not be easy, since primary kinetic forces resulting in musculoskeletal injury may also cause injury to the spine. Also, the fall following the initial impact and long bone injury may have injured the vertebral column.

The Airway, Breathing, and Circulation must be assessed as adequate or be corrected. If this cannot be achieved in the field, transport the patient immediately and give care focusing on the A-B-C's enroute. Identify any alteration in mental status or central nervous system depression before continuing with the assessment. Assess the head, neck, chest, and abdomen for signs of serious trauma, then complete the entire primary assessment.

While skeletal injury does not often account for life threatening hemorrhage, fracture of the pelvis or bilateral femur fractures may induce hypovolemia. If the mechanism of injury suggests either of these injuries, observe and palpate the pelvis and femurs early. If evidence of injury is found, PASG should be applied and all compartments inflated to a pressure immobilizing the pelvis and the lower extremities. Remember that femur fractures can account for blood loss in excess of 1,500 mL each, while the pelvis may account for more than 2,000 mL. Patients with these suspected injuries should be considered as candidates for immediate transport.

Secondary Assessment

Once the patient is felt to be without potential life threat and any serious problems have been attended to, secondary assessment should begin. The

✷ Muscular injury assessment and care must be deferred until the potential for life threat is ruled out.

✷ Patients with pelvic or femur fractures should be considered for immediate transport.

process may occur at the scene or enroute to the hospital. The head to toe exam will reevaluate the head, neck, chest and abdomen in more depth than the initial assessment did. It will examine for the signs and symptoms of internal or external injury or hemorrhage. Once the assessment reaches the pelvis, evaluation of the major musculoskeletal areas begins. The pelvis is assessed by applying gentle pressure to the iliac crests in a posterior direction, then medially. Posterior pressure may also be applied to the symphysis pubis. If there is any crepitus, pain or instability, stabilize the patient for a possible fractured pelvis.

Observe and palpate the extremities carefully for signs and symptoms of fracture, dislocation or other injury. Before any palpation occurs, however, the extremity should be exposed and visualized. Clothing should be removed carefully or cut away, whichever is most effective yet does not contribute to manipulation of a potential injury site. View the area entirely to locate any deformity, discoloration, or other signs of injury. Any unusual limb placement, asymmetry, or limb length inequality should arouse suspicion of musculoskeletal injury. Question the patient about pain, inability to move, or pain on attempted motion. The assessment must be gentle, yet complete, if any information suggests injury. If no specific injury is identified, palpate the extremity for instability, deformity, crepitation, false motion, or any regions of unusual warmth or coolness. The entire lateral and medial, then anterior and posterior surface should be palpated, with any abnormal signs recorded. As the assessment arrives at the foot, carefully examine the distal circulation. (See Figure 17-5.) Assess pulses for presence and then compare bilaterally. Test the skin for blanching, capillary refill, and warmth. Observe the skin for discoloration, whether it is erythema, ecchymosis, or any other abnormal hue. Approximate the level at which any deficit begins and note any relation to long bone injury.

Evaluate sensation and muscle strength distal to the injury. Check tactile (touch) response by stroking the bottom of the foot with the blunt end of a bandage scissors or other similar instrument. Ask the patient to describe the feeling. If the patient is responsive and there is no indication that the limb is injured, ask the patient to push down with the balls of both feet against your hands. Then ask the patient to pull upward with the top of the feet, again against your hands. If any unilateral weakness is felt, note it in the record and look for the cause.

The upper extremity should be similarly assessed. (See Figure 17-6.)

✱ Any unusual limb placement, asymmetry, or limb length inequality should arouse suspicion of musculoskeletal injury.

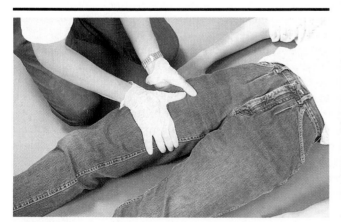

FIGURE 17-5 Assessment of the lower extremity.

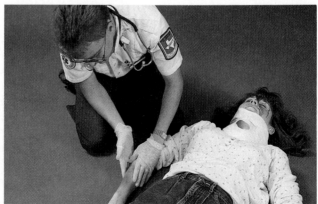

FIGURE 17-6 Assessment of the upper extremity.

Expose, observe, and then palpate it. Determine tactile response by using the back of the patient's hand. Test muscular strength by having the patient squeeze two of your fingers. Identify any deficit and attempt to locate the cause. Evaluate the upper extremity before using it for blood pressure determination.

When the assessment of an extremity yields results suggestive of injury, treat the limb as though a fracture or dislocation exists. The only way a fracture can be ruled out is by X-ray examination. Nothing more than slight discomfort will result from treating a soft tissue or muscular injury as a fracture. Failure to properly immobilize a fracture may lead to further soft, skeletal, connective, vascular or nervous tissue damage.

Reassess and record the distal pulse, skin temperature and capillary refill times during splint application, patient packaging, and transport. Give special attention to the pulse and sensation before, during and after splint application as well as periodically during transport and patient care. Any of these activities, or swelling of the affected limb, may cause an artery to be obstructed or a nerve to be compressed. If the compromise is undetected, the result may be prolongation of the healing process or loss of the limb.

If possible, find the exact site of injury and determine if it involves the joint area or long bone shaft. Make a mental image of the wound. This will enable you to describe it in the record and to the receiving physician. The splinting device (e.g., the PASG for a femur fracture) may hide the site from view, leaving the attending physician unable to determine what exists within. A good narrative description of the wound may delay the need to remove the splint to view the injury.

One complication of fractures and contusions is *compartment syndrome*. It results from bleeding into a closed space surrounded by membranes that will not stretch. Thus, blood vessels and nerves can be compressed, affecting circulation. Compartment syndrome should be suspected in any patient with an extremity injury who has lost the pulse or function in the hand or foot. Compartment syndrome most commonly occurs in the forearm or the leg.

During the physical exam, question the patient about the symptoms of injury. Determine the nature and location of pain, tenderness or dysfunction. The verbal investigation should be detailed and complete. Unless asked specifically about it, the patient may be unaware of a symptom. The description of the fracture or dislocation event may also be helpful. They may state that they felt the bone "snap" or the joint "pop out." Determined if the bone snapped causing the fall or vice versa. Examine the patient for the amount of pain and discomfort experienced with the injury. The elderly patient may present with a fractured hip and limited pain, usually related to a degenerative disease and secondary fracture. Such a presentation may suggest a less aggressive approach to care.

The mechanism of injury should be determined from the patient's explanation and observation of the environment. It is helpful for the paramedic to mentally relive the incident and determine what injury or injuries may have occurred. If any injury is suspected, the assessment may rule it out. If it doesn't, then treat the patient as though the injury exists.

As you conclude the trauma assessment, identify all injuries found, prioritize them, and establish the order of care. The moments taken to sort out what is wrong with the patient and to plan the care to follow will increase efficiency, reduce on-scene time, and ensure that the patient receives the proper care at the right time.

✳ At the conclusion of the trauma assessment, identify all injuries found, prioritize them, and establish the order of care.

MANAGEMENT

Some patients with musculoskeletal injuries require immediate transportation, while many will receive on-scene care. The care for these two types of patients however, differs greatly. In the seriously injured, fractures cannot be assessed or cared for as precisely as desired. Other priorities are more important. In contrast, patients with limited and isolated injuries must receive detailed splinting and packaging to ensure that no further harm occurs.

Immediate Transport

Once the decision to transport an unstable or potentially unstable patient has been made, long bone and muscle injury must also be considered. It is neither practical nor appropriate to splint each fracture while the patient exsanguinates from internal hemorrhage. You must, however, rapidly extricate the patient, using techniques of immobilization and movement to protect the body as a whole.

The use of axial traction for movement will cause the extremities to align. Axial traction moves the patient gently by applying the "pull" to the shoulders while stabilizing the head. As movement occurs, the travel of the patient will cause the upper extremities to align against the body, and the lower extremities to align together. Continuing movement will keep the limbs in position and limit their flailing about. While this procedure is certainly not ideal, it will minimize further trauma to the musculoskeletal system when rapid transport is the first priority.

If the use of axial traction is inappropriate, select other techniques that will minimize limb movement. For example, during removal from the auto or other accident scene, secure the upper extremities to the body and secure the legs to each other.

Securing the patient to the long spineboard will immobilize his or her extremities. Patient packaging can be adequately accomplished with the head secured in a cervical immobilization device. Straps should cross the shoulders and chest, encircling the pelvis (and hands), legs, and feet. The patient can be moved as a unit. Therefore, any fracture or dislocation will be minimally displaced during transport.

On-Scene Care

Should transport not be immediate, you can treat long bone and muscular injuries individually and according to the priorities established during the secondary assessment. Fractures of the pelvis, femur, and humerus generally take priority over other musculoskeletal injuries. Fractures or dislocations involving circulatory or nervous deficit should also be given a high priority.

Care of suspected fractures and dislocations usually includes frequent serial evaluation of the distal circulatory and nervous function before, during, and after splinting. Determine the presence of the pulse and compare its strength and rate with that of the opposite limb. Monitor distal temperature carefully and time capillary refill. Any deviation from baseline findings should be reason to check the splint for tightness and possible circumferential constriction. The adage "immobilize the adjacent joints," is appropriate for both fractures and dislocations. Whichever splint and splinting process the paramedic chooses must effectively im-

✱ It is neither practical nor appropriate to splint each fracture while the patient exsanguinates from internal hemorrhage.

✱ Should immediate transport not be required and the patient is stable, the long bone and muscular injuries can be cared for according to the priorities established during the secondary assessment.

mobilize the proximal and distal joint to prevent any transmitted motion. Transmitted motion can occur in many ways. The flexion/extension motion of the normal long bone joint is one way. Rotational and lateral motions also occur, especially once the joint structure has been damaged. The elbow demonstrates this well. In an elbow injury, if the palm of the hand can be rotated from supine to prone, the radius and ulna are moving at the injury site. This motion can induce further pain, if not further injury. This can only be eliminated if the joints proximal and distal to the injury are effectively immobilized.

Fractures, dislocations, and connective tissue injury affecting the long bones may be very difficult to differentiate from one another. If any question exists, err on the side of over-immobilization. Limb stabilization will rarely harm a patient, while failure to stabilize may allow significant soft tissue injury.

The extremity is best cared for if it can be placed in the neutral position. This will provide the least tension on the ligaments and tendons of the limb. The neutral position is closely approximated by leaving the various joints half-way between full extension and full flexion. While this position is physiologically ideal, it is sometimes difficult to obtain in the field.

A situation deserving special consideration is the hand injury. The hand's articulations are so sophisticated and essential to human function that care of such an injury is critical. The injured hand should be brought to the neutral position (also called the position of function) to ensure that patient comfort is maintained and that the limb receives no further damage. This position is obtained by placing the hand as if it were holding a softball. A roll of roller bandage surrounded by a trauma dressing and placed in the patient's palm will accomplish this position comfortably.

Shaft fractures are not as easy to immobilize as they might first seem. The major long bones are embedded within large muscle masses, such as the hamstring and the quadriceps of the thigh or the biceps and the triceps of the arm. These muscles make it difficult to splint the bone ends in any position other than aligned. If attempts are made to immobilize in an angulated position, the splint may be ineffective. Align a fracture gently and carefully. Explain to the patient what is about to happen. Tell him that the alignment will hurt, but pain will be reduced after the procedure. There will also be less pain during movement to the ambulance and travel to the hospital. Stabilize the proximal limb as found, while the distal limb is brought into alignment. This should occur with gentle traction. Once you align the limb, it should be immediately brought to its final position for transport. Assess the distal circulation and nervous function. If there is any noticeable resistance during the alignment process, discontinue. Assess the pulse and nervous function immediately, and if present, splint the limb in the position achieved. If the pulse or the innervation is compromised, gently manipulate the limb and splint it. If initial attempts do not restore the pulse or sensation, immobilize the limb and transport the patient.

* If distal pulses or innervation are compromised due to a skeletal injury, gently manipulate the limb to achieve its return and then splint.

While alignment is an uncomfortable process, it is necessary if splinting is to be effective. The splints most commonly used for fractures are the air splint, the PASG, and the traction splint. By their structure, they force alignment of the limb. The structure of the padded board splint and fracture straps performs the same function. The ladder and vacuum splints can conform to the limb angle without alignment. However, the ladder splints ability to immobilize firmly is limited.

Once the limb is positioned acceptably, immobilize it completely. One rescuer should hold the limb in position to monitor the distal pulse, as the other applies the splint. The gentle traction used to align the extremity should be continued while the limb is secured. The splint should maintain both limb immobilization and gentle traction during the entire prehospital period. At the conclusion of the splinting process, the pulse and sensation should be carefully reassessed.

Fractures within 3 inches of the joint or dislocations are splinted very differently than midshaft fractures. Since the danger of injury with such fractures through manipulation is great, and the initial position is easier to splint, it is recommended that the position of the skeletal injury be maintained. The exception is the patient with no circulation distal to the injury. In this case, gently move the limb while palpating the location of the distal artery for a returning pulse. If the pulse cannot be regained with a minimum of movement, splint the limb and transport the patient without delay. Many areas of the extremities call for special techniques of immobilization. It is essential to look at each injury separately and identify any special considerations of care.

Lower Extremities. The pelvis must be stabilized and care given to control hemorrhage. It is a standard practice to apply the PASG for stabilizing fractures because of the potential for severe blood loss and the difficulty in immobilizing the broken pelvic ring. Inflate the PASG until it affixes the pelvis and hip joint. Start two large-bore IVs and hang two 1,000 mL bags of lactated Ringer's solution or normal saline. Use trauma tubing and pressure infusion sets for rapid infusion. The lines need only run at a to-keep-open rate until the early signs of shock begin to display. Consider this patient a candidate for rapid transport.

Immobilize fractures and dislocations of the hip in the position found. Most often the long spineboard can be used to entirely splint the patient and accommodate the injury. Use pillows, blankets, and other padding to maintain the initial position and ensure patient comfort. Femur fractures can originate from two sources: severe trauma and degenerative disease. Patients with disease-induced fractures will present with a clouded history of trauma and the patient will be relatively comfortable. The patient is best cared for, as is the hip fracture patient, by immobilization as found and transport.

The patient with a femur fracture resulting from trauma will be in extreme discomfort. Often, the patient will be found writhing in pain. The protocol of care which will best reduce the pain and muscle spasm is distal traction. The traction splint is indicated for the isolated femur fracture of a patient who presents without hemodynamic embarrassment. If the early signs of shock are present or the history reflects that the patient has sustained enough trauma to induce shock, the PASG may be a better choice. Use only the amount of traction necessary to align or stabilize the limb and no more. Limited traction will begin a cycle of reduced pain, muscle relaxation, and limb lengthening. If mechanical traction is used (e.g., the traction splint), monitor and readjust the splint to ensure a constant gentle pull on the limb.

Fractures or dislocations of the knee are best immobilized as found. The common presentation is with the knee at an angle of or slightly greater than 90 degrees. It should be left in this position unless distal pulses are lost. Lateral and medial padded board splints effectively immobilize the injury. Anterior and posterior ladder splints or the vacuum splint will also accomplish fixation. Ankle and foot injuries can be easily cared for with either the full leg air, vacuum, or pillow splint. Each device

❋ Fractures in the vicinity of a joint, or dislocations, should generally be splinted in the position found.

will immobilize the injury. However, the pillow and vacuum splints will better conform to the position of the patient's extremity.

After the limb has been splinted, it is beneficial to tie the distal end to the uninjured leg. This will afford some protection against uncontrolled movement. It may also reassure the patient that he or she still has some control over the extremity.

Upper Extremities. Shoulder injuries, like all joint injuries, should be immobilized as found unless the pulse or innervation is absent. The anterior and posterior dislocation can be immobilized in place with a sling and swath and, if needed, a pillow under the arm and forearm. Any inferior dislocation calls for ingenuity by the paramedic. The arm is extended over the head and must be immobilized in that position. A long, padded splint tied with cravats to the torso, shoulder girdle, arm, and forearm may serve this purpose. Once the patient is moved to the long spineboard, the splint and patient can be affixed to the spineboard.

Humeral fractures can be splinted with the elbow either flexed or extended. If flexed, the patient should be seated and the arm slung with the elbow not included. The extremity is then swathed. If the extremity is extended, it is best secured with a padded board splint along the medial aspect of the limb and the splint and arm secured against the supine body. The paramedic should ensure that the splint is not pushed into the axilla. Such pressure may impinge the axillary artery and reduce circulation to the extremity.

The elbow can be splinted with a single padded board or ladder splint. Either way, it should be slung and swathed, with the wrist slightly above the elbow in the seated or supine patient. This position will increase venous return and reduce the swelling and pain.

Musculoskeletal injuries to the forearm, wrist, hand or fingers can be effectively immobilized with a padded board or air splint. Place a roll of bandage material or some similar object in the patient's hand to maintain the position of function. Then secure the extremity to the padded board or inflate the splint. It is necessary that the distal extremity be accessible to determine adequacy of perfusion and sensation. Placement of the wrist above the elbow will assist venous return and reduce distal swelling.

The fracture, dislocation, or other musculoskeletal injury is frequently accompanied by pain. Since patients with these isolated injuries do not also have respiratory or cardiovascular compromise, pain relief may be provided to increase comfort and reduce anxiety. Nitronox is the drug of choice because it is self-administered and has a short half-life. Morphine sulfate may also be considered. It is titrated to relief and halted immediately if any respiratory depression or hypotension develops. If the patient's response becomes severe, naloxone (Narcan) may be administered.

✱ Do not concentrate all efforts on the patient's injuries and neglect the emotional impact of the incident and the emergency care.

The trauma patient needs psychological as well as physiological support. Too often paramedics concentrate all efforts on the patient's injuries, forgetting the emotional impact of the incident and the emergency care. The paramedic can actually be very effective in treating the patient's emotional response to trauma. It is useful to remember that patients usually are not frequently exposed to traumatic injury. They do not know what effects the injury will have on their life, nor what to expect from medical care in the prehospital, emergency department, or the in-hospital setting. A concerned attitude, frequent and compassionate communication and a professional demeanor will go far to calm and reassure patients. Simple attention to the patient may make his experience with pre-hospital emergency medical service one they will remember positively.

SUMMARY

It is rare that musculoskeletal injury will threaten the life of the patient. The injuries and general care presented in this chapter take second priority to the many other life threatening injuries accompanying trauma. Once the patient is stable and found not to be a candidate for immediate transport, fractures, dislocations, strains, and sprains can be assessed and cared for appropriately.

The extremities cannot be assessed in detail and splinted if the patient's condition requires rapid transport to the hospital. The patient must be moved carefully and with consideration for possible extremity injury. A movement technique should be selected that transports the body as a unit, while limiting any movement of the limbs. Once the patient is on the spineboard, the legs and upper extremities should be immobilized to the spineboard and the body. The extremities should be assessed and cared for during transport as time permits. When you care for these injuries you must place the limb in the appropriate orientation for splinting. Circulation and sensation must be evaluated distally, and the adjacent joints firmly immobilized by the splint. Package the patient with consideration for possible musculoskeletal injuries and move him without aggravating these. Frequently reassess the distal circulation and sensation during transport.

As a paramedic you have the ability to greatly assist an injured patient by integrating the skills of musculoskeletal injury assessment and management with the other skills of trauma care. Always base the level of care you provide on the seriousness of the patient's overall condition.

FURTHER READING

AMERICAN COLLEGE OF SURGEONS, Committee on Trauma, *Advanced Trauma Life Support Course: Student Manual.* American College of Surgeons, 1989.

BUTMAN, A. M., AND PATURAS, J. L., *Pre-Hospital Trauma Life Support.* Akron, OH: Emergency Training, 1986.

CAMPBELL, J. E., *Basic Trauma Life Support.* 2nd ed. Englewood Cliffs, NJ: Prentice-Hall, Inc., 1988.

GRANT, H. D., MURRAY, R. H., AND BERGERON, J. D., *Emergency Care.* 5th ed. Englewood Cliffs, NJ: Prentice-Hall, Inc., 1990.

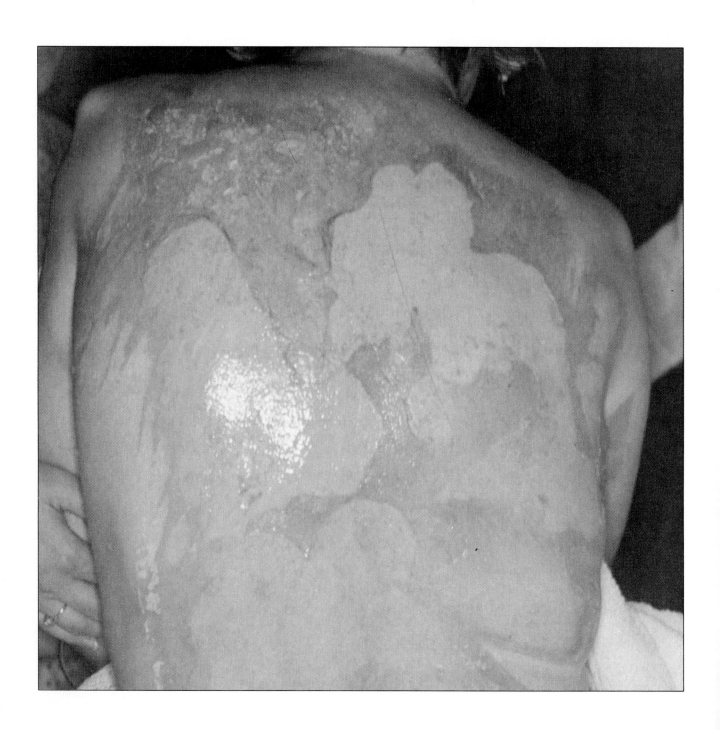

18

Soft Tissue Trauma And Burns

Objectives For Chapter 18

Upon completing this chapter, the student should be able to:

1. Identify the structure of skin, its layers and the functions they provide.

2. Describe contusion, abrasion, laceration, incision, avulsion, and amputation. Then describe the particular difficulties to assessment and care they represent.

3. List the advantages and the disadvantages of each method of bleeding control: direct pressure, elevation, pressure point, and the tourniquet. Identify the circumstances in which each or a combination might be best used.

4. Describe the three degrees of thermal burn as well as the depth and effects of these injuries.

5. Identify the two methods of burn surface area approximation and apply each to several burn patient descriptions.

6. List the anatomical areas which, if burned, will increase the overall severity of the burn.

7. Describe the precautions to take when approaching a possible radiological incident and the effect time, distance, and shielding have on the exposure.

8. List and explain the care steps for chemical burns and the special considerations given to lime and phenol burns.

Fire Rescue responds with trucks 23 and 56 to a working structure fire. Upon arrival, two fire units are already deployed, with firefighters engaging a wood frame home fully engulfed in flames. As you position your vehicle, the south wall of the structure collapses on a firefighter. Within minutes the burning wall is extinguished, and the firefighter freed. Removal of the turnout gear reveals relatively painless, dark, and discolored burns to his posterior thorax, lower back, and the left upper extremity circumferentially. The firefighter also has angulation, false motion, and pain in the right forearm. Respirations appear adequate, although he is coughing up sooty sputum and is slightly hoarse. Although extensively burned, he is conscious, alert, and without much pain. The firefighter's airway seems clear, except for the hoarseness. His breathing is normal in volume and rate, though he is coughing. His pulse is strong and regular at a rate of about 100. Distal pulses are also strong and capillary refill is timed at 2 seconds. The patient is fully conscious and oriented and is joking about the incident. All the clothing is cut away, including a still-smoldering belt. The burn site is covered with a dry, sterile sheet and an IV line is started, with normal saline running wide open. Oxygen is applied through a non-rebreathing mask and oximetry is recorded at 97%. The patient is quickly loaded into the ambulance and transport begins immediately. The blood pressure is taken (120/88). Respirations are at a rate of 26 and shallow, with some effort not previously noted. While the attending paramedic is splinting the right limb, the patient begins to cough deeply and to experience severe dyspnea. The dyspnea progresses, and the level of consciousness drops. Oxygen saturation falls to 76%. The paramedic begins to bag-valve-mask the patient with supplemental oxygen, while his partner prepares the intubation equipment. Orders are received by medical control to intubate and an attempt is made during transport. The airway is edematous, visualization of the vocal cords is difficult, and the tube is placed in the esophagus. Auscultation of breath sounds, failure to obtain chest rise, and a dropping oxygen saturation confirm this and the tube is withdrawn. The firefighter is hyperventilated, and another attempt is made to intubate. It is also unsuccessful. As the tube is withdrawn, the ambulance arrives at the emergency department. The physician places a large-bore catheter in the cricothyroid membrane and attempts transtracheal jet insuflation. It is successful and followed shortly by an emergency tracheostomy. The firefighter begins spontaneous respirations and maintains a strong pulse function. His level of consciousness does not, however, improve. He is transferred to the burn unit for definitive care.

INTRODUCTION

The skin is one of the largest, most important, and least appreciated organs of the human body. Containing the entire body, it protects us from fluid loss and bacterial invasion. It also provides a massive surface for sensation and a natural radiator to dissipate excess body heat. With all these responsibilities it still remains durable, flexible, and very able to repair itself.

Known collectively as the **integumentary system,** the skin is the first tissue of the human body to experience the effects of trauma. It covers the entire body surface and, therefore, every vital organ underneath. Any penetrating injury or the kinetic forces of blunt injury must pass through it. This transmission of energy will manifest with signs observable only by looking at the skin. Therefore, the skin is of great significance in both primary and secondary patient assessment.

■ **integumentary system** skin, consisting of the epidermis and dermis.

Trauma may manifest as abrasions, hematomas, lacerations, punctures, avulsions, and amputations. Such injuries infrequently cause threat to life, but may endanger blood vessels, nerves, connective tissue, and other important internal structures. Uncontrolled blood loss may lead to hypovolemia and shock, while the wound may provide a pathway for infection. Care for these injuries is easy to provide, although several objectives must be met.

Burns are a specific type of soft-tissue injury with a pathologic process all their own. While the term "burn" suggests combustion, the actual burn process is much different. The human body is predominantly water and will not support combustion. Instead, it changes chemically, evaporating the water and denaturing the proteins which make up cell membranes. The result can be widespread damage to the integumentary system.

Burn injury is often accompanied by inhalation injury. The products of combustion can cause severe respiratory burns from either thermal or chemical interaction with the airway tissue. Carbon monoxide may also "poison" the patient by reducing the red blood cells' ability to carry oxygen. It is in fact the most common source of poisoning in the United States. Burns also may be caused chemically. Chemicals can affect the body tissue at a molecular level in much the same way as the thermal burn. The insult may not cause the rapid evaporation of fluid, although it will destroy the cell's membranes. The resulting injury will present and affect the patient in a way similar to that of the thermal burn.

Paramedics must have a good understanding of the structure and function of the integumentary system and the pathologic processes possibly affecting it. This understanding will ensure that they can optimally assess and care for the patient who has sustained either wounds or burn injuries.

ANATOMY AND PHYSIOLOGY

The skin is the envelope within which the body is contained. If you will remember from Chapter 12, The Pathophysiology of Shock, the body is composed of about 60% water. Yet it survives in an atmosphere where the external humidity is relatively low. It also survives in an environment filled with microorganisms. They would raise havoc within the body if allowed to enter and grow freely.

The skin is really three layers of tissue designed to provide this protection and more. (See Figure 18-1.) The first and outermost layer is the **epidermis.** It is a layer of dying and dead cells being pushed outward by new cells growing from beneath. As these cells reach the surface, they are abraded away by everyday activity. The constant movement outward provides a barrier difficult for bacteria and other pathogens to penetrate.

■ **epidermis** outermost layer of the skin comprised of dead or dying cells.

To assist in making it watertight, the epidermis is moistened with an oil called **sebum.** It is secreted from glands in the tissue layer below. The sebum coats the outer layer of the epidermis, making it pliable. It also provides a barrier to the flow of water or other fluids either in-

■ **sebum** fatty secretion of the sebaceous gland. It helps keep the skin pliable and waterproof.

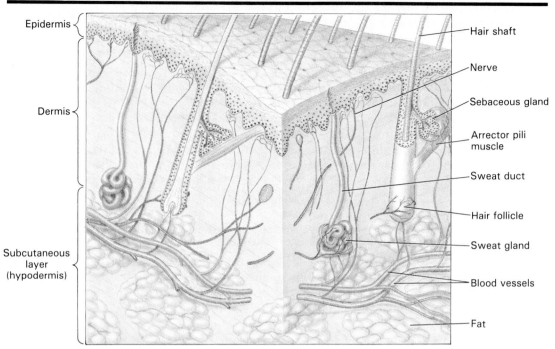

FIGURE 18-1 Anatomy of the skin.

Labels on image: Epidermis, Dermis, Subcutaneous layer (hypodermis), Hair shaft, Nerve, Sebaceous gland, Arrector pili muscle, Sweat duct, Hair follicle, Sweat gland, Blood vessels, Fat

■ **dermis** true skin, also called the corium. It is the layer of tissue producing the epidermis and housing the structures, blood vessels and nerves normally associated with the skin.

■ **sebaceous glands** glands within the dermis secreting sebum.

■ **tunica intima** interior layer of the blood vessels. It is smooth and provides for the free flow of blood.

■ **tunica media** the middle, muscular layer of the blood vessels. It controls the vessel lumen size.

■ **tunica adventitia** outer fibrous layer of the blood vessels. It maintains their maximum size.

ward or outward. Directly below the epidermis is the tissue layer called the **dermis.** It consists of many different structures, including blood vessels, glands, and nerve endings. It is here that sebum is produced in **sebacious glands** and secreted into hair follicles. Sweat is also secreted from this layer by sweat (sudoriferous) glands. Sweat is released on the surface of the skin. The water within it evaporates and is carried away by passing air, removing heat energy with it. The change of a fluid to a vapor (evaporation) is an efficient method of cooling. This process allows us to maintain a normal body temperature even in ambient temperatures of greater than 100 degrees (as long as evaporation is possible).

Additional regulation of body temperature occurs as warm blood from the body's core travels through the peripheral circulation. The blood is directed either to the dermal surface or beneath the subcutaneous tissue. Subcutaneous tissue is composed of adipose (fat) and connective tissues. Besides other functions, it serves as a strata of insulation. The shunting of blood into the deeper areas allows the skin's temperature to drop. This slows the movement of heat to the environment, thereby conserving heat energy. If the warm core blood is brought to the surface, skin temperature rises. Accordingly, the temperature difference between the body surface and the environment increases, as does the rate of heat exchange. This causes body cooling.

The skin varies in thickness from almost a centimeter on the heel to microscopic dimensions as it covers the surface of the eye. Extremely flexible, it ordinarily regenerates well. This protects the human body from many dangers of the environment.

Blood is an important medium traveling through the skin and becomes very important in understanding the wound and burn process. It is a fluid, consisting of water, electrolytes, proteins, and cells. Blood, of course, travels through arteries, arterioles, veins, venules, and capillaries. The arteries, arterioles, veins, and venules are made up of three layers: the **tunica intima,** the **tunica media,** and the **tunica adventitia.** The intima is the interior, smooth lining. It allows for the free flow of blood and prevents absorption of the blood's nutrients and oxygen as well as of waste products and carbon dioxide. The media is the muscular part of the tube. It allows the central nervous system to determine the vessel's internal diameter, called the **lumen.** The size of the lumen determines how much flow will pass to a particular organ or extremity. Muscle fibers of the tunica media are found in two orientations. Most are wrapped around the vessel circumferentially and cause lumen constriction when they contract. Others run lengthwise, with their function not well understood. The outer layer of the vessel is the adventitia. It consists of connective tissue defining the maximum lumen when the muscles relax. The final blood vessel is the capillary. Its wall is only one cell thick. It therefore allows the easy transfer of oxygen, carbon dioxide, nutrients, and waste products between the cardiovascular system, the interstitial spaces, and the body cells. The skin also functions as an organ of sensation. It perceives temperature, pressure (touch) and pain.

■ **lumen** opening, or space, within a needle, artery, vein, or other hollow vessel.

It's easy to see that the skin provides many essential services for the human body. We often take them for granted until the skin is significantly injured and no longer able to provide its fluid containment, infection barrier, temperature regulation, insulation from trauma, and sensory functions. A patient may then be subjected to severe blood and fluid loss, infection, hypothermia, as well as to further injury.

PATHOPHYSIOLOGY

Soft tissues can be injured through two very different mechanisms. One is trauma and the other is heat or chemical interaction. Trauma is a violently produced transfer of energy resulting in a wound. Extreme heat or chemical interaction induces a denaturing of the cell membrane and an injury called a burn. An understanding of these two injury mechanisms will allow the paramedic to better apply the assessment and management process.

Wounds

Wounds are soft-tissue injuries affecting the epidermis, dermis, and subcutaneous tissues. They can be either blunt or penetrating and include contusion, abrasion, laceration, avulsion, amputation, or puncture. Each wound is distinctly different and deserving of a special consideration.

Contusions are blunt, nonpenetrating injuries that crush and damage small blood vessels. Blood is drawn to the inflamed tissue, so contusions present with a reddening called **erythema.** Blood also leaks into the surrounding interstitial spaces through damaged vessels. As the stagnant blood loses its oxygen, it becomes dark red and then blue, resulting in **ecchymosis.** Since ecchymosis is a delayed sign in wound progression, trauma patients need to be carefully and serially evaluated. Contusions are more pronounced in areas where the skin has been trapped between the offending agent and skeletal structures such as the ribs or the skull. Occasionally, a chest injury will display an erythematous or ecchymotic outline of the ribs and sternum, reflecting the impact with the auto dashboard or other blunt object. Early evidence of the injury may be difficult to identify. But as time passes, it will become more distinct.

■ **contusion** closed wound in which the skin is unbroken, although damage has occurred to the immediate tissue beneath.

■ **erythema** general reddening of the skin due to dilation of the superficial capillaries.

■ **ecchymosis** blue-black discoloration of the skin due to leakage of blood into the tissues.

Soft-tissue bleeding can occur within the tissue and at times be significant. When a larger vessel is involved, most commonly an artery, the blood can actually separate tissue and pool in a pocket called a **hema-**

■ **hematoma** collection of blood beneath the skin or trapped within a body compartment.

toma. These injuries are very visible in head injury because of the unyielding skull underneath. They also occur in other areas and while less pronounced, can contain significant hemorrhage. A severe hematoma to the thigh, leg, or arm may contribute significantly to hypovolemia. The thigh has been known to contain over a liter of fluid before swelling becomes apparent.

Abrasions are typically the most minor of injuries that penetrate the epidermis and violate the protective envelope of the skin. They involve an abrasive action that removes layers of the epidermis and the upper reaches of the dermis. Bleeding is usually limited because only superficial capillaries are involved. If a large surface of the epidermis has been compromised, the injury carries the danger of secondary infection.

A **laceration** is an open wound penetrating more deeply into the dermis than the abrasion. A laceration tends to involve a smaller surface area, being limited to the immediate tissue surrounding the penetration. It endangers the deeper and more significant vasculature: arteries, arterioles, venules, and veins as well as nerves, tendons, ligaments and, possibly, underlying organs. Because of the potential for involvement of other structures, the paramedic should carefully evaluate the laceration site. (See Figure 18-2.) As with the abrasion, the protective barrier is broken, and a pathway exists for infection.

A specific laceration that is surgically smooth in nature is the **incision.** It is a wound normally caused by a knife, straight razor, or piece of glass and tends to bleed freely. In all other ways it is a laceration. A second special type of laceration is the **puncture.** It involves a small entrance wound with damage into the interior of the body. (See Figure 18-3.) The wound will normally seal itself and present in a way unreflective of the extent of injury. Besides the depth of damage, the puncture carries the danger of infection. Bacteria and other pathogens introduced into the wound may cause serious infection. The problem is compounded because low oxygen levels found in the wound do not retard bacterial growth as do high levels in the open wound.

Avulsion occurs when a flap of skin, although torn or cut, is not completely loose. Avulsion is frequently seen with blunt trauma to the skull where the scalp is torn and folded back. It may also occur with animal bites and machinery accidents. (See Figure 18-4.) Its seriousness depends on the area involved, the condition of the circulation to and distal to the injury site, and the degree of contamination.

A special type of avulsion is the degloving injury. The skin is torn

---

■ **abrasion** scraping or abrading away of the superficial layers of the skin. An open soft tissue injury.

■ **laceration** open wound, normally a tear with jagged borders.

■ **incision** very smooth or surgical laceration, frequently caused by a knife or scalpel.

■ **puncture** specific soft-tissue injury involving a deep, narrow wound to the skin and underlying organs. It carries an increased danger of infection.

■ **avulsion** forceful tearing away or separation of body tissue. The avulsion may be partial or complete.

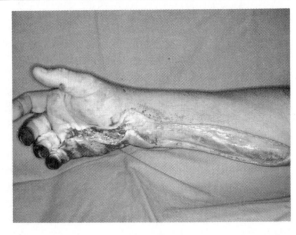

FIGURE 18-2 Severe hand injury resulting from contact with a high-pressure grease gun. The initial injury appeared very minor. (Courtesy of Scott and White Hospital and Clinic)

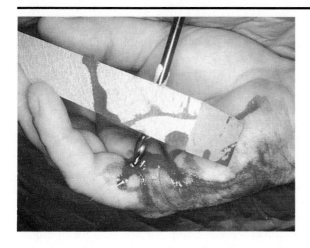

FIGURE 18-3 Penetrating injury with retained foreign body. (Courtesy of Scott and White Hospital and Clinic)

off the underlying muscle, blood vessels, and bone. It is a particularly gruesome injury, occurring occasionally with farm and industrial machinery. The skin is trapped in the device as the skeletal tissue underneath is pulled away with great force. The injury appears very grotesque and carries with it a poor prognosis. The wound exposes a large area of tissue and is often severely contaminated. If, however, the vasculature and the innervation remain, there may be some hope for use of the extremity or the digit.

A variation of the degloving process is the ring injury. As a person jumps or falls, the ring is caught, pulling the skin of the finger against the weight of the victim. The force may tear the upper layers of tissue away from the phalanges, exposing the tendons, nerves, and blood vessels. Although limited in the area involved, the ring injury is otherwise similar to the degloving injury.

The partial or complete severance of a digit or limb is referred to as an **amputation.** It will often result in the complete loss of the limb at the site of severance. The amputated part may be reattached or used as skin for grafting, as the remaining limb is repaired. If this skin is unavailable, the surgeon may be required to cut the bone and musculature back further to close the wound. This will reduce the length of the limb and its future usefulness.

■ **amputation** severance, removal, or detachment, either partial or complete, of a body part.

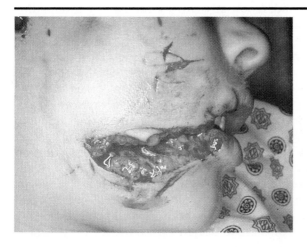

FIGURE 18-4 Laceration in a young child resulting from a dog bite. (Courtesy of Scott and White Hospital and Clinic)

Hemorrhage

Blood loss is frequently associated with soft-tissue injuries. It can range from inconsequential to life threatening and can be either easy or almost impossible to control. Blood loss is either arterial, venous, or capillary. The color of the hemorrhage is usually dark red in venous injury, red in capillary injury, and bright red in arterial injury. The rate of hemorrhage also progresses from capillary oozing to venous flowing to arterial pulsing. In practice, it may be hard to differentiate between the origins of hemorrhage. However, it is only important to determine the rate and quantity of blood loss and to stop it.

The blood itself may assist in the control of blood loss from an injured vessel, for it contains elements that assist in the clotting process. Proteins from the plasma and platelets are released at the site of disturbed flow and injury to the blood vessel. They form a matrix of fibers and capture the red blood cells, occluding flow. This clotting mechanism takes about ten minutes in the normal, healthy adult. It is more rapid if the blood vessel involved is small; it is less rapid if the vessel is a large artery or vein. The nature of the vessel injury may be more important than the size or type of vessel. If a moderately-sized vein or artery is cut cleanly, the muscles in its wall will contract. This will retract the severed vessel into the tissue. As the muscle is drawn back from the wound, it thickens and restricts the lumen. This tamponades flow, reduces the rate of loss, and assists the clotting mechanisms. Therefore, lacerations and amputations generally do not bleed profusely. If the vessel is not severed cleanly but laid open, the muscle contraction will open the wound, thereby increasing blood loss. Such an injury accompanies the laceration which parallels and involves a large vessel.

Another type of injury which may result in heavy, difficult to control bleeding is the crushing wound. It is a combination of lacerations and contusions that present with generalized bleeding from the wound. Because the vessels involved are not cleanly severed, they bleed without the natural control of retraction. The actual bleeding source is difficult to locate and control.

Burns

Burns are injuries to the soft tissues that may occur secondary to thermal, electrical, chemical, or radiation insult. While the result of the burn mechanism is much the same, the processes are very different.

Thermal Burns. The thermal burn actually causes damage by increasing the rate at which the molecules within an object move and collide with each other. At a temperature greater than absolute zero, the molecules of any object move about. The measure of the energy of this motion is called *temperature*. As the temperature of the object increases, the speed of the molecules and the incidence of collision with other molecules also increases. This changing internal energy causes many substances to expand with increased heat, such as steel. Others change in nature, such as water which changes from ice to water to steam. Heat energy may also cause chemical changes. As temperature increases, substances such as gasoline may combine with oxygen. Or matter may change its nature as, for example, when an egg is heated in a frying pan. Such a change in nature causes the physical injury in the burn patient. As molecular speed increases, the cell components, especially membranes and proteins, begin to break down. The result of exposure to extreme heat will be progressive injury and cell death.

The extent of burn injury is related to the amount of heat energy transferred to the patient's skin. That energy in turn is dependent upon three components of the burning agent: its temperature, the concentration of heat energy it possesses, and the length of contact time. Obviously, the greater the temperature of an agent the greater the potential for damage.

It is also important to consider the amount of heat energy the object or substance has. A blast of heated air from an oven at 350 degrees is much less damaging than hot cooking oil at the same temperature. Also, momentary contact with hot oil would result in less damage than if it were poured into one's shoe. The burn is a progressive process. Thus, the greater the heat energy transmitted to the body, the deeper the wound. Initially, the epidermis will be affected by the increase in temperature. As the contact with the substance continues, the heat energy will be transmitted further and deeper into the body tissue. It may involve the epidermis, dermis, subcutaneous, muscular, skeletal, and other internal tissue.

Degree Of Burn.   Burns are normally classified by degrees. (See Figure 18-5.) The *first-degree burn* involves only the upper layers of the epidermis and dermis. It is an irritation of the living cells in this region and results in some pain, minor edema, and erythema. It will normally heal without complication. (See Figure 18-6.)

The *second-degree burn* penetrates slightly deeper and produces blisters. The heat energy travels into the dermis, involving more of the tissue and resulting in greater destruction. The second-degree burn is similar to the first in that it is reddened, painful and edematous. (See Fig-

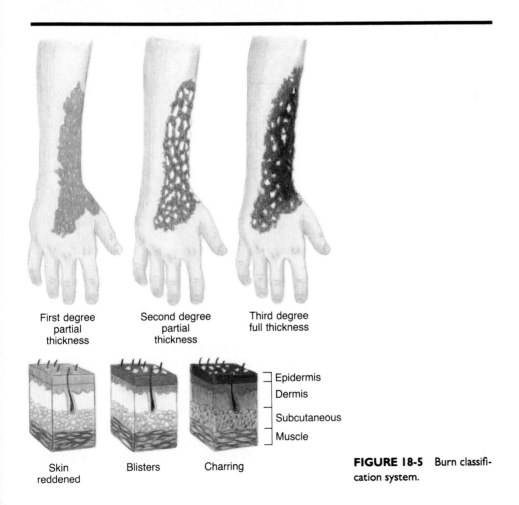

First degree
partial
thickness

Second degree
partial
thickness

Third degree
full thickness

Epidermis
Dermis
Subcutaneous
Muscle

Skin
reddened

Blisters

Charring

FIGURE 18-5   Burn classification system.

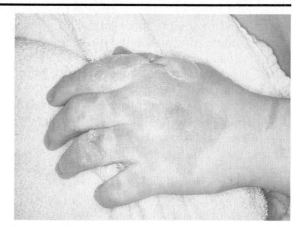

FIGURE 18-6 Hand injury with primarily first and second-degree burns. (Courtesy of Scott and White Hospital and Clinic)

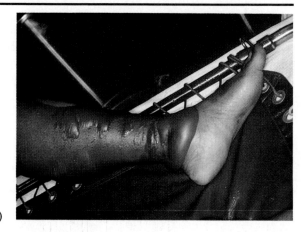

FIGURE 18-7 Second-degree burns are characterized by the formation of blisters. (Courtesy of Scott and White Hospital and Clinic)

ure 18-7.) It can be differentiated from the first-degree burn only after blisters have been formed. First- and second-degree burns are also referred to as partial-thickness burns because the dermis is still intact and complete regeneration of the skin is likely.

A special and common type of partial-thickness burn is the sunburn. It is caused by ultraviolet radiation rather than the normal thermal process. The radiation penetrates only superficially and damages the uppermost layers of the dermis. Although it may present as the classical first- or second-degree injury, it will be limited in its damage as compared to the thermal second-degree burn.

Third-degree, or full-thickness, burns penetrate the entire dermis destroying it, its regenerative properties, and the peripheral nerve endings. (See Figure 18-8.) The injury is painless because of the nerve destruction. The burn will take on various discolorations due to the nature of the burning agent and the damaged, dying, or dead tissue. Third-degree burn may involve injury to blood vessels, nerves, muscle tissue, bone, or internal organs. Because the entire dermis is destroyed, healing is difficult unless the wound is small or skin grafting is used. (See Figure 18-9.)

Burn Surface Area. Two methods are frequently applied to estimate burn surface area. The *rule of nines* is most commonly used in the pre-hospital setting and is a rather gross estimation. The less frequently used *palmar surface* (surface of the palm of the patient's hand) method is more accurate in the small burn.

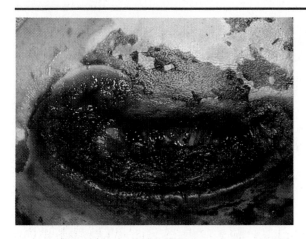

FIGURE 18-8 Third-degree burn. (Courtesy of Scott and White Hospital and Clinic)

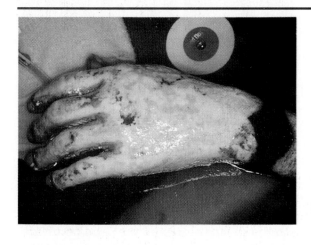

FIGURE 18-9 Third-degree burn results in complete loss of the skin. (Courtesy of Scott and White Hospital and Clinic)

Rule of Nines. The rule of nines identifies eleven topographical regions of the body surface, each of which occupies approximately 9% of body surface area. (See Figure 18-10.) The following are each given a 9% value: the entire head and neck, the front of the chest, the front of the abdomen, the posterior chest, the lower back (the posterior abdomen), the anterior surface of each lower extremity, the posterior surface of each lower extremity, and each upper extremity. The remaining 1% of surface area is assigned to the genitalia.

Since the anatomy of the infant and the child differs significantly from that of the adult, the rule of nines is modified for them. The head and neck area is divided into the anterior and posterior surface, with 9% awarded for each. Surface area of each lower extremity is reduced by 4 1/2% to ensure the total body surface area remains at 100%. This is at best a gross approximation of the area burned and should be regarded as such.

Palmar Surface. An alternate system for burn approximation, the palmar surface, uses the surface of the patient's hand to approximate the body area involved. The palm of one hand represents about 1% of the body surface area, whether the patient is an adult, a child, or an infant. If the paramedic can visualize the palmar surface area and apply it to the burned area mentally, he or she can obtain an estimate of the total skin surface affected. The system is easier to use for the local burn, while the rule of nines might be simpler and more appropriate for larger burns.

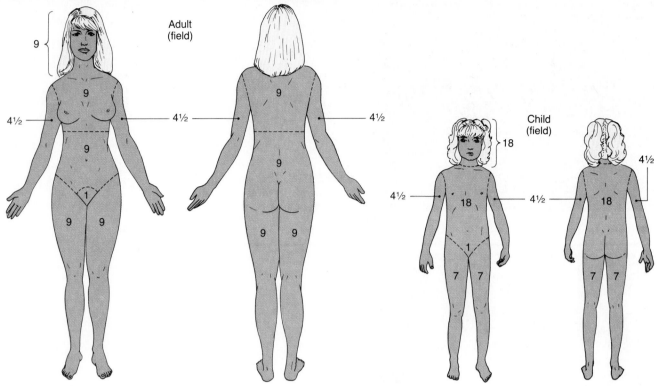

FIGURE 18-10   Rule of nines.

Many other burn approximation routines exist which are more specific to age and, in general, more accurate. They are, however, more complicated and time consuming to use. Both the rule of nines and the palmar surface method provide reasonable approximations of burn surface area if applied properly in the field.

Systemic Complications.   Burns are also associated with several systemic complications. These include hypothermia, hypovolemia, the formation of an **eschar,** inhalation injury, and infection. The burn environment may also produce chemical burns of the airway due to inhalation of the products of combustion and poisoning, secondary to carbon monoxide inhalation.

A burn may disrupt the body's ability to regulate core temperature. The destruction of tissue will reduce or eliminate the ability of the skin to contain fluid within. Plasma and other tissue fluids released by the burn process will seep into the wound. There they will evaporate, rapidly removing heat energy. If the burn is extensive, the uncontrolled loss of body heat may induce hypothermia.

Hypovolemia also may complicate the severe burn. The inability of damaged blood vessels to contain plasma will cause a shift of proteins and fluid into the burn tissue. Loss of plasma protein will reduce the blood's ability, via osmosis, to draw fluids from the uninjured tissues. This in turn will reduce the body's natural response to fluid loss and may produce a profound hypovolemia. (See Figure 18-11.) Although this is a serious complication of the extensive burn, it takes hours to develop. Modern aggressive fluid resuscitation can counteract this aspect of the burn process.

The third-degree thermal burn may be complicated by denaturing of the skin. As the burn destroys the dermal cells, they become hard and

■ **eschar** hard, leathery product of deep third-degree burn. It consists of dead and denatured skin.

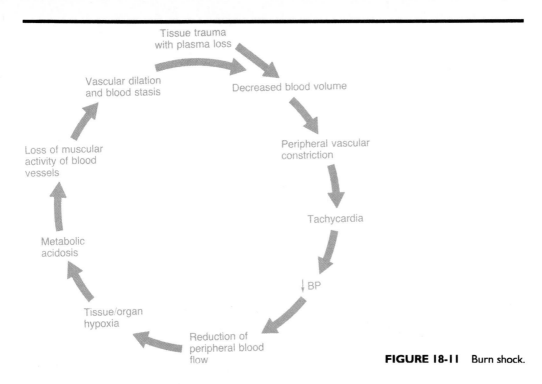

FIGURE 18-11 Burn shock.

leathery. The skin as a whole tightens over the wound site, restricting the flow of blood and increasing the pressure of any edema beneath. If the burn is **circumferential,** the constriction may be severe enough to occlude all blood flow into the distal extremity. In the case of a thoracic burn it may drastically reduce chest excursion and respiratory tidal volume. (See Figure 18-12.)

■ **circumferential** encircling or around the complete exterior.

Inhalation Injury. Inhalation injury is often associated with the burn environment. This is especially true if the injury occurred in a closed space or when the patient was unconscious. A patient who is unconscious or entrapped in a smoke-filled area will eventually breathe in the gases, heated air, flame, or steam and sustain airway and respiratory injury.

✱ Inhalation injury may be associated with burns, especially if the injury occurred in an enclosed space.

The synthetic resins and plastics used in modern construction are very dangerous as they burn. They can form such toxic compounds as potassium cyanide and hydrogen sulfide. If inhaled, they will react with the lung tissue, causing internal chemical burns or an actual systemic poisoning. The signs and symptoms of this injury may not display until an hour or two after inhalation.

Another, though less frequent, airway injury is the airway thermal burn. The airway is lined with very moist mucosa which insulates very well against heat damage. It takes great thermal energy to evaporate the fluid and injure the cells. The normal heat energy associated with hot air or flame inspiration is rarely enough to cause significant thermal airway burns.

An occasional cause of thermal burn is superheated steam. The steam is created under great pressure and heated well above 212°F. A common hazard to firefighters, it develops when a stream of water strikes a hot spot and vaporizes explosively. The blast may dislodge the firefighter's self-contained breathing apparatus and be inhaled. The superheated steam contains enough energy to severely burn the upper airway and may (though infrequently) damage the lower respiratory tract.

With any thermal or smoke-related chemical burn injury to the respiratory tract, there is the danger of airway restriction, severe dyspnea,

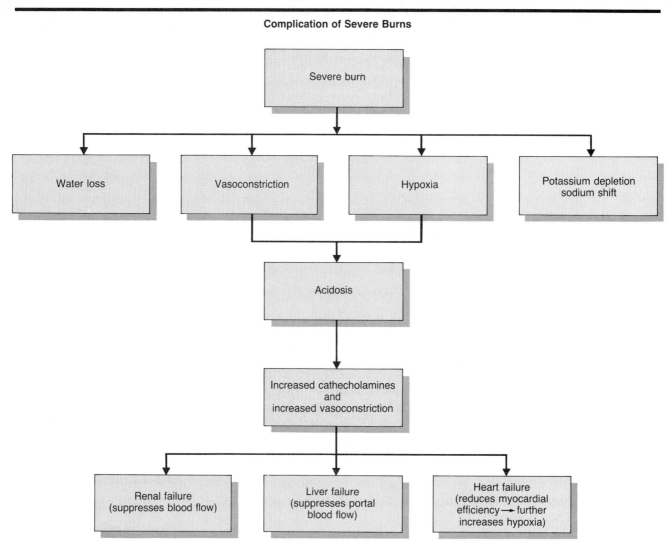

Severe burn

Water loss

Vasoconstriction

Hypoxia

Potassium depletion
sodium shift

Acidosis

Increased cathecholamines
and
increased vasoconstriction

Renal failure
(suppresses blood flow)

Liver failure
(suppresses portal
blood flow)

Heart failure
(reduces myocardial
efficiency ➝ further
increases hypoxia)

FIGURE 18-12 Complications of severe burns.

and possible respiratory arrest. The airway is a narrow tube, lined with extremely vascular tissue. If damaged, it will swell rapidly, seriously reducing the size of the airway lumen. (See Figure 18-13.) The patient may present with a minor hoarseness, followed precipitously by dyspnea. The injury may be so extensive as to induce complete respiratory obstruction and arrest.

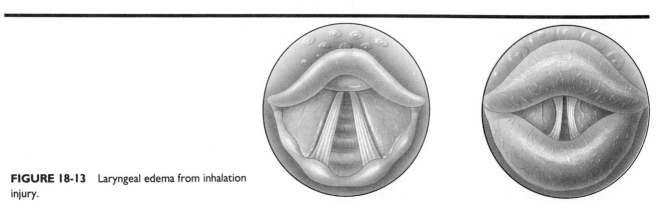

FIGURE 18-13 Laryngeal edema from inhalation injury.

Special Considerations

An additional concern associated with the burn injury environment is carbon monoxide poisoning. It is a frequent hazard that should be suspected in any patient who was within an enclosed space during combustion. Poisoning occurs because the hemoglobin of the blood has a much greater affinity for carbon monoxide than for the essential oxygen. If it is inhaled in even the smallest quantities, carbon dioxide will displace oxygen, subjecting the patient to hypoxemia. This problem is very difficult to detect, yet will subtly embarrass the patient's oxygen delivery to vital organs. If associated with airway burns, it will further compound the respiratory compromise.

Although infection is the most persistent killer of burn victims, it does not present as a problem to the paramedic. Pathogens invade the wound shortly after the burn occurs and up until the wound heals. Their hazard to life occurs as they grow to massive numbers, a process taking days or weeks to develop.

The extent of a burn injury must be considered in the context of the patient's overall health. The geriatric, pediatric, ill, or traumatized patient has greater difficulty handling the burn injury than does the healthy individual. The pediatric patient suffers from a high surface area to body weight ratio, which means the fluid reserves for the burn are low. Geriatric patients have reduced mechanisms for fluid retention, reduced reserves and are more apt to have underlying disease. Ill patients are already using body energy to fight their disease. With the burn, they will have two medical stresses to combat. Burn fluid loss will compound the blood loss of trauma patients, and they will have to recover from both injuries.

Electrical Burns And Injuries. The power of electricity is due to the flow of electrons from a point of high concentration to one of low concentration. The difference is called the *voltage* and the rate of flow (the current) is the *amperage*. A third variable is *resistance*. The copper of electrical wire allows free flow of electrons and has very little resistance. Tungsten (the filament in a light bulb) is moderately resistant and will heat, glow, and emit light as more and more current is applied.

The human body, like tungsten, is relatively resistant to the electricity flow. If it is subjected to a voltage differential, it will allow the current to pass. As it does, heat is created. For small voltages the energy is of little consequence. But if the voltage or current is high, the damage can be profound. A longer duration of contact will also increase the potential for injury.

Thermal injury due to electrical current will occur as the energy travels from the point of contact to the point of exit. (See Figure 18-14.) At both these points the concentration of electricity is great, as is the damage expected. The smaller the area of contact, the greater the concentration of current flow and the greater the injury. Between the entrance and exit points, the energy spreads out over a larger cross sectional area and generally causes less damage. The current of electricity may follow blood vessels and nerves since they offer less resistance than muscle and bone. This may lead to serious injury deep within the involved limbs.

Electrical contact may also cause some disruption of the control of muscle tissue. Muscles are controlled by complicated electrochemical reactions which are interrupted by the current, especially if it is alternating current. If the current continues for a period of time it may immobilize the muscles of respiration and lead to prolonged respiratory arrest,

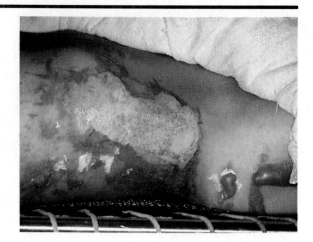

FIGURE 18-14 Electricity exit wound in a male who contacted 72,000-volt power lines. (Courtesy of Scott and White Hospital and Clinic)

anoxia, hypoxemia, and death. The electrical current may also disrupt the heart's electrical system and cause ventricular fibrillation, accompanied by ineffective pumping action.

At times, electrical energy may cause flash burns secondary to the heat of the current passing through adjacent air or by the ignition of clothing or other combustables. Air is very resistant to the passage of current. If the current is strong enough and the space is small, the electricity will arc, producing tremendous heat. If a patient's skin is close by, the heat may severely burn or vaporize the tissue. Additionally, the heat may ignite articles of clothing and result in the more common thermal burn.

Chemical Burns. Chemical burns denature the biochemical makeup of the cell membrane and destroy the cell. Such injury is not transmitted through the tissue as is the thermal injury. A chemical burn must destroy the tissue before chemically burning any deeper. This generally limits the "burn" process unless very strong chemicals are involved. (See Figure 18-15.)

Chemical burns may be caused by agents too numerous to mention. They are most commonly either strong acids or bases (alkali). Their interaction with the body tissue changes the tissue chemically, resulting in a breakdown of the membrane and cell death much like the burn. (See Figure 18-16.)

Chemical splashes that involve the eye should be irrigated with large volumes of water. Alkali burns are expecially damaging and should be flushed for at least 15 minutes. Acid burns should be irrigated for at least 5 minutes, while splashes of an unknown agent should be flushed for up to 20 minutes. Do not delay transport while flushing.

Radiation Injury. The earth has been bombarded with nuclear radiation since before recorded time. It is a daily, natural phenomenon. The danger becomes apparent with exposure to a synthetic source which greatly increases the intensity of radiation. Radioactive materials are used in industry and medicine for diagnostic testing and in energy production by power companies. The risk of injury occurs from accidents associated with improper handling, either in the transportation or on-site environment. Nuclear radiation damages through a process called **ionization.** An energy particle travels into a substance and changes an atom within. In the human body the cell affected either repairs the damage, dies, or goes on to produce damaged cells (cancer). The cells most sensitive to radiation

■ **ionization** the process of changing a substance into separate charged particles (ions).

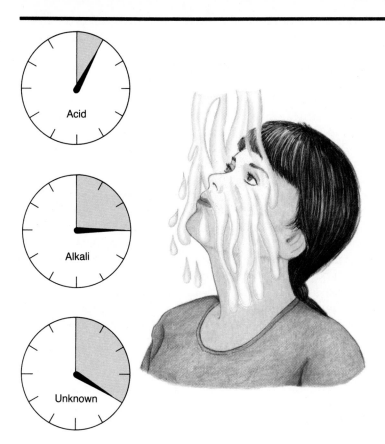

FIGURE 18-15 Treatment for chemical burns to the face and eye is copious, prolonged irrigation with water.

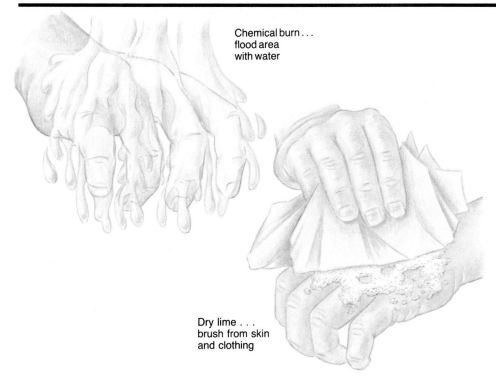

Chemical burn . . .
flood area
with water

Dry lime . . .
brush from skin
and clothing

FIGURE 18-16 Chemical burns should be flushed with water. Dry lime should be first brushed away before applying water.

injury are erythrocytes, those responsible for erythrocyte production (marrow), those lining the intestinal tract, and those involved in reproduction.

There are three types of radiation commonly encountered. **Alpha radiation** is emitted when the nucleus of a atom releases a neutron. It is a very weak energy source and travels only inches through air. Easily stopped by paper or clothing, alpha radiation will not penetrate the epidermis of the skin. It is really only a hazard if contaminated material is inhaled or ingested. The second radiological particle is **beta radiation.** Its energy is greater than that of alpha radiation and will travel 6 to 10 feet through air or a few layers of clothing. Beta particles will penetrate the first few millimeters of skin and hold the potential for external as well as internal contamination. **Gamma radiation,** also known as X-rays, is the most powerful ionizing radiation. It has the ability to travel through the entire body or ionize any atom within. Gamma radiation evokes the greatest concern for external exposure. It is the most dangerous and most feared type of radiation because it is difficult to protect against.

Exposure to radiation and the effects of ionization can occur through two mechanisms. A strong radioactive source, composed of an unstable material such as uranium, may expose the unshielded person to ionizing radiation. The second occurrence is contamination by dust, debris, or fluids that contain very small particles of active material. The contaminant gives off weaker levels of radiation, but because of its close proximity and greater length of contact time, the danger is great. Also, it should be noted that most substances, including human tissue, cannot be induced to give off radiation. The danger in the radiological incident is not caused by the patient. It comes from the source or contaminated material on the patient.

Three aspects of exposure to a radiation source are of importance to the paramedic. They are duration of exposure, distance from the source, and shielding between the rescuer, the patient, and the source. Knowledge of these three factors can limit the dose and potential for injury.

Duration: Radiation exposure is an accumulative danger. The longer a patient or the attending paramedic is exposed to the source, the greater the potential for injury.

Distance: Radiation strength is reduced quickly as you travel farther from the source. It is similar to the intensity of light from a light bulb. At a few feet we can easily read by it, while at a few hundred feet it becomes a point of light barely casting a shadow. Mathematically, the relationship is inverse and squared. As we double our distance from the source, its strength drops to one fourth. As we triple the distance its strength diminishes to one ninth, and so on.

Shielding: The more material between the source and the rescuers, the less radiation which penetrates. With alpha and beta radiation, shielding is very easy and reasonably effective. With gamma sources, dense objects such as earth, concrete, metal, and lead are needed to provide any real protection.

It is very difficult to determine when a radiological exposure has occurred. Radiation is invisible and cannot be felt. It will not present with any immediate side effects unless the exposure is extremely high. Instead, the results of an exposure may present serious medical problems years after the incident.

The injuries and side effects of exposure are dose related and occur in either the acute or delayed time parameters. The acute symptoms include nausea, vomiting, and malaise. If the dose was extremely high, it may lead to severe illness and death. In some cases burns may evolve,

- **alpha radiation** lowest level of nuclear radiation. A weak source of energy, it is stopped by clothing or the first layers of skin.

- **beta radiation** medium-strength radiation stopped with light clothing or the uppermost layers of skin.

- **gamma radiation** powerful electromagnetic radiation emitted by radioactive substances. It is stronger than alpha and beta radiation.

especially if a limb received very high doses of beta or gamma radiation. Moderate or prolonged exposure to radiation may produce long-term and delayed problems. Infertility is a potential injury since the cells producing the egg and sperm are very susceptible to ionization damage. Cancer is another delayed and severe side effect which may occur years and even decades after an incident.

ASSESSMENT

The evaluation of the skin tells more about the condition of the body than any other aspect of the assessment. Not only is the skin the first body organ to experience the effects of trauma, it is the first and often the only organ to display them. Therefore, the assessment of the skin, and the associated wounds and burns, must be deliberate, careful, and complete.

While the soft-tissue injury process is varied, assessment should be simple and well structured. It must be carefully applied and complete to ensure that the nature and extent of each injury is established, and they are placed in appropriate priority for care.

The assessment of patients with soft-tissue trauma follows the same general progression: survey the scene, primary assessment, and the elements of secondary assessment: the head to toe survey, vital signs, and patient history. The process is the same for wounds and burns, although they will be discussed separately.

* Wound assessment must be comprehensive to ensure that the extent of each injury is known so that care can be appropriately prioritized.

Primary Assessment—Wounds

Wound assessment plays a key role in the primary assessment. Often, wounds are the only or most apparent signs of internal injury. They may be accompanied by severe and life threatening hemorrhage. In either case, their evaluation begins after the A-B-C's have been assessed and secured, and the general neurologic status quickly determined.

Wounds to the face, head, neck, chest and abdomen are examined during the "Expose" aspect of the primary assessment. (See Figures 18-17 and 18-18.) Any discoloration, deformity, or open wound should be quickly investigated. The paramedic should ensure that the wound does

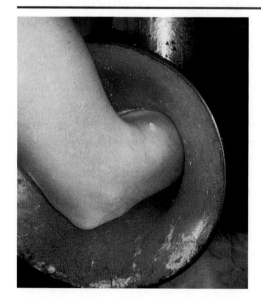

FIGURE 18-17 It is important to completely expose the patient and assess the wound. From this vantage point, the significance of this injury cannot be determined.

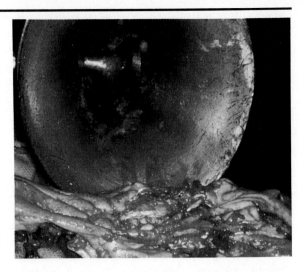

FIGURE 18-18 Removal from the machine reveals a significant crush injury from a commercial meat grinder.

not involve or endanger the airway or breathing, or contribute significantly to hypovolemia. Immediate care should focus on controlling severe blood loss or on the more serious injuries suggested by the soft-tissue trauma.

The entire body should be scanned for external bleeding. If the mechanism of injury suggests open wounds, the body areas hidden from sight should be swept with gloved hands. This action will quickly rule out otherwise unseen rapid and pooling blood loss. Moderate to severe hemorrhage should be controlled immediately. The control does not need to be definitive, but it should stop any continuing significant blood loss. When more time can be spent, the wound will be properly dressed and bandaged.

The bleeding wound should also be quickly surveyed to determine the type of bleeding: arterial, venous, or capillary. The volume of loss should be approximated and compared against the time since the accident. The result will be the overall rate of loss. At the conclusion of the primary assessment, the decision to immediately transport or remain and provide complete care must be made. The rate and volume of any blood loss and any uncontrollable bleeding must be considered in this decision.

Once the patient has been provided with the complete primary assessment and any emergent care actions are accomplished, the secondary survey may begin.

Secondary Assessment—Wounds

The head-to-toe evaluation of the skin will involve observation, inquiry, and palpation. It must follow a planned and comprehensive process, although the actual order is not critical.

Observe: Wound assessment should first observe a particular body region to identify any discoloration, deformity, or frank wounds. Discoloration should be identified as local, distal, or systemic. Local discoloration may include the erythema or ecchymosis of a limited area caused by a contusion, blood vessel injury, dislocation or long bone fracture. Distal discoloration may reflect the pale, cyanotic, or ashen color of a limb distal to the point of circulation loss. Systemic discoloration such as a pale, ashen, or gray hue may be found in all limbs, suggesting hypovolemia and shock. Any wound must be inspected in detail. Its depth should be visually determined. Also, the paramedic should evaluate the potential for damage to underlying structures: bones, muscle, or body organs. The paramedic should identify the offending agent if possible and determine the amount of transmitted force involved. Assessment should also include the nature and quantity of any wound contamination and the depth of its introduction. The wound should be observed in such a way that it can be described to the attending physician after the injury is dressed. This will help with prioritizing patient injuries and with their documentation in the run report.

✳ The wound should be observed in such a way that it can later be described to the attending physician.

Inquire: The patient needs to be questioned about the mechanism of injury, any pain or pain on movement, and the loss of function or sensation specific to an area. Additionally, the paramedic should attempt to determine what happened and the exact nature of any pain or sensory or motor loss. Question the patient about signs or symptoms before touching the area.

Palpate: Finally, the entire surface area is palpated. The process should attempt to locate any deformity, asymmetry, temperature variation, unexpected masses, and localized loss of skin or muscle tone. Also, any tenderness or loss of sensation should be noted. (Universal precautions should be observed during palpation.)

Soft tissue wounds should be prioritized to identify the order of care to follow. The few moments taken to sort injuries and to plan the management process will save time in the field. They will also ensure that the highest priority injuries are cared for early.

Primary Assessment—Thermal Burns

The scene must be secured before assessment and care can begin. In the thermal injury, fire must be controlled and no longer be a threat to the patient or paramedic. The patient's location must be free from the danger of structural collapse, contamination, electricity, and any other hazards.

Before assessment begins, the paramedic must ensure that the burning has stopped. Any overt flame must be extinguished, and the patient must be quickly surveyed for other sources that may continue the burn process. A quick survey of the patient's posterior surface should thus be included. Burn patients may be an actual source of hazard to the rescuer and to themselves. Leather articles will smolder for hours and continue to induce thermal injury. The paramedic should specifically look at any shoes, belts, or watchbands. Watches, rings, and other jewelry may also hold and transmit heat. Be careful as you check these items. They may be hot enough to burn you.

✳ Look for and extinguish smoldering shoes, belts, or watchbands early in the assessment of burn patients.

Except in the very local burn, the patient's entire body surface should be viewed. The paramedic should remove any clothing that was or could have been involved in the burn. If any of the clothing within the wound resists removal, it should be cut around as necessary. Once the scene is safe and the patient's clothing is not burning, examine the burn mechanism. Is there any possibility that the patient was unconscious during the fire or trapped within the building? If so, a special emphasis should be placed upon airway assessment and management. The paramedic should watch for any signs of airway restriction and be alert to the possibility of carbon monoxide poisoning.

Assessment of the burn patient must address the priorities of primary and secondary assessment. The danger of associated trauma and the possibility of spine injury must be ruled out. Otherwise, the patient must be protected from further cervical injury. The airway must be patent and protected. The burn patient must be given special consideration under this priority. The initial airway exam should look for the signs of any thermal or inhalation injury. Nasal hairs should be visualized to ensure that they have not been singed. Any sputum and the areas around the mouth and nose should be examined for carbonaceous material or any other evidence of inhalation. Airway sounds reflecting irritation or mucosal damage, such as hoarseness or coughing, should alert the paramedic to the potential for airway injury and progressive restriction to follow. A patient with any signs of respiratory involvement should be considered as a potential acute emergency and receive immediate transport and care. High flow oxygen should be instituted and the equipment for endotracheal intubation readied. These patients may progress rapidly from mild dyspnea to total respiratory arrest.

While the intubation of a respiratory burn patient may be difficult in the field, there are distinct advantages to performing it early. The edema is progressive and will gradually reduce the airway lumen. If intubation waits until the patient arrives at the emergency department, the airway may be so edematous that it is difficult if not impossible. On the other hand, cricothyrotomy or tracheostomy can be performed at the emergency department should intubation be unsuccessful. If field intubation is elected and approved by medical command, it must be done quickly and carefully. The airway is already swelling, so that even the normal trauma associated with intubation could make matters worse. The technique will also be complicated if the patient is conscious and fights the process. Under these circumstances, nasotracheal intubation may be useful. Oral intubation, using a topical lidocaine spray, may also be considered. In either case, the most experienced paramedic should attempt the procedure to ensure it is completed quickly. As with all intubation, it is best to maintain an airway using the largest endotracheal tube possible. The paramedic should have several smaller than normal-sized tubes ready, since the edema may limit the available size of the airway. He or she should select the largest one which may be easily passed through the cords.

The remainder of the primary assessment should progress as with any trauma patient. The level of patient consciousness or responsiveness should be established. Any circumferential burns of the head, neck, chest, extremity, or abdomen should be noticed as these areas are "Exposed" and examined. The signs and symptoms of the severe burn will not usually affect the patient within the prehospital environment. Pain may actually be paradoxical to the severity of the burn. The less severe first- and second-degree burns will be very uncomfortable, while the patient with extensive third-degree burns may be almost without pain. The other classical and deadly problems associated with extensive soft tissue burn will not develop until well after prehospital care has concluded. Hypovolemia may be delayed because the fluid loss is gradual and progressive. Infection, the greatest cause of delayed patient mortality, occurs days and often weeks after post-burn. If the patient is found to have third-degree burns over a large portion of the body, rapid transport is indicated. Patients with associated injury to the face, joints, hands, or feet are likewise immediate transport cases. Patients sustaining an inhalation of smoke, steam or flame or any geriatric, pediatric, ill, or trauma patient must be considered for immediate transport also.

Secondary Assessment—Thermal Burns

The head-to-toe examination and the rest of the secondary assessment should continue at the scene *only* if significant and life-threatening burns can be ruled out. Such assessment may also be instituted while the patient is being transported. During the assessment an accurate approximation of the depth and extent of the burn area is essential. This will guide the field paramedic in care. It will also guide the emergency department personnel in preparation for patient arrival.

The rule of nines should be applied to determine the total body surface area (BSA) burned. Nine percent should be added if an entire "rule of nines" region is involved. If only a portion is involved, that proportion of 9% should be added. For example, if 1/3 of the upper extremity were burned, the burn approximation would be 3% (1/3 of 9% = 3%).

The depth of a burn injury is also an important consideration. Areas of painful sensation identify *partial-thickness burns,* while those which present with limited or absent pain are most likely *full-thickness burns.* This differentiation may be difficult because the third-degree burn may be surrounded by partial thickness injury and pain. (See Table 18-1.)

The third consideration in determining the severity of a burn is the area affected. The face, hands, feet, joints, genitalia, and circumferential burns deserve particular consideration. Each present with special problems to patients and their recovery. The face has already been assessed and any burns considered because of respiratory involvement. However, this area also needs special consideration for aesthetic reasons. Facial damage and scarring may be more debilitating that any joint or limb burn. The area should be carefully assessed and given a high priority, even if respiratory involvement can be ruled out. Burns involving the feet or the hands are also considered serious. These areas are critical for much of the patient's daily activity. Serious burns and the associated scar tissue may make the injury very debilitating. These areas must be assessed carefully and the degree and specific area burned communicated to the receiving physician. Joints carry a similar danger. Scar tissue will replace the skin, with joint flexibility and mobility suffering. Any burn appearing as full thickness and involving the hands, feet, or joints should

> ✳ The head-to-toe examination should continue at the scene only if significant and life-threatening burns can be ruled out.

TABLE 18-1 Characteristics of Various Depths of Burns

	First degree	**Second degree**	**Third degree**
Cause	Sun or minor flash	Hot liquids, flashes, or flame	Chemicals, electricity, flame, hot metals
Skin color	Red	Mottled red	Pearly white and/or charred translucent and parchment-like
Skin surface	Dry with no blisters	Blisters with weeping	Dry with thrombosed blood vessels
Sensation	Painful	Painful	Anesthetic
Healing	3–6 days	2–4 weeks, depending on depth	Requires skin grafting

receive a higher priority than a burn of equal surface area and depth elsewhere.

Burns surrounding an extremity, the thorax, the abdomen or the neck are also of concern during assessment. Due to the nature of the third-degree burn, the area underneath may be drastically compressed as an eschar forms. Constriction may hinder respirations, restrict distal blood flow, or cause hypoxia of the tissues beneath. Any burn encircling a part of the body should be carefully assessed for distal circulation or other signs of vascular embarrassment. Finally, any burn affecting pediatric, geriatric, ill, or otherwise injured patients must be assigned a higher priority. The serious burn is a great stress on these patients. Massive fluid and heat loss as well as infection challenge the human system. The burn in the context of any other patient problem must be considered more serious. Once the depth, extent, and other contributing factors to burn severity have been determined, the patient may be categorized as either minor, moderate, or severely burned.

1. Minor
   ❑ Sunburns
   ❑ Limited Partial-Thickness Burn
2. Moderate
   ❑ Partial-Thickness Burn, over 15% BSA
   ❑ Limited Full-Thickness Burn
3. Severe
   ❑ Partial-Thickness Burn, over 30% BSA
   ❑ Full-Thickness Burn, over 5% BSA
   ❑ Inhalation Injury

Any involvement of a critical area, such as hands, feet, joints, face, or genitalia represent an increase in one level of severity. The same holds true for pediatric, geriatric, other trauma, or acute medical patients. Any signs or symptoms of respiratory involvement identify the patient as a severe emergency and require immediate transport to a Burn Center if possible. (See Table 18-2.)

Chemical Injury Assessment

❋ In dealing with the chemical burn, it is of the utmost concern that no one else is contaminated.

In dealing with the chemical burn, it is of the utmost concern that no one else is contaminated. The paramedic must be certain the source is isolated and no longer a danger to the patient or others. Any clothing possibly containing the agent must be removed and isolated from accidental con-

---

TABLE 18-2 Injuries that Benefit from Burn Center Care

A. Second-degree burn greater than 15% of body surface area (BSA)
B. Third-degree burn greater than 5% BSA
C. Significant face, feet, hands, perineal burns
D. High-voltage electrical injury
E. Inhalation injury
F. Chemical burns causing progressive tissue destruction
G. Associated significant injuries

Source: American Burn Association.

tact. It should be saved and disposed of properly. Personal protection is a priority. Gloves should be worn, though they should never be presumed to protect from the agent. Paramedics should take appropriate protective action against airborne dust or toxic fumes, both for themselves and the patient. The type of agent, its exact chemical name, the length of contact time, and the precise area affected should, if possible, be identified. The involvement of phenol, sodium, or dry lime should be ruled out. Any wound should be examined carefully to establish the depth, extent, and nature of the insult. First-aid given prior to the arrival of advanced life support personnel should be identified and recorded.

Electrical Injury Assessment

Before approaching the scene, the paramedic should be certain that the power has been shut off. Until it is, no one should be allowed to approach the patient or the proximity of the electrical source. Handling of live wires is a dangerous activity under the best of conditions, even for the specially trained personnel. It should not be attempted by paramedical personnel unless specially trained, equipped, and authorized. Once the scene is secure, the patient may be assessed and prepared for transport. Paramedics should search for both an entrance and an exit wound. They should look specifically at the possible points of contact with both the ground and the electrical source. In some circumstances multiple entrance and exit wounds will be present. As with thermal burns, the paramedic should look for smoldering shoes, belts, or other items of clothing. They may continue the burning process well after the current is shut off. Also, it is necessary to monitor the patient for possible cardiac disturbances. The heart's action may have been disrupted by the current. Thus, ventricular fibrillation, cardiac irritability, or other dysrhythmias may be present. If the patient is in respiratory arrest, ventilation should be initiated and continued. It will often take time until the normal muscular control of respirations begins. Any patient who has sustained a significant electrical shock should be examined by emergency department personnel. The damage caused by the current may be internal and undetermined during assessment. Such a patient must be considered a high priority for immediate transport.

✱ Until the power is off, no one should be allowed to approach the patient or the proximity of the electrical source.

Radiological Exposure Assessment

The potential radiation incident must be a concern during the dispatch and response phase of the emergency call. Because radiation can be neither seen nor felt, it can endanger EMS personnel unless the proper precautions are taken. If radiation exposure is expected, personnel should approach the scene very carefully. If the incident has occurred at a power generation plant, or in an industrial or a medical facility, persons knowledgeable in the substance being used and its degree of health hazard should be sought out. The paramedics should also ensure that the scene has been secured and bystanders, rescuers, and patients are protected from exposure. If patients are close to an unremovable source, they should be brought to the paramedic. If patients have been contaminated, they should be disrobed, washed with soap and water, then rinsed thoroughly before the assessment begins. It is necessary to document care-

✱ Because radiation can be neither seen nor felt, it can endanger EMS personnel unless proper precautions are taken.

fully the circumstances of exposure. The source must be identified. Also, the patients' proximity to the source during exposure as well as the length of exposure must be known. The actual assessment will be quite simple and reveal minimal signs or symptoms of injury. Only extreme exposure will result in the classical presentation of nausea, vomiting and malaise. Burns are extremely rare, although they may occur if the exposure was intense and long term. Even though the patient seems well, the consequences of high-dose radiation exposure can be devastating.

MANAGEMENT

* The management of wounds is a late priority in the care of the trauma patient, unless extensive bleeding is noted.

The management of wounds by dressing and bandaging is a late priority in the care of the trauma patient, unless extensive bleeding is noted. The paramedic should apply the appropriate objectives of wound care when higher-priority injuries have been cared for appropriately.

Objectives Of Bandaging. The objectives of bandaging are simple, straightforward, and essential to quality emergency care. They include hemorrhage control, sterility (or in the field, a degree of cleanliness), and immobilization. Any wound dressing and bandaging by the paramedic must employ and accomplish these objectives.

Hemorrhage Control. The control of severe blood loss from a soft tissue injury is often inadequate. If the bleeding continues despite initial attempts to use direct pressure, the wound should be examined to determine the exact site of blood loss. Then direct pressure should be applied to that point. Too often hemorrhage continues because the bandaging technique distributes the pressure over the entire wound site rather than focusing on the bleeding source. The pressure causing the hemorrhage is no greater than the patient's systolic blood pressure. Digital pressure can easily compress the vessel and hence should halt any blood loss. It may be necessary to maintain digital pressure for the duration of the care.

Elevation assists in controlling hemorrhage, although it is generally not as effective as direct pressure. Elevation may also benefit the wound by reducing extremity arterial pressure and increasing venous return. Both minimize potential edema and help maintain optimal circulation to the affected area. The use of pressure points may assist with bleeding control and the clotting process. The pulse point immediately proximal to the wound should be located and firm pressure applied. Pressure should be maintained for at least 10 minutes, if not for the entire prehospital time.

* A combination of techniques for hemorrhage control may be effective when bleeding is resistant to direct pressure.

A combination of techniques for hemorrhage control may be effective when bleeding is resistant to direct pressure. Direct pressure, elevation, and pressure points together will halt all but the most difficult bleeding. An exception to the effectiveness of normal blood loss techniques may be the severe crush injury. (See Figure 18-19.) In crush injury several blood vessels tear, making it difficult to pinpoint the bleeding. Even if the source can be found it is hard to apply direct pressure. In such cases the use of the tourniquet may be indicated.

The tourniquet is generally the last choice in controlling hemorrhage. If properly applied it will stop the flow of blood; however, it has serious risks:

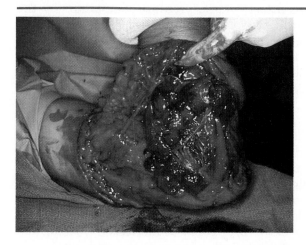

FIGURE 18-19 Crush injury to the elbow. This wound should be dressed and splinted. (Courtesy of Scott and White Hospital and Clinic)

1. If the pressure is insufficient, the tourniquet will halt venous return yet not affect arterial flow. The result will be an increase in the rate and the volume of blood loss.
2. When the tourniquet has been applied properly, the entire limb distal to the device is without circulation. The tissue beyond the tourniquet may be permanently damaged by hypoxia.
3. When the circulation is restored, highly hypoxic and acidic blood will be carried to the central circulation.

The tourniquet should not be used unless severe bleeding cannot be controlled by any other means. It must be applied in a way that does not injure the tissue beneath. During prehospital care, a readily-available and effective tourniquet may be a sphygmomanometer (regular for the upper extremity and high for the lower). It should be inflated to 20 to 30 mmHg above the patient's systolic blood pressure and beyond the pressure where the patient's hemorrhage ceases. Once applied, the tourniquet should be left in place until the patient arrives at the Emergency Department. The cuff pressure should be monitored during transport to ensure that it does not lose pressure. The staff should be alerted to it's application during transport as well as upon arrival.

✳ Once applied, the tourniquet should be left in place until the patient arrives at the emergency department.

Sterility. Once severe bleeding is halted, the wound should be kept as sterile as possible. Field conditions may limit this to keeping the wound as clean as is reasonably possible. Under normal circumstances, the wound need not be cleansed. But, if grossly contaminated, it may be irrigated with normal saline or lactated Ringer's solution. Larger particles: glass, debris, and so forth, may be carefully removed, if this can be accomplished swiftly without inducing further harm.

The dressing should appear as neat as allowed by time and the environment. The neat appearance will calm and reassure the patient, while the cleanliness will reduce contamination and, hopefully, post-trauma infection.

Immobilization. The last of the bandaging objectives is immobilization. Fixation of the wound site will help with the natural clotting mechanisms and reduce the patient's discomfort. Gentle pressure maintained by the bandage may offer the patient some comfort and will reduce swelling. The limb may be immobilized to the body or to a rigid splint such as a padded board or ladder splint. Use of elastic bandaging material is not recommended. The rapid edema immediately after an injury may cause increasing pressure to the tissue underneath. This pressure may well reduce or halt the circulation. Even soft roller gauze may cause pressure under the bandage.

Any limb bandaged circumferentially should be monitored frequently to ensure that the distal pulse remains strong. If a distal pulse cannot be located, the paramedic should monitor capillary refill, skin color, and temperature. If signs or symptoms suggest that the distal circulation is compromised, the bandaging should be checked and possibly loosened. Any circumferential pressure around a limb will retard the venous return of blood from the extremity. This will increase the edema and pain of the injury and reduce the circulation through the extremity.

Special Wound Care

Painful contusions or those with the potential for large or debilitating edema should be treated with cold and moderate-pressure bandages. Do not use ice. Ice will cool beyond the therapeutic value and possibly cause tissue freezing and further harm. In caring for any soft tissue injury, the paramedic is responsible for describing the wound in detail to the emergency department staff. This will avoid the need for them to remove the dressing and evaluate the wound until other more serious injuries are cared for. If the description of the wound is inaccurate, patient care and the paramedic's credibility will suffer.

✳ The current recommendation for management of separated body parts includes dry cooling and rapid transport.

The current recommendation for management of separated body parts includes dry cooling and rapid transport. (See Figures 18-20 and 18-21.) The amputated part should be placed in a plastic bag and kept cool by cold water immersion. The water in which the bag and body part sits may have a few ice cubes in it, but avoid direct contact between the ice and the injured part. Any avulsed or amputated part should be transported to the hospital receiving the patient. (See Figures 18-22 and 18-

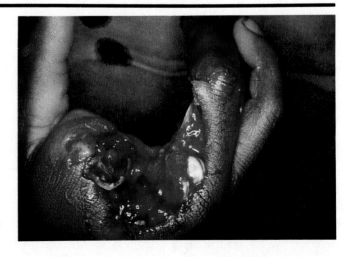

FIGURE 18-20 Amputation of the index and long fingers of the right hand. (Courtesy of Scott and White Hospital and Clinic)

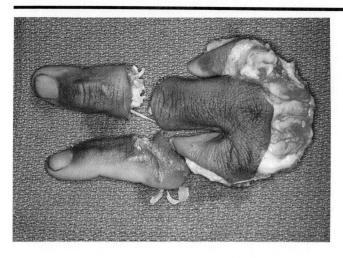

FIGURE 18-21 The amputated parts should be transported with the patient to the hospital. Even if replantation cannot be performed, the skin, blood vessels, and bone can be used in a repair. (Courtesy of Scott and White Hospital and Clinic)

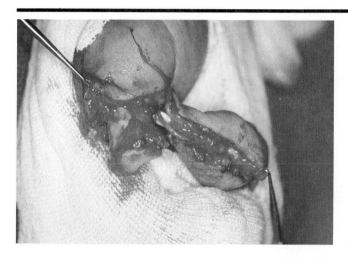

FIGURE 18-22 Near amputation of the thumb of the right hand. (Courtesy of Scott and White Hospital and Clinic)

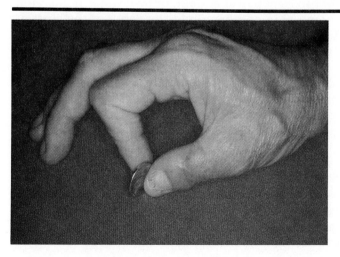

FIGURE 18-23 Using microsurgical techniques, plastic surgeons replanted the thumb, with good function preserved. (Courtesy of Scott and White Hospital and Clinic)

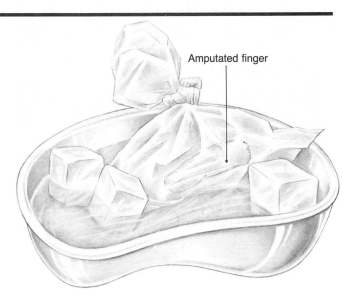

Amputated finger

FIGURE 18-24 Amputated parts should be put in a dry bag, sealed, and placed in cool water which contains a few ice cubes.

23.) If the situation dictates, the paramedic should not wait to find the part. The patient and the tissue when found or freed must be transported immediately. All body tissue should be transported. Even if the part cannot be totally reattached, the skin may be used to cover the limb end. (See Figure 18-24.)

Burns

Care of the burn patient can be divided into three categories: the soft-tissue burn, the inhalation burn, and the special burn.

Soft-Tissue Burns

Local And Minor Burns. Minor soft-tissue burns of partial thickness and involving only a small proportion of the body surface area can be treated with local cooling. Only burns of less than 10% of the body surface area should be cared for in this way, as larger surface area cooling might subject the patient to hypothermia. Cold, or cool water immersion, has some effect in reducing pain and may limit the depth of the burning process. If effective, it will be so immediately post-burn. It is also important to remove any article of clothing or jewelry which might possibly act to contain edema. As the injury site accumulates body fluid, it will increase in size. If any constriction is encountered, the swelling will induce an increase in tissue pressure. This may cause a tourniquet effect on the vasculature. The result may be loss of pulse and circulation distal to the burn.

Moderate To Severe Burns. Partial-thickness burns over 30% of the body or full-thickness burns over 5% should be treated with dry, sterile dressings. They will keep air movement past the sensitive first- and second-degree burn to a minimum. Sterile dressings will also provide padding against minor bumping. In the third-degree burn, they will provide a barrier to contamination. Intravenous routes should be established in any moderate to severely burned patient. Two large-bore catheters should be introduced and hung with 1000 mL bags of either normal saline or lactated Ringer's solution. Current fluid resuscitation formulas recommend 4 mL of fluid for every kilogram of patient weight multiplied by the percentage of body surface area burned. Half this fluid is needed in the first eight hours of care. This particular fluid resuscitation protocol is known as the Parkland formula and is most applicable to prehospital care. If the wound size is great, the paramedic may be asked to infuse two IV lines wide open. If all the normal IV access sites are burned, the catheter may be placed through the burned tissue. The paramedic must be careful with insertion. The skin may be leathery, yet the tissue underneath very delicate.

Special Burn Care

The patient who has come in contact with any chemical capable of tissue damage should be decontaminated early in the assessment/care process. Damage must be stopped with large volumes of cool water. Water will not only rinse away the offending material, it will dilute any water soluble agents. The cooling effect of the water will also reduce the heat and the rate of chemical reaction and, ultimately, its effects on the skin. The patient should be doused with large volumes of water. Use of a garden hose or low-pressure water from a fire truck is ideal. The water should be cool, not cold. Once the patient has been rinsed for a few minutes, the clothing can be removed. Care should be taken to ensure that the rescuers do not become contaminated and that all clothing, and all rinse water—if the agent is dangerous—is saved for proper disposal. The wound should be scrubbed. A mild soap and a gentle brush is best. Scrubbing should be rigorous enough to remove any remaining corrosive, though it should not cause further soft tissue damage. DO NOT USE ANY ANTIDOTE OR ANY NEUTRALIZING AGENT. Neutralizing agents may react violently with the chemical. They may ultimately increase the heat of the reaction and induce severe thermal burns. In some cases, the antidote or neutralizing agent is more damaging to the skin than the contaminant. After scrubbing has been completed, the wound should be gently irrigated with a constant flow of water. While the pain and the burning process may appear to subside, it is important to continue the irrigation until the patient arrives at the Emergency Department. If practicable, the corrosive container or a sample should be transported with the patient.

✱ Do not use any antidote or any neutralizing agent on chemical burns.

Some substances either do not dissolve in water or may react violently with it. These substances, most notably phenol, dry lime, and sodium should each be treated differently. Phenol is a gelatinous caustic used in industry as a powerful cleaner. It is very difficult to remove since it is sticky and insoluble in water. Alcohol, which will dissolve it, is frequently available where phenol is used. Alcohol should be used to remove the phenol. It should be followed by large volumes of water and the procedures just described.

A second agent is dry lime. It is a strong corrosive which will react with water, producing heat and both chemical and thermal injury. It should be brushed off gently but as completely as is possible. It should then be rinsed with large volumes of cool to cold water. While the water will react with the lime, it will also cool the area and remove any loose substance. In using water, the lime may react with it rather than with the fluid of the body's soft tissues.

Sodium is an unstable metal which reacts destructively with many substances, including human tissue. It will react vigorously with water, creating extreme heat, explosive hydrogen gas and possible ignition. It is normally stored under oil since it will react with the oxygen in air. If a patient has been contaminated with sodium, the wound should be decontaminated gently and quickly by gentle brushing and then covered with the oil used to store the substance.

Radiation Incidents

In radiation rescue, the source should be isolated, contained, and the scene tested for safety by professionals in the field. If this is impossible, the patient should be moved to a remote site where care can be given without danger to the rescuers. If this route is chosen, the persons providing patient removal should be the oldest ones available. The effects of radiation become evident many years after exposure. If older rescuers are used, it will be more likely that they will be past the reproductive years and have fewer years of life left if a problem does surface. The paramedic should be especially concerned for pregnant females and young adults of both sexes. Radiation damages the reproductive system very easily. The removal should be well planned, using as much shielding as possible and keeping exposure times to a minimum.

If the exposure is related to a contamination either by liquid or dust, the patient should be rinsed with copious amounts of water, carefully disrobed, scrubbed, and then rinsed again. All clothing and water used for decontamination must be saved for appropriate disposal. This activity should be performed before moving the patient to the ambulance. It should be accomplished by persons knowledgeable in the technique and well protected against contamination. Once decontaminated, the radiation patient is treated as any other patient. Because the human body alone cannot be a source of ionizing radiation, such a patient poses no threat to the paramedic. Any contaminated material on the patient, or any contamination transferred to the paramedic will provide a source of radiation exposure.

Patients who have been exposed to radiation should receive care for any other injuries sustained. It will be very rare that signs of patient exposure will be evident. Such patients may appear not to be in need of any care. Nevertheless, they must be seen by those with special knowledge of radiation sickness and injury.

SUMMARY

Soft-tissue injuries are not a frequent cause of patient mortality. They are, however, commonly found during assessment and do merit the paramedic's attention and care. In cases of severe hemorrhage or serious burn, the injury may be life threatening. The paramedic must understand the anatomy and physiology, the injury process, as well as the evaluation and management of soft-tissue injury.

The assessment of wounds is important to the overall care of the trauma patient, since the wounds may present the only overt signs that an internal injury has occurred. Their assessment must be careful and frequent as the signs of injury develop slowly over time. Wound care must address the three objectives of bandaging. The bleeding must be controlled with direct pressure, elevation, pressure point and, as a last resort, the tourniquet. The wound must be immobilized to assist the clotting mechanism. And, the wound must be kept as clean as practical (in the field) to reduce the danger of infection.

The burn must be assessed to determine the depth, the body surface area involved, and any respiratory, joint, hand, foot, or circumferential regions affected. Special consideration is given to the pediatric, geriatric, ill or injured patient who is also burned. Overall severity is determined from these factors and, if warranted, aggressive care is instituted. Aggressive burn care should include anticipation of airway compromise and fluid loss. The airway should be secured very early in care while IV access is initiated and fluids prepared to run. After stabilization has been accomplished, the wound should be covered and the patient transported.

Special burns such as chemical, radiation, or electrical burns, require special care and assessment. Chemical burns need rapid and effective decontamination. Radiation burns call for extreme care in removing the patient from the source and in providing decontamination and supportive aid. An electrical burn requires careful assessment to determine the area and depth of burn involvement, as well as wound site dressing, and cardiac monitoring.

While soft-tissue injuries often are not a high priority, they do represent a high incidence of patient injury and are significant to the overall assessment and care of the trauma victim.

FURTHER READING

American College of Surgeons, Committee on Trauma, *Advanced Trauma Life Support Course: Student Manual*. American College of Surgeons, 1989.

BUTMAN, A. M., and PATURAS, J. L., *Pre-Hospital Trauma Life Support*. Akron, OH: Emergency Training, 1990.

CAMPBELL, J. E., *Basic Trauma Life Support*, 2nd ed. Englewood Cliffs, NJ: Prentice-Hall, Inc., 1988.

GRANT, H. D., MURRAY, R. H., and BERGERON, J. D., *Emergency Care*, 5th ed. Englewood Cliffs, NJ: Prentice-Hall, Inc., 1990.

LODGE, D. W., and GRANT, H. D., *Handbook of Emergency Care Proceedures*. Englewood Cliffs, NJ: Prentice-Hall, Inc.,1989.

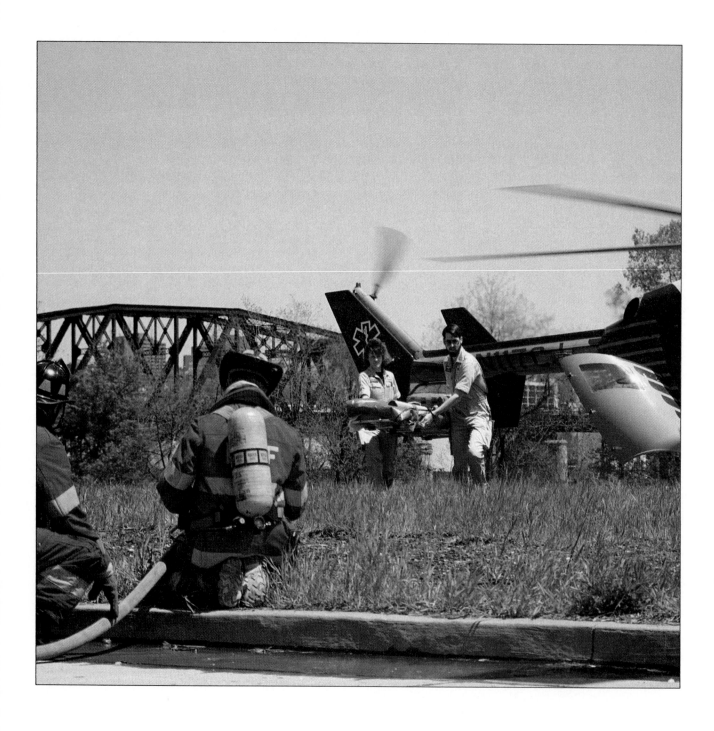

19

Shock Trauma Resuscitation

Objectives for Chapter 19

Upon completing this chapter, the student should be able to:

1. Identify the importance of rapid identification and treatment of shock in the trauma patient.

2. Define hypovolemic shock and explain how it affects the human body.

3. List the mechanisms which compensate for blood loss, and explain how each assists in compensation.

4. List the signs and symptoms of hypovolemic shock, and explain how they manifest themselves.

5. For each of the elements of the primary assessment, list the findings that relate to hypovolemic shock.

6. Compare and contrast compensated and decompensated shock.

7. Explain the effects of catheter length and diameter, and fluid pressure on the rate of intravenous infusion.

8. Identify the steps of care taken for a patient who is in hypovolemic shock.

9. Explain the physiologic action of the pneumatic antishock garment (PASG) in the hypovolemic patient.

10. List the signs and symptoms of circulatory overload in a patient receiving rapid crystalloid infusion.

CASE STUDY

An outlying basic life support unit has called for Metro-Rescue Unit 9, an advanced life support (ALS) unit, in order to help the victim of a farm accident who has been bleeding uncontrollably. Upon arrival, the ALS unit finds a young male patient with his leg trapped under an overturned tractor. The ground around the patient is soaked with blood, and the patient is pale with cool, moist skin. Assessment finds the patient conscious but anxious and somewhat combative. He is unsure of what happened, is breathing with shallow breaths (26 per minute), and has a weak carotid pulse of 120. Capillary refill is about 4 seconds and distal pulses are unobtainable. Primary assessment reveals no other injuries, except for those that might be found where his body is under the tractor. Extrication is expected in 3 minutes. The paramedic contacts medical control and obtains permission to start two large-bore IVs with pressure infusers at 300 mm Hg. Oxygen is applied via nonrebreather mask. Blood pressure is 80 by palpation, respirations are still 26 and shallow, oxygen saturation is 76%, and the patient's level of consciousness continues to diminish. The pneumatic antishock garment (PASG) is readied on a long spineboard.

Removal of the tractor reveals a crush wound to the patient's thigh with severe blood loss. Dressings are quickly applied and held with manual pressure while the patient is moved to the long board. The PASG is inflated, the patient is moved to the ambulance, and transport begins.

The patient's respirations and level of consciousness improve. The ambulance arrives at the Emergency Department. The 1,000 mL bags of fluid have been infused and a third bag has just been hung. The patient has blood drawn for typing and crossmatch and receives O negative blood immediately. X-ray determines that no fracture occurred, and the patient is taken to surgery for repair of a torn femoral artery. Three days later, the ambulance service receives a phone call from the patient's parents thanking the crew. Their son is doing fine and will be coming home this weekend.

INTRODUCTION

Trauma is the number three killer of persons in the United States today. However, it is the most common cause of death for persons under 44 years of age. Thus, trauma is the greatest killer of persons in their prime and a common reason for summoning emergency medical services. Trauma was the impetus which began the call for prehospital emergency medical care in the mid-1960s. Since then, it has taken a back seat in prehospital education to the cardiac and medical emergency response. The development of the Advanced Trauma Life Support (ATLS) course for physicians and Basic Trauma Life Support (BTLS) and the Prehospital Trauma Life Support (PHTLS) courses for paramedics have re-focused prehospital training on trauma management. Today, aggressive trauma care is the object of much study and is a strong emphasis in training.

The responsibility of the paramedic in the traumatic incident is great. Unlike the heart attack and other medical emergencies, trauma may affect several different body organs and structures. To understand the effects of this multisystem damage, one must understand the body's response to injury.

When responding to a patient who may be experiencing shock, the paramedic must evaluate the accident in an organized and deliberate pattern. He or she must begin a constant and consistent search for information about the nature and severity of the incident. Then the information must be sorted to determine what is wrong with the patient, or what may go wrong in the near future. The paramedic must render care either by meticulous attention at the scene or by expeditious transport to a definitive care facility. The responsibility is great, yet care often must be executed in the least ideal of conditions.

The paramedic follows an ordered progression in the response to trauma. This process includes:

1. Review of the dispatch information
2. Survey of the scene
3. Primary assessment
    Shock/trauma resuscitation
4. Secondary assessment
    Head-to-toe exam
    Vital signs
    Patient history
5. Management
6. Transportation

In the case of trauma, the paramedic should complete the first four steps in order. The elements of the secondary assessment—the head-to-toe exam, vital signs, and patient history—may occur simultaneously or in any sequence.

Once the existence, or even threat, of shock is recognized, the paramedic must aggressively treat the patient for it. The use of rapid transport coupled with invasive and noninvasive procedures can help combat hypovolemia and support the body's own compensatory mechanisms. Modalities of care include the PASG, advanced airway techniques, oxygen-supplemented positive pressure ventilation, and rapid intravenous infusion. These procedures, followed by the sophisticated approach of the Trauma Center, will help to improve the prognosis for the patient in shock.

In order to anticipate, recognize, and treat shock, the paramedic must understand its causes and manifestations. An appreciation of the body's compensatory mechanisms for blood loss provides this understanding. The dynamic response to hypovolemia is an important concept essential to providing care to the trauma patient.

ANATOMY AND PHYSIOLOGY OF THE CARDIOVASCULAR SYSTEM

The cardiovascular system plays the major role in compensation for blood loss. It consists of the blood, the vessels, and the heart. The blood, the substance most commonly lost in trauma, circulates through the body. It supplies the body cells with nutrients (including oxygen) and removes waste products (including carbon dioxide). The vessels (which lose fluid in trauma) make up the container and direct the flow of the blood to and from the vital organs. The heart is the pump that moves the fluid through the vessels. The heart, the vessels, and the blood work together to ensure that body cells receive their supply of nutrients.

Blood consists of two major components: the red blood cells (erythrocytes), and the fluid (plasma). The erythrocytes contain hemoglobin, an iron compound that carries oxygen from the lungs to the body cells. The **plasma** is the fluid that suspends the erythrocytes and carries them and the other blood components to the far reaches of the body. These two elements make up an essential fluid which accounts for 7 percent of the body weight, about 5 to 6 L in the normal adult.

Blood fills the vessels—the arteries, arterioles, capillaries, venules, and veins—to form a dynamic elastic container. Muscle fibers surround these vessels in order to change the lumen and, in concert, the size of the of the container. The vessels either constrict or dilate with the loss or retention of fluid. They also have the ability to increase or decrease the pressure of the walls inward against the fluid. This pressure is the blood pressure and is dependent upon cardiac output and blood vessel muscle tone.

Blood vessels further have the ability to open and close with a valve-like action. They determine where the blood, powered by the arterial pressure, will flow. This permits the body to direct blood through the organs that need it at a particular time and away from those that don't. The arterioles offer this control by changing their internal lumen by as much as a factor of five. The ability of the arterioles to constrict and reduce flow helps in the shock response. Through this action, the cardiovascular system can either draw fluid from, or pass fluid to, the interstitial spaces and body cells. If the arterioles constrict while the venules dilate, fluid leaves the tissues. If the arterioles dilate and the venules constrict, fluid redistributes into the interstitial spaces and cells. This control allows the body to regulate fluid placement and to use the body cells and spaces as a fluid reservoir.

The action of the arterioles can also affect and control blood pressure. If all the arterioles dilate, the resistance to blood flow on the arterial side would drop drastically. So would the blood pressure. If they all constrict, the blood pressure rises. The central nervous system can cause the arterioles leading to one organ to dilate and those before another organ to constrict. The body uses this system to maintain a rather stable pressure while controlling where blood flows.

The final component of the system is the heart. It is a two-sided, double-action pump that generates the major force and pressure of the system. It ejects its contents into the arterial side of the circulatory system. This outflow, in combination with the vessel valve function, creates the arterial pressure and directs blood flow to the desired body tissues.

The heart's pumping efficiency depends on several factors. The heart must receive blood from the venous system (**preload**) and have a moderate resistance to pump against (**afterload**). If the ventricle is forcefully filled through good venous return and atrial contraction, its walls stretch. This action increases the volume and pressure of the ejected blood.

The vascular system retains plasma through a complicated system of biochemical equilibrium. The protein and electrolyte concentrations are different in each of the vascular, interstitial, and intracellular spaces. However, the osmotic pressures they exert are equal. The system achieves a balance, and this balance continues even when intake and output of fluid are unequal.

Fluid loss from this container may be caused by various mechanisms. These include burns, diarrhea, reduced fluid intake, granulating

■ **plasma** the fluid portion of the blood consisting of serum and protein substances in solution.

■ **preload** the volume of blood delivered to the atria prior to ventricular diastole.

■ **afterload** the pressure or resistance against which the heart must pump.

wounds, sweating due to fever or environmental extremes, or hemorrhage. This chapter directs concern to the loss of blood through hemorrhage, be it external or internal.

PATHOPHYSIOLOGY

Shock is really the transition between normal body function and balance (called homeostasis) and death. Up to a point, the body's response to any insult is efficient and well designed. This portion of the response is termed **compensated shock.** After the body can no longer compensate and the compensatory mechanisms fail, the circulation then fails and the patient moves quickly to death. **Decompensated shock** is this final stage of the shock process. The objective of the paramedic is to recognize compensated shock early, treat it aggressively, and prevent it from becoming decompensated shock. (See Chapter 12.)

■ **compensated shock** a hemodynamic insult to the body in which the body responds effectively. Signs and symptoms are limited, and the human system functions normally.

■ **decompensated shock** a continuing hemodynamic insult to the body in which the compensatory mechanisms break down. The signs and symptoms become very pronounced, and the patient moves rapidly toward death.

Compensated Shock

The human system is able to adjust to varying levels of fluid intake and loss. A healthy young individual can drink a few liters of fluid at one sitting without experiencing the effects of fluid overload. He or she can lose large volumes of fluid due to sweating while working on a hot day, again without experiencing adverse effects. In either case, the body uses mechanisms that respond to fluid fluctuations and allow unimpeded body function. The body responds in a similar way to the loss of blood when the loss is minor and relatively uncomplicated.

As blood flows from a wound, the initial fluid adjustment mechanisms kick in. The veins are the first to respond. They contain about 60 percent of the circulating blood volume and have the ability to reduce their capacity drastically. By contraction of the muscles within their walls, the veins rapidly compensate for a blood loss of about 1 to 2 units (0.5 to 1 L). This mechanism allows for the donation of blood or a minor hemorrhage without major systemic consequences. If the blood loss is slowed, or stops, the body will draw fluid from the interstitial areas and body cells to replenish the volume. The arterioles will constrict and the venules will dilate. Interstitial and cell fluid is drawn into the circulation and assists in filling the vascular container. Since the body is over 60 percent water, there is a tremendous reservoir to draw from (about 40 L). While this mechanism is not as rapid as the venous constriction, it is reasonably quick and may return several liters to the active circulation.

In the short term, the body replaces lost fluid, but not red blood cells. Over time the system will regain erythrocytes from the areas where it manufactures or stores them. This process is slow and takes much longer than the body's system of plasma replacement. Erythrocyte loss reduces the oxygen-carrying capacity of the blood and its ability to supply oxygen to the cells. The greater and more rapid the blood loss, the more severe a problem this becomes.

If hemorrhage continues, the veins will constrict so much that their response is no longer adequate. The blood return to the heart begins to slow, and the heart does not pump with its normal force. The blood pressure drops as does the body's ability to direct the flow of blood. The central nervous system recognizes the problem and promptly orders the arterioles to constrict. This action decreases the blood flowing through the tissues and distributes the remaining blood to the vital organs. The circulation directs blood away from the skin and digestive tract and toward the heart, brain, and skeletal muscles.

The process of compensated shock presents a spectrum of signs and symptoms that may vary from occult to spectacular. They depend upon the health of the patient, the rate of blood loss, and the individual system's response. For the most part, the signs and symptoms of compensated shock will be subtle and difficult to identify. The observer must anticipate and search them out.

As the body begins to respond to blood loss, the preload and cardiac output begin to drop. The central nervous system increases the heart rate by reflex to increase cardiac output. Since preload remains low, the strength of the pulse becomes weak. In fact, the pulse may be diminished or absent in the distal extremities. The central nervous system calls for the arterioles to constrict, especially to nonvital organs like the skin. This vasoconstriction reduces the surface blood flow and the skin cools. It also becomes pale due to the reduced presence of erythrocytes, or ashen or cyanotic as they lose their oxygen. Capillary refill times are obviously slow, and the stagnation of blood causes the skin to seep fluid, becoming clammy.

As the pathology of shock becomes more severe, even the circulation to critical organs becomes reduced. Shock frequently affects the brain. The patient may show unusual anxiety or restlessness, the central nervous system's response to reduced oxygenated circulation. The patient may also display subtle and progressive lowering of the level of consciousness. This may be noted by observing the level of orientation to time, place (or event), person, and one's own person.

The effects of shock are also seen in the respiratory system. The muscles of respiration work less efficiently in a hypoxic state. They move less air while the central nervous system increases the rate of breathing. The result is a more rapid, less effective respiratory pattern: the rapid shallow respirations normally associated with shock states.

Another area where the early signs of developing shock may be present is in the eyes. The eyes are the windows into the brain. They accurately reflect the status of the critical brain circulation and, in shock, give the first hint that problems exist. The sparkle of the eye and the rate of pupillary response to light are dependent on good circulation. If the eyes are dull or pupillary response is diminished, it reflects a reduction in circulation quality or effectiveness.

As the body survives under the stress of compensation, several negative conditions develop. The low-flow condition and poor oxygen-carrying capacity of the blood leave much of the body in a hypoxic state. The body cells, deprived of energy, use inefficient, anaerobic biochemical processes to survive. In doing so, they produce lactic acid and accumulate other waste products. These contaminants build up in the noncritical body organs and compound the existing hypoxia. As the body's compensatory mechanisms reach their maximum response and hemorrhage continues, decompensation is imminent.

Decompensated Shock

If the blood loss continues, the system of compensation will eventually break down. The venous system, as with most systems during shock, is not well oxygenated. It loses its ability to constrict and subsequently relaxes. The container, which contracted in size to accommodate a reduced blood volume, now expands. The arterioles experience the same problem.

As the arterioles relax, the body loses its ability to maintain blood pressure and direct the flow of cardiac output.

The venous return to the heart all but ceases, the cardiac output drops, and the peripheral resistance and blood pressure fall precipitously. Circulation continues to slow as the patient becomes profoundly unconscious and the vital signs disappear. At this point the patient is moving irreversibly toward death. Immediate return of all the lost blood would not fill the vascular space. The muscles of the vessel walls are exhausted and relax. The lumen dilates, enlarging the container beyond its preshock state. Even if the vascular system could be filled, the hypoxic heart would have trouble maintaining a normal stroke volume, strength of contraction, blood pressure, and, ultimately, circulation. The arterioles lose their ability to constrict, support blood pressure, and direct circulation. The pulmonary muscles exhaust from working in an acidic and hypoxic environment. Finally, the entire human system is subject to poor circulation, oxygenation, and the build up of waste products. It becomes impossible to reverse the effects of shock once decompensation takes hold.

ASSESSMENT

Assessment of the trauma patient must look for the early indications of shock rather than wait for the classical signs and symptoms. (See Figure 19-1.) The body is able to adjust well to fluid loss with few signs or symptoms apparent. Should the assessment not discover these early signs of shock, the patient will deteriorate to the more obvious signs of serious circulatory insufficiency. The result of the missed assessment is the lost ability to intervene early in the shock process. The patient's condition and potential for survival will suffer. A careful assessment will reveal the early and subtle signs and symptoms well before the patient is close to decompensation. Deliberate anticipation and examination is the only way

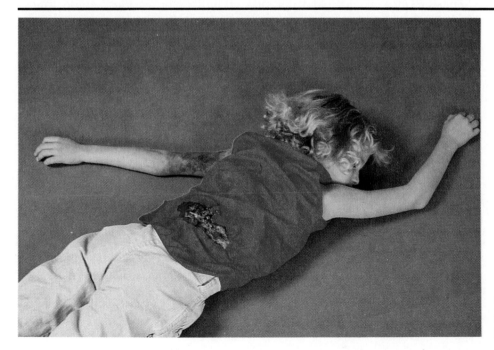

FIGURE 19-1 The victim of serious injury requires prompt and careful evaluation by the paramedic.

to ensure that you find the early signs and symptoms of shock. The patient is serially checked for any signs of shock compensation from the paramedics' arrival at the scene until delivery to the Emergency Department.

Review of Dispatch Information

The assessment process begins with evaluation of the dispatch information while the EMS unit is responding to the scene. The information allows the paramedic to plan the assessment and major steps of management before arrival. The general nature of the call location, reported number of injured persons, and other information will determine how the paramedic approaches the scene and patient. It also identifies what equipment is needed.

Survey of the Scene

Upon arrival, the paramedic quickly surveys the scene to exclude hazards and identify the mechanism of injury and the number of patients. The survey identifies the resources already at the scene and what will be needed. The paramedic must have a plan of approach to the incident and to the assessment and management of the patient before he or she leaves the ambulance.

The mechanism of injury may be the most revealing aspect of trauma patient assessment. It tells what injuries might have happened during the incident while patient signs and symptoms may not yet provide a clue. If the force, direction, and location of impact reflect substantial internal injury, treat the patient for such injury. Treatment occurs even if the vital signs and assessment do not support the suspicion. Head, chest, and abdominal injuries are notorious for silently causing shock and death.

Primary Assessment

C-Spine. Once at the patient's side, stabilize the cervical spine unless blunt trauma is ruled out. The kinetic forces that fracture any long bone, rib, or the skull demonstrate that the patient received enough trauma to fracture the vertebral column. Any large contusion or soft tissue injury, likewise, reflects spinal injury. The danger to the patient from proper spinal immobilization is negligible. The danger of an unstabilized spinal injury is life-threatening.

Airway. The airway needs rapid assessment to ensure it remains patent. (See Figure 19-2.) Quickly examine for any fluids (vomitus, blood, etc.) or any signs of trauma. Should the patient be unconscious, protect the airway with positioning, nasopharyngeal airway placement, or an endotracheal tube as necessary. If a management technique is chosen, the assessment continues while the paramedics are readying the equipment and preparing the patient.

Breathing. Evaluate breathing to determine the gross rate, depth, and minute volume. If you find significant trauma, the patient receives supplemental high-flow oxygen. If respiratory volume is not within normal limits, assist the patient's respirations. Ready any equipment and apply procedures while the assessment continues.

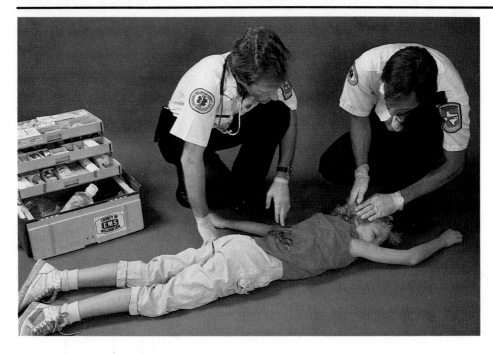

FIGURE 19-2 The first step in assessment of the shock trauma patient is completion of the primary survey.

Circulation. Check circulation by evaluating the pulse and peripheral perfusion. Palpate both the carotid and radial pulses. Evaluation will determine only if the pulse is slow, normal, or fast, not the exact rate. Assess pulse strength as either weak, normal, or strong. Compare the strength of the carotid and radial pulses to determine if the distal pulse is weaker. Finally, evaluate the blanching of the peripheral skin to determine capillary refill time. Should any sign point to developing hypovolemia, target the patient for PASG application. The patient should receive two large bore IVs, hung with two 1,000 mL bags of crystalloid solution and trauma tubing as the primary assessment is completed. Pressure infusers should be ready. (See Figure 19-3.) Prepare to provide rapid transport.

Disability. Evaluation of level of consciousness determines only the general cerebral function. The acronym AVPU represents the following levels:

A = conscious and alert
V = responsive to verbal stimuli
P = responsive to painful stimuli
U = completely unresponsive

Expose. As the primary assessment comes to a close, expose the patient for visual evaluation of the head, neck, chest, and abdomen. (See Figure 19-4.) The paramedic should observe for:

❑ *wounds:* contusions, abrasions, lacerations
❑ *deformities:* hematomas, subcutaneous emphysema, abnormal angulation or positioning
❑ *abnormal motion:* paradoxical respiration, use of accessory breathing muscles, sternal retraction, or abdominal pulsation

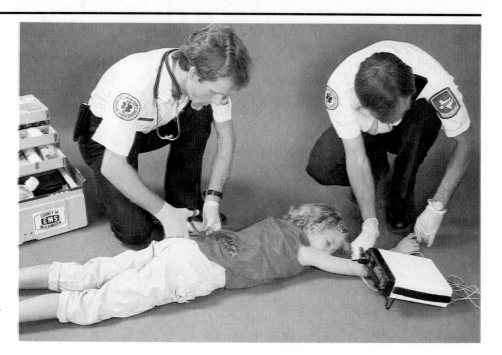

FIGURE 19-3 The paramedic should use every tool and skill available to assist the shock trauma patient.

✱ At the completion of the primary survey the decision to provide rapid transportation with care enroute or on-scene care should be made.

Scan the body for any signs of external hemorrhage. Sweep hidden areas with the hands for any unseen blood loss. Control any moderate to severe hemorrhage as it is found. (See Figure 19-4.)

At the completion of the primary survey, paramedics will have all the information they need to determine whether the patient is a candidate for immediate transport or for on-scene treatment. While the emphasis

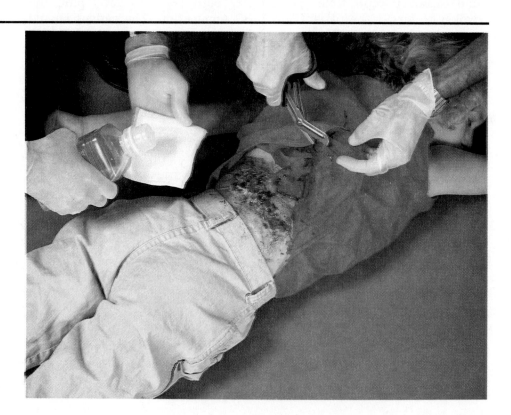

FIGURE 19-4 Exposure and treatment should be rapidly completed.

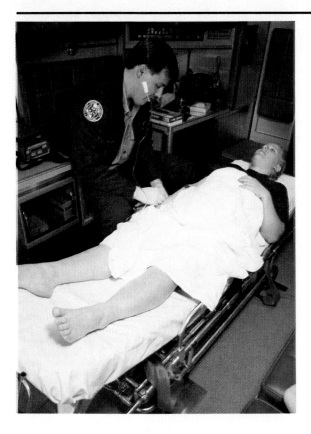

FIGURE 19-5 If shock is present the patient should be transported immediately with stabilization attempted enroute.

in this chapter is on rapid transport with care en route, the paramedic can best serve the vast majority of patients by providing care at the scene. Patients need the reduced risk of injury aggravation that results when on-scene care providers splint, bandage, and package the patient. If the patient is not a candidate for rapid transport, the assessment continues. This will include the head-to-toe exam, determination of vital signs, and a complete patient history, not necessarily in that order.

Certain injuries and patient conditions by themselves merit rapid transport and aggressive care. (See Figure 19-5.) They include:

❑ Cardiopulmonary arrest
❑ Uncorrectable airway problems
❑ Any embarrassment of the respiratory bellows system
❑ Any wounds that deform or penetrate the chest, head, or abdomen
❑ Significant external, or suspected internal, blood loss
❑ Signs and symptoms of compensatory shock
❑ Multiple fractures, especially pelvic ring or bilateral femur fractures
❑ Lowered or changing level of consciousness
❑ Mechanism of injury suggestive of severe trauma

Institute aggressive care and rapid transport to the trauma center if the patient is unstable or potentially unstable. Only when transport is underway and the skills of shock care have been applied does the complete evaluation of the patient begin. In the severely unstable patient, the paramedic may never have time to assess the patient completely. Repeat the primary assessment any time the patient receives significant intervention, a few minutes have passed, or a change is noted in the patient's pres-

✳ Repeat the primary assessment after any significant intervention, several minutes have passed or a patient condition change is noted.

entation. Serial assessment of the elements of the primary assessment will identify any sign or symptom of developing shock as well as alert the paramedic to any gradual deterioration of the patient.

Trauma Score

The trauma score (see Figure 10-18) is a numeric value placed upon the patient and determined through assessment. It consists of five components, including the results of the Glasgow Coma Scale. (See Chapter 15.) They are:

Respiratory Rate (per minute):

10–29	4
above 29	3
6–9	2
1–5	1
none	0

Respiratory Expansion:

Normal:	1
Retraction:	0

Blood Pressure (systolic):

above 89	4
76–89	3
50–75	2
0–49	1
no pulse	0

Capillary Return:

Normal:	2
Delayed:	1
None:	0

Coma Scale:

13–15	5
9–12	4
6–8	3
4–5	2
below 4	0

The range for patient evaluation is from 0 to 16 points. Research has found that patients with scores from 12 or above do relatively well while scores below 10 indicate a poor prognosis. Aggressive intervention has the greatest effect in patients who score between 4 and 12. The trauma score is used to communicate the patient's condition at the scene and during transport. It is an objective number that the receiving physician can use to determine the seriousness of the patient's condition and plan for care on arrival. Medical command may use it for quality control and research purposes. The advanced life support system may also use the trauma score to indicate the need for advanced life support within protocols.

SHOCK/TRAUMA RESUSCITATION

Suspect shock in any patient displaying the signs and symptoms of shock, who has a mechanism of injury that could produce it, or a series of injuries that may induce it. Once suspected, plan and execute shock management well. Time is of the essence. The human body can compensate only for so long and only for so much blood loss. The paramedic can use an electrolyte solution to compensate for blood loss only on a temporary basis. The patient needs definitive care as soon as possible. The effectiveness of prehospital care and eventual patient survival may depend more on the time between accident and arrival at the emergency department than on the skills and ability of the paramedic.

The paramedic should be at the critical patient's side at the accident scene for no more than 10 minutes. Spend those 10 minutes well. Assessment and care occur simultaneously. The paramedic team should work efficiently and quickly, applying what skills they can and preparing for rapid transport. Whenever possible, provide advanced level skills while en route to the hospital.

The airway is of first concern. If endangered by fluid, swelling, or collapse, secure it with the endotracheal tube. If the patient is unable to protect the airway, intubate. In potential cervical spine injury, immobilize the head firmly in the neutral position and attempt nasotracheal intubation (ideally with a directable tipped tube). If the technique seems ineffective or time consuming, attempt direct laryngoscope or digital placement. If endotracheal tube placement is not allowed by medical control or if other conditions prevent it, use the esophageal obturator or esophageal gastric tube airway. (See Chapter 11.)

After properly securing the tube, tape it firmly in place. Endotracheal tubes often become displaced in the patient during extrication and movement. The use of end-expiratory CO_2 detectors will verify that the tube is in the trachea and that respiratory exchange is removing CO_2.

When the airway is secure, ventilate the patient if the respirations are either too fast or too slow or do not move an adequate volume of air. Apply the bag-valve-mask to the endotracheal tube or tight sealing mask. Ventilations should be full and at a rate of about 20 to 25 times per minute. Provide the patient with supplemental oxygen at 15 L per minute via the reservoir attached to the bag-valve-mask. Remember that the hypovolemic patient may have erythrocytes and hemoglobin in short supply. The use of high flow oxygen and the positive pressure makes sure the patient is as well oxygenated as possible.

If pulse oximetry is available, gauge ventilation to keep the SaO_2 as high as possible. Any SaO_2 less than 90 percent is cause for concern and immediate attention. In low hemoglobin states, such as shock, pulse oximetry will give a false high reading. While the hemoglobin saturation is 98%, the red cell count (hematocrit) is very low, as is the available hemoglobin. This is due to the dilution of the whole blood with plasma and any prehospital crystalloid.

Stop any hemorrhage that is moderate to severe. Accomplish this immediately with digital pressure directly on the site of loss. Maintain pressure until control is assumed by dressing and bandage. Quickly check the hidden body areas and stop any blood loss found. If direct pressure is ineffective, try direct pressure and elevation or direct pressure, elevation, and pressure points. Only as a last resort, use the tourniquet. An effective and available bandage-dressing combination is a roll of roller dressing and a sphygmomanometer. Place the roller dressing at the site of hemorrhage, apply the cuff and inflate slowly until the bleeding ceases. Use this technique only as a rapid emergency approach under dire circumstances. If time permits, replace hemorrhage control with a more standard dressing and bandage.

In amputations, the hemorrhage is often easy to control. The severed vessels retract into the limb stump, thicken, and occlude the bleeding. This should occur during the first 10 minutes after an accident. On the other hand, crushing injuries may bleed severely from multiple locations and bleeding can be almost impossible to stop. Such injuries often require the use of the tourniquet.

Consider the pneumatic antishock garment to control blood loss and as a device that helps the body compensate for shock. Currently, its method of action and degree of benefit are being questioned; however, it is well established as being able to control lower extremity hemorrhage and to increase peripheral vascular resistance. The increase in vascular resistance will help maintain the blood pressure in shock states.

The PASG only **autotransfuses** around 250 mL of blood. While this is well below what was earlier thought, it is a significant contribution to the hypovolemic patient. The process that autotransfuses the blood also reduces the vascular container size, thus doubling the effect.

The only current contraindications to the application of the trousers are pulmonary edema and penetrating chest trauma. Pulmonary edema is rare in hypovolemic shock, but a paramedic should anticipate it in the patient with severe chest injury or underlying heart disease. Assess the chest and auscultate for breath sounds while applying and inflating the PASG. Check the chest frequently thereafter. If any rales or rhonchi appear, stop the inflation. The use of PASG in gunshot wounds, stab wounds, or other penetrating trauma has been shown to be of little value and may increase patient mortality.

Relative contraindications to the use of PASG include late pregnancy and impaled objects protruding from the area to be covered by the trousers. In such cases, apply the device and inflate the legs only. Head injury is also a relative contraindication because the garment may increase intracranial pressure. This contraindication only applies when the patient's systolic blood pressure is above 100 mm/Hg which is not normally associated with hypovolemic shock.

Apply the trousers and inflate them initially to at least 40 mm/Hg of pressure. Autotransfusion occurs at this level while increased peripheral resistance will progress from this point to the release valve pressures of around 105 to 110 mm Hg. Guide the inflation of the trousers by the patient's response: skin color, level of consciousness, pulse rate, and general appearance. Evaluate the blood pressure periodically, keeping in mind that it is only a relative measure of the circulatory status and somewhat time-consuming to monitor. Guide the application of the PASG using the patient's level of responsiveness, pulse rate and strength, and blood pressure together.

Do not release the PASG in the field for any reason. Deflation will reduce the circulating blood volume and the peripheral resistance rapidly. Such an insult to an already hypovolemic patient may have catastrophic results. Several associated deaths have resulted from deflation.

Fluid therapy begins very early in the care of the shock patient. In some circumstances the paramedic may wait until the patient is en route to the hospital to keep on-scene time under the 10-minute guideline. The initiation of an IV is an emergency procedure, not an elective one in the trauma patient. Execute it in a very short time (well under 1 minute).

■ **autotransfusion** a process that causes the displacement of the patient's blood from one region to another.

Often, an IV will be easier to initiate after PASG application because of increased venous pressure. The paramedic must be proficient at this skill through frequent practice.

The use of a pre-packaged trauma IV kit will help speed the procedure. The kit should contain packaged large bore catheters, tape, solution, trauma tubing, prep pads, bacteriostatic ointment, 1,000 mL bag of crystalloid solution, and a commercial pressure infuser. This packaging will ensure that set-up is easy, rapid, and complete.

The location of venipuncture is very important. In elective IV insertion select a vein that is as distal as possible. In the trauma patient it is important to select a vein large enough to pass a large bore catheter and peripheral enough so as not to require a long catheter. The most ideal locations are the antecubital fossa and the external jugular veins. Both locations provide good access to large veins which are rather close to the skin surface.

Central lines are not recommended because they are placed in deep veins, require longer catheters, are often in the way of other aggressive resuscitation techniques, and take much more time to complete. It is also much easier to obtain two or even three peripheral lines than to place one central line.

Catheter size is very important to the rate of administration of a fluid. The flow of a fluid is a factor of the radius of the lumen to a power of four (Poiseuille's law). By doubling the internal diameter of the catheter, the fluid will flow sixteen times faster. It is essential to pass the largest catheter into the vein as is reasonably possible.

Another factor that affects the flow of fluid into the trauma patient is catheter length. The longer the catheter the more resistance to flow. For this reason, a larger central line catheter (which must be reasonably long) may not infuse fluid as quickly as a short peripheral one.

The advantage of the peripheral line is increased with the placement of a large bore catheter. One such procedure is the **Seldinger technique,** which involves normal peripheral venipuncture using a moderately sized over-the-needle catheter. Thread the catheter and withdraw the needle. Introduce a guide wire through the catheter and hold it in place while withdrawing the catheter. With a scalpel nick the skin and enter the vein by threading the dilator over the wire. Remove the dilator and wire to leave a No. 8 or 9 French catheter in place. The technique is simple, quite effective, and allows the passage of a large catheter into a relatively small peripheral vein.

■ **Seldinger technique** a technique for guiding a larger catheter into a vein previously entered with a small catheter, using a wire dilator.

The same fluid administration principle holds true for administration sets. The smaller the diameter and the longer the set, the slower the flow of fluids. Administration sets for trauma use should be short in length and large in diameter. Trauma IV tubing is now available and suggested for advanced life support units. Blood tubing may also be used and can be used by emergency department staff to administer blood.

The last consideration regarding flow is the pressure used. One can easily demonstrate the effect of pressure on fluid flow through an IV administration set by simply raising the fluid bag. The drip rate and flow out of the needle will increase. In the trauma patient who needs large volumes of solution quickly, gravity may not create enough pressure. The use of a thigh blood pressure cuff or a commercially available pressure infusion device is necessary. Pressures of 200 to 300 mm Hg will double the rate of fluid delivery.

While there are obvious benefits to the rapid infusion of fluids in the prehospital setting, there are also some concerns. Rapid infusion in a patient who does not need it or in one who has underlying heart problems may precipitate pulmonary edema and congestive heart failure. Monitor the breath sounds, respiratory effort, and blood pressure carefully whenever fluids are rapidly infused. Slow or stop the IVs at the first sign of circulatory overload.

The standard of care for the patient who has lost or is losing a large volume of blood is two large-bore IV sites. Connect them to trauma tubing running from 1,000 mL bags of normal saline or lactated Ringer's solution. Apply pressure infusion devices and inflate to 200 to 300 mm Hg of pressure. Provide frequent serial vital signs and patient assessments. Place a special focus on breath sounds, pulse rate and quality, and the patient's level of consciousness.

There are limits to the effectiveness of crystalloid infusions. Not only does it take 3 L of crystalloid to expand the vascular volume by 1 L, the infusing fluid is not a complete replacement for blood. It does not contain hemoglobin needed to carry the oxygen to the body cells. The administration of crystalloid dilutes the remaining blood and compounds the problem already present as interstitial fluid is drawn into the vascular space. For these reasons, limit field infusion of crystalloid solutions to 3 L except in special circumstances such as prolonged extrications. Upon arrival at the emergency department the patient should receive typed and cross matched or O negative blood.

Certain circumstances, such as entrapment, may cause the paramedic to be at the scene for more than 10 minutes. In this situation, the paramedic must establish communication between the trauma scene and the hospital. While starting the IVs, consider drawing a tube of blood for typing and crossmatch. Send it to the hospital with a supervisor or the police, thus allowing the emergency department to obtain typed and crossmatched blood. Under dire circumstances, suggest bringing the blood and the emergency physician back to the scene.

The paramedic should administer oxygen, ventilate, start the needed IVs, and infuse crystalloids while the extrication continues. Prepare care equipment and movement devices for the patient's release. Communicate the patient's condition, injuries and the expected time before extrication to the Emergency Department.

SUMMARY

The critical trauma patient needs rapid assessment and aggressive care to obtain the best chance for survival. Use the dispatch information and the scene survey to plan the process of assessment and care. Provide a rapid and complete primary assessment and correct any problems as they are found. Determine the need for rapid transport or on-scene care. If the patient is displaying the signs and symptoms of shock, treat aggressively with PASG application and inflation, rapid infusion of fluids, and immediate transport to the trauma center.

In responding to the trauma emergency keep to the priorities of emergency care. They are:

A = Airway and cervical spine
B = Breathing
C = Circulation
D = CNS disability
E = Expose and correct any severe hemorrhage or any life threat detected by the primary survey

Keeping to these priorities will give the trauma patient the best chance to survive the syndrome called shock.

FURTHER READING

AMERICAN COLLEGE OF SURGEONS, Committee on Trauma. *Advanced Trauma Life Support Course: Student Manual.* American College of Surgeons, 1989.

BUTMAN, ALEXANDER M. AND PATURAS, JAMES L. *Pre-Hospital Trauma Life Support.* Akron, OH: Emergency Training, 1990.

CAMPBELL, JOHN E. *Basic Trauma Life Support.* 2nd ed. Englewood Cliffs, NJ: Prentice-Hall, Inc., 1988.

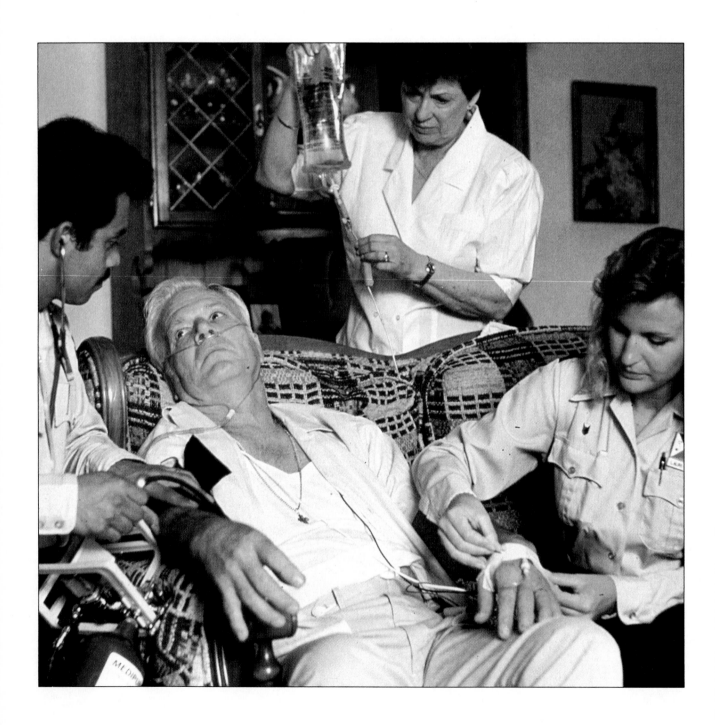

20

Respiratory Emergencies

Objectives for Chapter 20

Upon completing this chapter, the student should be able to:

1. Identify and describe the function of the structures of the upper airway.

2. Identify and describe the function of the structures of the lower airway.

3. Define the terms respiration and pulmonary ventilation.

4. Describe the physiology of the respiratory cycle.

5. Describe the pulmonary circulation.

6. Describe the process of gas exchange in the lungs.

7. Identify the normal partial pressures of oxygen and carbon dioxide in the alveolar, venous, and arterial blood.

8. Identify the systems involved in the process of regulation of respiration.

9. Describe the difference between the normal respiratory drive and the respiratory drive of the patient with chronic obstructive pulmonary disease.

10. Define and describe the modified forms of respiration including cough, sneeze, hiccough, sigh, and grunting.

11. List the normal respiratory rates for adults, children, and infants.

12. Identify the factors that affect respiratory rates.

13. Define the following terms:
   - dead space
   - tidal volume
   - minute volume
   - vital capacity

14. Identify the factors that alter carbon dioxide levels in the blood.

15. Identify factors that affect oxygen levels in the blood.

16. Identify the historical factors to be elicited when evaluating the respiratory system.

17. Identify specific observations and physical findings to be evaluated in the patient with a respiratory complaint.

18. Describe the techniques of inspection, auscultation, and palpation of the chest.

19. Define the following terms:
   - snoring
   - stridor
   - wheezing
   - rhonchi
   - rales
   - friction rub

20. Identify the basic principles of airway management.

21. Identify the causes of upper airway obstruction, and the pathophysiology, assessment, and management of each.

22. Review the pharmacology, action, dosage, side effects, contraindications, and routes of administration of the following drugs:
   - oxygen
   - epinephrine
   - terbutaline
   - racemic epinephrine
   - aminophylline
   - diphenhydramine
   - albuterol

23. Discuss the pathophysiology, assessment, and management of the following:
   - emphysema
   - chronic bronchitis
   - asthma
   - pneumonia
   - toxic inhalation
   - pulmonary embolism
   - hyperventilation syndrome
   - central nervous system dysfunctions

Ellis County EMS is dispatched on a "medical emergency" in a rural part of the county. The response time is approximately 12 minutes. Upon arrival at the rural farm house the paramedics are met by an EMT-Basic from the local volunteer fire department who reports they have a 55-year-old white male with difficulty breathing. The First Responder reports that oxygen is already being administered. The paramedics grab the drug box, monitor/defibrillator, airway kit, and stretcher and enter the small frame house.

Seated at the kitchen table is a 55-year-old male obviously short of breath. The paramedics quickly perform a primary assessment. The airway is clear, the patient is moving air, and has a strong pulse. The nasal cannula placed by the First Responders is replaced by a venti-mask which delivers an FiO_2 of 35%. The paramedics complete the secondary assessment. The patient has diminished breath sounds, occasional rhonchi, and is using the accessory muscles of respiration. There is a hint of cyanosis around the mouth. They learn the patient was diagnosed as having emphysema several years ago at the V.A. hospital. Over the last 24 hours he has had progressive dyspnea and didn't sleep at all the previous night. His vital signs are taken revealing a blood pressure of 140/78 mm/Hg, a pulse of 96, and a respiratory rate of 28. The monitor shows a sinus rhythm. His mental status is alert. He is currently taking theophylline and amoxicillin. He still smokes a pack of cigarettes per day and has a 30 pack/year history. The patient wants to be transported to the V.A. hospital. The paramedics contact medical control and provide the patient report. The medical control physician approves transport to the V.A. hospital as it is only 5 miles farther than the nearest hospital. The transport time will be approximately 40 minutes.

The medical control physician orders the placement of an IV of D5W at a "to keep open" rate. In addition, he orders a nebulizer treatment with 0.5 milliliters of albuterol (Ventolin) placed in 3 milliliters of normal saline. Because of the long transport time he also orders the administration of 125 milligrams of methylprednisolone (Solu-Medrol) by IV drip over 20 minutes. Halfway through the nebulizer treatment the patient is markedly improved. His respiratory rate slows to 20 and the transport to the hospital is uneventful. He remains in the hospital 2 days and is discharged home.

INTRODUCTION

The respiratory system is a vital body system responsible for the provision of oxygen to the tissues as well as for the removal of the metabolic waste product carbon dioxide. Oxygen is required for the conversion of essential nutrients into energy and must be constantly available to all body tissues.

Respiratory emergencies are some of the most common emergencies paramedics are called upon to deal with and must be promptly recognized and treated appropriately. This chapter will discuss respiratory emergencies. First, it describes their pathophysiology, then patient assessment, and, finally, management.

RESPIRATORY ANATOMY AND PHYSIOLOGY

The airway is divided anatomically into the *upper airway* and the *lower airway*. The upper airway is responsible for warming and humidifying incoming air. It is also very effective in air purification. Air entering the respiratory system does so through the nares into the nose, or through the mouth, into the oropharynx. The anterior nares are the openings in the front of the nose. Air is filtered by the hairs in the nose and subsequently heated and humidified as it enters into the nasopharynx. Structurally, the nose consists of the nasal bone, the nasal cartilage, and part of the maxilla. The nasal septum is the cartilaginous structure dividing the nose into the right and left cavity. Within the nose are shelf-like structures referred to as *turbinates* that create turbulent air flow as incoming air passes over them. This turbulent air flow aids in the precipitation of particulate matter into the nasal mucosa lining the entire nasal cavity. Blood supply to this area is generous because incoming air must be constantly warmed.

As just mentioned, air can also enter through the mouth, bypassing the nasopharynx. The mouth consists of the lips, cheeks, gums, tongue, and the hard and the soft palate. Like the nose, the mouth is lined by mucosa with good blood supply.

Either from the *nasopharynx* or the mouth, air then enters the *oropharynx*. The oropharynx is the portion of the pharynx extending from the soft palate to the base of the tongue. Located behind the mouth, the oropharynx receives air from the mouth and the nasopharynx. It also receives food from the mouth.

Immediately below the oropharynx is the *hypopharynx*. It contains such structures as the epiglottis and part of the tongue. The epiglottis is responsible for protecting the airway from food and water during swallowing.

The lowest portion of the upper airway is the *laryngopharynx*. It contains the larynx, the vocal cords, the arytenoid folds, and the trachea. (See Figure 20-1.) The esophagus is posterior to the larynx and the trachea. This area is protected by the thyroid cartilage, the cricoid cartilage, the arytenoid cartilage, and the hyoid bone.

The air enters the lower airway from the upper airway via the *trachea*. The trachea is a tube, 10-12 centimeters long, connecting the larynx with the mainstem bronchi in the lungs. It is maintained in an open position because of incomplete, C-shaped, cartilaginous rings extending throughout its length. The trachea is lined by respiratory epithelium which contain cilia (hairlike structures) and mucus-producing cells. This mucus tends to trap particulate matter not filtered out in the upper airway. The cilia move the trapped particulate matter up, out of the trachea and into the mouth, where it is swallowed or expelled. At the *carina,* the trachea divides into the right and the left mainstem *bronchi*. The right mainstem bronchus is almost straight, whereas the left mainstem bronchus angles more acutely to the left. The mainstem bronchi then divide into the secondary bronchi. These secondary bronchi ultimately divide into the *bronchioles,* or the small airways. The bronchioles contain smooth muscle which can contract, thus reducing the diameter of the airway. This ultimately decreases the amount of respiratory gases that can be transported. (See Figure 20-2.) After approximately 22 divisions, the bronchioles become *respiratory bronchioles*. They contain only muscular connective tissue and have a limited ability for gas exchange. The respiratory bronchioles then divide into the *alveolar ducts*. These terminate in the *alveolar sacs*. Most of the gas exchange occurs takes place in the alve-

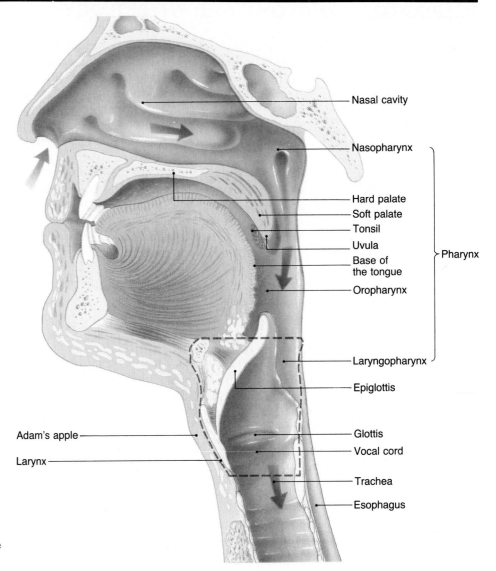

FIGURE 20-1 Anatomy of the upper airway.

oli, although limited gas exchange may occur in the alveolar ducts and respiratory bronchioles. (See Figure 20-3.)

The alveoli are the key functional unit of the respiratory system as this is the site of oxygen and carbon dioxide gas exchange. There is greater than 40 square meters of surface area in the alveoli. The alveoli are hollow and surrounded by the thin alveolar membrane often only one- to two-cell layers thick. The alveoli are kept open because of the presence of an important chemical called *surfactant* which tends to decrease the surface tension of the alveoli.

Although the alveoli are the terminal end of the respiratory tree, there is additional lung tissue, called *lung* **parenchyma,** present. The lung parenchyma is composed of primary pulmonary lobules. These are the functional units of the lung. The right lung contains three lobes, referred to as the upper lobe, middle lobe, and lower lobe. The left lung has only two lobes, the upper lobe and the lower lobe.

The lungs are covered by connective tissue called *pleura.* Unattached to the lung, except at the hilum (the point at which the bronchi enter the lungs), the pleura consists of two layers. The *visceral pleura* covers the lungs and does not contain nerve fibers. In contrast, the *parietal pleura*

■ **parenchyma** the principal or essential parts of an organ.

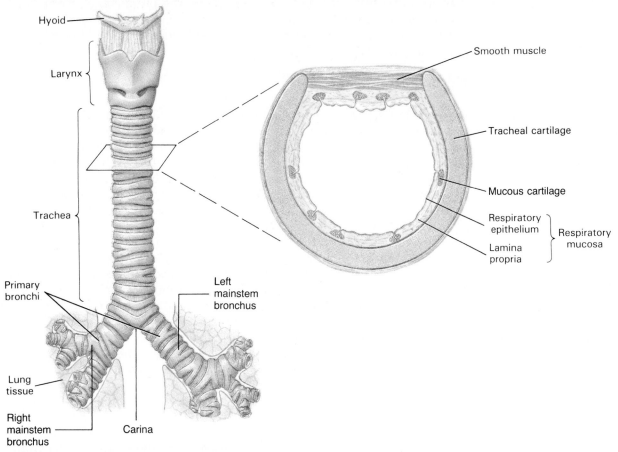

FIGURE 20-2 Anatomy of the lower airway.

Labels: Hyoid, Larynx, Trachea, Primary bronchi, Lung tissue, Right mainstem bronchus, Carina, Left mainstem bronchus, Smooth muscle, Tracheal cartilage, Mucous cartilage, Respiratory epithelium, Lamina propria, Respiratory mucosa

lines the thoracic cavity and contains nerve fibers. A small amount of *pleural fluid* usually can be found in the pleural space, a potential space between the two layers of pleura.

Blood supply to the lungs is through two systems, the pulmonary arteries and veins, and the bronchial arteries and veins. The *pulmonary artery* transports deoxygenated blood from the heart and presents it to the lungs for oxygenation. Oxygenated blood is then transported from the lungs back to the heart through the *pulmonary veins.* The lung tissue

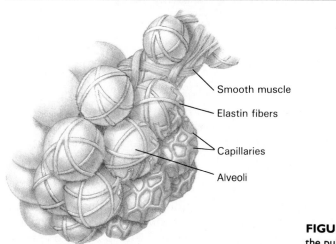

Labels: Smooth muscle, Elastin fibers, Capillaries, Alveoli

FIGURE 20-3 The alveoli and the pulmonary capillaries.

Respiratory Anatomy and Physiology   **551**

itself receives little of its blood supply from the pulmonary arteries and veins. Instead, *bronchial arteries* that branch from the aorta provide most of the blood supply. *Bronchial veins* return blood from the lungs to the superior vena cava.

Mechanics of Respiration

Respiration is defined as the exchange of gases between a living organism and its environment. *Pulmonary respiration* occurs in the lungs when the respiratory gases are exchanged between the alveoli and the red blood cells in the pulmonary capillaries through the capillary membranes. *Cellular respiration,* on the other hand, occurs in the peripheral capillaries and is the exchange of the respiratory gases between the red blood cells and the various tissues. *Ventilation* is the mechanical process whereby air is taken into and out of the lungs.

The lungs have no intrinsic capability to contract or expand. Pulmonary ventilation, therefore, depends upon changes in pressure within the thoracic cavity. The *respiratory cycle* requires coordinated interaction between the respiratory system, the central nervous system, and the musculoskeletal system. The respiratory cycle begins when the lungs have achieved a normal expiration. At this point the pressure inside the thoracic cavity is equal to atmospheric pressure. The thoracic cavity is a closed space, with the trachea as the only opening to the external environment. The size of the thoracic cavity can be made larger by contracting the diaphragm and the intercostal muscles in a process termed *inspiration.* Contraction of the diaphragm results in a downward motion, while contraction of the intercostal muscles results in outward expansion of the chest wall. In respiratory inadequacy this process can be augmented by the use of *accessory respiratory muscles* such as the strap muscles of the neck and the abdominal muscles. Both serve to increase the size of the thoracic cavity, thus further decreasing the intrathoracic pressure. The highly elastic lungs immediately assume the contour of the thoracic cavity due to negative pressure in the pleural space. As intrathoracic pressure decreases, air then rushes into the lungs through the trachea. When the pressure in the thoracic cavity again reaches that of atmospheric pressure, air exchange stops. Then, the respiratory muscles are allowed to relax, which causes the size of the chest cavity to decrease, resulting in *expiration.* This causes an intrathoracic pressure greater than the atmospheric pressure. Air then leaves the lungs through the trachea until pressure is again equalized. Normal expiration is a passive process compared to inspiration, which is an active, energy-utilizing process.

Pulmonary Circulation

An intact circulatory system is also required for respiration. Body cells take oxygen from red blood cells in the arterial system and return carbon dioxide to red blood cells in the venous system. Then the venous system presents this deoxygenated blood to the right side of the heart. The right ventricle pumps blood into the pulmonary artery. This artery immediately divides into the right and the left pulmonary arteries, each supplying the respective lung. Both branches quickly divide into smaller vessels that end in the pulmonary capillaries. The pulmonary capillaries are spread across the surface of the alveoli where the blood can pick up oxygen diffusing through the alveolar and pulmonary capillary membranes. After this occurs, the pulmonary capillaries recombine into larger veins, eventually terminating in the pulmonary veins. The pulmonary veins empty this oxygenated blood into the left atrium. It is then transported, via the ventricle, to the systemic arterial system.

Gas Exchange

As previously detailed, gas exchange in the lungs is opposite to that occurring in the periphery. Blood presented to the lungs is low in oxygen saturation and high in carbon-dioxide saturation, while blood presented to the tissues is high in oxygen saturation and low in carbon-dioxide saturation.

The amount of oxygen and carbon dioxide in the blood can be determined by measuring the *partial pressure* of those gases. Partial pressure is the pressure exerted by each of the components of a gas mixture. In other words, any partial pressure is a fractional concentration of the total gas mixture. Total gas pressure at sea level equals approximately 760 mm/Hg or 14.7 pounds per square inch. Since 1 millimeter of mercury pressure equals 1 Torr, the terms mm/Hg and Torr are interchangeable. Yet the latter is considered preferable. The partial pressure can be calculated by taking the total atmospheric pressure and multiplying it by the percentage of the desired gas present. For example, to calculate the partial pressure of oxygen at normal atmospheric pressure, multiply the percentage of oxygen present in atmospheric air (21%) by the atmospheric pressure (760 Torr). Thus:

$$760 \text{ Torr} \times 0.21 = 159.6 \text{ Torr}$$

Our atmosphere consists of four major respiratory gases: nitrogen (N_2), oxygen (O_2), carbon dioxide (CO_2), and water (H_2O). Nitrogen is metabolically inert, yet necessary for the inflation of gas filled body cavities such as the chest. These respiratory gases are present in the environment in the following partial pressures and concentrations:

Gas	Partial Pressure	Concentration
Nitrogen	597.0 Torr	78.62%
Oxygen	159.0 Torr	20.84%
Carbon Dioxide	0.3 Torr	0.04%
Water	3.7 Torr	0.50%
TOTAL	760.0 Torr	100.00%

If you look at these same gasses after the air has been taken into the alveoli, the partial pressures and concentrations are somewhat different:

Gas	Partial Pressure	Concentration
Nitrogen	569.0 Torr	74.9%
Oxygen	104.0 Torr	13.7%
Carbon Dioxide	40.0 Torr	5.2%
Water	47.0 Torr	6.2%
TOTAL	760.0 Torr	100.0%

Thus, since alveolar partial pressure and arterial partial pressure are essentially the same, normal arterial partial pressures are:

Oxygen (PaO_2) = 100 Torr (Average = 80 − 100)

Carbon Dioxide ($PaCO_2$) = 40 Torr (Average = 35 − 40)

Alveolar partial pressures are represented by the abbreviation PA (e.g., PA_{O_2}) while arterial partial pressures are represented by the abbreviation Pa (e.g., Pa_{O_2}). Since these values are almost always the same, the arterial gases are simply represented as PO_2 and PCO_2.

Diffusion

A function of diffusion is transfer of gases between the lungs and the blood and between the blood and the peripheral tissues. *Diffusion* is the movement of a gas from an area of higher partial pressure concentration to an area of lower partial pressure concentration. The rate of diffusion of a gas across the pulmonary membranes depends on its solubility in water. For example, carbon dioxide is 21 times more soluble in water than oxygen and readily crosses the pulmonary capillary membranes. In the lung, oxygen leaves the area of higher PO_2, the alveoli, and enters the area of lower PO_2, the arterial blood in the pulmonary capillaries. Concurrently, carbon dioxide leaves the area of higher PCO_2, the arterial blood, and enters the area of lower PCO_2, the alveoli. The blood then returns via the pulmonary vein to the heart, and then to the systemic circulation.

Oxygen Concentration in the Blood

Oxygen diffuses into the blood plasma, where it combines with hemoglobin. Hemoglobin approaches 100% saturation when the PaO_2 reaches 50–100 Torr. Each gram of saturated hemoglobin carries 1.34 milliliters of oxygen. Oxygen saturation is the ratio comparing the actual amount of oxygen available with the oxygen carrying capacity of the blood and is represented by the following equation:

$$\text{Oxygen Saturation} = O_2 \text{ content} / O_2 \text{ capacity} \times 100 \, (\%)$$

It is important to point out that the vast majority of oxygen in the blood is carried on the hemoglobin molecule (approximately 97%). Very little oxygen is available from the oxygen dissolved in the plasma. Since partial pressure measurements detect only the amount of oxygen dissolved in the plasma, and do not always reflect the total oxygen saturation, this often can be misleading. For example, a patient who has suffered carbon monoxide poisoning cannot transport enough oxygen to the peripheral tissues since carbon monoxide displaces oxygen from the hemoglobin molecule. But, if an arterial blood gas sample were taken, it might reveal a normal or high PaO_2. This indicates that adequate oxygen is reaching the blood, yet an inadequate amount of hemoglobin is available to transport the oxygen to the peripheral tissues.

Several factors can affect oxygen concentrations in the blood. These include:

❑ *Inadequate alveolar ventilation.* Inadequate alveolar ventilation is caused by many factors such as low-inspired oxygen concentration, respiratory muscle paralysis, and pulmonary conditions like emphysema, asthma, and pneumothorax.

❑ *Decreased diffusion across the pulmonary membrane.* Oxygen exchange is hampered when the distance it must diffuse is increased or if the membrane across which it must diffuse is altered. This occurs when fluid enters the space between the alveolar membrane and the pulmonary capillary membrane (pulmonary edema).

❑ *Ventilation/perfusion mismatch.* Additionally, ventilation-perfusion mismatch can occur when a portion of the alveoli collapses, as in **atelectasis.** Blood is then shunted past these collapsed alveoli without being oxygenated

■ **atelectasis** a collapse of the alveoli decreasing ventilatory effectiveness.

and without carbon dioxide being removed. Also, **pulmonary embolism**, a blood clot in the pulmonary artery, can halt blood flow through the vessel. Consequently, a significant volume of blood is prevented from reaching the alveolar/capillary membranes where gas exchange can occur.

Oxygen derangements are corrected by increasing ventilation, administering supplemental oxygen, using intermittent positive pressure ventilation (IPPV), or by administering drugs to correct underlying problems such as pulmonary edema, asthma, and pulmonary embolism. The desired **FiO_2** should be selected based on the emergency being treated.

Carbon Dioxide Levels in the Blood

Carbon dioxide is transported mainly in the form of bicarbonate (HCO_3^-). Approximately 66% of carbon dioxide is transported as bicarbonate, while 33% is transported combined with hemoglobin. Less than 1% is dissolved in the plasma.

Carbon dioxide levels in the blood are influenced by several factors including increased CO_2 production and/or decreased CO_2 elimination. Causes of CO_2 derangements include:

❑ *Increased CO_2 production.* Increased CO_2 production can result from several actions including:
   ❑ fever
   ❑ muscle exertion
   ❑ shivering
      metabolic processes resulting in the formation of acids
❑ *Decreased CO_2 elimination.* Decreased CO_2 elimination can result from alveolar hypoventilation. Common causes include:
   ❑ respiratory depression by drugs
   ❑ airway obstruction
   ❑ impairment of the respiratory muscles
   ❑ obstructive disease states such as asthma and emphysema

Raised CO_2 levels (**hypercarbia**) are usually treated by increasing the ventilation and by correcting the underlying cause.

Regulation of Respiration

Respiration is unique because it is under the control of both the voluntary and involuntary nervous systems. Most of respiratory control is, however, involuntary. Various chemical, physical, and nervous reflexes monitor body oxygen needs.

The main respiratory center is located in the medulla which is in the brainstem. Various neurons within the medulla initiate impulses that result in respiration. A rise in the frequency of these impulses results in an increase in respiratory rate. Conversely, a decrease in firing frequency results in a lowered respiratory rate. The medulla is connected to the respiratory muscles primarily via the vagus nerve. If the medulla fails to initiate respiration, an additional control center located in the pons, called the *apneustic center,* assumes respiratory control to ensure the continuation of respirations. Expiration, on the other hand, is controlled by a third center, the *pneumotaxic center,* also located in the pons.

While inspiration progresses, the thoracic cavity expands and the lungs fill with air, becoming distended. As the lungs become distended, stretch receptors in them become activated. As the degree of stretch increases, these receptors fire more frequently. The impulses they send to the brainstem inhibit the medullary cells, decreasing the inspiratory stimulus. Thus, the respiratory muscles relax, allowing the elastic lungs to recoil and expel air from the body. Then, as the stretch decreases, the stretch receptors stop firing. This is referred to as the *Hering-Breuer reflex,* and serves to prevent overexpansion of the lungs.

Additionally, there are central chemical receptors in the medulla and peripheral chemoreceptors in the carotid bodies and in the arch of the aorta. These chemoreceptors are stimulated by decreased PaO_2, increased $PaCO_2$, and decreased pH. Cerebrospinal fluid (CSF) pH is the primary control of respiratory center stimulation. A change in the CSF pH occurs very quickly in relation to arterial PCO_2. A rise in the CSF pH inhibits respiration, while a decrease in CSF pH stimulates it. Because arterial PCO_2 is inversely related to pH, including CSF pH, it is seen as the normal neuroregulatory control of respirations. Any increase in the arterial PCO_2 will stimulate the peripheral chemoreceptors. They will then send impulses to the brainstem to increase respirations. And, as indicated, any increase in $PaCO_2$ will decrease CSF pH, which will also stimulate the central chemoreceptors. The result will be increased respirations. Conversely, low $PaCO_2$ levels will decrease chemoreceptor stimulation, thereby effectively decreasing respiratory activity.

The body also constantly monitors the PaO_2 and the pH. In fact, **hypoxemia** is a profound stimulus of respiration in a normal individual. People with chronic respiratory disease such as emphysema and chronic bronchitis tend to retain CO_2 and therefore have a chronically elevated $PaCO_2$. Eventually becoming accustomed to this chronic condition, chemoreceptors in the periphery and the central nervous system will cease depending on $PaCO_2$ to regulate respiration. These individuals, then, have to depend on changes in PaO_2 to regulate respiration. This is termed *hypoxic drive.* The respiratory stimulation of such people is increased when PaO_2 falls and is inhibited when it climbs. This is the reason why high-volume oxygen administration can cause respiratory arrest in them. High-flow oxygen can quickly double or even triple the PaO_2. The peripheral chemoreceptors detect this increase and cease to stimulate the respiratory centers, causing apnea.

■ **hypoxemia** reduction in the oxygen content in the arterial blood or in the PaO_2.

Modified Forms of Respiration

There are several modified forms of respiration with various functions. They include:

❏ *Coughing*—forceful exhalation of a large volume of air from the lungs. This serves a protective function.
❏ *Sneezing*—sudden, forceful exhalation from the nose, usually caused by nasal irritation.
❏ *Hiccoughing*—sudden inspiration caused by spasmodic contraction of the diaphragm. It apparently serves no physiological purpose.
❏ *Sighing*—slow, deep inspiration followed by a prolonged expiration. Sighing hyperinflates the lungs and reexpands atelectatic areas.
❏ *Grunting*—grunting occurs primarily in neonates when the infant expires air against a partially closed epiglottis. It is usually an indication of respiratory distress.

Measures of Respiratory Function

The *respiratory rate* is the number of respirations per minute and is normally 12–20 in the adult. Infants breathe between 40–60 breaths per minute while children breathe at an average rate of 24 breaths per minute.

Several factors can affect respiratory rate. These include:

- ❑ fever—increases rate
- ❑ anxiety—increases rate
- ❑ hypoxia—increases rate
- ❑ depressant drugs—decreases rate
- ❑ sleep—decreases rate
- ❑ pain—increases rate

The capacity of the lungs and airways has been extensively studied and is important in emergency care. Maximum lung capacity in the average adult male is approximately 6 liters and is termed the *total lung capacity (TLC)*. There are some additional respiratory capacities and measurements paramedics must be familiar with. These are:

- ❑ *Tidal volume (V_T).* The tidal volume is the average volume of gas inhaled or exhaled in one respiratory cycle. In the adult male this is approximately 500 mL.
- ❑ *Dead space volume (V_D).* The dead space volume is the amount of gas in the tidal volume that remains in the passageways unavailable for gas exchange. It is approximately 150 mL in the adult male.
- ❑ *Alveolar volume (V_A).* The alveolar volume is the amount of gas in the tidal volume that reaches the alveoli for gas exchange. It is approximately 350 mL in the adult male. The following equation shows this relationship:

$$V_T - V_D = V_A$$

- ❑ *Minute volume (V_{min}).* The minute volume is the amount of gas moved in and out of the respiratory tract in one minute. It is represented in the following equation:

$$V_{min} = [V_T - V_D] \times \text{Respiratory rate}$$

or

$$V_{min} = V_A \times \text{Respiratory Rate}$$

- ❑ *Functional reserve capacity (FRC).* The amount of air that can be forcefully exhaled after a maximum inspiration is termed the functional reserve capacity. It is approximately 4,500 mL in an adult male.

ASSESSMENT OF THE RESPIRATORY SYSTEM

Assessment of the respiratory system is a vital aspect of prehospital care. The paramedic must be able to quickly assess the airway and ventilation status during the primary survey. Later, during the secondary survey, if the respiratory system appears to be involved in the patient's problem, the paramedic must concentrate on this aspect of the assessment.

History

The history and physical exam should be directed at problem areas as determined by the patient's chief complaint or primary problem. If the chief complaint is "shortness of breath," or **dyspnea,** the following should be ascertained:

■ **dyspnea** difficult or labored breathing.

- ❑ How long has the dyspnea been present?
- ❑ Was the onset gradual or abrupt?

❑ Is the dyspnea better or worse by position and is there associated **orthopnea**?
❑ Has the patient been coughing?
  ❑ If so, is the cough productive?
  ❑ What is the character and color of the sputum?
  ❑ Is there any **hemoptysis?**
❑ Is there any pain associated with the dyspnea?
  ❑ If so, what is the location of the pain?
  ❑ Was the onset of pain sudden or slow?
  ❑ What was the duration of the pain?
  ❑ Does the pain radiate to any area?
  ❑ Does the pain increase with respiration?
❑ What is the patient's past medical history?
❑ Identify current medications with particular emphasis on oxygen therapy,
  oral bronchodilators, and antibiotics.
❑ Are there any allergies?

Physical Examination

Physical examination of the respiratory system should follow the standard steps of patient assessment. They are inspection, palpation, percussion, and auscultation.

First, during the primary assessment the airway should be secured. If the airway is compromised, basic airway management techniques should be instituted. When assessing the airway the following principles should be kept in mind (see Figure 20-4):

❑ Noisy breathing nearly always means partial airway obstruction.
❑ Obstructed breathing is not always noisy.

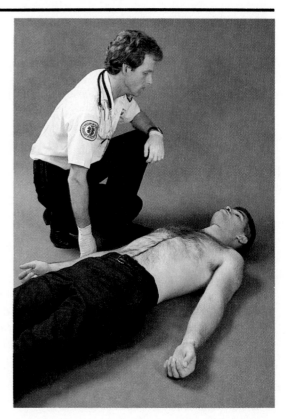

FIGURE 20-4 The first step in evaluating the respiratory emergency is to check the ABCs.

- The brain can survive only a few minutes in **asphyxia.**
- Artificial respiration is useless if the airway is blocked.
- A patient's airway is useless if the patient is apneic.
- If airway obstruction is noted do not waste time looking for help or equipment.

The primary assessment should be completed, and the paramedic should ensure adequate ventilation and circulation.

Following the primary assessment, the patient should be observed for any of the following:

- anxiety, discomfort, or stress—these may possibly indicate **hypoxia**
- difficulty in speaking due to dyspnea
- distraction from questioning due to the symptoms present
- alert replies versus confusion
- patient position
- obesity, which can result in hypoventilation

Following observation, the vital signs should be determined, including the rate and depth of the respiratory pattern. The paramedic should also determine if any abnormal respiratory patterns are present. A patient will occasionally exhibit *pulsus paradoxis,* a drop in the systolic blood pressure of 10 Torr or more with each respiratory cycle. Pulsus paradoxis is associated with **chronic obstructive pulmonary disease (COPD)** and cardiac tamponade. The paramedic should not take the time to look for pulsus paradoxis.

During the secondary assessment, attention should be turned to the respiratory system. First, inspection should be completed, after looking especially for signs of respiratory distress including:

- **nasal flaring**
- intercostal muscle retraction
- use of the accessory respiratory muscles
- **cyanosis**
- pursed lips
- **tracheal tugging**

The anterior-posterior dimensions and general shape of the chest should be inspected. (See Figure 20-5.) An increased anterior-posterior diameter is suggestive of chronic obstructive pulmonary disease. The chest should be inspected for symmetrical movement. Any asymmetry may be suggestive of trauma. A paradoxical movement is suggestive of flail chest. Any chest scars, lesions, wounds, or deformities should be also noted.

Following inspection, the chest should be palpated, both front and back, for any abnormalities. (See Figure 20-6.) Any tenderness, crepitus, subcutaneous emphysema, or air leakage should be noted. First, the anterior, then the posterior, chest should be palpated. The paramedic should inspect his or her gloved hands for blood each time they are removed from behind the patient's chest. In some instances, it may be appropriate to evaluate **tactile fremitus,** the vibration felt in the chest during speaking. The paramedic should compare one side of the chest with the other. Simultaneously, the trachea should be palpated for the presence of any deviation suggestive of a tension pneumothorax. (See Chapter 16.)

Following palpation, and if indicated, the chest should be quickly percussed. Percussion should be limited to suspected cases of pneumotho-

- **asphyxia** a decrease in the amount of oxygen and an increase in the amount of carbon dioxide as a result of some interference with respiration.

- **hypoxia** state in which insufficient oxygen is available to meet the oxygen requirements of the cells.

- **chronic obstructive pulmonary disease (COPD)** characterized by a decreased ability of the lungs to perform the function of ventilation.

- **nasal flaring** excessive widening of the nares with respiration.

- **cyanosis** bluish discoloration of the skin due to an increase in carboxyhemoglobin in the blood and directly related to poor ventilation.

- **tracheal tugging** retraction of the tissues of the neck due to airway obstruction or dyspnea.

- **tactile fremitus** vibratory tremors felt through the chest by palpation.

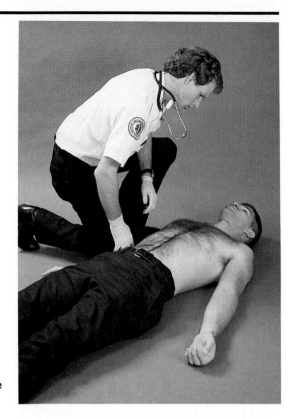

FIGURE 20-5 Inspection of the chest.

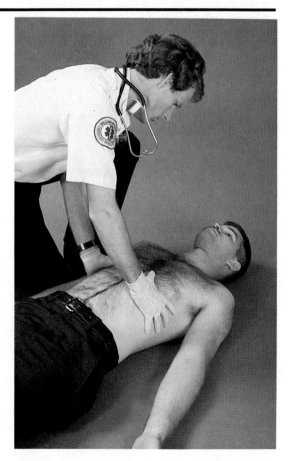

FIGURE 20-6 The chest should be palpated.

rax and pulmonary edema. (See Figure 20-7.) A hollow sound on percussion is often indicative of pneumothorax or emphysema. In contrast, a dull sound is indicative of pulmonary edema or pneumonia.

Finally, the chest should be auscultated. First, the paramedic should listen to the patient, without a stethoscope and from a distance. The paramedic should observe for loud stridor, wheezing, or cough. If possible, the patient should be in the sitting position, and the chest auscultated in a symmetrical pattern. (See Figure 20-8.) When the patient cannot sit up,

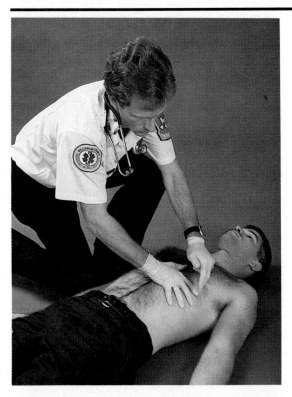

FIGURE 20-7 If indicated, the chest should be percussed.

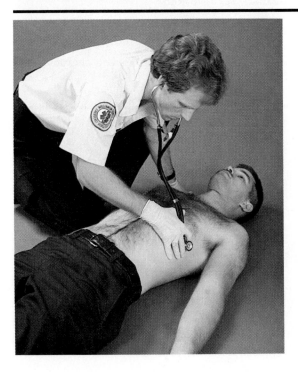

FIGURE 20-8 The chest should be auscultated.

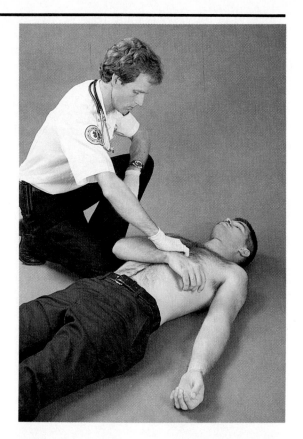

FIGURE 20-9 The respiratory rate should be counted. It is often helpful to take the pulse of patients when counting respirations. The patient will think that the paramedic is taking the pulse and will not consciously modify their respiratory rate.

the anterior and lateral parts of the chest should be auscultated. Each area should be auscultated for one respiratory cycle. While the patient breathes in and out deeply with the mouth open, the paramedic should note any abnormal breath sounds and their location. (See Figures 20-9 and 20-10.)

Many terms are used to describe abnormal breath sounds. The following are some of the more common terminology:

❑ *Snoring*—occurs when the upper airway is partially obstructed, usually by the tongue.
❑ *Stridor*—harsh, high-pitched sound heard on inspiration and characteristic of an upper airway obstruction such as croup.

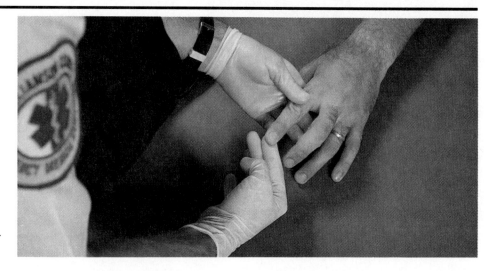

FIGURE 20-10 The fingers should be inspected. Any clubbing may indicate chronic respiratory or cardiac disease.

❑ *Wheezing*—whistling sound due to narrowing of the airways by edema, bronchoconstriction, or foreign materials.

❑ *Rhonchi*—rattling sounds in the larger airways associated with excessive mucus or other material.

❑ *Rales*—fine, moist crackling sounds associated with fluid in the smaller airways.

❑ *Friction rub*—occurs when the pleura become inflamed, as in pleurisy, and sounds like dried pieces of leather rubbing together.

Pulse Oximetry. Pulse oximetry offers a rapid and accurate means for assessing oxygen saturation. The device can be quickly applied to a finger. The pulse rate and oxygen saturation can be continously recorded. Use of the pulse oximeter, if available, is encouraged for any patient complaining of dyspnea or respiratory problems. (See Figures 20-11 through 20-13.)

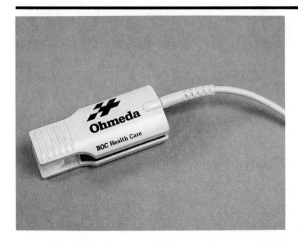

FIGURE 20-11 Sensing unit for pulse oximetry. This device transmits light through a vascular bed, such as in the finger, and can determine the oxygen saturation of red blood cells.

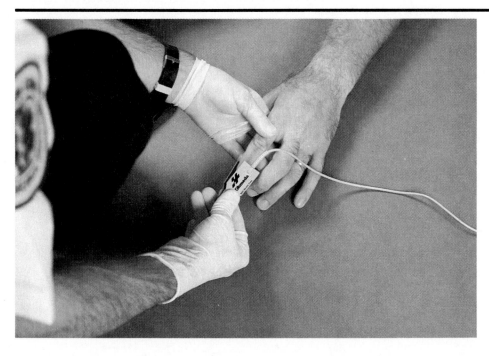

FIGURE 20-12 To use the pulse oximeter, it is only necessary to turn the device on and attach the sensor to a finger.

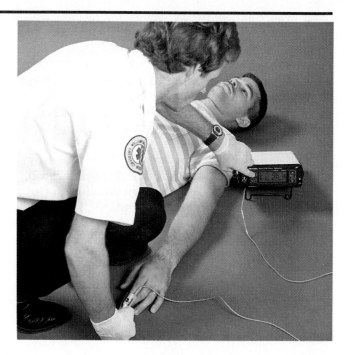

FIGURE 20-13 The desired graphic mode on the oximeter should be selected. The oxygen saturation and pulse rate can be continuously monitored.

MANAGEMENT PRINCIPLES OF RESPIRATORY EMERGENCIES

Several general principles should be employed in acute respiratory insufficiency. These include:

✱ In any respiratory emergency the first priority is to open and maintain the airway.

1. The airway always receives first priority. In trauma victims who may have associated cervical spine injuries the airway should be protected and maintained without extending the neck.
2. Any patient with respiratory distress should receive oxygen.
3. Any patient whose illness or injury suggests the possibility of hypoxia should receive oxygen.
4. If there is a question whether oxygen should be given, as in chronic obstructive pulmonary disease, the paramedic should administer it. *Oxygen should never be withheld from a patient suspected of suffering hypoxia.*

PATHOPHYSIOLOGY AND MANAGEMENT OF RESPIRATORY DISORDERS

The following sections will address the pathophysiology and management of the more common respiratory disorders encountered in prehospital care.

Upper-Airway Obstruction

The most common cause of upper-airway obstruction is the relaxed tongue. In an unconscious patient in the supine position, it can fall into the back of the throat, obstructing the upper airway. Additionally, the upper airway can become obstructed by such common materials as food, dentures, or other foreign bodies. A typical example of upper-airway obstruction is the "cafe coronary" which tends to occur in middle-aged or elderly patients who wear dentures. These people often are unable to sense how well they have chewed their food. Thus, they accidentally inhale a large piece of food, often meat, which obstructs their airway. Concurrent alcohol consumption is often implicated in the "cafe coronary." The upper airway can be obstructed in a variety of ways such as facial or neck trauma, upper-airway burns, and allergic reactions. It can also become blocked by swelling of the epiglottis or subglottic area because of epiglottitis or croup.

Assessment of the patient with an upper-airway obstruction varies, depending on the cause of the obstruction and the history of the event. The comatose patient should be evaluated for snoring respirations, possibly indicating tongue or denture obstruction. If confronted by a patient suffering a "cafe coronary," the paramedic should determine whether the victim can speak. If he or she can, this indicates that at present the obstruction is incomplete. But if the victim is unresponsive and had been eating, a food bolus lodged in the trachea should be strongly suspected. If a burn is present or suspected, laryngeal edema is assumed to exist until proven otherwise. Patients who may be having an allergic reaction to food will often report an itching sensation in the palate followed by a "lump" in the throat. The situation may progress to hoarseness, inspiratory stridor, and complete obstruction. Particular attention should be paid to the presence of urticaria (hives). Intercostal muscle retraction and use of the strap muscles of the neck for breathing suggest attempts to ventilate against a partially closed airway.

Management of the obstructed airway is based on the nature of the obstruction. Blockage by the tongue can be corrected by opening the airway, using either the head-tilt, chin-lift, jaw-thrust, or triple-airway maneuver. The airway can be maintained by employing either a nasopharyngeal or oropharyngeal airway. Obstructing foreign bodies should be removed, if possible, by the following basic airway maneuvers:

Conscious Adult Patient. In an adult patient who is conscious, the paramedic should (see Table 20-1):

1. Determine if there is a complete obstruction or poor air exchange. The paramedic should ask the patient, "Are you choking?" or "Can you speak?" If the patient can speak, he or she should be asked to produce a forceful cough to expel the foreign body.
2. If the patient has complete obstruction or poor air exchange, the paramedic should provide six to ten abdominal thrusts in rapid succession. If the thrusts are unsuccessful, they should be repeated until the obstruction is relieved or the patient becomes unconscious. In children or very obese or pregnant patients, chest thrusts should be used in lieu of abdominal thrusts.

Unconscious Adult Patient. If the patient is unconscious or loses consciousness, the paramedic should (see Table 20-2):

1. Use the head-tilt, jaw-thrust, or triple airway maneuver in an attempt to open the airway.
2. Pinch the patient's nostrils and attempt to give two ventilations. If the attempts to ventilate fail, the head should be repositioned and the attempt repeated. If this fails . . .
3. Straddle the patient and administer six to ten abdominal thrusts in quick succession. If this fails . . .

✱ An obstructed airway requires immediate intervention.

4. Try the tongue-jaw lift and, if the foreign body is seen, attempt finger sweeps. If successful, ventilation should be resumed. If unsuccessful . . .
5. While continuing the abdominal thrusts and finger sweeps, prepare the laryngoscope and the McGill forceps. The airway should be visualized with the laryngoscope. If the foreign body can be seen, it should be grasped with the McGill forceps and removed. Once removed, ventilations should begin as well as the supplemental administration of oxygen.

TABLE 20-1 OBSTRUCTED AIRWAY—ADULT CONSCIOUS

Step	Objective	Critical Performance
1. Assessment	Determine airway obstruction.	Ask "Are you choking?" Determine if victim can cough or speak.
2. Heimlich Maneuver	Perform abdominal thrusts.	Stand behind the victim. Wrap arms around victim's waist. Make a fist with one hand and place the thumb side against victim's abdomen in the midline slightly above the navel and well below the tip of the xiphoid. Grasp fist with the other hand. Press into the victim's abdomen with quick upward thrusts. Each thrust should be distinct and delivered with the intent of relieving the airway obstruction. Repeat thrusts until either the foreign body is expelled or the victim becomes unconscious (see below).
3. Positioning	Position the victim. Call for help.	Turn patient on back as a unit. Place face up, arms by side. Call out "Help!" or, if others respond, activate EMS system.
4. Foreign Body Check	Perform finger sweep.*	Keep victim's face up. Use tongue-jaw lift to open mouth. Sweep deeply into mouth to remove foreign body.
5. Breathing Attempt	Ventilate.	Open airway with head-tilt/chin-lift. Seal mouth and nose properly. Attempt to ventilate.
6. Heimlich Maneuver	(Airway is obstructed.) Perform abdominal thrusts.	Straddle victim's thighs. Place heel of one hand against victim's abdomen, in the midline slightly above the navel and well below the tip of the xiphoid. Place second hand directly on top of first hand. Press into the abdomen with quick upward thrusts. Perform 6–10 abdominal thrusts.
7. Foreign Body Check	(Airway remains obstructed.) Perform finger sweep.*	Keep victim's face up. Use tongue-jaw lift to open mouth. Sweep deeply into mouth to remove foreign body.
8. Breathing Attempt	Ventilate.	Open airway with head-tilt/chin-lift. Seal mouth and nose properly. Attempt to ventilate.
9. Sequencing	(Airway remains obstructed.) Repeat sequence.	Repeat Steps 6–8 until successful.†

Reproduced with permission of the American Heart Association.
* During practice and testing, simulate finger sweeps.
† After airway obstruction is cleared, ventilate twice and proceed with CPR as indicated.

TABLE 20-2   OBSTRUCTED AIRWAY—ADULT UNCONSCIOUS

Step	Objective	Critical Performance
1. Assessment	Determine unresponsiveness. Call for help. Position the victim. Open the airway. Determine breathlessness.	Tap or gently shake shoulder. Shout "Are you OK?" Call out "Help!" Turn on back as unit, if necessary, supporting head and neck (4–10 sec). Use head-tilt/chin-lift maneuver. Maintain open airway. Ear over mouth, observe chest: look, listen, feel for breathing (3–5 sec).
2. Breathing Attempt	Ventilate. (Airway is obstructed.) Ventilate. (Airway remains obstructed.) Activate EMS system.	Maintain open airway. Seal mouth and nose properly. Attempt to ventilate. Reposition victim's head. Seal mouth and nose properly. Reattempt to ventilate. If someone responded to call for help, send him/her to activate EMS system.
3. Heimlich Maneuver	Perform abdominal thrusts.	Straddle victim's thighs. Place heel of one hand against victim's abdomen in the midline slightly above the navel and well below the tip of the xiphoid. Place second hand directly on top of first hand. Press into the abdomen with quick upward thrusts. Each thrust should be distinct and delivered with the intent of relieving the airway obstruction. Perform 6–10 abdominal thrusts.
4. Foreign Body Check	Perform finger sweep.*	Keep victim's face up. Use tongue-jaw lift to open mouth. Sweep deeply into mouth to remove foreign body.
5. Breathing Attempt	Ventilate.	Open airway with head-tilt/chin-lift maneuver. Seal mouth and nose properly. Reattempt to ventilate.
6. Sequencing	Repeat sequence.	Repeat Steps 3–5 until successful.†

Reproduced with permission of the American Heart Association.
* During practice and testing simulate finger sweeps.
† After airway obstruction is cleared, ventilate twice and proceed with CPR as indicated.

In cases of airway obstruction caused by laryngeal edema, the airway should be established by the head-tilt, jaw-thrust, or triple airway maneuver. Supplemental oxygen should then be administered. Next, an IV with a crystalloid solution should be started and epinephrine administered. Then the patient should receive diphenhydramine (Benadryl). Transtracheal ventilation may be required if the patient does not respond to the treatments described.

Obstructive Lung Disease

Obstructive lung disease is common in our society. The most common obstructive lung diseases encountered in prehospital care are emphysema, chronic bronchitis, and asthma. This section will discuss each of these disease processes, detailing the pathophysiology, assessment, and treatment.

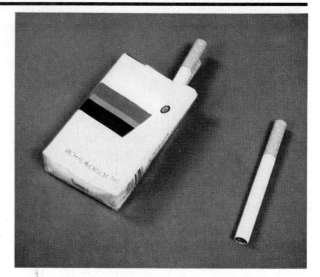

FIGURE 20-14 Cigarette smoking is a major factor in the development of emphysema and chronic bronchitis.

Emphysema. *Emphysema* results from destruction of the alveolar walls distal to the terminal bronchioles. It is more common in men than women and more common in rural settings. The major factor contributing to emphysema, in our society, is cigarette smoking. (See Figure 20-14.) Continued exposure to noxious substances, such as cigarette smoke, results in the gradual destruction of the walls of the alveoli. This process decreases the alveolar membrane surface area, thus lessening the area available for gas exchange. The loss of membrane results in an increased ratio of air to lung tissue in the lung. Additionally, the number of pulmonary capillaries in the lung is decreased, thus increasing resistance to pulmonary blood flow, which ultimately causes pulmonary hypertension. Pulmonary hypertension may ultimately lead to right heart failure, **cor pulmonale,** and death. (See Figure 20-15.) Emphysema also causes weakening of the walls of the small bronchioles. When the walls of the alveoli and small bronchioles are destroyed, the lungs lose their capacity to re-

■ **cor pulmonale** hypertrophy of the right ventricle resulting from disorders of the lung.

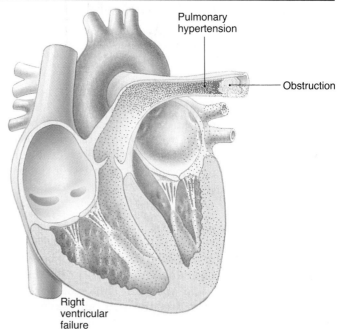

Pulmonary hypertension

Obstruction

Right ventricular failure

FIGURE 20-15 Chronic obstructive pulmonary disease of long standing can cause pulmonary hypertension, which, in turn, may lead to cor pulmonale.

coil and air becomes trapped in the lungs. Thus, residual volume increases, while vital capacity remains relatively normal. As the disease progresses, the PaO_2 further decreases, which may lead to increased red blood cell production and polycythemia (an abnormally high hematocrit). The $PaCO_2$ also increases and becomes chronically elevated, forcing the body to depend on hypoxic drive to control respirations. Patients with emphysema are more susceptible to acute respiratory infections, such as pneumonia, and to cardiac dysrhythmias. Chronic emphysema patients ultimately become dependent on bronchodilators, corticosteroids, and, in the final stages, supplemental oxygen.

Assessment of the Patient with Emphysema. The patient with emphysema may report a history of recent weight loss, increased dyspnea on exertion, and progressive limitation of physical activity. (See Figure 20-16.) Unlike chronic bronchitis, discussed in subsequent sections, emphysema is rarely associated with cough, except in the morning. The patient should be questioned about cigarette and tobacco usage. This is generally reported in pack/years. The patient should be asked the number of cigarette packs (20 cigarettes/pack) smoked per day and the number of years he or she has smoked. The number of packs smoked per day should be multiplied by number of years smoked. For example, a man who has smoked 2 packs per day for 15 years would have a 30 pack/year smoking history. Medical problems related to smoking, such as emphysema, chronic bronchitis, and lung cancer, usually begin after a patient has attained a 20 pack/year history, although this can vary significantly.

Physical exam of the patient with emphysema usually reveals a patient with a barrel chest as evidenced by an increase in the anterior/posterior chest diameter. Decreased chest excursion with a prolonged expiratory phase and a rapid resting respiratory rate may be present. Pa-

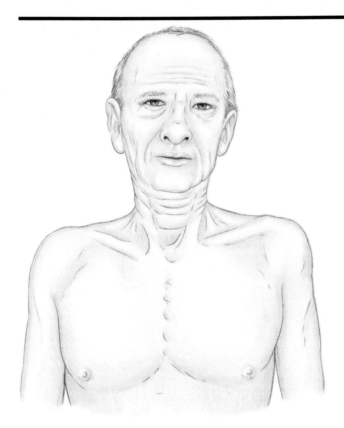

FIGURE 20-16 Typical appearance of patient with emphysema. There are well-developed accessory muscles and suprasternal retraction.

tients with emphysema are often thin since they must use a significant amount of the caloric intake for respiration. They tend to be pink in color due to **polycythemia** and are often referred to as "pink puffers." Emphysema patients often have hypertrophy of the accessory respiratory muscles. The patient will often involuntarily purse his or her lips to create increased airway pressure. Clubbing of the fingers is common. Breath sounds are usually diminished. Wheezes and rhonchi may or may not be present. The patient may exhibit signs of right heart failure as evidence by jugular venous distention, peripheral edema, and hepatic congestion.

Chronic Bronchitis. Although chronic bronchitis is a different disease process than emphysema, it shares several of the symptoms and the pathophysiology. Chronic bronchitis results from an increase in the number of the mucous-secreting cells in the respiratory tree. It is characterized by the presence of a large quantity of sputum. This often occurs after prolonged exposure to cigarette smoke. Unlike emphysema, the alveoli are not severely affected and diffusion remains normal. Gas exchange is decreased because there is lowered alveolar ventilation, which ultimately results in hypoxia and hypercarbia. (See Figure 20-17.) Hypoxia may increase red blood cell production and can result in polycythemia as occurs in emphysema. Increased $PaCO_2$ levels may lead to irritability, decreased intellectual abilities, headaches, and personality changes. Physiologically, an increased $PaCO_2$ causes pulmonary vasoconstriction, resulting in pulmonary hypertension and, eventually, cor pulmonale. Unlike emphysema, the vital capacity is decreased, while the residual volume is normal or decreased.

Assessment of the Patient with Chronic Bronchitis. The patient with chronic bronchitis often will have a history of heavy cigarette smoking. There may also be a history of frequent respiratory infections and these patients usually produce considerable quantities of sputum daily.

Patients with chronic bronchitis tend to be overweight and can be

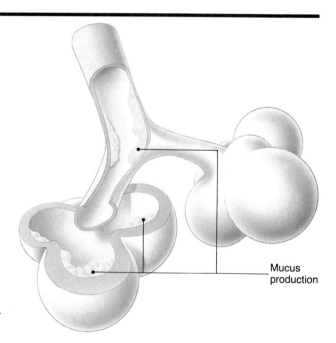

Mucus production

FIGURE 20-17 Chronic mucous production and plugging of the airways occurs in chronic bronchitis.

cyanotic. Because of this, they are often referred to as "blue bloaters." This can be contrasted with the "pink puffer" image of emphysema patients described above. Auscultation of the thorax often will reveal rhonchi due to occlusion of the larger airways with mucous plugs. The patient may also exhibit signs and symptoms of right heart failure such as jugular venous distention, ankle edema, and hepatic congestion.

Management of the Patient with Emphysema and Chronic Bronchitis. The primary goal in the emergency management of the patient with either emphysema or chronic bronchitis is to relieve hypoxia. Because many of these patients are dependent upon hypoxic respiratory drive, however, the supplemental administration of oxygen may decrease respiratory drive and inhibit ventilation. The paramedic must continually monitor the patient and be prepared to assist ventilations if signs of respiratory depression develop.

The first step in treating a patient suffering an exacerbation of emphysema or chronic bronchitis is to establish an airway. Then the patient may be placed in a seated or semiseated position to assist the accessory respiratory muscles. Supplemental oxygen should be administered at low flow, generally less than 2 liters per minute, or venti-mask. A nasal cannula should be used, with the paramedic constantly monitoring respiratory rate and depth. If hypoxia or respiratory failure is evident, then the concentration of delivered oxygen should be increased. An intravenous line should be established with 5% dextrose in water at a "to keep open" (TKO) rate. Then, if ordered by the medical control physician, the patient should be administered a bronchodilator medication such as aminophylline or a beta agonist.

Asthma. Asthma is a common respiratory disease that affects over 6 million Americans and accounts for over 5,000 deaths per year. It is usually detected before age 10 in approximately 50% of the cases and before age 30 in an additional 33%. There is a family tendency toward the disease. It is also often associated with atopic (allergic) conditions such as **eczema** and allergies. Prompt prehospital recognition and treatment of asthma is essential as it can quickly deteriorate, resulting in death.

Pathophysiology. Asthma is characterized by obstruction of the airway due to bronchospasm. In the acute attack, the patient will develop intense bronchospasm, frequently followed by swelling of the mucous membranes lining the bronchioles. Subsequently, there may be plugging of the bronchi by thick mucus, thus further obstructing the airway. Several factors have been identified that can trigger the attack including an allergic reaction to inhaled irritants, respiratory infection, emotional distress, and cold air. As bronchospasm develops, with an associated increase in sputum production, the lungs become progressively hyper-inflated, for air flow is more restricted on exhalation. This effectively reduces vital capacity and results in decreased gas exchange at the alveoli, causing hypoxemia. If allowed to progress untreated, hypoxemia will worsen and unconsciousness and death may ensue.

Assessment of the Patient With Asthma. Asthmatics will frequently report that they suffer from asthma. If this occurs, it is important to determine the frequency and the severity of attacks. The severity of the patient's asthma can often be determined by finding out how many times

✱ Do not deprive the COPD patient of oxygen.

■ **eczema** skin disorder seen commonly in allergic patients.

the patient has been hospitalized for the disease. Current medications may provide additional information. Asthmatics are usually taking one or two bronchodilator agents.

During the physical examination the patient is usually sitting up, leaning forward, and suffering from **tachypnea.** There is frequently an associated, unproductive cough. Accessory respiratory muscle usage is usually evident. Wheezing may be heard. In a severe attack, however, the patient may not wheeze at all. Thus the absence of wheezing is often an ominous finding. It indicates that air movement is absent or severely diminished. Tachycardia is usually present in an asthma attack and should be monitored since virtually all medications used to treat asthma increase the heart rate. The paramedic should remember that all wheezing is not a sign of asthma. For example, congestive heart failure and aspirated foreign bodies can also result in wheezing.

Management of the Asthmatic. The primary therapeutic goal in the asthmatic is to correct hypoxia and reverse bronchospasm. First, it is imperative that an airway be established. Supplemental, humidified oxygen should be administered. An IV of 5% dextrose in water should be initiated at a "to keep open" rate. A 0.3 mL to 0.5 mL subcutaneous injection of epinephrine 1:1000, or another injectable or inhaled β agonist should be admin-istered. This can be repeated in 30 minutes if required. Additionally, the medical control physician may order the administration of aminophylline. Many paramedic units have the capability of administering nebulized bronchodilator medications such as albuterol, terbutaline, or isoetharine.

During prolonged transports, the medical control physician may request that the paramedic administer a steroid. It may by in the form of methylprednisolone, hydrocortisone, or dexamethasone. Steroids decrease bronchial edema and inflammation, thus causing bronchodilation. It should be pointed out that the effects of steroids are delayed. Therefore, a steroid should not be used as the sole agent in the treatment of respiratory emergencies. Sedatives and aspirin should also never be administered. The patient should be calmly reassured throughout treatment as an asthmatic attack can be very frightening. Transport should be prompt.

Status Asthmaticus. *Status asthmaticus* is defined as a severe, prolonged asthma attack that cannot be broken by repeated doses of epinephrine. It is a serious medical emergency and prompt recognition, treatment, and transport are required. The patient suffering status asthmaticus frequently will have a greatly distended chest from continued air trapping. Breath sounds, and often wheezing, may be absent. The patient is usually exhausted, severely acidotic, and dehydrated. The management of status asthmaticus is basically the same as for asthma. The paramedic should recognize that respiratory arrest is imminent and be prepared for endotracheal intubation. Transport should be immediate, with aggressive treatment continued enroute.

Asthma in Children. Asthma in children is common. The pathophysiology and treatment are essentially the same as in adults, with altered medication dosages. Several additional medications are used in the treatment of childhood asthma. Asthma in children is discussed in greater detail in Chapter 30.

■ **tachypnea** rapid respiration.

✳ All wheezing is not asthma.

✳ In addition to oxygen, β agonists are the mainstay of emergent asthma therapy.

Pneumonia

Pathophysiology. Pneumonia is a common respiratory disease caused by infection of the lung by an infectious agent. Bacterial and viral pneumonias are the most frequent, although fungal and other forms of pneumonia do exist.

Assessment of the Patient with Pneumonia. The patient with pneumonia will generally appear ill. He or she may report a recent history of fever and chills. These chills are commonly described as "bed shaking." There is usually a generalized weakness and **malaise.** The patient will tend to complain of a deep, productive cough and may be able to expel yellow sputum, often streaked with blood. There is frequently associated chest pain. Therefore, pneumonia should be considered in any patient who presents complaining of chest pain. In pneumonias involving the lower lobes, patients may complain of nothing more than upper-abdominal pain.

■ **malaise** discomfort or uneasiness often associated with disease.

On physical examination there is often fever, tachycardia, and a cough. Respiratory distress may be present. Auscultation of the chest may reveal wheezes, rhonchi, or rales. There usually is decreased air movement in consolidated (filled with infection) areas.

Management. Pneumonia is generally diagnosed on the basis of physical examination, x-ray, and laboratory cultures, making diagnosis in the field unlikely. The primary treatment is antibiotics to which the causative organism is susceptible. In the field, however, antibiotics are not indicated and treatment is purely supportive. The patient should be placed in a comfortable position. Supplemental oxygen administration should be started. The medical control physician may sometimes order a breathing treatment with a β agonist because bronchospasm is often associated with pneumonia. Therefore, these drugs will often afford the patient some symptomatic relief.

Toxic Inhalation

Pathophysiology. The possibility of inhalation of products toxic to the respiratory system should be considered in any dyspneic patient. Causes of toxic inhalation include superheated air, toxic products of combustion, chemical irritants, and inhalation of steam. Each of these agents can result in upper airway obstruction due to edema and laryngospasm. Additionally, there often is associated bronchospasm and lower-airway edema. In severe inhalations, disruption of the alveolar/capillary membranes may result in life-threatening pulmonary edema.

Assessment. When assessing the patient with possible toxic inhalation exposure, it is important to determine the nature of the inhalant or the combusted material. Several products can result in the formation of corrosive acids or alkalis that irritate and damage the airway. These include:

❏ ammonia (ammonium hydroxide)
❏ nitrogen oxide (nitric acid)
❏ sulfur dioxide (sulphurous acid)
❏ sulfur trioxide (sulfuric acid)

It is also crucial to determine the duration of the exposure, whether the patient was in an enclosed area at the time of the exposure, or if he or she experienced a loss of consciousness. A history of loss of consciousness may mean that the airway became vulnerable due to loss of the airway protective mechanisms.

During physical examination particular attention should be paid to the face, mouth, and throat. Any burns or particulate matter should be noted. Next, the chest should be auscultated for the presence of any wheezes or rales. Wheezing may indicate bronchospasm, while rales may suggest pulmonary edema.

✶ The paramedic's first concern in any toxic inhalation situation is personal safety.

Management. After the safety of rescue personnel has been assured, the patient should be removed from the hazardous environment. Next, an airway should be established and maintained. The airway is often irritable and attempts at endotracheal intubation may result in laryngospasm, completely obstructing the airway. Laryngeal edema, as evidenced by hoarseness, brassy cough, and stridor, is ominous and may require prompt endotracheal intubation. Humidified oxygen at high concentration should be administered. An IV of a crystalloid solution also should be started to provide rapid venous access if required. Transport should be prompt.

Carbon Monoxide Inhalation

Pathophysiology. Carbon monoxide is an odorless, tasteless, colorless gas produced from the incomplete burning of fossil fuels. It is present in the environment in various concentrations primarily because of automotive exhaust emissions. Most poisonings occur from automobiles and home heating devices used in poorly ventilated areas. Carbon monoxide is often used in suicide attempts. It also is an occupational hazard for firefighters.

Carbon monoxide easily binds to the hemoglobin molecule. It has an affinity for hemoglobin 200 times that of oxygen. Once bound, receptor sites on the hemoglobin can no longer transport oxygen to the peripheral tissues. The result is hypoxia at the cellular level, and, ultimately, metabolic acidosis.

Assessment. When confronted by a patient suffering possible carbon-monoxide poisoning, the paramedic should determine the source of exposure, its length, and the location. Less time is required to develop a significant exposure in a closed space compared to one in an area that is fairly well ventilated.

Signs and symptoms of carbon-monoxide poisoning include headache, irritability, errors in judgment, vomiting, chest pain, confusion, agitation, loss of coordination, loss of consciousness, and even seizures. On physical examination, the skin may be cyanotic or it may be bright cherry red (a very late finding). There may be other signs of hypoxia such as peripheral cyanosis or confusion.

✶ The patient suffering carbon monoxide poisoning should initially receive as high a concentration of oxygen as possible.

Management. Upon detection of carbon-monoxide poisoning, the patient should be removed from the site of exposure. The airway should be assured and maintained. Supplemental oxygen should be administered at as high a concentration as possible. If respiratory depression is noted, respirations should be assisted. If shock is present, it should be treated. Prompt transport is essential. Hyperbaric oxygen therapy may be used in the treatment of severe carbon monoxide poisoning. Many EMS systems have protocols established whereby patients suffering carbon monoxide poisoning are transported to hospitals with hyperbaric oxygen therapy facilities. Hyperbaric oxygen increases the PaO_2, thus promoting increased oxygen uptake on parts of the hemoglobin molecule not yet bound by carbon monoxide.

Pulmonary Embolism

Pathophysiology. A pulmonary embolism is a blood clot or other particle that lodges in a pulmonary artery, effectively blocking blood flow through that vessel. Sources of pulmonary emboli include air embolism, such as can occur during the placement of a central line; fat embolism, such as can occur following a fracture; amniotic fluid embolism; and blood clots. Factors predisposing a patient to blood clots include prolonged immobilization, thrombophlebitis, use of certain medications, and atrial fibrillation.

When a pulmonary embolism occurs, the blocked blood flow through the affected artery causes the right heart to pump against increased resistance. This results in an increase in pulmonary capillary pressure. The area of the lung supplied by the occluded pulmonary vessel can no longer effectively function in gas exchange, although it is still ventilated.

Assessment. Signs and symptoms of a patient suffering a pulmonary embolism will vary, depending upon the size and location of the obstruction. The patient suffering acute pulmonary embolism may report a sudden onset of severe unexplained dyspnea which may or may not be associated with chest pain. There may be a recent history of immobilization such as hip fracture, surgery, or debilitating illness.

The physical examination may reveal labored breathing, tachypnea, and tachycardia. In massive pulmonary emboli there may be signs of right heart failure such as jugular venous distention and, in some cases, falling blood pressure.

Management. The patient suffering suspected pulmonary embolism should have an airway established and maintained. Ventilations should be assisted as required. Supplemental oxygen should be administered at the highest possible concentration. An IV of 5% dextrose in water should be established at a "to keep open" rate and immediate transport carried out.

The diagnosis of pulmonary embolism is often difficult and requires a high index of suspicion. Treatment in the hospital setting may include the use of various medications in an attempt to dissolve the clot.

Hyperventilation Syndrome

Pathophysiology. Hyperventilation syndrome is common and frequently occurs in anxious patients. The patient often senses that he cannot "catch his breath" and begins to breathe rapidly. Hyperventilation in a purely anxious patient results in the excess elimination of CO_2, causing a respiratory alkalosis.

Assessment. The paramedic may elicit a history of fatigue, nervousness, dizziness, chest pain, and numbness and tingling around the mouth, hands, and feet.

The physical examination will reveal an anxious patient with tachypnea and tachycardia. There may be spasm of the fingers and feet, the so called carpopedal spasm, also present. If the patient has a history of seizure disorder the hyperventilation episode may precipitate a seizure.

Management. The primary treatment for hyperventilation syndrome is reassurance. Mechanisms that will assist in decreasing the PCO_2, such as breath holding, or breathing into a paper bag, are discouraged in prehospital care. It is important to exclude other medical causes before determining that a patient is hyperventilating. Do not withhold oxygen.

The hyperventilating patient can often present a dilemma for prehospital personnel. Although anxiety is the most common cause of hyperventilation, other, more serious diseases, can present in exactly the same manner. For example, pulmonary embolism or acute myocardial infarction can present in much the same manner as hyperventilation syndrome. Hyperventilating patients require oxygen. Allowing them to rebreathe into a paper bag can be deadly. Many EMS systems permit paramedics to use rebreathing techniques only on physician order.

Central Nervous System Dysfunction

Pathophysiology. Central nervous system dysfunction can be a causative factor in respiratory depression and arrest. Causes include head trauma, stroke, brain tumors, and various drugs. Several medications, such as narcotics and barbiturates, make the respiratory centers in the brain less responsive to increases in $PaCO_2$. These agents also depress areas of the brain responsible for initiating respirations.

Management. In patients where central nervous system dysfunction is suspected an airway should be established and maintained. If respiratory depression is noted, or if respirations are absent, mechanical ventilation should be initiated. Supplemental oxygen should be administered. An IV of 5% dextrose in water should be established at a "to keep open" rate. Specific therapy should be directed at the underlying problem, if it is known.

Dysfunction of the Spinal Cord, Nerves, or Respiratory Muscles

Pathophysiology. Several disease processes can interfere with respiratory function. These include spinal cord trauma, polio, and myasthenia gravis. Certain tumors can also impinge on the spinal cord, depressing respiratory function. These disorders result in an inability of the respiratory muscles to contract normally, thus causing hypoventilation. Tidal and minute volume are decreased.

Management. Management of spinal cord and respiratory muscle dysfunction is purely supportive. An airway should be established and ventilatory support provided. If myasthenia gravis is present, and transport time is long, the physician may request the administration of one of several agents effective in treating such patients.

SUMMARY

Respiratory emergencies are commonly encountered in prehospital care. Recognition and treatment must be prompt. The primary treatment is to correct hypoxia. Necessary steps include establishing and maintaining the airway, assisting ventilations as required, and administering supplemental oxygen. Appropriate pharmacological agents may be subsequently ordered by the medical control physician.

FURTHER READING

GUYTON, A. C., *Textbook of Medical Physiology.* 7th ed. Philadelphia, PA: W.B. Saunders Company, 1987.

WALRAVEN, G., et. al., *Manual of Advanced Prehospital Care.* 2nd ed. Bowie, MD: Robert J. Brady Company, 1984.

21

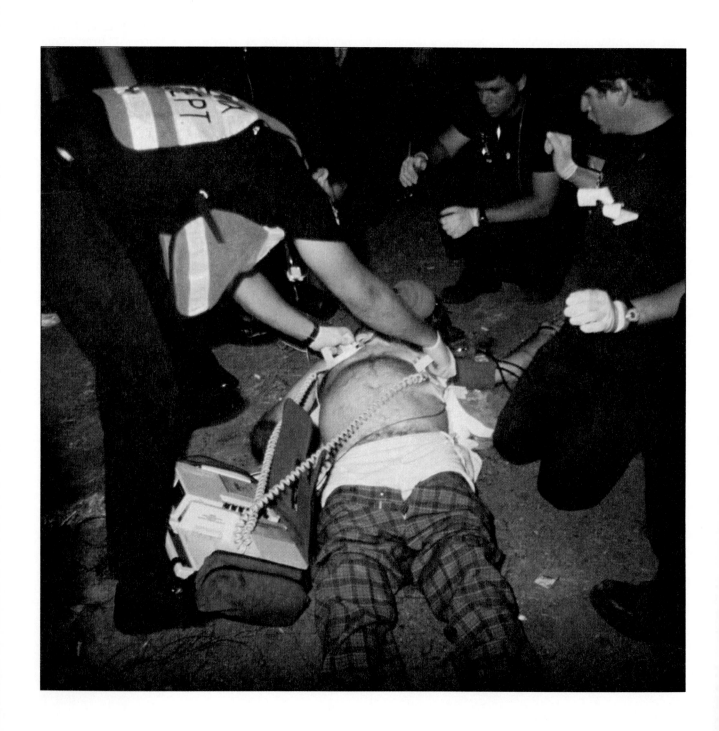

Cardiovascular Emergencies

Objectives for Chapter 21

Upon completing this chapter, the student should be able to:

1. Describe the size, shape, location, and orientation of the heart.

2. Describe the normal anatomy of the heart and peripheral circulatory system.

3. Describe the anatomy of the coronary arteries and veins.

4. Describe the differences between the structural and functional aspects of the arterial and venous systems.

5. Describe the structure and function of capillaries.

6. Describe the course of blood flow through the heart and lungs.

7. Name and describe the location of the cardiac valves.

8. Describe the cardiac cycle.

9. Define the following terms:
- afterload
- preload
- Starling's Law
- stroke volume
- cardiac output
- blood pressure

10. Describe the innervation of the heart.

11. Name major electrolytes that affect cardiac function.

12. Describe the electrical properties of the heart.

13. Describe the normal sequence of electrical conduction through the heart.

14. Describe cardiac depolarization and repolarization.

15. Define refractory period and describe the difference between the relative refractory period and the absolute refractory period.

16. Name three areas of the heart with pacemaking capabilities, and list the intrinsic rates of each.

17. Define the following:
- P wave
- QRS complex
- T wave
- U wave
- P-R interval
- QRS duration
- isoelectric line
- ST segment

18. Describe the basic concepts of ECG monitoring.

19. Explain what information can and cannot be obtained from the rhythm strip ECG.

20. Describe the grids and markings on ECG paper.

21. Name eight causes of dysrhythmias

22. Describe the etiology, ECG findings, clinical significance, and treatment for common dysrhythmias.

23. Name the common chief complaints of cardiac patients.

24. Describe appropriate history and physical assessment goals for cardiac patients.

25. Describe the pathophysiology of atherosclerosis.

26. List major risk factors for atherosclerosis.

27. Describe the pathophysiology, signs, symptoms, and management of the following patient problems:
- angina pectoris
- right ventricular failure
- pulmonary edema
- cardiac arrest
- abdominal aortic aneurysm
- acute arterial occlusion
- acute MI
- left ventricular failure
- cardiogenic shock
- electromechanical dissociation
- dissecting aortic aneurysm
- acute pulmonary embolus
- venous thrombophlebitis
- chronic peripheral arterial insufficiency
- ruptured varicose veins
- malignant hypertension

28. Describe three causes of cardiac arrest other than atherosclerotic heart disease.

29. Describe the indications for and use of:
- ECG monitoring
- rotating tourniquets
- carotid sinus massage
- defibrillation
- cardioversion
- basic life support

CASE STUDY

The crew of paramedic unit 428 was preparing to sit down to dinner when a car speeded into the station's driveway. A frantic woman ran around the parked ambulance yelling, "Help, Help!" The paramedics went to assist her. The woman saw them and yelled, "My husband is sick," pointing to the car. In the front seat of the car was an elderly man who was unresponsive and pulseless.

One paramedic pulled the patient from the car and began CPR. The other paramedic retrieved equipment from the ambulance and called the fire department for assistance. They learned that the 55-year-old patient and his wife started for the hospital when the man became nauseated. Approximately a block from the EMS station, the patient went into cardiac arrest.

Within 30 seconds, "quick look" paddles were applied to the patient's chest. The ECG revealed ventricular fibrillation. The paramedic charged the defibrillator and delivered a 200 joule shock. The ECG remained unchanged. A second 200 joule shock was delivered. The ECG still remained unchanged. A third shock was delivered at 360 joules, with the same results.

The engine company now arrived. With their help, CPR was continued, an IV started, an endotracheal tube placed, and the patient ventilated with 100 percent oxygen. The paramedic administered 1 mg of epinephrine intravenously. A fourth shock was delivered at 360 joules. This converted the patient to an idioventricular rhythm, which subsequently improved to a sinus tachycardia with a pulse. The patient's blood pressure was 110 by palpation. The ECG showed a few PVCs developing, and the paramedics administered 100 mg of lidocaine and began a lidocaine drip at 2 milligrams per minute.

The patient was subsequently transported to the hospital. He never regained spontaneous respirations in the ambulance. At the hospital, the patient was placed on a ventilator in the CCU. Cardiac enzyme studies and a 12-lead ECG confirmed the presence of an anterior wall myocardial infarction. The patient slowly improved and was weaned from the ventilator. He subsequently underwent cardiac rehabilitation and was discharged home on three different medications.

INTRODUCTION

■ **cardiovascular disease** diseases affecting the heart, peripheral blood vessels, or both.

✱ Cardiovascular disease is the number one cause of death in the United States.

Cardiovascular disease is a major cause of death and disability in the United States. It was with this in mind that emergency medical services, as we know it today, was developed. It has been shown that many patients suffering cardiovascular emergencies, especially heart attacks, die within the first hour after the onset of symptoms, many before they can arrive at the hospital. Prompt, definitive intervention has proven effective in preventing many of these deaths.

This chapter will discuss, in detail, advanced prehospital care of cardiovascular emergencies. First, we will review the pertinent anatomy and physiology. This will be followed by discussion of ECG monitoring, patient assessment, and recognition and treatment of cardiovascular disorders.

ANATOMY AND PHYSIOLOGY

The *cardiovascular system* includes two components, the heart and the peripheral blood vessels. Prehospital personnel must thoroughly understand the anatomy and physiology of each.

Anatomy of the Heart

The *heart* is a four-chambered muscular organ, approximately the size of a man's closed fist. It is located in the center of the chest in the mediastinum. (See Figure 21-1.) Approximately two-thirds of its mass is located to the left of the midline, with the remainder located to the right. It lies anterior to the spinal column and posterior to the sternum. The lower border of the heart, which forms a blunt point, is called the *apex.* The apex is positioned immediately above the diaphragm to the left of the midline. The top portion of the heart, referred to as the *base,* is located at approximately the level of the second rib. The great vessels enter the heart though the base.

The heart consists of several readily identifiable layers. (See Figure 21-2.) Surrounding the heart is a protective sac, the *pericardium.* The pericardium consists of two layers, the *visceral pericardium* and the *parietal pericardium.* The visceral pericardium is the layer in contact with the heart muscle itself, and the parietal pericardium is the outer, fibrous layer. Situated between the two layers is *pericardial fluid,* which acts as a lubricant during cardiac contraction. Generally, only a scant amount of pericardial fluid is present. However, during certain disease states, and with certain injuries, the pericardial sac becomes filled with blood or fluid, which can adversely affect cardiac output.

The outermost lining of the heart, the *epicardium,* is **contiguous** with the visceral pericardium. The thick middle layer of heart wall, con-

■ **contiguous** in contact or closely related.

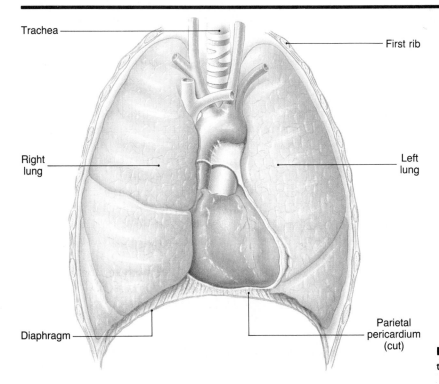

Trachea

First rib

Right lung

Left lung

Diaphragm

Parietal pericardium (cut)

FIGURE 21-1 Location of the heart within the chest.

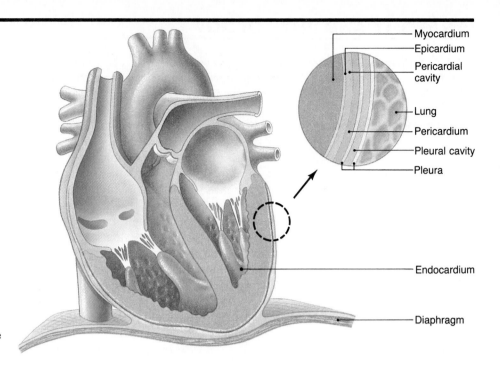

FIGURE 21-2 Layers of the heart.

taining the bulk of the muscle mass, is the *myocardium*. The innermost layer, which lines the chambers, is the *endocardium*.

The myocardial muscle cells are unique. They physically resemble skeletal muscle, but they have electrical properties like smooth muscle. Within the myocardial cells are specialized structures which promote the rapid spread of the myocardial electrical impulse from one muscle cell to another.

The heart contains four chambers. (See Figure 21-3.) The two superior chambers, which receive incoming blood, are called *atria*. The larger, inferior chambers are called the *ventricles*. The right and left atria are separated by the *interatrial septum*. The ventricles are separated by the *interventricular septum*. Both septa contain fibrous connective tissue as well as contractile muscle. The walls of the atria are much thinner than those of the ventricles and do not contribute significantly to the heart's pumping action.

The right atrium receives blood from the periphery of the body via the superior and inferior vena cavae. (See Figure 21-4.) The left atrium receives incoming oxygenated blood from the lungs via the pulmonary veins. The ventricles receive blood from the atria and in turn pump the blood out of the heart. The right ventricle receives blood from the right atrium and pumps it to the lungs through the pulmonary arteries. The right side of the heart is a low-pressure pump, because the pulmonary circulation does not offer a great deal of resistance. As a result, the *myocardial muscle mass,* or thickness, is significantly less on the right than on the left.

The left ventricle receives blood from the left atrium and pumps it out of the heart into the aorta. The left side of the heart is a high-pressure pump, because of the high level of resistance present in the peripheral circulation.

The heart contains two sets of valves. (See Figure 21-5.) Both sets are made of endocardial as well as connective tissue. The *atrioventricular (AV) valves* are those between the atria and the ventricles. The valve sepa-

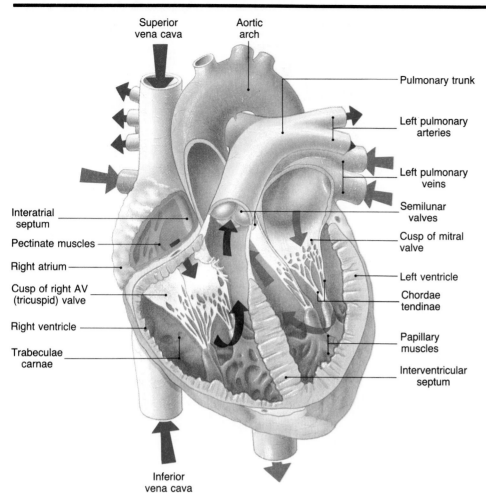

Superior
vena cava

Aortic
arch

Pulmonary trunk

Left pulmonary
arteries

Left pulmonary
veins

Semilunar
valves

Cusp of mitral
valve

Left ventricle

Chordae
tendinae

Papillary
muscles

Interventricular
septum

Interatrial
septum

Pectinate muscles

Right atrium

Cusp of right AV
(tricuspid) valve

Right ventricle

Trabeculae
carnae

Inferior
vena cava

FIGURE 21-3   Blood flow
through the heart.

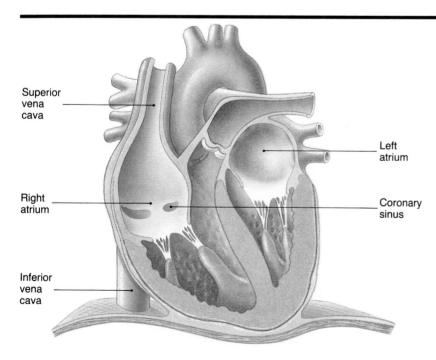

Superior
vena
cava

Right
atrium

Inferior
vena
cava

Left
atrium

Coronary
sinus

FIGURE 21-4   The chambers of the heart.

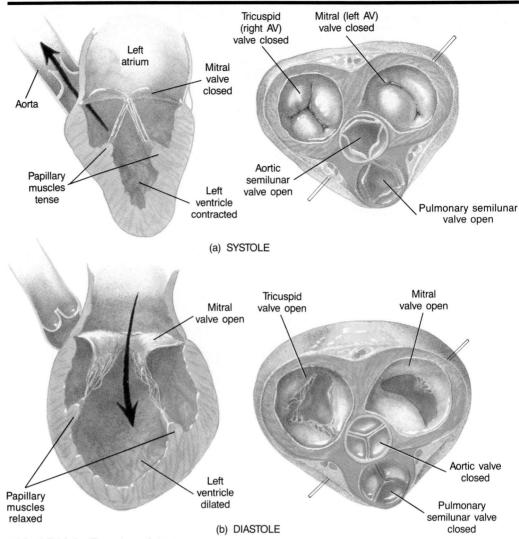

Tricuspid
(right AV)
valve closed

Mitral (left AV)
valve closed

Left
atrium

Mitral
valve
closed

Aorta

Papillary
muscles
tense

Aortic
semilunar
valve open

Left
ventricle
contracted

Pulmonary semilunar
valve open

(a) SYSTOLE

Tricuspid
valve open

Mitral
valve open

Mitral
valve open

Papillary
muscles
relaxed

Left
ventricle
dilated

Aortic valve
closed

Pulmonary
semilunar valve
closed

(b) DIASTOLE

FIGURE 21-5 The valves of the heart.

rating the right atrium from the right ventricle is the *tricuspid valve.*
The tricuspid valve contains three distinct leaflets. The *mitral valve* separates the left atrium from the left ventricle and contains only two leaflets.
The valve leaflets are connected to specialized muscles in the ventricles
called *papillary muscles.* These muscles, when relaxed, open the valves
and allow blood to flow between the two chambers. Specialized fibers called
chordae tendonae connect the leaflets to the papillary muscles. These fibers prevent the valves from prolapsing into the atria during ventricular
contraction.

The *semilunar valves* are located between the ventricles and the arteries into which they empty. The *pulmonic valve* is between the right
ventricle and the pulmonary artery. The *aortic valve* is between the left
ventricle and the aorta. These valves prevent the backflow of blood into
the ventricles during diastole.

The *great vessels* are the largest blood vessels in the body. They are
attached to the base of the heart and transport blood both to and from the
heart. Deoxygenated blood enters the heart through the *vena cava.* The
superior vena cava receives blood from the head and upper extremities,
and the *inferior vena cava* receives blood from areas below the heart. De-

oxygenated blood continues through the right side of the heart until it is emptied into the *pulmonary artery,* which transports it to the lungs for oxygenation. Oxygenated blood then returns to the heart, from the lungs, via the four *pulmonary veins.* The pulmonary veins deliver blood to the left atrium. Oxygenated blood ultimately leaves the heart via the aorta.

The heart is richly supplied with blood vessels, which transport nutrients and oxygen to the cardiac muscle and electrical conductive system. (See Figure 21-6.) These vessels, referred to as the *coronary arteries,* originate in the aorta just above the leaflets of the aortic valve. The main coronary arteries lie on the surface of the heart. Blood is supplied to the myocardial muscle mass through small penetrating arterioles. The *left coronary artery* supplies the left ventricle, the interventricular septum, and part of the right ventricle. The two major branches of the left coronary artery are the *anterior descending artery* and the *circumflex artery.* The *right coronary artery* supplies a portion of the right atrium and ventricle and part of the conduction system. The two major branches of the right coronary artery are the *posterior descending artery* and the *marginal artery.* The many **anastomoses** between the various branches of the coronary arteries allow for the development of collateral circulation. *Collateral circulation* is a protective mechanism which allows for an alternate path of blood flow in the event of vascular occlusion. The coronary vessels receive blood during diastole as the aortic valve leaflets cover the arterial openings during systole.

Deoxygenated blood is removed from the heart through the *coronary veins.* The major vein draining the left ventricle is the *coronary sinus.* The coronary veins roughly correspond to the coronary arteries and drain into the right atrium.

■ **anastomosis** a communication between two or more vessels.

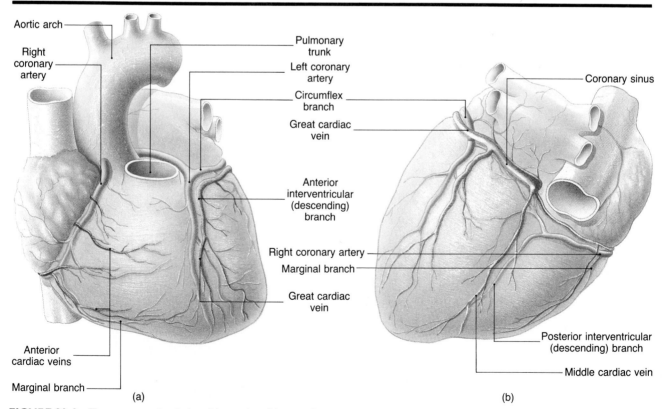

FIGURE 21-6   The coronary circulation: (a) anterior; (b) posterior.

Anatomy of Peripheral Circulation

The *peripheral circulation* transports oxygenated blood from the heart to the tissues and subsequently transports deoxygenated blood back to the heart. Oxygenated blood leaves the heart via the arterial system, while deoxygenated blood returns to the heart via the venous system.

The vessels of the peripheral circulation are made up of several layers. (See Figure 21-7.) The innermost lining of the blood vessels, the *tunica intima*, is a single cell layer thick. The middle layer, the *tunica media*, consists of elastic fibers and muscle. This layer gives blood vessels their strength and recoil, which results from the difference in pressure inside and outside the vessel. The tunica media is much thicker in arteries than in veins. The outermost lining is a fibrous tissue covering called the *tunica adventitia*. It provides the vessel with strength to withstand the pressures generated by the contraction of the heart. The *lumen* of a vessel is the cavity inside it. The diameter of vessels varies significantly. The amount of blood a vessel can transport is directly related to its diameter. The larger the diameter, the greater the blood flow. In fact, blood flow increases in direct proportion to the fourth power of the diameter of the vessel. For example, a vessel with a relative diameter of 1 would transport 1 mL per minute of blood at a pressure difference of 100 mmHg. If the vessel diameter was increased to 4, keeping the pressure difference constant, the flow would increase to 256 mL (4^4) per minute. This relationship is represented by **Poiseuille's Law,** which states that the blood flow through a vessel is directly proportional to the fourth power of the vessel's radius.

■ Poiseuille's Law a law of physiology that states that blood flow through a vessel is directly proportional to the radius of the vessel to the fourth power.

Arteries. The *arterial system*, which carries blood from the heart, functions under high pressure. The larger arterial vessels are called *arteries*. The arteries eventually branch into smaller structures called *arterioles*. The arterioles, the smallest branches of the arterial tree, control blood flow to various organs by their degree of resistance. The arterioles continue to divide until they become *capillaries*, which are the points of con-

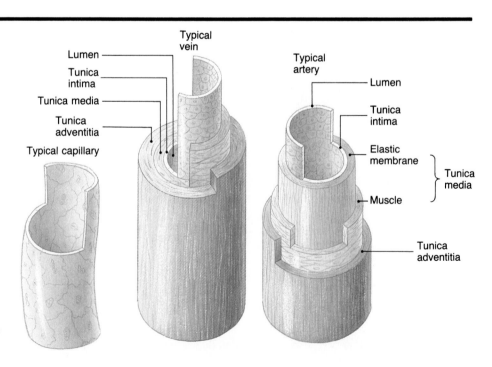

FIGURE 21-7 The layers of the peripheral arteries.

nection between the arterial and venous systems. The walls of the capillaries are a single cell layer thick, which allows for exchange of gasses, fluid, and nutrients between the vascular system and the tissues.

Veins. The *venous system* transports blood back to the heart from the peripheral tissues. It functions under low pressure. Blood flow is aided by the action of surrounding muscles and by the presence of one-way valves within the veins. Blood enters the venous system through the capillaries. The capillaries then drain into the *venules*. The venules then drain into the *veins,* which ultimately drain into the vena cava, which returns the blood to the heart.

Physiology of Circulation

It is important for the paramedic to understand the pathway of normal blood flow through the heart. The superior and inferior vena cava return blood from the body to the right atrium. The blood then leaves the right atrium, through the tricuspid valve, and enters the right ventricle. The right ventricle contracts, forcing blood through the pulmonary valve into the pulmonary arteries. The blood is transported, through the pulmonary arteries, to the lungs. The pulmonary arteries then divide, until they terminate as the pulmonary capillaries. In the pulmonary capillaries, the blood takes in oxygen and gives off carbon dioxide.

Oxygenated blood then leaves the pulmonary capillaries and enters the pulmonary veins, which ultimately deliver the blood to the left atrium. Blood leaves the left atrium through the mitral valve and enters the left ventricle. The left ventricle then contracts, forcing blood through the aortic valve and into the aorta. From the aorta, blood is supplied to the coronary arteries and peripheral circulation.

Although the heart is functionally divided into the right and left sides, it functions as a unit. For example, the right and left atria contract at the same time, filling both ventricles to their maximum capacities. Subsequently, both ventricles contract at the same time, ejecting blood into both the pulmonary and systemic circulations. The pressure of the contraction causes the tricuspid and mitral valves to close and the aortic and pulmonic valves to open at the same time.

The period from the end of one heart contraction until the end of the next is referred to as the **cardiac cycle.** The first phase of the cardiac cycle, **diastole,** is the phase at which ventricular filling begins. This is the relaxation phase. Diastole is much longer than systole, the contraction phase (0.52 second compared to 0.28 second). During diastole, most cardiac filling occurs and the coronary arteries are filled. As the heart rate increases, the length of diastole decreases and the length of systole decreases as well, although to a lesser degree. **Systole,** also referred to as *ventricular contraction,* is the phase during which blood is ejected from the heart.

The amount of blood ejected from the left and right ventricles is exactly the same. However, the resistance against which each ventricle must pump is different. The right ventricle pumps only against the resistance of the pulmonary system and is thus a low-pressure system. The left ventricle must pump against the entire systemic circulation and is a high-pressure system.

The amount of blood ejected from each ventricle during one contraction is called the **stroke volume.** (See Figure 21-8.) The average stroke volume is 60–100 mL, although this capacity can increase significantly in a healthy heart. The stroke volume is a reflection of three factors: pre-

■ **cardiac cycle** the period of time from the end of one cardiac contraction to the end of the next.

■ **diastole** the period of time when the myocardium is relaxed and cardiac filling and coronary perfusion occur.

■ **systole** the period of the cardiac cycle when the myocardium is contracting.

■ **stroke volume** the amount of blood ejected by the heart in one cardiac contraction.

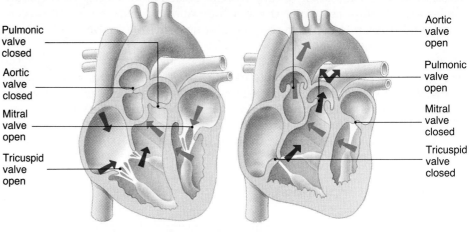

Pulmonic valve closed

Aortic valve closed

Mitral valve open

Tricuspid valve open

Aortic valve open

Pulmonic valve open

Mitral valve closed

Tricuspid valve closed

DIASTOLIC PHASE   SYSTOLIC PHASE

FIGURE 21-8 Relation of blood flow to cardiac contraction.

■ **preload** the pressure within the ventricles at the end of diastole, commonly called the end-diastolic volume.

■ **Starling's Law of the Heart** law of physiology which states that the more the myocardium is stretched, up to a certain amount, the more forceful the subsequent contraction will be.

■ **afterload** the resistance against which the heart must pump.

■ **cardiac output** the amount of blood pumped by the heart in 1 minute.

load, cardiac contractility, and afterload. Each ventricle can pump out only what it receives from the venous system. The ventricles fill during diastole. The pressure in the ventricle at the end of diastole is referred to as **preload,** or *end-diastolic volume.* Preload influences the force of the next contraction, which is based on **Starling's Law of the Heart,** which states that the more the myocardial muscle is stretched, up to a limit, the greater its force of contraction will be. In other words, the greater the volume of blood filling the chamber, the more forceful the cardiac contraction. Therefore, the greater the venous return, the greater the preload and the greater the stroke volume.

In addition, the pressure against which the ventricle must pump also affects stroke volume. The greater the resistance, the less the stroke volume. The resistance against which the ventricle must contract is called the **afterload.** An increase in peripheral vascular resistance will decrease stroke volume. Conversely, a decrease in peripheral vascular resistance, up to a point, will increase stroke volume.

Cardiac output is also related to stroke volume. **Cardiac output** can be defined as the volume of blood pumped by the heart in 1 minute. It is a function of stroke volume and heart rate, as shown in the following formula:

Stroke Volume (mL) × Heart Rate (bpm) = Cardiac Output (mL/min)

The normal heart rate is 60–100 beats per minute, and average stroke volume is 70 mL. Thus an average cardiac output is 5 L per minute:

Stroke Volume × Heart Rate = Cardiac Output
(70 mL)   ×   (70 bpm) = (4900 mL/min)

Blood pressure is directly related to cardiac output and peripheral resistance, as shown in this formula:

Blood Pressure = Cardiac Output × Systemic Vascular Resistance

In other words, if the peripheral resistance is kept constant and cardiac output is increased, blood pressure will increase. Conversely, if peripheral resistance is kept constant and cardiac output decreases, blood pressure will fall. Because of the body's compensatory mechanisms, these changes generally occur only in very sick patients. For example, if cardiac output falls, as can occur after myocardial infarction, the baroreceptors detect this change and increase peripheral vascular resistance to maintain blood pressure. In addition, the heart is stimulated to increase its rate, contractile state, or both to help correct the deficit in cardiac output.

Nervous Control of the Heart

The heart is regulated by both the sympathetic and parasympathetic components of the autonomic nervous system. (See Figure 21-9.) The sympathetic nervous system innervates the heart through the *cardiac plexus.* The sympathetic nerves arise from the thoracic and lumbar regions of the spinal cord. These nerves leave the spinal cord and form the sympathetic chain, which runs alongside the spinal column. The cardiac plexus arises from ganglia in the sympathetic chain and innervates both the atria and

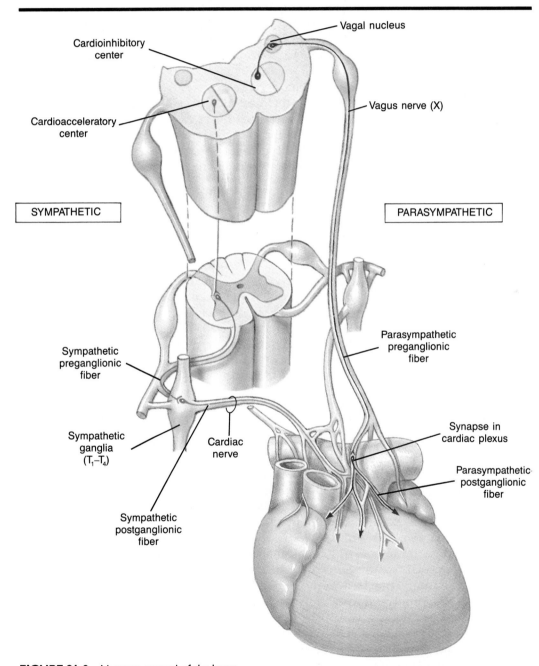

FIGURE 21-9 Nervous control of the heart.

ventricles. The chemical neurotransmitter for the sympathetic nervous system, and thus for the cardiac plexus, is *norepinephrine.* Release of norepinephrine causes an increase in heart rate and cardiac contractile force, primarily through its actions on beta receptors.

Parasympathetic control of the heart occurs through the *vagus nerve,* the tenth cranial nerve. The vagus nerve descends from the brain to innervate the heart and other organs. Vagal nerve fibers primarily innervate the atria, although some fibers innervate the upper portion of the ventricles. The neurotransmitter for the parasympathetic nervous system, and thus the vagus nerve, is *acetylcholine.* Release of acetylcholine slows the heart rate and slows atrioventricular conduction. Several maneuvers can cause stimulation of the vagus nerve. These include Valsalva (straining against a closed glottis), pressure on the carotid sinus, and distention of the urinary bladder.

The two cardiac control systems, the sympathetic and parasympathetic, are in direct opposition to one another. The normal state is a balance between the two. In stressful situations, the sympathetic system becomes dominant. However, parasympathetic control dominates during sleep.

■ **chronotropy** pertaining to heart rate.

The term **chronotropy** refers to heart rate. A drug or agent that is a *positive chronotropic agent* is one that increases heart rate. Conversely, a *negative chronotropic agent* decreases heart rate. The term **inotropy** refers to the strength of a muscular contraction of the heart. Thus, a *positive inotropic agent* is one that increases the strength of the cardiac contraction, and a *negative inotropic agent* is one that decreases it.

■ **inotropy** pertaining to cardiac contractile force.

Role of Electrolytes

Cardiac function, both electrical and mechanical, is strongly influenced by electrolyte imbalance. Electrolytes that affect cardiac function include sodium (Na^+), calcium (Ca^{++}), and potassium (K^+). Sodium plays a major role in depolarization of the myocardium. Calcium plays a role in myocardial depolarization and myocardial contraction. Hypercalcemia can result in increased contractility, whereas hypocalcemia has been associated with decreased myocardial contractility and increased electrical irritability. Potassium plays a major role in repolarization. Hyperkalemia results in decreased automaticity and conduction, whereas hypokalemia causes increased irritability.

Electrophysiology

The heart is composed of three types of cardiac muscle: atrial muscle, ventricular muscle, and specialized excitatory and conductive muscle fibers. The atrial and ventricular fibers contract in the same way as does skeletal muscle. However, there is a major difference. Within the cardiac muscle fibers are special structures, the **intercalated discs.** (See Figure 21-10.) These discs connect cardiac muscle fibers and conduct electrical impulses quickly from one muscle fiber to the next. The intercalated discs conduct electrical impulses 400 times faster than the standard cell membrane. This special feature allows cardiac muscle cells to function together in a **syncytium.** That is, when one cell becomes excited, the action potential spreads rapidly across the entire group of cells, resulting in a coordinated contraction.

■ **intercalated discs** specialized band of tissue inserted between myocardial cells that increase the rate in which the action potential is spread from cell to cell.

■ **syncytium** group of cardiac muscle cells which physiologically function as a unit.

Within the heart are two syncytia, the atrial syncytium and the ventricular syncytium. The *atrial syncytium* contracts in a superior-to-inferior direction, so that blood is expressed from the atria to the ventricles.

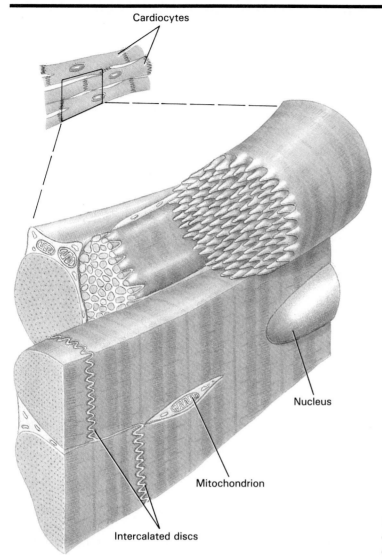

Cardiocytes

Nucleus

Mitochondrion

Intercalated discs

FIGURE 21-10 Microscopic appearance of cardiac muscle. The intercalated discs speed transmission of the electrical potential quickly from one cell to the next.

The *ventricular syncytium,* on the other hand, contracts in an inferior-to-posterior direction, expelling blood from the ventricles into the aorta and pulmonary arteries. The two syncytia are separated from one another by the fibrous structure which supports the valves and physically separates the atria from the ventricles. The only way an impulse can be conducted from the atria to the ventricles is through the *atrioventricular (AV) bundle.* Cardiac muscle functions according to an "all or none" principle. That is, if a single muscle fiber becomes depolarized, the action potential will spread through the whole syncytium. Stimulation of an atrial fiber will cause complete depolarization of the atria, and stimulation of a ventricular fiber will cause complete depolarization of the ventricles.

Cardiac Depolarization. The concept of *cardiac depolarization* is essential to the interpretation of electrocardiograms (ECGs). Normally, there is an ionic difference on the two sides of a cell membrane. Sodium (Na^+) is actively pumped out of the cell membrane by the sodium-potassium pump. This causes more negatively charged anions to remain inside the cell than positively charged cations, which results in a difference in voltage across the cell membrane. Thus the inside of the cell is more negatively charged than the outside. This difference, referred to as the **resting po-**

■ **resting potential** the normal electrical state of cardiac cells.

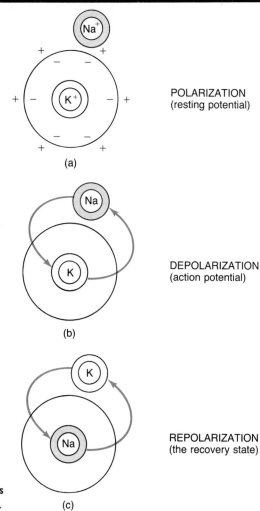

POLARIZATION
(resting potential)

(a)

DEPOLARIZATION
(action potential)

(b)

REPOLARIZATION
(the recovery state)

(c)

FIGURE 21-11 Schematic of ion shifts during depolarization and repolarization.

tential, can be measured experimentally by placing one probe inside the cell and another outside the cell and determining the difference in millivolts. In the resting myocardial cell, the difference is approximately —90 mV. (See Figure 21-11.)

When the myocardial cell is stimulated, the membrane surrounding the cell changes instantaneously to allow sodium ions to rush into the cell, bringing their positive charge. This charge is so strong that it causes the normal negative resting potential to disappear completely. In fact, it causes the inside of the cell to become positively charged at approximately +20 mV as compared to the outside. This influx of sodium and change of membrane polarity is referred to as the **action potential.** After the influx of sodium, there is a slower influx of calcium ions (Ca^{++}) through the calcium channels, which causes the inside of the cell to become even more positive. Once depolarization occurs in a muscle fiber, it is transmitted throughout the entire syncytium, via the intercalated discs, until the entire muscle mass is depolarized. Contraction of the muscle follows depolarization.

The cell membrane remains permeable to sodium for only a fraction of a second. Thereafter, sodium influx stops and potassium escapes from inside the cell, causing a change in the charge inside the cell back to a negative value. In addition, sodium is actively pumped outside, and the cell returns to its normal resting state. This return to the resting state is called **repolarization.**

■ **action potential** the stimulation of myocardial cells, as evidenced by a change in the membrane electrical charge, which subsequently is spread across the myocardium.

■ **repolarization** the return of the muscle cell to its pre-excitation resting state.

Cardiac Conductive System. The description above applies generally to cardiac muscle in both the atrial and ventricular syncytia. However, another type of cardiac muscle fiber has not yet been discussed: the conductive fibers. The *conductive fibers* of the heart are specialized muscle cells which are designed to transmit the depolarization potential quickly through the heart, much more quickly than the impulse could be conducted through regular myocardial cells. The conductive system stimulates the ventricles to depolarize in the proper direction. As mentioned above, the atria contract in a superior-to-inferior direction, and the ventricles contract in an inferior-to-superior direction. This allows blood to flow in the proper direction. If the depolarization impulse originated in the atria and was allowed to spread passively to the ventricles, then ventricular depolarization would occur in a superior-to-inferior direction and would be ineffective. The purpose of the conduction system, therefore, is to initiate an impulse, spread it through the atria, transmit it quickly to the apex of the heart, and there stimulate the ventricles to depolarize in an inferior-to-superior direction. (See Figure 21-12.)

The cells of the cardiac conductive system have several important properties. First, they have *excitability*. That is, they can respond to an electrical stimulus, like all other myocardial cells. Second, they have *conductivity*. They can propagate the electrical impulse from one cell to another. Finally, they have the unique property of *self-excitation*. That is, an individual conductive cell is capable of self-depolarization, without an impulse from an outside source. This property, shared by all cells of the conductive system, is called **automaticity**. Generally, the cell in the cardiac conductive system with the fastest rate of discharge, or automaticity, becomes the pacemaker of the heart. As a rule, the highest cell in the conductive system has the fastest rate of automaticity. Normally, this cell is in the *sinoatrial (SA) node,* which is located high in the right atrium. However, if a cell of the conductive system fails to discharge and depolarize, the cell with the next fastest rate becomes the pacemaker.

Knowledge of the anatomy of the cardiac conductive system is essential to understanding ECG readings. The SA node, located high in the right atrium, is connected to the AV node by the *internodal pathways.* The internodal pathways conduct the depolarization impulse to the atrial muscle mass and, through the atria, to the AV junction. The impulse is slowed at the AV junction to allow time for ventricular filling. Then, as

■ **automaticity** the capability of self-depolarization. Refers to the pacemaker cells of the heart.

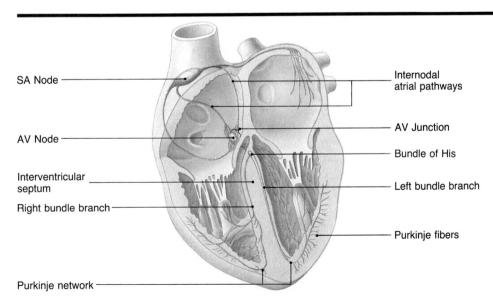

SA Node

Internodal atrial pathways

AV Node

AV Junction

Bundle of His

Interventricular septum

Left bundle branch

Right bundle branch

Purkinje fibers

Purkinje network

FIGURE 21-12 The cardiac conductive system.

the impulse passes through the AV junction, it enters the AV node. The AV node is connected to the AV fibers, which conduct the impulse from the atria to the ventricles. The AV fibers then become the *bundle of His,* which transmits the impulse through the interventricular septum.

The bundle of His subsequently divides into the right and left bundle branches. The *right bundle branch* delivers the impulse to the apex of the right ventricle, where it is spread across the myocardium by the *Purkinje system.* At the same time, the impulse is carried into the left bundle branch. The left bundle branch divides into the *anterior and posterior fascicles,* which ultimately terminate into the Purkinje system. At the same time the impulse is transmitted to the right ventricle, the Purkinje system spreads it across the mass of the myocardium. Repolarization predominantly occurs in the opposite direction.

Each component of the conductive system has its own intrinsic rate of self-excitation. These are:

SA node = 60–100 beats per minute

AV node = 40–60 beats per minute

Purkinje system = 20–40 beats per minute

RECOGNITION OF DYSRHYTHMIAS

Introduction to ECG Monitoring

Interpretation of ECGs is a fundamental paramedic skill. Although most EMS systems have the capability of telemetry, so that the ECG reading can be verified by the medical control physician, the paramedic is still the person who must interpret the tracing.

This section will address ECG monitoring and recognition and interpretation of dysrhythmias. This text presents basic information. ECG interpretation is a skill that can be mastered only through classroom instruction and repeated practice.

The Electrocardiogram. The **electrocardiogram (ECG),** is a graphic record of the electrical activity of the heart. It tells you nothing whatsoever about the heart's pumping ability. The heart is the largest generator of electrical energy in the body. The body acts as a giant conductor of electricity, and its electrical activity can be sensed by electrodes placed on the skin. These electrodes detect the total amount of electrical activity occurring within the heart at a given time.

The ECG machine records the positive and negative electrical impulses from the heart over time. Positive impulses are recorded as upward deflections on the paper, and negative impulses as downward deflections. The absence of any electrical impulse results in the recording of an *isoelectric line,* which is a flat line.

The electrical impulses present on the skin surface are of very low voltage. These impulses are amplified by the ECG machine and recorded on ECG graph paper or on an oscilloscope.

ECG Leads. The paramedic can obtain many views of the heart's electrical activity by monitoring the voltage change through various electrodes placed on the body surface. Each pair of electrodes is referred to as a lead. Normally, in the hospital, 12 leads are used. In the field, however, only 3 leads are generally available. One lead is adequate for detecting life-

✱ The paramedic must be capable of interpreting all rhythm strips, relying only on medical control when a question regarding interpretation arises.

■ **electrocardiogram (ECG)** the graphic recording of the heart's electrical activity. It may be displayed either on paper or on an oscilloscope.

threatening dysrhythmias. Discussion of the 12-lead ECG is not within the scope of this text, although the concept of 12-lead ECG monitoring will be briefly presented.

There are three types of ECG leads: bipolar leads, augmented leads, and precordial leads. A *bipolar lead,* the kind most frequently used, has 1 positive electrode and 1 negative electrode. On a bipolar lead, any electrical impulse within the body moving toward the positive electrode will cause a positive deflection on the ECG paper. Any electrical impulse moving toward the negative electrode will cause a negative deflection. The absence of a positive or negative deflection means either that there is no electrical impulse or that the impulse is moving perpendicular to the lead. Leads I, II, and III, commonly called *limb leads,* are bipolar leads and are the most frequently used in the field.

The electrodes of the three bipolar leads are placed in the following areas of the body:

Lead	Positive Electrode	Negative Electrode
I	left arm	right arm
II	left leg	right arm
III	left leg	left arm

These three leads form a triangle around the heart, referred to as *Einthoven's triangle.* (See Figure 21-13.) The direction from the negative

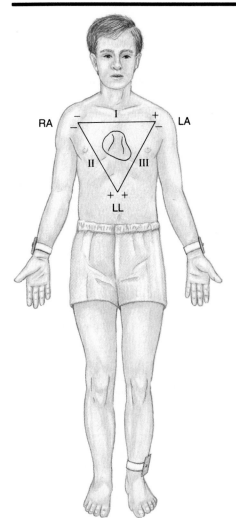

FIGURE 21-13 Einthoven's triangle as formed by Leads I, II, and III.

to the positive electrode is referred to as the *axis* of the lead. Each lead is designed to look at a different axis of the heart. Lead I forms the top of Einthoven's triangle and is said to have an axis of 0°. Lead II forms the right side of the triangle and has an axis of 60°, while Lead III forms the left side of the triangle and has an axis of 120°.

The bipolar leads provide only three views of the heart. Because additional views are sometimes useful, *augmented,* or *unipolar leads,* were developed. These leads evaluate different axes than the bipolar leads but utilize the same set of electrodes. They do this by electronically combining the negative electrodes of two of the bipolar leads to obtain an axis that is in between. The augmented leads are designated aVR, aVL, and aVF.

The six leads described so far can be obtained by using three standard electrodes. In addition, the *precordial leads* can be placed across the surface of the chest to measure electrical cardiac activity in a horizontal axis. These leads are helpful in viewing the left ventricle and septum. The precordial leads are designated V1 through V6.

Routine ECG Monitoring. In routine monitoring, whether in the ambulance, emergency department, or coronary care unit, only one lead is used, most commonly Lead II. (See Figure 21-14.) Considerable information can be obtained from a single monitoring lead. This includes:

❑ How fast the heart is beating.
❑ How regular the heartbeat is.
❑ How long it is taking to conduct the impulse through the various parts of the heart.

The following information CANNOT be obtained from a single lead:

❑ The presence or location of an infarct.
❑ Axis deviation or chamber enlargement.
❑ Right-to-left differences in conduction or impulse formation.
❑ The quality or presence of pumping action.

ECG Graph Paper. The ECG graph paper is standardized to allow comparative analysis of ECG patterns. (See Figure 21-15.) The paper moves across the stylus at a standard speed of 25 mm/sec. The amplitude of the ECG deflection is also standardized. When properly calibrated, the ECG stylus should deflect two large boxes when 1 mV of current is present.

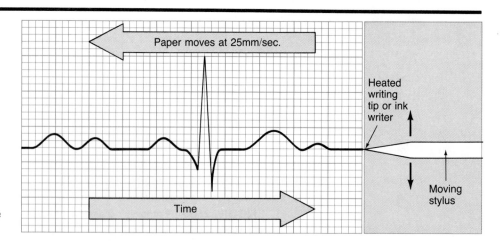

Paper moves at 25mm/sec.

Heated writing tip or ink writer

Moving stylus

Time

FIGURE 21-14 Recording of the ECG.

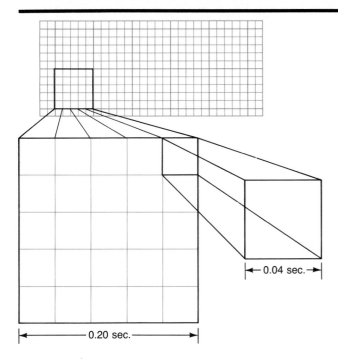

FIGURE 21-15 The ECG paper and markings.

Most machines have calibration buttons, and a calibration curve should be placed at the beginning of the first ECG strip.

The horizontal axis represents time, and the vertical axis represents voltage. The ECG paper is divided into small and large boxes. There are 5 small boxes in a large box. The following relationships hold for the horizontal axis:

$$1 \text{ small box} = 0.04 \text{ sec}$$

$$1 \text{ large box} = 0.20 \text{ sec } (0.04 \times 5 = 0.20)$$

These increments are used to measure the duration of the ECG complexes and time intervals. The vertical axis reflects the voltage amplitude in millivolts. Two large boxes equal 1 mV.

In addition to the grid, ECG paper has time interval markings at the top. These marks are placed at 3-second intervals. Each 3-second interval contains 15 large boxes (0.2 sec × 15 boxes = 3 sec). The time markings are used to calculate heart rate.

Relationship of the ECG to Electrical Events in the Heart. The ECG tracing has specific components which reflect electrical changes in the heart. (See Figure 21-16.) The first component of the ECG, corresponding to depolarization of the atria, is called the *P wave*. On Lead II it is a positive, rounded wave which precedes the QRS complex. The *QRS complex* reflects ventricular depolarization. The *Q wave* is the first negative deflection after the P wave. The *R wave* is the first positive deflection after the P wave, and the *S wave* is the first negative deflection after the R wave. All three waves are not always present, and the shape of the QRS complex can vary from individual to individual.

The next wave, which is normally positive in Lead II, is the *T wave*. The T wave is rounded and usually moves in the same direction as the QRS complex. The T wave reflects repolarization of the ventricles. Occasionally a *U wave* can be seen. This follows the T wave and is usually positive. The U wave may be associated with electrolyte abnormalities or may be a normal finding.

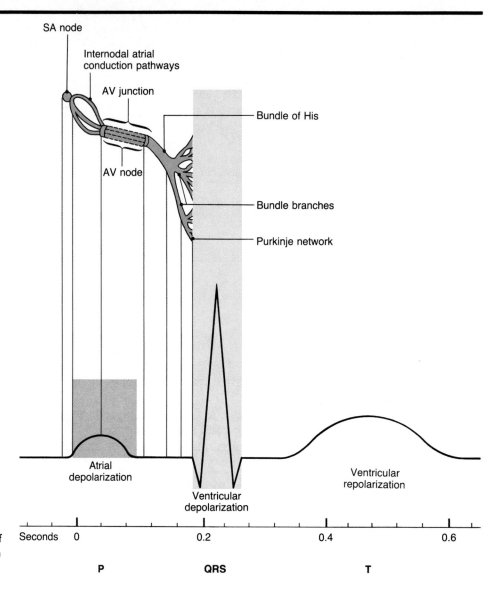

FIGURE 21-16 Relationship of the ECG to electrical activities in the heart.

SA node

Internodal atrial conduction pathways

AV junction

Bundle of His

AV node

Bundle branches

Purkinje network

Atrial depolarization

Ventricular depolarization

Ventricular repolarization

Seconds   0   0.2   0.4   0.6

P   QRS   T

■ **refractory period** the period of time when myocardial cells have not yet completely repolarized and cannot be stimulated again.

■ **absolute refractory period** the period of the cardiac cycle when stimulation will not produce any depolarization whatever.

■ **relative refractory period** the period of the cardiac cycle when a sufficiently strong stimulus may produce depolarization.

In addition to the wave forms described above, the ECG tracing reflects important time intervals. The distance from the beginning of the P wave to the beginning of the QRS complex is called the *P-R interval.* This represents the time necessary for the impulse to be transmitted from the atria to the ventricles. The *QRS duration* is the interval from the first deflection to the last deflection of the QRS complex. It represents the time interval necessary for ventricular depolarization. The *S-T segment* is the distance from the S wave to the beginning of the T wave. Usually this is an isoelectric line; however, it may be elevated or depressed in certain disease states, such as ischemia. (See Figures 21-17 to 21-24.)

Because of the all-or-none nature of myocardial depolarization, there is a time interval when the heart cannot be restimulated to depolarize. This **refractory period** is a period of time when the myocardial cells have not yet repolarized and cannot be stimulated again. (See Figure 21-25.) There are two aspects of the refractory period: the absolute refractory period and the relative refractory period. The **absolute refractory period** is the time when stimulation will not produce any depolarization whatsoever. This usually lasts from the beginning of the QRS complex to the apex of the T wave. The **relative refractory period** is a period when a

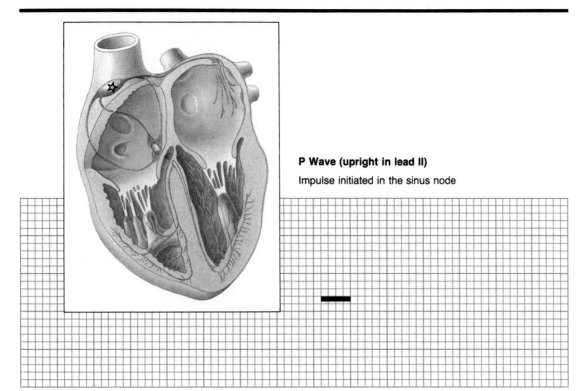

P Wave (upright in lead II)

Impulse initiated in the sinus node

FIGURE 21-17

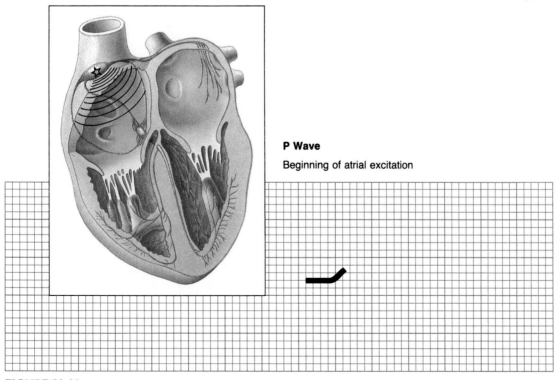

P Wave

Beginning of atrial excitation

FIGURE 21-18

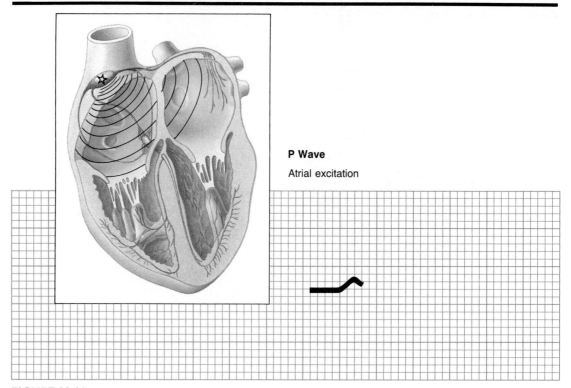

P Wave

Atrial excitation

FIGURE 21-19

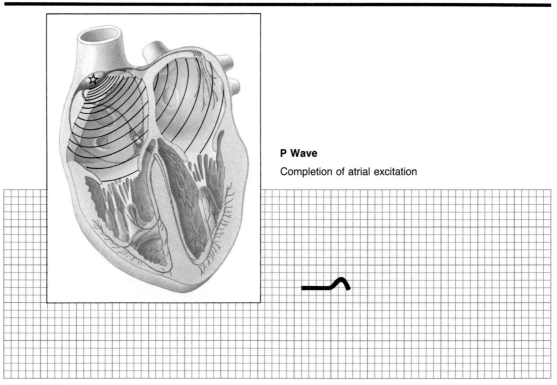

P Wave

Completion of atrial excitation

FIGURE 21-20

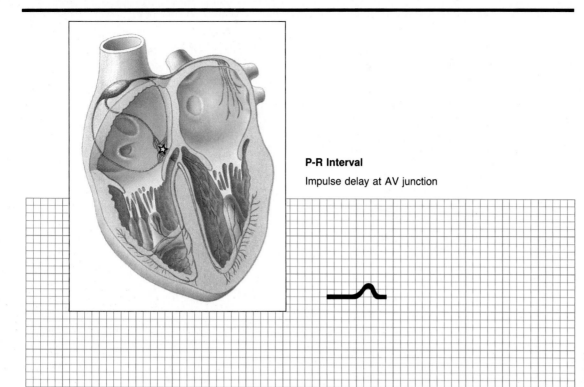

P-R Interval

Impulse delay at AV junction

FIGURE 21-21

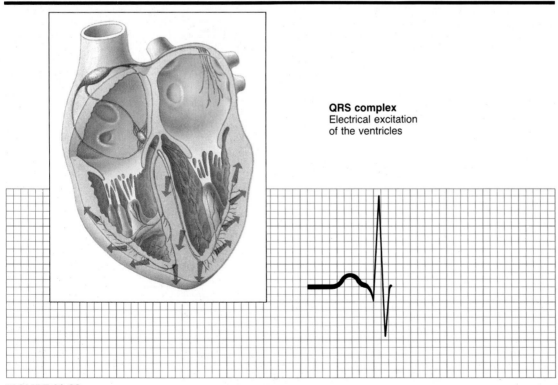

QRS complex
Electrical excitation
of the ventricles

FIGURE 21-22

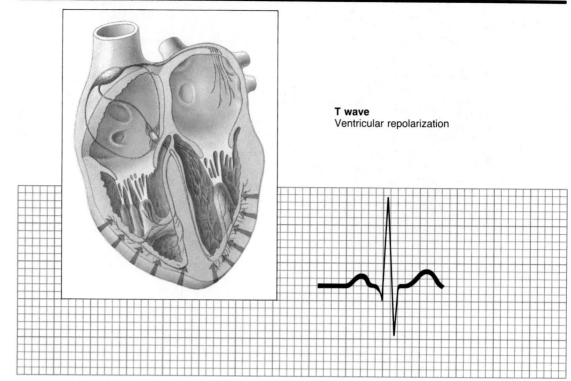

T wave
Ventricular repolarization

FIGURE 21-23

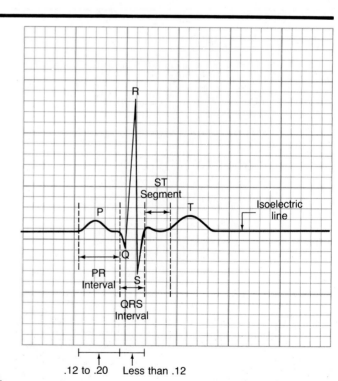

FIGURE 21-24 The ECG.

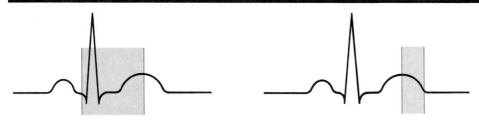

Absolute Refractory Period   Relative Refractory Period

FIGURE 21-25
Refractory periods.

sufficiently strong stimulus may produce depolarization. This usually corresponds to the down slope of the T wave.

As mentioned, the autonomic nervous system and the cardiac conductive system are closely interrelated. The vagus nerve provides parasympathetic (cholinergic) control to the SA node and, to a lesser degree, to the AV node. The cardiac plexus innervates the atria and the ventricle and provides sympathetic (adrenergic) control.

Artifacts are deflections on the ECG produced by factors other than the heart's electrical activity. Common causes of artifacts include:

❑ muscle tremors
❑ shivering
❑ patient movement
❑ loose electrodes
❑ 60 hertz interference
❑ machine malfunction

Interpretation of Rhythm Strips

The key to interpretation of rhythm strips is a logical, systematic approach to each strip. Attempting to "eyeball" the strip in a nonanalytical way often leads to an incorrect interpretation. The analytical approach to rhythm strip interpretation should include the following basic criteria:

✱ The key to interpretation of rhythm strips is to approach each in a logical, systematic manner.

1. Always use a consistent analytical approach.
2. Memorize the rules for each dysrhythmia.
3. Analyze a given rhythm strip according to a specific format.
4. Compare your analysis to the rules for each dysrhythmia.
5. Identify the dysrhythmia based on similarity to established rules.

There are several standard formats for ECG analysis. The format presented here includes the following items:

1. Rate
2. Rhythm
3. P waves
4. P-R interval
5. QRS complexes

Step 1: Analyze the Rate. The first step in ECG strip interpretation is to analyze the heart rate. Usually this means ventricular rate, but if the atrial and ventricular rates are different, you must calculate both.

■ **tachycardia** a heart rate greater than 100.

■ **bradycardia** a heart rate less than 60.

The normal heart rate is 60-100 beats per minute. A heart rate greater than 100 beats per minute is a **tachycardia.** A heart rate less than 60 beats per minute is a **bradycardia.**

The rate can be calculated in any of the following ways.

❑ *Six-Second Method.* The heart rate can be calculated by counting the number of complexes within a 6-second interval. Mark off a 6-second interval by noting two 3-second marks at the top of the ECG paper. Then multiply the number of complexes within the 6 second strip by 10, which will give the heart rate per minute.

❑ *Heart Rate Calculator Rulers.* Commercially available heart rate calculator rulers allow you to determine heart rate rapidly. Always use them according to the accompanying directions.

❑ *R-R Interval.* The R-R interval is directly related to heart rate. The R-R interval method is accurate only if the heart rhythm is regular. It can be calculated in the following ways:
  1. Measure the duration between R waves in seconds. Divide this number into 60, giving the heart rate per minute.
  2. Count the number of large squares within an R-R interval and divide the number of squares into 300.
  3. Count the number of small squares within an R-R interval and divide the number of squares by 1,500.

❑ *Triplicate Method.* Another method, also useful only with regular rhythms, is to locate an R wave that falls on a dark line bordering a large box on the graph paper. Then assign numbers corresponding to the heart rate to the next six dark lines to the right. The order is: 300, 150, 100, 75, 60, and 50. The number corresponding to the dark line closest to the peak of the next R wave is a rough estimate of the heart rate.

Step 2: Analyze the Rhythm. The next step is to analyze the rhythm. First, measure the R-R interval across the strip. Normally, the R-R rhythm is fairly regular. Some minimal variation, associated with respirations, should be expected. If the rhythm is irregular, note whether it is:

❑ occasionally irregular (only one or two R-R intervals on the strip are irregular)

❑ regularly irregular (patterned irregularity, or group beating)

❑ irregularly irregular (no relationship between R-R intervals)

Step 3: Analyze the P Waves. The P waves reflect atrial depolarization. Normally, the atria depolarize away from the SA node and toward the ventricles. In Lead II, this is seen as a positive, rounded P wave. The P wave analysis includes the following questions:

❑ Are P waves present?

❑ Are the P waves regular?

❑ Is there one P wave for each QRS complex?

❑ Are the P waves upright or inverted (compared to the QRS complex)?

❑ Do all the P waves look alike?

Step 4: Analyze the P-R Interval. The P-R interval represents the time necessary for atrial depolarization and conduction of the impulse up to the AV node. The normal P-R interval is 0.12–0.20 sec (3–5 small boxes). Any deviation is an abnormal finding. The P-R interval should be consistent across the strip.

Step 5: Analyze the QRS Complex. The QRS complex represents ventricular depolarization. When evaluating the QRS complex, ask the following questions:

❑ Do all of the QRS complexes look alike?
❑ What is the QRS duration?

The QRS duration is usually 0.04-0.12 sec. Anything longer than 0.12 sec (3 small boxes) is abnormal.

Analysis of a Normal Sinus Rhythm. On a normal ECG, the heart rate is between 60 and 100 beats per minute. The rhythm is regular (both P-P and R-R). The P waves are normal in shape, upright, and appear only before each QRS complex. The P-R interval lasts between 0.12 and 0.20 sec and is constant. The QRS complex has a normal morphology, and its duration is less than 0.12 sec. All of these factors indicate a normal sinus rhythm.

Introduction to Dysrhythmias

Any deviation from the heart's normal electrical rhythm is a **dysrhythmia.** The causes of dysrhythmias include:

❑ myocardial ischemia, necrosis, or infarction
❑ autonomic nervous system imbalance
❑ distention of the chambers of the heart (especially in the atria, secondary to congestive heart failure)
❑ blood gas abnormalities, including hypoxia and abnormal pH
❑ electrolyte imbalances (Ca^{++}, K^+, Mg^{++})
❑ trauma to the myocardium (cardiac contusion)
❑ drug effects and drug toxicity
❑ electrocution
❑ hypothermia
❑ CNS damage
❑ idiopathic events
❑ normal occurrences

Dysrhythmias that occur in the healthy heart are of little significance. NO MATTER WHAT THE ETIOLOGY OR TYPE OF DYSRHYTHMIA, THE PATIENT AND HIS OR HER SYMPTOMS ARE TREATED, NOT THE DYSRHYTHMIA.

Mechanism of Impulse Formation. Several physiologic mechanisms can result in cardiac dysrhythmias. The depolarization impulse is normally conducted through the conductive system and the myocardium. When the impulse is conducted normally, it is said to be conducted *antegrade.* However, in certain dysrhythmias, the depolarization impulse is conducted backwards. Backward conduction is said to be *retrograde.*

Ectopic Foci. One cause of dysrhythmias is *enhanced automaticity,* in which heart cells other than the pacemaker cells automatically depolarize, resulting in a contraction. Depolarizations that occur from cells other than the normal pacemakers are referred to as **ectopic beats.** Premature ventricular contractions and premature atrial contractions are examples of ectopic beats. The ectopic beat can be intermittent or sustained.

■ **dysrhythmia** any deviation from the normal electrical rhythm of the heart.

■ **arrhythmia** the absence of cardiac electrical activity, often used interchangeably with dysrhythmia.

✳ Always treat the patient, not the monitor.

■ **ectopic beats** cardiac depolarization resulting from depolarization of cells in the heart that are not a part of the heart's normal pacemaker.

Reentry. The phenomenon of reentry may be responsible for isolated premature beats, or *tachydysrhythmias. Reentry* occurs when two branches of a conduction pathway are altered by ischemia or other disease processes. Conduction is slowed in one branch, while the other has a unidirectional block. The depolarization wave is conducted slowly, in an antegrade fashion, through the branch with ischemia and is blocked in the branch with a unidirectional block. After the depolarization wave is conducted through the slowed branch, it enters the branch with the unidirectional block and is conducted retrograde back to the origin of the branch. By this time, the tissue is no longer refractory, and stimulation again occurs. This can result in the development of rapid rhythms, such as paroxysmal supraventricular tachycardia or atrial fibrillation.

Classification of Dysrhythmias

Dysrhythmias can be classified in any number of ways. Examples of classification methods include:

- ❑ Changes in automaticity versus disturbances in conduction
- ❑ Major versus minor dysrhythmias
- ❑ Life-threatening versus non-life-threatening dysrhythmias
- ❑ Site of origin

This text classifies dysrhythmias by site of origin. This approach is closely related to basic physiology and therefore easy to understand. The dysrhythmias addressed in this section include:

Dysrhythmias Originating in the SA Node
- ❑ Sinus bradycardia
- ❑ Sinus tachycardia
- ❑ Sinus dysrhythmia
- ❑ Sinus arrest

Dysrhythmias Originating in the Atria
- ❑ Wandering pacemaker
- ❑ Premature atrial contractions
- ❑ Atrial tachycardia
- ❑ Atrial flutter
- ❑ Atrial fibrillation

Dysrhythmias Originating in the AV Junction
- ❑ Premature junctional contractions
- ❑ Junctional escape complexes and rhythm
- ❑ Accelerated junctional rhythm
- ❑ Paroxysmal junctional tachycardia

Dysrhythmias Originating in the Ventricles
- ❑ Ventricular escape complexes and rhythm
- ❑ Premature ventricular complexes
- ❑ Ventricular tachycardia
- ❑ Ventricular fibrillation
- ❑ Asystole
- ❑ Artificial pacemaker rhythm

Dysrhythmias that are Disorders of Conduction

❏ AV blocks
  ❏ First-degree AV block
  ❏ Second-degree AV block (Mobitz I)—Wenkebach
  ❏ Second-degree AV block (Mobitz II)
  ❏ Third-degree AV block
❏ Disturbances of ventricular conduction
❏ Pre-excitation syndrome

DYSRHYTHMIAS ORIGINATING IN THE SA NODE

Dysrhythmias originating in the SA node most often result from changes in autonomic tone. However, disease can exist in the SA node itself. Dysrhythmias which originate in the SA node include:

- ❑ Sinus bradycardia
- ❑ Sinus tachycardia
- ❑ Sinus dysrhythmia
- ❑ Sinus arrest

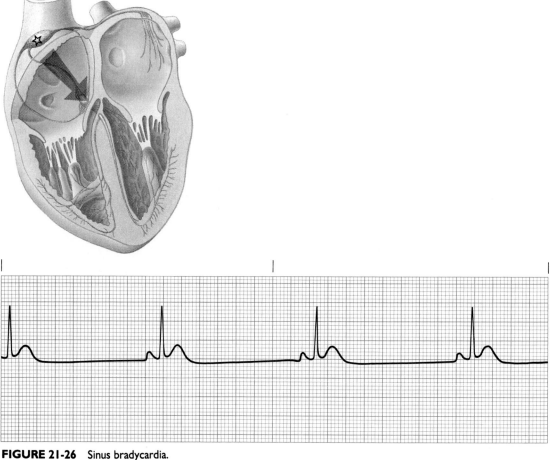

FIGURE 21-26   Sinus bradycardia.

Several ECG features are common to all dysrhythmias that originate in the SA node. These include the following:

❏ Upright P waves in Lead II
❏ Similar appearance in all P waves
❏ Normal P-R interval
❏ Normal QRS complex duration

Sinus Bradycardia

Description: *Sinus bradycardia* results from slowing of the SA node.

Etiology: Sinus bradycardia may result from any of the following:

❏ Increased parasympathetic (vagal) tone
❏ Intrinsic disease of the SA node
❏ Drug effects (digitalis, propranolol, quinidine)

Sinus bradycardia is a normal finding in healthy, well-conditioned persons.

Rules of Interpretation (Lead II Monitoring):
    Rate: Less than 60
    Rhythm: Regular
    Pacemaker Site: SA node
    P Waves: Upright and normal in morphology
    P-R Interval: 0.12–0.20 sec and constant (normal)
    QRS complex: 0.04–0.12 sec (normal)

Clinical Significance: The decreased heart rate can result in decreased cardiac output, hypotension, angina, or CNS symptoms. This is especially true for rates less than 50 beats per minute. Because of the slow heart rate, atrial ectopic or ventricular ectopic rhythms may occur.

Treatment: Treatment is unnecessary unless hypotension or ventricular irritability is present. If treatment is required, administer a 0.5 mg bolus of atropine sulfate. This can be repeated every 5 minutes until a satisfactory rate has been obtained or 2 mg of the drug has been given. Isoproteronel is rarely required. External pacing, if available, should be considered. If there is disease in the SA node, a pacemaker may be inserted in the hospital.

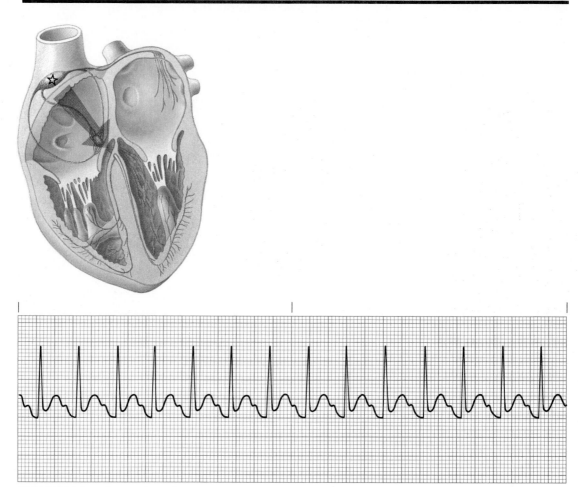

FIGURE 21-27 Sinus tachycardia.

Sinus Tachycardia

Description: *Sinus tachycardia* results from an increase in the rate of SA node discharge.

Etiology: Sinus tachycardia may result from any of the following:

- ❑ Exercise
- ❑ Fever
- ❑ Anxiety
- ❑ Hypovolemia
- ❑ Anemia
- ❑ Pump failure
- ❑ Increased sympathetic tone

Rules of Interpretation (Lead II Monitoring):
    Rate: Greater than 100
    Rhythm: Regular
    Pacemaker Site: SA node
    P Waves: Upright and normal in morphology
    P-R Interval: 0.12–0.20 sec and constant (normal)
    QRS complex: 0.04–0.12 sec (normal)

Clinical Significance: Sinus tachycardia is often a benign process. In some cases, it is a compensatory mechanism for decreased stroke volume. If the rate is greater than 140 beats per minute, cardiac output may fall because ventricular filling time is inadequate. Very rapid heart rates increase myocardial oxygen demand and can precipitate ischemia or infarct in diseased hearts. Prolonged sinus tachycardia accompanying acute MI is often an ominous finding suggestive of cardiogenic shock.

Treatment: Treatment is directed at the underlying cause. Hypovolemia or other cause should be corrected.

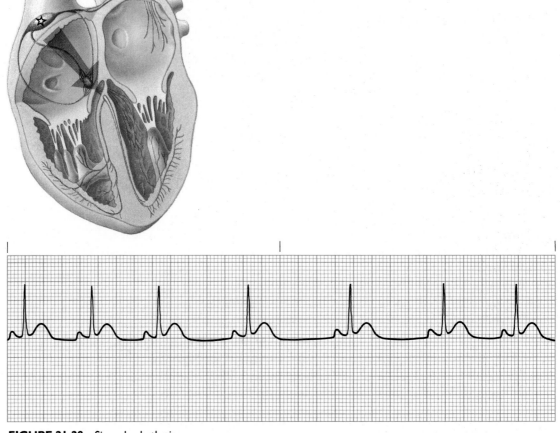

FIGURE 21-28 Sinus dysrhythmia.

Sinus Dysrhythmia

Description: *Sinus dysrhythmia* results from a phasic variation of the R-R interval.

Etiology: Sinus dysrhythmia is often a normal finding and is sometimes related to the respiratory cycle and changes in intrathoracic pressure. Pathologically, sinus dysrhythmia can be caused by enhanced vagal tone.

Rules of Interpretation (Lead II Monitoring):
    Rate: 60–100 (varies with respirations)
    Rhythm: Irregular
    Pacemaker Site: SA node
    P Waves: Upright and normal in morphology
    P-R Interval: 0.12–0.20 sec
    QRS complex: 0.04–0.12 sec

Clinical Significance: Sinus dysrhythmia is a normal variant, particularly in the young and the aged.

Treatment: Typically, none required.

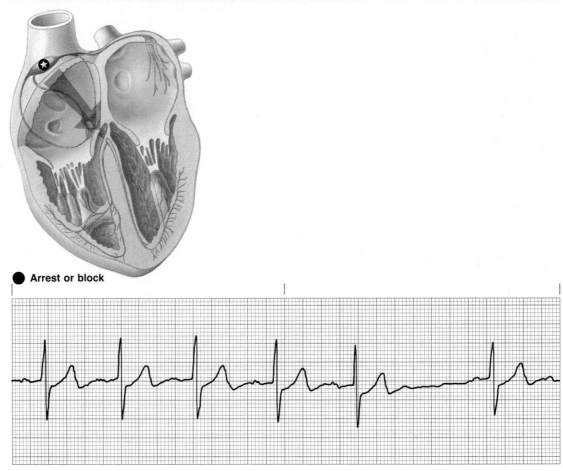

● Arrest or block

FIGURE 21-29 Sinus arrest.

Sinus Arrest

Description: Sinus arrest is an episode of failure of the sinus node to discharge, resulting in short periods of cardiac standstill. This standstill can persist until pacemaker cells lower in the conductive system discharge (escape beats) or until the sinus node resumes discharge.

Etiology: Sinus arrest can result from:

❑ Ischemia of the SA node
❑ Digitalis toxicity
❑ Excessive vagal tone
❑ Degenerative fibrotic disease

Rules of Interpretation (Lead II Monitoring):
  Rate: Normal to slow depending on the frequency and duration of the arrest
  Rhythm: Irregular
  Pacemaker Site: SA node
  P Waves: Upright and normal in morphology
  P-R Interval: 0.12–0.20 sec and constant
  QRS complex: 0.04–0.12 sec

Clinical Significance: Frequent or prolonged episodes may compromise cardiac output, resulting in syncope and other problems. There is always the danger of complete cessation of SA node activity. Usually, an escape rhythm develops. However, cardiac standstill can occasionally result.

Treatment: If the patient is asymptomatic, then observation is all that is required. If the patient is extremely bradycardic or symptomatic, adminster a 0.5 mg bolus of atropine sulfate. This can be repeated every 5 minutes until a satisfactory rate has been obtained or 2 mg of the drug has been administered. Isoproterenol is rarely required. External pacing, if available, should be considered. If sinus arrest is persistent, a pacemaker may be inserted in the hospital.

DYSRHYTHMIAS ORIGINATING IN THE ATRIA

Dysrhythmias can originate outside the SA node in the tissue of the atria or in the internodal pathways. Ischemia, hypoxia, atrial dilation, and other factors can cause atrial dysrhythmias. Dysrhythmias originating in the atria include:

- ❑ Wandering pacemaker
- ❑ Premature atrial contractions
- ❑ Atrial tachycardia
- ❑ Atrial flutter
- ❑ Atrial fibrillation

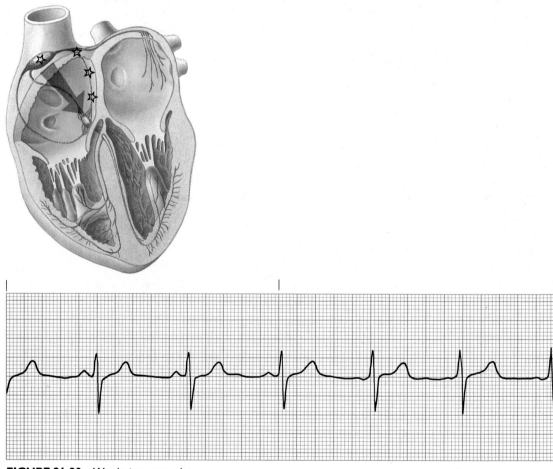

FIGURE 21-30   Wandering pacemaker.

Several ECG features are common to all dysrhythmias that originate in the atria. These are:

- ❑ P waves differ in appearance from sinus P waves
- ❑ The P-R interval may be normal, shortened, or prolonged
- ❑ Normal QRS complex duration

Wandering Pacemaker

Description: Wandering pacemaker, often called wandering atrial pacemaker, is the passive transfer of pacemaker sites from the sinus node to other latent pacemaker sites in the atria and AV junction. Often, more than one pacemaker site will be present, causing variation in P-R interval and P wave morphology.

Etiology: Wandering pacemaker can result from:

- ❑ A variant of sinus dysrhythmia
- ❑ A normal phenomenon in the very young or the aged
- ❑ Ischemic heart disease
- ❑ Atrial dilation

Rules of Interpretation (Lead II Monitoring):
  Rate: Usually normal
  Rhythm: Slightly irregular
  Pacemaker Site: Varies between the SA node, atrial tissue, and the AV junction.
  P Waves: Morphology changes from beat to beat; P waves may disappear entirely.
  P-R Interval: Varies. May be less than 0.12 sec, normal, or greater than 0.20 sec.
  QRS complex: 0.04–0.12 sec

Clinical Significance: Wandering pacemaker usually has no detrimental effects. Occasionally, it can be a precursor of other atrial dysrhythmias, such as atrial fibrillation. It is occasionally indicative of digitalis toxicity.

Treatment: If the patient is asymptomatic, observation is all that is required.

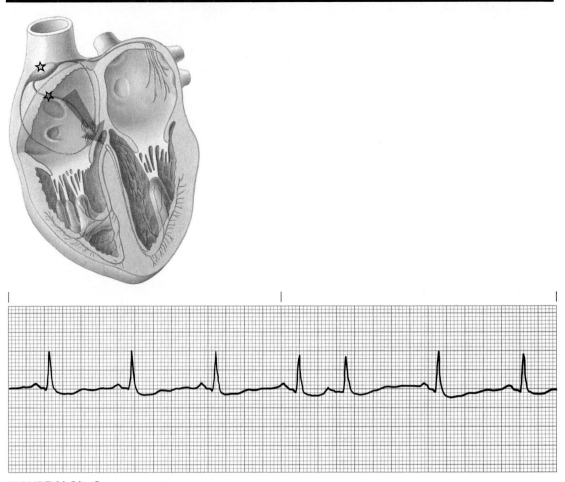

FIGURE 21-31 Premature atrial contractions.

Premature Atrial Contractions

Description: Premature atrial contractions (PAC) result from a single electrical impulse originating in the atria outside the SA node which causes a premature depolarization of the heart before the next expected sinus beat. Because it results in depolarization of the atrial syncytium, this impulse also depolarizes the SA node, interrupting the normal cadence. This creates a **noncompensatory pause** in the underlying rhythm.

Etiology: A premature atrial contraction can result from:

- ❏ Use of caffeine, tobacco, or alcohol
- ❏ Sympathomimetic drugs
- ❏ Ischemic heart disease
- ❏ Hypoxia
- ❏ Digitalis toxicity
- ❏ No apparent cause

Rules of Interpretation (Lead II Monitoring):
Rate: Depends on the underlying rhythm
Rhythm: Depends on the underlying rhythm, usually regular except for the PAC.
Pacemaker Site: Ectopic focus in the atrium.
P Waves: The P wave of the PAC differs from the P wave of the underlying rhythm. It occurs earlier than the next expected P wave and may be hidden in the preceding T wave.
P-R Interval: Usually normal. However, can vary with the location of the ectopic focus. Ectopic foci near the SA node will have a P-R interval of 0.12 sec or greater, whereas ectopic foci near the AV node will have a P-R interval of 0.12 sec or less.
QRS complex: Normal, 0.04-0.12 sec. However, may be greater than 0.12 sec if the PAC is abnormally conducted through partially refractory ventricles. In some cases, the ventricles are in the refractory period and will not depolarize in response to the PAC. In these cases, the QRS complex is absent.

Clinical Significance: Isolated PACs are of minimal significance. Frequent PACs may indicate organic heart disease and may be forerunners of other atrial dysrhythmias.

Treatment: If the patient is asymptomatic, observation is all that is required in the field.

■ **noncompensatory pause** the pause following an ectopic beat where the SA node is depolarized and the underlying cadence of the heart is interrupted.

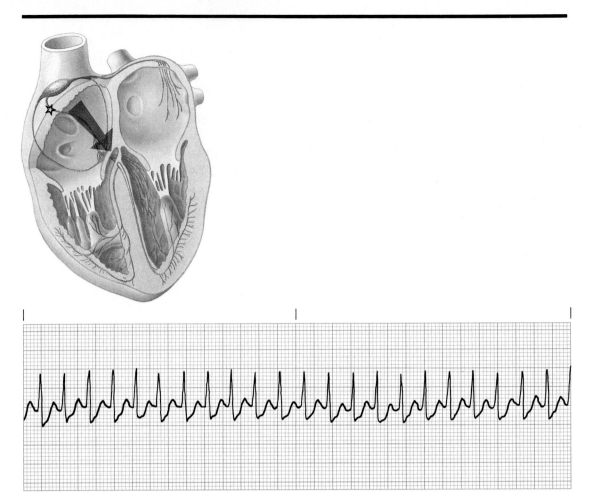

FIGURE 21-32 Paroxysmal atrial tachycardia.

Paroxysmal Atrial Tachycardia

Description: Paroxysmal atrial tachycardia (PAT) occurs when rapid atrial depolarization overrides the SA node. It often occurs in paroxysms with sudden onset, may last minutes to hours, and terminates abruptly. It may be caused by increased automaticity of a single atrial focus or by reentry phenomenon at the AV node. Paroxysmal atrial tachycardia is often more appropriately called *paroxysmal supraventricular tachycardia* (PSVT), because the rapid rate can make it indistinguishable from AV junctional tachycardia.

Etiology: Paroxysmal atrial tachycardia may occur at any age unassociated with underlying heart disease. It may be precipitated by stress, overexertion, smoking, or ingestion of caffeine. However, it is frequently associated with underlying atherosclerotic cardiovascular disease and rheumatic heart disease. PAT is rare in patients with myocardial infarction. It can occur with accessory pathway conduction, such as Wolff-Parkinson-White syndrome.

Rules of Interpretation (Lead II Monitoring):
Rate: 150–250 per minute
Rhythm: Characteristically regular, except at onset and termination.
Pacemaker Site: In the atria, outside the SA node.
P Waves: The atrial P waves differ slightly from sinus P waves. The P wave is often buried in the preceding T wave. The P wave may be impossible to see, especially if the rate is rapid. Turning up the speed of the graph paper or oscilloscope to 50 mm/sec spreads out the complex and can aid in the identification of P waves.
P-R Interval: Usually normal. However, can vary with the location of the ectopic pacemaker. Ectopic pacemakers near the SA node will have P-R intervals close to 0.12 sec, whereas ectopic pacemakers near the AV node will have P-R intervals of 0.12 sec or less.
QRS complex: Normal, 0.04–0.12 sec.

Clinical Significance: Young patients with good cardiac reserves may tolerate PAT well for short periods of time. Patients often sense PAT as palpitations. Rapid rates, however, can cause a marked reduction in cardiac output because of inadequate ventricular filling time. Coronary artery perfusion can also be compromised, since the diastolic phase of the cardiac cycle is reduced. PAT can precipitate angina, hypotension, or congestive heart failure.

(*continued*)

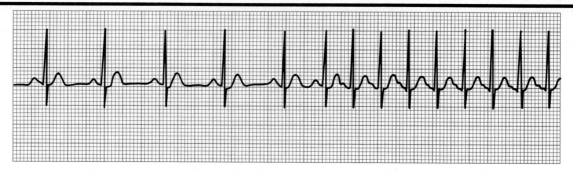

Paroxysmal supraventricular tachycardia (PSVT)

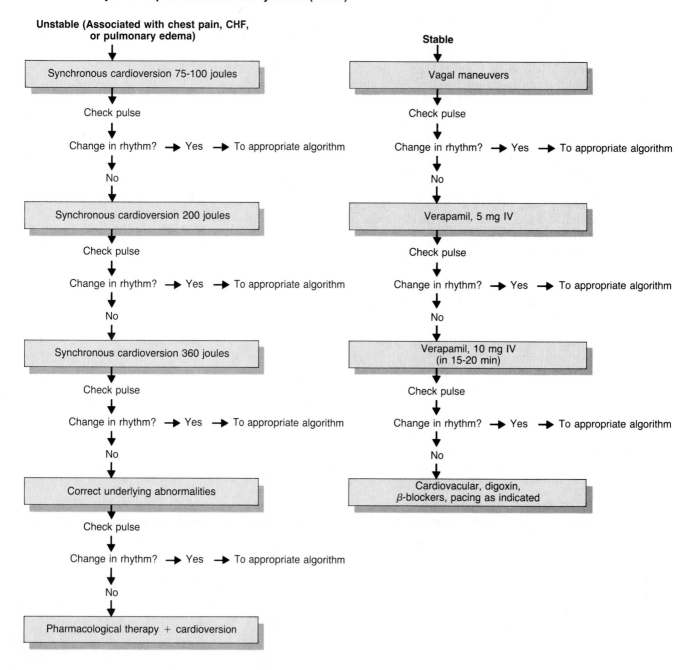

Unstable (Associated with chest pain, CHF, or pulmonary edema)

Synchronous cardioversion 75-100 joules
↓
Check pulse
↓
Change in rhythm? → Yes → To appropriate algorithm
↓
No
↓
Synchronous cardioversion 200 joules
↓
Check pulse
↓
Change in rhythm? → Yes → To appropriate algorithm
↓
No
↓
Synchronous cardioversion 360 joules
↓
Check pulse
↓
Change in rhythm? → Yes → To appropriate algorithm
↓
No
↓
Correct underlying abnormalities
↓
Check pulse
↓
Change in rhythm? → Yes → To appropriate algorithm
↓
No
↓
Pharmacological therapy + cardioversion

Stable

Vagal maneuvers
↓
Check pulse
↓
Change in rhythm? → Yes → To appropriate algorithm
↓
No
↓
Verapamil, 5 mg IV
↓
Check pulse
↓
Change in rhythm? → Yes → To appropriate algorithm
↓
No
↓
Verapamil, 10 mg IV
(in 15-20 min)
↓
Check pulse
↓
Change in rhythm? → Yes → To appropriate algorithm
↓
No
↓
Cardiovacular, digoxin,
β-blockers, pacing as indicated

FIGURE 21-33   If conversion occurs but PSVT recurs, repeated electrical cardioversion is *not* indicated. Sedation should be used as time permits.

Paroxysmal Atrial Tachycardia (*continued*)

Treatment: If the patient is not tolerating the rapid heart rate, as evidenced by hemodynamic instability, attempt the following techniques in the order they are given here (see Figure 21-33):

1. *Vagal Maneuvers.* Ask the patient to perform a Valsalva maneuver. This is a forced expiration against a closed glottis, or the act of "bearing down" as if to move the bowels. This results in vagal stimulation, which may slow the heart. If this is unsuccessful, attempt carotid artery massage if the patient is eligible. Do not attempt this in patients with carotid **bruits** or known cerebrovascular or carotid artery disease.

2. *Pharmacological Therapy.* Verapamil, the calcium channel blocker, is often effective in terminating PAT. This is especially true if the etiology of the dysrhythmia is reentry. Administer 5 mg of verapamil intravenously. If this is unsuccessful, administer another dose of 5–10 mg. Verapamil is contraindicated in patients with history of bradycardia, hypotension, or congestive heart failure. It should not be used with intravenous beta blockers and should be used with caution in patients on chronic beta blocker therapy. Hypotension that occurs following verapamil administration can often be reversed with 0.5–1.0 gm of calcium chloride administered intravenously.

3. *Electrical Therapy.* PAT that does not respond to vagal maneuvers or verapamil, or that becomes hemodynamically unstable, should be treated with synchronized cardioversion. If time allows, sedate the patient with 3–5 mg of diazepam IV. Apply synchronized DC countershock of 75–100 joules. If this is unsuccessful, repeat the countershock at increased energy as ordered by the medical control physician. DC countershock is contraindicated if digitalis toxicity is suspected as the cause of the PAT.

■ **bruit** the sound of turbulent blood flow through a vessel, often associated with atherosclerotic disease.

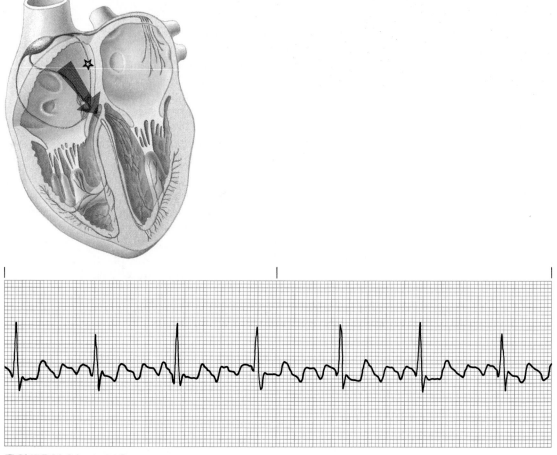

FIGURE 21-34 Atrial flutter.

Atrial Flutter

Description: *Atrial flutter* results from a rapid atrial reentry circuit and an AV node which, physiologically, cannot conduct all impulses through to the ventricles. The AV junction may allow impulses in a 1:1 (rare), 2:1, 3:1, or 4:1 ratio or greater, resulting in a discrepancy between atrial and ventricular rates. The AV block may be consistent or variable.

Etiology: Atrial flutter may occur in normal hearts, but it is usually associated with organic disease. It rarely occurs as the direct result of an MI. Atrial dilation, which occurs with congestive heart failure, is a cause.

Rules of Interpretation (Lead II Monitoring):
 Rate: Atrial rate is 250–350 per minute. Ventricular rate varies with the ratio of AV conduction.
 Rhythm: Atrial rhythm is regular. Ventricular rhythm is usually regular, but can be irregular if the block is intermittent.
 Pacemaker Site: Sites in the atria outside the SA node.
 P Waves: Flutter (F) waves are present, resembling a sawtooth or picket-fence pattern. This pattern is often difficult to identify in a 2:1 flutter. However, if the ventricular rate is greater than 150, 2:1 flutter should be suspected.
 P-R Interval: The P-R interval is usually constant but may vary.
 QRS complex: Normal, 0.04–0.12 sec.

Clinical Significance: Atrial flutter with normal ventricular rates is generally well tolerated. Rapid ventricular rates may compromise cardiac output and result in symptoms. Atrial flutter often occurs in conjunction with atrial fibrillation and is referred to as "atrial fib-flutter."

Treatment: Treatment is indicated for rapid ventricular rates with hemodynamic compromise. If treatment is required, atrial flutter often responds well to synchronized cardioversion with low energy. Verapamil is also effective. Vagal maneuvers are rarely effective and may transiently increase the AV block.

1. *Electrical Therapy.* Hemodynamically unstable atrial flutter should be treated with synchronized cardioversion. If time allows, sedate the patient with 3–5 mg of diazepam IV. Then apply synchronized DC countershock of 75–100 joules. If this is unsuccessful, repeat the countershock at increased energy as ordered by the medical control physician.

2. *Pharmacological Therapy.* Verapamil (Isoptin, Calan) is often effective in slowing the ventricular response to atrial flutter. Administer 5 mg of verapamil intravenously. If unsuccessful, give an additional dose of 5–10 mg. Verapamil is contraindicated in patients with history of bradycardia, hypotension, or congestive heart failure. It should not be used with intravenous beta blockers and should be used with caution in patients on chronic beta blocker therapy.

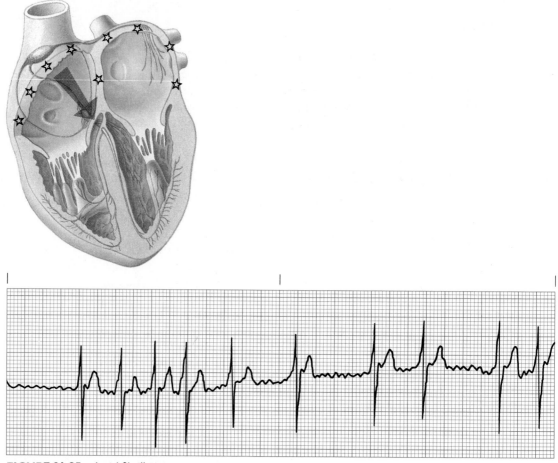

FIGURE 21-35 Atrial fibrillation.

Atrial Fibrillation

Description: Atrial fibrillation is a dysrhythmia that results from multiple areas of reentry within the atria or from multiple ectopic foci bombarding an AV node that physiologically cannot handle all of the incoming impulses. AV conduction is random and highly variable.

Etiology: Atrial fibrillation may be chronic and is often associated with underlying heart disease such as rheumatic heart disease, atherosclerotic heart disease, or congestive heart failure. Atrial dilation that occurs with congestive heart failure and is often the cause of atrial fibrillation.

Rules of Interpretation (Lead II Monitoring):
  Rate: Atrial rate is 350–750 per minute (cannot be counted). Ventricular rate varies greatly depending on conduction through the AV node.
  Rhythm: Irregularly irregular.
  Pacemaker Site: Numerous ectopic foci in the atria.
  P Waves: No discernible P waves are present. Fibrillation (f) waves are present, indicating chaotic atrial activity.
  P-R Interval: None
  QRS complex: Normal, 0.04–0.12 sec.

Clinical Significance: In atrial fibrillation the atria fail to contract and the so-called atrial kick is lost, thus reducing cardiac output by 20–25 percent. There is frequently a *pulse deficit* (a difference between the apical and peripheral pulse rates). If the rate of ventricular response is normal, as often occurs in patients on digitalis, the rhythm is usually well tolerated. If the ventricular rate is less than 60, cardiac output can fall. Digitalis toxicity should be suspected in patients with atrial fibrillation with ventricular rate of less than 60. If the ventricular response is rapid, coupled by the loss of "atrial kick," cardiovascular decompensation may occur, resulting in hypotension, angina, infarct, congestive heart failure, or shock.

Treatment: Treatment is indicated for rapid ventricular rates with hemodynamic compromise. If treatment is required, atrial fibrillation may respond well to synchronized cardioversion with low energy. Verapamil is also effective. Vagal maneuvers are rarely effective and may transiently increase the AV block.

1. *Electrical Therapy.* Hemodynamically unstable atrial fibrillation should be treated with synchronized cardioversion. If time allows, sedate the patient with 3–5 mg of diazepam IV. Apply synchronized DC countershock of 75–100 joules. If this is unsuccessful, repeat the countershock at increased energy as ordered by the medical control physician.

2. *Pharmacological Therapy.* Verapamil is often effective in slowing the ventricular response to atrial fibrillation. Administer 5 mg of verapamil intravenously. If this is unsuccessful, give a second dose of 5–10 mg. Verapamil is contraindicated in patients with history of bradycardia, hypotension, or congestive heart failure. It should not be used with intravenous beta blockers and should be used with caution in patients on chronic beta blocker therapy.

DYSRHYTHMIAS ORIGINATING IN THE AV JUNCTION

Dysrhythmias can originate within the AV node and the AV junction. The location of the pacemaker site will dictate the morphology of the P wave. Ischemia, hypoxia, and other factors have been identified as causes. Dysrhythmias originating in the AV junction include:

❑ Premature junctional contractions
❑ Junctional escape complexes and rhythm
❑ Accelerated junctional rhythm
❑ Paroxysmal junctional tachycardia

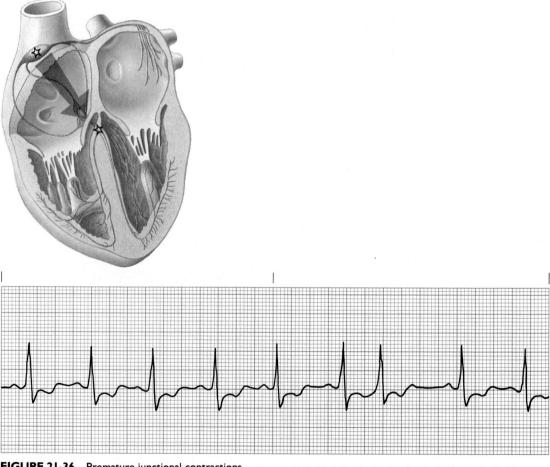

FIGURE 21-36 Premature junctional contractions.

Several ECG features are common to all dysrhythmias that originate in the AV junction. These are:

❑ Inverted P waves in Lead II as a result of retrograde depolarization of the atria. The relationship of the P wave to QRS depolarization is dependent on the relative timing of atrial and ventricular depolarization. The P wave can occur before the QRS complex if the atria depolarize first, after the QRS if the ventricles depolarize first, or during the QRS if the atria and ventricles depolarize simultaneously. Depolarization of the atria during ventricular depolarization masks the P wave. Some atrial complexes that originate near the AV junction can result in negative P waves as well.

❑ P-R interval of less than 0.12 sec.

❑ Normal QRS complex duration.

Premature Junctional Contractions

Description: Premature junctional contractions (PJCs) result from a single electrical impulse originating in the AV node which occurs before the next expected sinus beat. A PJC can result in either a compensatory pause or noncompensatory pause, depending on whether the SA node is depolarized. A **noncompensatory pause** occurs if the SA node is depolarized by the premature beat. The normal cadence of the heart is interrupted. A **compensatory pause** occurs only if the SA node discharges before the premature impulse reaches it.

Etiology: A premature junctional contraction can result from:

❑ Use of caffeine, tobacco, or alcohol
❑ Sympathomimetic drugs
❑ Ischemic heart disease
❑ Hypoxia
❑ Digitalis toxicity
❑ No apparent cause

■ **compensatory pause** the pause following an ectopic beat where the SA node is unaffected and the cadence of the heart is not interrupted.

Rules of Interpretation (Lead II Monitoring):
  Rate: Depends on the underlying rhythm.
  Rhythm: Depends on the underlying rhythm, usually regular except for the PJC.
  Pacemaker Site: Ectopic focus in the AV junction.
  P Waves: Inverted; may appear before or after the QRS complex. P waves can be masked by the QRS complex or be absent.
  P-R Interval: If the P wave occurs before the QRS complex, the P-R interval will be less than 0.12 sec. If the P wave occurs after the QRS complex, then technically it is an R-P interval.
  QRS complex: Normal, 0.04–0.12 sec. However, it can be greater than 0.12 sec if the PJC is abnormally conducted through partially refractory ventricles.

Clinical Significance: Isolated PJCs are of minimal significance. Frequent PJCs indicate organic heart disease and may be precursors to other junctional dysrhythmias.

Treatment: If the patient is asymptomatic, observation is all that is required in the field.

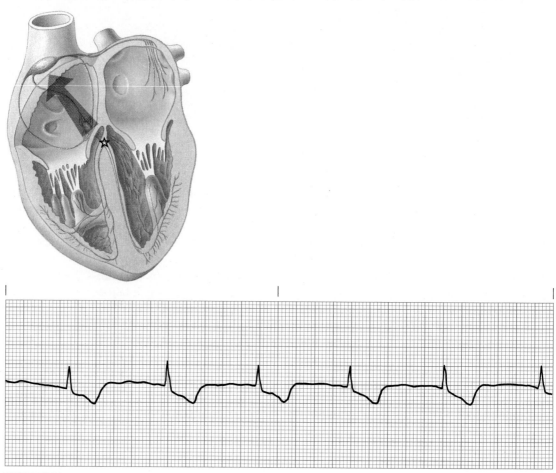

FIGURE 21-37 Junctional escape complex and rhythm.

Junctional Rhythm

Description: A *junctional escape beat,* or *junctional escape rhythm,* is a dysrhythmia that results when the rate of the primary pacemaker, usually the SA node, becomes less than that of the AV node. The AV node then becomes the pacemaker. The AV node usually discharges at its intrinsic rate of 40–60 beats per minute. This is a safety mechanism that prevents cardiac standstill.

Etiology: Junctional escape rhythm has several etiologies. These include increased vagal tone, which can result in SA node slowing, pathological slow SA node discharge, or heart block.

Rules of Interpretation (Lead II Monitoring):
    Rate: 40–60 per minute
    Rhythm: Irregular in single junctional escape complex; regular in junctional escape rhythm.
    Pacemaker Site: AV junction.
    P Waves: Inverted; may appear before or after the QRS complex. The P waves can be masked by the QRS or be absent.
    P-R Interval: If the P wave occurs before the QRS complex, the P-R interval will be less than 0.12 sec. If the P wave occurs after the QRS complex, technically it is an R-P interval.
    QRS complex: Normal, 0.04–0.12 sec. However, may be greater than 0.12 sec.

Clinical Significance: The slow heart rate can decrease cardiac output, possibly precipitating angina and other problems. If the rate is fairly rapid, the rhythm can be well tolerated.

Treatment: If the patient is asymptomatic, observation is all that is required in the field. Treatment is unnecessary unless hypotension or ventricular irritability is present. If treatment is required, administer a 0.5 mg bolus of atropine sulfate. This can be repeated every 5 minutes until a satisfactory rate has been obtained or a total of 2 mg of the drug has been given. Isoproterenol is rarely required. External pacing, if available, should be considered. If intrinsic disease is present in the SA node, a pacemaker may be inserted in the hospital.

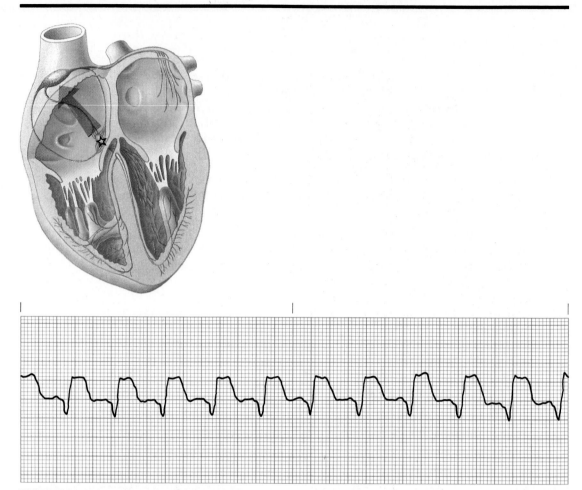

FIGURE 21-38 Accelerated junctional rhythm.

Accelerated Junctional Rhythm

Description: An *accelerated junctional rhythm* is one that results from increased automaticity in the AV junction, causing the AV junction to discharge faster than its intrinsic rate. If it is fast enough, the AV node can override the pacemaker. Technically, the rate associated with an accelerated junctional rhythm is not a tachycardia. However, when compared to the intrinsic rate of the AV junctional tissue (40–60 beats per minute), it is considered accelerated.

Etiology: Accelerated junctional rhythms often result from ischemia of the AV junction.

Rules of Interpretation (Lead II Monitoring):
    Rate: More than 60 per minute.
    Rhythm: Regular.
    Pacemaker Site: AV junction.
    P Waves: Inverted; may appear before or after the QRS complex. P waves may be masked by the QRS or be absent.
    P-R Interval: If the P wave occurs before the QRS complex, the P-R interval will be less than 0.12 sec. If it occurs after the QRS, technically it is an R-P interval.
    QRS complex: Normal, 0.04–0.12 sec.

Clinical Significance: An accelerated junctional rhythm is usually well tolerated. However, since ischemia is often the etiology, the patient should be monitored for other dysrhythmias.

Treatment: Prehospital treatment is generally unnecessary.

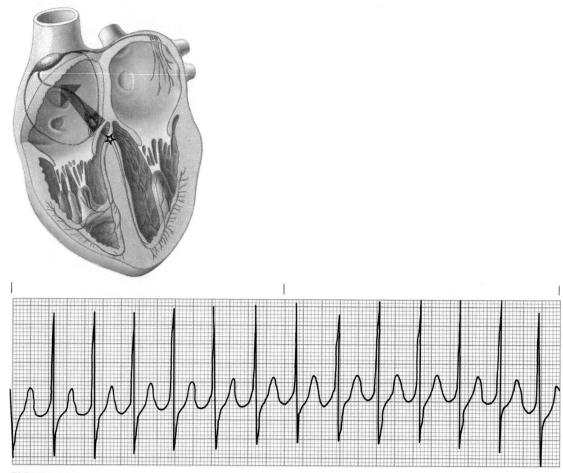

FIGURE 21-39 Paroxysmal junctional tachycardia.

Paroxysmal Junctional Tachycardia

Description: Paroxysmal junctional tachycardia (PJT) occurs when rapid AV junctional depolarization overrides the SA node. It often occurs in paroxysms with sudden onset, may last minutes to hours, and terminates abruptly. It may be caused by increased automaticity of a single AV nodal focus or by a reentry phenomenon at the AV node. Paroxysmal junctional tachycardia is often more appropriately called *paroxysmal supraventricular tachycardia* (PSVT), since it may be indistinguishable from paroxysmal atrial tachycardia because of the rapid rate.

Etiology: Paroxysmal junctional tachycardia may occur at any age unassociated with underlying heart disease. It may be precipitated by stress, overexertion, smoking, or ingestion of caffeine. However, it is frequently associated with underlying ASCVD and rheumatic heart disease. PJT rarely occurs with myocardial infarction. It can occur with accessory pathway conduction, as in Wolff-Parkinson-White syndrome.

Rules of Interpretation (Lead II Monitoring):

    Rate: 100–180 per minute

    Rhythm: Characteristically regular except at onset and termination of paroxysms.

    Pacemaker Site: AV junction

    P Waves: If present, P waves are inverted. They can occur before, during, or after the QRS complex. Turning up the speed of the graph paper or oscilloscope to 50 mm/sec spreads out the complex and aids in the identification of P waves.

    P-R Interval: If the P wave occurs before the QRS complex, the P-R interval will be less than 0.12 sec. If it occurs after the QRS complex, technically it is an R-P interval.

    QRS complex: Normal, 0.04–0.12 sec.

Clinical Significance: PJT may be well tolerated for a short period of time in young patients with good cardiac reserve. The patient will often sense it as palpitations. Rapid rates, however, can cause a marked reduction in cardiac output because of inadequate ventricular filling time. Coronary artery perfusion can also be compromised, since the diastolic phase of the cardiac cycle is reduced. PJT can precipitate angina, hypotension, or congestive heart failure.

Treatment: If the patient is not tolerating the rapid heart rate, as evidenced by hemodynamic instability, then the following techniques should be attempted in the order given here:

1. *Vagal Maneuvers.* Ask the patient to perform a Valsalva maneuver. This is a forced expiration against a closed glottis, or the act of "bearing down" as if to move the bowels. This results in vagal stimulation, which may slow the heart. If this is unsuccessful, attempt carotid artery massage if the patient is eligible. Do not attempt carotid artery massage in patients with carotid bruits or known cerebrovascular or carotid artery disease.

2. *Pharmacological Therapy.* Verapamil, the calcium channel blocker, is often effective in terminating PJT. This is especially true if the etiology of the dysrhythmia is reentry. Administer 5 mg of verapamil intravenously. If this is unsuccessful, administer an additional dose of 5–10 mg. Verapamil is contraindicated in patients with history of bradycardia, hypotension, or congestive heart failure. It should not be used with intravenous beta blockers and should be used with caution in patients on chronic beta blocker therapy. If verapamil causes hypotension, it can often be reversed with 0.5–1.0 gm of calcium chloride administered intravenously.

3. *Electrical Therapy.* Hemodynamically unstable PJT refractory to vagal maneuvers and verapamil should be treated with synchronized cardioversion. If time allows, sedate the patient with 3–5 mg of diazepam IV. Then apply synchronized DC countershock of 75–100 joules. If this is unsuccessful, repeat the countershock at increased energy as ordered by the medical control physician. DC countershock is contraindicated if digitalis toxicity is suspected as the cause of the PJT.

DYSRHYTHMIAS ORIGINATING IN THE VENTRICLES

Dysrhythmias can originate within the ventricles. The location of the pacemaker site will dictate the morphology of the QRS complex. Many factors, including ischemia, hypoxia, and medications have been identified as causes. Dysrhythmias originating in the ventricles include:

- ❑ Ventricular escape complexes and rhythms
- ❑ Premature ventricular contraction
- ❑ Ventricular tachycardia
- ❑ Ventricular fibrillation
- ❑ Asystole
- ❑ Artificial pacemaker rhythm

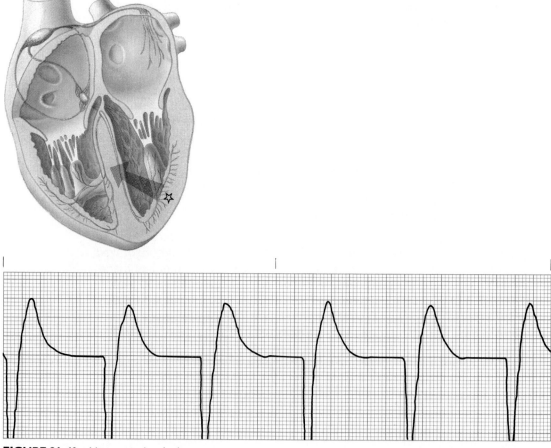

FIGURE 21-40   Idioventricular rhythm.

ECG features common to all dysrhythmias that originate in the ventricles include:

- ❏ QRS complexes of 0.12 sec or greater.
- ❏ Absent P waves.

Ventricular Escape Complexes and Rhythms (Idioventricular Rhythm)

Description: A *ventricular escape beat,* or *ventricular escape rhythm,* is a dysrhythmia that results when impulses from higher pacemakers fail to reach the ventricles, or when the rate of discharge of higher pacemakers becomes less than that of the ventricles (normally 15–45 beats per minute). Ventricular escape rhythms serve as safety mechanisms to prevent cardiac standstill.

Etiology: Ventricular escape complexes and ventricular rhythms have several etiologies. These include slowing of supraventricular pacemaker sites or high-degree AV block. They are frequently the first organized rhythms seen following defibrillation.

Rules of Interpretation (Lead II Monitoring):
Rate: 15–40 per minute (occasionally less)
Rhythm: The rhythm is irregular in a single ventricular escape complex. Ventricular escape rhythms are usually regular unless the pacemaker site is low in the ventricular conductive system, which makes regularity unreliable.
Pacemaker Site: Ventricle
P Waves: None
P-R Interval: None
QRS complex: Greater than 0.12 sec and bizarre in morphology.

Clinical Significance: The slow heart rate can significantly decrease cardiac output, possibly to life-threatening levels. The ventricular escape rhythm is a safety mechanism and should not be suppressed. Escape rhythms can be perfusing or nonperfusing and must be treated accordingly.

Treatment: If the escape rhythm is perfusing, the object of treatment is to increase the heart rate. Administer a 0.5 mg bolus of atropine sulfate. Repeat this every 5 minutes until a satisfactory rate has been obtained or 2 mg of the drug has been given. If atropine is unsuccessful, use isoproterenol as follows: place 1 mg of isoproterenol in 500 mL of D5W. The infusion should begin at 2–6 micrograms per minute. External pacing, if available, may be indicated. Epinephrine may also be used. Lidocaine is contraindicated until the heart rate is corrected. If the rhythm is nonperfusing, follow the EMD protocol. This includes airway stabilization and CPR. Place an IV line and administer epinephrine 1:10,000. Consider administering sodium bicarbonate. However, treatment should be directed at correcting the primary problem (cardiac tamponade, hypoxemia, acidosis, etc.). A fluid challenge should be considered.

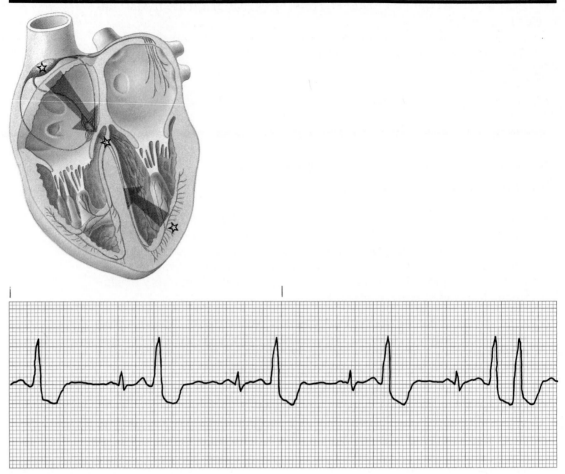

FIGURE 21-41 Premature ventricular contractions.

Premature Ventricular Contractions

Description: A *premature ventricular contraction* (PVC) is a single ectopic impulse, arising from an irritable focus in either ventricle, which occurs earlier than the next expected beat. It may result from increased automaticity in the ectopic cell or a reentry mechanism. The altered sequence of ventricular depolarization results in a wide and bizarre QRS complex. In addition, the altered sequence of ventricular depolarization can cause the T wave to occur in the opposite direction to the QRS complex.

A PVC does not usually depolarize the SA node and interrupt its rhythm. That is, the normal cadence of the heart is not interrupted. The pause following the PVC is fully compensatory. Occasionally a PVC falls between two sinus beats without interrupting the rhythm. This is called an **interpolated beat.**

If more than one PVC occurs, each one can be classified as unifocal or multifocal. The morphology of the PVC depends on the location of the ectopic pacemaker. Two PVCs of different morphologies imply two pacemaker sites (multifocal). PVCs with the same morphology are considered unifocal. If the coupling interval (the distance between the preceding beat and the PVC) is constant, the PVCs are most likely unifocal.

PVCs often occur in patterns of group beating. These include:

❑ bigeminy: every other beat is a PVC
❑ trigeminy: every third beat is a PVC
❑ quadrigeminy: every fourth beat is a PVC

These terms can be applied to PACs and PJCs as well.

Repetitive PVCs are two PVCs together without a normal complex in between. These can occur in groups of two (couplets) or groups of three (triplets). More than three PVCs in a row are often considered to be ventricular tachycardia.

PVCs can trigger lethal dysrhythmias such as ventricular fibrillation if they fall within the relative refractory period (the so-called R on T phenomenon). PVCs are often classified by their relationship to the previous normal complex.

Etiologies: Etiologies for PVCs include:

❑ myocardial ischemia
❑ hypoxia
❑ acid-base disturbances
❑ electrolyte imbalances

❑ increased sympathetic tone
❑ idiopathic causes
❑ normal variant

(continued)

■ **interpolated beat** a PVC that falls between two sinus beats without effectively interrupting this rhythm.

Premature Ventricular Contractions (*continued*)

Rules of Interpretation (Lead II Monitoring):

Rate: Depends on underlying rhythm and rate of PVCs.

Rhythm: Interrupts regularity of underlying rhythm (occasionally irregular).

Pacemaker Site: Ventricle.

P Waves: None, although a normal sinus P wave (interpolated P wave) can sometimes be seen before a PVC.

P-R Interval: None.

QRS complex: greater than 0.12 sec with bizarre morphology.

Clinical Significance: Patients often sense PVCs as "skipped beats." In a patient without heart disease, PVCs may be of no significance. In patients with myocardial ischemia, PVCs may indicate ventricular irritability and may trigger lethal ventricular dysrhythmias. PVCs are often classified as malignant or benign. Malignant PVCs have one of the following characteristics:

❑ more than 6 PVCs per minute
❑ R on T phenomenon
❑ couplets or runs of ventricular tachycardia
❑ multifocal
❑ associated with chest pain

With PVCs, the ventricles often do not fill adequately and there is often no pulse associated with them. If PVCs are frequent, then cardiac output may fall.

Treatment: If the patient has no history of cardiac disease and no symptoms and the PVCs are nonmalignant, no treatment is required. (See Figure 21-42.)

If the patient has a prior history of heart disease or symptoms, or the PVCs are malignant, administer oxygen and place an IV line. Administer lidocaine at a dose of 1 mg/kg of body weight. Give additional lidocaine every 5 minutes at a dose of 0.5 mg/kg until 3.0 mg/kg of the drug has been given. Concurrently, start a lidocaine drip beginning at a rate of 2 mg/min. Increase this with each additional bolus until 4 mg/min is being administered. If the patient is allergic to lidocaine or if a maximum dose of lidocaine (300 mg) has been given, procainamide or bretylium should be considered.

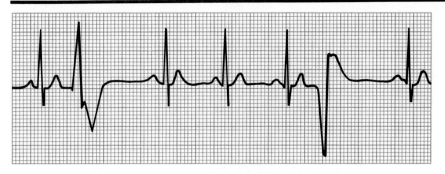

Ventricular ectopy

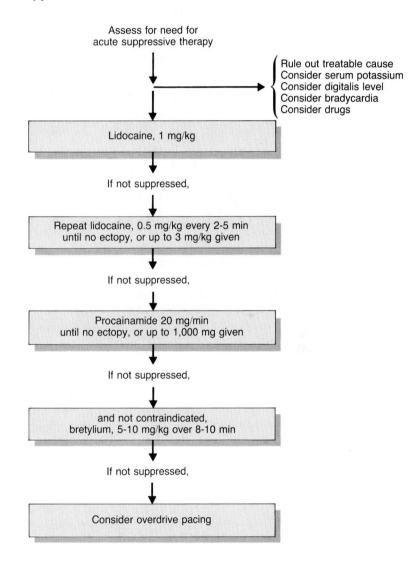

Assess for need for
acute suppressive therapy

Rule out treatable cause
Consider serum potassium
Consider digitalis level
Consider bradycardia
Consider drugs

Lidocaine, 1 mg/kg

If not suppressed,

Repeat lidocaine, 0.5 mg/kg every 2-5 min
until no ectopy, or up to 3 mg/kg given

If not suppressed,

Procainamide 20 mg/min
until no ectopy, or up to 1,000 mg given

If not suppressed,

and not contraindicated,
bretylium, 5-10 mg/kg over 8-10 min

If not suppressed,

Consider overdrive pacing

Once ectopy resolved, maintain as follows:
  After lidocaine, 1 mg/kg . . . lidocaine drip, 2 mg/min
  After lidocaine, 1-2 mg/kg . . . lidocaine drip, 3 mg/min
  After lidocaine, 2-3 mg/kg . . . lidocaine drip, 4 mg/min
  After procainamide . . . procainamide drip, 1-4 mg/min (check blood level)
  After bretylium . . . bretylium drip, 2 mg/min

FIGURE 21-42

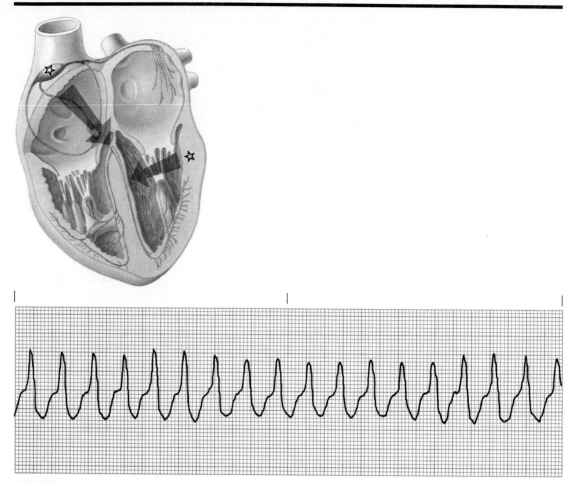

FIGURE 21-43 Ventricular tachycardia.

Ventricular Tachycardia

Description: *Ventricular tachycardia* is a rhythm which consists of three or more ventricular complexes in succession at a rate of 100 beats per minute or more. This rhythm overrides the normal pacemaker of the heart, and the atria and ventricles are asynchronous. Sinus P waves may occasionally be seen, dissociated from the QRS complexes.

Etiology: Several etiologies have been identified for ventricular tachycardia. As with PVCs, these include:

❑ myocardial ischemia
❑ hypoxia
❑ acid-base disturbances
❑ electrolyte imbalances
❑ increased sympathetic tone
❑ idiopathic causes

Rules of Interpretation (Lead II Monitoring):
    Rate: 100–250 (approximately).
    Rhythm: Usually regular; can be slightly irregular.
    Pacemaker Site: Ventricle.
    P Waves: If present, not associated with the QRS complexes
    P-R Interval: None.
    QRS complex: Greater than 0.12 sec and bizarre in morphology.

Clinical Significance: Ventricular tachycardia usually results in poor stroke volume. This, coupled with the rapid ventricular rate, may severely compromise cardiac output and coronary artery perfusion. Ventricular tachycardia may be either perfusing or nonperfusing, and this dictates the type of treatment. Ventricular tachycardia may eventually deteriorate into ventricular fibrillation.

Treatment: If the patient is perfusing, as evidenced by the presence of a pulse, administer oxygen and place an IV line. Administer lidocaine at a dose of 1 mg/kg body weight intravenously. Administer additional doses of 0.5 mg/kg until a total of 3.0 mg/kg has been administered. If this treatment is unsuccessful, attempt to administer procainamide. Use cardioversion if the patient becomes unstable, as evidenced by chest pain, dyspnea, or systolic blood pressure of less than 90 mm/hg.

If the patient's condition is unstable, as evidenced by an altered level of consciousness or falling blood pressure, then cardioversion should be the initial treatment after placement of an IV line and oxygen administration. If time allows, sedate the patient first. The treatment plan is illustrated in the protocol.

If the patient is nonperfusing, follow the protocol for ventricular fibrillation. (See Figure 21-63, page 680.)

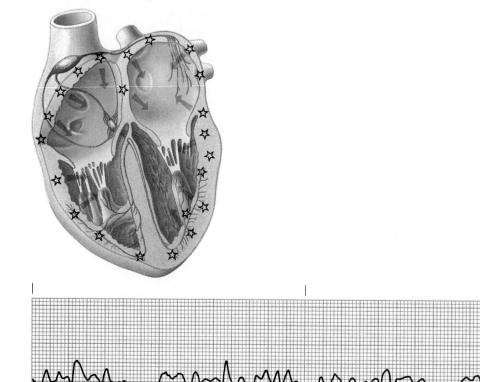

FIGURE 21-44 Ventricular fibrillation.

Ventricular Fibrillation

Description: Ventricular fibrillation is a chaotic ventricular rhythm usually resulting from the presence of many reentry circuits within the ventricles. There is no ventricular depolarization or contraction.

Etiology: A wide variety of causes have been associated with ventricular fibrillation. Most cases result from advanced coronary artery disease.

Rules of Interpretation (Lead II Monitoring):
   Rate: No organized rhythm.
   Rhythm: No organized rhythm.
   Pacemaker Site: Numerous ectopic foci throughout the ventricles.
   P Waves: Usually absent.
   P-R Interval: Absent.
   QRS complex: Absent.

Clinical Significance: Ventricular fibrillation is a lethal dysrhythmia. There is no cardiac output or organized electrical pattern, thus resulting in cardiac arrest.

Treatment: Ventricular fibrillation and nonperfusing ventricular tachycardia are treated identically. Initiate CPR. Follow this with DC countershock at 200 joules. If this is unsuccessful, repeat at 200–300 joules. If this is still unsuccessful, repeat at 360 joules. Subsequently, control the airway and establish an IV line. Epinephrine 1:10,000 is the drug of first choice. This can be administered every 5 minutes as required. If unsuccessful, lidocaine, bretylium, or possibly sodium bicarbonate should be considered. (See Figure 21-62, page 679.)

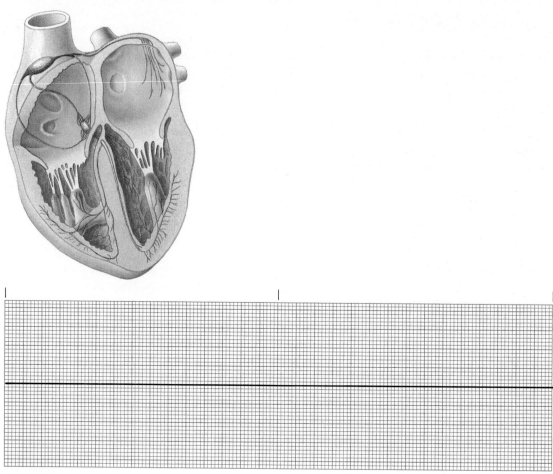

FIGURE 21-45 Asystole.

Asystole (Cardiac Standstill)

Description: *Asystole* is the absence of all cardiac electrical activity.

Etiology: Asystole may be the primary event in cardiac arrest. It is usually associated with massive myocardial infarction, ischemia, and necrosis. Asystole is often the end result of ventricular fibrillation. Asystole results from cases of heart block, in which no escape pacemaker takes over.

Rules of Interpretation (Lead II Monitoring):
    Rate: No electrical activity.
    Rhythm: No electrical activity.
    Pacemaker Site: No electrical activity.
    P Waves: Absent.
    P-R Interval: Absent.
    QRS complex: Absent.

Clinical Significance: Asystole results in cardiac arrest. The prognosis for resuscitation is very poor.

Treatment: Asystole is treated with CPR, airway management, oxygenation, and medications. If there is any doubt about the underlying rhythm, attempt defibrillation. Medications include epinephrine, atropine, and, in certain situations, sodium bicarbonate. (See Figure 21-64, page 681.)

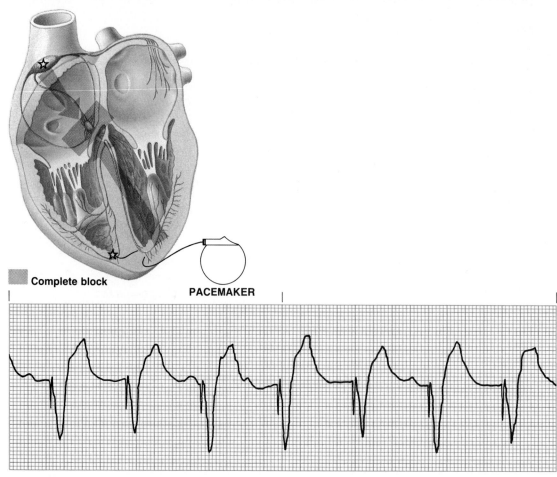

Complete block

PACEMAKER

FIGURE 21-46 Artificial pacemaker rhythm.

Artificial Pacemaker Rhythm

Description: An *artificial pacemaker rhythm* is a rhythm generated by regular electrical stimulation of the heart through an electrode implanted in the heart and connected to a power source. The pacemaker lead may be implanted in any of several locations in the heart, although it is most often placed in the right ventricle or in both chambers (dual-chambered pacemaker).

Pacemakers that fire continuously at a preset rate are called *fixed-rate pacemakers.* This firing occurs regardless of the electrical activity of the heart. *Demand pacemakers* contain a sensing device and fire only when the natural rate of the heart drops below the rate set for the pacemaker. In these cases, the pacemaker acts as an escape rhythm.

The ventricular pacemaker stimulates only the right ventricle, resulting in a rhythm that resembles an idioventricular rhythm. Dual-chambered pacemakers, commonly called *AV sequential pacemakers,* stimulate the atria first and then the ventricles. These are most beneficial for patients with marginal cardiac output who need the extra atrial "kick" to maintain cardiac output.

Pacemakers are usually inserted into patients with chronic high-grade heart block, sick sinus syndrome, or who have had episodes of severe symptomatic bradycardia.

Rules of Interpretation (Lead II Monitoring):

Rate: Varies with the preset rate of the pacemaker.

Rhythm: Regular if pacing constantly; irregular if pacing on demand.

Pacemaker Site: Depends on electrode placement.

P Waves: None produced by ventricular pacemakers. Sinus P waves may be seen but are unrelated to the paced QRS complexes. Dual-chambered pacemakers produce a P wave behind each atrial spike. A pacemaker spike is an upward or downward deflection from the baseline which is an artifact created each time the pacemaker fires. The *pacemaker spike* tells you only that the pacemaker is firing. It reveals nothing about ventricular depolarization.

P-R Interval: If present, varies.

QRS complex: The QRS complexes associated with pacemaker rhythms are usually longer than 0.12 sec and bizarre in morphology. They often resemble ventricular escape rhythms. Each pacemaker spike should be followed by a QRS complex. If this occurs, the pacemaker is said to be "capturing." In patients with demand pacemakers, some of the patient's own QRS complexes may be seen. A pacemaker spike should not be seen in these patients.

Problems with pacemakers: Problems, although rare, can arise from pacemakers. One cause is battery failure. Most pacemaker batteries have relatively long lives and can be checked by the cardiologist. Batteries are usually changed before problems arise. However, if a battery fails, no pacing will occur and the patient's underlying rhythm, which may be bradycardic or asystolic, may return.

Occasionally, a pacemaker can "run away." This condition, rarely seen with new pacemakers, results in a rapid rate of discharge. Runaway pacemaker usually occurs when the battery runs low. Newer models gradually increase their rate as their batteries run low.

Demand pacemakers can fail to shut down when the patient's heart rate exceeds the limit set for the device. Thus the pacemaker competes with the patient's own natural pacemaker. Occasionally, a paced beat can fall in the vulnerable period, precipitating ventricular fibrillation.

Finally, pacemakers can fail to capture. This can occur when the leads become displaced or the battery fails. In such cases, pacemaker spikes are usually present but are not followed by P waves or QRS complexes. Bradycardia often results.

Considerations for Management: Always examine any unconscious patient for a pacemaker. Battery packs are usually palpable under the skin, usually in the shoulder or axillary region. Bradydysrhythmias, asystole, and ventricular fibrillation resulting from pacemaker failure are treated as in any other patient. Ventricular irritability may be treated with lidocaine without fear of suppressing ventricular response to the pacemaker. Patients with pacemakers can be defibrillated as usual, but do not discharge paddles directly over the battery pack. External cardiac pacing, if available, can be used until definitive care is available. Patients with pacemaker failure should be promptly transported without prolonged field stabilization. Definitive care consists of battery replacement or temporary pacemaker insertion.

DYSRHYTHMIAS THAT ARE DISORDERS OF CONDUCTION

Several dysrhythmias result from improper conduction through the heart. The three general categories of conductive disorders are:

- ❑ Atrioventricular blocks
- ❑ Disturbances of ventricular conduction
- ❑ Pre-excitation syndromes

The dysrhythmias that will be discussed under this heading are:

- ❑ AV blocks
    - ❑ First-degree AV block
    - ❑ Second-degree AV block (Mobitz I)
    - ❑ Second-degree AV block (Mobitz II)
    - ❑ Third-degree AV block
- ❑ Disturbances of ventricular conduction
- ❑ Pre-excitation syndromes
    - ❑ Wolff-Parkinson-White Syndrome

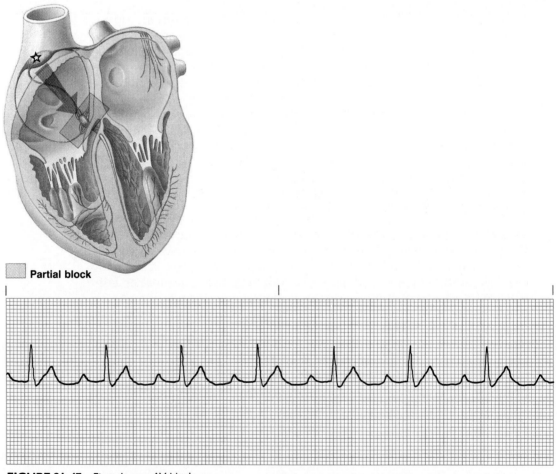

□ **Partial block**

FIGURE 21-47 First-degree AV block.

AV Blocks

An *AV block* is the delay or interruption of impulses between the atria and the ventricles. These dysrhythmias can be caused by pathology of the AV junctional tissue or by a physiological block, such as occurs with atrial fibrillation or flutter. Causes include AV junctional ischemia, AV junctional necrosis, degenerative disease of the conductive system, and drug toxicity (particularly digitalis).

AV blocks can be classified according to the site or according to the degree of the block. Blocks may occur at the following sites:

- ❏ At level of AV node
- ❏ At level of bundle of His
- ❏ Below bifurcation of bundle of His

The following discussion classifies AV blocks as the following degrees (traditional classification):

- ❏ First-degree AV block
- ❏ Second-degree AV block Type I
- ❏ Second-degree AV block Type II
- ❏ Third-degree AV block

First-Degree AV Block

Description: A *first-degree AV block* is a delay in conduction at the level of the AV node rather than an actual block. First-degree AV block is not a rhythm in itself, but a condition superimposed upon another rhythm. The underlying rhythm must also be identified (for example, sinus bradycardia with first-degree AV block).

Etiology: AV block can occur in the healthy heart. However, ischemia at the AV junction is the most common cause.

Rules of Interpretation (Lead II Monitoring):
Rate: Depends on underlying rhythm.
Rhythm: Usually regular. However, can be slightly irregular.
Pacemaker Site: SA node or atria.
P Waves: Normal.
P-R Interval: Greater than 0.20 sec (diagnostic).
QRS complex: Normally, less than 0.12 sec. May be bizarre in shape if conductive system disease exists in the ventricles.

Clinical Significance: First-degree block is usually no danger in itself. However, a newly developed first-degree block may be a forerunner of a more advanced block.

Treatment: Generally, no treatment is required except observation, unless the heart rate drops significantly. Drugs that slow AV conduction, such as lidocaine and procainamide, should be avoided if possible.

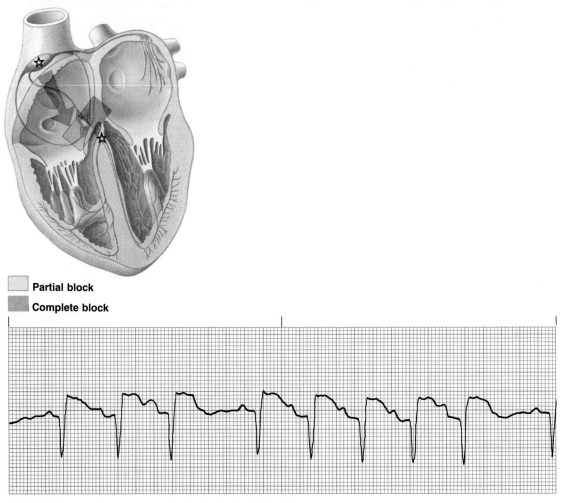

Partial block
Complete block

FIGURE 21-48 Second-degree AV block (Mobitz I) Wenkebach

Second-Degree AV Block (Mobitz I) Wenckebach

Description: A *second-degree AV block (Mobitz I)* is an intermittent block at the level of the AV node. It produces a characteristic cyclic pattern in which the P-R intervals become progressively longer until an impulse is blocked (not conducted). The cycle is repetitive. The P-P interval remains constant, whereas the P-R interval becomes progressively longer, until a beat is dropped. The ratio of conduction (P waves to QRS complexes) is commonly 5:4, 4:3, 3:2, or 2:1. The pattern may be constant or variable. Second-degree AV block (Mobitz I) is commonly called the *Wenckebach phenomenon.*

Etiology: AV blocks can occur in the healthy heart. However, ischemia at the AV junction is the most common cause. Increased parasympathetic tone and drugs are also common etiologies.

Rules of Interpretation (Lead II Monitoring):
  Rate: Atrial rate is unaffected. The ventricular rate may be normal or slowed.
  Rhythm: Atrial rhythm is typically regular and ventricular rhythm is irregular because of the nonconducted beat.
  Pacemaker Site: SA node or atria.
  P Waves: Normal; some P waves not followed by QRS complexes.
  P-R Interval: Becomes progressively longer until the QRS complex is dropped. The cycle is then repeated.
  QRS complex: Usually less than 0.12 sec. May be bizarre in shape if conductive system disease exists in the ventricles.

Clinical Significance: Second-degree block can compromise cardiac output by causing problems such as syncope and angina if beats are frequently dropped. This block is often a transient phenomenon that occurs immediately after an inferior wall myocardial infarction.

Treatment: Generally, no treatment, other than observation, is required. Drugs that slow AV conduction, such as lidocaine and procainamide, should be avoided if possible. If the heart rate falls and the patient becomes symptomatic, administer 0.5 mg of atropine IV every 5 minutes, as required, until a total of 2 mg has been given. Thereafter, isoproterenol may be required. If available, consider external pacing.

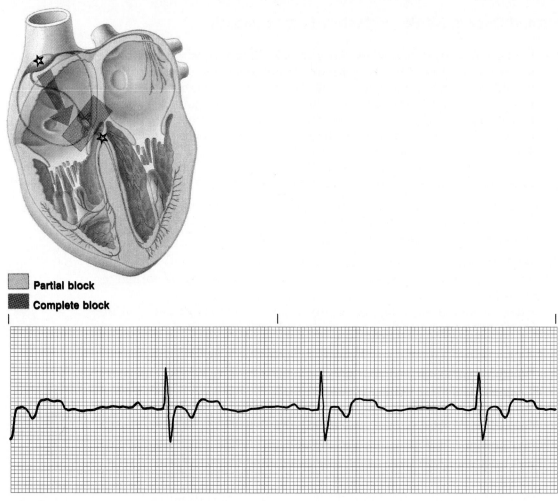

Partial block

Complete block

FIGURE 21-49 Second-degree AV block (Mobitz II).

Second-Degree AV Block (Mobitz II)

Description: A *second-degree AV block (Mobitz II)* is an intermittent block characterized by P waves that are not conducted to the ventricles, but without associated lengthening of the P-R interval before the dropped beats. The ratio of conduction (P waves to QRS complexes) is commonly 4:1, 3:1, or 2:1. The ratio may be constant or may vary. A 2:1 Mobitz II block is often indistinguishable from a 2:1 Mobitz I block.

Etiology: Second-degree AV block (Mobitz II) is usually associated with acute myocardial infarction and septal necrosis.

Rules of Interpretation (Lead II Monitoring):
Rate: Atrial rate is unaffected. Ventricular rate is usually bradycardic.
Rhythm: Regular or irregular depending, on whether the conduction ratio is constant or varied.
Pacemaker Site: SA node or atria.
P Waves: Normal; some P waves not followed by QRS complexes.
P-R Interval: Constant for conducted beats. May be greater than 0.21 sec.
QRS complex: May be normal. However, is often greater than 0.12 sec because of abnormal ventricular depolarization sequence.

Clinical Significance: Second-degree block can compromise cardiac output, causing problems such as syncope and angina if beats are frequently dropped. Since this block is often associated with cell necrosis resulting from myocardial infarction, it is considered much more serious than Mobitz I. Many Mobitz II blocks develop into full AV blocks.

Treatment: Pacemaker insertion is the definitive treatment. In the field, if stabilization is required, medications should be administered. If the heart rate falls and the patient becomes symptomatic, administer 0.5 mg of atropine IV every 5 minutes, as required, until a total of 2 mg has been given. Thereafter, isoproterenol may be required. Drugs that slow AV conduction, such as lidocaine and procainamide, should be avoided if possible. External pacing, if available, should be considered.

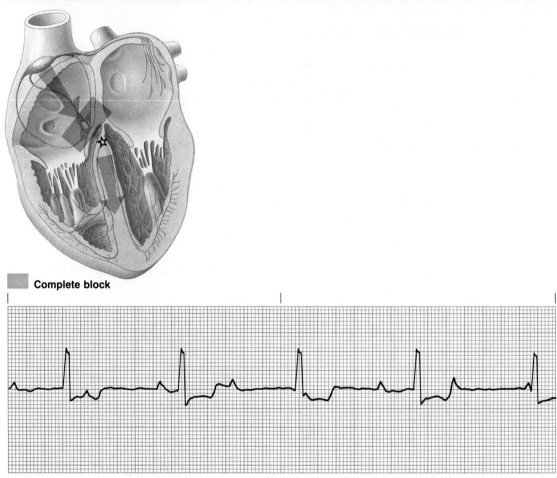

Complete block

FIGURE 21-50 Third-degree AV block.

Third-Degree AV Block

Description: A *third-degree AV block,* or complete block, is the absence of conduction between the atria and the ventricles resulting from complete electrical block at or below the AV node. The atria and ventricles subsequently pace the heart independent of each other. The sinus node often functions normally, depolarizing the atrial syncytium, while the escape pacemaker, located below the atria, paces the ventricular syncytium.

Etiology: Third-degree AV block can result from acute MI, digitalis toxicity, or degeneration of the conductive system, as occurs in the elderly.

Rules of Interpretation (Lead II Monitoring):
  Rate: Atrial rate is unaffected. Ventricular rate is 40-60 if the escape pacemaker is junctional or less than 40 if the escape pacemaker is lower in the ventricles.
  Rhythm: Both atrial and ventricular rhythms are usually regular.
  Pacemaker Site: SA node and AV junction or ventricle.
  P Waves: Normal. P waves show no relationship to the QRS complex, often falling within the T wave and QRS complex.
  P-R Interval: No relationship between P waves and R waves.
  QRS complex: Greater than 0.12 sec if pacemaker is ventricular. Less than 0.12 second if pacemaker is junctional.

Clinical Significance: Third-degree block can severely compromise cardiac output because of decreased heart rate and loss of coordinated atrial kick.

Treatment: Pacemaker insertion is the definitive treatment. In the field, if stabilization is required, medications should be administered. If the heart rate falls and the patient becomes symptomatic, administer 0.5 mg atropine IV every 5 minutes, as required, until a total of 2 mg has been given. Atropine not only increases SA node discharge but often increases AV conduction. Isoproterenol is often required as well. External pacing, if available, should be considered. Drugs that slow AV conduction, such as lidocaine and procainamide, should be avoided.

Disturbances of Ventricular Conduction. Disturbances in conduction of the depolarization impulse are not limited to the AV node. Problems can arise within the ventricles as well. Certain terms are frequently used in describing disturbances in ventricular conduction. **Aberrant conduction** is a single supraventricular beat that is conducted through the ventricles in a delayed manner. **Bundle branch block** is a disorder in which all supraventricular beats are conducted through the ventricles in a delayed manner. Either the left or right bundle branch can be involved. If both branches are blocked, then a third-degree AV block exists. These terms are used to describe complexes that originate above the ventricles and should be distinguished from pure ventricular rhythms, which can have a similar QRS morphology.

Two causes have been identified for ventricular conduction disturbances. One is ischemia or necrosis of either the right or left bundle branch, making it unable to conduct the impulse to the ventricle it supplies. The second cause occurs when a premature impulse, either a PAC or a PJC, reaches the ventricles when one of the bundle branches, usually the right, is still refractory and cannot conduct. This is often seen in atrial fibrillation as a result of the varying speed of repolarization related to the highly irregular rhythm.

The ECG features of ventricular conduction disturbances include a QRS complex longer than 0.12 sec. This happens because the blocked side of the heart is depolarized much more slowly than the unaffected side. The impulse passes much more slowly through the myocardium than through the rapid electrical conduction pathway. The QRS morphology is often bizarre. The QRS can be notched or slurred, reflecting rapid depolarization through the normal conductive system and slow depolarization through the myocardium on the blocked side.

The presence of a ventricular conduction disturbance sometimes complicates the interpretation of ECG rhythm strips. In these cases, supraventricular beats can have QRS complexes that are abnormally wide. Because of this, it may be impossible to distinguish between PVCs and aberrantly conducted PACs or PJCs on a lead II rhythm strip. Also, it is often difficult to distinguish supraventricular tachycardia with bundle branch block or aberrancy from ventricular tachycardia. A 12-lead tracing is often necessary to make the diagnosis. The presence of a bundle branch block or aberrancy does not affect management of the patient. When in doubt, treat all premature beats or rhythms with abnormally wide QRS complexes as ventricular in origin.

Pre-excitation Syndromes. The remaining category of cardiac dysrhythmias to be presented is the pre-excitation syndromes, the most common of which is *Wolff-Parkinson-White (WPW)* syndrome. WPW occurs in approximately 3 out of every 1,000 persons. It is characterized by a short P-R interval, generally less than 0.12 sec; and a prolonged QRS duration, generally longer than 0.12 sec. In addition, there is often a slur on the upstroke of the QRS, called the *delta wave*. (See Figure 21-51.) In WPW there is abnormal conduction of the depolarization impulse from the atria to the ventricles. An extra conduction pathway, the **bundle of Kent,** is present between the atria and ventricles. The AV node is effectively bypassed, resulting in a shortened P-R interval and prolonged QRS complex. Most WPW patients are asymptomatic. However, the disorder is associated with a high incidence of tachydysrhythmias, usually through a

■ **aberrant conduction** conduction of the electrical impulse through the heart's conductive system in an abnormal fashion.

■ **bundle branch block** a kind of interventricular heart block where conduction through either the right of left bundle branches is blocked or delayed.

■ **bundle of Kent** an accessory AV conduction pathway that is thought to be responsible for the ECG findings of pre-excitation syndrome.

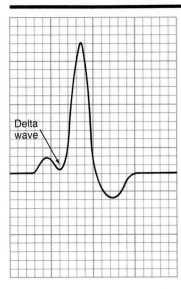

FIGURE 21-51   The delta wave of Wolf-Parkinson-White syndrome.

reentry mechanism. WPW is also frequently associated with organic heart disease, such as atrial septal defects, mitral valve prolapse, and other problems. Treatment is based on the underlying rhythm.

ASSESSMENT OF THE CARDIAC PATIENT

Common Chief Complaints and History

Cardiac disease can manifest itself in several ways. When assessing a patient suspected of suffering cardiac disease, the paramedic should note each presenting complaint and obtain a history appropriate to the presenting symptom. Common presenting symptoms of cardiac disease include:

❑ chest pain or discomfort
❑ shoulder pain
❑ neck pain
❑ jaw pain
❑ dyspnea
❑ syncope
❑ palpitations

This section addresses the common presenting symptoms of cardiac disease and highlights pertinent aspects of the history.

Chest Pain

Chest pain or chest discomfort are common presenting symptoms of cardiac disease. Chest pain is the most common presenting symptom of myo-

✱ Chest pain is the most common presenting symptom of cardiac disease.

cardial infarction. When confronted by a patient with chest pain, obtain the following essential elements of the history:

- ❑ specific location of the chest pain (midsternal, etc.)
- ❑ radiation of the pain, if present (e.g., to the jaw, back, or shoulders)
- ❑ duration of the pain
- ❑ factors that precipitated the pain (exercise, stress, etc.)
- ❑ type or quality of the pain (dull or sharp)
- ❑ associated symptoms (nausea, dyspnea)
- ❑ anything that aggravates or alleviates the pain (including medications)
- ❑ previous episodes of a similar pain (e.g., angina)

It is important to remember that chest pain has many causes other than cardiac disease. The history, therefore, is an important determining factor.

Shoulder, arm, neck, or jaw pain or discomfort may also be an indicator of cardiac disease. Any of these may occur with or without associated chest pain. If the patient has any of these symptoms and you suspect heart disease, obtain information similar to that described above for chest pain.

Dyspnea

Because of the close interrelationship between the heart and the pulmonary system, many cardiac patients have dyspnea. Dyspnea is often an associated symptom of myocardial infarction. In some patients it may be the only symptom of myocardial infarction. It may also be a primary symptom of pulmonary fluid congestion due to heart failure. Dyspnea is a subjective symptom and is often difficult to assess. When confronted by a dyspneic patient, try to determine the following:

- ❑ duration of dyspnea
- ❑ onset (sudden or rapid)
- ❑ anything that aggravates or relieves the dyspnea (including medications)
- ❑ previous episodes
- ❑ any associated symptoms
- ❑ prior cardiac problems

Many illnesses, other than cardiac disease, can cause dyspnea. Common causes include pneumonia, chronic obstructive pulmonary disease, asthma, and pulmonary embolism.

Syncope

Cardiac problems are a major cause of syncope. Syncope, which is caused by an interruption of blood flow to the brain, may be the only presenting symptom of cardiac disease, especially in the elderly. Cardiac causes of syncope usually result from dysrhythmias. These can include transient or prolonged bradycardia, causing decreased cardiac output and, subsequently, decreased cerebral perfusion. Very rapid heart rates, on the other hand, do not allow adequate time for ventricular filling. This also results in decreased cardiac output and can cause syncope. When the primary complaint is syncope, try to establish the following:

- ❑ circumstances of occurrence (for example, patient's position)
- ❑ duration of the episode
- ❑ any symptoms before the episode of syncope
- ❑ other associated symptoms
- ❑ previous episodes of syncope

Syncope will be discussed in detail in Chapter 23, Nervous System Emergencies.

Palpitations

Some patients with cardiac disease complain of an awareness of their own heartbeat. This is termed **palpitation** and is usually related to either an irregular beat ("skipping beats") or a rapid heart rate. Essential aspects of the history when assessing these patients include:

■ **palpitation** a sensation that the heart is pounding or racing.

- ❑ circumstances of occurrence
- ❑ duration of occurrence
- ❑ associated symptoms
- ❑ frequency of occurrence
- ❑ previous episodes

Significant Past Medical History in the Cardiac Patient

The paramedic should not spend a great deal of time obtaining the past medical history of a cardiac patient, because the patient will be treated based on current symptoms rather than the history. However, if the patient's condition permits, determine the following:

1. Is the patient taking prescription medications regularly, particularly cardiac medications? Examples include:

   - ❑ nitroglycerin
   - ❑ propranolol (Inderal)
   - ❑ digitalis (Lanoxin)
   - ❑ diuretics (Lasix, Maxzide, Dyazide)
   - ❑ antihypertensives (Vasotec, Prinivil, Capoten)
   - ❑ other antidysrhythmics (Mexitil, Quinaglute, Tambocor)

2. Is the patient currently under treatment for any serious illness?
3. Has the patient ever been known to have:

   - ❑ a heart attack or angina
   - ❑ heart failure

❑ hypertension
❑ diabetes
❑ chronic lung disease

4. Does the patient have any allergies?

Physical Examination of the Cardiac Patient

The physical examination of the suspected cardiac patient should begin like the examination of any patient. First, complete the primary survey. (See Figure 21-52.) This should include the mini-neuro examination. Subsequently, after addressing any life-threatening problems detected in the primary survey, begin the secondary assessment. Pay particular attention to the blood pressure, respiratory rate, rate and regularity of the pulse (an irregular pulse may be the first indication of a dysrhythmia), and level of consciousness. Any deviation from the normal level of consciousness may indicate inadequate cerebral perfusion, possibly caused by poor cardiac output.

The secondary survey of the cardiac patient should be systematic and complete. The paramedic should pay special attention to the following:

Look

Skin color and capillary refill. Both skin color and capillary refill are good indicators of red blood cell oxygenation. (See Figure 21-53.) They also indicate pump adequacy, since peripheral perfusion is among the first areas to become compromised in pump failure.

Jugular venous distention. The internal jugular veins are major vessels of the venous system. Thus, an increase in central venous pressure is

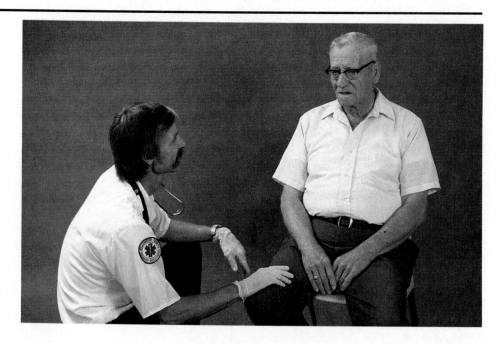

FIGURE 21-52 When treating a potential cardiac patient always begin with the primary assessment.

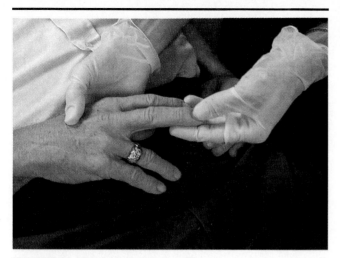

FIGURE 21-53 Assess capillary refill.

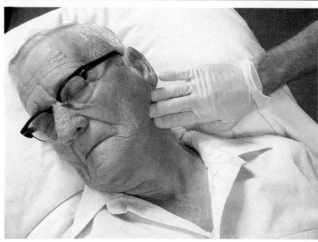

FIGURE 21-54 Look for the presence of jugular venous distension, ideally with the patient elevated at a 45 degree angle.

often evidenced by jugular venous distention. (See Figure 21-54.) Pump failure can cause backpressure in the systemic circulation and jugular vein engorgement. The patient should be examined while seated at a 45 degree angle, not lying flat. Jugular venous distention is often difficult to assess in the obese patient.

Peripheral/presacral edema. Peripheral and presacral edema are caused by chronic backpressure in the systemic venous circulation. They are most obvious in dependent parts, such as the ankles. (See Figure 21-55.) In bedridden patients, it is often necessary to inspect and palpate the sacral region for the presence of edema. Edema is generally classified as mild or pitting. The two types can be distinguished by pressing firmly on the edematous part. If, after removal of the pressure, the depression remains, then the edema is said to be pitting.

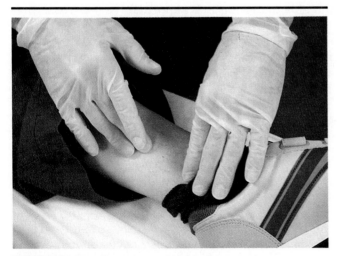

FIGURE 21-55 Check for peripheral edema.

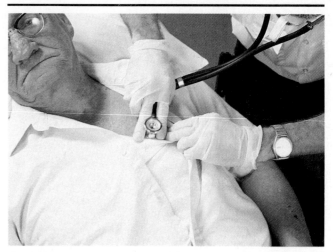

FIGURE 21-56 Auscultate the chest. Listen for heart sounds.

Subtle indicators of cardiac disease. Observe for things that indicate that a patient is being treated for cardiac problems. These include the presence of a midsternal scar from coronary artery bypass surgery, a pacemaker, or a nitroglycerin skin patch.

Listen

Breath sounds. Assessment of the breath sounds in the cardiac patient is just as important as it is in the patient with respiratory disease. Assess the lung fields for equality as well as for the presence of adventitious sounds (rales, wheezes, or rhonchi) that may indicate pulmonary congestion or edema.

Heart sounds. Do not spend a great deal of time auscultating heart sounds in the field, as the information obtained will generally not affect patient management. However, the paramedic should be familiar with normal heart sounds and able to distinguish abnormal from normal findings. (See Figure 21-56.) The first heart sound, referred to as S1, is produced by closure of the AV valves (tricuspid and mitral) during ventricular systole. The second heart sound, S2, is produced by closure of the aortic and pulmonary valves. S1 and S2 are normal findings. Extra heart sounds are abnormal findings. The third heart sound, S3, is associated with congestive heart failure. Occasionally, the skilled listener can hear the fourth heart sound, S4, which occurs immediately before S1. It is associated with increased contraction of the atria.

Carotid artery bruit. A bruit is a sign of turbulent blood flow through a vessel. Auscultation of the carotid arteries may reveal the presence of bruits. (See Figure 21-57.) A bruit indicates partial blockage of the vessel, most commonly from atherosclerosis. If a bruit is present, carotid sinus massage should not be attempted, as this may cause dislodgement of plaque, resulting in stroke or other mishap.

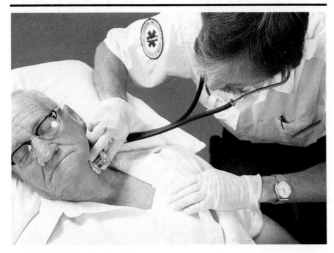

FIGURE 21-57 Listen to the carotid arteries. The presence of noisy blood flow is termed a bruit and may indicate underlying disease in the artery.

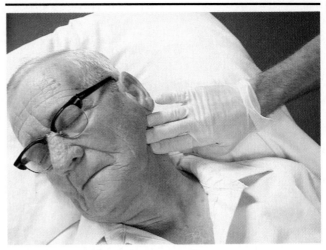

FIGURE 21-58 Check the pulse for both strength and character.

Feel

Pulse. As mentioned above, the pulse can tell a great deal about the status of the circulatory system. (See Figure 21-58.) Determine the rate and regularity of the pulse. Equality of the pulses should also be noted. Any pulse deficit can indicate underlying peripheral vascular disease and should be reported to the medical control physician.

Skin. Several changes in the skin can be associated with cardiovascular disease. A pale and diaphoretic skin is an indicator of peripheral vasoconstriction and sympathetic stimulation. It accompanies heart disease and other problems. A mottled appearance often indicates chronic cardiac failure.

PATHOPHYSIOLOGY AND MANAGEMENT

Atherosclerosis

Cardiovascular disease is the number one cause of death in the United States and in most developed countries. The major reason behind this is the disease atherosclerosis. **Atherosclerosis** is a progressive, degenerative disease of the medium-sized and large arteries. It affects the aorta and its branches, the coronary arteries, and the cerebral arteries, among others. It results from the deposition of fats (lipids and cholesterol) under the tunica intima layer of the involved vessels. After fat is deposited, an injury response occurs in the vessel wall which subsequently damages the tunica media as well. Over time, calcium is deposited, causing the formation of plaques. Small hemorrhages can occur in the plaques, causing scarring and fibrosis and further enlarging the plaques. The involved arteries can become completely blocked, either by additional plaque or by a blood clot.

■ **Atherosclerosis** a progressive, degenerative disease of the medium-sized and large arteries.

The risk factors for atherosclerosis include:

Modifiable risk factors:

❑ Hypertension
❑ Smoking
❑ Elevated blood lipids (cholesterol and triglycerides)
❑ Lack of exercise

Nonmodifiable risk factors:

❑ Male gender
❑ Advanced age
❑ Family history of heart disease and atherosclerosis
❑ Diabetes mellitus (good control reduces risk)

■ **arteriosclerosis** a thickening, loss of elasticity, and hardening of the walls of the arteries from calcium.

The results of atherosclerosis are evident in many disease processes. First, disruption of the intimal surface of the involved blood vessel causes loss of vessel elasticity. This condition, **arteriosclerosis,** can result in hypertension and other related problems. Second, blood flow through the affected vessel can be reduced. Common manifestations of this include angina pectoris and intermittent claudication. Frequently, thrombosis and complete obstruction occur, resulting in total obstruction of the vessel or the tissues it supplies. Myocardial infarction is a classic example of this process.

Specific Conditions Resulting From Atherosclerosis of the Coronary Arteries

Angina Pectoris. *Angina pectoris* literally means "pain in the chest." The condition is much more complicated than that, however. Angina occurs when the oxygen demands of the heart are transiently exceeded by the blood supply. In other words, during periods of increased oxygen demand, the coronary arteries cannot deliver an adequate amount of blood to the myocardium. This can result in ischemia of the myocardium and chest pain.

As a rule, the reduction in blood flow through the coronary arteries results from atherosclerosis. However, abnormal spasm of the coronary arteries, commonly called *vasospastic angina* or **Prinzmetal's angina,** can also lead to inadequate blood flow. It is important to remember that blood flow through a vessel is related to its diameter. Reducing the diameter of a vessel by one-half, such as can occur in atherosclerosis, causes a major reduction in the amount of blood that can be transported through that vessel.

■ **Prinzmetal's angina** variant of angina pectoris caused by vasospasm of the coronary arteries, not blockage *per se.*

Angina is generally divided into two types: stable angina and unstable, or preinfarction angina. *Stable angina* is angina that occurs during activity, when the oxygen demands of the heart are increased. Attacks of stable angina are usually precipitated by physical or emotional stress. They can be of relatively short duration, 3-5 minutes, or prolonged, lasting 15 minutes or more. The pain of stable angina can often be relieved by rest, nitroglycerin, or oxygen. *Unstable angina,* on the other hand, may not respond as readily. Unstable angina occurs at rest. Because the condition often indicates severe atherosclerotic disease, it is also called *preinfarction angina.*

The pain associated with angina is primarily caused by a buildup of lactic acid and CO_2 in the ischemic myocardium. The patient usually complains of substernal chest pain or epigastric discomfort. The patient may describe the discomfort as pain, pressure, squeezing, or tightness. Anginal pain is frequently mistaken for indigestion. One-third of angina patients feel pain only in the chest. Others have pain that radiates to the shoulder, arm, neck, jaw, or through to the back. Some patients have associated symptoms of anxiety, dyspnea, or diaphoresis.

Angina can be accompanied by dysrhythmias which are precipitated by ischemia. For this reason, all patients suspected of suffering angina should be placed on the cardiac monitor.

If a patient has a prior history of angina and is currently taking nitroglycerin, try to determine if the patient has taken nitroglycerin for the present attack, how much has been taken, and if it has relieved the discomfort. If the patient's nitroglycerin tablets are old, they may be ineffective. It is not uncommon for a patient's symptoms to be relieved by the time EMS arrives because of nitroglycerin therapy.

Management. The patient experiencing angina is often apprehensive. Place the patient at rest, physically and emotionally, to decrease myocardial oxygen demand. Administer oxygen, generally at a high flow rate, to increase oxygen delivery to the myocardium. Administer nitroglycerin sublingually, either as a tablet or spray. Nitroglycerin decreases myocardial work, and, to a lesser degree, dilates coronary arteries. If the patient's symptoms persist after the administration of one or two doses of nitroglycerin, assume that something more serious than angina, such as myocardial infarction, is occurring.

Nifedipine (Procardia) is now being used, in addition to nitroglycerin, in the management of angina. It is a vasodilator that works through a different mechanism than nitroglycerin.

Patients with first episodes of angina, or episodes that are not relieved by medication, are usually admitted to the hospital for evaluation.

Myocardial Infarction. **Acute myocardial infarction (MI)** is the death of a portion of the heart muscle from prolonged deprivation of arterial blood supply. MI can also occur when the oxygen demand of the heart exceeds its supply for an extended period of time. Myocardial infarction is most often associated with *atherosclerotic heart disease (ASHD)*. The precipitating event is most commonly the formation of a *thrombus,* or blood clot, in a coronary artery already diseased from atherosclerosis. In addition, myocardial infarction can result from coronary artery spasm, microemboli, acute volume overload, hypotension (from any cause), or from acute respiratory failure (acute hypoxia).

The actual location and size of the infarction depends on the vessel involved and the site of the obstruction. (See Figure 21-59.) Most infarctions involve the left ventricle. Obstruction of the left coronary artery may result in anterior, lateral, or septal infarcts. Right coronary artery occlusions usually result in inferior wall infarctions. The actual infarction is often classified as transmural or subendocardial. In a *transmural infarction,* the entire thickness of the myocardium was destroyed. This lesion is associated with Q wave changes on the ECG and is occasionally called *Q wave infarction.* In a *subendocardial infarction,* only the subendocardial layer is involved. This type of infarction is not usually accompanied by Q wave changes on the ECG. For this reason, it is often called a *non-Q wave infarction.*

The tissues affected by myocardial infarction can exhibit various degrees of damage. First, following occlusion of the coronary artery, the affected tissue develops ischemia. If the blockage is not relieved and collateral circulation is inadequate, the tissue will infarct and die. The in-

■ **acute myocardial infarction** death and subsequent necrosis of the heart muscle caused by inadequate blood supply.

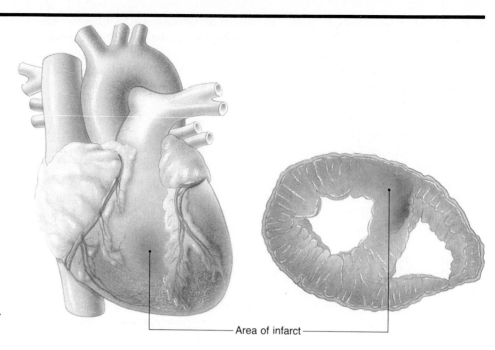

FIGURE 21-59 Myocardial infarction.

— Area of infarct —

farcted tissue becomes necrotic and, later, forms scar tissue. The area of myocardium which is infarcted is surrounded by a ring of ischemic tissue. This ischemic tissue survives, primarily because of collateral circulation. The ischemic area is often the site of origin of many dysrhythmias.

Myocardial infarction has several complications, the most common of which is dysrhythmias. Life-threatening dysrhythmias can occur almost immediately and can result in **sudden death,** or death within 1 hour after the onset of symptoms. This is the most common cause of death resulting from MI.

In addition to dysrhythmias, the patient can develop congestive heart failure because of destruction of a portion of the myocardial muscle mass. Such patients may have right heart failure, left heart failure, or both. *Heart failure* is present if the pumping ability of the heart is impaired, but the heart can meet the demands of the body. That is, the heart is inefficient but adequate. If the heart cannot meet the oxygen demands of the body, then *inadequate tissue perfusion* occurs, resulting in **cardiogenic shock.** In cardiogenic shock, the heart is both inefficient and inadequate. Another cause of death from MI is *ventricular aneurysm* of the myocardial wall. The damaged portion of the wall weakens. In some cases, it bursts, resulting in sudden death. *Pump failure,* resulting from extensive myocardial damage, can also result in death.

Signs and Symptoms of Myocardial Infarction. The most common presenting sign or symptom of myocardial infarction is substernal chest pain or epigastric pain. The pain generally has the same characteristics and location as anginal pain. It may be severe and is often described as crushing, but it may also be relatively mild. It frequently radiates to other areas, such as the arms, neck, jaw, and back. The pain is present when the patient is at rest and is not necessarily precipitated by exertion. The pain of myocardial infarction is not relieved by sublingual nitroglycerin or other home medications. Frequently, large doses of morphine, or a nitroglycerin drip, are required to alleviate it.

Patients with MI, especially elderly and diabetic patients, may not have chest pain. Instead, they may complain of pain in the shoulder, arm,

■ **sudden death** death within 1 hour after the onset of symptoms.

■ **cardiogenic shock** the inability of the heart to meet the metabolic needs of the body, resulting in inadequate tissue perfusion.

✳ The patient with MI may not have chest pain as a symptom.

neck, jaw, or back. Some patients with MI have no symptoms whatsoever. The MI is diagnosed by ECG changes or elevated cardiac enzyme levels.

Symptoms often associated with MI include:

- diaphoresis
- anxiety or apprehension
- dyspnea
- nausea or vomiting
- pallor
- general weakness or malaise

Many patients, especially the elderly, have no pain. Instead, they complain of general malaise or a history of syncope. Many MI patients deny the seriousness of the problem. This often causes them to delay seeking medical care during the first hours following onset, the most critical phase of the illness.

The vital signs associated with MI can vary with the extent of pump damage and the degree of autonomic nervous system response. The blood pressure can be normal, elevated due to increased sympathetic tone, or low due to increased parasympathetic tone or pump failure. The pulse rate depends on whether dysrhythmias are present. The rate may be fast or slow, regular or irregular, weak or bounding. Respirations may be either normal or increased.

Dysrhythmias are the most common complication of MI. Some dysrhythmias are warnings of life-threatening dysrhythmias and may require prehospital intervention. Life-threatening dysrhythmias such as ventricular fibrillation can result in sudden death. Non-life threatening dysrhythmias may not require prehospital intervention.

All patients with chest pain should be transported to the hospital. Any patient with chest pain and a compatible history should be presumed to have a myocardial infarction until proven otherwise. Age and other factors are not good discriminators.

Prehospital Management of Uncomplicated MI. Prehospital intervention can mean the difference between life and death to a patient with MI. Goals of prehospital intervention include:

- preventing pain and apprehension
- preventing serious dysrhythmias
- limiting the size of the infarct

Time is of the essence. Complete the primary assessment and begin the secondary survey quickly. Obtain the medical history while conducting the physical examination and initiating treatment. Place the patient physically at rest and reassure him, to decrease anxiety and to help alleviate apprehension. This will reduce heart rate and myocardial oxygen demand. In addition, place the patient in a position of comfort, ideally reclining with the head elevated 30 degrees. Do not allow the patient to walk. Get the stretcher as near the patient as possible.

Administer oxygen at high flow rate unless there is documented chronic obstructive pulmonary disease. This will increase myocardial oxygen delivery and can aid in the reduction of infarct size.

Determine baseline vital signs. A slow, fast, or irregular pulse may be the first indication of a dysrhythmia. Repeat the vital signs frequently.

As soon as possible, establish an IV with D5W at a "to keep open"

✱ With the advent of thrombolytic therapy (drugs that dissolve the blood clot causing a heart attack), prehospital care must be undertaken quickly, with expedient transport to the emergency department.

(TKO) rate to provide venous access. If the patient is diabetic, the medical control physician may request another fluid.

Place the ECG electrodes and record a baseline ECG. Cardiac monitoring should continue throughout patient assessment and transport. Record any dysrhythmias and attach the rhythm strip to the patient report.

Complete the history and physical examination, including auscultation of the lungs. The presence of basilar rales may indicate early heart failure.

Following patient assessment, administer medications according to written protocols or upon order of the medical control physician. Drugs commonly used for pain relief include:

- ❏ *nitroglycerin:* Nitroglycerin dilates peripheral arteries and veins, thus reducing preload and afterload and myocardial oxygen demand. Some coronary artery dilation may occur, increasing blood flow though the collaterals. Nitroglycerin administration often helps distinguish angina from MI. MI symptoms are not relieved by nitroglycerin.

- ❏ *morphine sulfate:* Morphine is an important medication in the management of MI. It reduces myocardial oxygen demand by reducing venous return (preload) and systemic arterial resistance (afterload). It acts directly on the central nervous system to relieve pain. Morphine also reduces sympathetic nervous system discharge, which can further decrease myocardial oxygen demand.

- ❏ *nitrous oxide (Nitronox):* Administration of the fixed combination of nitrous oxide and oxygen is useful in the management of MI. It is purely an analgesic without significant hemodynamic effects. However, delivery of 50 percent oxygen can increase myocardial oxygen supply.

- ❏ *diazepam (Valium):* Diazepam may be administered if the patient is extremely apprehensive or agitated. It is not an analgesic but will help relax the patient.

- ❏ *nalbuphine (Nubain):* Nalbuphine is used in some EMS systems instead of morphine. It is an effective analgesic but lacks the desirable hemodynamic effects of morphine.

Drugs used for dysrhythmias:

- ❏ *lidocaine (Xylocaine):* Lidocaine is the first-line antidysrhythmic agent for ventricular dysrhythmias. It can suppress warning dysrhythmias and may be given in the absence of dysrhythmias as a preventive measure.

- ❏ *procainamide (Pronestyl):* Procainamide can be used for dysrhythmias refractory to lidocaine or in patients allergic to lidocaine.

- ❏ *atropine sulfate:* Atropine is a parasympatholytic and is effective in bradycardias, especially of atrial origin. It is often useful in the management of asystole.

- ❏ isoproterenol (Isuprel): Isoproterenol may be used in bradycardias that are refractory to atropine to increase heart rate and cardiac output.

- ❏ *epinephrine:* Epinephrine is used in cardiovascular collapse and life-threatening dysrhythmias such as ventricular fibrillation and asystole.

- ❏ *verapamil (Isoptin, Calan):* Verapamil is used in the management of supraventricular tachycardias, particularly if the rate is so fast that it compromises cardiac output.

- ❏ *bretylium (Bretylol):* Bretylium is used in the management of life-threatening ventricular dysrhythmias. It is not a first-line agent.

Most patients suffering MI can be adequately stabilized in the field. After the patient is stabilized, he or she can be transported calmly, without lights or siren. This decreases apprehension and improves patient care. However, some patients may require Code 3 transport.

In-Hospital Management of MI. It is important that the paramedic understand the management of the MI patient after he or she has been delivered to the emergency department. This is especially true for paramedics who also staff emergency departments as a part of their regular duties. Myocardial infarction is usually diagnosed by ECG and by elevations in cardiac enzyme levels. The 12-lead ECG can indicate whether an infarction has occurred, its location, and its severity (transmural versus subendocardial).

Cardiac enzymes are muscle enzymes which are released from damaged myocardial cells. Elevated cardiac enzyme levels often indicate myocardial infarction. Commonly assayed enzymes include lactate dehydrogenase (LDH), creatine phosphokinase (CPK), and serum glutamic oxaloacetic transaminase (SGOT or AST). Paramedics should not administer any medication intramuscularly to a patient suspected of suffering MI. This can cause a release of muscle enzymes from the site of the injection, resulting in elevated enzyme levels. Such an elevation can hinder the emergency physician from determining whether an MI has occurred. Later, the source of the enzyme elevation can be detected in the laboratory, but this is not generally possible in the acute setting.

The current trend in the management of MI is *thrombolytic therapy,* or the administration of agents that can dissolve the blood clot responsible for the infarction and prevent death of a significant amount of myocardium. Commonly used thrombolytic agents are streptokinase, urokinase, and tissue plasminogen activator (tPA). These agents are administered intravenously or directly into the obstructed artery. If treatment is successful, blood flow is restored, and, in some cases, significant infarction is averted.

Other treatments used in the hospital include the placement of cardiac pacemakers, dilation of stenotic arteries with balloon angioplasty, emergency bypass surgery, and insertion of the aortic counterpulsation balloon pump.

Left Ventricular Failure with Pulmonary Edema

Left ventricular failure occurs when the left ventricle fails as an effective forward pump, causing back pressure of blood into the pulmonary circulation, often resulting in pulmonary edema. (See Figure 21-60.) This can be caused by various types of heart disease, including MI, valvular disease, chronic hypertension, and dysrhythmias. In left ventricular failure, the left ventricle cannot eject all the blood delivered to it from the right heart. Left atrial pressure rises and is subsequently transmitted to the pulmonary veins and capillaries. When pulmonary capillary pressure becomes too high, the serum (fluid) portion of the blood is forced into the alveoli, resulting in pulmonary edema. Progressive fluid accumulation in the alveoli decreases the oxygenation capacity of the lungs and can result in death from hypoxia. Since MI is a common cause of left ventricular failure, all patients with pulmonary edema should be assumed to have had an MI.

Signs and Symptoms. Signs and symptoms of left ventricular failure and pulmonary edema include:

❑ *Severe respiratory distress.* Severe respiratory distress is evidenced as orthopnea or dyspnea. Spasmodic coughing, which may be productive of pink, frothy sputum, is a characteristic finding. The patient may report a history of **paroxysmal nocturnal dyspnea (PND)** as well.

■ **paroxysmal nocturnal dyspnea (PND)** a sudden episode of difficult breathing occurring after lying down, most commonly caused by left heart failure.

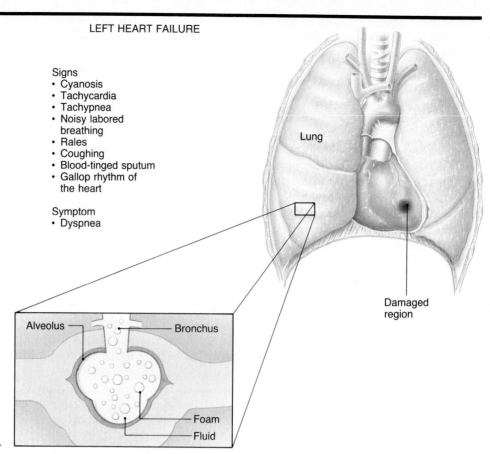

Signs
• Cyanosis
• Tachycardia
• Tachypnea
• Noisy labored
  breathing
• Rales
• Coughing
• Blood-tinged sputum
• Gallop rhythm of
  the heart

Symptom
• Dyspnea

Lung

Damaged
region

Alveolus   Bronchus

Foam
Fluid

FIGURE 21-60   Left heart failure.

✱ The most common
presenting symptom of left heart
failure is respiratory distress.

❑ *Severe apprehension, agitation, and confusion.* Left ventricular failure and pulmonary edema can result in hypoxia. The patient often has a smothering feeling. He or she becomes apprehensive and frightened. As hypoxia worsens, agitation and confusion can develop.

❑ *Cyanosis.* Cyanosis results from inadequate exchange of oxygen and carbon dioxide in the lungs, resulting from pulmonary edema. Thus the PaO_2 level falls and the $PaCO_2$ level increases.

❑ *Diaphoresis.* Diaphoresis often results from sympathetic stimulation, either from apprehension associated with pulmonary edema or from MI.

❑ *Adventitious lung sounds (pulmonary congestion).* Adventitious lung sounds are often present in pulmonary edema. These include rales, rhonchi, and wheezes:

  ❑ *Rales.* Rales, especially at the bases of the lungs, result from fluid in the alveoli. Severe rales can be heard all the way up to the scapulae and do not clear with coughing.

  ❑ *Rhonchi.* Rhonchi are associated with fluid in the larger airways and often indicate severe pulmonary edema.

  ❑ *Wheezes.* Wheezes occur in response to reflex airway spasm. The presence of fluid in the alveoli is misinterpreted by the protective mechanisms of the lungs, resulting in bronchoconstriction in an attempt to keep additional fluid from entering. The wheezing seen in pulmonary edema and congestive heart failure is often called "cardiac asthma," which is a confusing term that should be avoided.

❑ *Jugular venous distention.* Jugular venous distention does not result directly from left ventricular failure. However, it may be present when backpressure from left ventricular failure extends through the right heart to the venous circulation. Examine the patient for jugular venous distention with the patient seated and the head elevated at a 45 degree angle.

- *Vital signs.* There is usually a significant increase in sympathetic discharge to help the body compensate for the left heart failure. The blood pressure is often elevated. The pulse is rapid to compensate for the low stroke volume. The pulse may be irregular if dysrhythmias are present. Respirations are tachypneic and labored.
- *Level of consciousness.* The level of consciousness may vary. The patient may be extremely anxious or apprehensive. As cerebral perfusion decreases and hypoxia increases, the patient may become agitated, confused, and, finally, unconscious.
- *Chest pain.* The presence of chest pain depends on whether myocardial infarction has occurred. The pain may be masked by respiratory distress.

Prehospital Management of Left Ventricular Failure and Pulmonary Edema. Left ventricular failure and pulmonary edema is a true emergency. The patient can decompensate rapidly and unpredictably. The goals of management are to:

- decrease venous return to the heart (preload)
- decrease myocardial oxygen demands
- improve ventilation and oxygenation

Obtain pertinent medical history and complete the physical exam while initiating treatment.

Seat the patient with the feet dangling. This will promote venous pooling and thus decrease preload. DO NOT LIE THE PATIENT FLAT AT ANY TIME.

Administer high-flow oxygen. If necessary, provide positive-pressure assistance with either a demand valve or bag-valve-mask unit if the patient can assist or is comatose.

If possible, establish an IV of D5W at a TKO rate. It is imperative that fluids be limited. Therefore, use a minidrip set to avoid the accidental infusion of excessive amounts of fluid.

Place ECG electrodes. If the patient is extremely diaphoretic, apply tincture of benzoin first. Record a baseline ECG. Keep the monitor in place throughout care.

Administer medications according to written protocols or on the order of the medical control physician. Some cases of left ventricular failure result from very rapid dysrhythmias. If a dysrhythmia is suspected as a cause, it should be treated. Medications frequently used in left ventricular failure and pulmonary edema include:

- *Morphine sulfate:* Morphine is administered primarily for its hemodynamic properties, since the patient may not be in pain. Morphine decreases venous return (preload), reduces myocardial work, and helps alleviate anxiety.
- *Nitroglycerin:* Nitroglycerin may be used for peripheral vasodilation. This will decrease preload and afterload and can lessen the symptoms of left ventricular failure.
- *Furosemide (Lasix):* Furosemide is a potent loop diuretic with a relaxant effect on the venous system. Effects are often seen within 5 minutes. Also, through its diuretic effect, it decreases intravascular fluid volume. Increased doses of furosemide may be required if the patient has been taking this medication, or another diuretic, at home.
- *Aminophylline:* Aminophylline, commonly used in chronic obstructive pulmonary disease, also has a role in left ventricular failure and pulmonary edema. Bronchospasm is almost always present, and aminophylline can cause bronchodilation. Also, aminophylline can strengthen the respiratory muscles.

❏ *Dobutamine (Dobutrex):* Like dopamine, dobutamine increases cardiac output by increasing stroke volume. It has little effect on heart rate and is occasionally used in isolated left heart failure until other medications, such as digitalis, have taken effect. It is administered by intravenous infusion.

Apply rotating tourniquets to enhance venous pooling, especially if an IV cannot be established. This can decrease preload by trapping venous blood in the extremities. Use a constricting band or blood pressure cuff. Apply the tourniquet snugly to three of the four extremities, as high up on the extremity as possible. The constricting bands should interrupt venous flow only and should not interfere with arterial flow. Arterial pulses distal to the tourniquet should be palpable after application of the constricting bands. Rotate the bands every 5–10 minutes by releasing the band on one extremity and reapplying to another extremity. Do this systematically, in a clockwise rotation, so that a band does not remain on any one extremity for a prolonged period of time. Rotating tourniquets are contraindicated in patients who are in shock and are considered a secondary modality to pharmacological therapy. Rotating tourniquets are an optional skill. Consult your instructor regarding usage in your system.

Rapid transport to the hospital is essential.

Right Ventricular Failure

Right ventricular failure is failure of the right ventricle as an effective forward pump, resulting in backpressure of blood into the systemic venous circulation and venous congestion. (See Figure 21-61.) The most

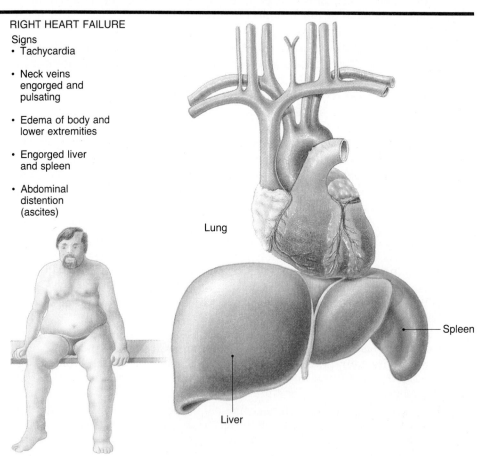

RIGHT HEART FAILURE

Signs
• Tachycardia

• Neck veins engorged and pulsating

• Edema of body and lower extremities

• Engorged liver and spleen

• Abdominal distention (ascites)

Lung

Spleen

Liver

FIGURE 21-61   Right heart failure.

common cause of right ventricular failure is left ventricular failure, because myocardial infarction is more common in the left ventricle than in the right and because the left ventricle is more adversely affected by chronic hypertension than is the right. However, right ventricular failure has other causes. Systemic hypertension can affect both sides of the heart and can cause pure right ventricular failure. Pulmonary hypertension and cor pulmonale result from the effects of chronic obstructive pulmonary disease (COPD). These problems are related to increased pressure in the pulmonary arteries. Increased pressure results in right ventricular enlargement, right atrial enlargement, and, if untreated, right heart failure.

Pulmonary embolism, the presence of a blood clot in one of the pulmonary arteries, is another cause of right heart failure. If the clot is large enough, a major vessel can be occluded, increasing the pressure against which the right ventricle must pump. This can throw the right ventricle into failure in much the same manner as pulmonary hypertension. In fact, it can be considered an acute form of pulmonary hypertension. Infarct of the right atrium or ventricle, although relatively rare, can also cause right ventricular failure.

From a pathophysiological standpoint, right heart failure develops when the right ventricle cannot keep up with venous return. As the stroke volume decreases, right atrial pressure rises and backpressure is transmitted to the vena cava and the rest of the venous system. When the systemic venous pressure becomes too high, the liquid portion of the blood (serum) is forced into the interstitial space, resulting in edema.

Signs and Symptoms. The signs and symptoms of right heart failure depend on the degree of failure and the patient's general condition. Common findings include:

❏ *Tachycardia.* Tachycardia results from the body's attempts to maintain cardiac output by increasing heart rate to compensate for the fall in stroke volume.

❏ *Venous congestion.* Systemic venous congestion is the hallmark of right heart failure. This results from the leakage of fluid into interstitial spaces. Symptoms of venous congestion include:
  ❏ *Peripheral edema.* Peripheral edema is usually noted in the ankles and the pretibial area. In the bedridden patient, it may be present only in the presacral region. Severe pitting edema may occur. Generalized edema affecting virtually the entire body, or *anasarca,* is often an ominous finding.
  ❏ *Jugular venous distention.* Jugular venous distention results directly from an increase in systemic venous pressure. Examine the patient for jugular venous distention with the patient seated and the head at a 45 degree angle.
  ❏ *Fluid accumulation in serous cavities.* The leakage of fluid out of the intravascular space can result in fluid accumulation in serous cavities. Fluid can accumulate in the abdominal cavity (ascites), the pleural space (pleural effusion), and in the pericardium (pericardial effusion). The amount of fluid in a serous cavity can be quite large. Patients often tolerate even large quantities of effusion that develop over an extended period.

❏ *Liver engorgement.* Increased venous pressure causes edema of the liver. This may be evident only to the skilled examiner. Liver enlargement is a common finding in right heart failure.

❑ *History.* Patients with right heart failure often have histories of prior MIs and may have chronic pump failure. Often, these patients are taking digitalis (Lanoxin) and furosemide (Lasix), and these medications will provide a clue to the patient's underlying problem. Occasionally, patients use lay terms such as "dropsy," "enlarged heart," or "weak heart" to describe their disease.

Management of the Patient With Right Heart Failure. Right heart failure is usually not an emergency unless it is accompanied by left heart failure and pulmonary edema. Administer high-flow oxygen. If possible, establish an IV of D5W at a TKO rate. It is imperative that fluids be limited. Use a minidrip set to avoid the accidental infusion of excessive amounts of fluid.

Place ECG electrodes. If the patient is extremely diaphoretic, apply tincture of benzoin first. Record a baseline ECG, and leave the monitor in place throughout care. Rapid transport to the hospital is usually not necessary unless left heart failure develops. Left heart failure should be treated as described above.

Cardiogenic Shock

■ **cardiogenic shock** the inability of the heart to meet the metabolic needs of the body, resulting in inadequate tissue perfusion.

Cardiogenic shock, the most severe form of pump failure, occurs when left ventricular function is so compromised that the heart cannot meet the metabolic demands of the body and compensatory mechanisms are exhausted. Cardiogenic shock is shock that remains after correction of existing dysrhythmias, hypovolemia, or altered vascular tone. It usually occurs after extensive myocardial infarction, often involving more than 40 percent of the left ventricle, or from diffuse ischemia.

✳ Cardiogenic shock is the most severe form of pump failure.

Signs and Symptoms. Myocardial infarction often precedes cardiogenic shock, and symptoms are initially the same as would be expected with MI. However, as cardiogenic shock develops and compensatory mechanisms fail, hypotension develops. The systolic blood pressure is often less than 80 mmHg. There may be an altered level of consciousness, ranging from restlessness and confusion to coma. The usual heart rhythm is sinus tachycardia, a reflection of the cardiovascular system's attempts to compensate for the decrease in stroke volume. If serious dysrhythmias are present, it may be difficult to determine whether the dysrhythmias are the cause of the hypotension or the result of the cardiogenic shock. Therefore, any major dysrhythmias must be corrected. The patient's skin is usually cool and clammy, reflecting peripheral vasoconstriction. Tachypnea is usually present, as pulmonary edema is a common complication.

✳ The mortality of cardiogenic shock approaches 80–90%, even with the best technology available.

Management. Management of cardiogenic shock is difficult, even in the hospital. The mortality rate approaches 80-90 percent, even with the best technology available. Therefore, prolonged stabilization in the field is not indicated. Transport should be expeditious. Carry out the primary assessment. Secure the airway and administer high-flow oxygen. Place the patient in a supine position. Initiate an IV of D5W, using a minidrip set. Place ECG electrodes and obtain a baseline ECG. On physical examination, pay particular attention to blood pressure, jugular venous distention, and breath sounds. Administer medications per written protocol or by order of the medical control physician. Remember, always treat the rate and rhythm first. Medications to be used include:

dopamine (Intropin): Dopamine increases cardiac output. It stimulates both the α and β receptors. It offers an advantage over other drugs in that it often maintains renal perfusion at recommended dosages.

norepinephrine (Levophed): For many years, norepinephrine was the standard vasopressor used for cardiogenic shock. With the advent of dopamine it has fallen into relative disuse, primarily because of its adverse effects on renal perfusion and its lack of significant β properties.

If left heart failure and pulmonary edema are present, as they often are, they should be treated concurrently. First-line medications include morphine, furosemide, and oxygen with positive pressure ventilation (see above). Some authors have recommended use of the PASG in cardiogenic shock. This device may have a role in treatment of patients without pulmonary edema. Its use is controversial and the paramedic is encouraged to follow local protocols.

The patient with cardiogenic shock should be transported rapidly. Do not wait to observe the effects of medications administered in the field.

Cardiac Arrest/Sudden Death

Cardiac arrest and sudden death accounts for 60 percent of all deaths from coronary artery disease. *Sudden death* is death that occurs within 1 hour after the onset of symptoms. At autopsy, actual infarction is often not present, but severe atherosclerotic disease is common, leading authorities to believe that a lethal dysrhythmia is the mechanism of death. The risk factors for sudden death are basically the same as those presented above for atherosclerotic cardiovascular heart disease (ASCVD). In a large number of patients, cardiac arrest is the first manifestation of heart disease. Causes of sudden death other than ASCVD include:

- ❏ drowning
- ❏ electrocution
- ❏ electrolyte imbalance
- ❏ hypothermia
- ❏ trauma
- ❏ acid-base imbalance
- ❏ drug intoxication
- ❏ hypoxia
- ❏ pulmonary embolism
- ❏ cerebrovascular accident

As mentioned above, dysrhythmias are often associated with cardiac arrest. The major offending dysrhythmia is ventricular fibrillation, which causes an estimated 60-70 percent of cases. The dysrhythmia may be the cause of the cardiac arrest (primary cause) or may result from another factor (secondary cause). In addition to ventricular fibrillation, cardiac arrest can result from ventricular tachycardia, asystole, severe bradycardias, severe heart blocks, and electromechanical dissociation.

Basic Considerations in the Management of Cardiac Arrest. The following section will present general, basic considerations of management of cardiac arrest. The actual protocol for each type of cardiac arrest is addressed later.

Basic life support is the mainstay of cardiac arrest therapy. Initiate basic life support promptly, during the primary survey. If basic life support is delegated to assisting personnel, the paramedic must continuously monitor its performance and effectiveness.

The airway can be managed by any number of methods. The most sophisticated method is not always the best. Individual circumstances should dictate the form of airway management utilized.

Primary ventricular fibrillation is easier to abolish than secondary ventricular fibrillation. To adequately treat **secondary ventricular fibrillation,** you must often find and correct the underlying cause. Defibrillation should occur as soon as possible, as this gives the best chance of successful resuscitation. External cardiac pacing may be used for bradycardias or asystole, or immediately after defibrillation of ventricular fibrillation.

Some cardiac arrests are managed differently from those occurring due to ASCVD because of the underlying mechanism of arrest. These include cardiac arrest caused by:

❑ drowning
❑ hypothermia
❑ traumatic arrest

The management of these problems is discussed elsewhere in the text.

Management of the Witnessed Cardiac Arrest. The management of witnessed cardiac arrest follows the guidelines for cardiopulmonary resuscitation and emergency cardiac care published by the American Heart Association. The algorithm for witnessed cardiac arrest is shown in Figure 21-62.

Management of Unwitnessed Cardiac Arrest. The management of unwitnessed cardiac arrest follows the guidelines for cardiopulmonary resuscitation and emergency cardiac care as published by the American Heart Association. The algorithm for unwitnessed cardiac arrest is shown in Figure 21-62.

Management of Cardiac Arrest Secondary to Ventricular Tachycardia. The management of cardiac arrest secondary to ventricular tachycardia follows the guidelines for cardiopulmonary resuscitation and emergency cardiac care as published by the American Heart Association. The algorithm for cardiac arrest secondary to ventricular tachycardia is shown in Figure 21-63.

Management of Cardiac Arrest Secondary to Asystole. Cardiac arrest secondary to asystole carries a poor overall prognosis for resuscitation. Asystole may be the end result of ventricular fibrillation or electromechanical dissociation. Asystole usually indicates extensive myocardial damage, a severe metabolic deficit, or markedly increased parasympathetic tone. Many authorities believe that asystole is a fine ventricular fibrillation. If there is any question whether the rhythm is asystole or fine ventricular fibrillation, then defibrillation should be carried out.

The management of asystole follows the guidelines for cardiopulmonary resuscitation and emergency cardiac care as published by the American Heart Association. The algorithm for asystole is shown in Figure 21-64.

Management of Cardiac Arrest Secondary to Electromechanical Dissociation. *Electromechanical dissociation* (EMD) is any organized ECG rhythm without a pulse. It, like asystole, carries a grave prognosis. Causes of electromechanical dissociation include massive myocardial damage, hypovolemia, cardiac rupture, cardiac tamponade, and acute pulmonary embolism. Most of these conditions cannot be diagnosed or managed in the field. Some, however, are treatable in the hospital if detected

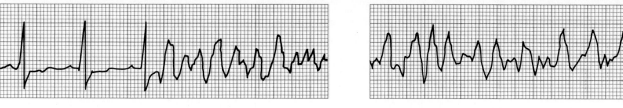

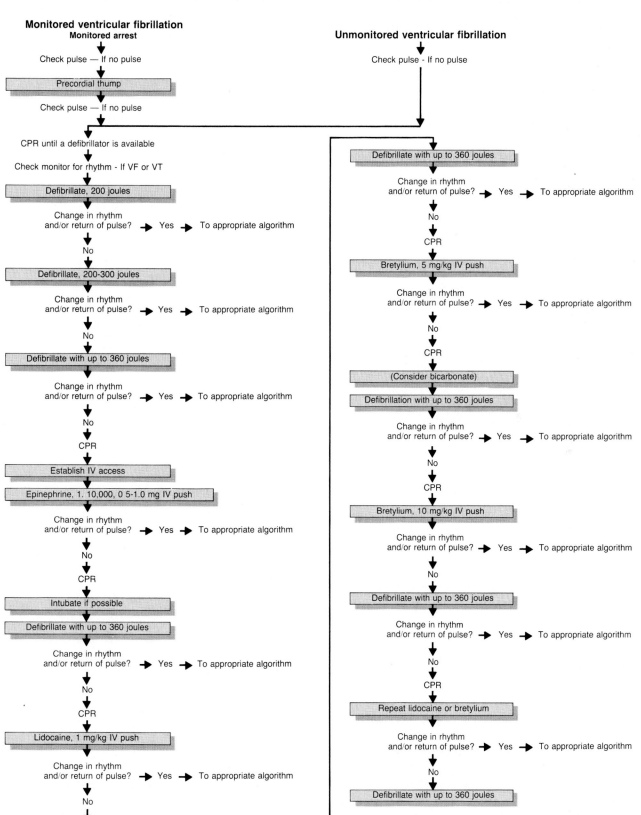

FIGURE 21-62 Management of witnessed and unwitnessed ventricular fibrillation.

679

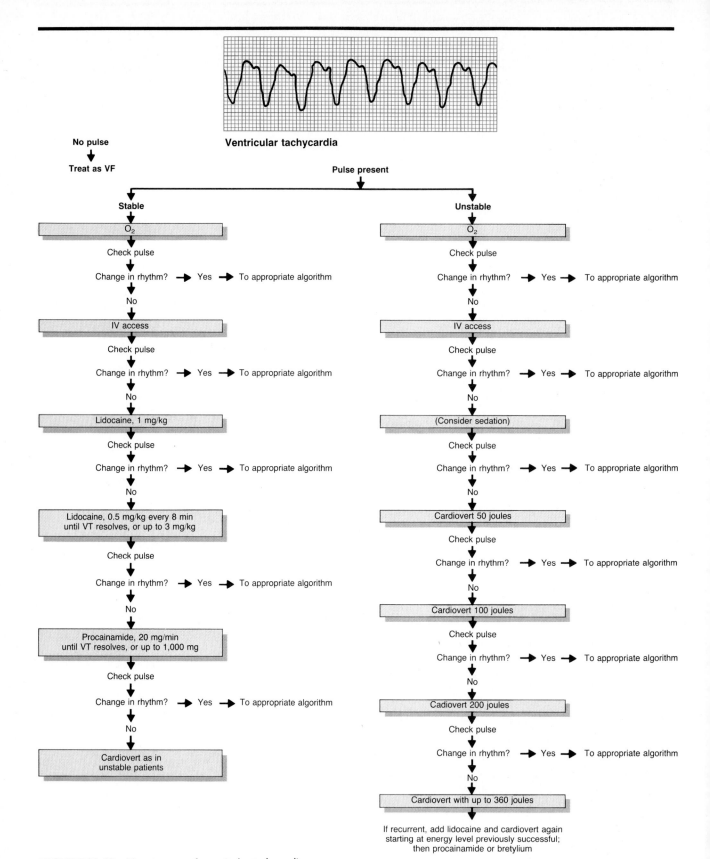

FIGURE 21-63 Management of ventricular tachycardia.

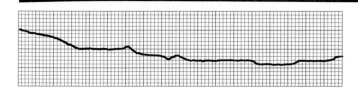

Asystole

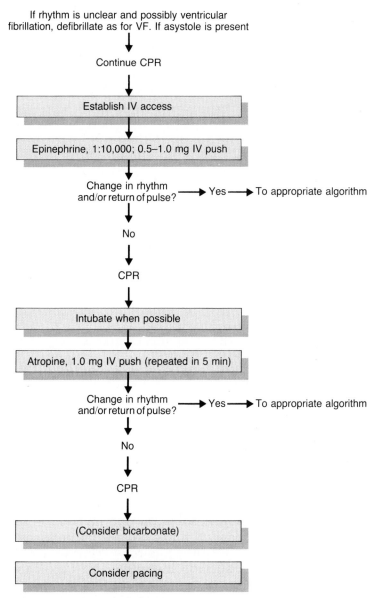

If rhythm is unclear and possibly ventricular fibrillation, defibrillate as for VF. If asystole is present

↓

Continue CPR

↓

Establish IV access

Epinephrine, 1:10,000; 0.5–1.0 mg IV push

Change in rhythm and/or return of pulse? → Yes → To appropriate algorithm

No

↓

CPR

↓

Intubate when possible

Atropine, 1.0 mg IV push (repeated in 5 min)

Change in rhythm and/or return of pulse? → Yes → To appropriate algorithm

No

↓

CPR

↓

(Consider bicarbonate)

Consider pacing

FIGURE 21-64 Management of asystole

early. When confronted by a patient in electromechanical dissociation, consider PASG, an IV fluid challenge, and transport immediately if there is a suspicion of any treatable etiology, such as hypovolemia.

The management of cardiac arrest secondary to electromechanical dissociation follows the guidelines for cardiopulmonary resuscitation and emergency cardiac care published by the American Heart Association. The algorithm for cardiac arrest secondary to electromechanical dissociation is shown in Figure 21-65.

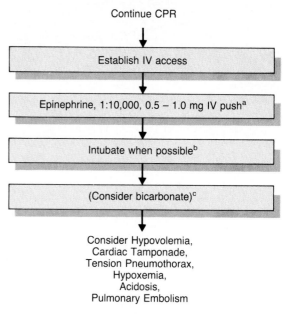

Electromechanical Dissociation

Continue CPR

↓

Establish IV access

↓

Epinephrine, 1:10,000, 0.5 – 1.0 mg IV push[a]

↓

Intubate when possible[b]

↓

(Consider bicarbonate)[c]

↓

Consider Hypovolemia,
Cardiac Tamponade,
Tension Pneumothorax,
Hypoxemia,
Acidosis,
Pulmonary Embolism

[a] Epinephrine should be repeated every 5 minutes.

[b] Intubation is preferable. If it can be accomplished simultaneously with other techniques, then the earlier the better. However, epinephrine is more important initially if the patient can be ventilated without intubation.

[c] Value of sodium bicarbonate is questionable during cardiac arrest, and is not recommended for routine cardiac arrest sequence. Consideration of its use in a dose of 1 mEq/kg is appropriate at this point. Half of original dose may be repeated every 10 minutes if it is used.

FIGURE 21-65 Management of electromechanical dissociation.

Peripheral Vascular and Other Cardiovascular Emergencies

Aneurysm. **Aneurysm** is a nonspecific term meaning dilation of a vessel. The types of aneurysms include:

- ❏ atherosclerotic
- ❏ dissecting
- ❏ infectious
- ❏ congenital
- ❏ traumatic

Most aneurysms result from atherosclerosis and involve the aorta. The aorta is the vessel most commonly involved because the pressure within it is the highest of that of any vessel in the body. This section discusses abdominal, dissecting, and traumatic aneurysms. Infectious aneurysms are most commonly associated with syphilis and are uncommon. Congenital aneurysms can occur with several disease states. One is *Marfan's syndrome,* a hereditary disease that affects the connective tissue. People with Marfan's syndrome are often slender and tall with long fingers. Aortic aneurysm occurs in people with Marfan's syndrome because of involvement of the connective tissue within the vessel wall. Those affected may experience sudden death, usually from spontaneous rupture of the aorta, often at a fairly young age.

Abdominal Aortic Aneurysm. *Abdominal aortic aneurysm* commonly results from atherosclerosis and occurs most frequently in the aorta, below the renal arteries and above the bifurcation of the common iliac ar-

■ **aneurysm** the ballooning of an arterial wall, resulting from a defect or weakness in the wall.

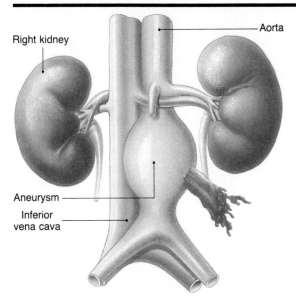

Right kidney

Aorta

Aneurysm

Inferior
vena cava

FIGURE 21-66 Rupture of an abdominal aortic aneurysm.

teries. It is 10 times more common in men than women and most prevalent between ages 60 and 70. (See Figure 21-66.)

Signs and symptoms of an abdominal aortic aneurysm include:

❑ abdominal pain
❑ back and flank pain
❑ hypotension
❑ urge to defecate, caused by the retroperitoneal leakage of blood
❑ pulsatile mass (the mass can usually be felt when it exceeds 5 cm in diameter)
❑ decreased femoral pulse
❑ GI bleeding if the aneurysm erodes into the bowel

Prehospital management consists of treating the patient for shock. Treatment should consist of oxygen, PASG, and intravenous volume replacement. Suspect abdominal aortic aneurysm when any of the above signs or symptoms are present. If ordered by medical control, palpate the abdomen gently to note the presence of a mass. Do not carry out additional palpation, as rupture can occur. Transport the patient rapidly.

Dissecting Aortic Aneurysm. A *dissecting aortic aneurysm* occurs after a small tear in the inner wall of the aorta allows blood to enter and create a false passage within the wall of the vessel. This can cause hematoma and, subsequently, aneurysm. The original tear often results from **cystic medial necrosis,** a degenerative disease of connective tissue often associated with hypertension, and, to a certain extent, aging. Predisposing factors include hypertension, which is present in 75–85 percent of cases. There is also a family tendency for this disease. It occurs more frequently in patients older than 40-50, although it can occur in younger individuals, especially pregnant women.

Of dissecting aortic aneurysms, 67 percent involve the ascending aorta. Once dissection has started, it can extend to all of the abdominal aorta as well as its branches, including the coronary arteries, aortic valve, subclavian arteries, and carotid arteries. The aneurysm can rupture at any time, usually into the pericardial or pleural cavity.

■ **cystic medial necrosis** a death or degeneration of a part of the wall of an artery.

The signs and symptoms of dissecting aortic aneurysm include pain, which is commonly characterized as ripping or tearing. The pain is usually substernal and may radiate to the back between the scapulae. The blood pressure is often elevated, yet the patient will often look "shocky" as a result of impaired perfusion. Dissection into other arteries and structures may cause the following:

❑ syncope
❑ stroke
❑ absent or reduced pulses
❑ heart failure
❑ pericardial tamponade
❑ acute myocardial infarction

Prehospital management consists of rapid transport for definitive care. Rupture can occur, even into another body cavity. Keep the patient quiet and administer high-flow oxygen. Start an IV of a crystalloid solution, such as lactated Ringer's solution, preferably en route to the hospital. If the diagnosis is fairly definite, the medical control physician may order the administration of morphine sulfate. Transport the patient rapidly. The survival rate is fairly good if the patient is treated promptly.

In-hospital management may be medical or surgical. Occasionally, the tear heals, creating a double lumen in the vessel.

Traumatic Aortic Rupture.   *Traumatic aortic aneurysm* or rupture can result from blunt or penetrating trauma to the vessel. If rupture occurs, the prognosis is grave. If the aneurysm is detected before it ruptures, it can occasionally be treated surgically. Additional discussion of traumatic aortic aneurysm and rupture is presented in the trauma chapters.

Acute Arterial Occlusion.   An *acute arterial occlusion* is the sudden occlusion of arterial blood flow to an area as a result of trauma, thrombosis, tumor, embolus, or idiopathic means. Embolus is probably the most common cause. Emboli can arise from within the chamber (*mural emboli*), a thrombus in the left ventricle, an atrial thrombus secondary to atrial fibrillation, or a thrombus from abdominal aortic atherosclerosis. Arterial occlusions most commonly involve vessels in the abdomen or extremities.

The signs and symptoms of an acute arterial occlusion include sudden, excruciating pain. Pain is present in 75-80 percent of cases and peaks within several hours. If pain is absent, there is usually paresthesia in the involved extremity. The area distal to the obstruction is often pale. The occluded extremity may have a mottled, cyanotic appearance. It is often cool to the touch because of loss of blood flow. The pulses distal to the occlusion are absent. An easy way to remember the signs and symptoms of arterial occlusion are the "5 P's":

❑ pallor
❑ pain
❑ pulselessness
❑ paralysis
❑ paresthesia

If the occlusion involve the mesentery, the blood supply to the intestines, shock can develop. The prehospital management of a mesenteric occlusion consists of typical shock treatment: oxygen, IV fluids, and PASG.

Morphine sulfate may be ordered by the medical control physician for relief of pain. Extremity occlusion is serious, but not life-threatening. Blood flow must be established within 4-8 hours. This is usually accomplished by surgical removal of the clot. If acute arterial occlusion is present, the affected extremity should be protected from injury. The patient should not be allowed to walk on it.

Acute Pulmonary Embolism. *Acute pulmonary embolism* is a blood clot or other particle that lodges in a pulmonary artery, blocking blood flow through that vessel. Sources of pulmonary emboli include air emboli, fat emboli, amniotic fluid emboli, and blood clots. Factors that predispose a patient to blood clots include prolonged immobilization, thrombophlebitis, use of certain medications, and atrial fibrillation.

When a pulmonary embolism occurs, the blood flow through the affected vessel is blocked, causing the right heart to pump against increased resistance. This results in increased pulmonary capillary pressure. The area of the lung supplied by the occluded vessel ceases to function, resulting in decreased gas exchange.

The signs and symptoms of pulmonary embolism depend upon the size of the obstruction. The patient suffering acute pulmonary embolism may report a sudden onset of severe and unexplained dyspnea which may or may not be associated with chest pain. There may be a recent history of immobilization, such as recent hip fracture, surgery, or other debilitating illness.

The physical examination may reveal labored breathing, tachypnea, and tachycardia. Patients with massive pulmonary emboli may have signs of right heart failure, such as jugular venous distention and, in some cases, falling blood pressure.

If you suspect that a patient has a pulmonary embolism, establish and maintain an airway. Assist the patient's ventilations as required. Administer supplemental oxygen at the highest possible concentration. Establish an IV of D5W at a TKO rate and transport the patient immediately.

Pulmonary embolism is often difficult to diagnose. Therefore, the paramedic should suspect this condition in patients with associated signs and symptoms. Patients with acute pulmonary embolism can present in a similar fashion to those with hyperventilation syndrome. Do not assume that all cases of hyperventilation are caused by anxiety. If in doubt, always administer oxygen.

Noncritical Peripheral Vascular Conditions

Deep Venous Thrombosis. *Deep venous thrombosis* is a blood clot in a vein. It most commonly occurs in the larger veins of the thigh and calf. Predisposing factors include a recent history of trauma, inactivity, pregnancy, or varicose veins.

The patient often complains of gradually increasing pain and calf tenderness. Often the leg and foot are swollen because of occlusion of venous drainage. The signs and symptoms may improve with leg elevation. In some cases, the patient may be asymptomatic. Gentle palpation of the calf and thigh may reveal tenderness and, on some occasions, cordlike clotted veins. Dorsiflexion of the foot may cause discomfort behind the knee. This is referred to as *Homan's sign* and is associated with deep venous thrombosis. The skin may be warm and red.

Prehospital management is primarily supportive. Deep vein thrombosis is not a life-threatening emergency, but patients are prone to develop pulmonary emboli. Palpate the calf and thigh gently. Do not allow the patient to walk, and elevate the leg.

Varicose Veins.   *Varicose veins* are the dilation of the superficial veins, usually in the lower extremity. Predisposing factors include pregnancy, obesity, and a genetic tendency. Signs and symptoms include the visible distention of the leg veins, lower leg swelling and discomfort (especially at the end of the day), and skin color and texture changes in the legs and ankles. If the condition is chronic, venous stasis ulcers can develop. Venous stasis ulcers are a noncritical condition. However, rupture can occur. The bleeding, which occasionally is significant, can usually be controlled by direct pressure.

Peripheral Arterial Atherosclerotic Disease.   Atherosclerosis, as discussed previously, can involve any of the major arteries. *Peripheral atherosclerotic disease* results from atherosclerosis of the aorta and its tributaries. It is a gradual, progressive disease, often associated with diabetes mellitus. Signs and symptoms include trophic changes in the feet, pretibial hair loss, and red skin color in the extremities when dependent. In extreme cases, there may be significant arterial insufficiency leading to ulcers and gangrene. *Intermittent claudication,* or pain and cramping in the affected leg when the tissue demands are in excess of the blood supply, occurs after exercise and is comparable to angina in the heart. Peripheral arterial disease is not a medical emergency unless arterial occlusion occurs.

Hypertensive Emergency.   A hypertensive emergency is a life-threatening elevation of blood pressure. It occurs in 1 percent or less of patients with hypertension, usually when the **hypertension** is poorly controlled or untreated. A **hypertensive emergency** is characterized by a rapid increase in diastolic blood pressure (usually > 130 mmHg), restlessness, confusion, somnolence, blurred vision, and nausea and vomiting. It is often accompanied by **hypertensive encephalopathy,** which is characterized by severe headache, vomiting, visual disturbances (including transient blindness), paralysis, seizures, stupor, and coma. On occasion, may cause left ventricular failure, pulmonary edema, or stroke.

Prehospital management varies with the patient. Keep the patient quiet and administer oxygen. In cases where frank hypertensive encephalopathy has not yet developed, the medical control physician may request the administration of sublingual nifedipine (Procardia). This is a calcium channel blocker that causes vasodilation of peripheral and coronary vessels and can reduce blood pressure. In severe cases, especially if hypertensive encephalopathy is present, the medical control physician may order one of the following medications:

❑ *Diazoxide (Hyperstat):* Diazoxide is a potent vasodilator that will lower blood pressure through vasodilation. It should be administered by rapid IV bolus with close observation of the blood pressure.
❑ *Sodium nitroprusside (Nipride):* Sodium nitroprusside is a popular agent for use in hypertensive crisis. It is a potent arterial and venous vasodilator. It is administered as an IV infusion, thus making administration more controlled and the patient's response more predictable.
❑ *Labetolol (Trandate, Normodyne):* Labetolol is a beta blocker that effectively decreases blood pressure. It is given by IV bolus and infusion.

If heart failure or pulmonary edema develops, the patient should be treated with appropriate medications.

■ **hypertension** a common disorder characterized by elevation of the blood pressure persistently exceeding 140/90 mmHg.

■ **hypertensive emergency** an acute elevation of blood pressure that requires the blood pressure be lowered within one hour, characterized by end-organ changes such as hypertensive encephalopathy, renal failure, or blindness.

■ **hypertensive encephalopathy** a cerebral disorder of hypertension indicated by severe headache, nausea, vomiting and altered mental status. Neurological symptoms may include blindness, muscle twitches, inability to speak, weakness, and paralysis.

Hypertension-Related Emergencies. Hypertension is a related factor in other emergencies. These include such things as pulmonary edema from left ventricular failure, dissecting aortic aneurysm, toxemia of pregnancy, and cerebrovascular accident. In these cases, hypertension often results from the primary problem. Treatment should be directed at the primary problem.

Drugs Used In Cardiovascular Emergencies

The medications used in the prehospital care of cardiovascular emergencies were discussed in detail in Chapter 13. This section reviews these medications briefly in preparation for the following sections on Advanced Cardiac Life Support.

Antidysrhythmics. *Antidysrhythmic medications* are those used to control or suppress cardiac dysrhythmias. They include:

❑ *Atropine sulfate.* Atropine sulfate is a parasympatholytic agent used in the treatment of symptomatic bradycardias, especially those arising from the atria. It also plays a role in the management of asystole. It is given by IV bolus or through an endotracheal tube.

❑ *Lidocaine.* Lidocaine is a first-line antidysrhythmic agent used in the treatment and prophylaxis of life-threatening ventricular dysrhythmias. It is administered by IV bolus, IV drip, or through an endotracheal tube.

❑ *Procainamide.* Procainamide is a second-line antidysrhythmic drug used for ventricular dysrhythmias refractory to lidocaine or in patients who are allergic to lidocaine. It is administered by slow IV bolus and IV drip.

❑ *Bretylium.* Bretylium is a second-line antidysrhythmic agent used in the treatment of life-threatening ventricular dysrhythmias, especially ventricular fibrillation. It is administered by IV bolus and IV drip.

❑ *Verapamil.* Verapamil is a calcium channel blocker that is effective in slowing heart rate in symptomatic atrial tachycardias. It is used to terminate paroxysmal supraventricular tachycardia and to control the rapid ventricular response often seen with atrial fibrillation or flutter. It is administered by slow IV bolus.

Sympathomimetic Agents. *Sympathomimetic agents* are drugs similar to the naturally occurring hormones epinephrine and norepinephrine. They duplicate or mimic stimulation of the sympathetic nervous system. They act either on alpha or beta adrenergic receptors. Stimulation of alpha receptors causes peripheral vasoconstriction. Stimulation of beta receptors causes an increase in heart rate, cardiac contractile force, bronchodilation, and peripheral vasodilation. Dopaminergic receptors are located in renal and mesenteric blood vessels. Stimulation of these receptors causes dilation.

❑ *Epinephrine.* Epinephrine is the mainstay of cardiac arrest resuscitation. It acts on both alpha and beta adrenergic receptors. It is used in ventricular fibrillation, asystole, and electromechanical dissociation. It is also sometimes used in bradycardias refractory to atropine. It is given by IV bolus, subcutaneously, and through the endotracheal tube.

❑ *Norepinephrine.* Norepinephrine is a sympathomimetic with enhanced alpha agonist properties as compared to epinephrine. It also acts, to a lesser degree, on beta receptors. It is used occasionally in hemodynamically significant hypotension and cardiogenic shock, although dopamine is considered the first-line agent for those conditions. It may be effective if total peripheral resistance is low, such as in neurogenic shock. It is administered by intravenous infusion.

- *Isoproterenol.* Isoproterenol is a potent beta agonist. It increases heart rate and cardiac contractile force. It is used in bradycardias refractory to atropine and in the management of asystole. It is administered by intravenous infusion.
- *Dopamine.* Dopamine is a vasopressor with both alpha and beta properties which are dose-related. In the appropriate dosage range, it maintains renal and mesenteric perfusion. It is used in the management of cardiogenic shock and given by intravenous infusion.
- *Dobutamine.* Dobutamine has a more pronounced effect on cardiac contractility than on heart rate. It is used in the treatment of significant left heart failure and administered by intravenous infusion.

Electrolyte Solutions

- *Sodium bicarbonate (NaHCO₃).* Sodium bicarbonate is used in the management of acidosis that cannot be corrected with ventilation alone. It provides a bicarbonate ion base (HCO_3^-) to buffer hydrogen ion. Its usage is currently under review because of side-effects. It is given intravenously.
- *Calcium chloride (CaCl₂).* Calcium chloride is rarely used in emergency care. It increases cardiac contractility and may play a role in certain electrolyte disorders. It is administered intravenously.

Drugs for Myocardial Ischemia and Pain

- *Oxygen.* Oxygen is an important agent in emergency cardiac care. It increases the oxygen content of the blood and aids in the oxygenation of peripheral tissues. It is indicated in any situation in which hypoxia or ischemia is possible.
- *Nitrous oxide (Nitronox).* Nitronox is a fixed 50%/50% combination of nitrous oxide and oxygen. It is an effective analgesic, at the same time providing 50 percent oxygen. The effects dissipate within 2–5 minutes after the cessation of administration.
- *Nitroglycerin.* Nitroglycerin is an arterial and venous vasodilator which decreases myocardial workload. It is used in the management of angina pectoris and MI. In addition, it can be used for pulmonary edema because of its vasodilatory effect. It is administered sublingually or intravenously.
- *Morphine sulfate.* Morphine is a narcotic and a potent analgesic. In addition to its sedative effects, it causes peripheral vasodilation. It is used in MI, pulmonary edema, and other cardiovascular emergencies. It is administered intravenously.

Other Prehospital Drugs

- *Furosemide.* Furosemide is a potent loop diuretic which inhibits sodium reabsorption in the kidneys. It is also thought to cause venous dilation, decreasing venous return (preload). Furosemide is used in the management of congestive heart failure and cardiogenic shock. It is administered by intravenous bolus.
- *Aminophylline.* Aminophylline is a bronchodilator which acts through a different mechanism than the sympathomimetic drugs. It is occasionally administered to cardiac patients if bronchospasm is suspected. It is administered by intravenous infusion.
- *Diazepam (Valium).* Diazepam is an anxiolytic. It is used to calm the extremely anxious patient suffering MI and as a sedative prior to cardioversion in the conscious patient. It is administered by slow intravenous bolus.

Important Cardiac Drugs Not Frequently Used in the Prehospital Setting. Many medications are not routinely used in the prehospital setting. These are described here because many paramedics also work in the emergency department. Also, many patients take these medications on a chronic basis.

- ❑ *Digitalis (digoxin, Lanoxin).* Digitalis is a cardiac glycoside. It increases the force of the cardiac contraction and cardiac output. It slows impulse conduction through the AV node and decreases the ventricular response to certain supraventricular dysrhythmias, such as atrial fibrillation, atrial flutter, and paroxysmal supraventricular tachycardia. It is used in the treatment of heart failure and the dysrhythmias mentioned above. Digitalis toxicity can result in almost any dysrhythmia which often is refractory to traditional antidysrhythmic drugs.
- ❑ *Beta blockers.* Beta blockers are frequently used to control dysrhythmias, high blood pressure, and angina. Many beta blockers, such as propranolol (Inderal), are nonselective, while others are selective for $\beta 1$ or $\beta 2$ receptors. Beta blockers may precipitate congestive heart failure, heart block, and asthma in patients who are predisposed to these conditions.
- ❑ *Calcium channel blockers.* The calcium channel blockers are a relatively new class of medication. They include verapamil (Isoptin, Calan), diltiazem (Cardizem), and nifedipine (Procardia). These agents are being used increasingly for angina pectoris, dysrhythmias, hypertension, and other cardiovascular problems.

Techniques of Management for Cardiovascular Emergencies

The following section will address, and in some cases review, management techniques frequently used in cardiac emergencies. The paramedic should become familiar with local protocols and procedures, as these can vary from system to system.

Basic Life Support. Basic life support is the primary skill for the management of serious cardiovascular problems. The techniques of basic life support are reviewed in Tables 21-1 through 21-3.

✱ Basic life support is the mainstay of prehospital cardiac care.

ECG Monitoring. ECG monitoring in the field is accomplished mainly with a combination ECG monitor/defibrillator which operates on a direct current (DC) battery source. (See Procedure 21-1, page 690.) The ECG monitor/defibrillator consists of several parts:

- ❑ paddle electrodes
- ❑ defibrillator controls
- ❑ synchronizer switch
- ❑ oscilloscope
- ❑ paper strip recorder
- ❑ patient cable and lead wires
- ❑ controls for monitoring
- ❑ special features (data recorders, etc.)

Monitoring requires the placement of three leads on the chest, corresponding to the bipolar leads described earlier in this chapter. One lead is positive, another negative, and the last a ground. The placement of the leads varies according to the brand of equipment used. As a rule, lead II is usually monitored. However, lead MCL_1 is occasionally used and is often better at determining the site of ectopic beats.

The patient can be monitored either through the defibrillator paddles ("quick-look") or through chest electrodes. The quick-look paddles are more frequently used in cases of cardiac arrest, in which there is no time to place chest electrodes. This system can also be used when the pa-

TABLE 21-1 Adult One-Rescuer CPR (Reproduced courtesy of the American Heart Association)

Step	Objective	Critical Performance	S	U
1. AIRWAY	Assessment: Determine unresponsiveness.	Tap or gently shake shoulder.		
		Shout "Are you OK?"		
	Call for help.	Call out "Help!"		
	Position the victim.	Turn on back as unit, if necessary, supporting head and neck (4–10 sec).		
	Open the airway.	Use head-tilt/chin-lift maneuver.		
2. BREATHING	Assessment: Determine breathlessness.	Maintain open airway.		
		Ear over mouth, observe chest: look, listen, feel for breathing (3–5 sec).		
	Ventilate twice.	Maintain open airway.		
		Seal mouth and nose properly.		
		Ventilate 2 times at 1–1.5 sec/inspiration.		
		Observe chest rise (adequate ventilation volume.)		
		Allow deflation between breaths.		
3. CIRCULATION	Assessment: Determine pulselessness.	Feel for carotid pulse on near side of victim (5–10 sec).		
		Maintain head-tilt with other hand.		
	Activate EMS system.	If someone responded to call for help, send him/her to activate EMS system.		
		Total time, Step 1—Activate EMS system: 15–35 sec.		
	Begin chest compressions.	Rescuer kneels by victim's shoulders.		
		Landmark check prior to hand placement.		
		Proper hand position throughout.		
		Rescuer's shoulders over victim's sternum.		
		Equal compression–relaxation.		
		Compress 1½ to 2 inches.		
		Keep hands on sternum during upstroke.		
		Complete chest relaxation on upstroke.		
		Say any helpful mnemonic.		
		Compression rate: 80–100/min (15 per 9–11 sec).		
4. Compression/Ventilation Cycles	Do 4 cycles of 15 compressions and 2 ventilations.	Proper compression/ventilation ratio: 15 compressions to 2 ventilations per cycle.		
		Observe chest rise: 1–1.5 sec/inspiration; 4 cycles/52–73 sec.		
5. Reassessment*	Determine pulselessness.	Feel for carotid pulse (5 sec).† If there is no pulse, go to Step 6.		
6. Continue CPR	Ventilate twice.	Ventilate 2 times.		
		Observe chest rise: 1–1.5 sec/inspiration.		
	Resume compression/ ventilation cycles.	Feel for carotid pulse every few minutes.		

* If 2nd rescuer arrives to replace 1st rescuer: (a) 2nd rescuer identifies self by saying "I know CPR. Can I help?" (b) 2nd rescuer then does pulse check in Step 5 and continues with Step 6. (During practice and testing only one rescuer actually ventilates the manikin. The 2nd rescuer simulates ventilation.) (c) 1st rescuer assesses the adequacy of 2nd rescuer's CPR by observing chest rise during ventilations and by checking the pulse during chest compressions.

† If pulse is present, open airway and check for spontaneous breathing: (a) If breathing is present, maintain open airway and monitor pulse and breathing. (b) If breathing is absent, perform rescue breathing at 12 times/min and monitor pulse.

TABLE 21-2 Adult Two-Rescuer CPR (Reproduced courtesy of the American Heart Association)

Step	Objective	Critical Performance	S	U
1. AIRWAY	**One rescuer (ventilator):** Assessment: Determine unresponsiveness.	Tap or gently shake shoulder.		
		Shout "Are you OK?"		
	Position the victim.	Turn on back if necessary (4–10 sec).		
	Open the airway.	Use a proper technique to open airway.		
2. BREATHING	Assessment: Determine breathlessness.	Look, listen, and feel (3–5 sec).		
	Ventilate twice.	Observe chest rise: 1–1.5 sec/inspiration.		
3. CIRCULATION	Assessment: Determine pulselessness.	Feel for carotid pulse (5–10 sec).		
	State assessment results.	Say "No pulse."		
	Other rescuer (compressor): Get into position for compressions.	Hands, shoulders in correct position.		
	Locate landmark notch.	Landmark check.		
4. Compression/Ventilation Cycles	**Compressor:** Begin chest compressions.	Correct ratio compressions/ventilations: 5/1.		
		Compression rate: 80–100/min (5 compressions/3–4 sec).		
		Say any helpful mnemonic.		
		Stop compressing for each ventilation.		
	Ventilator: Ventilate after every 5th compression and check compression effectiveness.	Ventilate 1 time (1–1.5 sec/inspiration).		
		Check pulse occasionally to assess compressions.		
	(Minimum of 10 cycles.)	Time for 10 cycles: 40–53 sec.		
5. Call for Switch	**Compressor:** Call for switch when fatigued.	Give clear signal to change.		
		Compressor completes 5th compression.		
		Ventilator completes ventilation after 5th compression.		
6. Switch	Simultaneously switch:			
	Ventilator: Move to chest.	Move to chest.		
		Become compressor.		
		Get into position for compressions.		
		Locate landmark notch.		
	Compressor: Move to head.	Move to head.		
		Become ventilator.		
		Check carotid pulse (5 sec).		
		Say "No pulse."		
		Ventilate once (1–1.5 sec/inspiration).†		
7. Continue CPR	Resume compression/ ventilation cycles.	Resume Step 4.		

* (a) If CPR is in progress with one rescuer (lay person), the entrance of the two rescuers occurs after the completion of one rescuer's cycle of 15 compressions and 2 ventilations. The EMS should be activated first. The two new rescuers start with Step 6. (b) If CPR is in progress with one healthcare provider, the entrance of a second healthcare provider is at the end of a cycle after check for pulse by first rescuer. The new cycle starts with one ventilation by the first rescuer, and the second rescuer becomes the compressor.

† During practice and testing only one rescuer actually ventilates the manikin. The other rescuer simulates ventilation.

TABLE 21-3 CPR Summary Performance Sheet (Reproduced courtesy of the American Heart Association)

	Objectives	Actions		
		Adult (over 8 yrs.)	**Child** (1 to 8 yrs.)	**Infant** (under 1 yr.)
A. Airway	1. Assessment: Determine unresponsiveness.	Tap or gently shake shoulder.		
		Say, "Are you okay?"		Observe
	2. Get help.	Call out "Help!"		
	3. Position the victim.	Turn on back as a unit, supporting head and neck if necessary. (4–10 seconds)		
	4. Open the airway.	Head-tilt/chin-lift		
B. Breathing	5. Assessment: Determine breathlessness.	Maintain open airway. Place ear over mouth, observing chest. Look, listen, feel for breathing. (3–5 seconds)		
	6. Give 2 rescue breaths.	Maintain open airway.		
		Seal mouth to mouth		mouth to nose/mouth
		Give 2 rescue breaths, 1 to 1½ seconds each. Observe chest rise. Allow lung deflation between breaths.		
	7. Option for obstructed airway	**a.** Reposition victim's head. Try again to give rescue breaths.		
		b. Activate the EMS system.		
		c. Give 6–10 subdiaphragmatic abdominal thrusts (the Heimlich maneuver).		Give 4 back blows.
				Give 4 chest thrusts.
		d. Tongue–jaw lift and finger sweep	Tongue–jaw lift, but finger sweep only if you see a foreign object.	
		If unsuccessful, repeat a, c, and d until successful.		
C. Circulation	8. Assessment: Determine pulselessness.	Feel for carotid pulse with one hand; maintain head-tilt with the other. (5–10 seconds)		Feel for brachial pulse; keep head-tilt.
	9. Activate EMS system.	If someone responded to call for help, send them to activate the EMS system.		
	Begin chest compressions: 10. Landmark check	Run middle finger along bottom edge of rib cage to notch at center (tip of sternum).		Imagine a line drawn between the nipples.
	11. Hand position	Place index finger next to finger on notch:		Place 2–3 fingers on sternum, 1 finger's width below line. Depress ½–1 in.
		Two hands next to index finger. Depress 1½–2 in.	Heel of one hand next to index finger. Depress 1–1½ in.	
	12. Compression rate	80–100 per minute		At least 100 per minute
CPR Cycles	13. Compressions to breaths.	2 breaths to every 15 compressions.	1 breath to every 5 compressions.	
	14. Number of cycles.	4 (52–73 seconds)	10 (60–87 seconds)	10 (45 seconds or less)
	15. Reassessment.	Feel for carotid pulse. (5 seconds)		Feel for brachial pulse.
		If no pulse, resume CPR, starting with 2 breaths.	If no pulse, resume CPR, starting with 1 breath.	
Option for entrance of 2nd rescuer: "I know CPR. Can I help?"	1st rescuer ends CPR.	End cycle with 2 rescue breaths.	End cycle with 1 rescue breath.	
	2nd rescuer checks pulse (5 seconds).	Feel for carotid pulse.		Feel for brachial pulse.
	If no pulse, 2nd rescuer begins CPR.	Begin one-rescuer CPR, starting with 2 breaths.	Begin one-rescuer CPR, starting with 1 breath.	
	1st rescuer monitors 2nd rescuer.	Watch for chest rise and fall during rescue breathing; check pulse during chest compressions.		
Option for pulse return	If no breathing, give rescue breaths.	1 breath every 5 seconds	1 breath every 4 seconds	1 breath every 3 seconds

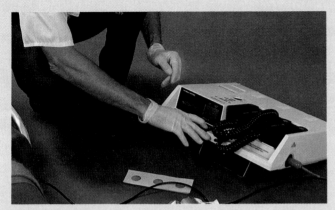

21-1A   Turn the machine on.

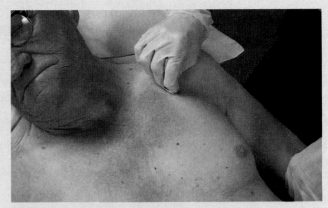

21-1B   Prep the skin.

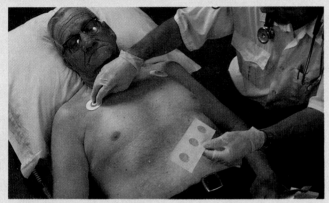

21-1C   Apply the electrodes.

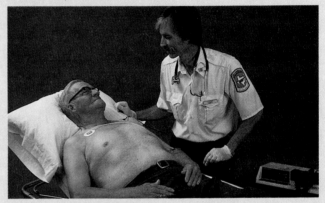

21-1D   Ask the patient to relax and remain still.

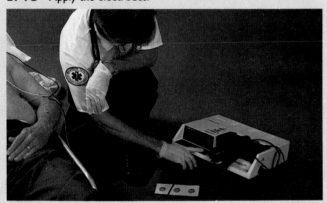

21-1E   Check the ECG.

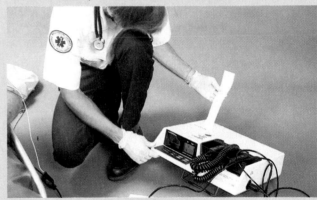

21-1F   Obtain tracing.

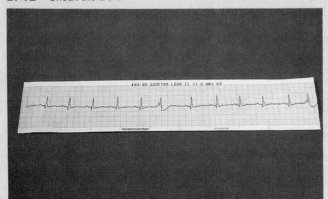

21-1G   ECG strip.

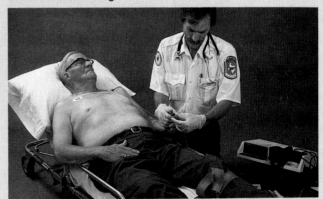

21-1H   Continue ALS care.

tient cable is inoperative. "Quick-look" paddle electrodes have several disadvantages. First, they tend to pick up more artifact than chest electrodes. Second, in order to monitor, they must be held in continuous contact with the chest.

The procedure for using quick-look paddles is as follows:

❑ Turn on oscilloscope power.
❑ Apply conducting gel or other medium liberally to the paddle surface.
❑ Hold the paddles firmly on the chest wall with the negative electrode on the right upper chest and the positive electrode on the left lower chest. This closely simulates lead II.
❑ Observe the monitor and obtain a tracing if desired.

The type of chest leads varies from manufacturer to manufacturer. Usually, to mimic lead II, the positive electrode is placed on the left lower chest and the negative electrode on the right upper chest. Placement of the ground wire varies. For MCL_1, the positive electrode is placed on the right lower chest wall and the negative electrode on the left upper chest wall. Placement of the ground wire varies.

Electrodes should be placed to avoid large muscle masses, large quantities of chest hair, or anything that keeps the electrodes from being flat on the skin. Also, avoid placing electrodes where defibrillator paddles would be placed if required. The procedure for placing electrodes is as follows:

1. Cleanse the skin with alcohol or abrasive pad. This removes dirt and body oil for better skin contact. If there is a lot of chest hair, shave small amounts before placing the electrodes. If the patient is extremely diaphoretic, tincture of benzoin may be applied.
2. Apply electrodes to the skin surface.
3. Attach wires to the electrodes.
4. Plug the cable into the monitor.
5. Adjust gain or sensitivity to the proper level.
6. Adjust the QRS volume. Be aware that the continual beep of the ECG may disturb the patient.
7. Obtain a baseline tracing.

A poor ECG signal is useless and should be corrected. The most common cause is poor skin contact. Check for:

❑ excessive hair
❑ loose or dislodged electrode
❑ dried conductive gel
❑ poor placement
❑ diaphoresis

An initially poor tracing may improve as the conductive gel breaks down skin resistance. Other causes of poor tracings include:

❑ patient movement or muscle tremor
❑ broken patient cable
❑ broken lead wire
❑ low battery
❑ faulty grounding
❑ faulty monitor

A paper printout should be obtained from each monitored patient. Be sure the stylus heat is adjusted properly. Each strip should be calibrated at the beginning of monitoring. A 1 mV calibration curve should deflect the stylus 10 mm (2 large boxes).

Precordial Thump.   The precordial thump still has a role in advanced prehospital care. The precordial thump is used to stimulate a depolarization within the heart and is sometimes effective in causing ventricular depolarization and resumption of an organized rhythm. Conversions from ventricular tachycardia, complete AV block, and, occasionally, ventricular fibrillation, have been reported. The technique should be used only in cases of monitored ventricular fibrillation or witnessed cardiac arrest when a defibrillator is not readily available. It is not recommended in pediatric patients.

The thump is delivered to the midsternum with the heel of the fist from a height of 10-12 in. (See Figure 21-67.) The arm and wrist should be parallel to the long axis of the sternum to avoid rib fractures and other problems.

Defibrillation.   **Defibrillation** is the process of passing a current through a fibrillating heart to depolarize the cells and allow them to repolarize uniformly, restoring an organized cardiac rhythm. A critical mass of the myocardium must be depolarized in order to suppress all of the ectopic foci. The critical mass is related to the size of the heart but cannot be calculated for a given individual or situation.

The *defibrillator* is an electrical capacitor which stores energy for delivery to the patient at a desired time. It consists of an adjustable high-voltage power supply, energy storage capacitor, and paddles. The capacitor is connected to the paddles by a current-limiting inductor.

Most defibrillators use direct current (DC). Alternating current (AC) models should not be used. Direct current is more effective, more portable, and causes less muscle damage. The electrical charge consists of sev-

■ **defibrillation** the process of passing a DC electrical current through a fibrillating heart to depolarize a "critical mass" of myocardial cells, allowing them to depolarize uniformly, resulting in an organized rhythm.

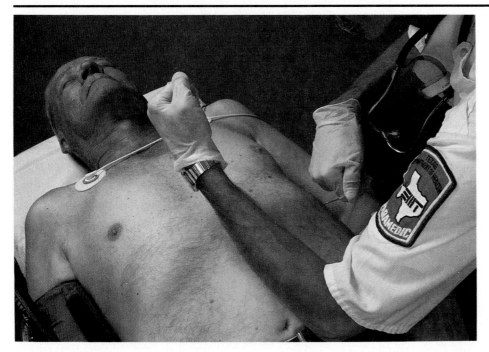

FIGURE 21-67   The precordial thump.

eral thousand volts delivered over a very short time interval, generally 4–12 milliseconds. The strength of the shock is commonly expressed in energy according to the following formula:

$$\text{Energy (joules)} = \text{power (watts)} \times \text{duration (seconds)}$$

The chest wall offers resistance to the electrical charge, which lowers the actual amount of energy delivered to the heart. Therefore, it is important to lower the resistance pathway between the defibrillator paddles and the chest. Factors that influence chest wall resistance include:

- paddle pressure
- paddle-skin interface
- paddle surface area
- number of previous countershocks
- inspiratory versus expiratory phase at time of countershock

The following factors influence the success of defibrillation:

- *Duration of ventricular fibrillation:* In conjunction with effective CPR, defibrillation begun within 4 minutes after the onset of fibrillation will yield significantly improved resuscitation rates, as compared with defibrillation begun within 8 minutes.
- *Condition of the myocardium:* It is more difficult to successfully convert ventricular fibrillation in the presence of acidosis, hypoxia, hypothermia, electrolyte imbalance, or drug toxicity. Secondary ventricular fibrillation (ventricular fibrillation that results from another cause) is more difficult to treat than primary ventricular fibrillation.
- *Heart size and body weight:* This is controversial. It is known that pediatric and adult energy requirements differ. However, it is not clear whether a relationship exists between size and energy level settings in adults.
- *Previous countershocks:* Repeated countershocks decrease transthoracic resistance, thereby allowing more energy to be delivered to the heart at the same energy level.
- *Paddle size:* Larger defibrillator paddles are thought to be more effective and cause less myocardial damage. The ideal size for adults, however, has not been established. It is recommended that the paddles be 10–13 cm in diameter. In infants, 4.5 cm paddles are adequate.
- *Paddle placement:* The placement of the paddles on the chest (transthoracic) is recommended for the emergency setting in both adults and children. One paddle is positioned to the right of the upper sternum, just below the clavicle. The other is placed to the left of the left nipple in an anterior axillary line, which is immediately over the apex of the heart. Paddles should not be placed over the sternum. The paddles may be marked as apex (positive electrode) and sternum (negative electrode). Reversing polarity does not affect defibrillation. It does, however, invert the ECG tracing.
- *Paddle-skin interface:* The paddle-skin interface should have as little electrical resistance as possible. Increased resistance decreases energy delivery to the heart and increases heat production on the skin. Many materials are available to decrease resistance. These include gels, creams, pastes, saline-soaked pads, and prepackaged gel pads. Any creams used should be made specifically for defibrillation, not for ECG monitoring. When using cream, make sure that the cream does not run, thus forming a bridge between paddles. NEVER use alcohol-soaked pads. These can cause fire.
- *Paddle contact pressure:* The paddle contact pressure is important. Firm, downward pressure decreases transthoracic resistance. Do not lean on the paddles; they may slip.
- *Properly functioning defibrillator:* The machine should deliver the amount of energy it indicates. Therefore, frequent inspection and testing are necessary. Change and cycle the batteries as directed by the manufacturer.

Procedure 21-2 shows the steps involved in defibrillation. See the description of emergency synchronized cardioversion below for further details.

Energy Recommendations. Defibrillation should initially be attempted at 200 joules in an adult. This should be increased to a maximum of 360 joules in 1-2 repeat countershocks. The pediatric dosage is generally 2 joules/kg initially, repeated at 4 joules/kg if required.

Emergency Synchronized Cardioversion. *Emergency synchronized* **cardioversion** is the delivery of an electrical shock to the heart, synchronized so as to coincide with the R wave of the cardiac cycle, thus avoiding the relative refractory period. Synchronization reduces the energy required and the potential for secondary complicating dysrhythmias.

Indications for emergency synchronized cardioversion include:

❑ perfusing ventricular tachycardia
❑ paroxysmal supraventricular tachycardia
❑ rapid atrial fibrillation
❑ 2:1 atrial flutter

■ **cardioversion** the passage of an electric current through the heart during a specific part of the cardiac cycle to terminate certain dysrhythmias.

The energy requirements are based on the type of dysrhythmia being treated. For ventricular tachycardia, 50 joules is recommended initially. This is progressively increased to 360 joules, as required. Some dysrhythmias, especially those of atrial origin, can be treated with as little as 10 joules.

The procedure for synchronized cardioversion is the same as for defibrillation. (See Procedure 21-3.) Conscious patients should be sedated with diazepam. The synchronizer switch must be turned on and the paramedic must verify that the machine is detecting the R waves. If it is not, the electrodes may need repositioning. The discharge buttons must be pressed and held until the machine discharges (on the next R wave). If ventricular fibrillation occurs, the synchronizer switch should be turned off and the machine used in the defibrillation mode. In ventricular fibrillation there is no R wave, so the machine will not discharge.

Rotating Tourniquets (optimal skill). Rotating tourniquets can be used in pulmonary edema and left heart failure. They tend to enhance venous pooling, especially if an IV cannot be established. This can decrease preload by trapping venous blood in the extremities. Constricting bands or blood pressure cuffs may be used. Apply the devices snugly to three of the four extremities as high up on the extremities as possible. The constricting bands should interrupt venous flow only. They should not interfere with arterial flow. Arterial pulses distal to the tourniquet should be palpable after application of the constricting bands. Rotate the bands every 5–10 minutes by releasing the band on one extremity and applying it to another extremity. Do this systematically, so that one extremity is not constricted for a long time. Use caution to avoid releasing all tourniquets at once. Rotating tourniquets are contraindicated in patients with shock and are considered a secondary modality to pharmacological therapy.

Carotid Sinus Massage (optional skill). Carotid sinus massage is used to convert paroxysmal supraventricular tachycardia into sinus rhythm by stimulation of the baroreceptors in the carotid bodies. This results in an increase in vagal tone and a decrease in heart rate.

PROCEDURE 21-2   Defibrillation.

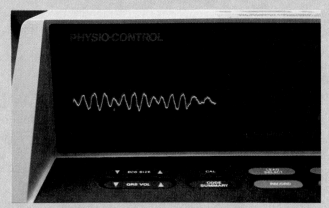

21-2A   Confirm rhythm.

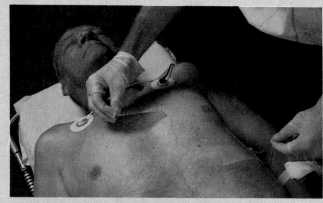

21-2B   Place conductive pads.

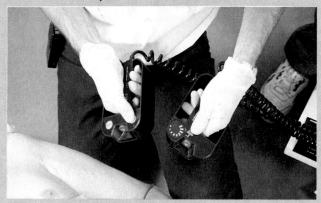

21-2C   Charge the defibrillator.

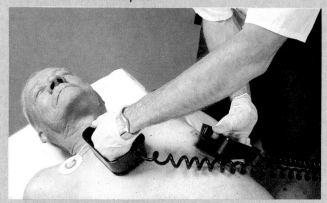

21-2D   Apply the paddles.

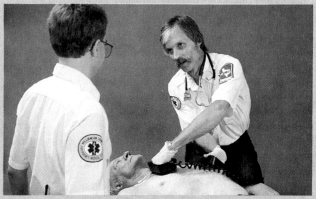

21-2E   Ensure that everyone is clear of the patient.

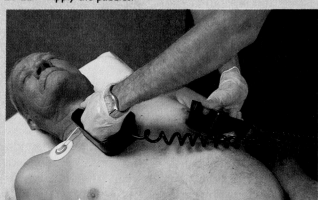

21-2F   Discharge the machine.

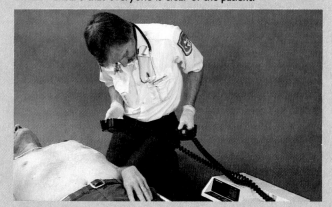

21-2G   Check the ECG.

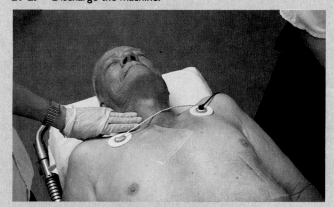

21-2H   Check the pulse.

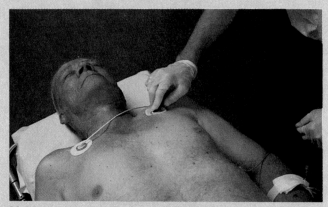

21-3A.   Place the patient on the monitor.

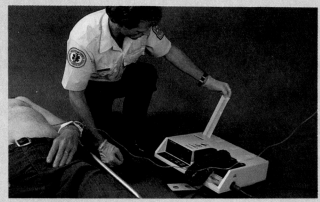

21-3B.   Confirm the rhythm.

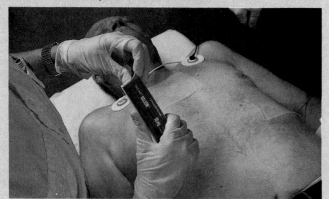

21-3C.   Sedate the patient, if necessary.

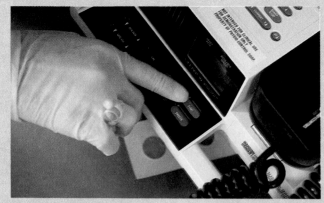

21-3D.   Activate the synchronizer.

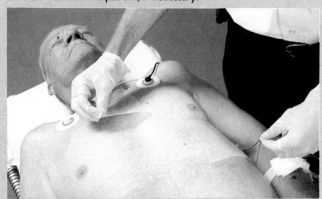

21-3E.   Place the conductive pads.

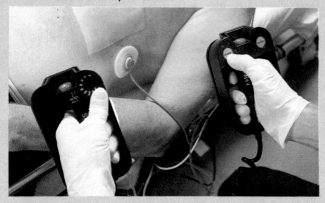

21-3F.   Select the appropriate energy level.

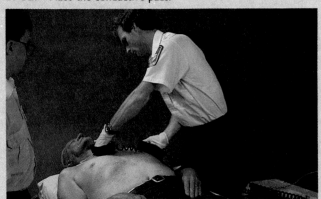

21-3G.   Discharge the machine.

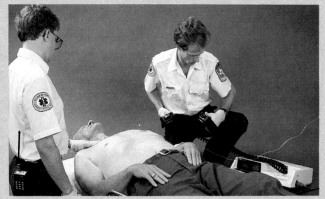

21-3H.   Monitor the patient.

The technique is as follows (see Procedure 21-4, page 701):

1. Initiate IV, oxygen, and ECG monitoring.
2. Position patient on the back, slightly hyperextending the head.
3. Gently palpate each carotid pulse SEPARATELY. Auscultate each side for the presence of carotid bruits. If the pulse is diminished, or if carotid bruits are present, DO NOT attempt carotid sinus massage.
4. Tilt the patient's head to either side and place your index and middle fingers over one artery below the angle of the jaw and as high up on the neck as possible.
5. Firmly massage the artery by pressing it against the vertebral body and rubbing.
6. Monitor the ECG and obtain a continuous readout. Terminate massage at the first sign of slowing or heart block.
7. Maintain pressure no longer than 15-20 seconds.
8. If it is ineffective, the massage may be repeated, preferably on the other side.
9. Have atropine sulfate readily available.

Complications include dysrhythmias, such as asystole, PVCs, ventricular tachycardia, or fibrillation. In addition, carotid sinus massage can interfere with cerebral circulation, causing syncope, seizure, or even stroke. Increased parasympathetic tone can cause bradycardias, nausea, or vomiting.

External Cardiac Pacing (optional skill). Many paramedic units now have the capability to perform external cardiac pacing. External cardiac pacing is beneficial in cases of symptomatic bradycardia such as that which occurs with high degree AV blocks, atrial fibrillation with slow ventricular response, and other significant bradycardias.

The technique for external cardiac pacing is as follows (See Procedure 21-5):

1. Initiate IV, oxygen, and ECG monitoring.
2. Place the patient in a supine position.
3. Confirm symptomatic bradycardia and confirm medical control order for external cardiac pacing.
4. Apply the pacing electrodes per the manufacturer's recommendations. Assure there is a good electrode/skin interface.
5. Connect the electrodes.
6. Set the desired heart rate on the pacemaker. This will typically be in the range of 60–80 beats per minute.
7. Turn the voltage setting down to 0.
8. Turn the pacer on.
9. Slowly increase the voltage until you note ventricular capture.
10. Check the pulse and blood pressure, and adjust the rate and voltage as ordered by medical control.
11. Monitor the patient's response to treatment.

Occasionally external cardiac pacing may cause patient discomfort. If this occurs the medical control physician may request the administration of an analgesic.

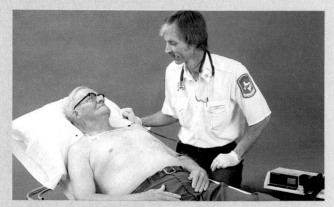

21-4A.   Assess the patient.

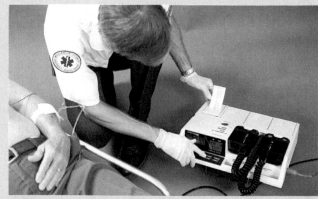

21-4B.   Turn on the monitor.

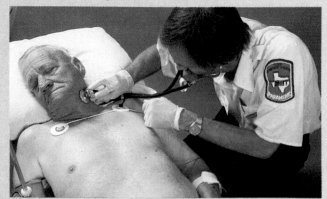

21-4C.   Listen to both carotids for the presence of bruits.

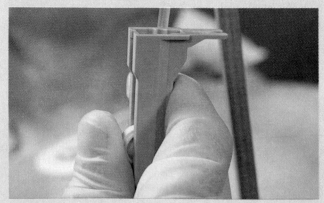

21-4D.   Start an IV line.

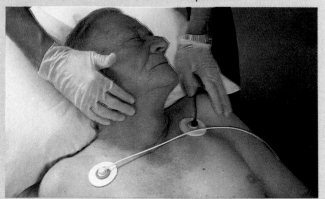

21-4E.   Rub the right carotid. Wait.

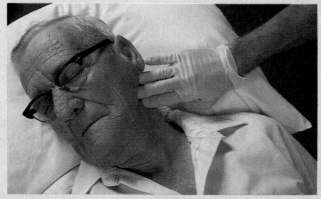

21-4F.   If unsuccessful, rub the left carotid.

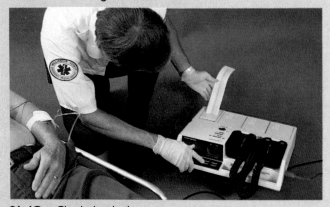

21-4G.   Check the rhythm.

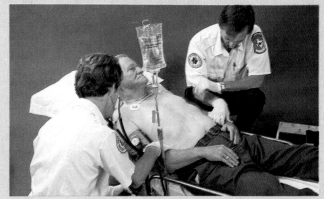

21-4H.   Re-evaluate the patient.

External cardiac pacing is now possible in the prehospital setting. External pacing is of benefit in bradycardias and heart blocks which are symptomatic. The electrodes are placed on the chest as shown. The desired heart rate is selected. The current is then adjusted until "capture" of the heart's conductive system is obtained.

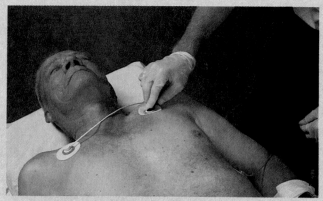

21-5A. Place ECG electrodes.

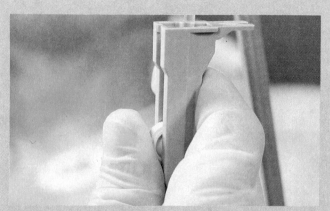

21-5B. Establish an IV line.

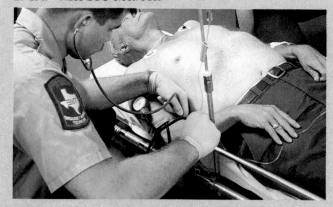

21-5C. Carefully assess vital signs and contact medical control.

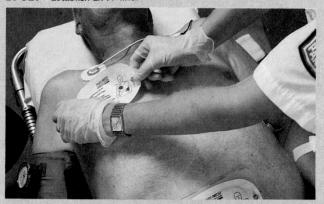

21-5D. If external pacing ordered, apply the pacing electrodes per the manufacturer's recommendations.

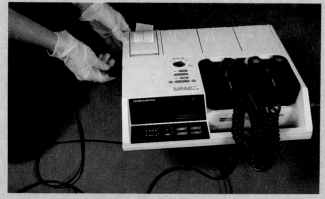

21-5E. Connect the electrodes.

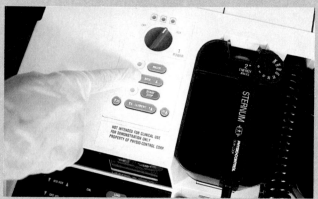

21-5F. Select the desired pacing rate and current.

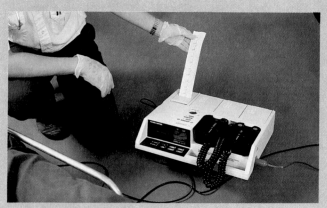

21-5G. Monitor the patient's response to treatment.

SUMMARY

Cardiovascular disease is the number one cause of death in the United States today. Many deaths from heart attack occur within the first 24 hours, many within the first hour. Therefore, prompt and efficient pre-hospital care can literally mean the difference between life and death.

FURTHER READING

AMERICAN HEART ASSOCIATION. *Textbook of Advanced Cardiac Life Support,* 2nd Ed. Dallas: American Heart Association, 1987.

AMERICAN HEART ASSOCIATION AND AMERICAN ACADEMY OF PEDIATRICS. *Textbook of Pediatric Advanced Life Support.* Dallas: American Heart Association, 1988.

AMERICAN HEART ASSOCIATION AND AMERICAN ACADEMY OF PEDIATRICS. *Textbook of Neonatal Resuscitation.* Dallas: American Heart Association, 1987.

BLEDSOE, BRYAN E. *Atlas of Paramedic Skills.* Englewood Cliffs, NJ: Prentice-Hall, 1987.

BLEDSOE, BRYAN E., BOSKER, GIDEON, AND PAPA, FRANK J. *Prehospital Emergency Pharmacology,* 2nd Ed. Englewood Cliffs, NJ: Prentice-Hall, 1988.

BRAUNWALD, EUGENE. *Heart Disease: A Textbook of Cardiovascular Medicine,* 2nd Ed. Philadelphia: W.B. Saunders 1984.

GUYTON, ARTHUR C. *Textbook of Medical Physiology,* 7th Ed. Philadelphia: W.B. Saunders, 1987.

HUSZAR, ROBERT J. *Emergency Cardiac Care,* 2nd Ed. Bowie, Md: Brady Communications, 1982.

SHADE, BRUCE, ET AL. *Advanced Cardiac Life Support: Certification, Preparation, and Review.* Englewood Cliffs, NJ: Brady Communications, 1988.

WALRAVEN, GAIL. *Basic Arrhythmias,* 2nd Ed., Rev. Englewood Cliffs, NJ: Prentice-Hall, 1986.

WALRAVEN, GAIL, ET. AL. *Manual of Advanced Prehospital Care,* 2nd Ed. Bowie, Md: Robert J. Brady Company, 1984.

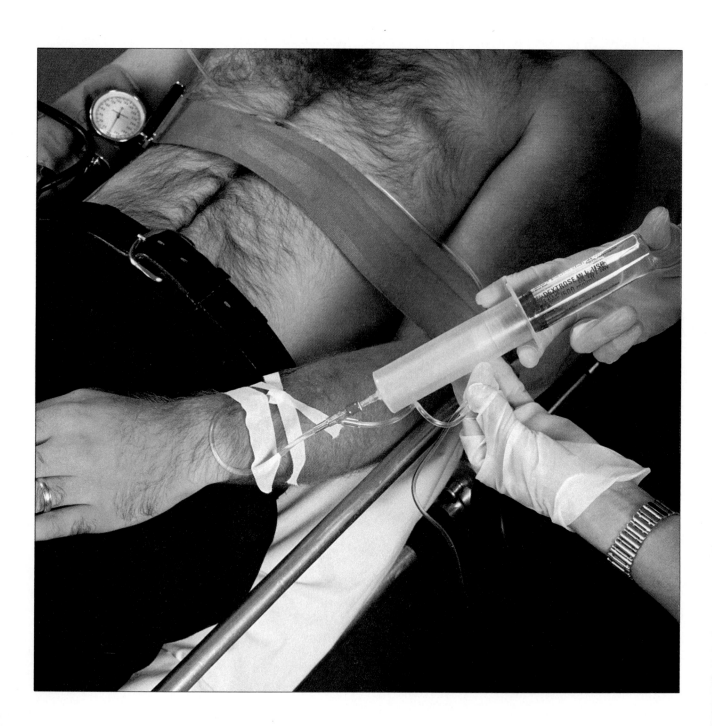

22

Endocrine and Metabolic Emergencies

Objectives for Chapter 22

Upon completing this chapter, the student should be able to:

1. Define the term hormone.

2. Discuss the location and function of the following endocrine glands:
   - pituitary
   - parathyroid
   - pancreas
   - ovaries
   - thyroid
   - adrenal
   - testes

3. Discuss the function of insulin and its relation to glucose metabolism.

4. List two of the functions of the islets of Langerhans.

5. Discuss the function of glucagon.

6. Define diabetes mellitus.

7. Compare and contrast juvenile (Type I) and adult-onset (Type II) diabetes.

8. Discuss the osmotic diuresis occurring in diabetes.

9. Discuss the pathophysiology, presentation, and management of hypoglycemia.

10. Discuss the pathophysiology, presentation, and management of diabetic ketoacidosis.

Rescue 21 is dispatched on a "medical emergency" in the suburb where they are stationed. Upon arrival they find a 31 year old white male unconscious on the couch. His wife says that she discovered him on returning home to pick up her clothes after a domestic quarrel. The last time she saw her husband was four days ago. Stating that he is diabetic, she brings his insulin from the refrigerator. While one paramedic obtains the patient's history, the other completes the primary assessment. He is breathing deeply and has a pulse rate of 100. His skin is warm and dry. He is unresponsive. The secondary assessment is completed, with no other problems identified. The patient has, however, a sweet odor on his breath. ECG reveals sinus tachycardia. Pulse oximetry shows an oxygen saturation of 96%. The paramedics contact medical control. The physician orders an IV of normal saline established. He directs them to administer one ampule of 50% dextrose, 100 milligrams of thiamine, and 1 milligram of Narcan. One paramedic places an oxygen mask while the other starts the IV. Blood is drawn for the hospital and for glucose determination. Then the drugs are administered. The glucometer reading is too high to be determined by the machine. The patient's status remains unchanged. The paramedics again contact medical control and update the physician as they prepare to transport. Medical control orders them to increase the IV flow rate to 250 mL/hour and transport. The patient's status remains the same en route. At the hospital he is admitted to MICU. His blood glucose was 680 mg% in the sample drawn by the paramedics (normal: 70–110). The attending physician begins an insulin drip and continues fluids. Ultimately, the patient recovers. The paramedics learn later that he was intoxicated virtually the entire time after his wife's departure and forgot to take his insulin.

INTRODUCTION

Closely associated with the nervous system, the *endocrine system* is an important body system responsible for controlling many body functions. It exerts its control by releasing special chemical substances called **hormones.** Hormones are chemicals which, when secreted by **endocrine glands** into the blood stream, affect other endocrine glands or body systems. The endocrine system derives its name from the fact that the hormones produced by the various glands are released directly into the blood which transports them to their target tissue. The exocrine system, on the other hand, transports its hormones to target tissues via ducts. Emergencies involving the endocrine system range from the very common, such as diabetes, to the unusual, such as **thyrotoxicosis.**

ANATOMY AND PHYSIOLOGY

The endocrine system consists of several glands located in various parts of the body. They include the following (see Figure 22-1):

■ **hormone** chemical substance released by a gland that controls or affects other glands or body systems.

■ **endocrine gland** gland that secretes hormones directly into the blood.

■ **thyrotoxicosis** toxic condition characterized by tachycardia, nervous symptoms, and rapid metabolism due to hyperactivity of the thyroid gland.

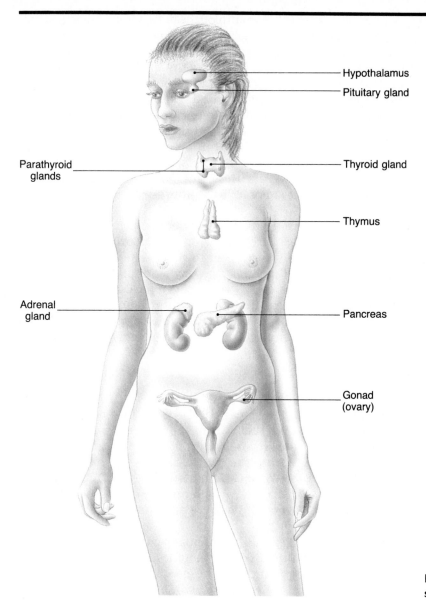

FIGURE 22-1 The endocrine system.

Pituitary

The *pituitary gland* is a small gland located on a stalk hanging from the base of the brain. Sometimes referred to as the "master gland," its primary function is to control the other endocrine glands. Many hormones are produced by the pituitary. Their secretion is controlled by the hypothalamus in the base of the brain. The pituitary gland is divided into two areas, differing both structurally and functionally. Each area has separate types of hormone production. The *posterior pituitary* produces the hormones oxytocin and antidiuretic hormone (ADH). The *anterior pituitary* produces thyroid-stimulating hormone (TSH), growth hormone (GH), adrenocorticotropin (ACTH), follicle-stimulating hormone (FSH), luteinizing hormone (LH), and prolactin. The function of these hormones is discussed below.

Posterior Pituitary. *Oxytocin,* the naturally occurring form of the drug pitocin, stimulates contraction of the gravid uterus and "let down" of milk from the breast. *ADH,* sometimes called vasopressin, causes the kidney to retain water. The interrelationship of these two hormones is significant in emergency medicine. For example, women suffering preterm labor are often administered a bolus of IV fluid to suppress their labor. When the IV fluid is administered, it increases the intravascular fluid volume. Detecting this increase, the kidney sends a message to the pituitary that there is now adequate intravascular fluid volume, and therefore, it is time to release some fluid by filtration through the kidney. The kidney's message causes the pituitary to decrease secretion of ADH, thereby allowing the kidney to produce more urine. Inhibition of ADH by the fluid bolus, however, also causes inhibition of oxytocin, as the two hormones are quite similar and secreted from the same portion of the pituitary. Thus, by using a fluid bolus, it is possible to suppress preterm labor.

Anterior Pituitary. The anterior pituitary hormones primarily regulate other endocrine glands and are rarely a factor in endocrinological emergencies. *TSH* stimulates the thyroid gland to release its hormones, thus increasing metabolic rate. When released by the pituitary, growth hormone has several effects. In adults, the most important is to decrease glucose usage and to increase consumption of fats as an energy source. *ACTH* stimulates the adrenal cortex to release its hormones. *FSH* and *LH* each have specific roles in stimulating maturation and release of eggs from the ovary.

Thyroid Gland

The *thyroid gland* is in the anterior part of the neck just below the larynx. It has two lobes, located on either side of the trachea, connected by a narrow band of tissue called the *isthmus.* Sacs inside the gland contain a thick material called *colloid.* Within the colloid are the thyroid hormones *thyroxine* and *triiodothyronine.* When stimulated, either by TSH from the anterior pituitary or by cold, the thyroid gland releases these two hormones into the circulatory system. Their release increases the overall metabolic rate.

Inadequate levels of the thyroid hormones produce *hypothyroidism* or myxedema. Symptoms of this disorder include facial bloating, weakness, cold intolerance, lethargy, and altered mental states. Additionally, the skin and hair are quite oily. Treatment is by replacement of thyroid hormone.

Increased thyroid hormone release causes *hyperthyroidism,* commonly called *Graves' disease.* Signs and symptoms include insomnia, fatigue, tachycardia, hypertension, heat intolerance, and weight loss. If the hyperthyroidism has existed fairly long, there will be exophthalmos, or bulging of the eyeballs. In severe cases, a medical emergency, called *thyrotoxicosis,* can result. Discussion of these conditions is not within the scope of this text.

Parathyroid Glands

The *parathyroid glands* are small, pea shaped glands, located in the neck near the thyroid. There are usually four of them, although the number can vary. The parathyroid glands regulate the level of the mineral calcium in the body. They produce a hormone called *parathyroid hormone* which, when released, causes the level of calcium in the blood to increase.

The parathyroid glands rarely cause problems. Sometimes they are accidentally removed with the thyroid or sometimes destroyed when it is irradiated. Removal or destruction of the parathyroid glands causes loss of parathyroid hormone and hypocalcemia may then occur.

Pancreas

The *pancreas* is a key gland located in the folds of the duodenum within the abdominal cavity. It has both exocrine and endocrine functions. (See Figure 22-2.) Exocrine functions include responsibility for secreting several digestive enzymes. Within the pancreas are specialized tissues, referred to as the *islets of Langerhans,* where pancreatic endocrine function occurs. Within the islets of Langerhans are three types of cells. Alpha (α) cells secrete the hormone *glucagon,* beta (β) cells secrete the hormone *insulin,* and delta (δ) cells secrete the hormone *somatostatin.*

Glucagon, a very important hormone, is released when the blood glucose level falls. It, in turn, increases the level of glucose in the blood by stimulating the liver to release glucose stores from glycogen and additional glucose storage sites. Glucagon also stimulates the liver to manufacture glucose from other substances in a process called *gluconeogenesis.* Together, both processes effectively raise the blood glucose level.

Insulin is antagonistic to glucagon and causes the various cells in the body to take up glucose. Thus, insulin effectively lowers the blood glucose level. Insulin is rapidly broken down by the liver and must be secreted constantly. The role of insulin in the disease diabetes mellitus will be discussed later in this chapter.

The third endocrine hormone of the pancreas, somatostatin, inhibits glucagon and insulin. Its role in regulating the blood glucose level is incompletely understood.

Adrenal Glands

The *adrenal glands* are two small glands that sit atop both kidneys. These glands have two distinct divisions, each with different functions. The *adrenal medulla,* closely related to the sympathetic component of the autonomic nervous system, secretes the catecholamine hormones *norepinephrine* and *epinephrine.* The *adrenal cortex* secretes three classes of hormones, all of them steroid hormones. They include the *glucocorticoids,* the *mineralocorticoids,* and the *androgenic hormones.*

The glucocorticoids account for 95% of adrenal cortex hormone production. Like glucagon, they increase the level of glucose in the blood. But they perform many other functions, such as anti-inflammatory actions and immune suppression. They are released—like the hormones from the adrenal medulla—in response to stress, trauma, or serious infec-

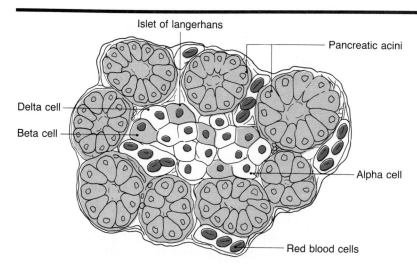

Islet of langerhans

Pancreatic acini

Delta cell

Beta cell

Alpha cell

Red blood cells

FIGURE 22-2 The internal anatomy of the pancreas.

tion. The mineralocorticoids play an important role in regulating the concentration of potassium and sodium in the body.

A prolonged increase in adrenal cortex hormone secretion results in *Cushing's disease.* Patients with it typically have increased blood sugar levels, unusual body fat distribution, and rapid mood swings. Additionally, if there is an associated increase in mineralocorticoids, there will be a serious electrolyte imbalance due to the greater secretion of potassium by the kidney, causing hypokalemia. Sodium also may be retained by the kidney, resulting in hypernatremia. This can result in dysrhythmias, coma, or even death. A tumor is usually responsible, and treatment generally consists of removing it.

Gonads

The gonads are the endocrine glands associated with human reproduction. The female's ovaries produce eggs, and the male's testes produce sperm. However, both ovaries and testes also have endocrine functions.

Ovaries.   The *ovaries,* or the female gonads, are located in the abdominal cavity adjacent to the uterus. As described, they produce eggs for reproduction. Under the control of LH and FSH from the anterior pituitary, they also manufacture *estrogen* and *progesterone.* These hormones have several functions, including sexual development and preparation of the uterus for implantation of the egg.

Testes.   The *testes,* or the male gonads, are located in the scrotum and, as indicated, produce sperm for reproduction. They also manufacture *testosterone* which promotes male growth and masculinization. Like the female ovary, the testes are controlled by the anterior pituitary hormones FSH and LH.

ENDOCRINE EMERGENCIES

By far the most common endocrine emergencies paramedics will be called upon to treat are complications of the disease diabetes mellitus.

Diabetes Mellitus

Introduction.   **Diabetes mellitus** is one of the most common diseases in North America. It is characterized by decreased insulin secretion by the beta cells of the islets of Langerhans in the pancreas. The complications of this disease are numerous. Among others it contributes to heart disease, kidney disease, and blindness.

Diabetes mellitus is generally divided into two different categories. Type I diabetes, or insulin dependent diabetes, usually begins in the early years. Patients who have Type I diabetes must take insulin. Type II, or non-insulin dependent diabetes, usually begins later in life and tends to be associated with obesity. Type II diabetes can often be controlled without using insulin. It is important for paramedics to understand the difference between these two forms of diabetes.

Type I Diabetes.   *Type I diabetes mellitus* is a serious disease. Because it is characterized by inadequate production of insulin by the endocrine pancreas, the patient must take daily supplemental doses. In the normal state, the intake of glucose, such as in a meal, results in the release of insulin. Insulin promotes the uptake of glucose by the cells. Type I diabe-

■ **diabetes mellitus** endocrine disorder characterized by inadequate insulin production by the beta cells of the islets of Langerhans in the pancreas.

tes generally begins with decreased insulin secretion which subsequently leads to elevated blood glucose levels. However, since insulin is required to get glucose into the various body cells, they become starved despite increased blood glucose levels.

Insulin acts as a messenger. When released by the pancreas, it travels through the blood to the target tissues. On reaching its destination, insulin combines with specific insulin receptors on the surface of the cell membrane, allowing glucose to enter the cell. Without insulin, glucose entry cannot occur. Since glucose is the primary energy source for the cells adequate insulin is an absolute necessity for cellular survival.

In diabetes, a drop in insulin levels is accompanied by a steady accumulation of glucose in the blood. As the cells become starved for glucose, they begin to use other sources of energy. Various harmful by-products, such as ketones and organic acids, are, therefore, produced. When these start to accumulate, several of the classic findings of diabetic **ketoacidosis** appear. If the various acids and ketones continue to collect in the blood, severe metabolic acidosis occurs and coma ensues. Severe acidosis can result in serious brain damage or death.

As the concentration of glucose in the blood continues to rise, the kidneys will begin excreting glucose in the urine. When glucose is spilled into the urine, it takes water with it, resulting in an osmotic diuresis, which dehydrates the patient.

Type II Diabetes Mellitus. *Type II diabetes mellitus* occurs more commonly than Type I does. Like Type I, it is characterized by decreased insulin production by the endocrine pancreas. As indicated, Type II diabetes typically begins in later life and is usually associated with obesity. Increased body weight causes a general decrease in the number of available insulin receptors. There is also decreased insulin production, which ultimately leads to increased blood glucose levels. Type II diabetes can generally be managed by diet, oral medication, or a combination of both. If diet and oral agents fail, insulin may be required.

The first approach in treating Type II diabetes is to reduce the intake of carbohydrates by encouraging the patient to lose weight. Physicians may also prescribe oral hypoglycemic agents. These medications tend to stimulate increased insulin secretion from the pancreas and to promote an increase in the number of insulin receptors on the cells. Both actions tend to lower blood glucose levels.

Type II diabetes does not usually result in diabetic ketoacidosis. It can, however, develop into a life-threatening emergency termed *non-ketotic hyperosmolar coma*. In Type II diabetes, when blood glucose levels exceed 600 mg/dL, the high osmolality of the blood causes an osmotic diuresis and dehydration of body cells. In non-ketotic hyperosmolar coma sufficient insulin is produced which prevents the manufacture of ketones and the complications of metabolic acidosis. In this respect, it differs from diabetic ketoacidosis.

Diabetic Ketoacidosis (Diabetic Coma)

Pathophysiology. *Diabetic ketoacidosis* develops as blood glucose levels increase and individual cells become starved. The body begins spilling sugar into the urine. This causes a significant osmotic diuresis and serious dehydration as shown by dry, warm skin and mucous membranes. As cellular starvation continues, ketone and acid production occur. Subsequently, blood becomes acidotic. Deep respirations begin as the body tries to compensate for the metabolic acidosis. If the ketoacidosis is uncorrected, coma will follow.

■ **ketoacidosis** complication of diabetes due to decreased insulin secretion or intake. It is characterized by high levels of glucose in the blood, metabolic acidosis, and, in advanced stages, coma. Ketoacidosis is often called diabetic coma.

Clinical Presentation. The onset of diabetic ketoacidosis is slow, lasting from 12 to 24 hours. In its early stages, the signs and symptoms include increased thirst, excessive hunger, urination, and malaise. Increased urination results from the osmotic diuresis accompanying glucose spillage into the urine. Intensified thirst is caused by the body's attempt to replace the fluids lost by increased urination. Diabetic ketoacidosis is characterized by nausea, vomiting, marked dehydration, tachycardia, and weakness. The skin is usually warm and dry. Coma is not uncommon. The breath may have a sweet or acetone-like character due to the increased ketones in the blood. Very deep, rapid respirations, called *Kussmaul's respirations,* also occur. (See Figure 22-3.) Kussmaul's respirations represent the body's attempt to compensate for the metabolic acidosis produced by the ketones and organic acids present in the blood.

Diabetic ketoacidosis is often associated with infection or decreased insulin intake and may be complicated by several electrolyte imbalances. The most significant is decreased potassium. Decreased potassium (hypokalemia) can lead to serious dysrhythmias or even death.

Ketoacidosis can occur in patients who fail to take their insulin or who take an inadequate amount over an extended period. Persons not previously diagnosed as diabetic will occasionally present in ketoacidosis.

Assessment. The approach used with the patient suffering from diabetic ketoacidosis is essentially the same as with any unconscious patient. First, the paramedic should complete the primary assessment of airway, breathing, and circulation. Next, secondary assessment should be completed. Pay particular attention to the presence of Medic-Alert bracelets and of insulin in the refrigerator. A history should also be taken from bystanders. The fruity odor of ketones occasionally can be detected on the breath. The rapid test for blood glucose should, if available, be completed. (See Procedure 22-1.)

Emergency Intervention. If the blood glucose can be estimated in the field, and a high blood glucose is found to be present, the classical signs and symptoms of diabetic ketoacidosis may be evident. Treatment should consist of drawing a red top tube (or the tube specified by local protocols) of blood. Following this, the paramedic should administer one to two liters of 0.9% sodium chloride. If transport time is lengthy, the medical control physician may request intravenous or subcutaneous administration of regular insulin.

If the blood glucose level cannot be quickly determined, the patient should have a red top tube of blood taken for analysis and an IV of 5% dextrose in water started. Following this, the paramedic should administer 50 mL of 50% dextrose solution, 1–2 mg Narcan, and 100 mg of

Type of respiration	Diagram	Discussion
Normal		16-20/min; regular in rhythm; ratio of respiratory rate to pulse rate is 1:4
Kussmaul's respiration		Increase in both rate and depth; hyperpnea is an increase in depth only. Associated with diabetic ketoacidosis

FIGURE 22-3 Kussmaul's respirations.

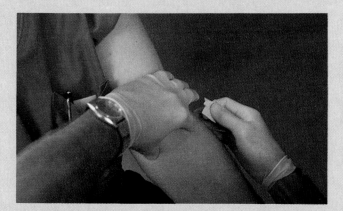

22-1A. Choose a vein and prep the site.

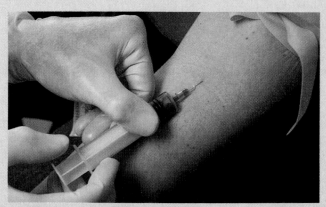

22-1B. Perform the venipuncture.

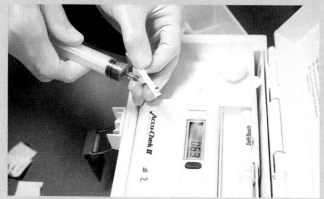

22-1C. Place a drop of blood on the reagent strip. Activate the timer.

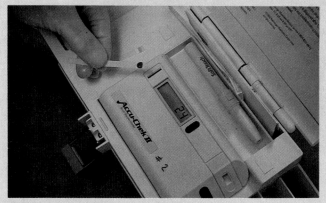

22-1D. Wait until the timer sounds.

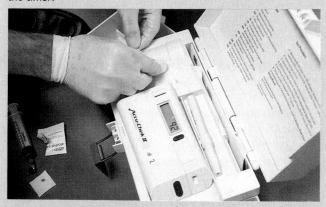

22-1E. Wipe the reagent strip.

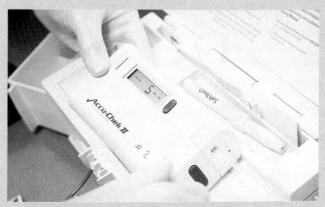

22-1F. Place the reagent strip in the glucometer.

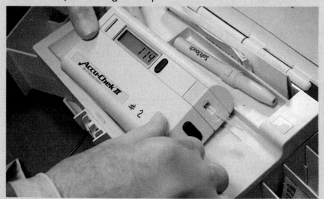

22-1G. Read the blood glucose level.

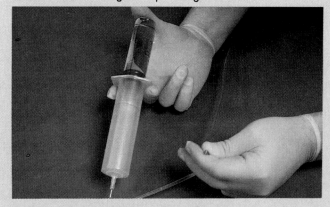

22-1H. Administer 50% dextrose intravenously if the blood glucose level is less than 80 mg.

thiamine. This additional glucose load will not adversely affect the keto-acidotic patient because it is negligible compared to the total quantity present in the body.

Hypoglycemia (Insulin Shock)

Pathophysiology.   At the other end of the spectrum from diabetic keto-acidosis is **hypoglycemia,** sometimes called insulin shock. Hypoglycemia can occur if a patient accidentally or intentionally takes too much insulin or eats an inadequate amount of food after taking insulin. If the patient is untreated, the insulin will cause the blood glucose level to drop to a very low level. THIS IS A TRUE MEDICAL EMERGENCY. If the patient is not treated quickly, he or she can sustain serious injury to the brain since it receives most of its energy from glucose metabolism.

Clinical Presentation.   The clinical signs and symptoms of hypoglycemia are many and varied. An abnormal mental status is the most important. In the earliest stages of hypoglycemia the patient may appear restless or impatient or complain of hunger. As the blood sugar falls lower, he or she may display inappropriate anger (even rage) or display a variety of bizarre behaviors. Sometimes the patient may be placed in police custody for such behaviors or be involved in an automobile accident.

Physical signs may include diaphoresis and tachycardia. If the blood sugar falls to a critically low level, the patient may sustain a **hypoglycemic seizure** or become comatose.

In contrast to diabetic ketoacidosis, the changes of hypoglycemia come on quickly. A change in mental status can occur without warning. When encountering a patient behaving bizarrely, the paramedic should always consider hypoglycemia. (See Table 22-1.)

Assessment.   The primary assessment should be quickly performed. The patient must be inspected for Medic-Alert bracelets. If possible, blood glucose level should be determined. Most paramedic units need to have the capability to quickly estimate the blood glucose level.

Emergency Intervention.   If the blood glucose level is noted to be less that 45 mg/dl, then a red top tube of blood should be drawn and an IV of normal saline started. Then, 50–100 milliliters of 50% dextrose should be administered intravenously. If the patient is conscious and able to swallow, then glucose administration can be completed with orange juice, sodas, or commercially available glucose pastes.

But if the blood glucose cannot be obtained, and the patient is unconscious, then the paramedic should start an IV of normal saline and administer 50–100 milliliters 50% dextrose, 1–2 mg Narcan, and 100 mg thiamine. Transport to a medical facility is also indicated. (See Table 22-1.)

SUMMARY

Like the nervous system, the endocrine system is extremely important in regulating many body functions. With the exception of complications from diabetes mellitus, endocrine emergencies tend to be quite rare and probably would be undetected in the prehospital setting.

Prehospital personnel should always suspect diabetes. Hypoglycemia, the most urgent diabetic emergency, must be quickly treated to prevent serious nervous system damage. When the exact type of diabetes is

---

■ **hypoglycemia** complication of diabetes characterized by low levels of blood glucose. This often occurs from too high a dose of insulin or from inadequate food intake following a normal insulin dose. Sometimes called insulin shock, hypoglycemia is a true medical emergency.

■ **hypoglycemic seizure** seizure that can occur when blood glucose levels fall dangerously low, seriously altering the brain's energy supply.

✳ Hypoglycemia is a true medical emergency that requires prompt intervention to prevent permanent brain injury.

TABLE 22-1 Diabetic Emergencies

Diabetic Ketoacidosis	Hypoglycemia
Causes	**Causes**
Patient has not taken insulin.	Patient has taken too much insulin.
Patient has overeaten, flooding the body with carbohydrates.	Patient has overexerted, thus reducing glucose levels.
Patient has infection which disrupts glucose/insulin balance	
Signs and Symptoms	**Signs and Symptoms**
Polyuria, polydypsia, polyphagia	Weak, rapid pulse
Nausea/ vomiting	Cold, clammy skin
Tachycardia	Weakness/uncoordination
Deep, rapid respirations	Headache
Warm, dry skin	Irritable, nervous behavior
Fruity odor on breath	May appear intoxicated
Abdominal pain	Coma (severe cases)
Falling blood pressure	
Fever (occasionally)	
Decreased LOC	

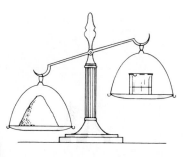
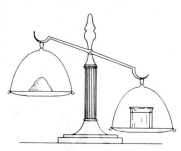

Diagnostic Signs by System		
	Diabetic Ketoacidosis	Hypoglycemia
Cardiovascular		
Pulse	Rapid	Normal (may be rapid)
Blood Pressure	Low	Normal
Respiratory		
Respirations	Exaggerated air hunger	Normal or shallow
Breath odor	Acetone (sweet, fruity)	
Nervous		
Headache	Absent	Present
Mental state	Restlessness → unconsciousness	Apathy, irritability → unconsciousness
Tremors	Absent	Present
Convulsions	None	In late stages
Gastrointestinal		
Mouth	Dry	Drooling
Thirst	Intense	Absent
Vomiting	Common	Uncommon
Abdominal pain	Frequent	Absent
Vision	Dim	Double vision (diplopia)
Management	Fluids, insulin	Dextrose

undetermined, prehospital personnel should treat the emergency as if it were hypoglycemia. Treatment of diabetic ketoacidosis is primarily a hospital procedure.

FURTHER READING

HAMBURGER S., RUSH, D.R., and BOSKER, G., *Endocrine and Metabolic Emergencies.* Bowie, MD:Brady Communications, 1984.

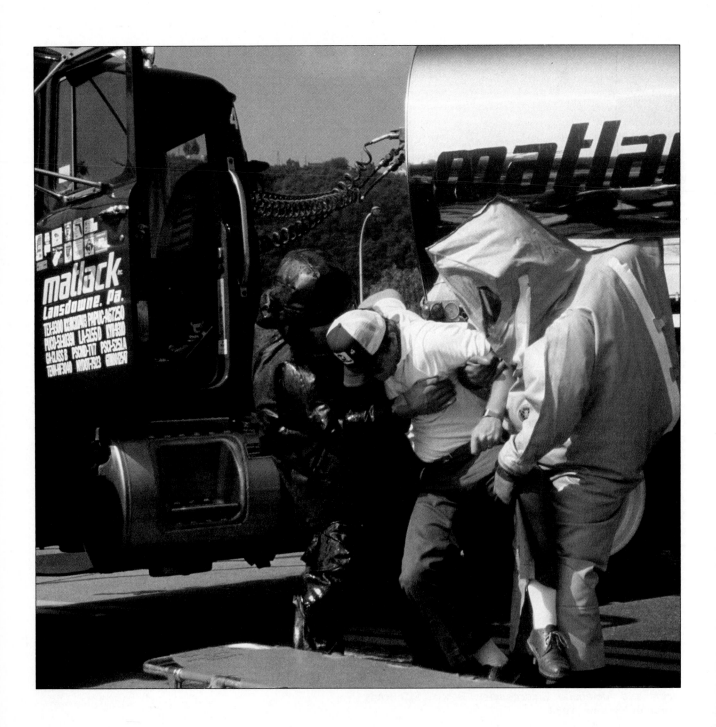

23

Nervous System Emergencies

Objectives for Chapter 23

Upon completing this chapter, the student should be able to:

1. Identify the parts of the neuron and give their function.
2. Describe the process of nerve impulse transmission.
3. Identify the protective structures of the brain and the spinal cord.
4. List the parts of the brain and briefly give the function of each.
5. Identify the functions of the spinal cord.
6. Identify the divisions of the spinal cord and the spinal column.
7. Identify the location of the brachial plexus.
8. Identify the factors to be elicited when evaluating the nervous system including trauma and non-trauma related problems.
9. Identify the following specific observations and physical findings to be evaluated in a patient with a nervous system disorder:
   a. primary assessment
   b. vital signs
   c. neuro evaluation
   d. secondary assessment
      i. pupils
      ii. extraocular movements
      iii. spinal evaluation

10. Describe the Glasgow Coma Scale.
11. Describe the pathophysiology, assessment, and management of the following:
    a. coma
    b. status epilepticus
    c. TIA
    d. seizure
    e. CVA
12. Describe the use of the following drugs in relation to CNS problems:
    a. D-50-W
    b. naloxone
    c. diazepam
    d. dexamethasone
    e. mannitol
    f. thiamine
13. List the possible causes of coma.
14. Differentiate between syncope and seizures.
15. Describe and differentiate the major types of seizures.
16. Describe the different phases of a generalized seizure.

Paramedic Engine Company 10 and Ambulance 17 are dispatched to a "seizure" at a run-down hotel usually frequented by the homeless. The response time is approximately 3 minutes. Upon arrival emergency personnel are led to a ramshackle room where an elderly white male is lying on a mattress on the floor. The room smells of urine and feces. Paramedics quickly perform a primary assessment. The patient has a good airway. Respirations are adequate, and the pulse is strong. The secondary survey reveals a cachectic male with many of the stigmata of alcoholism. As paramedics attempt to arouse the patient to assess the level of consciousness, his body goes into intense spasm. This is followed by alternating contraction and relaxation of the skeletal muscles. This seizure lasts approximately 45 seconds. Following the seizure the patient remains postictal. Paramedics quickly administer oxygen to the patient with a non-rebreathing mask. An IV of D5W is established. Per standing orders, 100 mg of thiamine and 50 mL of 50% dextrose in water are administered. As the paramedic is pushing the dextrose, the patient has another seizure, within 2 minutes of the last. The paramedics then administer 5 mg of diazepam intravenously, and the seizure is terminated. The patient remains postictal and is transported to the hospital. Upon arrival at the emergency department the patient's condition remains unchanged. A routine laboratory profile (SMA-7) is normal. Blood levels of the patient's seizure medications (Dilantin and phenobarbital) are subtherapeutic. Because the patient was sluggish in arousing from the seizure, the emergency department physician orders a CT scan of the brain. The CT scan reveals a rather large subdural hematoma on the left side. The patient is taken to the operating room where a neurosurgeon evacuates the subdural hematoma. The patient's postoperative course is unremarkable. He is later transferred to the Veterans Administration hospital where his rehabilitation continues.

INTRODUCTION

Emergencies involving the nervous system are often difficult to recognize and to treat. Nervous system emergencies are generally categorized as traumatic or medical. This chapter will address the relevant anatomy and physiology of the nervous system. It will also present common medical neurological emergencies as well as the recommended prehospital management.

ANATOMY AND PHYSIOLOGY

✱ The nervous system is the body's control system.

The *nervous system* is the body's control system, regulating nearly all body functions. It exerts this control via electrical impulses transmitted through nerves. The endocrine system, another key system, is closely related to the nervous system, and exerts its control via hormones. The circulatory system serves as an assistant communication system, aiding in the distribution of hormones and other chemical messages.

The nervous system is customarily divided into the central nervous system, the peripheral nervous system, and the autonomic nervous system. The *central nervous system* consists of the *brain* and the *spinal cord*. In contrast, the *peripheral nervous system* is composed of the cranial nerves and the peripheral nerves. The **autonomic nervous system** is functionally divided into the *sympathetic* and the *parasympathetic* nervous systems.

Anatomy and Physiology of the Central Nervous System

The fundamental unit of the nervous system is the nerve cell, or **neuron.** The neuron consists of the cell body, containing the nucleus; the dendrites, which carry nervous impulses to the cell body; and the axons, which transmit nervous impulses away from the cell body.

The transmission of nervous impulses in the nervous system resembles the conduction of electrical impulses through the heart. In its resting state, the neuron is positively charged on the outside and negatively charged on the inside. When stimulated, sodium rapidly enters the cell, and potassium rapidly leaves it, producing a positive charge at the entry site. This positive charge, called the *action potential,* is subsequently transmitted down the neuron at extremely high velocity. The neuron joins with other neurons at junctions called *synapses.* (See Figure 23-1.) The neurons do not come into contact with each other at these synapses. Instead, on reaching the synapse, the axon causes the release of a chemical neurotransmitter. This **neurotransmitter,** either *acetylcholine* or *norepinephrine,* then crosses the gap and stimulates the connecting nerve. Acetylcholine is the neurotransmitter of the parasympathetic and voluntary nervous systems. (See Figure 23-2.) Norepinephrine is found in the synaptic terminals of sympathetic nerves.

■ **autonomic nervous system** part of the nervous system controlling involuntary bodily functions. It is divided into the sympathetic and the parasympathetic systems.

■ **neuron** the nerve cell, the fundamental component of the nervous system.

■ **neurotransmitter** a substance that is released from the axon terminal of a presynaptic neuron upon excitation that travels across the synaptic cleft to either excite or inhibit the target cell. Examples include acetylcholine, norepinephrine, and dopamine.

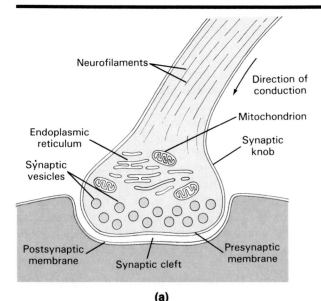
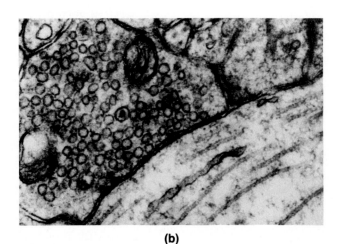

(a)

(b)

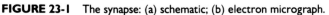

FIGURE 23-1 The synapse: (a) schematic; (b) electron micrograph.

Labels on figure (a): Neurofilaments; Direction of conduction; Mitochondrion; Synaptic knob; Endoplasmic reticulum; Synaptic vesicles; Postsynaptic membrane; Synaptic cleft; Presynaptic membrane

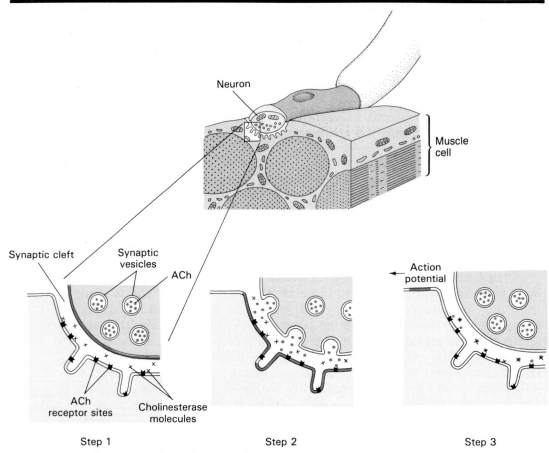

FIGURE 23-2 The motor end plate (connection between nerve and muscle).

Synaptic cleft
Synaptic vesicles
ACh
Neuron
Muscle cell
Action potential
ACh receptor sites
Cholinesterase molecules
Step 1
Step 2
Step 3

Most of the central nervous system is protected by bony structures. Protected by the skull, the brain lies in the cranial vault. Covered by the scalp, the cranium consists of the bones of the head, excluding the facial bones. Bones composing the cranium include the *frontal* and *occipital* bones, each a single bone. Additionally, the *parietal, temporal, sphenoids,* and *ethmoids*—all paired bones—contribute to the structure of the cranium. (See Figure 23-3.)

Protecting the spinal cord are the 33 bones of the spine. There are 7 cervical vertebra, 12 thoracic vertebra, 5 lumbar vertebra, 5 sacral vertebra, and 3 to 5 coccygeal vertebra. The spinal cord is housed inside the spinal canal.

The entire central nervous system is covered by protective membranes called the **meninges.** There are three layers of meninges. The outermost layer is referred to as the *dura mater.* The middle layer is known as the *arachnoid membrane.* The innermost layer, directly overlying the central nervous system, is called the *pia mater.* The space between the pia mater and the arachnoid membrane is referred to as the subarachnoid space. That space between the dura mater and the arachnoid membrane is called the *subdural space.* And the space outside the dura mater is known as the *epidural space.* Both the brain and the spinal cord are bathed in **cerebrospinal fluid.**

The brain is the largest part of the nervous system. Filling the cranial vault, it can be anatomically divided into six major parts. (See Figure 23-4.) These parts are described next. The midbrain, pons, and the medulla oblongata are collectively called the brainstem.

■ **meninges** membranes covering and protecting the brain and spinal cord. They consist of the pia mater, arachnoid membrane, and dura mater.

■ **cerebrospinal fluid** watery, clear fluid that acts as a cushion, protecting the brain and spinal cord from physical impact. The cerebrospinal fluid also serves as an accessory circulatory system for the central nervous system.

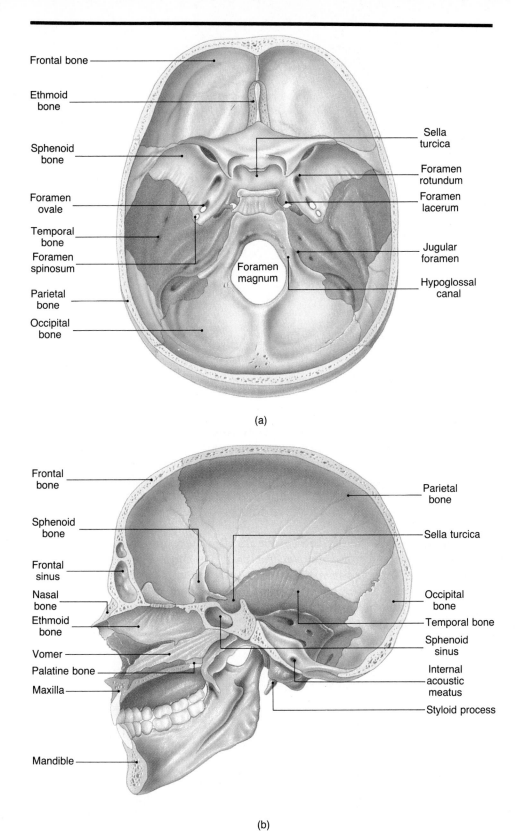

Frontal bone

Ethmoid
bone

Sphenoid
bone

Foramen
ovale

Temporal
bone

Foramen
spinosum

Parietal
bone

Occipital
bone

Sella
turcica

Foramen
rotundum

Foramen
lacerum

Jugular
foramen

Hypoglossal
canal

Foramen
magnum

(a)

Frontal
bone

Sphenoid
bone

Frontal
sinus

Nasal
bone

Ethmoid
bone

Vomer

Palatine bone

Maxilla

Mandible

Parietal
bone

Sella turcica

Occipital
bone

Temporal bone

Sphenoid
sinus

Internal
acoustic
meatus

Styloid process

(b)

FIGURE 23-3 The bones of the skull.

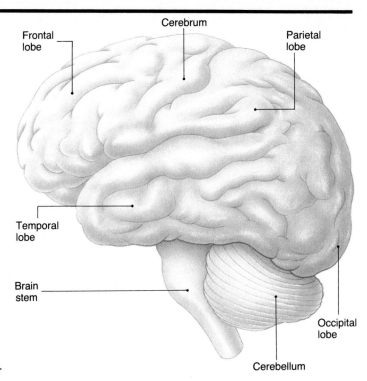

FIGURE 23-4 External anatomy of the brain.

■ **cerebrum** largest part of the brain. It consists of two hemispheres separated by a deep longitudinal fissure. The cerebrum is the seat of consciousness and the center of the higher mental functions such as memory, learning, reasoning, judgment, intelligence, and the emotions.

■ **midbrain** portion of the brain connecting the pons and cerebellum with the cerebral hemispheres.

■ **pons** process of tissue connecting two or more parts of an organ.

■ **medulla oblongata** lower portion of the brainstem.

■ **cerebellum** portion of the brain located dorsally to the pons and medulla oblongata. It plays an important role in the fine control of voluntary muscular movements.

Cerebrum. The **cerebrum,** occasionally referred to as the telencephalon, is in the anterior and middle fossa of the cranium. Containing two hemispheres, it is joined by a structure called the *corpus callosum.* The cerebrum governs all sensory and motor actions. It is the seat of intelligence and responsible for learning, analysis, memory, and language. The *cerebral cortex* is the outermost layer of the cerebrum.

Diencephalon. Covered by the cerebrum, the diencephalon is the superiormost portion of the brain stem. Inside it are the *thalamus, hypothalamus,* and the *limbic system.* This area is responsible for many involuntary actions such as temperature regulation, sleep, water balance, stress response, and emotions. It plays a major role in regulating the autonomic nervous system.

Mesencephalon. The mesencephalon is the **midbrain.** Located between the diencephalon and the pons, it is responsible for certain aspects of motor coordination. The mesencephalon is the major region controlling eye movement.

Pons. Between the midbrain and the medulla oblongata, the **pons** contains connections between the brain and the spinal cord.

Medulla Oblongata. The **medulla oblongata** is located between the pons and the spinal cord. It marks the division between the spinal cord and the brain. Major centers controlling respiration, cardiac activity, and vasomotor activity are located here.

Cerebellum. The **cerebellum** is located in the posterior fossa of the cranial cavity. It consists of two hemispheres closely related to the brainstem and higher centers. The cerebellum coordinates fine motor movement, posture, equilibrium, and muscle tone.

Areas of Specialization

Several areas of specialization are recognized within the brain and have clinical application. These include:

- ❑ *speech center*–located in the temporal lobe
- ❑ *vision*–located in the occipital cortex
- ❑ *personality*–located in the frontal lobes
- ❑ *balance and coordination*–located in the cerebellum
- ❑ *sensory*–located in the parietal lobes
- ❑ *motor*–located in the frontal lobes

Vascular Supply

Blood flow to the brain is provided by two systems. The *carotid system* is anterior and the *vertebrobasilar system* is posterior. Both join at the *Circle of Willis* before entering the substance of the brain. The system is designed so that interruption of any part will not cause significant loss of blood flow to the tissues. Venous drainage of the brain is through the venous sinuses and the internal jugular veins.

    Besides blood flow, the brain and spinal cord are bathed in cerebrospinal fluid which circulates throughout. Several chambers within the brain, called *ventricles,* contain this fluid.

✱ Blood flow to the brain is supplied by two separate systems.

Spinal Cord

The *spinal cord* is 17–18 inches long. It leaves the brain at the medulla and proceeds, through the *foramen magnum,* down the spinal canal. The spinal cord, ending at about the level of the first lumbar vertebra, is responsible for conducting impulses to the peripheral nervous system and for reflexes. *Reflexes* are protective. If a peripheral sensory nerve senses harm, such as intense heat, it sends an impulse to the spinal cord. The spinal cord can then stimulate the appropriate muscles to remove the part of the body closest to the perceived threat. This process saves time as impulses do not have to go to the brain for processing. Because they are mediated in the spinal cord, reflexes lack fine control. Thirty-one pairs of nerve fibers exit the spinal cord as it descends and enters the peripheral nervous system. The dorsal roots contain **afferent** fibers, while the ventral roots contain **efferent** fibers. Afferent fibers transmit impulses from the body to the brain. Efferent fibers carry impulses from the brain to the body.

    Each nerve root has a corresponding area of the body, called a **dermatome,** to which it supplies sensation. The amount of paralysis incurred in a spinal cord injury depends on the location of the injury. The nearer the **brainstem,** the more serious it is.

■ **afferent** fibers carrying impulses toward the center of the body. Sensory nerves send messages toward the brain and are thus afferent.

■ **efferent** fibers carrying conducted impulses away from the brain or spinal cord to the periphery.

■ **dermatome** areas of the skin innervated by spinal nerves.

■ **brainstem** that part of the brain connecting the cerebral hemispheres with the spinal cord. It is comprised of the medulla oblongata, the pons, and the midbrain.

ANATOMY AND PHYSIOLOGY OF THE PERIPHERAL NERVOUS SYSTEM

Consisting of the cranial and the peripheral nerves, the peripheral nervous system has both voluntary and involuntary components. The cranial nerves originate in the brain and supply nervous control to the periphery. The peripheral nerves, as described above, originate in the spinal cord and also supply nervous control to the periphery.

The four categories of peripheral nerves are:

1. *Somatic Sensory.* These nerves transmit sensations involved in touch, pressure, pain, temperature, and position (proprioception).
2. *Somatic Motor.* These fibers carry impulses to the skeletal muscles.
3. *Visceral Sensory.* These tracts transmit sensations from the visceral organs. Sensations such as a full bladder or the need to defecate are mediated by visceral sensory fibers.
4. *Visceral Motor.* These fibers leave the central nervous system and supply nerves to the viscera, such as glands and other organs.

Many of the nerves innervating the upper extremity come from the cervical and thoracic portion of the spinal cord. They enter a network of nerves at the posterior part of the neck called the brachial plexus. This system can be injured at birth or with trauma to the upper extremity, causing permanent disability.

The involuntary component of the peripheral nervous system, commonly called the *autonomic nervous system,* is responsible for the unconscious control of many body functions. There are two functional divisions of the autonomic nervous system. The **sympathetic nervous system,** often referred to as the "fight or flight" system, prepares the body for stressful situations. It is located in the thoracic and lumbar part of the spinal cord. Stimulation causes increased heart rate and blood pressure, pupillary dilation, rise in the blood sugar, as well as bronchodilation. The neurotransmitters epinephrine and norepinephrine mediate its actions. The sympathetic nervous system is closely associated with the adrenal gland of the endocrine system.

The **parasympathetic nervous system,** sometimes called the "feed and breed" system, is responsible for controlling vegetative functions. Associated with the cranial nerves and the sacral plexus, it is mediated by the neurotransmitter acetylcholine. When stimulated it causes a decrease in heart rate, an increase in digestive activity, pupillary constriction, and a reduction in blood glucose.

The sympathetic and parasympathetic systems are antagonistic. In their normal state, they exist in balance with each other. During stress, the sympathetic system dominates. During rest, the parasympathetic system dominates.

■ **sympathetic nervous system** division of the autonomic nervous system that prepares the body for stressful situations.

■ **parasympathetic nervous system** division of the autonomic nervous system that is responsible for controlling vegetative functions.

ASSESSMENT OF THE NEUROLOGICAL SYSTEM

Assessment of the neurological system is frequently difficult. One of the first steps in assessment involves attempting to establish whether the CNS problem is traumatic or medical. Clarification will help determine the plan for subsequent prehospital treatment. The initial history may be hard to obtain because of the patient's impaired mental functioning. In these cases, information from bystanders, if available, becomes critical.

If the neurological injury is due to trauma, the following information should be obtained:

❑ When did the incident occur?
❑ How did the incident occur and what is the mechanism of injury (kinetics)?
❑ Was there any loss of consciousness?

❑ What is the patient's chief complaint?

❑ Has there been any change in symptoms?

❑ Are there any complicating factors?

If the neurological injury is due to nontraumatic problems, the following information should be obtained:

❑ What is the chief complaint?

❑ What are the details of the present illness?

❑ Is there a pertinent underlying medical problem such as:

    ❑ cardiac disease

    ❑ chronic seizures

    ❑ diabetes

    ❑ hypertension

❑ What is the previous history of the same symptoms?

❑ Are there any environmental clues? They include:

    ❑ evidence of current medications

    ❑ Medic-Alert identification

    ❑ alcohol bottles or drug paraphernalia

The procedure for performing a primary and secondary assessment is the same regardless of the injury. The following discussion focuses on particular aspects related to CNS problems.

The first step in performing the patient assessment is to check for responsiveness. Here the greatest emphasis should be placed on maintenance of cervical spine alignment and of the airway. If the patient is unconscious, the paramedic should assume that a cervical spine injury exists and treat it appropriately. The chin-lift and jaw-thrust maneuvers should be used to open the airway. Once it is opened, the appropriate airway adjunct should be inserted.

In any patient with CNS injury it is essential to observe for respiratory arrest which can result from increased intracranial pressure. The paramedic should be alert for an absent gag reflex and vomiting. In addition, blood from facial injuries and possible aspiration of gastric contents further threaten the patient's airway.

Respiratory derangement may occur with CNS illness or injury. The following respiratory patterns may be observed in patients with CNS injury (see Figure 23-5):

Cheyne-Stokes Respiration: a breathing pattern characterized by a period of apnea lasting 10–60 seconds, followed by gradually increasing depth and frequency of respirations.

Central Neurogenic Hyperventilation: hyperventilation caused by a lesion in the central nervous system, often characterized by rapid, deep, noisy respirations.

Ataxic Respirations: poor respirations due to CNS damage, causing ineffective thoracic muscular coordination.

Apneustic Respirations: breathing characterized by prolonged inspiration unrelieved by expiration attempts. This is seen in patients with damage to the upper part of the pons.

Diaphragmatic Breathing: breathing due to intercostal muscle dysfunction.

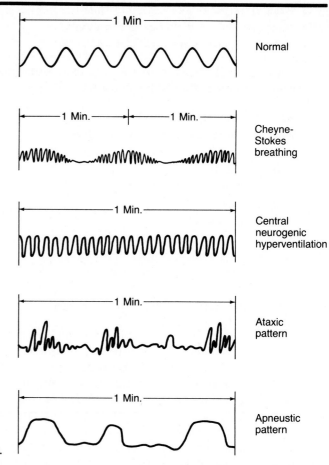

FIGURE 23-5 Respiratory patterns seen with CNS dysfunction.

There may be several other respiratory patterns depending on the injury. As a terminal event, the patient may present with central neurogenic hyperventilation. His or her respirations can be affected by so many factors (fear, hysteria, chest injuries, spinal cord injuries, diabetes), that they are not as useful as other signs in monitoring the course of CNS problems.

The blood level of carbon dioxide (CO_2) has a critical effect on cerebral vessels. The normal blood $PaCO_2$ is 40 mmHg. Increasing the $PaCO_2$ causes cerebral vasodilatation, while decreasing it results in cerebral vasoconstriction. If the patient is poorly ventilated, the CO_2 will increase, causing even further vasodilatation with a subsequent increase in intracranial pressure. Hyperventilation can decrease the $PaCO_2$ to nearly 25 mm/Hg, effectively causing vasoconstriction of the cerebral vessels. Therefore, any patient suspected of having increased intracranial pressure should be hyperventilated at a rate of 24 breaths per minute or greater.

Vital signs are crucial to following the course of CNS problems. Such signs can indicate changes in intracranial pressure. Patients suspected of having a CNS injury should have vital signs taken and recorded every five minutes. Increased intracranial pressure can affect them in the following ways:

❑ Increased blood pressure
❑ Decreased pulse
❑ Decreased respirations
❑ Increased temperature

Dysrhythmias are common with increased intracranial pressure. Thus, the patient should be monitored accordingly.

The following compares vital signs of the patient with shock versus those of the head injury patient with increased intracranial pressure:

Vital Signs	Shock	Increased ICP
Blood Pressure	Decreased	Increased
Pulse	Increased	Decreased
Respirations	Increased	Decreased
LOC	Decreased	Decreased

A patient in the early stages of increased intracranial pressure usually shows a decrease in pulse rate and a rise in blood pressure and temperature. Later, if the intracranial pressure continues to rise without correction, the pulse will increase, the blood pressure will fall, and the temperature will remain elevated.

Neurological Evaluation

Prehospital assessment of the patient with a CNS injury cannot be comprehensive. An effective neurological examination depends, nevertheless, on a thorough knowledge of the range of normal responses. An orderly neurologic examination will provided the most information in the briefest time. To document the progress of the neurologic deficit, the examination must be repeated frequently. A baseline neurological examination is necessary during the initial patient assessment for comparison with later examinations to determine whether the patient's condition is improving or worsening.

The most significant sign in the evaluation of the patient with a CNS injury is the level of consciousness. Assessing this is best performed by using the "AVPU" method. AVPU is rapid and easy to understand.

A = *Patient is alert.* The patient is orientated to person, time, and place, can recall the event as well as relate it to the paramedic.

V = *Patient responds to verbal stimuli.* Note whether he or she can respond appropriately to questions, or if he or she answers normally or sluggishly. The paramedic should also observe whether the patient has purposeful or uncoordinated movements.

P = *Patient responds to painful stimuli.* If the patient is not alert, the paramedic should note the degree of stimulation required for response (sternal rub, squeeze trapezius muscle, or pin prick).

U = *Patient is unresponsive.*

Sensation and motor function should be noted in each extremity. Does the patient have feelings in the hands and the feet? Can he or she wiggle fingers and toes? Compare both sides. If the patient is unconscious, pain response should be observed. If the unconscious patient withdraws or localizes to the pinching of fingers and toes, there is intact sensation and motor function. This is a sign of normal or only minimally impaired cortical function.

Both **decorticate posturing** (arms flexed, legs extended) and **decerebrate posturing** (arms and legs extended) are ominous signs of deep cerebral or upper brainstem injury. (See Figures 23-6 and 23-7.) Flaccid paralysis usually indicates spinal cord injury.

■ **decorticate posture** characteristic posture of a patient with a lesion at or above the upper brainstem. He or she presents with the arms flexed, fists clenched, and legs extended.

■ **decerebrate posture** sustained contraction of extensor muscles of the extremities resulting from a lesion in the brain stem. The patient presents with stiff and extended extremities and retracted head.

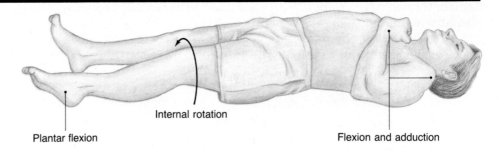

FIGURE 23-6 Decorticate posturing.

Internal rotation

Plantar flexion

Flexion and adduction

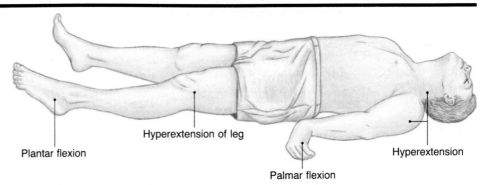

FIGURE 23-7 Decerebrate posturing.

Hyperextension of leg

Plantar flexion

Hyperextension

Palmar flexion

Glasgow Coma Scale

■ **Glasgow Coma Scale** tool used in evaluating and quantifying the degree of coma by determining the best motor, verbal, and eye-opening response to standardized stimuli.

The **Glasgow Coma Scale** offers a simple way to evaluate and monitor the patient who is in a coma due to a CNS injury. The three components of the Glasgow Coma Scale (see Figure 23-8) are:

1. Eye Opening
2. Verbal Response
3. Motor Response

Scoring is as follows:

    Eye Opening:
        Spontaneous.... 4
        To voice.... 3
        To pain.... 2
        None.... 1
    Verbal Response
        Oriented.... 5
        Confused.... 4
        Inappropriate.... 3
        Incomprehensible sounds.... 2
        None.... 1
    Best Motor Response
        Obeys commands.... 6
        Localizes to pain.... 5
        Withdraws to pain.... 4
        Decorticate.... 3
        Decerebrate.... 2
        None.... 1

The total score can serve as an indicator of survival. For example:

Total Scores:
        8 or better . . . . 94% favorable outcome
        5,6,7 . . . . 50% favorable (adult), 90% (children)

Glasgow Coma Scale

Eye opening	Spontaneous	4	
	To voice	3	
	To pain	2	
	None	1	
Verbal response	Oriented	5	
	Confused	4	
	Inappropriate words	3	
	Incomprehensible words	2	
	None	1	
Motor response	Obeys command	6	
	Localizes pain	5	
	Withdraw (pain)	4	
	Flexion (pain)	3	
	Extension (pain)	2	
	None	1	
Glasgow coma score total			

FIGURE 23-8 The Glasgow Coma Scale.

3 and 4 . . . . 10% favorable outcome
5,6,7 who drop a grade . . . . 100% unfavorable outcome
5,6,7 who improve to more than 7 . . . . 80% favorable outcome

The lowest GCS score possible is 3.
The highest possible score is 15.

Head to Toe Survey

Pupils.   The pupils are controlled by the third cranial nerve. This nerve follows a long course through the skull and is easily compressed by brain swelling. Thus, it can be an early indicator of increasing intracranial pressure. If both pupils are dilated and do not react to light, the patient probably has a brainstem injury or has suffered serious brain anoxia. If the pupils are dilated but still react to light, the injury may be reversible if the patient is transported quickly to an emergency facility capable of treating CNS injuries. A unilaterally dilated pupil that remains reactive to light may be the earliest sign of increasing intracranial pressure. The patient who presents with or develops a unilaterally dilated pupil is in the "immediate transport" category. Slight pupillary inequality is normal.

A common method of assessing extraocular movement is to have the patient follow finger movements. The patient is asked to follow the examiner's finger to the extreme left, then up, down, then extreme right, then up, and down. These positions are referred to as the *Cardinal Positions of*

Gaze. Inability to look in all directions with both eyes can indicate CNS problems.

When examining a patient's pupils, it is important to check for contact lenses.

Spinal Evaluation.   The purpose of spinal evaluation is to document loss of sensation and/or motor function. The spinal evaluation does not have to be detailed in the field. Initial assessment of the patient with a possible spinal injury should include the following:

1. Evaluate for pain and tenderness.
2. Observe for bruises.
3. Observe for deformity.
4. Check for motion, sensation, and position (proprioception) in each extremity. The patient should be asked to move the toes and push them against resistance. The paramedic should also check bilateral grip strength.
5. If the patient is unconscious, the paramedic needs to check the response to pain.

If there is a suspected spinal injury, the patient should be placed on a long spine board with the PASG in place since he or she may develop spinal shock. A patient with a spinal injury is likely to vomit. Therefore, it must be possible for the patient on the long spine board to be rolled to the side to prevent aspiration of vomitus.

PATHOPHYSIOLOGY AND MANAGEMENT OF CENTRAL NERVOUS SYSTEM EMERGENCIES

■ **coma** a state of unconsciousness from which the patient cannot be aroused.

Stupor and Coma.   The pathological depressions of consciousness are stupor and coma. *Stupor* is a partial or nearly complete unconsciousness or reduced responsiveness. **Coma,** whatever its cause, is an abnormally deep state of unconsciousness from which the patient cannot be aroused, even by powerful external stimuli. There are generally only two mechanisms capable of producing stupor or coma:

1. structural lesions that depress consciousness by destroying or encroaching upon the substance of the brain
2. toxic-metabolic states, involving either the presence of circulating toxins or metabolites, or the lack of metabolic substrates (oxygen, glucose, or thiamine); these states produce diffuse depression of both cerebral hemispheres, with or without depression within the brainstem.

Within the two general mechanisms, there are many difficult-to-classify causes of stupor or comma. Some of the more common causes are listed in the six following general categories:

Structural: Trauma
Brain tumor
Epilepsy
Intracranial hemorrhage
Other space-occupying lesions

Metabolic:	Anoxia
	Hypoglycemia
	Diabetic ketoacidosis
	Hepatic failure
	Renal failure
	Thiamine deficiency
Drugs:	Barbiturates
	Narcotics
	Hallucinogens
	Depressants (including alcohol)
Cardiovascular:	Hypertensive encephalopathy
	Shock
	Anaphylaxis
	Dysrhythmias
	Cardiac arrest
	CVA
Respiratory:	COPD
	Inhalation of toxic gas
Infectious:	Meningitis
	Encephalitis
	AIDS Encephalitis

When evaluating a patient, many paramedics find mnemonic devices useful as assessment aids. A mnemonic that may be helpful for some common causes of coma is "AEIOUTIPS."

A = Acidosis, alcohol

E = Epilepsy

I = Infection

O = Overdose

U = Uremia (kidney failure)

T = Trauma

I = Insulin (hypoglycemia or diabetes ketoacidosis)

P = Psychosis

S = Stroke

An initial assessment must be made as to the severity and cause of the CNS disorder. Of primary importance is the patient's breathing and cardiovascular status. Information should be gathered simultaneously from the patient's relatives, friends, or bystanders. Data on the patient's past history is especially valuable, including whether he or she is a diabetic, drug or alcohol user, or if there was a fall or head trauma involved. The history should include any medications used by the patient and information on previous episodes of a similar nature. The patient should be checked for a Medic-Alert identification. Clues about the mechanism of the problem may be obtained by quickly surveying the environment.

Initial evaluation of the patient should include:

❑ breathing
❑ response to stimuli
❑ eye response
❑ pupil response

Further examination of the patient may explain why he or she is comatose. Questions to be asked include:

✱ The primary concern in any CNS emergency is always the airway, breathing, circulation, and C-spine control.

- ❏ Is the patient jaundiced?
- ❏ Is there respiratory failure?
- ❏ Is there an odor on the patient's breath consistent with alcohol or ketones?
- ❏ Are there medications nearby such as sedatives or insulin?
- ❏ Are there needle tracks on the patient's limbs suggesting possible drug abuse?

While performing an assessment on the patient presenting with a CNS problem, particular focus should be on the following:

Pupillary Reflexes. Constriction of the pupils is controlled by parasympathetic fibers. These originate in the midbrain and accompany the oculomotor nerve. Dilatation of the pupils involves fibers that descend the entire brainstem and ascend in the cervical sympathetic chains. Failure in the midbrain interrupts both pathways, usually resulting in fixed, midsized pupils. Lesions within the pons can interfere with sympathetic tone alone, producing pinpoint pupils barely reactive to light. Third-nerve compression interrupts parasympathetic tone. This is shown by a unilateral fixed and dilated pupil. Fixed or asymmetric pupils tend to strongly imply structural lesions. In contrast, reactive pupils generally indicate toxic-metabolic states.

Extraocular Movements. Dysconjugate gaze at rest usually implies the patient has received a structural brainstem injury.

Motor Findings. Motor responses to noxious stimuli are markers of the level and asymmetry of brain dysfunction. Asymmetry generally implies structural lesions. Appropriate responses by the patient which localize or withdraw from pain indicate normal or minimally impaired cortical function. Decorticate and decerebrate posturing are ominous signs of deep cerebral hemispheric or upper brainstem injury. Flaccid paralysis usually indicates spinal injury.

Respiratory Patterns. Respiratory patterns can be confusing and are not as clinically useful as pupillary reactivity, extraocular movements, and motor responses. For example, Kussmaul respirations are virtually indistinguishable from central neurogenic hyperventilation. Kussmaul respirations are commonly seen with deep bilateral dysfunction of the cerebral hemispheres. In contrast, central neurogenic hyperventilation results from dysfunction at a level anywhere from the forebrain to the upper pons. Apnea places the CNS dysfunction in the medulla.

Assessment. Assessment of the patient suffering stupor or coma should include the following:

1. *Obtain history.*
2. *Observe the environment.*
3. *Obtain information from bystanders, family, friends.*
   Ask specific questions such as:
   - ❏ What is the length of the coma?
   - ❏ Was it of sudden or gradual onset?
   - ❏ Is there a history of recent head trauma within the last four weeks?
   - ❏ Is the patient under medical care?
   - ❏ Is there any alcohol or drug use or abuse?
   - ❏ Were there any preceding symptoms or complaints?
   - ❏ What medications is the patient taking?
   - ❏ Is there Medic-Alert identification?

4. *Physical examination:* the physical examination should consist of primary and secondary assessment:

- ❏ *Primary Assessment.* During the primary assessment the paramedic should pay special attention to the cervical spine and airway. Next, a complete neurological evaluation should be carried out.
- ❏ *Secondary Assessment.* The secondary assessment should begin with determination of the vital signs. Observe for:

> Hypertension
> Bradycardia
> Abnormal respiratory patterns
> Elevation or depression of body temperature
> Ketone breath
> Tongue trauma (indicating seizure activity)
> Cyanosis
> Alcohol breath
> Neck rigidity
> Flaccid extremities on one side
> Posturing
> Needle tracks
> Jaundice
> Head trauma

Management. The initial priority is to ascertain if the patient has an immobilized cervical spine (in cases of suspected head/neck injury). Following this, his or her airway should be secured. If the patient is breathing inadequately, then respirations should be supported. A comatose patient requires an appropriate airway adjunct.

After the airway is secured, management should include the following:

1. Draw blood and use reagent strip for blood glucose determination. A serum glucose determination tells if the coma is due to hypoglycemia.

2. Establish an IV of D5W at a keep open rate. If shock is present, an IV of lactated Ringer's should be established.

3. Monitor cardiac rhythm.

4. Administer 50% dextrose. This will correct hypoglycemia, which may be the cause of the coma. Even if the patient is an uncontrolled diabetic, hyperglycemia produced by administration of glucose will not do any harm. If, however, the patient is hypoglycemic from too much insulin, the administration of glucose can be life-saving and he or she may immediately respond. For the alcoholic patient who is hypoglycemic, the glucose may be lifesaving as well. The field dosage for 50% dextrose is (see Table 23-1):

    Adult: 50 mL (25 gm) IVP. May be repeated as necessary.

    Pediatric: 0.5 to 1.0 gm/kg IVP Dilute D-50-W 1:1 with sterile water to yield a 25% (D-25-W) solution.

5. Administer naloxone (see Table 23-2) in the patient suspected of having a narcotic overdose. Naloxone, a narcotic antagonist, has proven effective in the management and reversal of overdose caused by narcotics or synthetic narcotic agents. Recent studies have shown that naloxone may also help reverse coma associated with alcohol ingestion. Field dosage for naloxone is:

    Adult: 1–2 mg IV, ET, IM, or SQ. This may be repeated at 2–3-minute intervals for 2–3 doses if no response is noted. Darvon overdoses may require larger doses of naloxone.

    Pediatric: 0.01 mg/kg/dose. Maximum dose = 0.8 mg IV or ET. If no response in 10 minutes, 2 mg should be given

6. Thiamine (vitamin B1) should be administered to the suspected alcoholic patient. (See Table 23-3.) It is required for the conversion of pyruvic acid to acetyl-coenzyme-A. Without this step a significant amount of energy available in glucose cannot be obtained. The brain is extremely sensitive to thiamine deficiency.

✳ In coma of unknown cause always consider the administration of thiamine, 50% dextrose, and naloxone.

TABLE 23-1   50% Dextrose

Class:	Carbohydrate
Actions:	Elevates blood glucose level rapidly
Indications:	Hypoglycemia
	Coma of unknown origin
Contraindications:	None in the emergency setting
Precautions:	Dextrostix must be performed and blood sample drawn before administration
Side Effects:	Local venous irritation
Dosage:	25 grams (50 ml)
Route:	IV
Pediatric Dosage:	0.5–1 gm/kg slow IV

TABLE 23-2   Naloxone (Narcan®)

Class:	Narcotic antagonist
Action:	Reverses effects of narcotics
Indications:	Narcotic overdoses including:
	morphine Demerol® heroin
	Dilaudid® Paregoric Percodan®
	fentanyl methadone
	Synthetic analgesic overdoses including:
	Nubain® Talwin®
	Stadol® Darvon®
	Alcoholic coma
	To rule out narcotics in coma of unknown origin
Contraindication:	Patients with a history of hypersensitivity to the drug
Precautions:	Should be administered with caution to patients dependent on narcotics as it may cause withdrawal effects
	Short-acting, should be augmented every 5 minutes
Side Effects:	None
Dosage:	1–2 mg up to a total dose of 10 mg (larger doses may be required to reverse effects of Darvon®)
Routes:	IV
	IM
Pediatric Dosage:	0.005 mg/kg

■ **Wernicke's syndrome** condition characterized by loss of memory and disorientation, associated with chronic alcohol intake and a diet deficient in thiamine.

■ **Korsakoff's syndrome** psychosis characterized by disorientation, muttering delirium, insomnia, delusions, and hallucinations. Symptoms include painful extremities, bilateral wrist drop (rarely), bilateral foot drop (frequently), and pain on pressure over the long nerves.

Chronic alcoholism interferes with the absorption, intake, and use of thiamine. A significant percentage of alcoholics have thiamine deficiency which can cause Wernicke's syndrome or Korsakoff's psychosis. **Wernicke's syndrome** is an acute and reversible encephalopathy characterized by ataxia, eye muscle weakness, and mental derangement. Of even greater concern is Korsakoff's psychosis, characterized by memory disorder. Once established, **Korsakoff's psychosis** may be irreversible. Therefore, comatose patients, especially those who are suspected alcoholics, should receive intravenous thiamine as well as 50% dextrose and naloxone. The field dosage of thiamine is 100 mg IV push. When an IV cannot be started, thiamine can be given IM.

TABLE 23-3   Thiamine (Vitamin BI)

Class:	Vitamin
Action:	Allows normal breakdown of glucose
Indications:	Coma of unknown origin (especially if alcohol or malnourishment may be involved)
	Delirium tremens
Contraindications:	None
Precaution:	Occasional anaphylactic reactions have been reported
Side Effects:	Rare, if any
Dosage:	100 mg
Route:	IV
Pediatric Dosage:	Rarely used

✱ Always consider the administration of thiamine in the alchoholic patient.

If an increase in intracranial pressure is likely, as occurs in a closed head injury, many physicians may request administration of a steroid. The most commonly used steroid is dexamethasone (Decadron) (see Table 23-4) which may help reduce cerebral edema. Many systems also use the osmotic diuretic mannitol (Osmotrol). Mannitol causes diuresis, eliminating fluid from the intravascular space through the kidneys. Many authorities feel that its oncotic effect also causes a fluid shift from the substance of the brain to the circulation, thus reducing brain edema. Paramedics are encouraged to follow local protocols for these medications.

Seizures.   A **seizure** is a temporary alteration in behavior due to the massive electrical discharge of one or more groups of neurons in the brain. Seizures can be clinically classified as generalized or partial. *Generalized seizures* include grand mal and petit mal. *Partial seizures* may be either simple or complex (psychomotor) and may remain confined to a limited portion of the brain or spread, thereby becoming generalized.

■ **seizure** a disorder of the nervous system due to a sudden, excessive, disorderly discharge of brain neurons.

■ **convulsion** a sudden, violent, uncontrollable contraction of a group of muscles.

TABLE 23-4   Dexamethasone (Decadron®, Hexadrol®)

Class:	Steroid
Actions:	Decreases cerebral edema
	Anti-inflammatory
	Suppresses immune response (especially in allergic/anaphylactic reactions)
Indications:	Cerebral edema
	Possibly effective as an adjunctive agent in the management of shock
Contraindications:	None in the emergency setting
Precautions:	Should be protected from heat
	Onset of action may be 2–6 hours and thus should not be considered to be of use in the critical first hour following an anaphylactic reaction
Side Effects:	GI bleeding
	Prolonged wound healing
Dosage:	4–24 mg
Route:	IV
Pediatric Dosage:	1 mg/kg

Seizures may occur in any individual when placed under the "right" stress, such as hypoxia, sudden elevation of temperature, or a rapid lowering of blood sugar. Seizures also are caused by structural diseases of the brain such as tumors, head trauma, eclampsia, and vascular disorders. The most common cause is due to *idiopathic epilepsy*. The terms epilepsy or epileptic indicate nothing more than the potential to develop seizures in circumstances that would not induce them in most individuals.

Major Seizure Types

■ **grand mal** form of seizure characterized by tonic-clonic muscle contractions. It may occur with or without coma.

Grand Mal. A **grand mal** seizure is a generalized major motor seizure, producing a loss of consciousness. The grand mal seizure also causes alternating **tonic** (contractions) and **clonic** (successive contractions and relaxations) movements of the extremities, beyond the patient's control. During the seizure episode, his or her intercostal muscles and diaphragm become temporarily paralyzed, interrupting respirations and producing cyanosis. The patient's neck, head, and face muscles may also jerk. Once respirations resume, there will be copious amounts of oral secretions (frothing). Incontinence and mental confusion is also common during the seizure episode, followed by coma or drowsiness.

■ **tonic phase** phase of a seizure characterized by tension or contraction of muscles.

■ **clonic** alternating contraction and relaxation of muscles.

Focal Motor. Focal motor seizures are characterized by dysfunction of one area of the body. When there is electrical discharge from a small portion of the brain, only those functions served by that area will have dysfunction. Focal seizures begin as localized tonic/clonic movements. They frequently spread and appear as generalized major motor seizures. It is crucial that the paramedic document how such seizures begin and the course they take.

■ **psychomotor** mental processes causing or associated with physical activity.

Psychomotor. **Psychomotor** seizures, occasionally called temporal lobe seizures, are characterized by distinctive auras. They include unusual smells, tastes, sounds, or the tendency of objects to look very large and near, small and distant, or scenes to appear, that seem familiar (*deja vu*) or strange. A metallic taste in the mouth is a common psychomotor seizure aura. These are focal seizures, lasting approximately 1–2 minutes. The patient experiences a loss of contact with his or her surroundings. Additionally, the patient may be confused, may stagger, perform purposeless movement, and make unintelligible sounds. He or she may not understand what is said, and may even refuse medical aid. Some may develop automatic behavior, or show a sudden change in personality, or abruptly begin to rage.

■ **petit mal seizure** form of seizure where consciousness may or may not be lost.

Petit Mal. **Petit mal** seizures are brief, generalized seizures which usually present with a 10 to 30-second loss of consciousness, eye or muscle fluttering, and occasionally, with loss of muscle tone. Unconsciousness may be so brief that the patient or observers may be unaware of the episode. Petit mal seizures are an idiopathic disorder of early childhood and rarely begin after age twenty. They may not respond to normal treatment modalities.

Hysterical. Hysterical seizures stem from psychological disorders. The patient presents with sharp and bizarre movements which curt commands often can interrupt. The seizure is usually witnessed and there will not be a postictal period. Very rarely do patients experiencing an hysterical seizure injure themselves. Aromatic ammonia may help differentiate an hysterical from a true seizure.

Progression of a Grand Mal Seizure. Grand mal seizures have a specific progression of events. It is descriptively convenient to refer to this progression as ranging from warning phase to period of recovery.

1. *Aura.* An aura is a subjective sensation preceding seizure activity. The aura may precede the attack by several hours or only by a few seconds. An aura may be of a psychic or a sensory nature, with olfactory, visual, auditory, or taste hallucinations. Some common types include hearing noise or music, seeing floating lights, smelling unpleasant odors, feeling an unpleasant sensation in the stomach, or experiencing tingling or twitching in a given body area. Not all seizures are preceded by an aura.

2. *Loss of consciousness.* The patient will become unconsciousness after the aura sensations.

3. *Tonic phase.* This is a phase of continuous motor tension, characterized by tension and contraction of the patient's muscles.

4. **Hypertonic phase.** The patient experiences extreme muscular rigidity including hyperextension of the back.

5. *Clonic phase.* The patient experiences muscle spasms marked by muscular rigidity and then relaxation.

6. *Post-seizure.* The patient progresses into a coma.

7. *Postictal.* The patient will awaken confused, fatigued, may complain of a headache, and experience some neurological deficit.

■ **hypertonic phase** phase of a seizure when muscles are in a state of greater than normal tension or of incomplete relaxation.

Assessment. The paramedic's initial contact with the patient and bystanders offers a unique opportunity to obtain a history which may influence management. What was called a seizure may be a simple fainting spell. Therefore, exactly what was observed is of key importance.

Many other problems can suggest that a seizure has occurred. For example, migraine headaches, cardiac dysrhythmias, hypoglycemia after exercise or drug ingestion, and the tendency to faint due to orthostatic hypotension may mimic seizure activity. Stiffness of the extremities can be caused by hyperventilation, meningitis or intracranial hemorrhage, certain tranquilizers, and decerebrate movements associated with increased intracranial pressure. If it is unclear whether the patient has had a seizure, administration of an anticonvulsant medication may be more harmful than beneficial. When obtaining a history, the paramedic should remember to include the following:

❑ History of seizures. This should include length of the seizure, if it was generalized or focal, if there were any aura, incontinence, or trauma to the tongue.
❑ Recent history of head trauma.
❑ Any alcohol and/or drug abuse.
❑ Recent history of fever, headache, or stiff neck.
❑ History of diabetes, heart disease, or CVA.

It is also important to try to distinguish between syncope and true seizure. **Syncope** is caused by insufficient blood flow to the brain, resulting from ineffective cardiac activity, relaxation of peripheral blood vessels, or insufficient blood volume. The most common cause of fainting is vasovagal syncope associated with fatigue, emotional stress, or cardiac disease.

■ **syncope** transient loss of consciousness due to inadequate flow of blood to the brain; fainting.

The physical examination of the seizure patient should include the following:

❑ Note any signs of head trauma or injury to the tongue.
❑ Note any evidence of alcohol and/or drug abuse.
❑ Document dysrhythmias.

Differentiation between Syncope and Seizure

Syncope	Seizure
Usually begins in a standing position. Patient will usually remember a warning or fainting.	May begin in any position. Begins without warning.
Patient regains consciousness almost immediately on becoming supine.	Results in jerking during unconsciousness.
Patient initially has a slow, weak pulse, and is clammy and pale.	Often preceded by an aura.

Management. Seizures have a tendency to provoke anxiety in patients, families, and paramedics. However, from a medical standpoint most of these situations only require nasal oxygen and turning the patient to the side to prevent aspiration. Because the patient may become hypo- or hyperthermic if exposed, protecting body temperature is also crucial. Field management of the seizure patient generally includes the following:

❋ Airway maintenance, administration of supplemental oxygen, and protection of the patient from injury are the principle treatments for an uncomplicated seizure.

- ❑ Airway maintenance. Objects should not be forced between the patient's teeth—this includes padded tongue blades. Pushing objects into the patient's mouth may cause him or her to vomit, or aspirate. It can also cause laryngospasm.
- ❑ Administer oxygen.
- ❑ Never attempt to restrain the patient. This may injure him or her. The patient should, however, be protected from hitting objects in the environment.
- ❑ Maintain body temperature.
- ❑ Position the patient on his or her side after the clonic-tonic phase.
- ❑ Suction if appropriate.
- ❑ Monitor cardiac rhythm.
- ❑ Provide a quiet, reassuring atmosphere.
- ❑ Transport the patient in the supine or lateral recumbent position.

■ **status epilepticus** act of having two or more successive seizures without intervening periods of consciousness.

❋ Status epilepticus can be life-threatening.

Status Epilepticus. **Status epilepticus** is a series of two or more generalized motor seizures without an intervening return of consciousness. The most common cause in adults is failure to take prescribed anticonvulsant medications. Status epilepticus is a major emergency since it involves a prolonged period of hypoxia of vital brain tissues. These seizures may result in respiratory arrest, extreme hypertension, increased intracranial pressure, serious elevations in body temperature, fractures of the long bones and spine, necrosis of the cardiac muscle, and severe dehydration.

The most valuable intervention is to protect the patient from airway obstruction and deliver 100% oxygen at high-flow rates. This should preferably be accomplished by bag-valve-mask assistance, since the normal ventilatory mechanisms of the patient are seriously impaired and air exchange is generally ineffective. Once the airway is maintained and ventilations are being assisted, patient management should continue as follows:

1. Begin an IV of D5W at a TKO rate.
2. Monitor cardiac rhythm.
3. Administer 25 gms of 50% dextrose IV push.
4. Administer diazepam IV push. (See Table 23-5.) Diazepam is a sedative and anticonvulsant that depresses the spread of seizure activity across the motor cortex of the brain. It also acts as a skeletal muscle relaxant. The dosage for diazepam in the field is:

TABLE 23-5   Diazepam (Valium®)

Class:	Tranquilizer
Actions:	Anticonvulsant Skeletal muscle relaxant Sedative
Indications:	Major motor seizures Status epilepticus Premedication prior to cardioversion Skeletal muscle relaxant Acute anxiety states
Contraindications:	Patients with a history of hypersensitivity to the drug
Precautions:	Can cause local venous irritation Has short duration of effect Do not mix with other drugs because of possible precipitation problems
Side Effects:	Drowsiness Hypotension Respiratory depression
Dosage:	Status epilepticus: 5–10 mg IV Acute anxiety: 2–5 mg IM or IV Premedication prior to cardioversion: 5–15 mg IV
Routes:	IV (care must be taken not to administer faster than 1 milliliter/minute) IM
Pediatric Dosage:	Status epilepticus. 0.5–2.0 mg

Adult: 5–10 mg IV push.

Pediatric (infants 30 days to children 5 years): 0.2–0.5 mg IV push every 2-5 minutes to a maximum of 2.5 mg.

Pediatric (children > 5 years): 1.0 mg IV push every 2–5 minutes to a maximum of 5.0 mg.

Stroke (Cerebrovascular Accident).   CVA, or stroke, is a general term that describes injury or death of brain tissue usually due to interruption of cerebral blood flow from either ischemic or hemorrhagic lesions. These lesions are commonly secondary to atherosclerotic disease, hypertension, or both. The patient tends to experience a sudden loss of consciousness followed by paralysis. (See Figure 23-9.) This may be caused by hemorrhage into the brain tissue, an embolus in the cerebral blood vessels, or thrombus formation which occludes arterial supply to the brain. Additionally, a rupture of an artery causing hemorrhage, usually in the subarachnoid space, can cause stroke.

Strokes are the third most common cause of death and, in the middle-aged and older patient, are a frequent cause of disability. They can be divided into the following two broad categories:

1. *Infarction.* An infarction occurs when the blood supply to a limited portion of the brain is inadequate and death of nervous tissue follows. Infarction may be caused by an embolism or by blood vessel occlusion due to atherosclerosis (thrombus). Emboli are usually small clots arising from diseased blood vessels in the neck (carotid) or from clots originating in the heart. Atrial fibrillation often causes atrial dilation, a precursor to the formation of clots. Other types of emboli that may cause occlusion in cerebral blood vessels are air, tumor tissue, and fat.

■ **CVA (cerebrovascular accident)** caused by either ischemic or hemorrhagic lesions to a portion of the brain, resulting in damage or destruction of brain tissue. CVA is commonly referred to as "stroke."

✱ Thrombotic strokes often occur during sleep or are present when the patient arises in the morning. A warning is common to thrombotic strokes.

✱ Embolic strokes usually occur during waking hours, and often occur without warning.

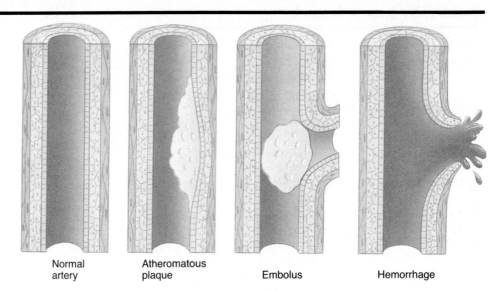

FIGURE 23-9 Etiologies of stroke.

Normal artery   Atheromatous plaque   Embolus   Hemorrhage

✳ Intracerebral hemorrhage usually occurs during waking hours and may develop slowly, over minutes to hours.

2. *Hemorrhages.* Hemorrhages are usually categorized as being either intra-cerebral or subarachnoid. (See Figure 23-10.) Onset is usually sudden and marked by a severe headache and stiff neck. Most intracranial hemorrhages occur in the hypertensive patient when a small vessel deep within the brain tissue ruptures. Subarachnoid hemorrhages most often result from congeni-tal blood vessel abnormalities or are caused by head trauma. The congenital abnormalities are known as aneurysms (weakened vessels) and arteriov-enous malformations (collections of abnormal blood vessels). Aneurysms tend to be on the surface and may hemorrhage into the brain tissue or the subarachnoid space. Arteriovenous malformations may be within the brain, subarachnoid space, or both.

Hemorrhage inside the brain often tears and separates normal brain tissue. The release of blood into the spinal fluid-containing cavities within the brain may paralyze vital centers. If blood in the subarachnoid space impairs drainage of cerebrospinal fluid, it may cause a rise in the intracranial pressure. Herniation (protrusion) of brain tissue through a narrow opening in the skull may then occur.

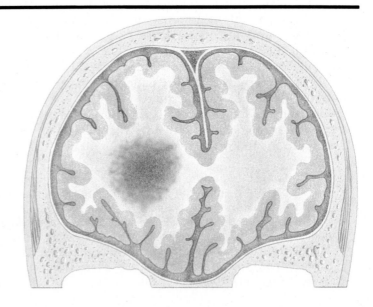

FIGURE 23-10 Intracerebral hemorrhage.

In infarction, the tissue that has died will swell causing further damage to nearby tissue that only has a marginal blood supply. If swelling is severe, herniation may result.

Clinical Presentation. Symptoms of the patient who has experienced a stroke will depend on the area of the brain damaged. Those areas commonly affected are the motor, speech, and sensory centers. The onset of symptoms will be acute, and the patient may experience unconsciousness. There may be stertorous breathing (laborious breathing accompanied by snoring) due to paralysis of a portion of the soft palate. Respiratory expiration may be puffs of air out of the cheeks and mouth. The patient's pupils may be unequal, with the larger pupil on the side of the hemorrhage. Paralysis will usually involve one side of the face, one arm, and one leg. The eyes often will be turned away from the side of the body paralysis. The patient's skin may be cool and clammy. Speech disturbances also may be noted.

Predisposing factors possibly contributing to the stroke are hypertension, diabetes, abnormal blood lipid levels, oral contraceptives, sickle cell disease, and some cardiac dysrhythmias.

Transient Ischemic Attacks (TIAs). Some patients may have small emboli that cause transient strokelike symptoms known as **TIAs,** or **transient ischemic attacks.** These emboli temporarily interfere with the blood supply to the brain, producing symptoms of neurological deficit. These symptoms may last for only a few minutes or several hours. After the attack the patient will show no evidence of residual brain or neurological damage. The patient who experiences a TIA may, however, be a candidate for an eventual CVA.

■ **TIA (transient ischemic attack)** temporary interruption of blood supply to the brain.

The onset of a transient ischemic attack is usually abrupt with the patient experiencing giddiness or a light-headed sensation. The specific signs and symptoms depend on the area of the brain affected. Any one or a combination of the following may be present:

❑ monocular blindness (blindness in one eye)
❑ hemiplegia (paralysis on one side)
❑ inability to recognize by touch
❑ staggering
❑ difficulty in swallowing
❑ hemiparesis (weakness on one side)
❑ aphasia (inability to speak)
❑ dizziness
❑ numbness
❑ paresthesia (numbness or tingling)

Probably the most common cause of a TIA is carotid artery disease. Other causes can be decreasing cardiac output, hypotension, overmedication with antihypertensive agents, or cerebrovascular spasm.

While obtaining the history of the patient suspected of sustaining a TIA, the paramedic should pay special attention to the following:

❑ previous neurological symptoms
❑ initial symptoms and their progression
❑ changes in LOC
❑ precipitating factors
❑ dizziness
❑ palpitations

❑ history of:
    hypertension
    cardiac disease
    sickle cell disease
    previous TIA or CVA

During the physical examination, attention should focus on the following:

❑ neurologic exam—note hemiparesis or hemiplegia
❑ speech disturbances including dysarthria (impairment of the tongue and
❑ muscles essential to speech), motor and receptive aphasia
❑ confusion and agitation
❑ gait disturbances or uncoordinated fine motor movements
❑ vision problems
❑ inappropriate behavior with excessive laughing or crying
❑ coma

✱ The prehospital
management of stroke and TIA is
primarily supportive.

Management of CVA and TIA.   Because of impaired blood flow to the patient's brain, he or she should be kept supine with the head elevated approximately 15 degrees. This allows for adequate venous drainage. If the patient has congestive heart failure, he or she should be maintained in a semiupright position.

Other important points during management of the CVA or TIA patient include the following:

❑ Assure patient safety.
❑ Establish and maintain cervical spine support if trauma is suspected.
❑ Establish and maintain an adequate airway. Suction equipment should be readily available.
❑ Administer oxygen and assist ventilation when required. If the patient's airway is adequate and air exchange is present, oxygen flow rates of 6 l/min. via face mask or nasal cannula are appropriate.
❑ Hyperventilate if unresponsive.
❑ Draw blood sample for glucose determination.
❑ Start an IV of D5W at a TKO rate.
❑ Monitor cardiac rhythm.
❑ If it appears that hypoglycemia may be a factor, the physician may order 25 gm of 50% dextrose.
❑ Protect paralyzed extremities.
❑ Give the patient reassurance—all procedures should be explained to him or her. The patient may be unable to speak, but may be able to hear.
❑ Transport without excessive movement or noise. Otherwise, the patient may feel nauseated and vomit.

SUMMARY

Nervous system emergencies include a complex variety of injuries and illnesses. The paramedic's assessment and neurologic checks are invaluable for subsequent hospital management. Initial field management is directed at ensuring an adequate airway and ventilation. The brain requires a constant supply of oxygen, glucose, and vitamins. After 10–20 seconds without blood flow, the patient becomes unconscious. Significant loss of oxygen (anoxia) or low blood sugar (hypoglycemia) can cause coma or seizures. In patients with brain disorders, adequate blood, glucose, and oxygen supplies must be ensured.

CNS injuries need treatment as soon as possible to prevent progressive damage. Signs of central nervous system compromise include headache, dizziness, fainting, vomiting, partial to full loss of consciousness, personality, pupillary, and respiratory changes, loss of motor function, and altered response to pain. Elevated blood pressure, bradycardia, and convulsions may also occur.

Treatment of CNS injuries includes: airway maintenance, support of the neck and spine, control of hemorrhage, careful neurologic exam, care for any other injuries, and transport to the appropriate emergency facility.

FURTHER READING

LANGFITT, D.E., *Critical Care: Certification Preparation and Review.* Bowie, MD: Robert J. Brady Company, 1984.

LANROS, N.E., *Assessment and Intervention in Emergency Nursing* (3rd ed.). Norwalk, CT: Appleton and Lange, 1988.

TINTINALLI, J.E., KROME, R.L., and RUIZ, E., *Emergency Medicine: A Comprehensive Study Guide* (2nd ed.). New York, NY: McGraw-Hill Book Company, 1988.

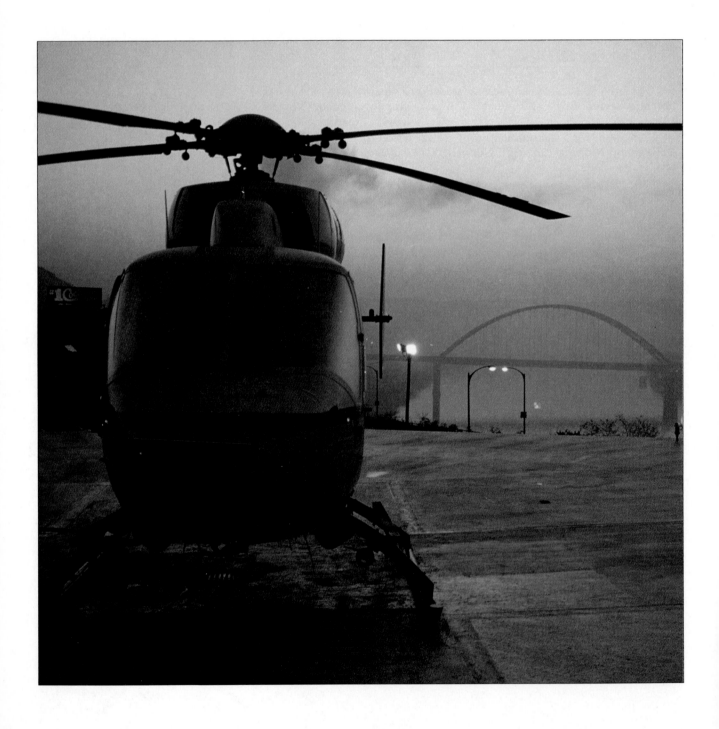

24

The Acute Abdomen

Objectives for Chapter 24

Upon completing this chapter, the student should be able to:

1. Discuss the topographical anatomy of the abdomen and describe which organs lie within each quadrant.

2. Describe the organs of the gastrointestinal system.

3. Describe the organs of the genitourinary system.

4. Describe the organs of the male and the female reproductive systems.

5. Describe two borders of the abdominal cavity.

6. Name the two major blood vessels found within the abdominal cavity.

7. Discuss the nonhemorrhagic causes of acute abdominal pain.

8. Discuss the hemorrhagic causes of acute abdominal pain.

9. Describe the signs and symptoms of upper and lower gastrointestinal hemorrhage.

10. Discuss the field management of acute abdominal pain.

11. Discuss the general causes of genitourinary disorders.

12. Discuss pathophysiology, causes, and complications of the following:
   - Acute renal failure
   - Urinary stones
   - Chronic renal failure
   - Urinary tract infection

13. Discuss the general assessment and management of genitourinary problems.

14. Discuss hemodialysis.

15. Discuss assessment, management and complications of the dialysis patient.

16. Discuss the management of the following:
   - Epididymitis
   - Testicular torsion
   - Pelvic inflammatory disease
   - Ectopic pregnancy

CASE STUDY

Steve Fletcher, EMT-P, was at home watching Sunday afternoon baseball. When Steve awoke earlier, he "just wasn't feeling right." Nevertheless, he completed his planned activities for the morning. But shortly after noon Steve began to detect a vague abdominal pain around the navel. He initially attributed it to the beer and nachos he had consumed the evening before with some fellow paramedics. As Steve watched the game, the pain worsened. Although he hadn't eaten all day, he found himself running to the bathroom to vomit. After throwing up twice, Steve began to feel feverish. He noticed that the pain was moving toward the lower right abdominal quadrant. He sat on the couch, leaning forward, and thought about what could be wrong. The idea that he might be having acute appendicitis suddenly hit him. "No," he reassured himself, "I'm not that sick." But, as he continued to watch the game, Steve became increasingly ill. Finally, he called the EMS station to see if anybody else who had been out with him was sick. Steve described his symptoms to Glen, one of his fellow paramedics. Glen said, "Hey buddy, you've got appendicitis. Don't go anywhere, we'll be right over." Steve lay down on the couch to wait. Soon he heard a siren. "Surely they didn't respond code 3," he said to himself, as the ambulance, with siren on, arrived. The next minute Glen strode into the room and immediately took charge of the situation, treating Steve like any other patient. In his own ambulance, Steve was transported to the hospital. That afternoon he underwent an appendectomy. After three days in the hospital he returned home. Ten days later he was allowed to return to light duty. And he didn't get an ambulance bill.

INTRODUCTION

■ **acute** having a rapid onset and a short course.

■ **guarding** voluntary or involuntary contraction of the abdominal muscles in response to severe abdominal pain.

Abdominal pain is a frequent complaint and one of the most difficult problems in medicine to diagnose and treat. The paramedic usually will be unable to determine the cause of most abdominal pain in the field. An understanding of medical conditions possibly resulting in the acute abdomen is, nevertheless, essential. The term **acute abdomen** refers to abdominal pain of relatively sudden onset. It is often accompanied by nausea and vomiting, tenderness, **guarding** (voluntary or involuntary contraction of the abdominal muscles in response to severe abdominal pain), rigidity, and, in some cases, shock. Emergency surgical intervention is frequently required.

Most cases of abdominal pain arise from problems within the abdomen itself. However, approximately 10–15% result from pathology elsewhere in the body. Other conditions such as a fracture of the lumbar spine, myocardial infarction, pulmonary embolism, and pneumonia may present with abdominal pain as the primary symptom.

The primary responsibility of the paramedic in dealing with a patient suffering an abdominal emergency consists of detection and stabilization. The patient with an acute abdomen can deteriorate quite rapidly. Therefore, the patient must be constantly reassessed and managed accordingly.

This chapter will discuss pathophysiology, patient assessment, and specific management of conditions that can produce acute abdominal emergencies. Additionally, genitourinary disorders, complications associated with hemodialysis, and disorders of the reproductive system will be presented as well.

ANATOMY AND PHYSIOLOGY OF THE ABDOMEN

The **abdomen** is the largest body cavity. It is separated from the chest by the diaphragm and from the pelvis by an artificial plane extending through the pelvic inlet. It is bordered posteriorly by the spine and back, and anteriorly by the abdominal wall.

The anterior surface of the abdomen is divided topographically into four divisions, or quadrants. They are delineated by drawing a vertical line from the symphysis pubis to the xiphoid process and a horizontal line through the umbilicus. Each quadrant contains the following organs (see Figure 24-1):

- ❑ *Left Upper:* Spleen, tail of the pancreas, stomach, left kidney, and splenic flexure of the colon.
- ❑ *Right Upper:* Liver, gall bladder, head of the pancreas, part of the duodenum, right kidney, and hepatic flexure of the colon.
- ❑ *Right Lower:* Appendix, ascending colon, small intestine, and the right ovary and fallopian tube.
- ❑ *Left Lower:* Small intestine, descending colon, left ovary, and fallopian tube.

The lateral portion of the abdomen, often referred to as the *flank,* is associated with the kidneys. Immediately inferior to the xiphoid process is the **epigastrium.** A common location of abdominal pain, the epigastrium is frequently associated with peptic ulcer disease and esophagitis.

The abdomen is lined with a membrane called the **peritoneum.** Most organs are located within the peritoneum. Some, however, are located behind it and are referred to as being *retroperitoneal.* These include the kid-

■ **abdomen** portion of the body located between the thorax and the pelvis; the superior portion of the abdominopelvic cavity.

■ **epigastrium** portion of the abdomen immediately below the xiphoid process.

■ **peritoneum** serous membrane covering the viscera of the abdomen and lining the interior of the abdominal cavity.

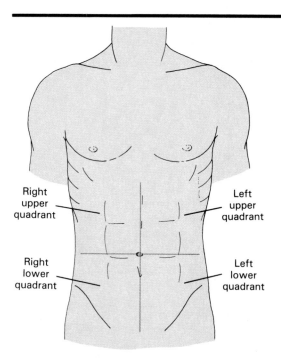

Right upper quadrant

Left upper quadrant

Right lower quadrant

Left lower quadrant

FIGURE 24-1 Topographical anatomy of the abdomen.

neys and portions of the duodenum. In certain disease states the peritoneum can become inflamed, a condition known as *peritonitis*. Generalized abdominal pain and **rebound tenderness** are characteristic.

Anatomically, the organs of the abdominal cavity can be divided into two categories, solid and hollow:

❏ *Solid Organs*: liver, spleen, pancreas, kidneys, adrenals, and ovaries (in the female)
❏ *Hollow Organs*: stomach, intestines, gall bladder, urinary bladder, and uterus (in the female)

Gastrointestinal System

Most of the organs in the abdomen are part of the gastrointestinal system. The gastrointestinal system is responsible for converting raw food into an energy form the body can use. The gastrointestinal system includes (see Figure 24-2):

❏ *Mouth*: The mouth, or oral cavity, consists of the lips, cheeks, gums, teeth, and tongue. It plays an essential role in digestion, breaking down food into smaller particles. Also, through salivary gland secretions, primarily amylase, digestion is begun.
❏ *Esophagus:* A hollow, muscular tube, the esophagus transports food between the mouth and the stomach.
❏ *Stomach:* The stomach is a hollow organ in the left upper quadrant of the

■ **rebound tenderness** tenderness on release of the examiner's hands, allowing the patient's abdominal wall to return to its normal position. Rebound tenderness is associated with peritoneal irritation.

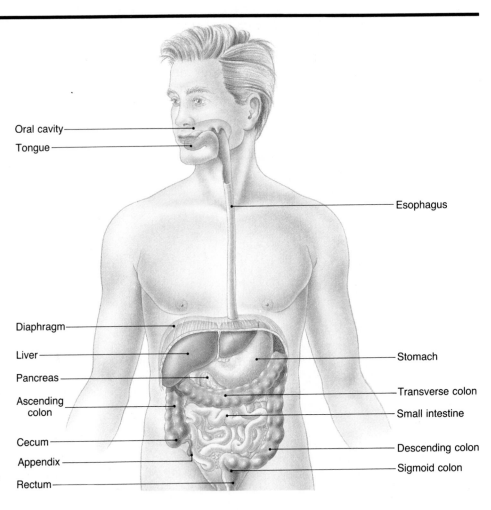

FIGURE 24-2 The gastrointestinal system.

abdomen. After receiving food from the esophagus, it continues the process of digestion. Covered by a mucous membrane to protect itself from the low pH, the stomach secretes hydrochloric acid.

❑ *Intestines:* The intestines are the major sites of digestion and absorption. Partially digested food enters from the stomach and is absorbed, primarily in the small intestine. Waste products are also cleared through this system, which has two major intestinal divisions. The longer division, and more proximal, is the *small intestine,* which receives food from the stomach. The small intestine itself has three anatomical divisions: the *duodenum, jejunum,* and *ileum.* The food leaves the ileum, through the *ileocecal valve,* and enters the large intestine, which is also divided into three sections. The proximal division is called the *cecum.* The middle division is the *colon.* And the terminal division is the *rectum,* connecting to the outside via the anus.

Besides these major organs, a number of accessory organs play a part in digestion. These include:

❑ *Salivary Glands.* Located in the head, the salivary glands produce saliva to lubricate food passage and amylase to initiate digestion.

❑ *Teeth.* The teeth play a major role in processing food into a form usable by the digestive system.

❑ *Liver.* Located in the right, upper quadrant, the liver is the largest organ in the body. It secretes bile which is necessary for the digestion of fats. Additionally, the liver produces essential proteins, detoxifies many substances, and stores glucose, in the form of glycogen, for immediate use.

❑ *Pancreas.* The pancreas lies in both the right and left upper abdominal quadrants. It secretes several digestive enzymes. The pancreas also has endocrine function, secreting glucagon, insulin, and somatostatin.

❑ *Appendix.* The appendix is a hollow, fingerlike structure attached to the cecal area of the large intestine. Virtually without any function, it is probably a remnant from an earlier stage of evolutionary development.

Vascular Supply

Major blood vessels travel through the abdomen. The descending *aorta* is the largest artery in the abdomen and supplies blood to all of the abdominal viscera. The superior mesenteric and inferior mesenteric arteries supply blood to most of the intestines. The aorta divides into the iliac arteries to supply the lower extremities. The *inferior vena cava,* the largest vein in the abdomen, drains the lower extremities and certain abdominal viscera. The **portal system** is a specialized circulatory system within the abdomen. This system drains blood from parts of the intestines and transports it to the liver where it is filtered and processed.

■ **portal system** circulatory system that collects blood from parts of the abdominal viscera and transports it to the liver.

ABDOMINAL PATHOPHYSIOLOGY

The "acute abdomen" refers to the relatively sudden onset of abdominal pain. It is often associated with other signs and symptoms such as nausea, vomiting, guarding, and rebound tenderness. Many conditions producing the acute abdomen are potentially fatal unless treated promptly by surgery. Therefore, it is essential to assess the severity of the patient's complaints. Every patient with abdominal pain should be transported to the emergency department for evaluation by a physician.

Abdominal emergencies can be divided into *nonhemorrhagic* and *hemorrhagic* causes. Nonhemorrhagic causes result from inflammation or infection and may include the following:

Disease Processes Related to Nonhemorrhagic Abdominal Emergencies

Peptic Ulcer Disease. Peptic ulcer disease is caused by ulcers (erosions) in the lining of the esophagus, stomach, or duodenum. It often results from excess secretion of hydrochloric acid from glands in the lining of the stomach. The breakdown of the protective mucous lining of these organs by drugs, alcohol, and other agents is another cause. Aspirin and the non-steroidal anti-inflammatory class of drugs (Motrin, Advil, Naprosyn) are common offending agents. Abdominal pain associated with peptic ulcer disease is usually located in the epigastrium or the left upper quadrant. It is often improved following meals or following usage of antacids such as Maalox, Mylanta, or Riopan. Severe ulceration can cause significant gastrointestinal bleeding. The ulcer can sometimes erode through the wall of the organ, resulting in an acute abdomen.

Appendicitis. Appendicitis is the inflammation of the vermiform appendix. A piece of hard stool (fecalith) or a similar substance will occasionally obstruct the **lumen** of the appendix. This can result in inflammation of the appendix itself. Often, however, no identifiable cause can be found. The patient suffering appendicitis will usually complain of right, lower quadrant abdominal pain. The onset of the pain is usually acute, often beginning in the area around the umbilicus. As the process develops, the pain migrates to the right lower quadrant. Nausea, vomiting, fever, and **anorexia** are common. The peritoneum will generally become inflamed and rebound tenderness will be present. Treatment is surgical removal of the appendix.

Diverticulitis. Diverticuli are pouches which develop, usually with age, on the large intestine, particularly on the descending segment (left side). These diverticuli can become inflamed in much the same manner as the appendix. Most cases of diverticulitis in fact present like a left-sided appendicitis. The patient has abdominal pain, fever, vomiting, anorexia, and tenderness. Treatment includes antibiotics, dietary modifications, and, in certain cases, surgery.

Kidney Stone. A kidney stone is the result of crystal aggregation in the collecting system of the kidney. Sometimes these stones will break loose and enter the ureter. Since their diameter is usually greater than that of the ureter, the passage is quite painful. Some kidney stones will not pass completely through the ureter and will obstruct urine flow from the kidney on the involved side. The kidney stone is one of the most painful conditions known to humans. The pain typically starts acutely as the stone enters the ureter. Initially colicky (intermittent), the pain is either in the back or in the flank. As the stone moves down the ureter, the pain also appears to move down. When the stone approaches the bladder the pain may actually seem as though it is in the testicle (in male patients). Initial therapies for kidney stones are intravenous fluids, which often facilitate stone movement into the bladder, and analgesics. Kidney stones unable to pass remain lodged in the ureter and require surgical removal. Sometimes they can be broken up by sound waves generated through extracorporeal shock wave lithotripsy.

Pelvic Inflammatory Disease (PID). PID is an infection of the female reproductive organs, most commonly the fallopian tubes. It usually presents as lower abdominal pain, pain on walking, pain with intercourse, and, in

■ **lumen** the cavity or channel within a tube or organ.

■ **anorexia** lack of or loss of appetite.

Signs and Symptoms of Nonhemorrhagic Abdominal Pain

Local Inflammation	Pain
	Vomiting
	Diarrhea
	Guarding
Peritoneal Inflammation	Localized pain
	Vomiting
	Diarrhea
	Guarding
	Rebound tenderness
Generalized Inflammation	Pain throughout abdomen
	Rigid abdomen
Vital Signs	Increased heart rate
	Decreased B/P
	Orthostatic changes
	Normal to increased respirations

certain cases, vaginal discharge. Chapter 31 discusses PID in greater detail.

Pancreatitis. Pancreatitis, an inflammation of the pancreas, is frequently associated with chronic alcohol abuse. It can also occur in persons with marked elevations of blood lipids (cholesterol and triglycerides). In some cases the cause is unclear. Patients with pancreatitis will often complain of abdominal pain which begins abruptly. Located in the mid-abdomen, the pain tends to radiate through to the back and shoulders. Nausea and vomiting are common. Treatment of this condition includes IV fluids, pain medications, and placement of a nasogastric tube to rest the digestive system and control vomiting.

Cholecystitis. Inflammation of the gall bladder is called cholecystitis. It usually occurs when gall stones lodge in the duct draining the gall bladder. A stone may lodge in the common bile duct, causing congestion of the liver, inflammation of the gall bladder, and, in severe cases, pancreatitis. The usually colicky pain of cholecystitis is located in the upper right quadrant. It generally worsens following meals, especially those containing high amounts of fats (fried foods, cheeses, etc.). Antacids usually do not lessen this pain. Treatment generally consists of surgical removal of the gall bladder.

Pyelonephritis. Pyelonephritis is infection of the kidney. Because of ascending infection from the bladder, it appears more commonly in women than men. Women's bladders are more prone to infection because of the shortness of the urethra. The patient will typically be febrile and complain of flank or low back pain. Chills are also common. There may be tenderness at the area below where the 12th rib attaches to the 12th thoracic vertebra (costovertebral angle). Urinary burning and frequency may or may not be present. Treatment usually requires intravenous antibiotics.

Ovarian Cyst. An ovarian cyst is a fluid-filled sac that forms intermittently on the ovaries. Such cysts occasionally cause lower abdominal pain.

Hepatitis. Hepatitis is an inflammation or infection of the liver. It can result from viral infection, alcohol or other substance abuse, and other causes. The patient will often complain of dull right upper quadrant abdominal tenderness usually unrelated to digestion of food. There is usually associated malaise, decreased appetite, clay colored stools, and jaundice (yellow tint to sclera and skin). Paramedics working with any patient suspected of having hepatitis, regardless of the probable cause, should wear protective gloves. In nonviral cases, treatment of hepatitis involves removing the offending agent. But, in viral-induced hepatitis, the patient is simply observed and treated sympathetically.

Disease Processes Related to Hemorrhagic Abdominal Emergencies

Hemorrhagic causes of abdominal pain include the following:

Esophageal Varices. Esophageal varices are swollen veins in the lower third of the esophagus. They result from increased pressure in the portal circulation (portal hypertension). The portal circulation drains from the intestines to the liver. Diseases of the liver, such as alcoholic cirrhosis, can slow portal circulation, causing engorgement of the veins in the lower esophagus and the rectum (hemorrhoids). The most common presentation is painless gastrointestinal bleeding. Massive quantities of blood can be vomited. Treatment consists of fluid replacement and transfusion. If bleeding does not stop, the veins can be injected—via a scope passed into the esophagus—with an agent to constrict them. A specialized tube (Sengstaken-Blakemore) may occasionally be placed to tamponade the bleeding vessels. Patients with significant bleeding esophageal varices tend to do poorly.

Perforated Abdominal Viscus. Perforation of a hollow abdominal organ, most commonly the stomach or duodenum, can cause loss of the stomach or intestinal contents into the abdominal cavity. This can result in inflammation and infection of the peritoneum and other abdominal organs. Common causes of perforation include perforated ulcers or a perforated diverticulum. The patient will present with sudden onset of abdominal pain and generalized tenderness. Rebound is often present. In many cases the abdomen is rigid from sympathetic contraction of the muscles of the abdominal wall. Treatment includes IV fluids, antibiotics, and emergency surgery to repair the perforation.

■ **diverticuli** small finger-like pouches on the colon associated with degeneration of the muscular layer of the organ.

Diverticulosis. Diverticulosis is bleeding from **diverticuli** on the large intestines. It usually presents as painless rectal bleeding. Left-sided abdominal pain, however, can be present. The primary concern is prevention of shock.

Carcinoma of the Colon. Carcinoma of the colon is a malignant growth occurring anywhere in the colon. Presentation may be diverse. It may begin as painless rectal bleeding, weight loss, or abdominal pain. Prevention of shock is the primary concern if the bleeding is severe.

Ectopic Pregnancy. An ectopic pregnancy is the implantation of a developing fetus outside of the uterus, and must be considered in any female of childbearing age with lower abdominal pain. The most common location is in the fallopian tube (hence the name "tubal pregnancy"). The fetus continues to grow until it exerts pressure on the wall of the fallopian tube. If the pregnancy is allowed to progress, the fallopian tube can rupture,

Upper Gastrointestinal Hemorrhage	**Hematemesis** (vomiting of blood) Bright red = fresh blood Coffee ground = old blood	■ **hematemesis** the vomiting of blood.
Lower Gastrointestinal Hemorrhage	Rectal bleeding Bright red = low location (hemorrhoid/rectum) Wine color = colon or rapid upper GI bleed **Melena** = upper GI bleed	■ **melena** black, tarlike feces due to gastrointestinal bleeding.
Vital Signs	Increased heart rate Decreased B/P Orthostatic changes Normal to increased respirations	

causing significant bleeding into the abdomen and pelvis. The patient often will report a missed menstrual period or irregular periods. The pain tends to be low in the abdomen and can occur on either side. Associated vaginal bleeding is common. Chapter 31 discusses ectopic pregnancy in more detail.

Aortic Aneurysm. Weakness in the wall of the descending aorta can occur with age and result in a ballooning of the wall of the vessel. This ballooning may increase in size and eventually rupture. The patient with an abdominal aortic aneurysm is usually an older person who complains of diffuse abdominal pain. Such patients will occasionally report a tearing sensation if the artery is dissecting (loosening of the layers of the artery wall, allowing blood to flow in between). A pulsatile abdominal mass may be noted. Treatment consists of surgical repair or replacement of the diseased vessel.

ASSESSMENT OF THE ACUTE ABDOMEN

The paramedic should not attempt to discern the cause of abdominal pain in the prehospital setting. This is a difficult enough process for the emergency department with laboratory, x-ray, and other diagnostic facilities available. A complete assessment is, however, indicated to detect obvious threats to life including impending shock.

Assessment should begin with the primary assessment. Any threats to life should be immediately dealt with. If the patient is stable, the paramedic should proceed with the secondary assessment, including the standard head to toe examination. Particular attention should be paid to the abdomen. First, it needs to be inspected, and any obvious asymmetry or distention noted. (See Figure 24-3.) The position of the patient should also be observed. Patients presenting with acute abdominal pain will frequently have the knees drawn up toward the chest to lessen tension on the peritoneum and to decrease intra-abdominal pressure. (See Figure 24-4.)

The abdomen should be gently palpated. First, the patient should be asked to point to where the pain is located. (See Figure 24-5.) Palpation should begin away from the site of the pain. Each quadrant must be lightly palpated and any tenderness noted. (See Figure 24-6.) Also, the

✱ The paramedic should not attempt to discern the cause of abdominal pain in the prehospital setting.

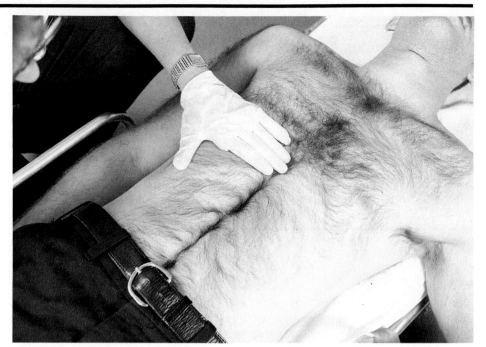

FIGURE 24-3 Inspection of the abdomen.

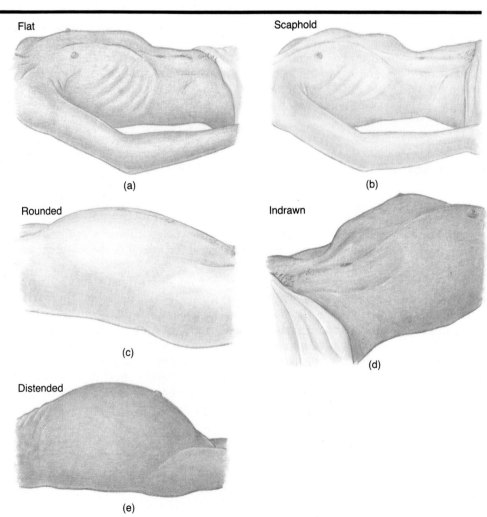

Flat

(a)

Scaphold

(b)

Rounded

(c)

Indrawn

(d)

Distended

(e)

FIGURE 24-4 Various abdominal appearances.

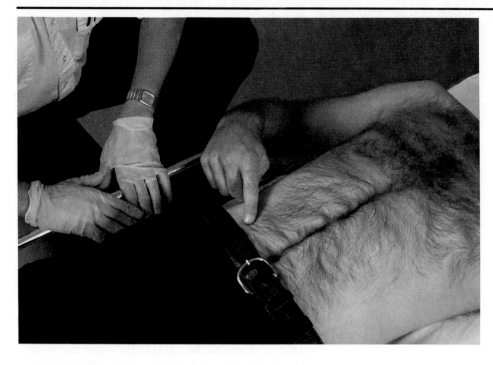

patient should be tested for the presence of rebound tenderness. This can be done by slowly palpating each abdominal quadrant. Then, the examiner should quickly withdraw his or her hand, allowing the abdominal wall to return to its normal position. If this causes pain, the patient has rebound tenderness, usually suggestive of peritoneal irritation. If a pulsatile mass is located, palpation should stop and the patient should be transported. Prolonged or vigorous palpation of an abdominal aortic aneurysm can result in rupture with disastrous results. Auscultation and percussion of the abdomen should not be attempted in the prehospital setting.

✴ Rebound tenderness should NOT be tested in the prehospital setting unless ordered by medical control.

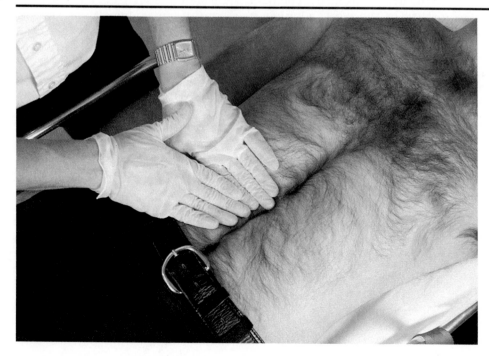

FIGURE 24-6 Soft palpation.

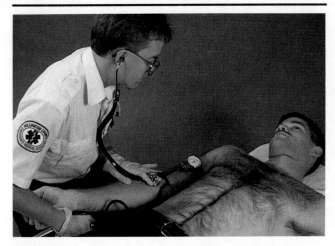

FIGURE 24-7 The tilt test should be performed. First, determine the pulse and blood pressure with the patient supine.

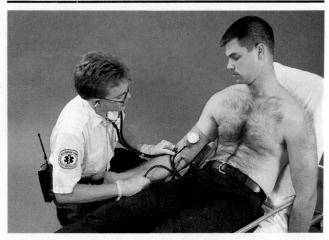

FIGURE 24-8 Then, elevate the patient and repeat the pulse and blood pressure. A fall in the systolic blood presure of 15 mm/Hg or a rise in the pulse of 15 beats per minute is considered positive.

■ **tilt test** A drop in the systolic blood pressure of 15mmHg or an increase in the pulse rate of 15 beats per minute when a patient is moved from a supine to a seated position is considered positive and suggestive of a relative hypovolemia. Also called orthostatic vital signs.

Determination of vital signs is extremely important in the patient suffering abdominal pain. The pulse, blood pressure, respiration, and, if possible, the temperature should be taken. Additionally, a **tilt test** needs to be performed on all patients with abdominal pain. It is accomplished by first taking the patient's blood pressure and pulse in the supine position and then repeating it with the patient in a seated position. A positive tilt test is an increase in the pulse rate of 15 beats per minute or a drop in the systolic blood pressure of 15 mm/Hg when the patient is moved from the supine to the sitting position. A positive tilt test indicates a relative hypovolemia and necessitates further intervention. (See Figures 24-7 and 24-8.)

After the primary and secondary assessment, the paramedic should obtain a pertinent and brief history. Pain is the most common presentation of the acute abdomen. The paramedic should elicit information about the quality of the pain, whether it is continuous, intermittent, or constant, or increases, then decreases, and subsequently increases again.

The patient should be asked where in the abdomen the pain began and whether it radiates or is referred to another area of the body. If the pain moves, it should be determined whether it penetrates through to the back or goes around the abdomen to the back. The patient should be asked if the pain is associated with or aggravated by food intake, physical activity, or any increase in intra-abdominal pressure (breathing, coughing, or straining). The occurrence of related symptoms such as nausea, vomiting, or diarrhea can be of assistance in localizing the source of the symptoms to a specific site or organ. Many paramedics find the PQRST method useful for evaluation of pain. It is:

P = provocation:	What initiates or aggravates the pain, makes it worse or better?
Q = quality:	What is the patient's own description of the pain?
R = region:	In what area of the body is the pain located?
radiation:	Does the pain travel to other body areas?
referred:	Is the pain felt in another body area?

S = severity: What is the patient's degree of discomfort?

T = time: When and how frequently does the pain occur, and is it intermittent or constant?

It is crucial to obtain a history of menstrual activity of female patients who present with abdominal pain. The date of the last menstrual period (LMP) should be recorded. Also, the patient should be asked whether her periods have been regular. She should also be questioned about whether she is taking oral contraceptives (birth control pills) and, if so, whether she has missed any pills. If the LMP was abnormal, duration, time of onset, estimated amount of blood loss, or unusual pain associated with menstruation should also be noted. If the patient's menses are late, she should be questioned about possible pregnancy.

Appropriate past medical history is also significant in assessing the patient presenting with abdominal pain. Information concerning any previous illnesses, particularly any abdominal condition or prior surgery, should also be obtained during the patient assessment.

MANAGEMENT OF THE ACUTE ABDOMEN

If the patient shows no evidence of active hemorrhage and vital signs are stable without signs of shock, the following should be considered:

- ❑ Keep the patient supine.
- ❑ Supply oxygen via nasal cannula.
- ❑ Monitor vital signs and cardiac rhythm.
- ❑ Administer IV, using crystalloid solution at a TKO rate.
- ❑ Provide immediate transport.

If the patient is actively hemorrhaging (bloody stools or vomiting blood), or if signs of impending shock are present (positive tilt test), the following treatment should be initiated (see Figure 24-9):

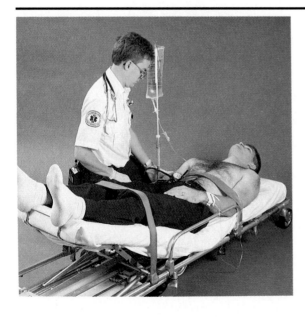

FIGURE 24-9 Management of the patient with an acute abdomen and positive tilt test.

□ Keep patient in the shock position (feet elevated).
□ Maintain high flow 100% oxygen.
□ Start IV(s), using a crystalloid solution wide open.
□ Monitor vital signs and cardiac rhythm.
□ PASG (have them in position if needed later).
□ Provide rapid transport.

GENITOURINARY SYSTEM

Anatomy of the Genitourinary System

Much of the genitourinary system is also located in the abdominal cavity. The system is composed of the following (see Figure 24-10):

Kidneys. The kidneys are paired organs located in the retroperitoneal space. They filter blood and produce urine. Additionally, they perform several endocrine functions, are a major regulator of blood pressure, and maintain fluid and electrolyte balance.

Ureters. The ureters are tubes connecting the kidneys with the urinary bladder. They also are retroperitoneal. A kidney stone can sometimes enter a ureter, causing intense pain. These stones often lodge at the pelvic brim where the ureter enters the pelvis.

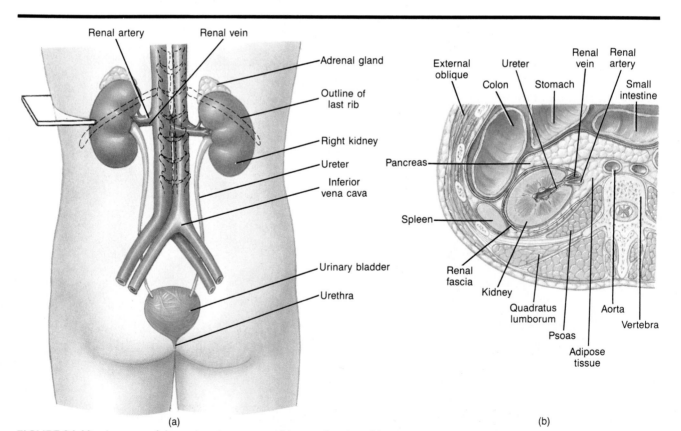

(a)   (b)

FIGURE 24-10 Anatomy of the genitourinary system: (a) posterior view; (b) cross-section.

Urinary Bladder. Located in the pelvis, the bladder receives and stores urine from the kidneys.

Urethra. The urethra is the tube connecting the bladder to the outside. It is considerably shorter in the female than in the male.

Pathophysiology of the Genitourinary System

There are four general causes of genitourinary disorders: inflammation, infection, obstruction, and hemorrhage. The kidneys can also either quit working or work less efficiently. This condition is often referred to as renal failure or renal insufficiency. Depending on its duration and potential reversibility, renal failure can be classified as acute or chronic.

Acute Renal Failure. The kidneys normally maintain body fluid volume, blood pH, and the composition of the body fluids within a very narrow range. They also continuously eliminate metabolic waste products.

Acute renal failure is characterized by rapid and potentially reversible deterioration of kidney function. Acute renal failure can be caused by several conditions. These include:

❑ *Prerenal:* Reduced renal blood flow (shock, dehydration, and use of vasopressor agents)
❑ *Renal:* Injury to the substance of the kidney itself (trauma, nephrotoxic drugs, or infection)
❑ *Postrenal:* Obstruction to the flow of urine (enlarged prostate or tumor obstructing the ureters or bladder)

As renal failure progresses, metabolic waste products accumulate. These can have a toxic effect on virtually every body organ. Urea is an end-product of protein metabolism and is usually cleared by the kidneys. In renal failure the level of urea in the blood increases and is termed **uremia.**

■ **uremia** toxic condition caused by the retention of nitrogen-based substances (urea) in the blood, normally excreted by the kidneys.

Chronic Renal Failure. **Chronic** renal failure refers to long-standing renal failure associated with loss of the nephron (kidney cell) mass and is not usually reversible. Many disease processes can destroy the kidneys or the renal arteries and result in chronic renal failure.

Renal failure can produce fluid overload, hyperkalemia, uremic pericarditis and pericardial tamponade, as well as uremic encephalopathy. In patients with severe renal failure and low urine output, the ability to excrete electrolytes and water is markedly diminished, predisposing them to fluid overload and episodes of noncardiac pulmonary edema. These patients present with severe dyspnea, neck vein distention, **ascites,** and rales at the lung bases.

■ **chronic** of long duration.

Many medications are eliminated through the kidneys. Because patients with renal failure do not clear medications as rapidly as normal patients do, they are susceptible to toxic drug concentrations despite relatively low medication doses.

■ **ascites** accumulation of fluid within the peritoneal cavity.

Signs and Symptoms of Renal Failure. Patients with chronic renal failure will often appear wasted. Their skin will be pasty yellow skin and their extremities thin. The latter is due to the protein loss accompanying chronic renal failure and poor nutrition. In the later stages, urea crystals may form on the skin, producing a frostlike appearance (uremic frost). Edema (due to decreased protein, jaundice, and low urine output) is frequently present.

■ **calculus** a stone, usually formed from crystalline urinary salts.

Kidney Stones.   Urinary stone (renal **calculus**) formation is a common problem of undetermined cause. Such stones may appear anywhere in the urinary tract including:

❑ the kidney,
❑ the renal pelvis,
❑ the ureter,
❑ the bladder, or
❑ the prostate gland.

Kidney stones are crystallized urinary salts held together by organic matter.

Urinary stone formation is more common in men than women. The usual age range is 20–50 years, although it can occur at any age. Although they can form anytime during the year, they are more often seen in the spring and the fall. Many factors predispose a patient to kidney stone formation. These include:

❑ urinary tract infections
❑ immobilization
❑ metabolic disorders (increased calcium)
❑ gout (increased uric acid)
❑ tumors

Complications from urinary stone formation include inflammation, infection, and partial or total urinary obstruction.

Symptoms of a kidney stone include:

excruciating flank pain (may radiate to the groin)
difficulty in urination
hematuria (presence of blood in the urine)
nausea and vomiting

■ **hematuria** presence of blood in the urine.

Urinary Tract Infections.   Urinary tract infections (UTI) are common. The most common UTI is bladder infection (cystitis), seldom a medical emergency. UTI occurs more frequently in females because of the relatively short urethra compared to that in males. Such infections are extremely rare in the male and less common in the female who is sexually inactive. The UTI can sometimes infect the kidney, causing pyelonephritis. This is usually characterized by fever, chills, and flank pain.

Symptoms of urinary tract infection include:

❑ dysuria (painful or burning urination)
❑ hesitancy (difficulty starting urine stream)
❑ discolored urine
❑ lower abdominal pain (especially during urination)

Assessment of the Genitourinary System

Performing an assessment on the patient suspected of having a genitourinary system problem is basically no different than for any other medical problem and should include:

- ❑ Primary assessment
- ❑ Secondary assessment
- ❑ Determine chief complaint
- ❑ History of present illness
    - ❑ When and how it occurred
    - ❑ Character
    - ❑ Onset
    - ❑ Location
    - ❑ Duration
    - ❑ Alleviation/aggravation
- ❑ Appropriate past medical history
    - ❑ Similar incident
    - ❑ Recent illness
    - ❑ Medications

If a genitourinary emergency is highly suspected, specific information must also be ascertained:

- ❑ Does the patient receive renal dialysis?
- ❑ Does the patient have a history of kidney transplant?
- ❑ Is the patient experiencing flank pain?
- ❑ Has the patient ever had a similar incident?

Management of Genitourinary Disorders

The paramedic generally can not do much in the field for the patient experiencing a genitourinary emergency except provide assessment and supportive care. There are, however, conditions which develop that can be treated in the field. For example:

- ❑ Renal Failure
    - ❑ Treat pulmonary edema, if present.
    - ❑ Treat dysrhythmias.
    - ❑ Transport to facility with **dialysis** capabilities, if possible.
    - ❑ Control shunt bleeding, if present.
- ❑ Urinary Stones
    - ❑ Transport only, unless medical control orders specific medications.
- ❑ Urinary Tract Infections
    - ❑ No specific field treatment is usually indicated.

■ dialysis process of exchanging various biochemical substances across a semipermeable membrane to remove toxic substances.

Renal Hemodialysis. **Hemodialysis** is a medical procedure whereby waste products, normally excreted by the kidneys, are removed by a machine. Patients with renal failure must undergo dialysis two to three times a week. Many patients now have home dialysis units and paramedics may be called on to assist them.

■ hemodialysis a medical procedure whereby waste products and fluid, normally excreted by the kidneys, are removed by a machine.

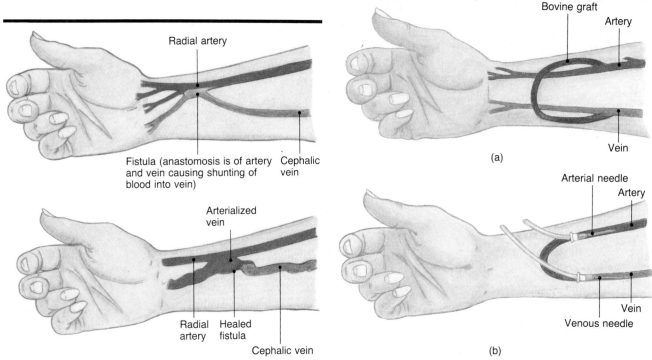

FIGURE 24-11 Fistula for dialysis access.

FIGURE 24-12 Dialysis cannula in place.

Radial artery

Fistula (anastomosis is of artery and vein causing shunting of blood into vein)

Cephalic vein

Arterialized vein

Radial artery

Healed fistula

Cephalic vein

Bovine graft

Artery

Vein

(a)

Arterial needle

Artery

Vein

Venous needle

(b)

■ **dialysate** physiologic solution used in renal dialysis.

The basic principle of dialysis is the diffusion of water and solutes across semipermeable membranes separating two fluid compartments. Solutes tend to migrate from areas of higher concentrations to ones of lower concentrations. Over time, these solutes will equilibrate. This equilibration is the basis for dialysis treatment. During dialysis, the patient's blood comes in contact with a physiologic solution called **dialysate** across a semi-permeable membrane. Equilibration of the patient's blood with dialysate normalizes the patient's electrolyte composition and eliminates undesirable waste products which his or her kidneys cannot excrete.

Vascular access must exist to dialyze the patient. The two most common routes of access are external arteriovenous shunts or internal fistulae. An arteriovenous shunt is a surgical connection between the arterial and venous systems. It provides the high flow required for dialysis and to prevent clotting. External arteriovenous shunts are usually placed in the patient's forearm, groin, or ankle. Between treatments, the shunt is wrapped and protected by a dressing to prevent dislodgment or injury. The internal fistula, located in the subcutaneous tissue of the forearm, groin, or upper arm, will have a bruit which can be palpated. It results from turbulent blood flow from the high pressure arterial system to the low pressure venous system. (See Figures 24-11 and 24-12.)

Another method for dialysis is via the peritoneum. Peritoneal dialysis uses the lining of the peritoneal cavity as the dialysis membrane. Dialysate is introduced into the patient's peritoneal cavity, where it is allowed to remain for 1–2 hours before removal. If needed, the procedure can be repeated as often as necessary. The major complication of peritoneal dialysis is the development of peritonitis. Therefore, this procedure must be done under aseptic conditions. (See Figure 24-13.)

Complications of Dialysis:

❑ HYPOTENSION: Hypotension due to dialysis is caused by dehydration, sepsis, or blood loss. The patient who becomes hypotensive will present with lightheadedness, dizziness, weakness, pallor, cold sweats, and syncope. The hypotension is treated by reducing the blood flow rate through the dialysis machine, lowering the patient's head, elevating the legs, and infusing IV saline.

❑ CHEST PAIN/DYSRHYTHMIAS: Dysrhythmias produced in response to dialysis can be caused by potassium intoxication. Yet, frequently, no specific electrolyte derangement can be identified. Dysrhythmias sometimes may be related to the development of transient myocardial ischemia which may also cause the patient to experience chest pain. The most common cardiac abnormalities seen are PVCs. The dialysis procedure must be discontinued if the dysrhythmia is considered severe or does not respond to treatment.

❑ DISEQUILIBRIUM SYNDROME: Disequilibrium syndrome is characterized by cerebral symptoms in patients with severe renal failure which can occur at the beginning, during, or immediately following hemodialysis. These patients may present with headache, lethargy, convulsions, and may even lapse into coma. Disequilibrium syndrome may be caused by rapid changes of body fluids, sodium concentrations, and osmolalities. With a rapid decline in the level of blood urea, time is insufficient for an equal lowering of urea across the "blood-brain barrier." This may cause an osmotic diuresis of water from the cerebral blood and from the extracellular fluid in the central nervous system, resulting in cerebral edema and increased intracranial pressure. The major concern is the development of convulsions. Diazepam may be given to the patient with seizures.

❑ AIR EMBOLISM: An air embolism can occur when negative pressure develops in the venous side of the dialysis tubing. This negative pressure sucks air in and carries it to the right ventricle of the heart where it mixes with blood, creating a foam. The foam is pumped into the pulmonary artery, blocking the passage of blood to the left side of the heart. This will cause the

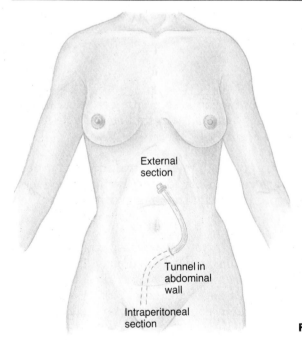

External
section

Tunnel in
abdominal
wall

Intraperitoneal
section

FIGURE 24-13 Peritoneal dialysis.

patient to experience severe dyspnea, cyanosis, hypotension, and respiratory distress. When this problem is recognized, the dialysis machine must be immediately shut off and the patient turned on the left side, with feet elevated, and head down. Oxygen should be administered via nasal cannula.

Complications Related to Vascular Access:

☐ CLOTTING: Clotting of the shunt or fistula can occur spontaneously. A clotted shunt is easy to recognize because, in an internal shunt, the bruit will be lost. In an external shunt clots will be visible in the tubing. Clotting poses no immediate emergency.

☐ HEMORRHAGE: Massive external hemorrhage can occur with separation of arteriovenous fistulas. Rupture of internal fistulas is possible if an aneurysm has formed and the shunt ruptures through the skin. For the external shunt, clamps are secured to the dressing covering it and are there to clamp the shunt when necessary. If an internal shunt ruptures, the hemorrhage can be frightening to the patient, and difficult for the paramedic to stop. The best method to end the hemorrhage is by direct pressure and rapid transport to the emergency department.

Management of the Dialysis Patient. In most EMS systems the paramedic rarely has an opportunity to deal with a dialysis patient on a regular basis. Listed below are treatment guidelines specific to the dialysis patient:

☐ Intravenous therapy; IV access may be difficult. The shunt SHOULD NOT be used. Fluid administration should be at the direction of the medical control physician.

☐ Monitor ECG.

☐ Treat medical emergencies the same as for any patient.

☐ Remove patient from dialysis machine:
   1. Turn off dialysis machine.
   2. Clamp shunt tubing ends.
   3. Control shunt hemorrhage (internal or external) with either direct pressure or by pinching the shunt ends.

REPRODUCTIVE SYSTEM

Anatomy and Physiology

Female. Certain parts of the reproductive system are located in the abdominal and abdominopelvic cavity, especially in the female. The female reproductive organs include (see Figure 24-14):

Ovaries. The ovaries, or female gonads, are small, walnut-sized organs adjacent to the uterus. They are responsible for producing a portion of the female hormones and for production of the female component of reproduction, the ovum.

Fallopian Tubes. The fallopian tubes are hollow tubes connecting the ovary to the uterus. They transport the ovum to the uterus. Fertilization usually occurs in the fallopian tube, which is open at the end adjacent to the ovary. This provides direct access to the abdominal cavity and to the uterus. The fallopian tube is a frequent source of infection (salpingitis), especially in pelvic inflammatory disease.

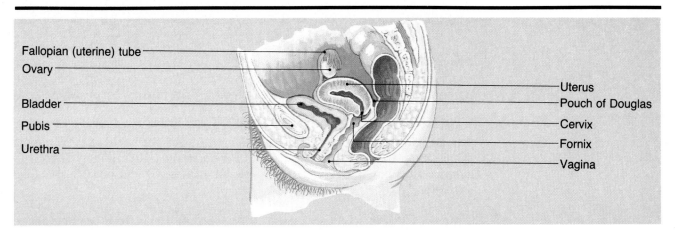

FIGURE 24-14 The Female Reproductive system.

Uterus. The uterus is a hollow, muscular organ, situated low in the pelvis. A portion of it, the cervix, extends into the vagina. The superior part of the uterus is called the fundus. The uterus is the site of implantation and development of the fetus.

Vagina. The vagina extends from the uterus to the vulva. It is the female organ of copulation and the birth canal.

Vulva. The vulva is the external female genitalia. It consists of the labia majora, labia minora, introitus, and accessory glands.

Male. Most of the male reproductive organs are located in the low pelvis, and outside the pelvic cavity in the scrotum. They include (see Figure 24-15):

Testes. The testes, or male gonads, lie in the scrotum. They are responsible for production of the male hormones and sperm. To facilitate sperm production, the scrotum maintains the testes at a temperature slightly lower than that of the body.

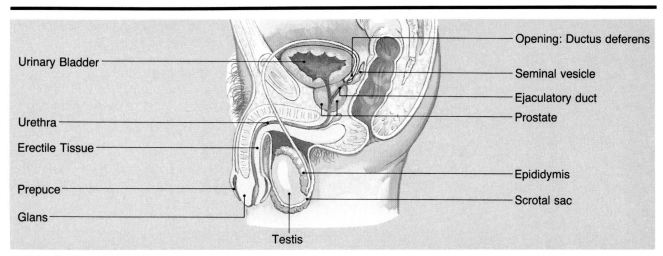

FIGURE 24-15 The Male Reproductive System.

Epididymis. The epididymi are small appendages on the testes acting as a reservoir for sperm.

Prostate. A small gland at the base of the bladder, the prostate is responsible for production of fluid to transport sperm. In older men, it can become enlarged (benign prostatic hypertrophy) and, at certain times, obstruct urine flow.

Vas Deferens. The vas deferens are small muscular tubes that transport sperm from the testes to the urethra for discharge during ejaculation. To achieve sterility in the male, they are sometimes cut in a procedure called *vasectomy.*

Urethra. The urethra is a canal that releases urine from the bladder to the outside. In the male, it also discharges sperm during ejaculation.

Penis. The male organ of copulation, the penis is covered by a loose skin allowing for erection. The skin overlying the end of the penis (glans) is frequently surgically removed in a procedure called *circumcision.* Because of its location, the penis is vulnerable to trauma.

Pathophysiology and Management of Reproductive System Disorders

Female:

Pelvic Inflammatory Disease (PID). Pelvic inflammatory disease results from a sexually transmitted disease. An ascending infection, PID spreads from the vagina or cervix to the uterus, the fallopian tubes, and the broad ligaments. The patient usually presents with fever, chills, abdominal pain, and vaginal bleeding. (See Chapter 31.)

Ectopic Pregnancy. An ectopic pregnancy occurs when the fertilized ovum is implanted outside of the uterine cavity. The patient will usually present with tenderness on the affected side. She will often show pallor, weak pulse, and signs of shock or hemorrhage. Pain may be referred to the shoulder, and the umbilicus may appear bluish in color. (See Chapter 31.)

Ruptured Ovarian Cyst. The patient will present with abdominal pain which may have rapid or gradual onset. On rare occasions, the patient may experience syncope and develop shock. (See Chapter 31.)

Mittelschmerz. Mittelschmerz is abdominal pain that may accompany ovulation. It occurs half-way through the menstrual cycle and is associated with release of the ovum from the ovary. In rare cases, pain can be severe.

Management. Female reproductive emergencies tend to be more serious than male reproductive emergencies with the exception of testicular torsion. Specific field management of female emergencies includes the following:

❑ Airway management and supplemental oxygen.
❑ IV of lactated Ringer's solution as indicated for a patient with hemorrhage.
❑ Monitor vital signs and cardiac rhythm.

❑ Have PASG ready.

❑ Transport in the position of comfort.

Male:

Epididymitis. Epididymitis is the inflammation of the epididymis. It may occur secondary to gonorrhea, syphilis, tuberculosis, mumps, prostatitis, urethritis, or following prolonged use of an indwelling catheter. The patient with epididymitis will present with fever and chills, pain in his inguinal region, and have a swollen epididymis.

Testicular Torsion. Torsion of testes occurs when part of a blood vessel within them becomes twisted or rotated. The patient will present with severe testicular pain, and may feel as though he has received a traumatic injury to his testicles. Testicular torsion tends to occur in younger males and children.

Management. Field management for the patient with epididymitis or torsion of testes is mostly supportive. The paramedic should, however, monitor the following:

❑ patient's airway status

❑ vital signs

❑ the possible development of shock.

Patients should be transported in the position of comfort.

SUMMARY

Determining the origin of an abdominal disorder can be extremely difficult, not only for the paramedic in the field, but for the emergency physician. Most field procedures required for abdominal emergencies can be performed while enroute to the emergency department. Excessive time should not be spent in the field since many of these patients may require abdominal surgery.

Sometimes the paramedic will have to treat the patient on renal hemodialysis. Therefore, the paramedic should be familiar with complications and management of dialysis such as hypotension, dysrhythmias, chest pain, disequilibrium syndrome, air embolism, clotting, and hemorrhage.

FURTHER READING

BLEDSOE, B. E., *Atlas of Paramedic Skills.* Englewood Cliffs, NJ: Prentice-Hall, Inc., 1987.

LANGFITT, D. E., *Critical Care: Certification Preparation and Review.* Bowie, MD: Robert J. Brady Company, 1984.

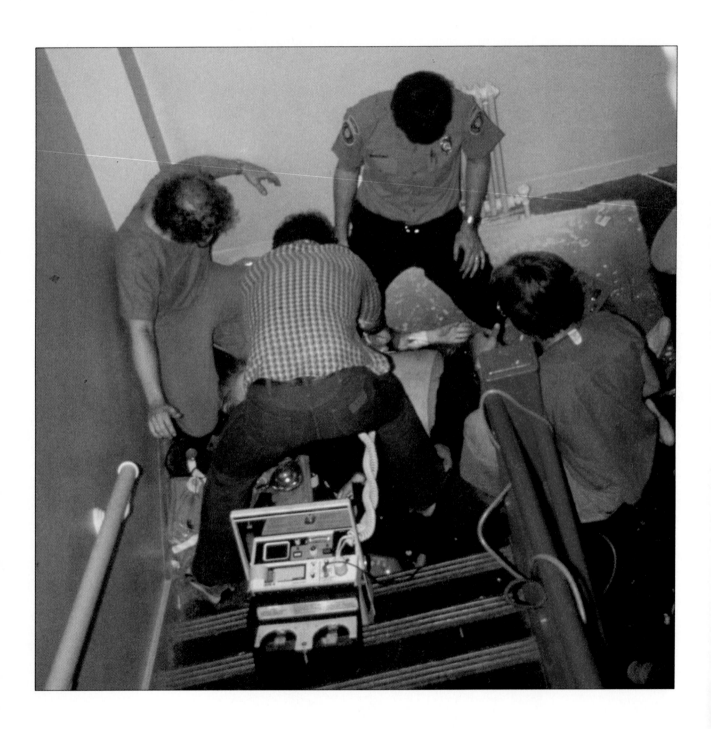

25

Anaphylaxis

Objectives for Chapter 25

Upon completing this chapter, the student should be able to:

1. Define antigen.

2. List four ways an antigen can be introduced into the body.

3. Define antibody.

4. Define anaphylaxis.

5. Describe the pathophysiology of anaphylaxis.

6. Discuss the effects of anaphylaxis on the following body systems:

    *   respiratory
    *   cardiovascular
    *   gastrointestinal
    *   nervous
    *   skin

7. Describe the clinical presentation of the patient suffering anaphylaxis.

8. Discuss the assessment of the patient suffering anaphylaxis.

9. Describe the actions of the following medications and relate their usage in the management of anaphylaxis:

    *   oxygen
    *   epinephrine
    *   diphenhydramine
    *   aminophylline

The Parker Township volunteer paramedic squad dispatcher receives a call from a distressed woman who states, "My husband was just stung by several bees. He fell off the ladder and can't breathe. Please come quickly." Within 3 minutes of receiving the call the ambulance is dispatched. A police officer has already arrived at the scene and is "administering oxygen."

Upon arrival the crew finds the patient supine on the ground next to a ladder leaning against the house. A few angry bees are still patrolling the area. The oxygen mask is quickly moved back and the primary assessment completed. The airway is open, and the patient is moving air. His attempts to speak result only in a stridorous, scratchy groan. The carotid pulse is present at 120 per minute. The radial pulse is absent. The oxygen mask is replaced and the flow rate increased to 10 L/min. One of the EMTs responding on the call begins to take the vital signs. The paramedic opens the airway kit and selects a laryngoscope, a #3 MacIntosh blade, a stylet, and an 8.0-mm endotracheal tube. Lidocaine jelly is placed on the endotracheal tube wrapper.

The secondary assessment reveals a 55-year-old white male in severe distress. The blood pressure is 70 mm/Hg by palpation. Pulse is 130. Respirations are 32 and shallow. The patient is diaphoretic and pale. He is confused and is attempting to speak. Each breath shows increasing stridor. Breath sounds are virtually absent. A 16-gauge IV catheter is placed in the right antecubital fossa. An infusion of lactated Ringer's is started wide open. The EMT is allowed to tape the line in place. Immediately, following local standing orders, 0.5 mg of epinephrine 1:10,000 is administered intravenously. While the paramedic is drawing up an ampule of diphenhydramine (Benadryl), the EMTs attach the monitor electrodes. The ECG shows a sinus tachycardia. Almost immediately the patient's stridor improves. Next 50 mg of diphenhydramine is injected intravenously. The patient's respiratory status, as evidenced by improved air movement and decreased stridor, improves. The senior paramedic feels that endotracheal intubation is, at present, not worth the risk of laryngospasm in light of the patient's improved respiratory status.

The medical control physician is contacted. A second set of vital signs shows the blood pressure up to 110/60 and the pulse up to 140. The on-line medical control physician requests that the paramedics administer 125 mg of methylprednisolone intravenously while en route.

The patient is packaged and taken to the ambulance. Transport is Code 3 with all of the intubation equipment remaining at the patient's head. By the time the ambulance arrives at the hospital the patient's stridor and mental status is much improved. His blood pressure appears stable. His pulse rate is down because the effects of the initial dosage of epinephrine are wearing off. A physician from the Department of Anesthesiology evaluates the patient and determines that elective intubation will probably not be necessary because of the patient's marked improvement.

INTRODUCTION

Anaphylaxis is an acute, generalized, and violent antigen-antibody reaction that may be rapidly fatal even with prompt and appropriate emergency medical care. Anaphylaxis develops in seconds to minutes after the ingestion, injection, inhalation, or absorption of an antigenic substance. This chapter will address the pathophysiology and management of anaphylaxis and related disorders.

■ **anaphylaxis** acute, generalized, and violent antigen-antibody reaction that can be rapidly fatal.

PATHOPHYSIOLOGY

As mentioned above, anaphylaxis develops following exposure to a certain antigenic substance. An **antigen** is any substance capable of inducing an immune response. Examples of antigens include drug molecules, serum or other secretions from animals, blood from an individual of a different blood type, and many others. Most antigens are proteins. Antigens can enter the body through the skin, the respiratory tract, or the gastrointestinal tract. Following the entrance of the antigen into the body, the immune system responds by manufacturing special proteins called **antibodies.** There are five classes of antibodies. They include:

■ **antigen** any substance capable of inducing an immune response.

1. IgM: the antibody that responds immediately.
2. IgG: the antibody that "has memory" and recognizes a repeat invasion of the same infection.
3. IgA: the antibody that is present in the mucous membranes.
4. **IgE:** the antibody that contributes to allergic and anaphylactic responses.
5. IgD: the antibody present in the lowest concentration.

■ **antibodies** proteins, produced by plasma cells, released in response to an antigen. Antibodies bind to antigens to facilitate their removal by scavenger cells such as macrophages and neutrophils.

Once released, antibodies find the offending antigen and combine with it to form the so-called "antigen-antibody complex." This bulky complex is then taken up by cells of the immune system, such as neutrophils and macrophages, and eliminated from the body.

■ **immunoglobulin E (IgE)** antibody responsible for mediating allergic and anaphylactic reactions.

The immune system can "remember" an antigen. That is, once an antigen has provoked an antibody response, the body will remember this antigen and will respond with the production of antibody much more quickly. This is the principle behind immunity. For example, all viruses and bacteria have highly antigenic proteins on their surface. Once a person becomes infected by these organisms, the immune system will then produce antibodies and other substances to aid the body in eliminating the infectious agent. In addition, the body will store in memory the configuration of the antigen. If the same antigen or a closely similar antigen again enters the body, the immune system will "remember" this antigen and immediately release the appropriate antibody to eliminate the substance from the body before infection can develop.

Most vaccines are inactivated, or **attenuated,** versions of the original infectious virus or bacteria. The vaccine contains the same antigens that were present on the original organism but these antigens are incapable of causing infection. When the vaccine is administered to a patient, the immune system is stimulated to produce the antibody to the antigen. If the person later comes into contact with a disease for which he or she has been vaccinated, the immune system will quickly respond by releasing the appropriate antibody thus preventing infection. Sometimes the

■ **attenuated** diluted or weakened. Applied to organisms that are weakened, so as not to be infectious, so that they can be administered to provoke an immune response.

memory of the antigen lasts for a lifetime, as in the case of chicken pox; in other cases, for example, tetanus, the effect of vaccination will last only 5 to 10 years.

Most responses to an antigen are not noticed by the patient. Occasionally, however, a patient becomes sensitized to the antigen, and the body's immune response is much more profound. What is called an **allergic reaction** occurs. Allergic reactions are usually not life-threatening, merely uncomfortable for the patient. Anaphylaxis, in contrast, is the most severe form of allergic reaction and is an immediate threat to life.

Allergic patients are said to be **"atopic."** That is, they tend to exhibit several similar conditions such as asthma, eczema, and allergies. Many of these "atopic" patients have a higher tendency to develop anaphylaxis.

Anaphylaxis is primarily caused by release of the antibody IgE, which finds and attaches to *mast cells,* specialized cells of the immune system. Mast cells, along with basophils, release several substances, the most important of which is **histamine.** Histamine is a potent biochemical agent that causes several different actions. First, histamine is released into the blood where it finds histamine receptors on which to bind. Among these receptors are H1 receptors in the lungs and in the peripheral blood vessels and H2 receptors in the stomach. When histamine attaches to the H1 receptors, it causes bronchoconstriction and peripheral vasodilation. When it attaches to the H2 receptors, it increases gastric acid secretion and speeds transport of material through the intestines. In addition, histamine causes the peripheral capillaries to become "leaky," resulting in edema. All of these responses serve to aid the immune system in ridding the body of the antigenic substance and in preventing entry of additional antigen into the body. Bronchoconstriction decreases intake of the antigen through the respiratory system. Increased gastric acid secretion and the speed-up of intestinal transport aid the body in deactivating and eliminating antigenic material taken into the digestive tract. Histamine is the most important mediator of anaphylaxis.

Several agents can cause anaphylaxis. One of the more common is antibiotics. Another frequent cause of anaphylaxis was the iodine-based contrast dyes formerly used in radiology. Newer dyes generally do not have this effect. Any medication administered by the paramedic must be considered capable of causing anaphylaxis. (See Figure 25-1.)

Some people can become overly sensitized to the venom of insects, especially bees, wasps, and ants, as was illustrated in the case study that opened this chapter.

CLINICAL PRESENTATION

Anaphylaxis can occur within seconds or even hours after the event that caused it. Common symptoms include dyspnea, sneezing, coughing, or upper airway stridor. This is due to the release of histamine, which causes bronchoconstriction. In addition, edema of the lungs, larynx, or trachea can develop quite rapidly due to the leaking of fluid out of the capillaries into the interstitial spaces of the respiratory system.

From a cardiovascular standpoint, anaphylaxis is manifested by massive vasodilation, increased heart rate, and decreased blood pressure. The presence of all three of these constitutes anaphylactic shock and must be promptly recognized.

The gastrointestinal system also responds violently to histamine release. Abdominal cramping and significant nausea and vomiting may be

■ **allergic reaction** hypersensitivity to a given antigen. A reaction more pronounced than would occur in the general population.

■ **atopy** patients with a group of diseases of an allergic nature. Included in these are asthma, eczema, and allergic rhinitis. These diseases have a strong hereditary component.

■ **histamine** a chemical released by mast cells and basophils upon stimulation. It is one of the most powerful vasodilators known and a major mediator of anaphylaxis.

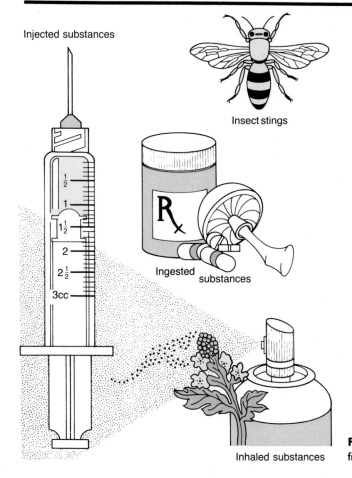

Injected substances

Insect stings

R
x

Ingested substances

Inhaled substances

FIGURE 25-1 Anaphylactic reactions can result from several items.

present. Many patients will experience diarrhea. All of these responses are the body's attempt to rid the gastrointestinal tract of the offending antigen. (See Figure 25-2.)

The nervous system is also affected. The most common complaint related to this system is headache, but in severe circumstances, convulsions may be present. Unconsciousness occurs early in severe anaphylaxis.

The skin is highly involved in an anaphylactic reaction. Peripheral vasodilation may cause swelling of the face and mucous membranes (angioedema). It is important to recognize this symptom, because often these patients will develop laryngeal edema and, in severe cases, complete airway obstruction.

ASSESSMENT

The primary assessment should be aimed at correcting life-threatening situations such as airway obstruction, respiratory compromise, and cardiac arrest. Stridor can indicate a life-threatening condition. The time interval from the onset of stridor to complete occlusion of the airway can be very short.

The paramedic needs to determine, if possible, the offending antigen and when the contact occurred. It is essential to inquire about prior reactions. It is also important to determine whether or not the patient is

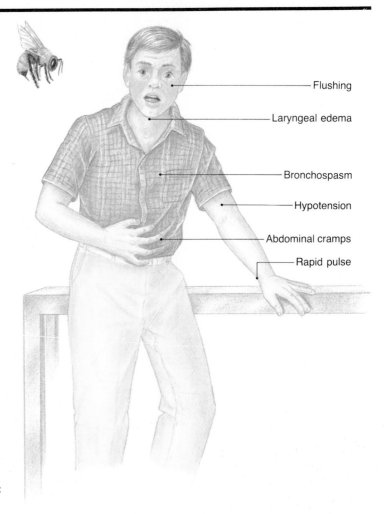

Flushing

Laryngeal edema

Bronchospasm

Hypotension

Abdominal cramps

Rapid pulse

FIGURE 25-2 Clinical presentation of anaphylactic reaction.

atopic. If time permits, the patient should be questioned about asthma, eczema, and allergies.

The secondary survey begins with assessment of vital signs. Vital signs MUST be monitored closely. In addition, the level of consciousness must be reassessed. Often, the appearance of the skin will indicate anaphylaxis. The skin will turn red and may exhibit wheals (**urticaria**), commonly called "hives."

■ **urticaria** name given the raised areas that occur on the skin associated with vasodilation due to histamine release. Commonly referred to as "hives."

MANAGEMENT

The first component of the management of anaphylaxis is that of airway management. The patient should be administered supplemental oxygen in a high concentration. If necessary, ventilations should be initiated with bag-valve-mask or demand valve. Endotracheal intubation, or even transtracheal ventilation, may be required should airway compromise be evident. The most experienced member of the EMS team should perform the endotracheal intubation. This is because the airway is very sensitive, and often, you will only have one attempt at placing the tube. Once the tube contacts the larynx, the vocal cords can spasm, completely shutting off the airway.

If the site of antigen entry is known, and if it is on an extremity, then a venous constricting band can be applied between the site and the heart. This should not be so tight that it interrupts arterial flow.

An IV with a crystalloid solution, such as lactated Ringer's solution or 0.9% sodium chloride, should be initiated. Following this the patient should be administered 0.3 to 0.5 mg of epinephrine 1:1,000 subcutaneously. If the reaction is life-threatening, then 3 to 5 mL of epinephrine 1:10,000 should be administered very slowly intravenously. Some EMS systems may want the initial bolus followed by an epinephrine drip if the reaction is severe and the transport time long.

Epinephrine reverses many of the effects of histamine. Through its action on β_1 receptors it causes bronchodilation and an increase in heart rate and contractile force. Through its α_1 properties it causes in some reversal of the vasodilation. *Epinephrine is the primary drug for management of anaphylaxis.* (See Table 25-1.)

✳ Epinephrine is the primary drug for management of anaphylaxis.

Following the administration of epinephrine the patient should receive diphenhydramine (Benadryl) intravenously. Diphenhydramine blocks both H1 and H2 histamine receptors, thereby limiting the further release of histamine. (See Table 25-2.)

Following the administration of both epinephrine and diphenhydramine, the medical control physician may request the administration of aminophylline. Aminophylline is a potent bronchodilator whose mechanism of action is different than that of epinephrine. (See Table 25-3.)

Some physicians may request the administration of a corticosteroid solution such as methylprednisolone (Solu-Medrol), hydrocortisone (Solu-Cortef), or dexamethasone (Decadron). (See Table 25-4.) These drugs slow histamine release and the leakage of fluid from capillaries, reducing edema. These steroids do not have an immediate effect and should not be considered a first-line medication. They are mentioned here only because some systems have prolonged transport times.

TABLE 25-1 Epinephrine 1:1,000

Class:	Sympathomimetic
Actions:	Bronchodilation
	Positive chronotrope
	Positive inotrope
Indications:	Bronchial asthma
	Exacerbation of some forms of chronic obstructive pulmonary disease (COPD)
	Anaphylaxis
Contraindications:	Patients with underlying cardiovascular disease
	Hypertension
	Pregnancy
	Patients with tachydysrhythmias
Precautions:	Should be protected from light
	Blood pressure, pulse, and EKG must be constantly monitored
Side Effects:	Palpitations
	Anxiousness
	Headache
Dosage:	0.3–0.5 mg
Route:	Subcutaneously
Pediatric Dosage:	0.01 mg/kg up to 0.3 mg

TABLE 25-2 Diphenhydramine (Benadryl®)

Class:	Antihistamine
Actions:	Blocks histamine receptors
	Has some sedative effects
Indications:	Anaphylaxis
	Allergic reactions
Contraindications:	Asthma
	Nursing mothers
Precautions:	Hypotension
Side Effects:	Sedation
	Dries bronchial secretions
	Blurred vision
	Headache
	Palpitations
Dosage:	25–50 mg
Routes:	Slow IV push
	Deep IM
Pediatric Dosage:	2–5 mg/kg

TABLE 25-3 Aminophylline

Class:	Xanthine bronchodilator
Actions:	Smooth muscle relaxant
	Causes bronchodilation
	Has mild diuretic properties
	Positive chronotrope
Indications:	Bronchial asthma
	Reversible bronchospasm associated with chronic bronchitis and emphysema
	Congestive heart failure
	Pulmonary edema
Contraindications:	Patients with history of hypersensitivity to the drug
	Hypotension
	Patients with peptic ulcer disease
Precautions:	Monitor for arrhythmias
	Monitor blood pressure
Side Effects:	Convulsions
	Vomiting
	Palpitations
Dosages:	Method 1: 250–500 mg in 90 or 80 mL of D5W respectively infused over 20–30 minutes (approximately 5–10 mg/kg/hr)
	Method 2: 250–500 mg (5–7 mg/kg) in 20 ml of D5W infused over 20–30 minutes
Route:	Slow IV
Pediatric Dosage:	Status asthmaticus: 3–4 mg/kg loading dose to be infused over 20–30 minutes. Maximum dose not to exceed 12 mg/kg per 24 hours.

TABLE 25-4 Methylprednisolone (Solu-Medrol®)

Class:	Steroid
Actions:	Anti-inflammatory
	Suppresses immune response (especially in allergic/anaphylactic reactions)
Indications:	Severe anaphylaxis
	Possibly effective as an adjunctive agent in the management of shock
Contraindications:	None in the emergency setting
Precautions:	Must be reconstituted and used promptly
	Onset of action may be 2–6 hours and thus should not be expected to be of use in the critical first hour following an anaphylactic reaction
Side Effects:	GI bleeding
	Prolonged wound healing
	Suppression of natural steroids
Dosage:	125–250 mg
Routes:	IV
	IM
Pediatric Dosage:	30 mcg/kg

SUMMARY

Anaphylaxis is a serious medical emergency that must be promptly recognized and treated appropriately. Anaphylaxis occurs when an antigen to which a patient has been previously sensitized enters the body. This causes a chain of events which begins with the release of IgE. This subsequently causes the mast cells to release histamine. Histamine causes the systemic symptoms associated with the disease. Therapy is aimed at supporting respiration and circulation and at reversing, pharmacologically, the effects of histamine using epinephrine and diphenhydramine.

✱ Anaphylaxis can rapidly kill. It must be promptly recognized and treated accordingly.

FURTHER READING

American Heart Association. *Textbook of Advanced Cardiac Life Support,* 2nd ed. Dallas, TX: American Heart Association, 1987.

Bayer, Mark J., Rumack, Barry H., and Wanke, Lee A. *Toxicological Emergencies.* Bowie, MD: Brady Communications, 1984.

Bledsoe, Bryan E., Bosker, Gideon, and Papa, Frank J. *Prehospital Emergency Pharmacology,* 2nd ed. Englewood Cliffs, NJ: Prentice-Hall, Inc., 1988.

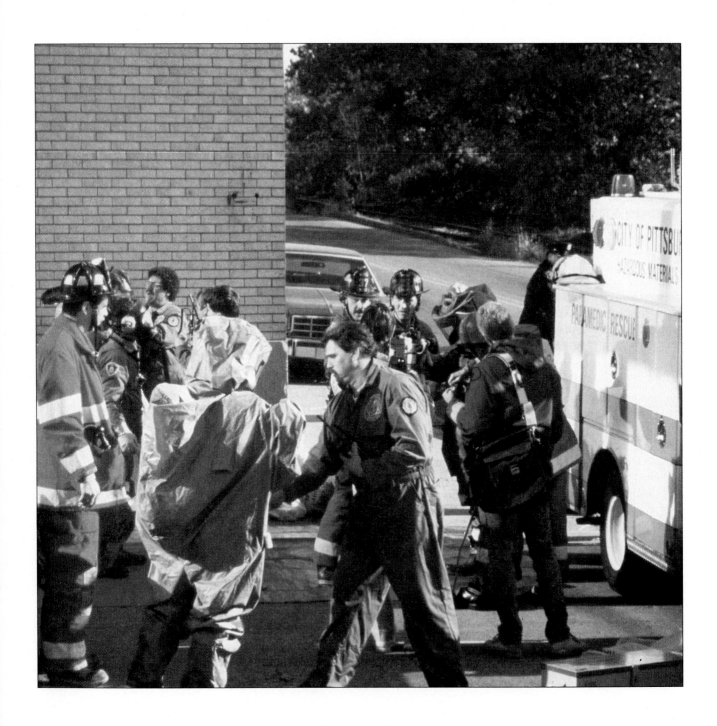

26

Toxicology and Substance Abuse

Objectives for Chapter 26

Upon completing this chapter, the student should be able to:

1. Discuss the importance of toxicologic emergencies in prehospital care.

2. Describe the various routes of entry of toxic substances into the body.

3. Discuss the role of poison control centers within the EMS system.

4. Describe the aspects of the patient history and general principles of management for a patient who has ingested poison.

5. Discuss the factors affecting whether to induce vomiting in a patient who has ingested poison.

6. Describe the signs, symptoms, and management of patients who have:

- ingested poisons
- injected poisons
- inhaled poisons
- surface absorbed poisons

7. Discuss the presentation and management of bites or stings of the following:

- bees, hornets, wasps, or yellow jackets
- brown recluse spider
- black widow spider
- scorpion
- rattlesnakes, copperhead or cotton-mouth water moccasin
- coral snake
- marine animals

8. Discuss the general principles regarding the recognition and management of substance abuse.

Rescue 190 is dispatched to 1311 E. Rosedale on an unconscious-person call. The paramedics, upon hearing the dispatcher, recognize the address. It is in a run-down part of town where drug use is rampant. The paramedics arrive at the scene within a few minutes. They are met by police officers who direct them to a young male lying face down on the pavement. Evidently the police were making a drug raid when they found the patient.

The paramedics quickly complete the primary assessment. The patient is alive but unresponsive. Supportive ventilations are started with a demand valve. The secondary assessment reveals pin-point pupils and needle tracks on both arms. The paramedics establish an IV and contact medical control. The medical control physician orders 1 mg of naloxone given intravenously at a slow rate. If the naloxone is unsuccessful in arousing the patient, the paramedics are told to give him 25 g of 50% dextrose and 100 mg of thiamine. However, shortly after administration of the naloxone the patient begins to arouse. At first he moans and then, later, pushes the demand valve away. He awakens and sees the police officers and tries to get up, as if to run away. He is quickly subdued by the officers and elects to go to the hospital instead of jail. He refuses any additional care including oxygen. The transport to the hospital is uneventful. The patient remains in the emergency department for 4 hours before being discharged.

INTRODUCTION

toxicology medical and biological science that studies the detection, chemistry, pharmacological actions, and antidotes of toxic substances.

Toxicological emergencies result from the ingestion, inhalation, injection, or surface absorption of toxic substances. The study of poisons and their antidotes is referred to as **toxicology.** Physicians or scientists who specialize in the field of toxicology are called *toxicologists*.

Toxicological emergencies are becoming more prevalent in society for many various reasons. Virtually every emergency call has the potential for involvement of a toxic substance. For example:

❑ Over 1 million persons are poisoned annually.
❑ 10% of all emergency department visits and EMS responses involve toxic exposures.
❑ 70% of accidental poisonings occur in children under the age of 6 years.
❑ A child who has experienced an accidental ingestion has a 25% chance of another, similar ingestion within one year.
❑ 80% of all attempted suicides involve a drug overdose.

poisoning taking a substance into the body that interferes with normal physiological functions.

overdose a dose of a drug in excess of that usually prescribed. It can adversely affect the patient's health.

Theoretically all toxicological emergencies can be classified as **poisoning.** However, in this discussion, the term "poisoning" will be used to describe exposure to non-pharmacological substances. The term **overdose** will be used to describe exposure to pharmacological substances, whether the overdose is accidental or intentional. Substance abuse, although technically a form of poisoning, will be addressed separately.

In this chapter we will discuss various aspects of toxicologic emergencies as they apply to prehospital care. Rather than cover specific poisons in great detail, we will establish general treatment guidelines for each type of toxic exposure. Because the field of toxicology is rapidly changing, it is virtually impossible for a paramedic to remain up-to-date on treatment protocols for each type of toxic exposure. Specific treatment should be directed by medical control in association with a **poison control center.** This system will ensure the patient is receiving the most current level of care available.

■ **poison control center** information center staffed by trained personnel which provides up-to-date toxicologic information.

POISONING

The term "poisoning" usually refers to the accidental exposure of the body to toxic substances in an amount sufficient to have a damaging or destructive effect on the body. In order to have a destructive effect poisons must gain entrance into the body. The four portals of entry are ingestion, inhalation, injection, and surface absorption. (See Figure 26-1.)

INHALATION

Cleaning fluid

Sprays

INJECTION

Spiders

Snakes

Drugs

INGESTION

Lye

Rat poison

Drain cleaners

ABSORPTION

Household cleaners

Insecticides

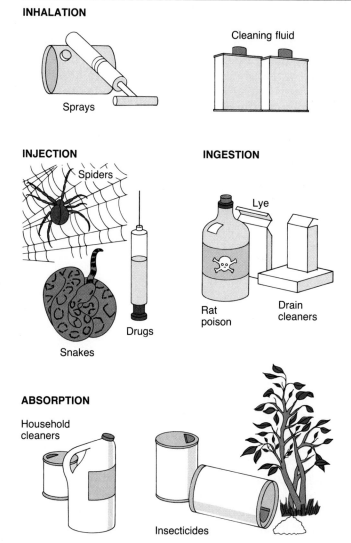

FIGURE 26-1 Routes of toxic exposure.

Ingestion

Ingestion is the most common route of entry for toxic exposure. Commonly ingested poisons include:

❑ household products
    petroleum based agents (gasoline, paint)
    cleaning agents (alkalis and soaps)
    cosmetics
❑ medications
❑ plants
❑ foods

The toxic effects following ingestion can be both immediate and delayed. Immediate effects include such things as burns to the lips, tongue, throat, and esophagus from passage of corrosive substances such as strong acids or alkalis. Delayed effects result from absorption of the poison from the gastrointestinal tract. Most absorption occurs in the small intestine, with only a small amount being absorbed from the stomach. Some poisons may remain in the stomach for up to several hours because the intake of a large bolus of poison can retard absorption.

Inhalation

Inhalation of a poison results in rapid absorption of the toxic agent through the alveolar-capillary membrane. Inhaled toxins can irritate pulmonary passages and destroy tissue. When these toxins are absorbed, wider systemic effects can occur. Causative agents can include gases, vapors, fumes, or aerosols. Common inhalation poisons include:

Toxic Gases

❑ carbon monoxide
❑ ammonia
❑ chlorine
❑ freon

Toxic Vapors, Fumes, or Aerosols

❑ carbon tetrachloride
❑ methyl chloride
❑ tear gas
❑ mustard gas

Injection

Injection of a toxic agent under the skin, into muscle, or into the circulatory system can result in both immediate and delayed effects. The immediate local reaction is at the site of the injection. Later, as the toxin is distributed throughout the body by the circulatory system, delayed systemic reactions can occur. In addition, an anaphylactic reaction can also result.

Other than intentional injection of illicit drugs, most poisonings by injection result from the bites and stings of insects and animals. Most insects that can sting and bite belong to the class *hymenoptera,* which includes bees, hornets, yellow jackets, wasps, and ants. Only the females in this group can sting. In addition spiders, ticks, and other arachnids, such as scorpions, are notorious for causing poisonings by injection. Higher animals that bite and sting include the snakes and marine animals. Among the marine animals are the jellyfish, Portuguese men-of-war, stingrays, anemones, coral, hydrae, and certain spiny fish.

Surface Absorption

Surface absorption is entry of a toxic substance through the skin. This most frequently occurs from contact with poisonous plants, including poison ivy, poison sumac, and poison oak. Many toxic chemicals may also be absorbed through the skin.

Poison Control Centers

Poison control centers have been set up across the United States and Canada to assist in the treatment of poison victims and to provide information on new products and new treatment recommendations. They are usually based in major medical centers and teaching hospitals and serve a large population. Most poison control centers now have computer capabilities to rapidly access information.

Poison control centers are usually staffed by physicians, pharmacists, or nurses with special training in toxicology. Information is provided to callers 24 hours a day. Paramedics should routinely access their local poison control center. There are several advantages to this. First, there can be an immediate determination of the potential toxicity based on the type of agent, amount, time of exposure, and physical condition of the patient. Second, in about four out of five cases, definitive treatment can be started in the field. Finally, the poison control center can notify the receiving hospital of current treatment even before arrival of the patient.

GENERAL PRINCIPLES OF POISONING MANAGEMENT

Although there are specific protocols for managing various types of poisoning, there are certain principles common to all types. First, the call to assist the poisoned patient should begin with the standard primary assessment. Particular attention should be paid to the airway and respiratory status. Following the primary assessment, the secondary assessment and the history should be completed. Then, appropriate measures should be taken to limit absorption and enhance elimination of the poison. In addition, supportive care should be provided, and, if indicated, the appropriate antidote should be administered.

Absorption can be prevented or limited by decontamination, usually of the gastrointestinal tract. This minimizes the extent of toxicity and can be carried out by administering an emetic agent, such as syrup of ipecac, to empty the stomach. If the patient is unconscious or uncooperative, emptying of the stomach can be carried out by inserting a nasogastric tube and aspirating stomach contents. This is often followed by repeatedly irrigating and aspirating the stomach with water or a similar solution. Another agent useful in gastrointestinal decontamination is activated charcoal. Activated charcoal has a large surface area and can absorb the molecules of the offending poison, thereby inhibiting their absorption. Finally, gastrointestinal decontamination can be carried out using a cathartic agent. Cathartics speed up passage of the poison through the gastrointestinal system, thereby decreasing absorption.

Following decontamination attention should be turned to supportive care. Respiratory complications are common and should be managed accordingly. Cardiovascular and neurological complications can also occur.

Finally, if indicated, the appropriate **antidote** should be administered. Most poisonings will not require the administration of an antidote.

■ **antidote** a substance that neutralizes a poison or the effects of a poison.

INGESTED POISONS

General Principles of Assessment

When a person has been poisoned, rapid assessment is necessary. However, half of poisoning histories are inaccurate because of drug-induced confusion, misinformation, or deliberate attempts at deception. Still, an attempt should be made to ascertain the type and route of intoxication, the quantity of poison involved, and the time elapsed since ingestion. The victim should also be asked about chronic drug habituation or abuse, underlying medical illnesses, and allergies.

Relevant History Questions

❑ What was ingested? Obtain poison container and remaining contents. Obtain sample of ingested substance. Obtain sample of vomitus.
❑ When was substance taken? Affects decisions as to emesis, gastric lavage, the use of activated charcoal, and whether to administer an antidote.
❑ How much was taken?
❑ Has an attempt been made to induce vomiting?
❑ Has an antidote or activated charcoal been administered?
❑ Does the patient have a psychiatric history? (Pertinent to suicide attempts.)

✱ The history in an overdose patient may be unreliable.

Since the history can be unreliable, the physical examination assumes an important role. The physical examination of the poisoned patient has two purposes: (1) to provide physical evidence of intoxication, and (2) to find any underlying illnesses that may account for the patient's symptoms or that may affect the outcome of the poisoning.

First, the primary and secondary assessments should be completed. Particular attention should be paid to the skin. Are cyanosis, pallor, wasting, or needle marks present? Flushing of the skin may indicate poisoning with an anticholinergic substance. Staining of the skin may occur from chronic exposure to mercuric chloride, bromine, or similar chemicals.

Examination of the eyes may reveal pupillary constriction or dilation, which can occur with various types of poisons. During eye examination inquire about impaired vision, blurring of vision, or coloration of vision. Inspection of the mouth should be carried out to look for signs of caustic ingestion, presence of the gag reflex, the amount of salivation, any breath odor, or the presence of vomitus. Examination of the patient's chest may reveal evidence of aspiration, atelectasis, or excessive pulmonary secretions. The cardiac examination may give clues as to the type of toxin ingested. For example, the presence of tachydysrhythmias or bradydysrhythmias may suggest specific toxins. The patient who shows abdominal pain may be suffering poisoning from salicylates, methyl alcohol, caustics, or botulism toxin. Stool examination may show blood resulting from salicylate, iron, caustic, or phosphorus ingestion.

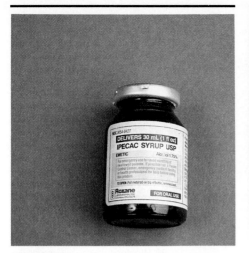

FIGURE 26-2 Syrup of ipecac is an important medication in the management of poisoning by ingestion.

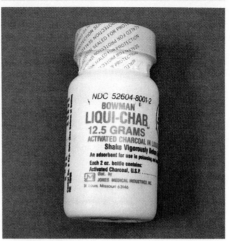

FIGURE 26-3 Activated charcoal is effective in decreasing absorption by binding the poison in the gastrointestinal system.

General Principles of Management

As mentioned previously, priorities in the treatment of the poisoned patient are maintenance of airway, breathing, and circulation. Prevention of aspiration is one of the major objectives of prehospital care. The adequacy of the patient's airway is assessed by observation of ventilatory effort, estimation of force and volume of expiration, and recognition of the sound of obstructed breathing. In cases where more definitive airway management is needed, insertion of an endotracheal tube may be necessary. Generally, nasotracheal intubation is preferred if the patient has a gag reflex. Oxygen supplementation should be routinely performed.

If the toxic substance was ingested within the past 3 to 6 hours, vomiting should be induced before arrival at the hospital emergency department. Vomiting must NOT be induced in the following circumstances:

❑ stuporous or comatose patient
❑ in the presence of seizures
❑ pregnant patient
❑ patient with possible MI
❑ patient who has ingested **corrosive substances** (strong **acids** or **alkalis**)
❑ patient who has ingested hydrocarbon substances (petroleum products)

However, there are exceptions even in the above circumstances. Vomiting SHOULD be induced if the patient has ingested:

❑ pesticides
❑ heavy metals
❑ halogenated hydrocarbons
❑ camphor-based hydrocarbons
❑ aromatic hydrocarbons

Because these substances have such a high toxicity, the risk of aspiration can be justified. However, if there is still uncertainty, the poison control center should be contacted for assistance.

■ **corrosive substances** acids, alkalis, or antiseptics.

■ **acid** a chemical substance that liberates hydrogen ions (H^+) when in solution.

■ **alkali** a strong base; a substance that liberates hydroxyl ions (OH^-) when in solution.

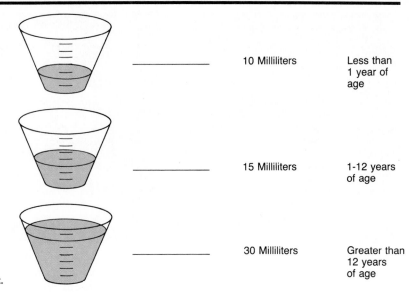

FIGURE 26-4 Dosage of syrup of ipecac.

Vomiting should be initiated as soon as possible unless contraindicated. Syrup of ipecac should be administered in the following doses (see Figure 26-4):

❑ 10 mL in patients under 1 yr. of age.
❑ 15 mL in patients 1–12 yrs.of age.
❑ 30 mL in patients over 12 yrs. of age.

Water should be given in a dose of 15 mL/kg (2–3 glasses in the adult) following the ipecac. If vomiting has not occurred within 20 to 30 minutes, the ipecac can be readministered. The patient should be appropriately positioned to prevent aspiration. Some toxicologists advocate giving the patient a carbonated beverage after the ipecac because this may stimulate vomiting more rapidly. Also, if water is not available, any acceptable beverage may be given after the ipecac (fruit juice, soda, etc.).

Activated charcoal can often be administered in the field. If administered, activated charcoal should be given as follows (see Table 26-2):

❑ *Adult:* 50–100 g mixed in tap water to make a slurry. The use of premixed preparations—for example, Actidose—is encouraged.
❑ *Pediatric:* 20–50 g (1 g/kg) mixed in tap water to make a slurry. The use of premixed preparations—for example, Actidose—is encouraged.

Maintenance of blood pressure requires adequate intravascular volume, cardiac function, and systemic vascular resistance. In addition to volume replacement with a crystalloid solution, cardiac monitoring is necessary. An IV of D5W is adequate if cardiovascular compromise is not present. Repeated assessments, including frequent monitoring of vital signs, are mandatory.

As airway, breathing, and circulation are assured, the unresponsive patient should receive 25–50 g of D50W IV push. If opiate intoxication is suspected, naloxone should be administered at 1–2 mg IV push. The administration of 100 mg of thiamine IV should also be considered if chronic alcoholism is suspected.

TABLE 26-1   Ipecac

Class:	Emetic
Actions:	Irritates the enteric tract
	Stimulates vomiting center
Indications:	Poisoning in conscious patient
Contraindications:	Vomiting should not be induced in any patient with impaired consciousness
	Poisonings involving strong acids, bases, or petroleum distillates
	Antiemetic poisonings, especially of the phenothiazine type
Precautions:	Monitor and assure a patent airway
Side Effects:	Rare
Dosage:	30 ml (1 ounce) followed by several glasses of warm water
Route:	Oral
Pediatric Dosage:	Less than 1 year of age: 5–10 mL
	Greater than 1 year of age: 15 mL repeated in 20 minutes

TABLE 26-2   Activated Charcoal

Class:	Absorbent
Action:	Adsorbs toxins by chemical binding and surface area
Indications:	Poisoning following emesis or where emesis contraindicated
Contraindications:	None in severe poisoning
Precautions:	Should only be administered following emesis in cases where it is so indicated
Side Effects:	Rare
Dosage:	Two tablespoons (50 grams) mixed with a glass of water to form a slurry
Route:	Oral
Pediatric Dosage:	Two tablespoons (50 grams) mixed with a glass of water to form a slurry

INHALED POISONS

Signs and Symptoms of Toxic Inhalations

The principal effects of inhaled toxic substances are seen in the respiratory system and include tachypnea, cough, hoarseness, stridor, dyspnea, chest pain, chest tightness, chest retraction, and wheezing, rales, or rhonchi.

1. *CNS:* dizziness, headache, confusion, seizures, hallucinations, coma
2. *Respiratory:* tachypnea, cough, hoarseness, stridor, dyspnea, retractions, wheezing, chest pain or tightness, rales or rhonchi
3. *Cardiac:* dysrhythmias

The first priority for treatment of a patient who has inhaled toxic gases or powders should be the removal of the patient from the source as soon as it is safe to do so. Below are the general principles for management of the patient exposed to an inhalational poison.

General Management: Inhalation Emergencies

✱ Your first concern in any inhalational emergency is personal safety.

1. Remove patient from poisonous environment:
   - ❑ wear protective clothing
   - ❑ use appropriate respiratory apparatus
   - ❑ remove patient's contaminated clothing
2. Perform primary and secondary assessment.
3. Perform the following management actions:
   - ❑ establish and maintain airway
   - ❑ administer oxygen
   - ❑ intubate and assist ventilations if appropriate
   - ❑ administer CPR, if necessary
   - ❑ use bag-valve-mask or demand valve
   - ❑ establish venous access
   - ❑ contact poison control

INJECTED POISONS

General Principles of Management

Bites and stings of insects, reptiles, and animals are among the most common injuries sustained by humans. The patient who has been bitten or stung can receive additional injury from bacterial contamination or from a reaction produced by an injected substance. The general principles of field management for bites and stings include:

1. Protect rescue personnel.
2. Remove the patient from danger of repeated injection.
3. If possible, identify the insect, reptile, or animal that caused the injury and bring it to the emergency center along with the patient.
4. Perform primary and secondary assessment.
5. Prevent or delay further absorption of poison.
6. Watch for anaphylactic reaction.
7. Transport the patient as rapidly as possible.
8. Contact poison control.

Insect Bites and Stings

Insect Stings.   Many people die from allergic reactions to the stings of insects from the class *hymenoptera*. As mentioned earlier, hymenoptera is the class of insects which includes the wasps, bees, hornets, and ants.

In most cases of insect bite, local treatment is all that is necessary. However, the major problem resulting from a hymenoptera sting is anaphylaxis. Signs and symptoms include the following:

- ❑ localized pain, redness, swelling
- ❑ allergic reactions (itching or flushing of skin, rash tachycardia, hypotension, bronchospasm, or laryngeal edema)

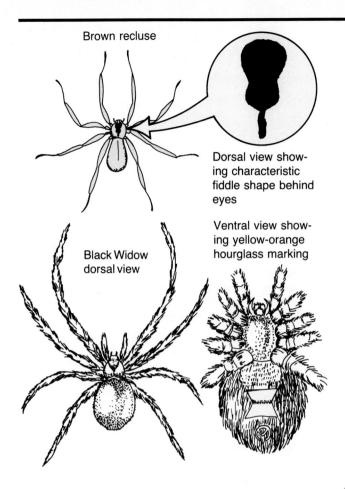

Brown recluse

Dorsal view showing characteristic fiddle shape behind eyes

Ventral view showing yellow-orange hourglass marking

Black Widow dorsal view

FIGURE 26-5 Poisonous spiders.

Management: Insect Stings

- ❑ Wash the area.
- ❑ Gently remove the stinger, if present, by scraping without squeezing the venom sac.
- ❑ Apply cool compresses to injection site.
- ❑ Observe for and treat anaphylaxis.

Brown Recluse Spider Bite. The brown recluse spider is approximately 15 mm in length and lives in the midwestern and mid-southern states. Its habitat is generally dark locations, and the brown recluse is often found in and around the house. There is a characteristic violin marking on the back, giving the spider its name of "fiddleback spider." (See Figure 26-5.)

The site of the brown recluse spider bite can become ischemic and ulcerate. Most patients are unaware that they have been bitten until after symptoms develop. Severe local symptoms include the following (see Figures 26-6 and 26-7):

- ❑ Small bleb surrounded by a white ring. This can progress to a blue necrotic lesion after a few days.
- ❑ Localized pain, redness, swelling 2-8 hours after the bite
- ❑ Localized tissue necrosis
- ❑ Chills

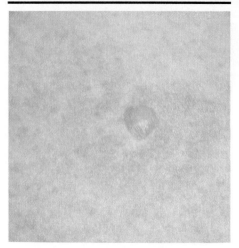

FIGURE 26-6 Brown recluse spider bite 24 hours after bite. Note the bleb and surrounding white halo. (Courtesy of Scott and White Hospital and Clinic.)

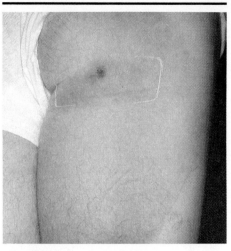

FIGURE 26-7 Brown recluse spider bite 4 days after the bite. Note the spread of erythema and early necrosis. (Courtesy of Scott and White Hospital and Clinic.)

❏ Fever
❏ Nausea and vomiting
❏ Joint pain
❏ Bleeding disorders

Prehospital treatment for the bite of the brown recluse spider is mostly supportive. No antivenom is available. However, if the patient is treated in the emergency department within 24 hours, the prognosis is usually good. Prompt administration of antihistamines may reduce systemic reactions. The patient may require surgical excision of the necrotic tissue.

Black Widow Spider Bites. Black widow spiders live in virtually all parts of the continental United States. They are commonly found in brush or wood piles. The female black widow spider is responsible for bites and is black with an orange or red hourglass figure on her abdomen. The venom of the black widow spider is very potent, producing the effects of ascending motor paralysis. The severity of the symptoms can be influenced by the patient's age, weight, and general health.

Signs and symptoms of the patient bitten by a black widow spider include the following:

❏ immediate localized pain, redness and swelling
❏ progressive muscle spasms (usually in the back or abdomen)
❏ progressive spasms of all large muscle groups
❏ severe back, chest, or shoulder pain (bite on upper extremity)
❏ severe abdominal pain (bite on lower extremity)
❏ nausea and vomiting
❏ sweating
❏ seizures
❏ paralysis
❏ hypertension
❏ diminished LOC

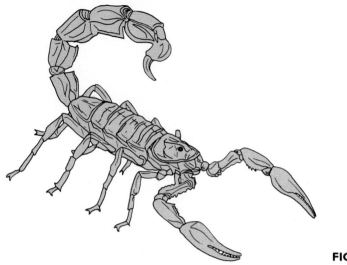

FIGURE 26-8   Scorpion.

Management: Black Widow Spider Bites

- ❑ Reassure the victim.
- ❑ Administer muscle relaxant per physician order if muscle spasms are severe: diazepam, 2.5–10 mg IV or calcium gluconate, 10 mL of a 10% solution IV.
- ❑ Transport to emergency department for antivenom.

Scorpion Stings.   Scorpions are nocturnal arachnids. (See Figure 26-8.) They hide during the day, staying beneath debris and buildings, and move at night. The poisonous scorpions live in the arid southwestern United States and Mexico. The scorpion's venom is located in a bulblike enlargement at the tip of its long tail. The scorpion stings only when provoked and injects only a small quantity of venom. Thus, fatal scorpion stings are infrequent. The scorpion's venom acts on the patient's central nervous system, by affecting the cardiac and respiratory centers.

Signs and symptoms of scorpion stings include the following:

- ❑ mild to sharp localized pain, which often progresses to numbness
- ❑ restlessness
- ❑ slurred speech
- ❑ salivation
- ❑ muscle twitching
- ❑ abdominal pain and cramps
- ❑ nausea and vomiting
- ❑ seizures

Management: Scorpion Bites

- ❑ Reassure the victim.
- ❑ Apply a constricting band above the wound site.
- ❑ Avoid the use of analgesics, which may increase the toxicity of the venom
- ❑ If systemic symptoms develop, transport to emergency department for possible administration of scorpion antiserum

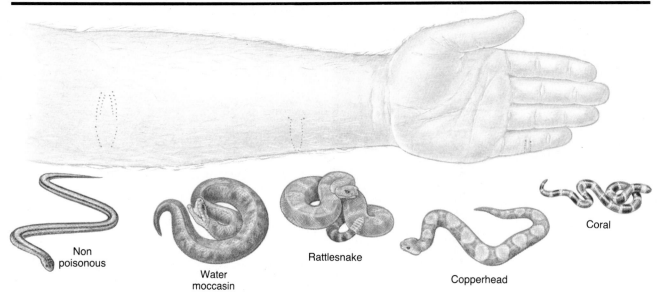

FIGURE 26-9 Types of poisonous snakes.

Labels within figure: Non poisonous, Water moccasin, Rattlesnake, Copperhead, Coral

Snake Bites

There are several thousand snake bites each year in the United States. Fortunately, these bites result in very few deaths. The signs and symptoms of snake bites depend upon the snake, the location of the bite, and the type and amount of venom injected.

There are two families of poisonous snakes native to the United States. (See Figure 26-9.) One family (*Crotalidae*) includes the pit vipers. Common pit vipers are rattlesnakes, cottonmouths (water moccasins), and copperheads. Pit vipers are so named because of the distinctive pit between the eye and the nostril on each side of the head. These snakes have elliptical pupils, two well-developed fangs, and a triangular shaped head. Only the rattlesnake, the most common pit viper, has rattles on the end of its tail.

The second family of poisonous snakes is the *Elapidae,* or coral snake, which is a distant relative of the cobra. Several varieties of coral snakes are found in the United States, primarily the southwest. Because it is a small snake and has small fangs, the coral snake cannot readily attach itself to a large surface, such as an arm or leg. The coral snake has round eyes, a narrow head, and no pit. It has characteristic yellow-banded red and black rings around its body.

■ **hydrolytic** splits compounds when in the presence of water.

Pit Vipers. Pit viper venom contains **hydrolytic** enzymes that are capable of destroying proteins and most other tissue components. These enzymes may produce destruction of red blood cells and other tissue components and may affect the body's blood clotting system within the blood vessels. This will produce infarction and tissue necrosis, especially at the site of the bite.

A severe bite of a pit viper can result in death from shock within 30 minutes. However, most deaths from pit-viper bites occur from 6 to 30 hours after the bite. Signs and symptoms of pit viper bite include the following:

❑ fang marks
❑ swelling and pain at wound site

- continued oozing at the wound site
- weakness, dizziness, or faintness
- sweating and/or chills
- thirst
- nausea and vomiting
- diarrhea
- tachycardia and hypotension
- bloody urine and gastrointestinal hemorrhage (late)
- shallow respirations progressing to respiratory failure
- numbness and tingling around face and head (classic)

Management: Pit Viper Bites.   In treating a person who has been bitten by a pit viper, the primary goal is to slow absorption of venom.

- Apply constricting band between bite and heart.
- Keep patient supine.
- Immobilize limb with splint.

Supportive care:

- Start IV with crystalloid fluid.
- Transport to Emergency Department for management which may include the administration of antivenom.

DO NOT apply ice, cold pack, or freon spray to the wound. DO NOT apply an arterial tourniquet.

Coral Snake.   The venom of the coral snake contains some of the enzymes found in pit viper venom. However, because of the presence of neurotoxin, coral snake venom primarily affects nervous tissue. The classic, severe coral snake bite will result in respiratory and skeletal muscle paralysis.

After the bite of a coral snake, there may be no local manifestations or even any systemic effects for as long as 12–24 hours. Signs and symptoms of a coral snake bite include the following:

- localized numbness, weakness, and drowsiness
- ataxia
- slurred speech and excessive salivation
- paralysis of tongue and larynx (produces difficulty breathing and swallowing)
- drooping of eyelids, double vision, dilated pupils
- abdominal pain
- nausea and vomiting
- loss of consciousness
- seizures
- respiratory failure
- hypotension

Management: Coral Snake Bite

- Wash wound with copious amounts of water.
- Apply constricting band between bite and heart.

✱ Use common sense with snake bites. Apply constricting band, keep the patient supine, splint the affected limb, administer oxygen, and start an intravenous lifeline.

☐ Immobilize limb with splint.

☐ Start IV using crystalloid fluid.

☐ Transport to emergency department for administration of antivenin.

DO NOT apply ice, cold pack, or freon sprays to the wound. DO NOT incise the wound.

Marine Animal Injection

✱ Heat will relieve pain and help inactivate the venom of many marine animals.

Injection of toxins from marine life can result from stings of jellyfish and corals or from punctures by the bony spines of animals such as sea urchins and sting-rays. All venoms of marine animals contain substances that produce pain out of proportion to the size of the injury. These poisonous toxins are unstable and heat labile. Heat will relieve pain and inactivate the venom.

Both fresh water and salt water contain considerable bacterial and viral pollution. Therefore, secondary infection is always a possibility in injuries from marine animals. Signs and symptoms of marine animal injection include the following:

☐ intense local pain and swelling

☐ weakness

☐ nausea and vomiting

☐ dyspnea

☐ tachycardia

☐ hypotension or shock (severe cases)

Management: Marine Animal Injection

☐ Establish and maintain airway.

☐ Apply constricting band between wound and heart.

☐ Apply heat.

☐ Inactivate or remove any stingers.

SURFACE ABSORBED POISONS

Many poisons can be absorbed through the skin. These include the organophosphates, cyanide, and others. Treatment includes the following:

1. Remove patient from poisonous environment:
   ☐ Wear protective clothing.
   ☐ Use appropriate respiratory apparatus.
   ☐ Remove patient's contaminated clothing.
2. Perform primary and secondary assessment.
3. Take the following management actions:
   ☐ Establish and maintain airway.
   ☐ Administer oxygen.
   ☐ Intubate and assist ventilations if appropriate.
   ☐ Administer CPR, if necessary.
   ☐ Use bag-valve-mask or demand valve.
   ☐ Establish venous access.
   ☐ Contact poison control.

DRUG OVERDOSE

In general terms, drug overdose refers to poisoning from a pharmacological substance, either legal or illegal. This can occur by accident, miscalculation, changes in the strength of a drug, suicide, polydrug use, or recreational drug usage. Many overdose emergencies seen in the field occur in the habitual drug abuser. It is most difficult to obtain a good history in these cases. However, if the paramedic is familiar with street-drug slang, a more accurate history may be obtained. It is imperative that the paramedic maintain a nonjudgmental attitude in these cases, even though this may be difficult. (See Tables 26-3 and 26-4.)

TABLE 26-3 Common Drugs of Abuse

Drug	Symptoms	Routes	Prehospital Management
Alcohol Beer whiskey gin vodka wine tequila	-CNS depression -slurred speech -disordered thought -impaired judgement -diuresis -stumbling gait -stupor -coma	-oral	-ABC's -provide respiratory support -oxygenate -establish intravenous access -Administer 100 mg thiamine intra- venously -ECG monitor -Dextrostix -administer D50W if hypoglycemic
Cocaine crack rock	-euphoria -hyperactivity -dilated pupils -psychosis -twitching -anxiety -hypertension -tachycardia -chest pain -seizures	-snorting -injection -smoking (freebasing)	-ABC's -provide respiratory support -oxygenate -ECG monitor -establish intravenous access -treat life-threatening dysrhythmias -seizure precautions
Opiates heroin morphine methadone codeine Darvon Demerol Dilaudid	-altered mental status -constricted pupils -depressed respira- tions -hypotension -bradycardia -pulmonary edema -hypothermia	-injection -oral	-ABC's -provide respiratory support -oxygenate -establish intravenous access -administer 1–2 mg Narcan intra- venously or endotracheally until respirations improve -cardiac monitor
Marijuana grass weed hashish	-euphoria -dry mouth -dilated pupils -altered sensation	-smoked	-ABC's -reassure the patient -speak in a quiet voice -ECG monitor if indicated

(continued)

TABLE 26-3 Common Drugs of Abuse (*continued*)

Drug	Symptoms	Routes	Prehospital Management
Amphetamines Benzedrine Dexedrine Ritalin "speed"	-exhilaration -hyperactivity -dilated pupils -hypertension -psychosis -tremors -seizures	-oral -injected	-ABC's -oxygenate -ECG monitor -establish intravenous access -treat life-threatening dysrhythmias
Hallucinogens LSD STP mescaline psilocybin	-psychosis -nausea -dilated pupils -rambling speech -headache -dizziness -suggestibility -distortion of sensory perceptions -hallucinations	-oral -smoked	-ABC's -reassure the patient -"talk down" the "high" patient -protect the patient from injury -provide a dark, quiet environment -speak in a soft, quiet voice
Sedatives Seconal Valium Librium Xanax pentobarbital Halcion Restoril Dalmane	-altered mental status -hypotension -slurred speech -respiratory depres- sion -shock -bradycardia -seizures	-oral	-ABC's -respiratory suppoprt -oxygenate -establish intravenous access -ECG monitor -medical control may order Narcan

TABLE 26-4 Common Drug Overdoses

Drug	Signs and Symptoms	Prehospital Management
Acetaminophen Tylenol Tempra	-anorexia -nausea -vomiting -malaise -diaphoresis -RUQ pain	-ABC's -respiratory support -establish intravenous access -administer ipecac and activated charcoal as ordered by medical control -ECG monitor -contact poison control as indicated
Alcohol beer wine whiskey gin vodka tequila	-altered mental status -coma -seizures -hallucinations -delirium tremens -coma -death	-ABC's -respiratory support -oxygenate -establish intravenous access -administer 100 mg thiamine IV -Dextrostix -administer D50W if hypoglycemic -administer Valium IV for seizures

TABLE 26-4 Common Drug Overdoses (*continued*)

Drug	Signs and Symptoms	Prehospital Management
Salicylates Bayer Excedrin Bufferin Oil of Winter- green Aspirin	-nausea -vomiting -confusion -lethargy -seizures -dysrhythmias -coma -death	-ABC's -respiratory support -oxygenate -establish intravenous access -ECG monitor -fluid challenge as ordered -treat life-threatening dysrhythmias -ipecac and activated charcoal as ordered by medical control -administer sodium bicarbonate as ordered by medical control
Benzodiazepines Valium Librium Xanax Halcion Restoril Dalmane Centrax Ativan Serax	-altered mental status -slurred speech -dysrhythmias -coma	-ABC's -respiratory support -oxygenate -ipecac and activated charcoal as ordered by medical control -establish intravenous access -ECG monitor -contact poison control
Narcotics heroin codeine Demerol morphine Dilaudid Talwin Darvon Darvocet methadone	-CNS depression -constricted pupils -respiratory depression -hypotension -bradycardia -pulmonary edema -coma -death	-ABC's -respiratory support -oxygenate -establish intravenous access -administer 1–2 mg Narcan intrave- nously or endotracheally as ordered by medical control until res- pirations improve -ECG monitor
Tricyclic *Antidepressants* Elavil Triavil Norpramin Doxepin Asendin Pamelor Sinequan Tofranil	-CNS depression -tachycardia -dilated pupils -respiratory depression -slurred speech -twitching, jerking -seizures -ST and T wave changes -AV blocks -shock	-ABC's -respiratory support -oxygenate -establish intravenous access -ECG monitor -ipecac and activated charcoal as ordered by medical control -administer sodium bicarbonate if ordered by medical control -contact poison control

■ **benzodiazepines** general term to describe a group of tranquilizing drugs with similar chemical structures.

The presentation of the drug overdose will vary based on the substance used. Management should be the same as for any ingested, inhaled, or injected poison. *Poison control should be contacted for additional direction.*

ALCOHOL

Alcohol (ethyl alcohol, or ethanol) depresses the central nervous system, potentially to the point of stupor, coma, and death. In patients with severe liver disease, metabolism of alcohol may become impaired, which increases the course and severity of intoxication. At low doses, alcohol has excitatory and stimulating effects, thus depressing inhibitions. At higher doses alcohol's depressive effect is more obvious. Abuse of, and dependence on alcohol is called *alcoholism* and is a major problem in our society.

Many highway traffic fatalities involve an alcohol-intoxicated driver. Alcohol is also a major factor in drownings, burns, trauma, and drug overdoses.

Alcohol is completely absorbed from the stomach and intestinal tract in approximately 30 to 120 minutes after ingestion. Once absorbed, alcohol is distributed to all body tissues and fluids, with concentrations of alcohol in the brain rapidly approaching the alcohol level in the blood.

Alcohol should always be considered a CNS depressant despite the initial increased activity as seen with lower doses. In addition, alcohol causes a peripheral vasodilator effect on the cardiovascular system, resulting in flushing and a feeling of warmth. Therefore, in extreme cold conditions, alcohol may cause the blood vessels to dilate, resulting in an increased loss of body heat. The diuretic effect seen when large amounts of alcohol are ingested is due to the inhibition of vasopressin, which is the hormone responsible for the conservation of body fluids. Without vasopressin, an increase in urine flow occurs. The "dry mouth" syndrome experienced after alcohol consumption may be the result of alcohol-induced cellular dehydration.

General Alcoholic Profile

- ❑ Drinks early in the day.
- ❑ Prone to drink alone and secretly.
- ❑ Periodic binges (may last for several days).
- ❑ Partial or total loss of memory during period of drinking.
- ❑ Unexplained history of gastrointestinal problems (especially bleeding).
- ❑ "Green Tongue Syndrome" (using chlorophyll-containing substances to disguise the odor of alcohol on the breath).
- ❑ Cigarette burns on clothing.
- ❑ Chronically flushed face and palms.
- ❑ Tremulousness.
- ❑ Odor of alcohol on breath under inappropriate conditions.

Consequences of Chronic Alcohol Ingestion

- ❑ Poor nutrition.
- ❑ Alcohol hepatitis.
- ❑ Liver cirrhosis.
- ❑ Loss of sensation in hands and feet.
- ❑ Loss of cerebellar function (balance and coordination).

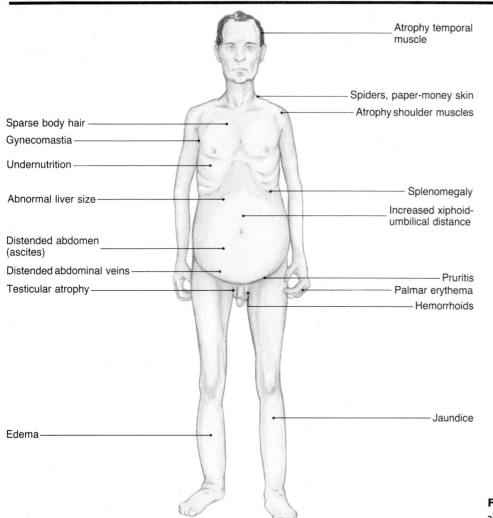

Atrophy temporal muscle

Spiders, paper-money skin

Atrophy shoulder muscles

Sparse body hair

Gynecomastia

Undernutrition

Abnormal liver size

Splenomegaly

Increased xiphoid-umbilical distance

Distended abdomen (ascites)

Distended abdominal veins

Testicular atrophy

Pruritis

Palmar erythema

Hemorrhoids

Jaundice

Edema

FIGURE 26-10 The chronic alcoholic.

❑ Pancreatitis.
❑ Upper gastrointestinal hemorrhage (often fatal).
❑ Hypoglycemia.
❑ Subdural hematoma (due to falls).
❑ Rib and extremity fractures (due to falls). (See Figure 26-10.)

Symptoms of alcohol intoxication can be produced by some drugs and by many medical conditions such as diabetic coma and subdural hematoma. The odor of the patient's breath should be considered a poor indicator of alcohol intoxication.

Withdrawal Syndrome. The alcoholic may suffer a withdrawal reaction either because of abrupt discontinuation of the ingestion after prolonged use or as the blood alcohol level falls after acute intoxication. Withdrawal symptoms can occur several hours after sudden abstinence and can last up to 5 to 7 days. Seizures (sometimes called "rum fits") may occur within the first 24–36 hours of abstinence. **Delirium tremens** (**DT's**) usually develops on the second or third day of the withdrawal. Delirium tremens is characterized by a decreased level of consciousness, and the patient hallucinates and misinterprets nearby events. Seizures and delirium tremens are ominous signs. There is a significant mortality from delirium tremens. Medical control may order diazepam in severe cases.

Signs and symptoms of withdrawal syndrome include the following:

- ❑ coarse tremor of hands, tongue, and eyelids
- ❑ nausea and vomiting
- ❑ general weakness
- ❑ increased sympathetic tone
- ❑ tachycardia
- ❑ sweating
- ❑ hypertension
- ❑ orthostatic hypotension
- ❑ anxiety
- ❑ irritability or a depressed mood
- ❑ hallucinations
- ❑ poor sleep

Some alcoholics will drink methanol (wood alcohol) or ethylene glycol (a component of antifreeze) if ethanol is unavailable. Ingestion of these chemicals can cause blindness or death. Alcohol intoxication, whether acute or chronic, should not be underestimated as a toxic emergency problem.

Management: Alcohol Ingestion

- ❑ Establish and maintain airway
- ❑ Induce emesis using ipecac, depending on age of victim, amount of alcohol ingested, and vital signs (check local protocols)
- ❑ Start IV using D5W
- ❑ Administer 100 mg of thiamine
- ❑ Administer 25 g of D50W
- ❑ Reassure the patient

SUMMARY

The effective treatment of poisoning is based on two factors: (1) prompt recognition of the poisoning and (2) an accurate and thorough initial patient evaluation. The basic concept for prehospital treatment is the prompt removal of the poison and the prevention of further absorption. In addition, supportive and specific management should be carried out as indicated based on the route of toxic exposure. Often the initial prehospital treatment will include the administration of syrup of ipecac and of activated charcoal. If these steps are completed promptly, the need for additional measures will be minimized.

FURTHER READING

BAYER, MARK J., RUMACK, BARRY H., and WANKE, LEE A. *Toxicological Emergencies.* Bowie, MD: Brady Communications, 1984.

BEHRMAN, RICHARD and VAUGH, V.C. *Nelson's Textbook of Pediatrics,* 13th ed. Philadelphia, PA: W. B. Saunders, 1987.

BLEDSOE, BRYAN E., BOSKER, GIDEON, and PAPA, FRANK J. *Prehospital Emergency Pharmacology,* 2nd ed. Englewood Cliffs, NJ: Prentice Hall, Inc., 1988.

GOODMAN, L.S., GILMAN, A. *The Pharmacological Basis of Therapeutics,* 7th ed. New York, NY: Macmillan, 1985.

GRANT, HARVEY D., MURRAY, ROBERT H., and BERGERON, J. DAVID. *Emergency Care,* 5th ed. Englewood Cliffs, NJ: Prentice Hall, Inc., 1990.

WALRAVEN, GAIL, et al. *Manual of Advanced Prehospital Care,* 2nd ed. Bowie, MD: Robert J. Brady Company, 1984.

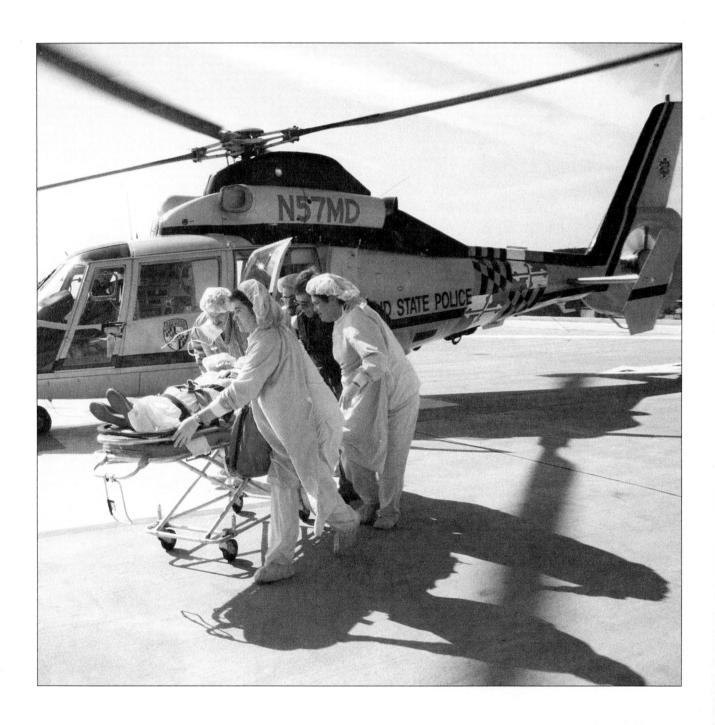

27

Infectious Diseases

Objectives for Chapter 27

Upon completing this chapter, the student should be able to:

1. Define the following terms:
   - virus
   - fungus
   - antibody
   - bacteria
   - antigen
2. Briefly discuss the body's immune system.
3. Define toxin and give example of endotoxins and exotoxins.
4. Describe the difference between bacterial and viral infections.
5. Define the following:
   - leukocytes
   - humoral immunity
   - cell-mediated immunity
   - macrophages
6. Describe important factors in the transmission of disease.
7. Describe meningitis, its presentation, prehospital care, and appropriate safety precautions.

8. Describe tuberculosis, its presentation, prehospital care, and appropriate safety precautions.
9. Describe gastroenteritis, its presentation, prehospital care, and appropriate safety precautions.
10. Describe hepatitis, its presentation, prehospital care, and appropriate safety precautions.
11. Define common sexually transmitted disease and prehospital management.
12. Define acquired immune deficiency syndrome (AIDS).
13. Differentiate AIDS and ARC.
14. Describe methods of HIV transmission.
15. List precautions that should be employed to protect prehospital personnel from AIDS and HIV.
16. Define "Universal Precautions."
17. Describe scabies and lice.
18. Describe common childhood diseases and their implication for prehospital care.

Sunday morning begins uneventfully as it usually does for the paramedics of Station 10. The ambulance and fire engine have been washed and returned to the bay. Also, the patient compartment of the ambulance has been cleaned, as is usually required following a Saturday night. The paramedics now on duty are always particularly careful about cleaning those surfaces that patients frequently contact.

At approximately 10:30 AM the alarm sounds. The watch officer hands the computer printout to the driver stating, "Your day isn't off to a bang." The printout gives the patient's address and the cross street. Under the comments section is the statement, "Patient states his cigarettes don't taste good anymore." The crew of Medic 10 go en route leaving the laughs and comments of the crew from Engine 10 behind.

The trip to the scene takes approximately 2 minutes. The house is a rundown structure, with all of the windows open and the curtains blowing freely in the Texas summer breeze. The paramedics find the patient sitting on the couch, in the dark, with a package of cigarettes beside him. "I just ain't feeling worth a damn," the man says. He explains that he hasn't felt like working and hasn't wanted to drink a beer. Even his cigarettes don't taste good anymore.

The paramedics open the curtains to let in some light. They notice immediately that the patient has a definite yellow hue to his eyes and skin. Both paramedics now don gloves, follow universal precautions, and complete the patient assessment. The physical examination is essentially unremarkable, except for multiple needle tracks on both forearms and the neck. There is also some tenderness in the upper right quadrant of the abdomen. When questioned, the patient states that he has been "shooting up" for several years. He primarily uses heroin and occasionally crack. He states his urine has been dark brown for over a week. His live-in girlfriend, who has left for work at the restaurant where she is a waitress, has had dark urine as well.

The paramedics suspect hepatitis and transport the patient to the hospital. No advanced skills are needed. After delivering the patient, the paramedics immediately wash their hands and disinfect the ambulance with bleach and water. Linen used on the call is left at the hospital in the infectious linen bag. A communicable disease exposure report is completed.

Approximately a week later the paramedics receive a report that the patient did indeed have hepatitis B. His liver enzymes were markedly elevated and his blood showed the hepatitis B surface antigen, indicating acute infection. Both paramedics had fortunately received the hepatitis B vaccine while in school.

INTRODUCTION

Infectious diseases are those illnesses caused by infection or infestation of the human body by various biological agents. These diseases, which account for most of the known human and animal diseases, generally are not life threatening. Paramedics must, however, recognize several infectious diseases in the emergency setting either to begin emergency treatment of the patient or to protect emergency personnel. Because of acquired immune deficiency syndrome (AIDS) these procedures have become even more important. This chapter will first address the fundamental principles of infectious disease as they apply to prehospital care. Next it examines the various infectious diseases that emergency personnel may encounter.

PATHOGENESIS OF INFECTIOUS DISEASE

Several biological agents can cause human infection. These include bacteria, viruses, fungi, and parasites. Since treatment and management of the different infections vary significantly, paramedics need to recognize the causative agent of the more commonly encountered infectious diseases.

Many infections are caused by bacteria. **Bacteria** are small, unicellular organisms that live throughout the environment. Smaller than human red blood cells, they can only be viewed through the microscope. Bacteria are capable of living without the presence of another organism. Many of the common infections in medicine are caused by bacteria, including middle ear infections in children, many cases of tonsillitis, and meningitis. Most bacterial infections respond to treatment with drugs called **antibiotics.** Once administered, antibiotics kill or inhibit the growth of invading bacteria by one of several mechanisms. Bacteria can usually be cultured and identified readily in most hospital laboratories.

Many bacteria are categorized according to their appearance under the microscope after staining with several dyes referred to as a Gram stain. Some bacteria are blue in color after Gram staining, while others are red. Bacteria that stain blue are referred to as Gram positive bacteria. They are somewhat similar to each other in their composition. Bacteria that stain red are referred to as Gram negative. They are also somewhat similar to each other in their structure.

Simple infection is not the only consequence of a bacterial infection. Many bacteria release poisonous chemicals, or **toxins.** There are two general categories of toxins: exotoxins and endotoxins. *Exotoxins* are released from living bacteria during infection. They travel through the blood or lymph throughout the body, ultimately causing problems. The life-threatening consequences of tetanus infection is an example of the effects of an exotoxin. Tetanus is caused by the bacteria *Clostridium tetani.* The actual infection by the bacteria is mild and may be limited, for example, to a puncture wound in the foot. Yet, on entering the body, the bacteria releases its toxin, called *tetanospasmin.* This toxin then travels through the blood to the skeletal muscles, causing the spastic rigidity classically seen in tetanus. Other bacteria release toxins referred to as endotoxins. *Endotoxins* are usually released upon the death and destruction of the bacterial cell. Septic shock, for example, is caused by the release of an endotoxin from several Gram-negative bacteria.

Most infections are caused by biological agents called **viruses.** Viruses are much smaller than bacteria and cannot grow without the assistance of another organism. In fact, viruses are referred to as intracellular parasites, since they must invade the cells of the organism they infect. Once inside a cell they take over, using the various cellular enzymes to replicate and produce more viruses. Viruses cannot reproduce outside of the host cell, and, unlike bacteria, they are very difficult to treat. Once a virus infects a cell it can only be killed by destroying the infected cell. Drugs have not yet been developed that can selectively destroy cells infected by viruses, while simultaneously leaving uninfected cells unharmed. This partially explains the dilemma facing researchers attempt-

■ **bacteria** small, unicellular organisms present throughout the environment. They are capable of life independent of other organisms.

■ **antibiotics** medications effective in inhibiting the growth or killing of bacteria. They have no impact on viruses.

■ **toxins** poisonous chemicals secreted by bacteria or released following destruction of the bacteria.

■ **virus** microscopic organism, smaller than the bacteria, which require the assistance of another organism for their survival. Viruses are a common cause of human disease.

ing to find a cure for AIDS. Most viral illnesses, fortunately, are mild and fairly self-limited. But severe viral infections cannot be treated, at present, with other than symptomatic care.

■ **fungi** class of organisms containing yeast and molds.

Another biological agent that can cause human infection are **fungi** (the plural of fungus). More like plants than animals, they include yeasts and molds. Fungi rarely cause human disease other than minor skin infections, such as athlete's foot and some of the more common vaginal infections. Fungi infections are commonly called *mycoses.* Patients whose immune system is impaired are much more vulnerable to fungal infection than healthy people. In such patients the fungi can invade the lungs, blood, and several organs. Treatment of complicated, deep fungal infections is difficult.

Finally, *parasites* are also responsible for human infection. They can range from small unicellular organisms, not much larger than bacteria, to large intestinal worms. Parasites are relatively rare in the United States. Treatment depends on the organism and the location.

IMMUNITY

The body has a very complicated system for fighting disease called the *immune system.* Our white blood cells, or *leukocytes,* are primarily responsible for fighting infection. Once a bacterial or viral infection begins, the immune system immediately responds to suppress and kill it. Most viruses and bacteria have proteins on their surface called **antigens.** The human immune system detects these antigens as being foreign and responds.

■ **antigens** proteins capable of eliciting an immune response.

There are two general parts to the immune response. One is called *cell-mediated immunity* and the other *humoral immunity.* Cell-mediated immunity is derived from special leukocytes called *T lymphocytes.* They originate in the thymus, a gland located in the upper part of the chest. T cells are primarily responsible for fighting infections of biological agents living in certain body cells. Examples of such infections include tuberculosis, many viral infections, and most fungal infections. Such infections result in movement of white cells to the site of infection, which then attack and eliminate the infection.

■ **antibody** protein complex produced by the immune system in response to an antigen. An antibody marks the antigen for removal by other components of the immune system.

In contrast, humoral immunity derives from *B lymphocytes* and results in the formation of special proteins called **antibodies.** There are five classes of human antibodies. They include:

- ❏ IgM: the antibody that responds immediately.
- ❏ IgG: the antibody that has "memory" and recognizes a repeatedly invading infection.
- ❏ IgA: the antibody present in the mucous membranes.
- ❏ IgE: the antibody contributing to allergic and anaphylactic responses.
- ❏ IgD: the antibody present in the lowest concentration.

■ **lymphatic system** a complex network of small thin vessels, valves, ducts, lymph nodes and organs which helps to protect and maintain the fluid environment of the body and plays a major role in fighting disease. The lymph is restored to the regular circulation by the thoracic duct and the lymphatic duct.

Antibodies are produced in response to antigens. The two combine, forming what is commonly called the *antigen-antibody complex.* This large complex is then removed by scavenger cells such as *macrophages.*

Cells in the body are surrounded by fluid referred to as interstitial fluid. Along with killed or inactivated infectious agents, water and solutes filter out of the capillaries into the **lymphatic system.** A separate circulatory system, the lymphatic system filters the fluid, called lymph, before returning it to the venous system. A key organ in the lymphatic system is the *spleen.* Located in the left upper quadrant of the abdomen,

on any mucous membrane. If untreated, the chancre will ultimately disappear and the patient may become asymptomatic.

Secondary Stage: Approximately six to eight weeks after the appearance of the chancre, the patient will develop headache, malaise, anorexia, fever, and often a sore throat. A reddish rash develops on both the palms of the hands and the soles of the feet. Often referred to as the *latent stage*, this stage, if untreated, will end and the patient may again become asymptomatic.

Tertiary Stage: Months or years after the secondary stage, the patient will enter the tertiary phase of syphilis. In this stage the bacteria invade various blood vessels, especially the aorta and the central nervous system. The spinal cord is particularly vulnerable, and a syndrome called tabes dorsalis develops. *Tabes dorsalis* is characterized by a wide gait, slapping of the feet on the ground, and ataxia. In addition, tertiary syphilis is also characterized by psychosis. If untreated, especially in the tertiary stage, the disease will be fatal. A common cause of death is rupture of the aorta due to weakening of the aortic wall from infection by syphilis bacteria.

Gonorrhea and Chlamydia.   Gonorrhea is another common sexually transmitted disease which has been a public health problem for many years. Caused by the bacteria *Neisseria gonorrhea,* it exists throughout the world. In the male, gonorrhea is characterized by burning urination and yellowish penile discharge. In the female, it is not always symptomatic. Recently, gonorrhea has been surpassed in frequency of infection by Chlamydia. Caused by the bacteria *Chlamydia trachomatis,* chlamydia has symptoms quite similar to those of gonorrhea. Both gonorrhea and chlamydia are common causes of pelvic inflammatory disease in the female.

Herpes.   Herpes is a sexually transmitted disease caused by the herpes virus. The herpes class of viruses is a common source of human disease. There are two general categories of herpetic infections. They include:

Herpes Simplex, Type I: Herpes simplex Type I causes thin-walled vesicles, usually around the mouth and lips. Commonly called "cold sores," these infections tend to be self-limited.

Herpes Simplex, Type II: Herpes simplex, Type II causes genital herpes. This infection is quite painful, resulting in thin-walled vesicles on the genitalia. Other signs and symptoms include burning, itching, tingling, and tenderness. In some cases these may be accompanied by fever, swollen lymph glands, and general malaise. The infection is recurrent and no curative treatment is available. If the patient is pregnant she should be asked when the most recent recurrence of the infection occurred. This information should be noted on the patient report form and relayed to emergency department personnel. Women who have active herpes lesions at the time of delivery are typically delivered by Caesarean section to prevent the baby from becoming infected as it passes through the birth canal.

✱ Herpes Whitlow, a herpes infection of the finger, can occur following contact with a person who has an active herpes lesion.

Paramedic Protection.   When treating or transporting a patient suspected of having a sexually transmitted disease, paramedics should follow these precautions:

❑ Wear gloves at all times.
❑ Wash hands following contact with any body secretion.
❑ Notify emergency department personnel.
❑ Dispose of or sterilize all instruments used.
❑ Bag and label all linen.

■ **acquired immune deficiency syndrome (AIDS)** fatal illness caused by infection with the Human Immunodeficiency Virus (HIV). Because AIDS destroys the ability of the immune system to fight infection, patients die from overwhelming infection. Also called HIV infection.

HIV Infection. **Acquired immune deficiency syndrome (AIDS)** was virtually unheard of ten years ago. Today it is a world-wide epidemic and a virtual threat to every individual.

AIDS is caused by the *Human Immunodeficiency Virus (HIV)*. This virus, formerly called HTLV-III, has only recently been identified. The HIV virus is transmitted through body secretions, including:

❑ blood
❑ vaginal secretions
❑ semen

Although not common, transmission of the virus is theoretically possible through:

❑ Tears
❑ Cerebrospinal fluid
❑ Saliva
❑ Breast milk
❑ Amniotic fluid
❑ Urine

People at high risk are those who have increased exposure to blood or body secretions. Initial high-risk groups included homosexual and bisexual males, IV drug abusers, and hemophiliacs. But now AIDS is occurring with increasing frequency in the heterosexual population. Health care workers are conceivably at increased risk because of potential contact with contaminated blood or body secretions. Yet infection of those who work with AIDS patients has been exceedingly rare.

The HIV virus can enter the body via breaks in the skin, through mucous membranes or the eyes, or by transmission through the placenta from an infected mother to her fetus. Once in the blood, the virus affects the T lymphocytes of the immune system. Following the incubation period—lasting from six months to several years—the virus destroys certain T lymphocytes. This weakens the entire immune system, making the body susceptible to infection.

AIDS-Related Complex (ARC). The HIV infected patient may first develop vague symptoms such as fatigue, fever, chronic diarrhea, and weight loss. This group of symptoms is a pre-AIDS state referred to as *AIDS-Related Complex (ARC)*. Most patients develop full-blown AIDS although others, for some unknown reason, remain in the ARC stage.

Advanced Disease (AIDS). Many ARC patients progress to AIDS and most will ultimately die. Initially, the patient presenting with ARC symptoms will show generalized swelling of the lymph nodes which becomes quite striking in conjunction with the weight loss. Many patients will develop unusual, purplish skin tumors, known as *Kaposi's sarcoma,* anywhere on the body. They will also develop severe pneumonia. Most pneumonia associated with AIDS is due to infection with the parasite *Pneu-*

mocystis carinii. There may also be secondary infection with bacteria related to the causative agent of tuberculosis. As the disease progresses, the central nervous system becomes involved and a psychosis, commonly called *AIDS encephalopathy,* will develop. Death usually results from overwhelming infection, loss of respiratory function due to pneumonia, and, often, suicide. (See Figure 27-1.)

At present there is no cure or vaccine for AIDS. There are several drugs, such as AZT, which are being used in treatment. These drugs alleviate many of the symptoms, but have little effect on the overall course of the disease.

AIDS patients are obviously difficult to treat. Despite some recent changes in societal attitudes, they are often shunned and condemned. Even if medicine has little to offer them in terms of treatment, it is tremendously important for prehospital personnel to be compassionate, understanding, and nonjudgmental. While paramedics must take precautions to prevent disease transmission, they need to do this in a humane and compassionate manner.

Paramedic Precautions. The Centers for Disease Control in Atlanta, Georgia, has recommended the following **universal precautions** for persons, such as EMS personnel, who are at increased risk for exposure to

■ **universal precautions** set of procedures and precautions published by the Centers for Disease Control to assist health care personnel in protecting themselves from infectious disease.

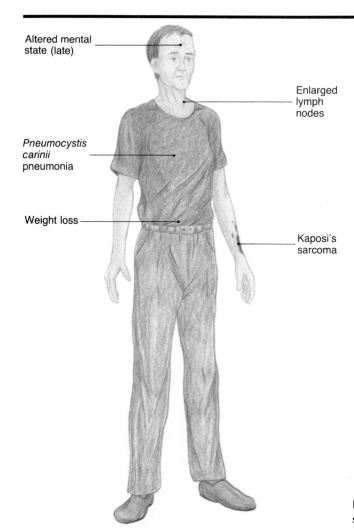

Altered mental state (late)

Enlarged lymph nodes

Pneumocystis carinii pneumonia

Weight loss

Kaposi's sarcoma

FIGURE 27-1 The patient with acquired immune deficiency syndrome (AIDS).

all blood-borne infections including AIDS. Since it is impossible to determine reliably which patients have a blood-borne infection, the following precautions are recommended *FOR ALL PATIENTS:*

1. All health-care workers should routinely use appropriate barrier precautions to prevent skin and mucous membrane exposure when contact with blood, or other body fluids, of ANY patient may be anticipated. Gloves should be worn when touching blood and body fluids, mucous membranes, or nonintact skin, in handling items or surfaces soiled with blood or body fluids, and for performing venipuncture or other vascular access procedures. (See Figure 27-2.) After contact with each patient, gloves should be changed and disposed of. To prevent exposure of mucous membranes of the mouth, nose, and eyes, masks and protective eye wear, or protective face shields should be worn during procedures that are likely to generate droplets of blood or other body fluids. (See Figure 27-3.) If, during a procedure, a glove is torn or a needle stick occurs, the glove should be removed and replaced as soon as possible. The needle or instrument should also be discarded and another obtained. Gowns or aprons should be worn during any procedure likely to generate splashes of bloods or other body fluids.

2. Hands and other skin surfaces should be washed immediately and thoroughly if contaminated with blood or other body fluids. After gloves are removed, hands also should be washed immediately.

3. All health-care workers should take precautions to prevent injuries caused by needles, scalpels, or other sharp instruments or devices during procedures, cleaning of instruments, or during disposal of instruments. To prevent needle stick injuries, needles SHOULD NOT be recapped, purposely bent, broken by hand, removed from disposable syringes, or otherwise manipulated by hand. After they are used, disposable syringes and needles, scalpel blades, and other sharp items should be placed in puncture-resistant containers for disposal. These containers should be placed as close as possible to work areas.

4. Although saliva has not been directly implicated in HIV transmission, mouth pieces, resuscitation bags, or ventilation devices should be

✱ Universal precautions should be just that; you should assume every patient is infected and follow the universal precautions detailed here.

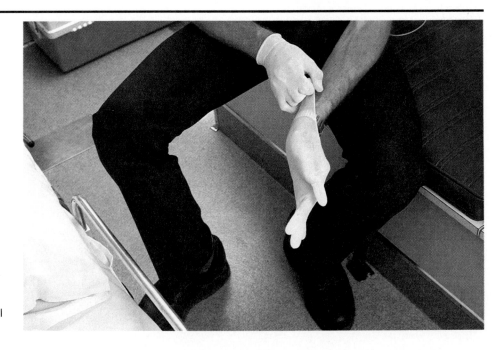

FIGURE 27-2 Wear gloves at all times.

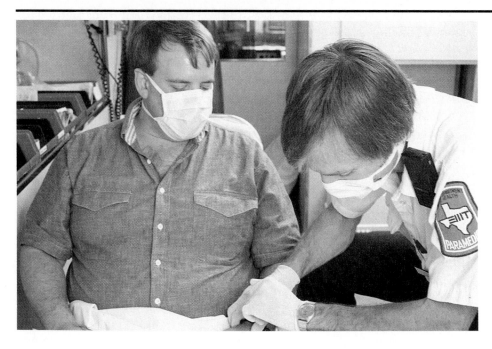

FIGURE 27-3 Use respiratory protection if a respiratory infectious disease, such as tuberculosis, is suspected.

immediately available for use in areas in which the need for resuscitation is predictable to avoid the need for mouth-to-mouth ventilation.

5. Health-care workers who have exudative or weeping skin lesions should refrain from direct patient care and from handling patient care equipment until the condition resolves.

6. Pregnant health care workers are not known to be at greater risk of contracting HIV infection than health care workers who are not pregnant. If, however, a health care worker develops HIV infection during pregnancy, the infant is at risk from perinatal transmission. Therefore, pregnant health care workers should be especially familiar with, and strictly adhere to, precautions to minimize the risk of HIV transmission.

Skin Infections

There are many skin infections and most are not a threat to health care workers. It is, however, important that EMS personnel be familiar with the common skin parasites, scabies and lice.

Scabies. Scabies is a highly communicable skin disease caused by a species of mite. This infection, commonly called "the seven year itch," results from burrowing of the mite into the skin. The webs of the fingers and toes are among the most common sites of infections. Close inspection may reveal the small mite burrows. Besides these burrows, papules may be present. Both are associated with intense itching.

Lice. Lice are parasites slightly larger than mites. Becoming attached to hair follicles, they ultimately lay their eggs, or "nits," there. Patients infested with lice usually experience severe itching and have small white specks in the hair. Close inspection will frequently reveal the parasite itself. As with scabies, lice infestation is highly communicable and precautions should be taken.

Paramedic Precautions. When treating or transporting patients suspected of having scabies or lice, paramedics should follow these precautions:

- ❑ Wear gloves at all times.
- ❑ Wash hands following contact with the patient.
- ❑ Notify emergency department personnel.
- ❑ Dispose of or sterilize all instruments used.
- ❑ Bag and label all linen.

Childhood Diseases

Most children are required by law to have vaccination against the common childhood diseases. Vaccines are now available for mumps, measles, German measles, polio, diphtheria, whooping cough, and tetanus. Some children also receive a vaccine against *Haemophilus influenza* meningitis. Nevertheless, most children are not vaccinated against chicken pox.

Measles. Measles, commonly called red measles, is not common due to widespread vaccination. Caused by the measles (rubeola) virus, the infection is primarily transmitted through the respiratory tract. In rare epidemic situations, persons born since 1956 and not vaccinated after 1968 are at risk for developing measles due to changes that have occurred in the vaccine.

The incubation period is eight to thirteen days. Usually the initial fever is then accompanied by a reddish rash which typically first appears on the face before spreading to the rest of the body. Measles is usually self limited and treatment is symptomatic. The high fever occasionally may cause febrile seizures.

Mumps. Like measles, mumps is relatively uncommon today due to widespread vaccination. Mumps is caused by the mumps virus. Transmission usually occurs through the saliva of an infected person. The incubation period is twelve to twenty-six days. The disease begins as a fever, and later is accompanied by swelling of the salivary glands under the jaw and around the cheek area. In males, the testes can sometimes become involved. In females the ovaries are subject to involvement. The disease is self limited and treatment is symptomatic.

Varicella. Chicken pox, or varicella, is still quite common. Technically, varicella is a herpes infection. Although a vaccine is now available, it has not been used extensively in this country. The Varicella zoster virus, a member of the herpes class, causes the infection. Transmission is primarily through the respiratory tract. The incubation period is approximately ten to twenty-one days. Chicken pox initially begins as a fever. Shortly afterwards, "crops" of reddish skin eruptions appear over the body. The lesions first appear on the trunk and usually move to the extremities. Several crops will typically appear, each associated with itching. While the eruptions are still oozing, transmission is possible. Treatment is symptomatic and the infection is self limited. Once a person has been infected, he or she is usually immune for life. But the virus may remain in the body dormant for many years, generally living in nerves along the back. In later life, or during periods of stress, the virus may become active. Spreading through the distribution of the nerve in which it resides, it causes the illness known as "shingles." Unlike chicken pox, shingles is not contagious.

Paramedic Precautions. When treating or transporting a patient suspected of having a childhood infectious disease the following precautions are recommended:

- ❑ Wear gloves at all times.
- ❑ Wash hands following contact with any body secretions.
- ❑ Notify emergency department personnel.
- ❑ Dispose or heat sterilize all instruments used.
- ❑ Bag all linen and trash for protection of others.
- ❑ Always follow-up with the emergency department to determine what sort of infection the child had.

SUMMARY OF PREHOSPITAL PRECAUTIONS

Hand washing should be performed after each patient contact. All jewelry should be removed and all surfaces of the hand lathered with an antimicrobial soap for at least 30 seconds. If water is unavailable, an alcohol-based scrub should be used.

A general wipe-down of the ambulance floor, walls, and stretcher, should be done at least once every 24 hours. A hospital-grade disinfectant and water or a 1:10 solution of household bleach and water should be used. High contact items such as stethoscopes, radios, kits, monitors, and stretcher railings should be wiped after each run. Contaminated trash should be emptied into the appropriate container. Soiled linen must be discarded at least once each shift. (See Figure 27-4.)

When cleaning EMS equipment, the following general precautions are recommended for paramedics:

Blood spillage. Clean blood spillage while wearing eye protection and disposable gloves. Use paper towels or disposable linen to clean excessive amounts of blood. The area where the blood is found should be cleaned

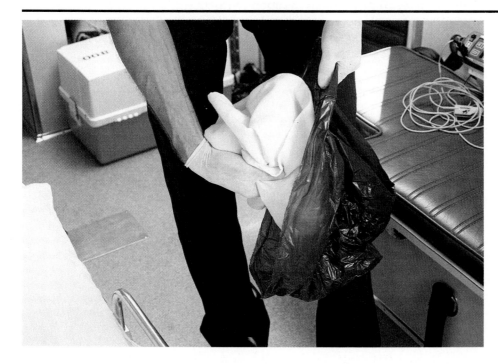

FIGURE 27-4 Bag all linen and label if infectious.

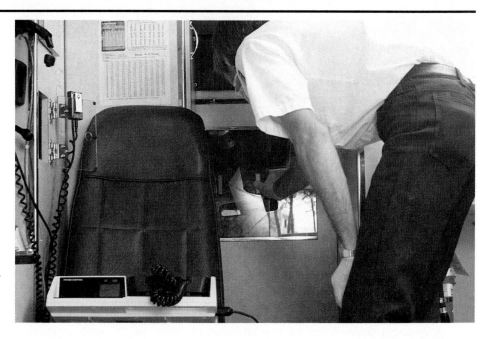

FIGURE 27-5 Keep the ambulance well ventilated, if weather permits, when transporting a patient with suspected respiratory infectious disease.

with a bleach (Chlorox) solution. When using the bleach, remember to make sure there is good ventilation.

✳ Needles should never be recapped.

Needles and sharp instruments. Approved containers for disposal of sharp items should be available in the rear of the ambulance. Dispose of these containers frequently, following local rules and regulations for disposal of hazardous wastes. (See Figure 27-6.)

Respiratory equipment. Most respiratory equipment should be disposable. Wear disposable gloves to disconnect nondisposable parts such as laryngoscopes. Then sterilize these parts following the manufacturer's recommendations. Afterwards, allow them to air dry.

Suction equipment. Most suction equipment should be disposable. Parts that are not disposable should be disconnected, while wearing disposable gloves, and sterilized following the manufacturer's recommendations. Following this they should be allowed to air dry.

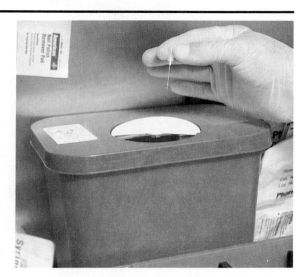

FIGURE 27-6 Dispose of needles and other sharp objects properly.

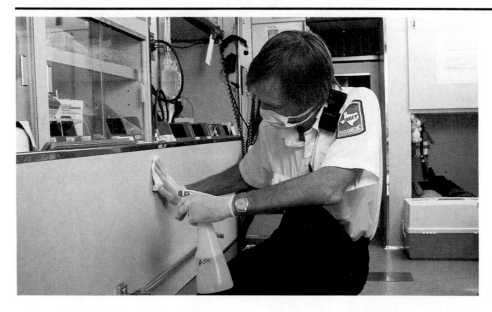

FIGURE 27-7 Clean the ambulance daily with an antiseptic solution.

General cleaning. Use a 10% solution of household bleach (Clorox) for general cleaning. Ensure that the area is well ventilated during this process. A good general cleaning should be conducted daily. Also, once each week the ambulance should be taken out of service for extensive cleaning, followed by air drying. (See Figures 27-7 and 27-8.)

Backboards and straps. Use hot, soapy water to scrub these items. Rinse them with water and air dry before use.

Cervical collars. Cervical collars should be scrubbed with hot, soapy water. Then rinse them with water and air dry before use. If they are excessively soiled, discard them.

✱ Never reuse equipment labeled as disposable.

PASG. The PASG should be cleaned following each use. Remove organic material and scrub the garment with warm, soapy water. Rinse with water and air dry. Never store the device unless it is completely dry.

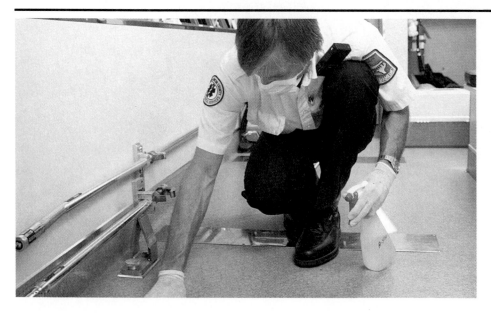

FIGURE 27-8 Finally, mop the floor with an antiseptic solution.

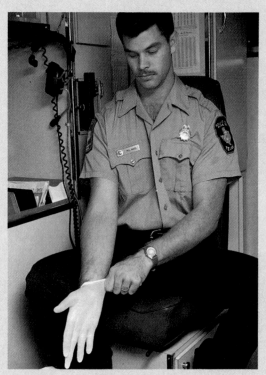

27-1A.   Always wear protective gloves.

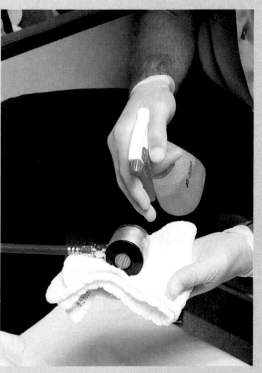

27-1B.   Using an approved antiseptic solution, clean any equipment that potentially contacted the patient.

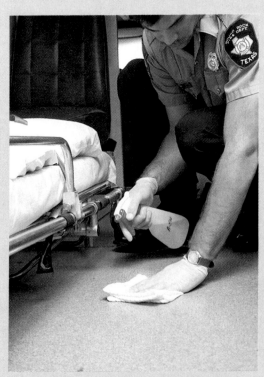

27-1C.   Clean the ambulance compartment.

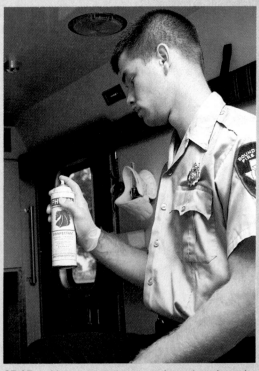

27-1D.   Use antiseptic sprays and ventilate the ambulance.

SUMMARY

Prehospital personnel generally will not be directly involved in the treatment of infectious disease. Nevertheless, they should suspect infectious disease and take proper precautions. Appropriate protective devices should be immediately available for every paramedic, such as disposable gloves, eye protection, face mask, and a gown or apron. A mouth shield, or mouth to mask ventilation device should also always be immediately available. Moreover, because the spectrum of infectious disease is changing rapidly, paramedics must keep up to date with the latest recommendations on prevention of infectious disease. The key to infectious disease management is prevention. (See Figures 27-9, 27-10, and 27-11.)

✱ Infectious diseases, such as hepatitis B and HIV infection, are the number one threat to the health and safety of prehospital personnel today.

✱ Each EMS system must have a mechanism for tracking exposure to infectious disease and must include post-exposure follow-up.

COMMUNICABLE DISEASE EXPOSURE REPORT

SECTION I (EMS personnel completes at time of incident)

NAME _____ TITLE _____

ADDRESS _____ PHONE _____

DATE OF INCIDENT_____ EMS # _____

LOCATION _____

EXPOSURE DESCRIPTION

A.   Blood or Body Fluids

1. _____ Needlestick with contaminated needle
2. _____ Blood/body fluids into natural body openings
3. _____ Blood/body fluids into cut/wound less than 24 hrs old
4. _____ Blood/body fluids on intact skin
5. _____ Other (describe) _____

B.   Respiratory

1. _____ Mouth to mouth resuscitation
2. _____ Resuscitation using airway
3. _____ Present at scene, but no resuscitation effort
         involving breathing
4. _____ Other (describe) _____

Type of Fluid to which you were exposed

1. _____ Blood   2. _____ Emesis   3. _____ Saliva   4. _____ Amniotic
5. _____ Other (describe) _____

How could this incident have been prevented _____
_____
_____

Source of Contamination

Patient name _____

Address _____

Male/Female _____ Phone _____

Receiving Hospital _____

Signature of EMS Personnel _____

FIGURE 27-9   A communicable disease exposure report should be completed on each case of suspected communicable disease exposure.

COMMUNICABLE DISEASE EXPOSURE REPORT

SECTION II EXPOSURE INFORMATION   (Hospital staff completes)

Patient Diagnosis _____

Does the patient have a communicable disease which would put the

EMS personnel at risk of occupational exposure? _____ Yes _____ No

Exposure Evaluation

Hepatitis B Surface Antigen (patient)   _____ Pos _____ Neg _____ Not Done
HIV Antibody (patient)   _____ Pos _____ Neg _____ Not Done

Exposure significant   _____ Yes _____ No
Further Follow-up needed   _____ Yes _____ No

Recommended treatment follow-up

_____
_____
_____
_____
_____

_____
Signature of hospital infection control representative

FIGURE 27-10   The hospital should complete part II of the form, relating to patient test results.

FURTHER READING

BEHRMAN, R. and VAUGHN, V. C., *Nelson's Textbook of Pediatrics.* 13th ed. Philadelphia, PA: W.B. Saunders, 1987.

CENTERS FOR DISEASE CONTROL, Guidelines for Prevention of Transmission of Human Immunodeficiency Virus and Hepatitis B Virus to Health-Care and Public Safety Workers, *MMWR,* June 23, 1989, vol. 38, No. 5–6.

GRANT, H. D., MURRAY, R. H ., and BERGERON, J.D., *Emergency Care.* 5th ed. Englewood Cliffs, NJ: Prentice-Hall, Inc., 1989.

U. S. DEPARTMENT OF LABOR, OSHA, *Worker Exposure to AIDS and Hepatitis B.* 1988.

COMMUNICABLE DISEASE EXPOSURE REPORT

SECTION III EXPOSURE INFORMATION   (EMS completes)

EMS Personnel Hepatitis B History

Treated for exposure to Hep B within past 6 months _____ Yes _____ No

Is EMS Personnel immune to Hepatitis B _____ Yes _____ No

If yes, _____ Had vaccine _____ Had disease

Hep B Surface Antibody (EMS Personnel)   _____ React _____ NonR _____ Not Done

HIV Antibody (EMS Personnel)   _____ React _____ NonR _____ Not Done

SECTION IV ACTION PLAN

_____ No further follow-up necessary

Employee RX _____ Td/T _____ HBIG _____ ISG   _____ Hep B Vaccine
                                                          _____ Date 1st dose
                                                          _____ Date 2nd dose
                                                          _____ Date 3rd dose

_____ Medication: Type & dosage _____

HIV Surveillance Started (0, 3, 6 months)

_____ Date Results _____
_____ Date Results _____
_____ Date Results _____

Medical Program Director _____

FIGURE 27-11   A post-exposure action plan should be prepared and supervised by the system medical director.

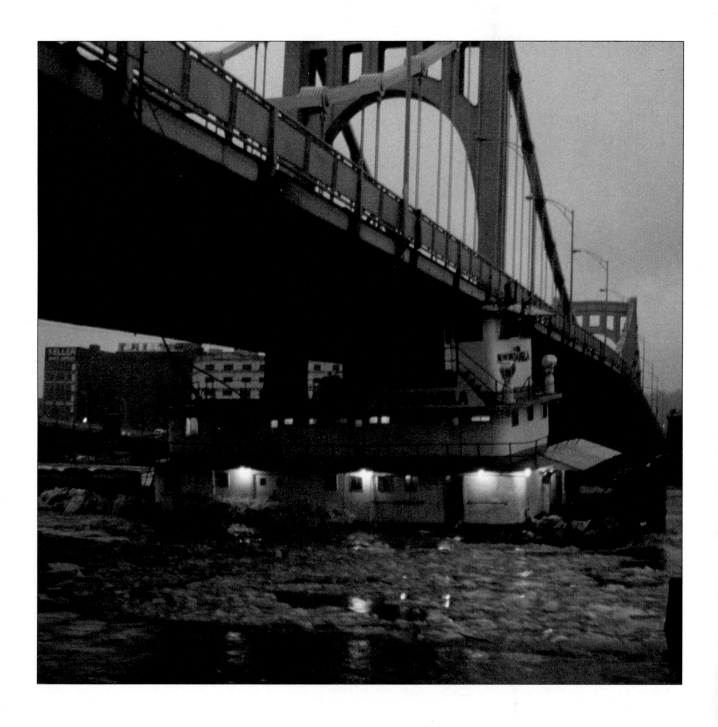

28

Environmental Emergencies

Objectives for Chapter 28

Upon completing this chapter, the student should be able to:

1. List and describe the four mechanisms by which the body loses heat.

2. Describe the mechanisms which the body uses to maintain body temperature in warm and cold environments.

3. Define the respective pathologies for the three heat disorders that affect the human system.

4. Identify the signs, symptoms and recommended management techniques for heat cramps, heat exhaustion and heat stroke.

5. List the predisposing factors for the common heat disorders.

6. Define the pathologies associated with hypothermia and cold-related injuries.

7. Identify the stages of systemic hypothermia and the physical signs and symptoms associated with them.

8. Relate the physiologic affects hypothermia may have on resuscitation attempts.

9. Discuss the concerns and considerations regarding field rewarming of the hypothermia patient.

10. Identify the sources of ionizing radiation and relate their relative penetrating potential.

11. Relate the considerations which can serve to reduce the exposure to a radiation source.

12. Identify the care considerations for the patient who was exposed to ionizing radiation.

13. Describe the events which occur during the near-drowning emergency.

14. List and describe the pathologies of the various diving/hyperbaric emergencies.

15. Describe the signs and symptoms of diving-related emergenies.

16. Describe the management of the patient with the various diving-related emergencies.

Engine 21, Rescue 10, and EMS 10 are dispatched to a "possible drowning" at a local apartment complex. En route the dispatcher reports that telephone CPR instructions are being given by another dispatcher. Upon arrival at the scene paramedics find a 15-year-old male, lying beside the pool, in cardiac arrest. Two bystanders are attempting CPR, yet are being deterred by vomiting. With the aid of the EMTs, the paramedics quickly perform a primary survey. The quick look paddles reveal fine ventricular fibrillation. A 200 joule shock is applied and CPR resumed. Ventricular fibrillation persists and the paddles are again charged and another 300 joule shock is delivered. This is unsuccessful and repeated a third time at 360 joules. CPR is initiated with 100% oxygen via demand valve. With the patient still in ventricular fibrillation, an IV is established and an endotracheal tube placed. One milligram of epinephrine is administered intravenously. Defibrillation is again attempted and the patient converted to an idioventricular rhythm. A carotid pulse is detected afterwards. Respirations are continued during the patient's immediate transport to the hospital. There he remains alive for three days before dying from multiple organ failure, without ever regaining consciousness.

INTRODUCTION

Paramedics are frequently called upon to treat medical emergencies related to environmental conditions. Most of these types of emergencies occur during the summer or winter. Understanding their causes and underlying pathophysiologies should help paramedics recognize and manage these emergencies. Although many environmental factors can result in medical emergencies, this chapter will primarily focus on problems related to the extremes of heat and cold, nuclear radiation, and diving accidents.

The *environment* can be defined as all of the surrounding external factors that affect the development and functioning of a living organism. Human beings obviously require the environment for life. But they also must be protected from its extremes.

THERMOREGULATION

The human body functions within a very small temperature range. The body temperature of the deep tissues, commonly called the *core temperature,* usually does not vary more than a degree or so from its normal 37 degrees Celsius (98.6 degrees Fahrenheit). This characteristic of warm-blooded animals is called *steady-state metabolism.* The various biochemical reactions occurring within the cell are most efficient when the body temperature is within this narrow temperature range. A naked person can be exposed to an external environment ranging anywhere from 55–140 degrees F. and still maintain a fairly constant internal body temperature. Extrinsic (environmental) thermal stressors, such as extreme heat or cold, may exceed the body's thermal compensatory mechanisms, causing thermal disorders such as hypothermia or hyperthermia.

The body must maintain a balance between heat generated internally and the external environment. Nervous or negative feedback mechanisms almost entirely regulate the body's temperature. Most of these mechanisms operate through temperature-regulating centers located in the **hypothalamus** at the base of the brain. This area acts like a thermostat. It produces neurosecretions important in the control of many metabolic activities, including temperature regulation.

Although the hypothalamus plays a key role in body temperature regulation, temperature receptors in other parts of the body also have a major effect on temperature regulation. Temperature receptors in the skin, certain mucous membranes, and selected deep tissues of the body are especially significant. The skin has both cold and warm receptors. Because cold receptors outnumber warm receptors, peripheral detection of temperature consists mainly of detecting cold instead of warm. Deep body temperature (afferent) receptors are mostly in the spinal cord, abdominal viscera, and in or around the great veins. These receptors are exposed to the body's core temperature rather than the surface temperature. Deep body temperature receptors also respond mainly to cold rather than warmth. Both skin and deep temperature receptors act to prevent hypothermia.

Heat Generation

The human body gains heat through either internal or external sources. Internal heat comes from routine cellular metabolism and thermogenesis. In producing energy, the cell gives off heat. The body can also stimulate certain cells to generate heat in a process called **thermogenesis.**

Sympathetic stimulation, including an increase in circulating norepinephrine and epinephrine, can cause an immediate increase in the rate of cellular metabolism, which, in turn, increases heat production. Besides routine cellular metabolism, the body can expend energy to generate heat through thermogenesis. This primarily occurs in fatty tissue. Shivering can also occur, further generating heat through skeletal muscle contraction.

Environmental Heat

Our body receives external heat from the environment via the thermal gradient. The **thermal gradient** is the difference in temperature between the environment and the body. The environment is usually at a different temperature than the body. If the environment is warmer than the body, heat flows from it to the body. If the body is warmer than the environment, heat flows from the body to it. Several factors affect the thermal gradient. They include ambient air temperature, infrared radiation, and relative humidity. Ambient air temperature is simply the temperature of the surrounding air. Infrared radiation is radiation with a wavelength longer than that of visible light. Relative humidity is the percentage of water vapor present in air.

Although the peripheral receptors are largely responsible for temperature detection, they also help control body temperature mainly through the hypothalamus. The heat-controlling mechanism of the hypothalamus is referred to as the *hypothalamic thermostat.* When body heat becomes too great, the hypothalamic thermostat and associated compensatory mechanisms attempt to eliminate body heat through five mechanisms. They include:

■ **hypothalamus** portion of the diencephalon producing neurosecretions important in the control of certain metabolic activities including body temperature regulation

■ **thermogenesis** the production of heat, especially within the body.

■ **thermal gradient** the difference in temperature between the environment and the body.

1. *Vasodilatation.* The blood vessels in the skin become dilated due to the inhibition of the sympathetic centers in the hypothalamus. Heat is then lost through the skin through sweating and other mechanisms.

2. *Perspiration.* Perspiration occurs when the core temperature rises above "normal" (98.6 degrees F. or 37 degrees C.). This mechanism is ineffective if the relative humidity is 75% or greater due to decreased evaporation of perspiration from the skin surface.

3. *Decrease in heat production.* Shivering and chemical thermogenesis are inhibited, causing decreased heat production.

4. *Increased cardiac output.* Increased cardiac output aids in increasing blood flow through the skin, thus aiding in the elimination of heat.

5. *Increased respiratory rate.* An increase in respiratory rate results in elimination of warm air and in water evaporation.

Heat Loss

As discussed above, heat is a by-product of metabolism and is always being lost to the environment. This occurs because the body is usually warmer than the environment. The body can lose heat due to the following methods (see Figure 28-1):

Radiation. An unclothed person will lose approximately 60% of total body heat by radiation at normal room temperature. This heat loss is in the form of infrared rays. All objects not at absolute zero temperature will radiate heat.

■ **conduction** moving electrons, ions, heat, or sound waves through a conductor or conducting medium.

Conduction. Direct contact of the body's surface to another, cooler object causes the body to lose heat by **conduction**. Heat flows from higher temperature matter to lower temperature matter. The law of thermodynamics states that if **ambient** air temperature is higher than the skin temperature, then heat will flow from the air to the skin.

■ **ambient** surrounding on all sides.

■ **convection** transferring of heat via currents in liquids or gases.

Convection. Heat loss to air currents passing over the body is called **convection**. Heat, however, must first be conducted to the air, and then carried by convection currents.

Evaporation. Evaporative heat loss occurs as water evaporates from the skin. Additionally, a great deal of heat loss occurs through **evaporation** of fluids in the lungs. Water evaporates from the skin and lungs at approximately 600 mL/day.

■ **evaporation** change from liquid to a gaseous state.

Heat Preservation

When the body becomes too cold, the hypothalamic thermostat reacts in exactly the opposite fashion in order to preserve body heat. The body has several mechanisms which it can engage in order to maintain heat. These include:

1. *Vasoconstriction.* Caused by stimulation of the hypothalamic sympathetic centers, *vasoconstriction* causes diversion of blood flow from the skin to the body's core to maintain heat.

2. *Piloerection (hairs standing on end).* This is a response which was present millions of years ago when humans had a great deal more body hair than

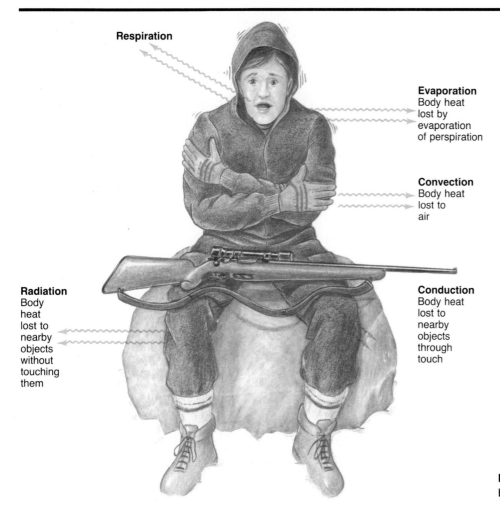

Respiration

Evaporation
Body heat
lost by
evaporation
of perspiration

Convection
Body heat
lost to
air

Radiation
Body
heat
lost to
nearby
objects
without
touching
them

Conduction
Body heat
lost to
nearby
objects
through
touch

FIGURE 28-1 Heat loss by the body.

now. Standing the hair on end increased the insulating ability and decreased heat loss.

3. *Increase in heat production.* Heat production is increased by the metabolic systems in the following ways:

❑ *Thermogenesis (shivering)*—The hypothalamus has an area called the *primary motor center* which controls shivering. It is excited by cold signals from the skin and spinal cord.

❑ *Sympathetic excitation of heat production*—Norepinephrine and epinephrine are released following sympathetic stimulation, which causes an immediate increase in the rate of cellular metabolism and generates heat.

In summary, if the body temperature gets too high the various cooling mechanisms discussed above are engaged. If the body becomes too cool, heat-preserving mechanisms are engaged. An increase in the body temperature is called **hyperthermia** while a decrease is called **hypothermia**. Hyperthermia and fever are different. Fever occurs when the hypothalamus "resets" the "thermostat" in the brain. This purposeful increase in body temperature helps the body's various defense mechanisms clear itself of the infectious agent (i.e. bacteria or virus).

■ **hyperthermia** unusually high body temperature.

■ **hypothermia** having a body temperature below normal.

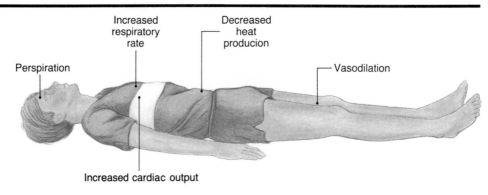

FIGURE 28-2 The victim of a heat emergency.

Labels in figure: Increased respiratory rate · Decreased heat producion · Perspiration · Vasodilation · Increased cardiac output

HYPERTHERMIA

Hyperthermia is an increase in the body temperature caused by heat transfer from the external environment. It can manifest either as heat cramps, heat exhaustion, or heat stroke. (See Figure 28-2.)

Heat (Muscle) Cramps

■ **heat cramps** acute painful spasms of the voluntary muscles following strenuous activity in a hot environment without adequate fluid or salt intake.

Heat cramps are extremely common in hot climates. They result in intermittent, painful contractions of various skeletal muscles. Heat cramps are caused primarily by a rapid change in extracellular fluid osmolarity resulting from sodium and water losses. Sweating occurs as sodium is transported to the skin. Water follows sodium and is deposited on the skin surface, where it evaporates, thereby aiding in the cooling process. Sweating not only involves the loss of water, but of electrolytes, such as sodium, as well.

The patient with heat cramps will present with cramps in the fingers, arms, legs, or abdominal muscles. He or she will be mentally alert, with hot sweaty skin, tachycardia, normal blood pressure, and a normal core temperature.

Prehospital Management—Heat Cramps. The treatment of heat cramps is usually easily accomplished by removing the patient from the hot environment. Fluid and sodium intake should be increased. Severe cases of heat cramps may require IV fluid replacement with a salt solution.

Heat Exhaustion

■ **heat exhaustion** acute reaction to heat exposure. Blood pools in the vessels as the body attempts to give off excessive heat. It can lead to collapse due to inadequate blood return to the heart.

Heat exhaustion is the most common heat-related illness seen clinically by prehospital personnel. Excessive water and salt loss due to sweating accounts for the presenting symptoms, which include the following:

❑ Weakness
❑ Vertigo
❑ Nausea
❑ Syncope
❑ Pallor
❑ Thirst
❑ Anxiety or apathy
❑ Profuse sweating
❑ Tachycardia

- ❏ Elevated or normal respiratory rate
- ❏ Elevated or depressed blood pressure
- ❏ Core temperature normal or 1–2 degrees elevated

Since the above symptoms are not exclusive to heat exhaustion, the history of patient exposure to hot, humid weather is needed to reach a correct diagnosis.

Each liter of perspiration contains anywhere from 20 to 50 mEq of sodium chloride. Therefore, a deficiency in water and sodium combine to cause electrolyte, volume, and vasomotor regulatory disturbances. This fluid and electrolyte loss, combined with generalized vasodilatation, leads to low circulating blood volume, venous pooling, a reduction in cardiac output, and hypotension.

Prehospital Management—Heat Exhaustion. Prehospital treatment for heat exhaustion consists of removing the patient from the hot environment and providing intravenous replacement of sodium and water. A crystalloid solution of normal saline or lactated Ringer's is preferred. If untreated, heat exhaustion can progress to heat stroke.

Heat Stroke

Heat stroke occurs when the body's hypothalamic temperature regulation is lost causing uncompensated hyperthermia, which in turn causes cell death and physiologic collapse. Heat stroke is generally characterized by a body temperature of at least 105 degrees F. (40.6 degrees C.), CNS disturbances, and usually the cessation of sweating. Sweating is thought to stop due to destruction of the sweat glands or when sensory overload causes them to temporarily dysfunction. The patient's skin may, however, be dry or may be covered with sweat. If the patient has not been exercising, the skin will be dry. However, if the heat stroke occurred during strenuous exercise, sweating may be profuse. The patient may also present with the following signs and symptoms:

- ❏ Increased core temperature
- ❏ Tachycardia followed by bradycardia
- ❏ Hypotension with low or absent diastolic reading
- ❏ Rapid, shallow respirations, which may later slow
- ❏ Confusion or disorientation
- ❏ Seizures
- ❏ Coma

If the patient develops heat stroke due to exertion, he or she may go into severe metabolic acidosis caused by lactic acid accumulation. Hyperkalemia may also develop because of the release of potassium from injured muscle cells, renal failure, or metabolic acidosis.

Prehospital Management—Heat Stroke

1. *Rapid patient cooling.* This can be accomplished en route to the hospital by removing the patient's clothing and covering the patient with ice-water soaked sheets. Body temperature must be lowered to 102 degrees F. (39 degrees C.). A target of 102 degrees is used to avoid an overshoot. Ice packs and fans may also be used.
2. *Administer oxygen.*

■ **heat stroke** acute, dangerous reaction to heat exposure, characterized by a body temperature usually above 106 degrees F. (41.1 degrees C.). The body ceases to perspire.

✳ The patient with heat stroke should be cooled as soon as possible.

3. *Establish IV(s).* Begin 1–2 IVs, using lactated Ringer's or normal saline wide open.

4. *Monitor ECG.* Cardiac dysrhythmias may occur at any time. S-T segment depression, non-specific T wave changes with occasional PVCs, and supraventricular tachycardias are common.

5. *Avoid vasopressors and anticholinergic drugs.* These agents may potentiate heat stroke by inhibiting sweating. They can also produce a hypermetabolic state in the presence of high environmental temperatures and relatively high humidity.

6. *Monitor core temperature.* EMS systems operating in extremely warm climates should carry some device to record the body temperature, whether a simple rectal thermometer or a sophisticated electronic device. Simple glass thermometers generally do not measure above 106 degrees or below 95 degrees. This may become significant when transport times may be long and it essential that changes in the patient's condition be detected. (See Procedure 28-1).

FEVER (PYREXIA)

■ **pyrexia** above normal body temperature, fever.

A fever (**pyrexia**) is the elevation of the body temperature above the normal temperature (0.5–1.0 degree higher for rectal temperatures) for that person. In other words, fever is essentially a resetting of the hypothalamic thermostat. The body develops a fever when pathogens enter and cause infection, which in turn stimulates the production of pyrogens. **Pyrogens** are any substances that cause fever. They reset the "hypothalamic pointer" to a higher level. Metabolism is therefore increased, producing a fever. The increased body temperature is a defense mechanism, for it makes the body a less hospitable environment for the invading organism. The hypothalamic thermostat will reset to normal when pyrogen production stops, or when pathogens end their attack on the body.

■ **pyrogen** any substance causing a fever.

Prehospital Management—Pyrexia

The underlying cause of the fever must be treated before the fever can be arrested. The paramedic should not attempt to treat fever unless it is very high (> 105 degrees), mental status changes are present, or if febrile seizures appear imminent. If requested by medical control, prehospital treatment of fever includes the oral or rectal administration of acetaminophen (Tylenol). Additional cooling may be obtained by removing all extra clothing and allowing the patient to lose heat to the environment by convection. Sponge baths are generally not recommended as these can drop the body core temperature too much causing shivering and additional heat production.

✱ Sponge baths are not recommended in the management of fever.

HYPERPYREXIA

■ **hyperpyrexia** elevation of body temperature, due to fever, above 106 degrees F. (41.1 degrees C.).

Hyperpyrexia is the elevation of body temperature above 106 degrees F. (41.1 degrees C.). It can be produced by physical agents such as hot baths or hot air, or by reaction to infection caused by microorganisms. Some people develop hyperpyrexia in the hospital within 24 hours after surgery. A rare cause of hyperpyrexia is *malignant hyperthermia,* which can occur following a general anesthetic in patients genetically predisposed. This, however, is rarely seen outside of the hospital setting.

Condition	Muscle Cramps	Breathing	Pulse	Weakness	Skin	Perspiration	Loss of Consciousness
Heat cramps	Yes	Varies	Varies	Yes	Moist-warm No change	Heavy	Seldom
Heat exhaustion	No	Rapid Shallow	Weak	Yes	Cold Clammy	Heavy	Sometimes
Heat-stroke	No	Deep, then shallow	Full Rapid	Yes	Dry-hot	Little or none	Often

1 HEAT CRAMPS

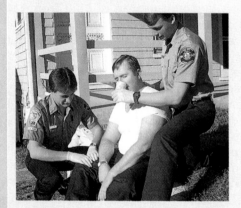

SYMPTOMS AND SIGNS:
Severe muscle cramps (usually in the legs and abdomen), exhaustion, sometimes dizziness or periods of faintness.

EMERGENCY CARE PROCEDURES:
• Move patient to a nearby cool place
• Give patient salted water to drink or half-strength commercial electrolyte fluids
• Massage the "cramped" muscle to help ease the patient's discomfort, massaging with pressure will be more effective than light rubbing actions. (Optional in some EMS systems).
• Apply moist towels to the patient's forehead and over cramped muscles for added relief
• If cramps persist, or if more serious signs and symptoms develop, ready the patient and transport

2 HEAT EXHAUSTION

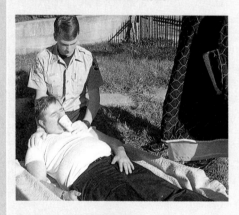

SYMPTOMS AND SIGNS:
Rapid and shallow breathing, weak pulse, cold and clammy skin, heavy perspiration, total body weakness, and dizziness that sometimes leads to unconsciousness.

EMERGENCY CARE PROCEDURES:
• Move the patient to a nearby cool place.
• Keep the patient at rest.
• Remove enough clothing to cool the patient without chilling him (watch for shivering)
• Fan the patient's skin.
• Give the patient salted water or half-strength commercial electrolyte fluids. Do not try to administer fluids to an unconscious patient.
• Treat for shock, but do not cover to the point of overheating the patient.
• Provide oxygen if needed
• If unconscious, fails to recover rapidly, has other injuries, or has a history of medical problems, transport as soon as possible.

3 HEATSTROKE

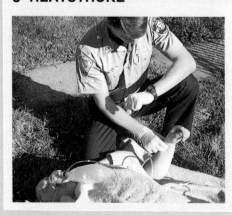

SYMPTOMS AND SIGNS:
Deep breaths, then shallow breathing; rapid strong pulse, then rapid, weak pulse; dry, hot skin; dilated pupils; loss of consciousness (possible coma); seizures or muscular twitching may be seen.

EMERGENCY CARE PROCEDURES:
• Cool the patient—in any manner—rapidly, move the patient out of the sun or away from the heat source. Remove patient's clothing and wrap him in wet towels and sheets. Pour cool water over these wrappings. Body heat must be lowered rapidly or brain cells will die!
• Treat for shock and administer a high concentration of oxygen.
• If cold packs or ice bags are available, wrap them and place one bag or pack under each of the patients armpits, one behind each knee, one in the groin, one on each wrist and ankle, and one on each side of the patient's neck.
• Transport as soon as possible.
• Should transport be delayed, find a tub or container—immerse patient up to the face in cooled water. Constantly monitor to prevent drowning.
• Monitor vital signs throughout process.

HYPOTHERMIA

Hypothermia is a state of low body temperature, specifically low body core temperature. When the core temperature of the body drops below 95 degrees F. (35 degrees C.), an individual is considered to be in a hypothermic state. Hypothermia can be attributed to either a decrease in heat production, an increase in heat loss, or a combination of both.

Exposure to cold normally causes shivering and increased muscle tone, resulting in increased metabolism to maintain the body temperature. Initial signs of hypothermia are peripheral vasoconstriction with an increase in cardiac output and respiratory rate. When this additional heat production can no longer keep up with heat lost from the body surface, body temperature falls. As body temperature falls, so does metabolic rate and cardiac output. Hypovolemia results from the shift of fluid from the vascular to the extravascular compartment, allowing the body to preserve energy and prevent cell death. However, if the hypothermic state is not corrected, cell ischemia and necrosis eventually result in death.

As discussed, the major sources of heat production are exercise and cold-weather shivering. The major sources of body heat loss are conduction, radiation, evaporation, and convection. Heat loss can be increased by the removal of clothing, the wetting of clothing by rain or snow, increased air movement around the body (increased convection), or increased conduction such as cold-water immersion.

Hypothermia patients can be divided into two categories, mild or severe hypothermia. An arbitrary core temperature of 90 degrees F. (32 degrees C.) has been accepted as a reasonable dividing line to differentiate between mild and severe hypothermia. Patients who experience body temperatures above 90 degrees F. will usually have a favorable prognosis. Those with temperatures below 90 degrees F. show a significant increase in mortality rate. Remember that most thermometers used in medicine do not register below 96 degrees. EMS systems in colder areas should carry special thermometers for recording subnormal temperature readings.

Patients experiencing mild hypothermia (core temperature > 90 degrees F.), will generally exhibit shivering. The patient may be lethargic and somewhat dulled mentally. (But, in some cases, they may be fully oriented.) Muscles may be stiff and uncoordinated, causing the patient to walk with a stumbling, staggering gait.

Patients experiencing severe hypothermia (core temperature < 90 degrees F.) may be disoriented and confused. As their temperature contin-

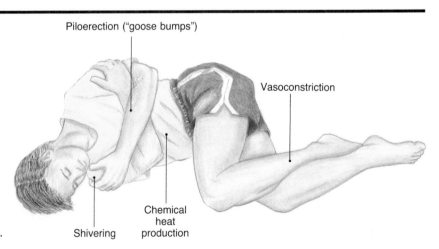

Piloerection ("goose bumps")

Vasoconstriction

Chemical heat production

Shivering

FIGURE 28-3   The victim of hypothermia.

ues to fall, they will proceed into stupor and complete coma. Shivering will usually stop, and physical activity becomes uncoordinated. Muscles may be stiff and rigid. Continuous cardiac monitoring is indicated for anyone experiencing hypothermia. The ECG will frequently show pathognomonic (indicative of a disease) **J waves** associated with the QRS complexes. Atrial fibrillation is the most common presenting dysrhythmia seen in hypothermia. As the body cools, however, the myocardium becomes progressively more irritable and may develop a variety of dysrhythmias. In severe hypothermia, bradycardia is inevitable. Ventricular fibrillation becomes more probable as the body's core temperature falls below 85 degrees F. The severely hypothermic patient requires assessment of pulse and respirations every 1–2 minutes.

■ **J wave** ECG deflection found at the junction of the QRS complex and the ST segment. It is associated with hypothermia and seen at core temperatures below 32°C, most commonly in leads II and V$_6$.

Rewarming of the hypothermic patient is best carried out by a team using a prearranged protocol in the hospital. Most patients who die during rewarming die from ventricular fibrillation. Rewarming should not be attempted in the field unless travel to the Emergency Department will take more than 15 minutes.

External application of heat by warmed blankets is a safe and effective means of rewarming the hypothermic patient. Application of external heat, however, results in peripheral vasodilatation. This, in turn, may cause the blood pressure to fall, especially when there is also volume depletion. An IV volume expander should be used to manage volume depletion. Another excellent means of rewarming the hypothermic patient is by administering heated and humidified oxygen. The hypothermic patient should be moved gently. Unnecessary rough handling may stimulate the return of cool blood and acids from the extremities to the core. This causes an "afterdrop" core temperature decrease and may induce cardiac dysrhythmias.

Prehospital Management—Hypothermia

Mild Hypothermia. Care should follow these recommendations:

❑ Handle patient gently. The ventricular fibrillation threshold is lowered in the hypothermic patient. Even mild physical trauma may cause the heart to develop dysrhythmias such as ventricular fibrillation.

❑ Insulate the patient from the cold.

❑ Add heat to the patient's head, neck, chest and groin. Respiratory warmers may also be used.

❑ Do not give alcohol, coffee, and nicotine.

❑ Warm oral fluids and sugar sources can be given AFTER uncontrolled shivering stops and the patient exhibits evidence of rewarming.

Severe Hypothermia (Vital Signs Present). Care should follow these recommendations:

✱ Rewarming of the hypothermic patient should be deferred until the patient is in the emergency department unless transport time is long and rewarming is ordered by medical control.

❑ Handle patient gently

❑ Insulate the patient from the cold.

❑ Add heat to the patient's head, neck, chest and groin. Respiratory warmers may also be used.

❑ Give nothing by mouth.

❑ Do not administer oxygen unless it is heated to > 99 degrees F. If warmed oxygen is unavailable, use the mouth-to-mask technique for ventilations.

❑ Establish an IV of D5W or D5NS at 75 mL/hr (with warm fluids if possible).

❑ Monitor the ECG.

❑ Do not administer medications. They are poorly metabolized in hypothermia, due to the hypometabolic state. Administration may cause medications to persist in the body resulting in toxic drug levels upon patient rewarming.

✱ The hypothermic patient is not dead until he or she is warm and dead.

Severe Hypothermia (Vital Signs Absent). Care should follow these recommendations:

❑ Assess pulse and respirations for 1-2 minutes.
❑ If pulse and respirations are absent, begin CPR.
❑ Observe the ECG rhythm. If the patient is in ventricular fibrillation, defibrillate immediately at 400 joules.
❑ Measure the rectal core temperature.
❑ If defibrillation is unsuccessful and core temperature is 85 degrees F. or greater, repeat defibrillation. Do not attempt to defibrillate again if the core temperature is below 85 degrees.
❑ If defibrillation is successful, administer lidocaine 1 mg/kg, followed by 0.5 mg/kg IV in 15 minutes.
❑ Warm oxygen and intubation are appropriate for the pulseless, apneic patient.
❑ PASG may be used for hypovolemia
❑ Rewarming should not be attempted unless the patient is more than 15 minutes from a medical facility

Metabolic Factors in Hypothermia

Not all hypothermia cases are caused by environmental conditions. For example, hypothyroidism depresses the body's heat-producing mechanisms. Brain tumors or head trauma can depress the hypothalamic temperature control center, causing hypothermia. Other conditions such as myocardial infarction, diabetes, hypoglycemia, drugs, poor nutrition, sepsis, or old age, can also contribute to metabolic and circulatory disorders that predispose to hypothermia.

Any patient thought to have hypothermia, but with no history of exposure to the environment, should be assessed for any predisposing factors which may have led to it. The patient should be assessed for level of consciousness, cool skin, and shivering. Also, a rectal temperature should be assessed. A rectal temperature of less than 95 degrees F. indicates hypothermia.

Frostbite

Frostbite is environmentally induced freezing of body tissues. As the tissues freeze, ice crystals form within and water is drawn out of the cells into the extracellular space. These ice crystals expand, causing the destruction of cells. During this process, intracellular electrolyte concentration increases, further destroying cells. Damage to blood vessels from ice crystal formation causes loss of vascular integrity, resulting in tissue swelling and loss of distal nutritional flow.

Generally there are two types of frostbite. *Superficial frostbite* affects the dermis and shallow subcutaneous layers. *Deep frostbite* affects the dermal and subdermal layers of tissue.

Assessment. Frostbite mainly occurs in the extremities and in areas of the head and face exposed to the environment. Subfreezing temperatures are required for frostbite to occur, although they are not necessary to produce hypothermia. Many patients who experience frostbite will also have hypothermia.

Most patients will describe the clinical sequence of events for frostbite in the following order: extremities become cold → then become painful → pain gradually changes to numbness. The skin may initially have the appearance of reddening. This will change to a white or gray with full freezing. There can be tremendous variation of how an individual can present with frostbite. For example, some patients do not feel a great deal of pain at onset. Others will report severe pain. A certain degree of compliance may be felt beneath the frozen layer in superficial frostbite. But in deep frostbite, the frozen part will be hard and noncompliant.

Prehospital Management—Frostbite.   Care should follow these recommendations:

❏ Do not thaw affected area if there is any possibility of refreezing.
❏ Do not massage the frozen area or rub with snow. Rubbing the affected area may cause ice crystals within the tissues to seriously damage the already injured tissues.
❏ Administer analgesia prior to thawing.
❏ Thaw frozen part by immersion rewarming in a 100–106 degree F. water bath. Water temperature will fall rapidly, requiring additional warm water throughout the process.
❏ Cover the thawed part with loosely applied dry, sterile dressings.
❏ Elevate the thawed part.
❏ Do not puncture or drain the blisters.

✳ Frostbite should be rewarmed in water between 100°F and 106°F.

NEAR-DROWNING AND DROWNING

It is estimated that in the United States, approximately 8,000 persons die annually due to drowning, and approximately 40% of these (3,200) are under 5 years of age. Drowning is the second leading cause of accidental death in the 1–44 year-old age group. Approximately 85% of near-drowning victims are male and two-thirds of these do not know how to swim. There has been an attempt made to differentiate between the terms drowning and near-drowning. It seems to be accepted that the term *drowning* means that death occurred within 24 hours of submersion. In contrast, the term *near-drowning* indicates that death either did not occur or occurred more than 24 hours after submersion.

The paramedic needs to understand the sequence of events in drowning or near-drowning. Following submersion, if the victim is conscious, he or she will undergo a period of complete apnea for up to three minutes. This apnea is an involuntary reflex as the victim strives to keep the head above water. During this time, blood is shunted to the heart and brain, in a fashion similar to the primitive "diving reflex" present in certain lower animals.

When the victim is apneic, the $PaCO_2$ in the blood rises to greater than 50 mmHg. Meanwhile, the PaO_2 of the blood falls below 50 mmHg. The stimulus from the hypoxia ultimately overrides the sedative effects of the hypercarbia, and central nervous system stimulation results. There is associated panic during this stage up until unconsciousness ensues. During this stage the victim makes violent inspiratory and swallowing efforts. At this point, copious amounts of water enter the mouth, posterior pharynx, and stomach, stimulating severe laryngospasm and bronchospasm. In approximately 10% of drowning victims, and in a much greater percentage of near-drowning victims, this laryngospasm prevents the influx of water into the lungs. If a significant amount of water

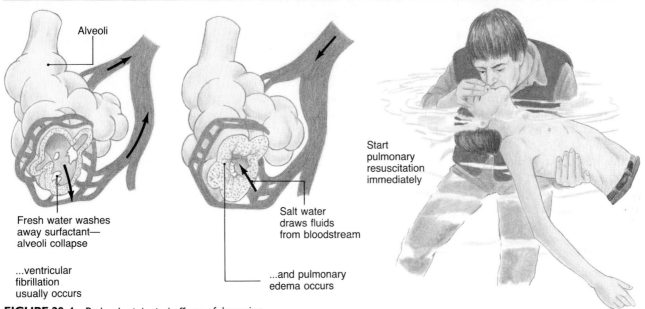

Alveoli

Fresh water washes
away surfactant—
alveoli collapse

...ventricular
fibrillation
usually occurs

Salt water
draws fluids
from bloodstream

...and pulmonary
edema occurs

Start
pulmonary
resuscitation
immediately

FIGURE 28-4 Pathophysiological effects of drowning.

■ **surfactant** a compound secreted by cells in the lungs which
contributes to the elastic properties of the pulmonary tissue.

does not enter the lungs it is referred to as a *dry drowning*. Conversely,
if a laryngospasm does not occur, and a significant quantity of water
does enter the lungs, it is referred to as a *wet drowning*. The laryngospasm, or airway obstruction due to aspirated water, further aggravates the hypoxia, with coma ultimately ensuing. Persistent anoxia
results in a deeper coma. Following unconsciousness, reflex swallowing
occurs which results in gastric distention and increased risk of vomiting
and aspiration. If untreated, hypotension, bradycardia, and death result
in a short period.

Drowning and near-drowning are primarily due to asphyxia from
airway obstruction in the lung secondary to the aspirated water or laryngospasm. If, in a near-drowning episode this process does not end in
death, the fluid may cause lower airway disease.

In fresh water near-drowning, the large surface area of the alveoli
and small airways allows a massive amount of hypotonic water to diffuse
across and into the vascular space. This results in a thickening of the
alveolar walls with inflammatory cells, hemorrhagic pneumonitis, and
destruction of surfactant. **Surfactant** is a substance in the alveoli responsible for maintaining the alveoli open. When the capillaries of the alveoli
are damaged, plasma proteins leak back into the alveoli, resulting in the
accumulation of fluid in the small airways, in turn leading to multiple
areas of atelectasis with shunting and hypoxemia. (See Figure 28-4.)

In saltwater drowning, the hypertonic nature of the fluid draws
water from the bloodstream into the alveoli. In sea water near-drowning,
the hypertonic nature of sea water, which is 3—4 times more hypertonic
than plasma, draws water from the bloodstream into the alveoli. This produces pulmonary edema leading to profound shunting. The result is failure of oxygenation, producing hypoxemia, since the blood is traveling
through the lung tissues without being oxygenated. Additionally, respiratory and metabolic acidosis develop due to the retention of CO_2 and
developing anaerobic metabolism. Since all of the above factors disrupt
normal pulmonary function, initial field treatment must be directed toward correcting the profound hypoxia.

There are other factors which may have an impact on drowning and near-drowning survival rates. These include such things as the cleanliness of the water, the length of time submerged, and the age and general health of the victim. Children have a longer survival time and a greater probability of a successful resuscitation. Even more significant is the water temperature. The concept of developing brain death after four to six minutes without oxygen is not applicable in cases of near-drowning in cold water. Some patients in cold water (below 68 degrees F.) can be resuscitated after 30 minutes or more in cardiac arrest. However, persons under water 60 minutes or longer usually cannot be resuscitated. A possible contribution to survival may be the **mammalian diving reflex.** When a person dives into cold water, he or she reacts to the submersion of the face. Breathing is inhibited, the heart rate becomes bradycardic, and vasoconstriction develops in tissues relatively resistant to asphyxia, while cerebral and cardiac blood flow is maintained. In this way, oxygen is sent and used only where it is needed to immediately sustain life. The colder the water, the more oxygen is diverted to the heart and brain. A common saying in emergency medicine is that the cold water drowning victim is not dead until he or she is warm and dead.

■ **mammalian diving reflex (diving reflex)** a complex cardiovascular reflex, resulting from submersion of the face and nose in water, that constricts blood flow everywhere except to the brain. It decreases cardiac output and rate, and produces stable or slightly increased arterial blood pressure.

Prehospital Management

The patient should be removed from the water as soon as possible by a trained rescue swimmer. Ventilation should be initiated while the patient is still in water. Rescue personnel should wear protective clothing if water temperature is less than 70 degrees F. In addition, a safety line should be attached to the rescue swimmer. In fast water it is essential to use personnel specifically trained for this type of rescue.

Head and neck injury should be suspected if the patient experienced a fall or was diving. The victim should be rapidly placed on a long backboard and should be removed from the water. (See Figure 28-5).

The near-drowning victim should be initially examined for airway patency, breathing, and pulse. If indicated, begin CPR. Airway management should include proper suctioning and use of airway adjuncts. C-spine injury should be considered and treated accordingly. Oxygen should be administered at a 100% concentration. If available, and if transport time is longer than 15 minutes, respiratory rewarming should take place. The Heimlich maneuver is *contraindicated.*

An IV of D5W should be established for venous access and run at 75 mL/hour. If indicated, defibrillation should be carried out. ACLS protocols should be carried out if the patient is normothermic. If the patient is hypothermic, he or she should be treated as described in the hypothermic protocol presented earlier in the chapter

Resuscitation is not indicated if there is evidence of putrefaction (decomposition) or if immersion has been extremely prolonged, unless hypothermia is present.

More than 90% of near-drowning patients survive without sequelae. All near-drowning patients should be admitted to the hospital for observation. Some of these patient have problems with pulmonary parenchymal injury, destruction of surfactant, aspiration pneumonitis, or pneumothorax. A number require an extended hospital stay due to hypoxia, hypercarbia, and mixed metabolic and respiratory acidosis. Treatment of the effects of cerebral hypoxia occasionally continues through and after hospitalization.

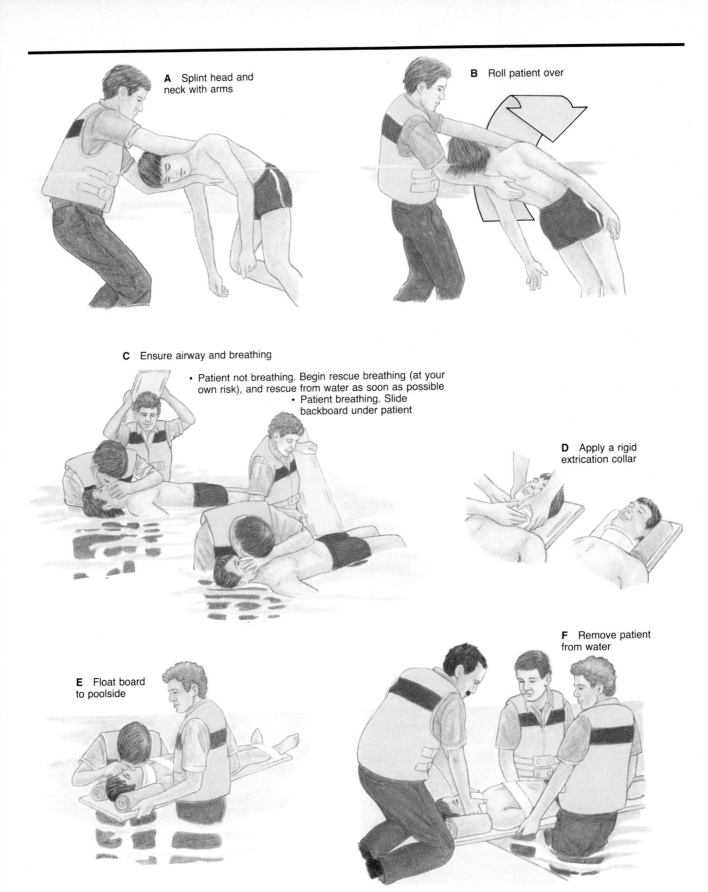

A Splint head and neck with arms

B Roll patient over

C Ensure airway and breathing

- Patient not breathing. Begin rescue breathing (at your own risk), and rescue from water as soon as possible
  - Patient breathing. Slide backboard under patient

D Apply a rigid extrication collar

E Float board to poolside

F Remove patient from water

NOTE: The use of gloves and protective breathing masks or units is not practical for patients receiving in-water care.

FIGURE 28-5 Care of the drowning victim, with possible cervical spine injury.

NUCLEAR RADIATION

Injury due to exposure to ionizing radiation occurs infrequently. However, the incidence of radiation emergencies is, however, becoming more frequent due to the expansion of nuclear medicine procedures and commercial nuclear facilities.

Radiation is a general term applied to the transmission of energy. This energy can include nuclear energy, ultraviolet light, visible light, heat, sound, and X-rays. A radioactive substance emits ionizing radiation, and is referred to as a *radionuclide* or *radioisotope.*

To understand nuclear radiation, it is best to first look at the atomic and nuclear structure, and define some of the basic terms. The atom consists of various sub-atomic particles. Among these are:

- ❏ *Protons*—positively charged particles which form the nucleus of hydrogen, and are present in the nuclei of all elements. The atomic number of the element indicates the number of protons present.
- ❏ *Neutrons*—subatomic particles which are equal in mass to a proton, but without an electrical charge. As a free particle, a neutron has an average life of less than 17 minutes.
- ❏ *Electrons*—minute particles with negative electrical charge, revolving around the nucleus of an atom. When emitted from radioactive substances, electrons are called *beta particles.*

Other terms associated with nuclear medicine the paramedic should be familiar with include:

- ❏ *Isotopes* (*radioisotope*)—atoms in which the nuclear composition is unstable. That is, they give off **ionizing radiation.**
- ❏ **Half-life**—the time required for half the nuclei of a radioactive substance to lose their activity due to radioactive decay.

A radioactive substance is one that emits ionizing radiation. There are four types of radiation:

1. *Alpha particles.* Alpha particles are slow moving, low energy particles that usually can be stopped by such things as clothing and paper. When they contact the skin they only penetrate a few cells deep. Because they can be absorbed (stopped) by a layer of clothing, a few inches of air, or the outer layer of skin, alpha particles constitute a minor hazard. They can produce serious effects if taken internally by ingestion or inhalation.

2. *Beta particles.* Smaller than alpha particles, beta particles are higher in energy. Although beta particles can penetrate air, they can be stopped by aluminum and similar materials. Beta particles generally cause less local damage than alpha particles, but can be harmful if inhaled or ingested.

3. *Gamma rays.* Gamma rays are more highly energized and penetrating than alpha and beta particles. The origin of gamma rays is related to that of x-rays. Gamma radiation is extremely dangerous, carrying high levels of energy which is able to penetrate thick shielding. Gamma rays easily pass through clothing and the entire body, inflicting extensive cell damage. They also cause indirect damage by causing internal tissue to emit alpha and beta particles. Lead shielding is necessary to protect from gamma radiation.

4. *Neutrons.* Neutrons are more penetrating than the other types of radiation. The penetrating power of neutrons is estimated to be 3-10 times greater than gamma rays, but less than the internal hazard associated with ingestion of alpha and beta particles. Exposure to neutrons causes direct tissue damage. However, in nuclear accidents, neutron exposure is not normally a

■ **ionizing radiation** electromagnetic radiation (e.g., X-ray) or particulate radiation (e.g., alpha particles, beta particles, and neurons) capable of producing ions by direct or secondary processes.

■ **half-life** time required for half of the nuclei of a radioactive substance to lose activity by undergoing radioactive decay.

✱ Radiation emergencies should only be handled by those with proper protective equipment and adequate training.

problem for paramedics because neutrons tend to be present only near a reactor core.

Ionizing radiation cannot be seen, felt, or heard. Therefore, a detection instrument is required to measure the radiation given off by the radiation source. The most commonly used device is the Geiger counter. The rate of radiation is measured in roentgens per hour (R/hr) or milliroentgens per hour (mR/hr) (1,000 mR = 1R).

The unit of local tissue energy deposition is called *radiation absorbed dose (RAD)*. *Roentgen equivalent in man (REM)* provides a gauge of the likely injury to the irradiated part of an organism. For all practical purposes, RAD and REM are equal in clinical value. When neutrons or other high energy radiation sources are used, a *quality factor (QF)* is applied to determine the equivalent dose.

Simply stated, ionizing radiation causes alterations in the body's cells, primarily the genetic material (DNA). Depending on the dosage received, the changes can be in cell division, cell structure, and cellular biochemical activities. Cell damage due to ionizing radiation is cumulative over a lifetime. If a person is exposed to ionizing radiation long enough, there will be a decreased number of white blood cells. Additionally, there may be defects in offspring, an increased incidence of cancer, and various degrees of bone marrow damage.

The time it takes for the first biological effects of exposure to ionizing radiation to become detectable varies. These effects are:

❑ *Acute*: effects appearing in a matter of minutes to weeks.
❑ *Long-term*: effects appearing years to decades later.

✱ Limiting radiation exposure is based on three principles: time, distance, and shielding.

There are three basic principles which allows rescue personnel and patients to limit exposure to ionizing radiation. These are time, distance, and shielding. Determining exposure, absorption, and damage done by radiation requires specialized training. How much radiation a person receives depends on the source of radiation, the length of time exposed, the distance from the source, and the shielding between the exposed person and the source. For example, the amount of radiation at the patient's initial location may be 300 R/hr. If exposure is for 20 minutes, this is the same radiation equivalent as working one hour at a 100 R/hr scene. The amount of radiation may drop off rapidly as the patient is decontaminated and moved away from the exposure. The distance from an ionizing radiation source is crucial since exposure is determined by the inverse square relationship. Doubling the distance away from a radiation source reduces the exposure by a factor of four. Conversely, halving the distance to a radiation source, increases exposure by a factor of four.

There are basically two types of ionizing radiation accidents: clean and dirty accidents. In a *clean accident,* the patient is exposed to radiation but is not contaminated by the radioactive substance, particles of radioactive dust, or radioactive liquids, gases, or smoke. If he or she is properly decontaminated before arrival of rescue personnel, there will be little danger, provided the source of the radiation is no longer exposed at the scene. After exposure to ionizing radiation, the patient is not radioactive and therefore poses no hazard to rescue personnel. In contrast, the *dirty accident*—often associated with fire at the scene of a radiation accident—not only exposes the patient to radiation, but contaminates him or her with radioactive particles or liquids. The scene may be highly contaminated, although the primary source of ra-diation is shielded when rescue

Whole Body Exposure Dose (RAD)	Effect
5–25	Asymptomatic. Blood studies are normal.
50–75	Asymptomatic. Minor depressions of white blood cells and platelets in a few patients.
75–125	May produce anorexia, nausea and vomiting, and fatigue in approximately 10–20% of patients within two days.
125–200	Possible nausea and vomiting. Diarrhea, anxiety, tachycardia. Fatal to less than 5% of patients.
200–600	Nausea and vomiting, diarrhea first several hours, weakness, fatigue. Fatal to approximately 50% of patients within six weeks without prompt medical attention.
600–1,000	Severe nausea and vomiting, diarrhea first several hours. Fatal to 100% of patients within two weeks without prompt medical attention.
1,000 or more	"Burning sensation" within minutes, nausea and vomiting within 10 minutes, confusion, ataxia, and prostration within one hour, watery diarrhea within 1–2 hrs. Fatal to 100% within short time without prompt medical attention.

Whole Body Exposure Dose (RAD)	Effect
50	Asymptomatic.
500	Asymptomatic (usually). May have risk of altered function of exposed area.
2,500	Atrophy, vascular lesion, and altered pigmentation.
5,000	Chronic ulcer, risk of carcinogenesis.
50,000	Permanent destruction of exposed tissue.

personnel arrive. Unless the arriving paramedics are properly trained in dealing with this type of emergency, rescue procedures may have to wait until properly trained technical assistance arrives. (See Figure 28-6.)

Prehospital Management—Radiation Emergencies

1. *Park rescue vehicle upwind:* Minimize contamination
2. *Look for signs of radiation exposure:* Radioactive packages are marked by clearly identifiable color-coded labels. (See Figure 28-7.)
3. *Use portable instruments to measure the level of radioactivity:* If dose estimates are significant, rotate rescue personnel.
4. *Normal principles of emergency care:* ABCs; shock management; trauma care.
5. *Externally radiated patient:* No danger to paramedic; normal care procedures for injuries other than radiation.
6. *Internally radiated patient (Ingested or inhaled):* No danger to paramedic; normal care procedures; collect body wastes; use bag-valve-mask or demand valve if artificial respiration required; if inhaled, swab nasal passages and save the swabs.

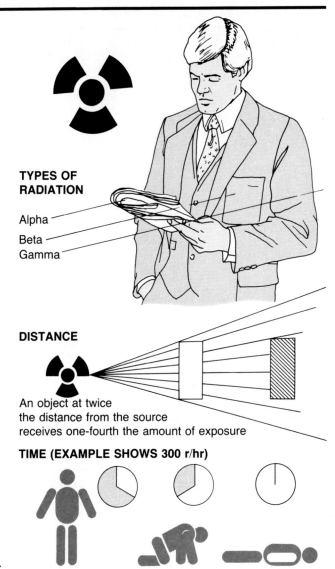

TYPES OF RADIATION

Alpha

Beta

Gamma

DISTANCE

An object at twice
the distance from the source
receives one-fourth the amount of exposure

TIME (EXAMPLE SHOWS 300 r/hr)

FIGURE 28-6 Nuclear radiation.

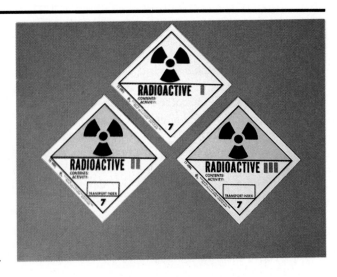

FIGURE 28-7 Radioactive warning labels.

7. *Externally radiated patient (Liquids, dirt, smoke)*: Decontamination of patient required; Normal emergency care procedures; Decontamination of paramedic required after call complete.

8. *Patient with open, contaminated wounds*: Normal emergency care procedures; Avoid cross-contamination of wounds

DIVING EMERGENCIES

SCUBA (Self-Contained Underwater Breathing Apparatus) diving has become an extremely popular recreational sport. SCUBA diving accidents are fairly uncommon, but more prevalent among inexperienced divers. Scuba diving emergencies can occur on the surface, in three feet of water, or at any depth. The more serious emergencies usually follow a dive.

Water is an incompressible, colorless liquid. Fresh water has a density, or weight per unit of volume of 62.4 pounds per cubic foot. Salt water has a density of 64.0 pounds per cubic foot. This density is pressure, which is defined as a weight or force acting on a unit area. Thus, the weight of a cubic foot of fresh water exerts a pressure (weight) of 62.4 pounds over an area of one square foot. This measurement is typically measured in pounds per square inch (psi).

Humans at sea level live in an atmosphere of air weighing and exerting a pressure of 14.7 pounds per square inch. This may vary within the environment. For example, ascending to an altitude of 1 mile decreases the weight of air (the atmospheric pressure) by 17% to approximately 12.2 pounds.

Certain laws explaining the behavior of gases are applicable to diving. First, *Boyle's Law* states that the volume of a gas is inversely proportional to its pressure if the temperature is kept constant. For example, doubling the pressure of a gas mixture will decrease its volume by one-half. The pressure of air at sea level is 14.7 lb./sq.in. or 760 mmHg. This pressure is called one atmosphere absolute or 1 "ata." Two ata occurs at a depth of 33 feet of water, and 3 ata occurs at a depth of 66 feet of water, and so on. Therefore, one liter of air at the surface is compressed to a 500 mL at 33 feet. At 66 feet 1 liter of air would be compressed to 250 mL.

Henry's law states that the amount of gas dissolved in a given volume of fluid is proportional to the pressure of the gas with which it is in equilibrium. The body is primarily made up of liquid. Therefore, gases that are inhaled will be dissolved in the body in proportion to the partial pressure of each breath. The body uses oxygen, but does not use nitrogen. Therefore, the primary gas dissolved in the body is nitrogen because it is inert and not used by the body. At 33 feet below the surface, the quantity of oxygen and nitrogen dissolved in the tissues will be twice that at sea level. Gas molecules will be absorbed into a given quantity of liquid until a condition of equilibrium is reached where the gas in the liquid reaches a value equal to the partial pressure of the gas (saturation). A diver's body can also become saturated if he or she breathes gases long enough under pressure. As long as the pressure is maintained, gases dissolved in liquids will remain in solution. However, if the pressure is gradually reduced, the gases in the solution can escape with no noticeable effect. For example, carbon dioxide is held in solution in a carbonated soda by pressure of that gas in the space above the liquid. When the soda can or bottle is opened, the carbon dioxide is released from the solution into the atmosphere. Gases are dissolved in the diver's blood under pressure. During controlled ascent dissolved gases escape through respiration or else bub-

■ **SCUBA** abbreviation for Self-Contained Underwater Breathing Apparatus.

bles can form within the body. The ascending diver who comes to the surface too rapidly, not adhering to safety measures, is at risk of becoming a veritable "living" can or bottle of soda.

Scuba diving injuries are due to either *barotrauma* (mechanical effect of the pressure differential), cerebral air embolism, compression illness, cold, panic, or a combination of the above. Accidents generally occur at four stages of the dive. These stages include the following:

Injuries on the Surface. This can involve entanglement of lines or entanglement in kelp fields while swimming to the area of the dive. Divers in these situations may panic, become fatigued, or drown. Additionally, the water may be cold producing shivering and blackout. Boats in the area are another potential source of injury to the diver. To prevent such accidents, divers will usually mark the area of their dive with a flag. Maritime rules require boat operators to stay clear of the area.

Injuries During Descent. Barotrauma, commonly called the "squeeze," becomes a concern during the descent. If the diver is unable to equilibrate the pressure between the nasopharynx and the middle ear through the eustachian tube, he or she can experience middle ear pain. Besides pain, signs and symptoms include ringing in the ears, dizziness, and hearing loss. In severe cases rupture of the ear drum can occur. A diver who has an upper respiratory infection and therefore cannot clear the middle ear through the eustachian tube should not dive. A similar lack of equilibration can occur in the sinuses, producing severe frontal headaches or pain beneath the eye in the maxillary sinuses.

Injuries on the Bottom. Major diving emergencies while at the bottom of the dive involve nitrogen narcosis, commonly called "raptures of the deep." This is due to nitrogen's effect on cerebral function. The diver may appear to be intoxicated and may take unnecessary risks. If the diver runs low or out of air, he or she may suddenly panic, causing increased oxygen consumption and further carbon dioxide production.

Injuries During Ascent. Serious and life-threatening emergencies can occur during the ascent. The causes may be related to barotrauma and the diver's inability to equilibrate his or her inner ear pressure with nasopharyngeal pressure. Dives below 40 feet require staged ascent to prevent the bends. The most serious barotrauma which occurs during the ascent is injury to the lung. This can occur in as little as three feet below the surface or it can occur during a deep dive. The injury results from the diver holding his or her breath during the ascent. As the diver ascends, the air in the lung, which has been compressed, expands. If it is not exhaled, the alveoli may rupture. If this occurs, the result will be structural damage to the lung and **air embolism.** There may also be mediastinal and subcutaneous emphysema due to diffusion of the gas through the lung into the mediastinum and the neck. Pneumothorax is possible if the alveoli rupture into the pleural cavity. Air embolism can occur if the air ruptures into the pulmonary veins or arteries and returns to the left atrium and finally into the left ventricle and out the systemic circulation.

In the early management of diving accidents all symptoms of air embolism and decompression sickness are considered together. Early assessment and treatment of a diving injury is of more importance than trying to distinguish the exact problem. The initial history from divers presenting with a diving-related injury is the *diving history* or *profile.*

■ **air embolism** presence of an air bubble in the circulatory system.

General Assessment—Diving Emergencies

- ❏ Time relationship of signs and symptoms:
    - ❏ Before surfacing
    - ❏ During surfacing
    - ❏ After surfacing
- ❏ Type of breathing apparatus:
    - ❏ SCUBA
    - ❏ Other
- ❏ Type of hypothermia protective garment:
    - ❏ Wet suit
    - ❏ Dry suit
- ❏ Dive parameters:
    - ❏ Depth of dive
    - ❏ Number of dives
    - ❏ Duration of dive
    - ❏ Aircraft travel following dive
- ❏ Rate of ascent:
    - ❏ Panic?
    - ❏ Student diver
    - ❏ Depth gauge working?
- ❏ Previous medical diseases
- ❏ Old injuries
- ❏ Previous decompression illness
- ❏ Medications
- ❏ Use of alcohol

From a quick assessment of the patient's diving profile, it can be rapidly determined if the diver is an excellent candidate for decompression sickness.

Decompression Sickness (Caisson Disease or "Bends")

Decompression sickness is a condition that develops in divers subjected to rapid reduction of air pressure after ascending to the surface following exposure to compressed air. Nitrogen bubbles enter the tissue spaces and small blood vessels. Symptoms present when a diver, exposed to a depth of 33 feet or greater for sufficient time for the body's tissues to be saturated with nitrogen, ascends to the surface rapidly. The effects of nitrogen bubbles on the body can be direct or indirect.

■ **decompression sickness** condition, commonly known as "the bends," in which nitrogen bubbles develop within the tissues due to a rapid reduction of air pressure after a diver returns to the surface following exposure to compressed air.

Direct:

- ❏ *Intravascular.* Blood flow will be decreased, leading to ischemia or infarct.
- ❏ *Extravascular.* Tissues will be displaced, which further results in pressure on neutral tissue.
- ❏ **Audiovestibular.** Air can diffuse into the vestibular system, causing vertigo.

■ **audiovestibular system** the organs and structure of the inner ear associated with hearing and balance.

Indirect:

- ❏ Surface of air emboli may initiate platelet aggregation and intravascular coagulation.
- ❏ Extravascular plasma loss may lead to edema.

❑ Electrolyte imbalances.
❑ Lipid emboli are released.

The bubbles produced by rapid decompression are thought to produce obstruction of blood flow and lead to local ischemia, subjecting tissues to anoxic stress. In some cases, this stress may lead to tissue damage.

Decompression sickness can be divided into types I and II based on the presenting signs and symptoms.

Type I. The historical term for type I decompression sickness is the "bends." Patients with it experience extremity pain, usually localized to larger joints, such as the shoulders or elbows. The bends is caused by expansion of gases present in the joint space. Skin manifestations of type I decompression sickness usually consists only of pruritus (the itch), although a rash, spotted pallor or cyanosis, or pitting edema may also occur. The treatment for type I decompression sickness mainly consists of oxygen inhalation, occasional **recompression,** and observation for signs of more serious decompression sickness. Prognosis for type I decompression sickness is good.

Type II. Patients who develop type II decompression sickness may present with a broad spectrum of complaints. The patient can present with any of the signs and symptoms of type I decompression sickness plus any one or more of the following:

❑ Paresthesia
❑ Dizziness or vertigo
❑ Nausea
❑ Auditory disturbances
❑ Vestibular disturbances
❑ Paralysis
❑ Headache
❑ Dyspnea
❑ Chest pain
❑ Loss of consciousness
❑ Hemoptysis

Decompression sickness has been called the "Great Imitator" due to its variety of presentations. The pulmonary complications of decompression sickness, referred to as "the chokes," are extremely serious.

■ **recompression** the restoration of pressure, often used in the treatment of diving emergencies so that a patient can be slowly decompressed.

General and Individual Factors Relating to the Development of Decompression Sickness

General Factors	Individual Factors
Cold water dives	Age—older individuals
Diving in rough water	Obesity
Strenuous diving conditions	Fatigue—lack of sleep prior to dive
History of previous decompression dive incident	Alcohol—consumption before or after dive
Overstaying time at given dive depth	History of medical problems
Dive at 80 feet or greater	
Rapid ascent—panic, inexperience, unfamiliarity with equipment	
Heavy exercise before or after dive to the point of muscle soreness	
Flying after diving (24 hour wait is recommended)	
Driving to high altitude after dive	

General Symptoms—Decompression Sickness. In summary, the general symptoms of decompression sickness include:

- ☐ Extreme fatigue (early sign)
- ☐ Joint pain
- ☐ Headache
- ☐ Lower abdominal pain
- ☐ Chest pain
- ☐ Urinary dysfunction
- ☐ Vertigo and ataxia
- ☐ Pruritus (severe itching)
- ☐ Nausea/vomiting
- ☐ Back pain
- ☐ Priapism
- ☐ Paresthesias (numbness/tingling)
- ☐ Paralysis
- ☐ Dysarthria (difficult speech)
- ☐ Frothy, reddish sputum
- ☐ Dyspnea

Patients with decompression sickness usually seek medical treatment within 12 hours of ascent from a dive. Some patients may not seek treatment for as long as 24 hours after the last dive. It is generally safe to assume that signs or symptoms developing more than 36 hours after a dive cannot reasonably be attributed to decompression sickness.

Decompression sickness may require urgent recompression for complete treatment. However, prompt stabilization at the nearest emergency department should be accomplished before transportation to a recompression chamber.

Early oxygen therapy may reduce symptoms of decompression sickness substantially. Divers who are administered high concentrations of oxygen have a considerably better treatment outcome. The following lists the prehospital management of decompression sickness.

Prehospital Management—Decompression Sickness*

1. Assess ABCs.
2. Administer CPR if required.
3. Administer oxygen at 100% concentration with a non-rebreathing mask. An unconscious diver should be intubated.
4. Keep the patient in left-side-head-low position (10–15 degrees) if possible (considered optional).
5. Protect the patient from excessive heat, cold, wetness, or noxious fumes.
6. Give the conscious, alert patient nonalcoholic liquids such as fruit juices or oral balanced salt solutions.
7. Evaluate and stabilize the patient at the nearest emergency department prior to transport to a recompression chamber. Begin IV fluid replacement with electrolyte solutions for unconscious or seriously injured patients. Ringer's lactate, normal saline, or 5% dextrose in normal saline may be used. *Do not use 5% dextrose in water.*

* Diving physician can be contacted at Divers Alert Network (919) 684-8111. Call collect if necessary in an emergency.

8. If there is evidence of CNS involvement, administer dexamethasone, heparin, Dextran, or Valium as ordered by medical control.*

9. If air evacuation is used, do not expose the patient to decreased barometric pressure. Cabin pressure must be maintained at sea level, or fly at the lowest possible safe altitude.

10. Send diving equipment with the patient for examination. If impossible, arrange for local examination and gas analysis.

Pulmonary Overpressure Accidents

Lung overinflation due to rapid ascent is the common cause of a number of emergencies. A pressure buildup in the lung can damage the lung and allow air to escape into the circulation leading to air embolism. Air expansion on ascent can rupture the alveolar membranes. This can result in hemorrhage, reduced oxygen and carbon dioxide transport, and capillary and alveolar inflammation. Air can also escape from the lung into other nearby tissues and cause pneumothorax and tension pneumothorax, subcutaneous emphysema, or **pneumomediastinum.**

■ **pneumomediastinum** the presence of air in the mediastinum.

Air Embolism. If any person using scuba equipment presents with neurologic deficits during or immediately after ascent, an air embolism should be suspected. As death or serious disability can result, prompt medical treatment is crucial.

Air embolism is a form of barotrauma of ascent. It is a very serious condition in which air bubbles enter the circulatory system through rupture of small pulmonary vessels. Air can also be trapped in blebs, or air pockets, within the pulmonary tissue. These bubbles can then be transported to the heart and the brain, where they may lodge and obstruct blood flow, causing ischemia and possibly infarct.

Signs and symptoms of air embolism include a rapid and dramatic onset, sharp, tearing pain, paralysis (frequently hemiplegia), cardiac and pulmonary collapse, unequal pupils, and wide pulse pressure. Prehospital management of air embolism and should include:

1. Assess ABCs
2. Administer oxygen by non-rebreathing mask at 12 lpm.
3. Place patient in left lateral Trendelenburg position
4. Frequent monitoring of vital signs
5. Administer IV fluids at a TKO rate
6. Dexamethasone (Decadron) may be ordered by medical control
7. Transport to recompression chamber ASAP

If air transport is utilized it is very important to use pressurized aircraft or fly at a low altitude.

Pneumomediastinum. A *pneumomediastinum* is the release of gas (air) through the visceral pleura into the mediastinum and pericardial sac. Signs and symptoms of a pneumomediastinum include substernal chest pain, irregular pulse, abnormal heart sounds, reduced blood pressure and narrow pulse pressure, and a change in voice. There may or may not

* Give drugs only under the direction of a physician familiar with diving medicine.

be evidence of cyanosis. The field management of pneumomediastinum includes administering high concentration oxygen via non-rebreathing face mask, IV lactated Ringer's or normal saline as per physician order, and transport to the emergency department. Treatment generally ranges from observation to recompression to relieve acute symptoms. The patient should be observed for 24 hours for any other signs of lung overpressure. He or she should not be recompressed unless air embolism or decompression sickness are also present.

SUMMARY

Basic knowledge of common environmental, recreational, and exposure injuries is necessary for the paramedic to administer prompt and proper treatment in the prehospital setting. Familiarity with such subjects as hyperthermia, hypothermia, near-drowning, diving, and radiation emergencies is not easy to retain since they are not usually encountered on a daily basis. There are too many cases where paramedics have lost their lives when attempting a rescue for which they were not properly trained. Rapid action is always necessary when performing an environmental rescue. However, common sense must prevail.

FURTHER READING

BLEDSOE, B. E., BOSKER, G., and PAPA, F. J., *Prehospital Emergency Pharmacology. 2d ed.* Englewood Cliffs, NJ: Prentice-Hall, Inc., 1988.

DANZL, D. F., POZOS, R. S., and HAMLET, M. P., "Accidental Hypothermia," from Auerbach and Geehr: Management of Wilderness and Environmental Emergencies, 2d ed, St. Louis, MO: C. V. Mosby Co., 1989.

GAZZANIGA, A. B., ISERI, L. T., and BAREN, M., *Emergency Care: Principles and Practices for the EMT-Paramedic. 2d ed.* Reston, VA: Reston Publishing Company, 1982.

GRANT, H. D., MURRAY, R. H., and BERGERON, J. D., *Emergency Care. 4th ed.* Englewood Cliffs, NJ: Prentice-Hall, Inc., 1986.

GUYTON, A. C., *Textbook of Medical Physiology. 7th ed.* Philadelphia, PA: W.B. Saunders Company, 1987.

TINTINALLI, J. E., KROME, R. L., and RUIZ, E., *Emergency Medicine: A Comprehensive Study Guide. 2d ed.* New York, NY: McGraw-Hill Book Company, 1988.

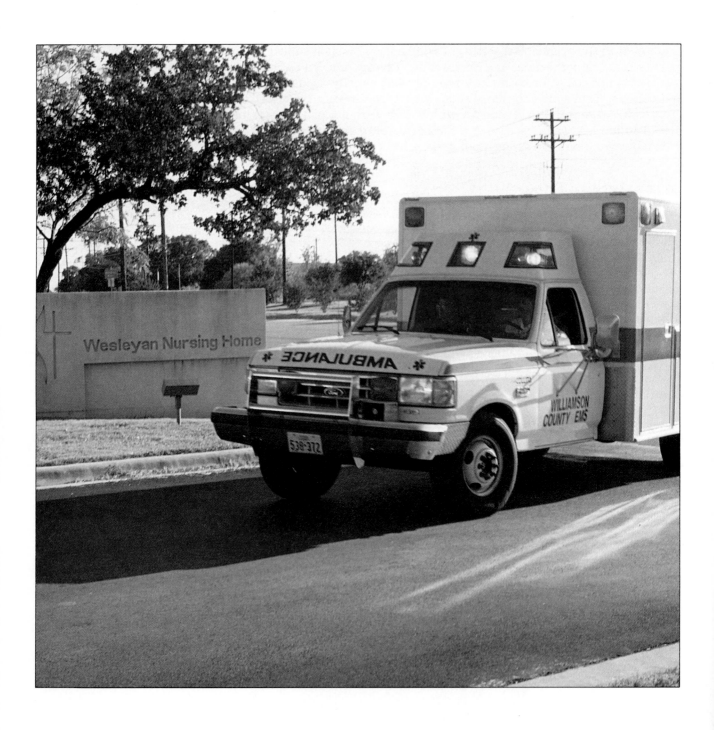

29

Emergencies in the Geriatric Patient

Objectives for Chapter 29

Upon completing this chapter, the student should be able to:

1. Discuss statistics on aging and the geriatric population.

2. Discuss the general age-related organ-system decline as it relates to the following body systems:
   - respiratory system
   - cardiovascular system
   - renal system
   - nervous system
   - musculoskeletal system
   - gastrointestinal system

3. List four factors that complicate the clinical evaluation of the geriatric patient.

4. List some common complaints of geriatric patients as related to the medical history.

5. Be able to distinguish the chief complaint from the primary problem.

6. Define syncope.

7. Discuss the following kinds of syncope:
   - vasodepressor syncope
   - orthostatic syncope
   - cardiac syncope

8. Define seizure and discuss the progression of events.

9. Define vertigo and discuss the progression of events.

10. Define dementia as it applies to the elderly.

11. Define Alzheimer's Disease.

12. List two causes of cardiac dysrhythmias in the elderly.

13. Discuss gastrointestinal bleeding.

14. Discuss the general management of gastrointestinal bleeding.

15. Discuss the impact of environment on the elderly.

16. Discuss why the elderly are more susceptible to trauma.

17. Discuss elderly abuse and neglect, and determine what resources are available and what laws concerning these problems are available in your community.

Mrs. Robertson is a 76-year-old white female who lives alone. Her husband died several years ago and her children look in on her occasionally. When her daughter comes in to check on her, Mrs. Robertson says she hasn't been feeling well. Her daughter notes that she is quite pale. As the patient starts to get up, she faints and falls to the floor. She soon comes to, but is still quite weak. Her daughter summons EMS.

Within five minutes, a paramedic ambulance arrives. The paramedics complete the primary and secondary assessment. The patient is indeed pale. Her blood pressure is 100/60 and pulse is 110. ECG shows atrial fibrillation. The paramedics repeat the vitals signs with the patient seated. The blood pressure drops to 80/60 and the pulse increases to 130. A brief review of the history reveals the patient has been having diarrhea, with black stools. She has had some occasional epigastric pain. Also, her arthritis has been acting up and she has been taking a lot more aspirin.

The paramedics apply oxygen and begin an IV of lactated Ringer's. The patient is placed on the PASG, but it is not inflated. Transport to the hospital goes without problem. In the emergency department, a nasogastric tube is inserted and bloody material aspirated. The patient's hemoglobin is 6.6 grams (normal 12–14). A bleeding duodenal ulcer is found. The patient is transfused with blood and placed on anti-ulcer medications. She is discharged seven days later and does well.

INTRODUCTION

The elderly are rapidly becoming the fastest-growing segment of our population. Among the reasons for this trend are:

- ❑ an increased mean survival of older persons
- ❑ a declining birth rate
- ❑ the absence of major wars and other catastrophes
- ❑ improved health care

It is important to realize that there has been a 53% increase in life-expectancy for all persons since 1900. For example, average life-expectancy in 1900 was 49 years; in 1986, it was up to 75 years.

Generally, the elderly are persons over age 65 years. Though arbitrary, this age is often used because it is the age at which people become eligible for Medicare and retirement. Over the last several years there has been a trend for physicians and other health care workers to specialize in care of the elderly. This aspect of medicine, commonly called **geriatrics,** is an important and necessary one to care for the aging population.

■ **geriatrics** the study and treatment of diseases of the old.

There are several important considerations in providing health care to the elderly. This chapter will present the fundamental principles of geriatrics, and will address the needs and problems of persons in this age group, especially in the area of advanced prehospital care.

ANATOMY AND PHYSIOLOGY

Many anatomical and physiological changes occur as we enter **senescence.** Overall, there is a general decline in organ system function, affecting virtually every organ system. The decline and change begin at the cellular level. As an overview, it is important to note that the amount of total body water is decreased. In addition, total body fat decreases as much as 15%–30%. Although the metabolic rate remains fairly constant, there is often a decrease in the total number of body cells, often up to 30%, by age 65. Most important, there is a progressive reduction in the efficiency of the body's homeostatic control systems. The homeostatic systems are those body control systems that keep the internal environment of the body constant. These systems play a major role in aiding the body in recovery from illness or injury, as well as in the prevention of illness and injury. Inhibition of these control systems results in delayed healing and delayed recuperation.

No body system is spared the effects of age. (See Figure 29-1.) Age-related changes in the respiratory system begin as early as age 30. By the time we reach age 65 years, vital capacity may decrease as much as 50%. The maximum breathing capacity may decrease as much as 60%, while the maximum work capacity and the maximum oxygen uptake may decrease up to 70%. This is often complicated by the presence of underlying pulmonary disease, such as emphysema.

■ **senescence** the process of growing old.

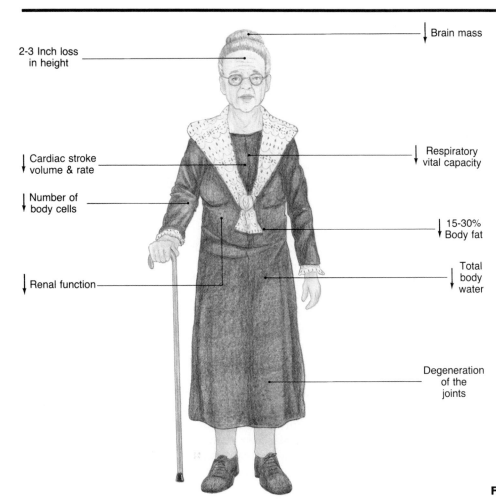

FIGURE 29-1 Age-related changes.

hypertrophy an increase in the size or bulk of an organ.

fibrosis the formation of fiber-like connective tissue, also called scar tissue, in an organ.

nerve conduction velocity the rate at which a nervous impulse is transmitted along a nerve.

osteoporosis softening of bone tissue due to the loss of essential minerals, principly calcium.

kyphosis exaggeration of the normal posterior curvature of the spine.

The cardiovascular system is affected as well. Stroke volume declines and heart rate slows. The conductive system of the heart degenerates, resulting in dysrhythmias and various degrees of heart block. The wall of the left ventricle can thicken (**hypertrophy**), often as much as 25%. This is even more pronounced if there is associated hypertension. In addition, **fibrosis** develops in the heart and peripheral vascular system, resulting in hypertension, arteriosclerosis, and decreased cardiac function.

The effects of aging are also evident in the renal system, where the number of functioning nephrons, the functional units of the kidney, may be decreased 30%–40%. Renal blood flow may decrease as much as 45%, thus increasing the amount of waste products in the blood.

The brain can lose as much as 45% of its cells in certain areas of the cortex. Overall, there is an average 6%–7% reduction in the weight of the brain. Blood flow to the cerebral areas is decreased as well, due to increased resistance and the presence of arteriosclerosis. The amount of oxygen the brain uses, especially in the cortical areas, may decrease. Peripherally, there may be up to a 15% reduction in **nerve conduction velocity,** thus slowing reflexes, as well as sensory and motor function.

A steady deterioration of hearing and vision is also associated with aging. Although the degree varies between individuals, impairment can contribute significantly to dementia and confusion.

An aging person may lose as much as 2–3 inches of height from narrowing of the intervertebral discs and **osteoporosis.** Osteoporosis is the loss of minerals from the bone, resulting in softening of the bones. This is especially evident in the vertebral bodies, thus causing a change in posture. The posture of the aged individual often reveals an increase in the curvature of the thoracic spine, commonly called **kyphosis,** and slight flexion of the knee and hip joints. The demineralization of bone often makes the patient much more susceptible to hip and other fractures. In addition to skeletal changes, a decrease in skeletal muscle weight often occurs with age.

The gastrointestinal system is affected in various ways. The volume of saliva may decrease as much as 33%. Gastric secretions may decrease to as little as 20% of the quantity present in youth. Esophageal motility decreases, thus making swallowing less effective and more difficult.

ASSESSMENT OF THE GERIATRIC PATIENT

The assessment of the geriatric patient is essentially the same as that for any adult. However, several factors complicate the clinical evaluation. It is often difficult to separate the effects of aging from the consequences of disease. For example, it is hard to discern whether a patient's subjective dyspnea is due to normal age-related changes in the respiratory system, or to underlying disease, such as emphysema.

Often, the chief complaint of the geriatric patient may be trivial or vague, and the patient may fail to report important symptoms. The paramedic should try to distinguish the patient's chief complaint from the patient's primary problem. The chief complaint is the symptom the patient is most concerned about, whereas the primary problem may be entirely different. A patient may complain about nausea, which is the chief complaint. The primary problem, however, may be the rectal bleeding the patient forgot to mention.

Another complicating factor is that the geriatric patient is more apt to suffer from more than one disease at a time. The presence of chronic problems may make it more difficult to assess an acute problem. Often, it is easy to confuse symptoms of a chronic illness with those of an acute problem. When confronted with an elderly patient who has chest pain, for example, it is difficult to determine whether the presence of frequent premature ventricular contractions is acute or chronic. Lacking access to the patient's medical record, paramedics must treat the patient on a "threat-to-life" basis.

Another important complication in managing the elderly patient is that aging changes an individual's response to illness and injury. Pain may be diminished or absent, thus causing both the patient and the paramedic to underestimate the severity of the illness. In addition, the temperature-regulating mechanism may be altered, or depressed. This can result in the absence of fever, or a minimal fever, even in the face of severe infection. The alteration in the temperature-regulating mechanism makes the elderly more prone to environmental thermal problems. Social and emotional factors may have a greater impact on health in the elderly than in any other age group. A common example is that of a previously healthy elderly person, who becomes seriously ill, or dies, soon after the death of his or her spouse.

Remember that while the chief complaint of the geriatric patient may seem trivial, it often indicates more serious underlying disease. Common complaints in the elderly include:

❏ fatigue and weakness
❏ dizziness, vertigo, or syncope
❏ falls
❏ headache
❏ insomnia (trouble sleeping)
❏ dysphagia (difficulty in swallowing)
❏ loss of appetite
❏ inability to void
❏ constipation or diarrhea

When presented with these complaints, the paramedic must probe for significant symptoms and, ultimately, the primary problem.

Communications often become more difficult when dealing with the aged. Their sight is often diminished, due to **cataracts** and **glaucoma**. Blindness, often resulting from diabetes and stroke, is more common in the elderly. There is often an increased level of anxiety in the patient, caused by his or her inability to control the situation, and complicated by the inability to see his or her surroundings. When dealing with the patient whose vision is decreased, it is important to talk calmly. Yelling is unnecessary and unhelpful. The paramedic should position himself or herself to be easily seen by the patient.

■ **cataracts** medical condition where the lens of the eye loses its clearness.

■ **glaucoma** medical condition where the pressure within the eye increases.

Hearing, too, is affected by age. Diminished hearing or deafness can make it virtually impossible to obtain a history. With truly deaf patients, you can often determine the history from a friend or family member. Do not assume a patient is deaf without inquiring. Do not shout at the patient. This will not help if the patient is deaf, and it may distort sounds and make it difficult for the patient who has some hearing to understand you. Write notes if necessary. If the patient can lip-read, speak slowly and directly toward the patient. Whenever possible, verify the history with a reliable friend or relative.

There often is a decrease in mental status that makes communications more difficult. The patient can be confused and unable to remember details. In addition, the noise of radios, ECG equipment, and strange voices may add to the confusion. Both senility and organic brain syndrome may manifest themselves similarly. Common symptoms include:

❑ delirium
❑ confusion
❑ distractibility
❑ restlessness
❑ excitability
❑ hostility

✱ Never assume that a confused elderly patient is "just senile." Always assess for an underlying problem.

When confronted with a confused patient, try to determine whether the patient's mental status represents a significant change from normal. DO NOT assume that a confused, disoriented patient is "just senile" and fail to assess for an underlying problem. Alcoholism is more common in the elderly than is generally recognized. It can further complicate taking the history.

✱ Depression is more common in the elderly than once thought.

Depression is fairly common in the elderly and can be mistaken for many other diseases. It can often mimic senility and organic brain syndrome, and can inhibit patient cooperation. The depressed patient may be malnourished, dehydrated, overdosed, contemplating suicide, or simply imagining physical ailments for attention. If depression is suspect, the patient should be questioned regarding drug ingestion or suicidal ideation. It is important to remember that suicide is now the fourth-leading cause of death among the elderly in the United States.

The paramedic should obtain a pertinent, yet brief, medical history from the geriatric patient. The history may be quite complicated, because of multiple diseases and multiple medications. The medication history is also important and can be an indicator of the patient's diseases. It is important to find all of the patient's medications and take them with the patient to the hospital. The paramedic should try to determine which of

TABLE 29-1   Risk Factors For Suicide

- Age over 55
- Male
- Presence of a painful or disabling physical illness, especially in a man who was robust and energetic
- Alone
- History of prior suicide attempts
- Family history of suicide
- History of drug or alcohol abuse
- Depression, especially associated with agitation, hypochondriasis, excessive guilt or self-reproach, and insomnia
- Decreased income, or debt
- Bereavement
- Suicidal preoccupation and talk
- Toward the end of a depressive illness, when energy returns but low mood persists
- Well-defined plans for suicide

the medications, including over-the-counter ones, are current. The elderly patient is often on multiple medications, thus causing an increased chance of medication errors, drug interactions, and noncompliance.

After obtaining the history, and if time allows, try to verify the patient's history with a reliable family member or neighbor. This will often be less offensive to the patient if done out of his or her presence. While at the scene, it is important to observe the surroundings for indication of the patient's ability to care for himself or herself. Look for evidence of drug or alcohol ingestion and for Medic-Alert and Vial-of-Life items. It is also important to look for signs of abuse or neglect.

Physical Examination

Certain considerations must be kept in mind when examining the geriatric patient. It is important to remember that the patient is often easily fatigued and cannot tolerate a long examination. Also, because of the problems with temperature regulation, the patient may be wearing several layers of clothing, which can make examination difficult. Be sure to explain all actions clearly before initiating the examination, especially in patients with decreased sight. Be aware that the patient may minimize or deny symptoms because he or she fears being bedridden or institutionalized, or being forced to give up self-sufficiency.

Peripheral pulses may be difficult to evaluate, because of peripheral vascular disease and arthritis. The paramedic must try to distinguish signs of chronic disease from an acute problem. For example, the elderly may have non-pathological rales. There is often an increase in mouth breathing, and a loss of skin elasticity, which may be easily confused with dehydration. Dependent edema may be caused by varicose veins and inactivity, not congestive heart failure. Only experience and practice will allow the paramedic to distinguish acute from chronic physical findings.

PATHOPHYSIOLOGY AND MANAGEMENT

Trauma in the Elderly

The elderly are more at risk from trauma than younger people, especially from falls. Contributing factors include:

* ❏ slower reflexes
* ❏ failing eyesight and hearing
* ❏ arthritis
* ❏ loss of elasticity in the peripheral blood vessels, making them more subject to tearing
* ❏ tissues and bones that are more fragile

The elderly, because of their physical state and vulnerability, are at high risk from trauma caused by criminal assault.

The elderly are more prone to head injury, even from relatively minor trauma, than their younger counterparts. A major factor is the difference in proportion between the brain and the skull. As mentioned ear-

✳ The elderly are at increased risk for more serious injuries due to trauma than their younger counterparts.

lier, the brain decreases in size and weight with age. The skull, however, remains constant in size, allowing the brain more room to move, thus increasing the likelihood of brain injury. Because of this, signs of brain compression may develop more slowly in the elderly, sometimes over days and weeks. In fact, the patient may often have forgotten the offending injury.

■ **spondylolysis** a degeneration of the vertebral body.

The cervical spine is also more susceptible to injury, from osteoporosis and **spondylolysis.** Spondylolysis is a degeneration of the vertebral body. The elderly often have a significant degree of this disease. In addition, arthritic changes can gradually compress the nerve rootlets or spinal cord. Thus, injury to the spine in the elderly makes the patient much more susceptible to spinal-cord injury. In fact, sudden neck movement, even without fracture, may cause spinal-cord injury. This can occur with less than normal pain, due to the absence of fracture.

Trauma Management Considerations in the Geriatric Patient

The priorities of care for the geriatric trauma patient are similar to those for any trauma patient, but they require the consideration of organ system decline and the presence of chronic disease. This is especially true of the cardiovascular, respiratory, and renal systems. Recent or past myocardial infarctions may contribute to the risk of dysrhythmia or congestive heart failure in the trauma patient. In addition, there may be a decreased response of the heart, in adjusting heart rate and stroke volume, to hypovolemia. The geriatric trauma patient may require higher than usual arterial pressures for perfusion of vital organs, due to increased peripheral vascular resistance and hypertension. Care must be taken in intravenous fluid administration, because of decreased myocardial reserves. As a result, hypotension and hypovolemia are poorly tolerated. In addition, the geriatric patient's physical response to drugs may be altered.

Physical changes in the elderly can decrease chest wall movement and vital capacity. Higher PaO_2's are required with each passing decade. To complicate matters, with age, all organs have a much lower tolerance for anoxia. Chronic obstructive pulmonary disease is common, thus requiring airway management and ventilation to be properly attuned to provide adequate oxygenation and appropriate CO_2 removal. It is important to remember that use of 50% nitrous oxide (Nitronox®) for persons of this age group may result in more respiratory depression than would occur in a younger person. Positive pressure ventilation should be used cautiously in the geriatric patient—there is an increased danger of resultant alkalosis and rupture of emphysematous bullae, resulting in pneumothorax. The decreased ability of the kidney to maintain normal acid/ base balance, and to compensate for fluid changes, can further complicate the management of the geriatric trauma patient. Any pre-existing renal disease can further decrease the kidney's ability to compensate. The decrease in renal function, along with a decreased cardiac reserve, places the injured elderly patient at risk for fluid overload and pulmonary edema.

Positioning, immobilization, and packaging of the geriatric patient before transportation may have to be modified to accommodate physical deformities such as arthritis, spinal abnormalities, and frozen limbs.

RESPIRATORY DISTRESS IN THE GERIATRIC PATIENT

Many factors can cause respiratory distress in the elderly patient. Pulmonary embolism should always be considered as a possible etiology of respiratory distress. This is most apt to follow a period of immobilization or develop from atrial fibrillation. This should be suspected in any patient with the acute onset of dyspnea.

Acute pulmonary edema, which often accompanies acute myocardial infarction, can present as acute dyspnea. This is often accompanied by the presence of moist rales on physical examination.

It is not uncommon for an older patient to suffer a silent myocardial infarction and have dyspnea as the only symptom. The paramedic should be particularly aware of this and listen carefully for physical signs of pulmonary edema.

Chronic obstructive pulmonary diseases—emphysema, chronic bronchitis, and, to a lesser degree, asthma—are frequent causes of respiratory distress in the elderly. Pneumonia, as well as other respiratory infections, is a frequent cause of dyspnea, and many times death, in elderly persons. It should always be suspect, especially in the face of fever or chills.

Cancer occurs more frequently in the geriatric population. Often, progressive dyspnea will be the first presentation of a cancerous lesion. Cancerous tissue does not have to be present in the lung to present as dyspnea.

The management of respiratory distress in the geriatric patient is essentially the same as for all age groups. However, the paramedic should be familiar with the altered respiratory function of older patients and plan management accordingly. Many geriatric patients with respiratory disease also have underlying cardiac disease. With this in mind, drugs such as theophylline and the beta agonists should be used with extreme caution.

Syncope

Cardiovascular conditions are more common in older persons, primarily due to progressive atherosclerotic disease. **Syncope** is a common presenting complaint, yet a difficult one to assess. However, syncope has a much higher morbidity in the patient over 60 years of age than in younger individuals. Syncope results when blood flow to the brain is temporarily interrupted or decreased. It is most often caused by problems with either the nervous system or the cardiovascular system. Common causes of syncope include:

■ **syncope** a transient loss of consciousness, caused by inadequate blood flow to the brain.

Vasodepressor Syncope. Vasodepressor syncope is the common faint. It may occur following emotional distress; pain; prolonged bed rest; mild blood loss; prolonged standing in warm, crowded rooms; anemia; or fever.

Orthostatic Syncope. Orthostatic syncope occurs when a person rises from a seated or supine position. There are several possible causes. First,

- **varicosities** an abnormal dilation and distention of a vein.

- **autonomic dysfunction** an abnormality of the involuntary aspect of the nervous system.

- **Valsalva's maneuver** forced exhalation against a closed glottis. This maneuver increases intra-abdominal and intra-thoracic pressure, causing slowing of the pulse.

- **Stokes-Adams syndrome** a series of symptoms resulting from heart block, most commonly syncope, which results from decreased blood flow to the brain caused by the sudden decrease in cardiac output.

- **transient ischemic attack** reversible interruption of blood flow to the brain. Often seen as a precursor to major stroke.

there may be a disproportion between blood volume and vascular capacitance. That is, there is a pooling of blood in the legs reducing blood flow to the brain. Causes of this include hypovolemia, venous **varicosities,** prolonged bed rest, and **autonomic dysfunction.** Many drugs, especially blood pressure medicines, can cause drug-induced orthostatic syncope due to the effects of the medications on the capacitance vessels.

Vasovagal Syncope. Vasovagal syncope occurs when the patient **valsalva's,** as occurs during defecation, coughing, or similar maneuvers. This effectively slows the heart rate and cardiac output, thus decreasing blood flow to the brain.

Cardiac Syncope. Cardiac syncope results from transient reduction in cerebral blood flow, due to a sudden decrease in cardiac output. It can result from several mechanisms. Syncope can be the primary symptom of silent myocardial infarction. In addition, many dysrhythmias can cause syncope. Dysrhythmias that have been shown to cause syncope include bradycardias, **Stokes-Adams syndrome,** heart block, tachyarrhythmias, and sick sinus syndrome.

Seizures. Seizures, unlike most cases of syncope, tend to occur without warning and are unpredictable. The differentiation of seizures from syncope is often hard to determine in the prehospital setting.

Transient Ischemic Attacks. **Transient ischemic attacks** occur more frequently in the elderly. They are a frequent cause of syncope.

TABLE 29-2 Differentiation Between Syncope, Stokes-Adams, And Seizures

History	Syncope	Stokes-Adams	Seizure
Position	Usually upright	Upright or supine	Upright or supine
Skin color	Pale	Pallor then cyanosis	No change
Injury	Rare	Frequent	Frequent
Duration of episode	Short	Variable	Long
Tonic/Clonic movements	Few clonic jerks	Few clonic jerks	Frequent
Tongue biting	Rare	Rare	Occasional
Incontinence	Rarely urinary	Rarely urinary	Frequent; urinary or fecal
Post-ictal	Promptly lucid	Promptly lucid	Return to consciousness slow, headache, confusion, and weakness prolonged

Myocardial Infarction

The elderly patient with myocardial infarction is less likely to present with classic symptoms than a younger counterpart. Atypical presentations that may be seen in the elderly include confusion, syncope, dyspnea, abdominal pain, epigastric pain, and fatigue.

Stroke

Stroke is a common problem in the elderly. Occlusive stroke is statistically more common in the elderly and relatively uncommon in younger individuals. Older patients are at higher risk of stroke because of atherosclerosis, hypertension, immobility, limb paralysis, congestive heart failure, and atrial fibrillation. Transient ischemic attacks, commonly called TIAs, are more common in older patients. More than one-third of patients suffering TIAs will go on to develop a major, permanent stroke. TIAs are a common cause of syncope in the elderly.

■ **stroke** an interruption of blood flow—from emboli, thrombus, or hemorrhage—to an area of the brain.

Congestive Heart Failure

Congestive heart failure, both acute and chronic, is also common in the elderly patient. It results from myocardial changes that normally occur with age, as well as disease factors such as hypertension, arteriosclerotic disease, and diabetes. It commonly presents with confusion or an alteration in mental status. Congestive heart failure may be hard to diagnose in the elderly, as chronic pedal edema and basilar rales may be normal findings.

Dysrhythmias

Many cardiac dysrhythmias develop with age. These occur primarily as a result of degeneration of the heart's conductive system. To complicate matters, the elderly patient does not tolerate extremes in heart rate as well as a younger person would. For example, a heart rate of 140 in an older patient may cause syncope, while a younger patient can often tolerate a heart rate greater than 180.

Aortic Dissection

Aortic dissection is a degeneration of the wall of the aorta, either in the thoracic or abdominal cavity. It can result in an aneurysm or in rupture of the vessel. In younger persons, it is associated with syphilis, connective-tissue diseases, and congenital defects. In older patients, it is almost always due to arteriosclerosis. These patients will often present with tearing chest or abdominal pain or, if rupture occurs, cardiac arrest.

■ **aortic dissection** a degeneration of the wall of the aorta.

Managing the Geriatric Patient with Cardiovascular Disease

The geriatric patient with cardiovascular disease is managed in much the same manner as a younger patient. However, due to the increased prevalence of congestive heart failure, liver disease, and metabolic problems, the medical control physician may often modify medication dosages, as well as fluid administration orders.

NEUROLOGICAL DISORDERS IN THE GERIATRIC PATIENT

Coma in the elderly patient can have many causes. These include stroke, myocardial infarction, seizures, drug interactions, drug overdose, and metabolic disturbances. It is often impossible in the field to distinguish the cause of coma. The approach to management, however, is the same as with any patient presenting in coma.

Stroke is primarily a disease of the elderly. The signs and symptoms can present in many ways—coma, paralysis, slurred speech, a change in mood, and seizures among them. The disease should be highly suspect in any patient with a sudden change in mental status. If stroke is suspect, it is essential that the paramedic complete a Glasgow Coma Scale for later comparison in the emergency department.

Seizures may be easily mistaken for stroke in the elderly. Often, the difference cannot be distinguished in the field. Also, a first-time seizure may occur due to damage from a previous stroke. Not all seizures occurring in the elderly are of the major motor type; many are more subtle. Many etiologies of seizure activity in the elderly have been identified. Common causes include:

- ❑ seizure disorder
- ❑ recent or past head trauma
- ❑ mass lesion (tumor or bleed)
- ❑ alcoholic withdrawal
- ❑ diabetic hypoglycemia
- ❑ stroke

■ **vertigo** the sensation of faintness or dizziness which may cause a loss of balance.

Dizziness is a frightening experience and a frequent complaint of older persons. The complaint of dizziness may actually mean the patient has suffered syncope, pre-syncope, light-headedness, or true **vertigo.** There are so many causes of syncope that it is often hard, even for the physician, to determine the right one. Any factor that impairs visual input, inner-ear function, peripheral sensory input, or the central nervous system can cause dizziness. In addition, alcohol and many prescription drugs can cause dizziness. It is virtually impossible to distinguish dizziness, syncope, and pre-syncope in the prehospital setting.

■ **Meniere's disease** a disease of the inner ear characterized by vertigo, nerve deafness, and a roaring or buzzing in the ear.

Vertigo is a specific sensation of motion perceived by the patient as spinning or whirling. Many patients will report that they feel as though they are spinning, while others report they feel that the room around them is spinning. Vertigo is often accompanied with sweating, pallor, nausea, and vomiting. **Meniere's disease,** a disease of the inner ear, can cause severe, **intractable** vertigo. It is often, however, associated with a constant "roaring" sound in the ears, as well as ear "pressure."

■ **intractable** resistant to cure, relief, or control.

Senile Dementia

■ **senile dementia** general term used to describe an abnormal decline in mental functioning seen in the elderly.

Unfortunately, many older patients experience a decrease in mental functioning along with physical deterioration. This mental deterioration is often called "organic brain syndrome," "**senile dementia,**" or "senility." It is important to find out whether a **dementia** is acute or chronic. Causes of chronic senile dementia include:

■ **dementia** a deterioration of mental status.

- ❑ small strokes
- ❑ atherosclerosis of the cerebral blood vessels

- aging
- neurological diseases
- certain hereditary diseases (e.g., Huntington's chorea)

Etiologies of acute senile dementia include:

- subdural hematoma
- tumors and other mass lesions
- drug-induced changes or alcohol intoxication
- CNS infections
- electrolyte abnormalities
- cardiac failure

Alzheimer's Disease is a particular type of senile dementia. It is a progressive, degenerative disease that attacks the brain and results in impaired memory, thinking, and behavior. It affects an estimated 2.5 million American adults.

General Management of Neurological Disorders

Again, management techniques for the geriatric patient are similar to those for all other age groups. When confronted with a confused, dangerous, or violent patient, it is important to determine whether the behavior is acute or chronic. In the syncope patient, it is essential to try to obtain historical information in order to help determine the type of syncope. Factors to determine include:

- position of the patient at time of attack
- any associated symptoms
- the duration of the attack
- vital signs, including evaluation of orthostatic changes.

Psychiatric Disorders in the Geriatric Patient

Psychiatric problems are common in the geriatric population. There is more dementia and depression, and less schizophrenia and alcoholism, than in younger patients. It is important to remember that emotional disorders are common, due to isolation, loneliness, loss of self-dependence, loss of strength, and fear of the future. Any of these may present as physical disorders. Conversely, many physical disorders can present as psychiatric disorders.

There are several methods of classifying psychiatric disease. The following is a simple scheme for classifying psychiatric disorders of old age:

- organic brain syndrome
- affective disorders (depression)
- neurotic disorders (anxiety, hypochondriasis, phobias)
- personality disorders (dependent personality)
- paranoid disorders (schizophrenia)
- alcoholism

It is important to keep in mind that individuals over 65 years of age account for 25% of all suicides reported.

Management of psychiatric disturbances in the elderly is essentially the same as for other age groups. The older patient may have increased susceptibility to the depressant effects, as well as the side-effects, of neuroleptic medications such as Haldol and Thorazine.

Environmental Emergencies

The elderly and infants are highly susceptible to extreme variations in environmental temperature. This occurs in the elderly because of altered or impaired thermoregulating mechanisms. Predisposing factors for hypothermia in the elderly include:

- ❏ accident exposure
- ❏ drugs that interfere with heat production
- ❏ CNS disorders
- ❏ endocrine disorders
- ❏ poor nutrition
- ❏ chronic illness and debilitation
- ❏ low or fixed income

Similar factors tend to predispose these same patients to the other extreme, hyperthermia. These factors include:

- ❏ decreased functioning of the thermoregulatory center
- ❏ commonly prescribed medications that inhibit sweating
- ❏ low or fixed income
- ❏ altered sensory input, which would normally warn a person of overheating
- ❏ inadequate liquid intake

The management technique for the elderly is the same as for other patients, with special precautions against accidental fluid overload resulting in pulmonary edema or congestive heart failure.

Gastrointestinal Emergencies in the Geriatric Population

Older people seem overly concerned with bowel function. However, gastrointestinal complaints—such as nausea, poor appetite, diarrhea, and constipation—are often the presenting complaint of more serious disease.

Gastrointestinal bleeding is one of the most common gastrointestinal complaints of the elderly. Major causes of gastrointestinal hemorrhage include:

Upper GI Bleed
- ❏ **peptic ulcer disease**
- ❏ **gastritis**
- ❏ **esophageal varices**
- ❏ **Mallory-Weiss tear**

Lower GI Bleed
- ❏ **diverticulosis** (causes 70% of life-threatening lower GI bleeds).
- ❏ **tumors**
- ❏ **ischemic colitis**
- ❏ **arterio-venous malformations**

■ **peptic ulcer disease** injury to the mucus lining of the upper part of the gastrointestinal tract due to stomach acids, digestive enzymes, and other chemicals.

■ **gastritis** an inflammation of the lining of the stomach.

■ **esophageal varices** an abnormal dilation of veins in the lower esophagus, a common complication of cirrhosis of the liver.

■ **Mallory-Weiss tear** a tear in the lower esophagus which is often caused by severe and prolonged retching.

■ **diverticulosis** the presence of bleeding from small pouches on the colon, which tend to develop with age.

■ **ischemic colitis** an inflammation of the colon due to impaired or decreased blood supply.

■ **arterio-venous malformations** an abnormal link between an artery and a vein.

Signs of significant gastrointestinal blood loss include the presence of "coffee ground" emesis; black, tarry stools (**melena**); frank blood in the emesis or stool; orthostatic hypotension; pulse greater than 100 (unless on beta blockers); and confusion. Gastrointestinal bleeding in the elderly may result in such complications as a recent increase in angina symptoms, congestive heart failure, weakness, or dyspnea.

Prompt recognition and management of the GI bleed are essential, regardless of the age group. There is a tendency to take such patients less seriously than those suffering moderate or severe external hemorrhage. This is a serious mistake; these patients should be aggressively treated. Management should include:

❑ airway management
❑ support of breathing and circulation, if compromised
❑ high-flow oxygen therapy
❑ IV fluid replacement with a crystalloid
❑ PASG garment
❑ rapid transport

It is important to remember that the elderly tolerate hypotension and anoxia less than younger patients.

PHARMACOLOGY IN GERIATRICS

Most older patients are on some form of medication. Elderly persons use 25% of all prescribed and over-the-counter drugs sold in the United States. Many patients are on multiple medications, thus causing drug interactions to be fairly common. Adverse drug reactions may be more easily missed in the elderly, because of the overall increase in medical problems and symptoms attributed to normal aging.

✱ The dosage of emergency medications administered to elderly patients may need to be reduced. For example, elderly patients should receive 50% of the regular dose of lidocaine due to slower elimination.

The pharmacokinetics of drugs are altered in the older patient. Because of decreased excretion, and poor nutritional state, many drugs tend to accumulate in the blood with prolonged usage. In addition, the various compensatory mechanisms that help buffer against medication side-effects are less effective in the elderly than in younger patients.

Approximately 30% of all hospital admissions are related to drug-induced illness. More than 30% of these persons are over the age of 60 years. Overdose, usually accidental, may occur more frequently in the aged, due to confusion, vision impairment, self-selection of medication, and forgetfulness. Intentional drug overdose also occurs in attempts at self-destruction.

Underdose of medication is also more common in the elderly. In fact, underdosing of medication accounts for about half of all medication errors. This can be attributed to forgetfulness (the patient forgot to take the medication) or to limited income (the patient cannot afford the prescribed medication). Drugs that have been identified as commonly causing toxicity in the elderly include:

❑ digitalis [leading cause] (Lanoxin®, Lanoxicaps®, etc.)
❑ antiParkinson medications (Symmetrel®, carbidopa, etc.)
❑ diuretics (furosemide, hydrochlorthiazide, etc.)
❑ anticoagulants (Coumadin®)

- lidocaine (very important to prehospital care)
- quinidine (Quinaglute®, etc.)
- propranolol (Inderal®)
- theophylline (Theo-Dur®, Slow-Bid®, etc.)
- narcotic analgesics and acetaminophen (meperidine, etc.)
- phenothiazines (Haldol®, Thorazine®, Mellaril®, etc.)
- tricyclic antidepressants (Elavil®, Limbitrol®, etc.)

GERIATRIC ABUSE/NEGLECT

■ **geriatric abuse** a syndrome in which an elderly person has received serious physical or psychological injury.

Geriatric abuse and neglect is as big a problem in our society as child abuse and neglect. **Geriatric abuse** is defined as a syndrome in which an elderly person has received serious physical or psychological injury from his or her children or other care providers. Abuse of the elderly knows no socioeconomic bounds. It often occurs when an older person is no longer able to be totally independent, and the family has difficulty upholding their commitment to care for the patient. It can also occur in nursing homes and other health care facilities. The profile of the potential geriatric abuser may often show a great deal of life stress. There is often sleep deprivation, marital discord, financial problems, and work-related problems. As the abuser's life gets in further disarray, and as the patient further deteriorates, abuse may be the outcome.

Signs and symptoms of geriatric abuse or neglect are often obvious. Unexplained trauma is often the primary presentation. The average abused patient is older than 80 and has multiple medical problems, such as cancer, congestive heart failure, heart disease, and incontinence. Senile dementia is often present. In these cases, it is hard to determine whether the dementia is chronic or acute, especially if there is an increased likelihood of head trauma from abuse.

✱ Many states have laws which require prehospital personnel to report suspected cases of geriatric abuse.

When geriatric abuse is suspect, the paramedic should obtain complete patient and family history, paying particular attention to inconsistencies. *Do not* confront the family. Your suspicions should be reported to the emergency department and the appropriate governmental authority. Many states have very strong laws protecting the geriatric patient from abuse or neglect. In fact, many states consider it a criminal offense not to report suspected geriatric abuse. These states also offer legal immunity to those who report geriatric abuse, as long as the report was made in good faith.

SUMMARY

The paramedic of today will be treating an increasing number of aged patients. It is important to remember that many changes occur—anatomical, physiological, emotional—as we enter senescence. It is important to keep these changes in mind when treating elderly patients. Also, certain illnesses and injuries tend to occur more frequently in the older patient. Elderly patients are much more susceptible to medication side-effects and toxicity. They are also more susceptible to environmental stressors. Abuse of the elderly occurs and should always be kept in mind, especially when injuries do not match the history. Any suspected abuse or neglect of an elderly patient should be reported to the emergency department and the appropriate governmental authorities.

FURTHER READING

KAPLAN, HAROLD I., and BENJAMIN J. SADLOCK. *Modern Synopsis of Comprehensive Textbook of Psychiatry/ III*. 3d ed. Baltimore: Williams and Wilkins, 1981.

SCHWARTZ, GEORGE R., GIDEON BOSKER, and JOHN W. GRIGSBY. *Geriatric Emergencies*. Bowie, MD: Brady Communications, 1984.

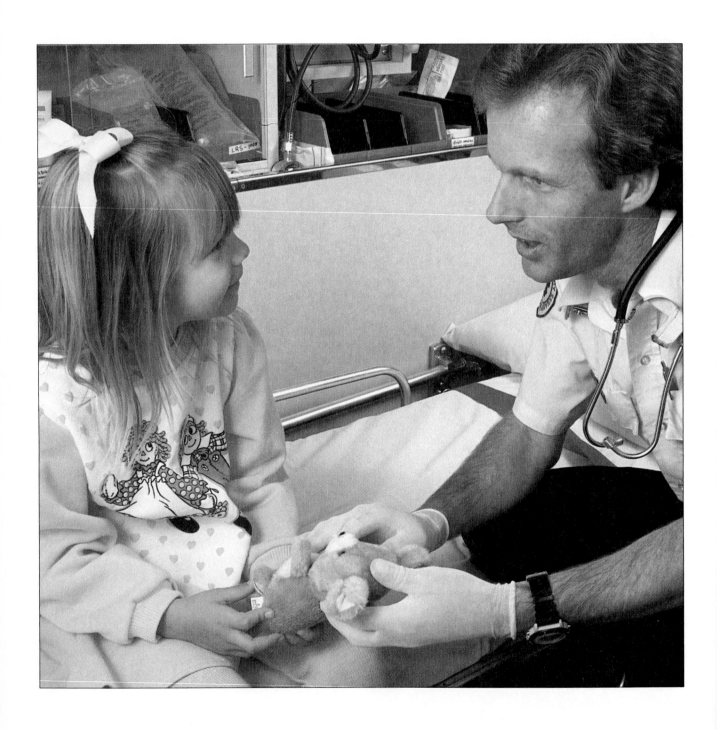

30

Pediatric Emergencies

Objectives for Chapter 30

Upon completing this chapter, the student should be able to:

1. Identify the general goals of management of the pediatric patient.

2. Identify normal age-related vital signs in the pediatric patient.

3. Describe the normal and abnormal appearance of the anterior fontanelle in the infant.

4. List appropriate developmental milestones for each age group of children and relate the appropriate approach to patient assessment.

5. Define Sudden Infant Death Syndrome (SIDS), the theories of etiology, and management in the prehospital setting.

6. Describe the characteristics of the abused child and of the child abuser.

7. Describe signs and symptoms suggestive of child abuse or neglect.

8. Discuss pediatric seizures with emphasis on febrile seizures.

9. Discuss the pathophysiology, assessment, and prehospital management of meningitis.

10. Discuss the pathophysiology, assessment, and prehospital management of septicemia.

11. Discuss the pathophysiology, assessment, and prehospital management of dehydration.

12. Discuss the pathophysiology, assessment, and prehospital management of Reye's syndrome.

13. Discuss the pathophysiology, assessment, and prehospital management of:

    a. croup
    b. bronchiolitis
    c. epiglottitis
    d. asthma
    e. aspirated foreign bodies

14. Describe the modifications required of ACLS for pediatric patients, including drug dosage, endotracheal intubation, defibrillation, and IV therapy.

15. Describe the concept of Pediatric Advanced Life Support (PALS).

The crew of Medic 1 is awakened at 5:45 AM and dispatched to assist "a child with difficulty breathing." The morning is cold but clear. The response time is three minutes. Arriving at the suburban residence, the paramedics enter the living room. The patient is a 2-year-old girl sitting on her mother's lap. The child looks ill and has a barking cough. When she coughs she becomes somewhat cyanotic. The mother reports they have tried the usual remedies (steamy shower, humidifier), and the child is getting worse.

Paramedics complete a primary and secondary survey. The child's axillary temperature is 101.2 degrees. Paramedics do not examine the throat because of the possibility of epiglottitis. The lungs are clear. The brassy stridor is obvious. The child is bundled up in a blanket and taken to the ambulance. The mother holds the child and humidified oxygen is administered as she is transported to the pediatric emergency room. Arriving at the hospital, the paramedics note the presence of three other children with a similar cough in the emergency room. The emergency physician completes a soft-tissue X-ray of the neck, which excludes epiglottitis. The child is treated and admitted.

INTRODUCTION

✱ Children are not small adults.

The ill or injured child presents special problems for the paramedic. First, children often may not be able to describe what is bothering them, or what happened. Second, in addition to the sick or injured child, the paramedic must deal with the parents. Finally, the child's size often makes routine procedures more difficult. These and other factors in pediatric emergencies often cause a great deal of stress and anxiety for both parents and paramedics. Children are not simply "small adults." They have special considerations and needs. This chapter will present the topic of pediatric emergencies as it applies to advanced prehospital care.

APPROACH TO THE PEDIATRIC PATIENT

The approach to the pediatric patient will vary with the age of the patient and the nature of the problem. When obtaining the medical history of the pediatric patient, gather information as quickly and as accurately as possible. The parents are usually the primary source of information. However, as the child becomes older, he or she can also be a good source. The paramedic should try to establish a good relationship with the child. Children can often give accurate descriptions of symptoms or details. It is important to let the child express his or her opinion.

General Approach to Pediatric Assessment

Priorities of management in the pediatric patient, as with all patients, are established on a threat-to-life basis. However, if life-threatening problems are not present, the following approach is recommended.

Questioning of the child should be specific and direct, keeping in mind the developmental stages described below. The paramedic should

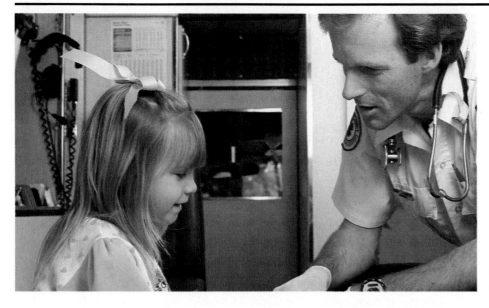

FIGURE 30-1 The approach to the pediatric patient should be gentle and slow.

focus on the observed behavior, as well as on what the child or parent says. Visual assessment is very important. Approach the child slowly and gently to encourage cooperation and to gain confidence. (See Figure 30-1.) The approach should be kind, yet firm. The child should not be separated from the parent unnecessarily. Get down to the same visual level as the child. Remember, if the child did something that he or she felt was forbidden, he or she may distort the facts. In addition, children may imagine fantasy as reality, and reality as fantasy. Always be honest with the patient. Never tell the child that it "won't hurt" if you know it will. Instead, say "This might hurt a little bit and you can cry if you want to." Children respond to calm reassurance. Converse with the patient in a soft voice, using simple words.

✳ Always be honest with a child.

After the pertinent patient history has been obtained, attention should be turned toward the physical examination. Avoid touching any injured or painful areas until the child's confidence has been gained. (See Figure 30-2.) Begin your examination without instruments. If possible, allow the child to determine the order of the examination.

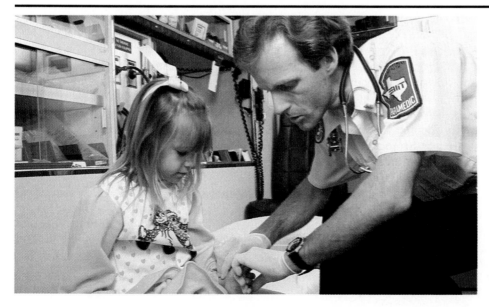

FIGURE 30-2 As confidence is gained, proceed with the secondary survey.

TABLE 30-1 Normal Pediatric Vital Signs By Age

Age	Respirations	Pulse	Blood Pressure (Systolic)
Newborn	30–60	100–160	50–70
1–6 Wks.	30–60	100–160	70–95
6 Months	25–40	90–120	80–100
1 Year	20–30	90–120	80–100
3 Years	20–30	80–120	80–110
6 Years	18–25	70–110	80–110
10 Years	15–20	60–90	90–120

Pediatric Vital Signs. Poorly-taken vital signs in the pediatric patient are of less value than no vital signs at all. The following are general guidelines for obtaining accurate pediatric vital signs:

❑ Vital signs should be taken with the patient in as close to a resting state as possible. If necessary, allow the child to calm down before attempting vital signs. Vital signs in the field should include pulse, respiration, blood pressure, and, if equipment is available, temperature.

❑ The blood pressure should be obtained with an appropriate-sized cuff. The cuff should be two-thirds the width of the upper arm. Table 30-1 illustrates normal blood pressure readings for children.

❑ The pulse should be determined at the brachial artery, carotid artery, or wrist, depending on the size of the child. There is often a significant variation in pulse rate in children, due to respirations. Therefore, it is important to monitor the pulse for at least 30 seconds, a full minute if possible. The range of normal pulse rates is shown in Table 30-1.

❑ It is generally not possible to weigh the child. However, if medications are required, it is important to make a good estimate of the child's weight. Often the parents can provide a fairly reliable weight from a recent visit to the doctor. Table 30-2 lists the average weight for age in pediatric patients.

❑ Observe respiratory rate before beginning the examination. After the examination is started, the child will often begin to cry, and it will be impossible to determine respiratory rate. For an estimate of upper limit of respiratory rate, subtract the child's age from 40. It is also important to identify respiratory pattern, as well as retractions, nasal flaring, or paradoxical chest motion.

❑ Observe the child for level of consciousness. There may be a wide variability in levels of consciousness and activity.

The physical examination of the child should be systematic and should follow the same format used for adults. Special attention should be paid to the anterior fontanelle. The **fontanelles** are areas of the skull that have not yet fused. They allow for compression of the head during childbirth and for the rapid growth of the brain that occurs in early life. The posterior fontanelle is generally closed by 4 months of age. The anterior fontanelle diminishes after 6 months of age and is generally closed by 9–18 months of age.

The anterior fontanelle should be inspected in all infants. Normally, it should be level with the surface of the skull, or slightly sunken, and it may pulsate. With increased intracranial pressure, such as what occurs with meningitis or head trauma, the fontanelle may become tight and bulging. Pulsations may diminish or disappear. With dehydration, the anterior fontanelle may often fall below the level of the skull and appear sunken.

■ **fontanelles** areas in the infant skull where bones have not yet fused. Posterior and anterior fontanelles are present at birth.

TABLE 30-2 Pediatric weights and pound-kilogram conversion.

Age	Weight (lb)	Weight (kg)
Birth	7	3.5
3 mo	10	5
6 mo	15	7
9 mo	18	8
1 yr	22	10
2 yr	26	12
3 yr	33	15
4 yr	37	17
5 yr	40	18
6 yr	44	20
7 yr	50	23
8 yr	56	25
9 yr	60	28
10 yr	70	33
11 yr	75	35
12 yr	85	40
13 yr	98	44

Pounds	→	Kilograms	Pounds	→	Kilograms	Pounds	→	Kilograms
2.2		1	35.2		16	68.2		31
4.4		2	37.4		17	70.4		32
6.6		3	39.6		18	72.6		33
8.8		4	41.8		19	74.8		34
11		5	44		20	77		35
13.2		6	46.2		21	79.2		36
15.4		7	48.4		22	81.4		37
17.6		8	50.6		23	83.6		38
19.8		9	52.8		24	85.8		39
22		10	55		25	88		40
24.2		11	57.2		26	90.2		41
26.4		12	59.4		27	92.4		42
28.6		13	61.6		28	94.6		43
30.8		14	63.8		29	96.8		44
33		15	66		30	99		45

Gastrointestinal disturbances are common in children and can occur with virtually any disorder. When confronted with a child who has been vomiting, it is important to determine how many times the child has vomited, the color of the vomitus, and other associated symptoms. The same holds true for diarrhea.

Developmental Stages. The child progresses through several developmental stages on the way to adulthood. These stages of development are often significantly different and the approach to the pediatric patient should relate to the appropriate developmental stage.

Neonates (ages birth to 1 month). The **neonate** is generally defined as an infant up to 1 month of age. (See Figure 30-3.) This a major stage of

■ **neonate** an infant up to one month of age.

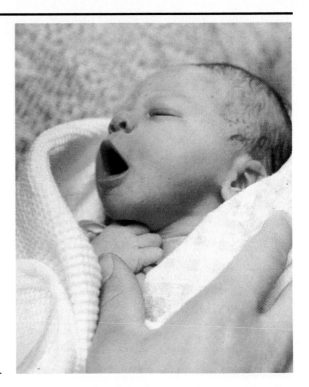

FIGURE 30-3 The neonate.

development. Often, congenital problems and other illnesses will be noted during this stage. Initially, following birth, there is a weight loss as the neonate adjusts to extrauterine life. It is not uncommon for the infant to lose up to 10% of his or her birth weight. This weight loss, however, is routinely recovered in 10 days. Gestational age affects early development. Children born at term (40 weeks) should follow accepted developmental guidelines. Infants born prematurely will not be as developed, both neurologically and physically, as their term counterparts.

This stage of development is one of reflexes. Personality development begins. The infant is close to the mother. He or she may stare at faces and smile. The mother, and occasionally the father, can comfort and quiet the child. Obviously, the history must be obtained from the parents. However, it is also important to observe the child. Common illnesses in this age group include jaundice, vomiting, and respiratory distress. Children of this age generally do not develop fever with minor illnesses. Therefore, the documented presence of fever should raise concern. In fact, many authorities feel that fever in a child under 3 months of age is meningitis, until proven otherwise.

The approach to this age group should include several factors. First, the child should always be kept warm. It is important to observe skin color, tone, and respiratory activity. The absence of tears when crying may indicate dehydration. The lungs should be auscultated early during the exam while the infant is quiet. It is often helpful to have the child suck on a pacifier during the examination. Often, allowing the infant to remain in the parent's lap will keep him or her quiet.

Ages 1 to 5 Months. Children in this age group should have doubled their birth weight by 5 to 6 months. They should be able to follow the movements of others with their eyes. Muscle control develops in a cephalo-caudal fashion. That is, development of muscular control begins at the head and moves toward the tail, and also begins at the trunk and moves toward the extremities. The personality of the child at this stage is still closely centered on the parents. The history must be obtained from the parents, with close observation of illnesses and accidents, including SIDS, vomiting, diarrhea, dehydration, meningitis, child abuse, and household accidents. The approach to these patients should include keeping the child warm and comfortable. The child should be allowed to remain in the parent's lap. (See Figure 30-4.) A pacifier or bottle can be used to keep the child quiet during the examination.

Ages 6 to 12 Months.   Children of this age group may stand, or even walk with assistance. They are active and explore their world with their mouths. The personality continues to develop. They have considerable anxiety toward strangers. They don't like lying on their backs. Children in this age group tend to cling to the mother, although the father will "do" most of the time. Common illnesses and accidents include febrile seizures, vomiting, diarrhea, dehydration, bronchiolitis, car accidents, croup, child abuse, ingestions, falls, foreign bodies, and meningitis. These children should be examined in the mother's lap. The exam should progress in a toe-to-head order, since the child may become disturbed if you begin the exam at the face. If time and conditions permit, allow the child to become accustomed to you before beginning the examination.

Ages 1 to 3 Years.   Great strides occur in gross motor development during this stage. Children are invariably upon or under everything. They can run and walk and are always on the move. Language development has begun. They can often understand better than they speak. At this stage of development, the child still clings to the parent but begins to stray. The parent is still the only person who can comfort them. The older they become, the more brave, curious, or stubborn they also become. The majority of the medical history should come from the parents. However, the child can also be asked certain questions.

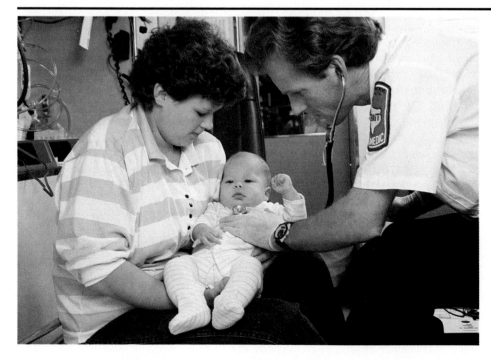

FIGURE 30-4 Young children should be allowed to remain in their mother's arms.

Accidents of all types are the leading cause of death between the ages of 1 and 15 years. Common illnesses and accidents in this age group include auto accidents, vomiting, diarrhea, febrile seizures, ingestions, falls, child abuse, croup, meningitis, and ingestion of foreign bodies. The approach to children in this age group should be more cautious. Approach the child slowly and try to gain his or her confidence. Conduct the exam in a toe-to-head order. The child may be difficult to examine and may resist being touched. Avoid asking questions that allow the child to say "no." Be sure to tell the child if something will hurt.

Ages 3 to 5 Years. Children in this age group show a tremendous increase in fine and gross motor development. Language development continues. Children in this age group know how to talk, but often won't, especially to strangers. They may be afraid, and they always have a vivid imagination. Monsters are a part of their world. They often will have a temper and will express it. During this stage of development, they have a fear of mutilation and may view treatment procedures as hostile. Children of this age group are close to either one parent or the other on different occasions. They will stick up for the parents and are openly loving. They still look to parents for comfort and support.

When evaluating children in this age group, you should first question the child, keeping in mind that imagination may interfere with facts. The child's time frame is often distorted and you must rely on the parents to fill in the gaps. Common illnesses and accidents in this age group include croup, asthma, ingestions, auto accidents, burns, child abuse, ingestion of foreign bodies, drowning, epiglottitis, febrile seizures, and meningitis. The approach to children of this age requires tact. Often, the use of a doll or stuffed animal will assist in the examination. Allow the children to hold equipment and use it. Let them sit on your lap. Start the examination with the chest and do the head last. Don't trick or lie to the child; always explain what you are going to do.

Ages 6 to 12 Years. The children of this age group are active and carefree. There are growth spurts that sometimes lead to clumsiness. The personality continues to develop. Children of this age are protective and proud of their parents, and they like their parents' attention. Peers are important, but the child also needs home support. When examining children of this age group, it is important to give them the responsibility of providing the history. If an injury was sustained while the child was doing something forbidden, he or she may be reluctant to provide information. The parents can fill in the pertinent details. When assessing children in this age group, it is important to be honest, to protect their modesty, and to tell the child what is wrong. A small toy may help to calm the child. (See Figure 30-5.) Common illnesses and injuries of this age group include drowning, auto accidents, bicycle accidents, fractures, falls, sports injuries, child abuse, and burns.

Ages 12 to 15 Years. Youngsters in the 12–15 age group vary significantly in their development. Some are fully mature, while others are not. They are not necessarily adults, but believe that they are. They have a tremendous desire to be liked and included. Teenagers are very concerned with their body image. The relationship between children and their parents is also changing. This is a time for more independence. Peers are important, as are adolescents of the opposite sex. Generally, these patients are good historians. Their perception of events often differs from that of their parents.

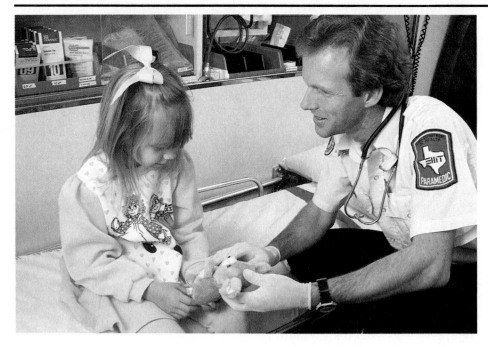

FIGURE 30-5 A small toy may calm a child in the 6–12 years age group.

Common illnesses and injuries in this age group include mononucleosis, asthma, auto accidents, sports injuries, drug and alcohol problems, suicide gestures, sexual abuse, and pregnancy. When assessing teenagers, it is important to be honest. Be factual and address the patient's questions. Often, it may be wise to interview the child outside of the parent's presence. Pay attention to what they are saying, as well as to what they are not saying. Some are very comfortable with their bodies, while others are not. The paramedic should provide support and reassurance.

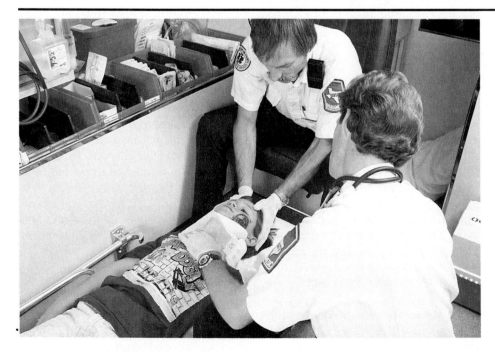

FIGURE 30-6 Injuries account for the majority of pediatric EMS calls.

PROBLEMS SPECIFIC TO THE PEDIATRIC PATIENT

Sudden Infant Death Syndrome (SIDS)

Sudden Infant Death Syndrome (SIDS) is defined as the sudden death of an infant during the first year of life from an illness of unknown etiology. The incidence of SIDS in the United States is approximately 2 deaths per 1,000 births. SIDS is the leading cause of death between 1 week and 1 year of age in the United States, responsible for a significant number of deaths between 1 month and 6 months of age. The peak incidence occurs at 2–4 months.

Death usually occurs during sleep. The incidence seems to be greater during winter and is more common in males than females. It is more prevalent in families with younger mothers and in those from low socioeconomic groups. A higher incidence is also reported in infants with a low birth weight. Occasionally, a mild upper respiratory infection will be reported prior to the death. SIDS is not caused by external suffocation from blankets or pillows. Neither is it related to child abuse, regurgitation and aspiration of stomach contents, or allergies to cow's milk. It is not hereditary, but does tend to recur in families.

Current theories vary about the etiology. Some authorities feel it may result from an immature respiratory center in the brain, and the child simply stops breathing. Others feel there may be an airway obstruction in the posterior pharynx, as a result of pharyngeal relaxation during sleep, a hypermobile mandible, or an enlarged tongue. There are many other theories and investigation continues.

Infants suffering SIDS have similar physical findings. From an external standpoint, there is a normal state of nutrition and hydration. The skin may be mottled. There are often frothy, occasionally blood-tinged, fluids in and around the mouth and nostrils. Vomitus may be present. Occasionally, the infant may be in an unusual position, due to muscle spasm at the time of death. Common findings noted at autopsy include intrathoracic petechia (small hemorrhages) in 90% of cases. There is often associated pulmonary congestion and edema. Sometimes, stomach contents are found in the trachea. Microscopic examination of the trachea often reveals the presence of inflammatory changes.

The immediate needs of the family with a SIDS baby are many. Active and aggressive care of the infant should be undertaken to assure the parents that everything possible is being done. A first responder, or other personnel, should be assigned to assist the parents and to explain what is being done. After arrival at the hospital, the management and care are directed at the parents, since there is often nothing that can be done for the child. If the infant is dead, the family should be allowed to see the child. A normal grief reaction from the parents should be expected. Initially, there may be shock, disbelief, and denial. Other times, the parents may express anger, rage, hostility, blame, or guilt. Often, there is a feeling of inadequacy as a parent, as well as helplessness, confusion, and fear. The grief process may last as long as 1–2 years. SIDS has major long-term effects on family relationships.

Child Abuse and Neglect

Child abuse should always be suspected, especially if injuries are not consistent with the history. There are several characteristics common to abused children. Often, the child is seen as "special" and different from others. Premature infants or a twin are at higher risk of abuse. Many abused children are less than 5 years of age. Handicapped children, as well as those with special needs, are also at greater risk. Uncommunicative (i.e. autistic) children are also more apt to be abused than other children. Boys are abused more often than girls. A child who is not what the parents wanted (e.g., the wrong sex) is at increased risk for abuse.

The child abuser can come from any geographic, religious, ethnic, occupational, educational, or socio-economic group. There are, however, certain characteristics common to people who abuse children. The abuser is usually a parent or someone in the role of a parent. The mother is the most frequently identified abuser when she is the parent who spends the most time with the child. Most abusers of children were themselves abused as children.

The three elements necessary for abuse to occur are:

❑ Parent or adult with potential to abuse.
❑ A particular child at risk from abuse.
❑ The presence of a crisis.

Common crises that may precipitate abuse include financial stress, marital or relationship stress, and physical illness in a parent or child.

Assessment of the Potentially Abused Child. There are several findings that should make the paramedic highly suspicious of child abuse. These are (see Figures 30-7 to 30-10):

✱ In many states prehospital personnel are required by law to report suspected child abuse or neglect to the appropriate authorities.

❑ Any obvious or suspected fractures in a child under 2 years of age.
❑ Injuries in various stages of healing, especially burns and bruises.
❑ More injuries than usually seen in children of the same age.
❑ Injuries scattered on many areas of the body.
❑ Bruises or burns in patterns that suggest intentional infliction.
❑ Increased intracranial pressure in an infant.
❑ Suspected intra-abdominal trauma in a young child.
❑ Any injury that does not fit with the description of the cause given.

Information in the medical history that should raise the index of suspicion for child abuse includes:

❑ History that does not match the nature or severity of the injury.
❑ Parent's account is vague, or changes during the interview.
❑ Accusations that the child injured himself intentionally.
❑ Delay in seeking help.
❑ Child dressed inappropriately for the situation.

Child neglect should be suspected if any of the following are present:

❑ Extreme malnutrition
❑ Multiple insect bites
❑ Longstanding skin infections
❑ Extreme lack of cleanliness

Sexual abuse can occur at any age. The sexual abuser is almost always someone in the family, someone known to the family, or someone the child trusts. Stepchildren are often more at risk for sexual abuse by a parent than natural children. When child abuse is suspected, the genita-

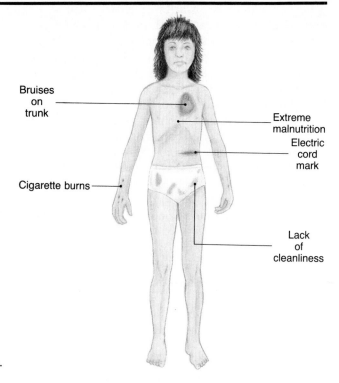

FIGURE 30-7 The stigmata of child abuse.

Bruises on trunk

Extreme malnutrition

Electric cord mark

Cigarette burns

Lack of cleanliness

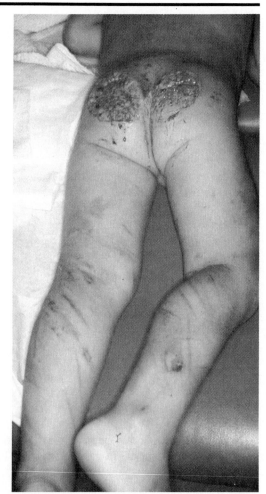

FIGURE 30-8 An abused child. Note the marks on the legs associated with beatings with an electrical wire. The burns on the buttocks are from submersion in hot water. (Courtesy of Scott and White Hospital and Clinic)

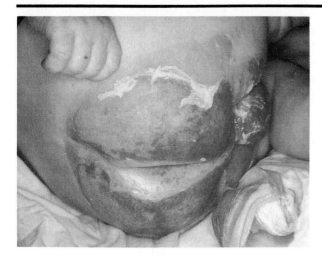

FIGURE 30-9 Burn injury from placing child's buttocks in hot water as a punishment. (Courtesy of Scott and White Hospital and Clinic)

lia should be examined externally for serious injury. Touching of the child, or disturbing the clothing, should be avoided—this might disturb the later gathering of evidence by police. The approach to the child who has been sexually abused should be supportive.

Management. The goals of management of the child who is suspected of being abused or neglected are to treat his or her injuries appropriately, protect the child from further abuse, and to notify the appropriate authorities. The paramedic should obtain as much information as possible, in a non-judgmental manner, and document it in the patient report. The parents should not be "cross-examined"; this is the role of the police. The attitude of the paramedic toward the parents should be supportive and non-judgmental. The child should be transported to the hospital in the ambulance or by another dependable person. The alleged abuser should not be left with the task of transporting the child.

Upon arrival at the emergency department, your suspicions should be reported to the emergency department personnel and the proper au-

✱ Do not confront the parents (or other caregiver) about your suspicion of child abuse. Instead, report it to emergency department personnel or law enforcement officers.

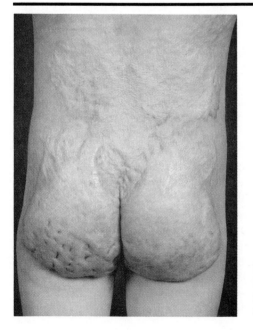

FIGURE 30-10 The effects of child abuse, both physical and mental, can last a lifetime. (Courtesy of Scott and White Hospital and Clinic)

thorities. The patient report, and all available documentation, should be completed at that time, since delay may inhibit the accurate recall of data. Child abuse and neglect are a particularly stressful aspect of emergency medical services. The paramedic must recognize and deal with his or her own feelings.

Seizures

The topic of seizures has been presented in earlier chapters. However, seizures can and do occur in children. They are a frequent reason for summoning EMS. Several factors have been identified as causing seizures. These include:

❑ fever
❑ hypoxia
❑ infections
❑ idiopathic epilepsy
❑ electrolyte disturbances
❑ head trauma
❑ hypoglycemia
❑ toxic ingestions or exposure
❑ tumors
❑ CNS malformations

Often, however, the etiology is not known. Status epilepticus can also occur in children. Status epilepticus is a prolonged seizure, or multiple seizures with no regaining of consciousness between them. This is a serious medical emergency. Most pediatric seizures that involve EMS personnel are febrile seizures.

✱ The diagnosis of febrile seizure should not be made in the field.

Febrile Seizures. *Febrile seizures* are those seizures that occur as a result of a sudden increase in body temperature. They occur most commonly between the ages of 6 months and 6 years. Febrile seizures seem related to the rate at which the body temperature increases, not to the degree of fever. Often, the parents will report the recent onset of fever or cold symptoms. The diagnosis of febrile seizure should not be made in the field. All pediatric patients suffering a seizure must be transported to the hospital so that other etiologies can be excluded.

Assessment. The history is a major piece of information in determining seizure type. Febrile seizure should be suspected if the temperature is above 103 degrees F (39.2 degrees C). (See Figure 30-11.) The history of a previous seizure may suggest idiopathic epilepsy or other CNS problem. However, there is a tendency for recurrence of febrile seizures in children who are predisposed.

When confronted with a seizing child, it is important to determine if there is a history of seizures, or seizures with fever. Has the child had a recent illness? Also, it is important to determine how many seizures occurred during the incident. If the child is not seizing upon arrival, a description of the seizure activity should also be sought. The condition and position of the child when found should be noted. Parents or bystanders should be questioned about the possibility of head injury. A history of irritability or lethargy prior to the seizure may indicate CNS infection. It should be determined, if possible, whether the child suffers from diabetes or has recently complained of a headache or a stiff neck. Any current medications should be noted, as well as possible ingestions.

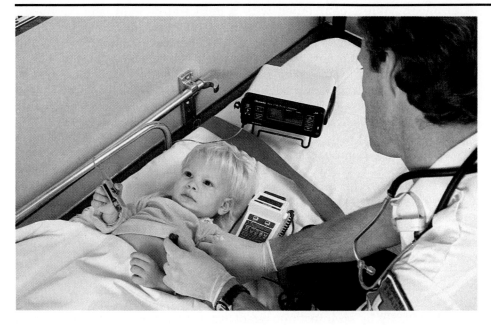

FIGURE 30-11 If possible, temperature determination in the field should be carried out.

The physical examination should be systematic. Particular attention should be paid to the adequacy of respirations, the level of consciousness, neurological evaluation, and signs of injury. The child should also be inspected for dehydration. Dehydration may be evidenced by the absence of tears or, in an infant, by the presence of a sunken fontanelle.

Management. Management of the pediatric seizure is essentially the same as for the seizing adult. The patient should be placed on the floor or on the bed, on his or her side, away from the furniture. The patient should not be restrained, but should be protected from injury. The airway should be maintained, but nothing, such as a bite stick, should be forced between the teeth. Supplemental oxygen should be administered. The vital signs should be taken and recorded. If the child is febrile, excess layers of clothing should be removed. If status epilepticus is present, the following should be instituted:

❑ Start an IV of D5NS or D5RL
❑ Administer diazepam according to the following:
   Children 1 month to 5 years: 0.2–0.5 mg slowly IV push every 2–5 minutes to a maximum of 2.5 milligrams.
   Children 5 years or older: 1 mg slowly IV push every 2–5 minutes to a maximum of 5 milligrams.

Contact medical control for additional dosing. Diazepam can be administered rectally if an IV cannot be established.

✱ Diazepam can be administered rectally to a seizing child when an IV cannot be started.

As mentioned previously, all pediatric seizure patients should be transported. The parents should be supported and reassured. This is a very stressful and frightening situation for them.

Dehydration

The child is very vulnerable to dehydration. Among the causes are diarrhea, vomiting, poor fluid intake, fever, and burns. Children have a high body-surface-area-to-weight ratio and are thus very vulnerable to heat loss, and along with it, dehydration. They also have a higher percentage of water to body tissues than adults.

Assessment. When confronted with a dehydrated child, the paramedic should question the parents about recent infection, diarrhea, vomiting, or fever. They should also be asked about decreased urination. Many parents will notice that their children are wetting fewer diapers than usual.

Physical examination may show decreased skin turgor, weight loss, and absent tears. Urine may be quite concentrated. The eyes may be dull and sunken-looking. Infants may exhibit a depressed anterior fontanelle. The child may have altered mental status or poor pain response.

✱ The dose of fluids for the dehydrated or volume-depleted child is 20 mL/kg.

Management. The management of dehydration should first include the primary survey: airway, breathing, and circulation. The vital signs should be determined and monitored. If the child is in shock, an IV of LR should be started. An initial fluid bolus of 20 mL/kg should be administered and repeated as indicated. Transport, however, should not be delayed if there is difficulty in starting the IV.

Infectious Disease

Infectious diseases are those illnesses caused by the infection or infestation of the body by an infectious agent, such as a virus, bacteria, fungus, or parasite. Childhood is a time of frequent infectious illness due to the relative immaturity of the immune system. Most children will have 5–6 upper respiratory infections per year. Most infections are minor and self-limited. There are, however, several infections that can be life-threatening. These include meningitis and bacterial septicemia.

■ **meningitis** infection and inflammation of the meninges, the covering of the brain and spinal cord.

Meningitis. **Meningitis** is an infection of the meninges, the lining of the brain and spinal cord. Meningitis can result from both bacteria and viruses. Viral meningitis is frequently called *aseptic meningitis,* since an organism cannot be routinely cultured from CSF fluid. Aseptic meningitis is generally less severe than bacterial meningitis and self-limited. Bacterial meningitis most commonly results from *Streptococcus pneumoniae, Haemophilus influenza,* and *Neisseria meningitides.* These infections can be rapidly fatal if not promptly recognized and treated appropriately.

✱ Documented fever in a child less than 3 months of age is meningitis until proven otherwise.

Assessment. Meningitis is more common in children than adults. Findings in the history suggestive of meningitis include a child who has been ill for one day to several days, recent ear or respiratory tract infection, high fever, lethargy or irritability, a severe headache, or a stiff neck. The child with meningitis may present in various ways. Infants generally do not develop a stiff neck. They will generally become lethargic and will not feed well. Some babies may simply develop a fever. Documented fever in a child less than 3 months of age is considered meningitis until proven otherwise.

On physical examination, the child with meningitis will appear very ill. With an infant, the fontanelle may be bulging or full unless accompanied by dehydration. Extreme discomfort with movement, due to irritability of the meninges, may be present.

Management. Prehospital care of the infant or child with meningitis is supportive. The primary survey and secondary assessment should be rapidly completed. The infant should be transported to the emergency department. If shock is present, it should be treated with intravenous fluids and oxygen.

Septicemia. **Septicemia** is the presence of an infectious agent, usually bacteria, in the bloodstream. It is a systemic infection and usually severe. It occurs more commonly in children than in adults. The etiology can be varied, as can the presenting signs and symptoms. Often there is a focus of infection, such as pneumonia, ear infections, or wound infections, that is seeding the blood with bacteria.

Septicemia should be suspected in any child who becomes ill or who has been ill for several days, especially if accompanied by fever, lethargy, irritability, or shock. The fontanelle in infants with septicemia is usually flat.

Assessment. Management of septicemia includes the standard primary survey and secondary assessment. Supplemental oxygen should be administered. IV access should be established with LR. Shock can develop and should be anticipated and treated appropriately. Septicemia is a very serious condition that can deteriorate quickly. It must be promptly recognized and treated appropriately. The goal is to prevent the development of septic shock.

Reye's Syndrome. **Reye's syndrome** is a disease that was undescribed until 1963. The etiology of Reye's syndrome has not been clearly established. Reye's syndrome affects all ages, with peak incidence between ages 5–15 years. It tends to occur more frequently in younger children. The frequency is higher in fall and winter. After 1 year of age, there is a higher incidence in the suburban and rural populations.

Although no single etiological factor has been identified, several possible toxic and metabolic causes have been postulated. Outbreaks tend to cluster during epidemics of Influenza B. Occasionally, it has been associated with the chicken pox (varicella) virus. Infants often will have a recent history of gastroenteritis. There has also been a correlation between the use of aspirin and the disease, particularly after the flu.

The typical presentation is a healthy child who develops severe nausea and vomiting during an unremarkable viral illness. Within hours, the patient may begin to display hyperactive or combative behavior. In addition, there may be personality change, irrational behavior, progressive stupor, restlessness, convulsions, and coma. The sudden onset of vomiting often marks the early stages of the disease. In approximately 10–20% of cases, there is a recent history of chicken pox. Other children may have had a recent upper-respiratory infection. Infants may have recently had gastroenteritis.

On physical examination, there may be rapid deep respirations, which may be irregular. The pupils can be dilated and react sluggishly. There also may be signs of increased intracranial pressure, such as deviations in gaze. Unfortunately, Reye's syndrome cannot be diagnosed in the field. The diagnosis is difficult enough to make in the hospital.

Complications that can occur with Reye's syndrome include respiratory failure, cardiac arrhythmias, and acute pancreatitis. Death usually results from CNS complications such as herniation of the brainstem.

Management. Management is general and supportive. The primary survey should be completed, with particular attention on the respiratory status. Ventilations should be supported, if necessary. Supplemental oxygen should be administered. Transport should be rapid.

■ **septicemia** the presence of an infectious agent, usually bacteria, in the bloodstream.

✱ Septicemia in a child is a medical emergency.

■ **Reye's syndrome** illness of uncertain etiology that results in alteration of mental function in children. Often associated with viral infections and the use of aspirin.

Respiratory Emergencies

Respiratory problems are common in childhood. Children are susceptible to many of the respiratory problems that occur in adults. In addition, there are several problems that are unique to children. Respiratory problems should be identified in the primary assessment and treated appropriately. First, the airway should be assessed. If the airway is obstructed, it should be cleared, if possible, using the techniques of basic life support. Second, breathing should be assessed. If the child is not breathing, artificial ventilations should be initiated.

Pediatric respiratory emergencies that deserve special attention include bronchiolitis, croup, epiglottitis, asthma, and aspiration of foreign bodies. Children with any of these disorders can suffer respiratory arrest. This is most often due to airway obstruction or exhaustion.

Bronchiolitis. Wheezing in a child under 1 year of age is frequently due to bronchiolitis. **Bronchiolitis** is a respiratory infection of the medium-sized airways, the bronchioles, that occurs in early childhood. It should not be confused with bronchitis, which is an infection of the larger bronchi. Bronchiolitis is caused by a viral infection, most commonly *respiratory syncytial virus,* which affects the lining of the bronchioles. Characterized by prominent expiratory wheezing, it clinically resembles asthma.

■ **bronchiolitis** viral infection of the medium-sized airways, occurring most frequently during the first year of life.

✱ Wheezing in a child under one year of age, especially in the fall and winter months, is often bronchiolitis.

Assessment. The history is necessary to distinguish bronchiolitis from asthma. Often, with bronchiolitis, there is a family history of asthma or allergies, although neither is yet present in the child. In addition, there often is a low-grade fever. A major distinguishing factor is age. Asthma rarely occurs before the age of 1 year, whereas bronchiolitis is more frequent in this age group.

The physical examination should be systematic. Particular attention should be paid to the presence of rales or wheezes. Also, evidence of infection or respiratory distress should be noted.

Management. Prehospital management of suspected bronchiolitis is much the same as with asthma. The child should be placed in a semi-sitting position, if old enough, and given humidified oxygen by mask. Ventilations should be supported as necessary. Equipment for intubation should be readily available. If bronchospasm is present, epinephrine 1:1,000 should be administered. If ordered, epinephrine should be given by subcutaneous injection. The cardiac rhythm should be constantly monitored.

■ **croup** laryngotracheobronchitis, a common viral infection of young children, resulting in edema of the sub-glottic tissues. Characterized by barking cough and inspiratory stridor.

Croup. **Croup,** medically referred to as *laryngotracheobronchitis,* is a viral infection of the upper airway. It most often occurs in children 6 months to 4 years of age and is most prevalent in the fall and winter. The infection causes edema to develop beneath the larynx and glottis, narrowing the lumen of the airway. Severe cases of croup may result in complete airway obstruction.

Assessment. The history for croup is fairly classic. Often, the child will have a mild cold or other infection and be doing fairly well until dark. After dark, however, a harsh, barking cough develops. The attack may subside in a few hours, but can persist for several nights.

The physical exam will often reveal inspiratory stridor. There may be associated nasal flaring, tracheal tugging, or retraction. The para-

TABLE 30-3 Symptoms of Croup and Epiglottitis

Croup	Epiglottitis
Slow onset	Rapid onset
Generally wants to sit up	Prefers to sit up
Barking cough	No barking cough
No drooling	Drooling; painful to swallow
Fever approx. 100–101°F	Fever approx. 102–104°F
	Occasional stridor

medic SHOULD NEVER examine the oropharynx. Often, in the prehospital setting, it is difficult to distinguish croup from epiglottitis. (See Table 10-3.) If epiglottitis is present, examination of the oropharynx may result in laryngospasm and complete airway obstruction may occur. If the attack of croup is severe and progressive, the child may develop restlessness, tachycardia, and cyanosis. Complete airway obstruction can occur, resulting in respiratory arrest.

Management. Management of croup should consist of appropriate airway maintenance. The child should be placed in a position of comfort and administered humidified oxygen by face mask. The process of transporting the child from the house to the ambulance will often allow him or her to breathe the cool air. Because this cool air causes a decrease in subglottic edema, the child may be clinically improved by the time he or she reaches the ambulance. If the attack of croup is severe, the medical control physician may order the administration of racemic epinephrine. Some physicians advocate the use of steroids in croup because they feel these drugs shorten the course of the illness. The child should be transported to the hospital.

Epiglottitis. **Epiglottitis** is an acute infection and inflammation of the epiglottis and is potentially life-threatening. The epiglottis is a flap of cartilage that protects the airway during swallowing. Epiglottitis, unlike croup, is caused by a bacterial infection, usually *Haemophilus influenza.* It tends to occur in older children, generally 4 years and older, and is characterized by a swollen, cherry red epiglottis.

Assessment. The child with epiglottitis is acutely ill. The presentation is similar to croup. Often, the child will go to bed feeling relatively well, usually with what the parents consider to be a mild infection of the upper respiratory tract. Later, the child awakens with a high fever and a brassy cough. The progression of symptoms can be dramatic. There is often pain upon swallowing, sore throat, high fever, shallow breathing, dyspnea, inspiratory stridor, and drooling.

On physical examination, the child appears toxic. The paramedic SHOULD NEVER attempt to visualize the airway. Often, however, when the child is crying, the tip of the epiglottis can be seen posterior to the base of the tongue. In epiglottitis it is red and swollen. As airway obstruction develops, the child will exhibit retractions, nasal flaring, and pulmonary hyperexpansion. (See Figure 30-12.)

Management. Management of epiglottitis should consist of appropriate airway maintenance. The child should be placed in a position of comfort and administered humidified oxygen by face mask. (See Figure 30-13.)

■ **epiglottitis** bacterial infection of the epiglottis, usually occurring in children older than age 4. A serious medical emergency.

✱ Epiglottitis is a serious medical emergency.

✱ Never attempt to visualize the pharynx in a child who might have epiglottitis.

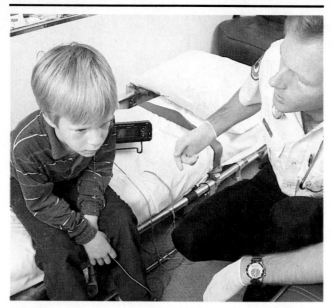

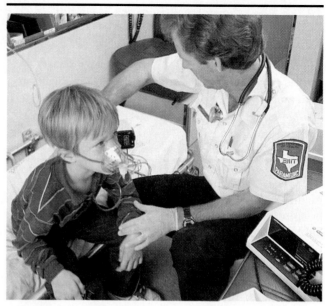

FIGURE 30-12 Posturing of the child with epiglottitis. Often, there will be excessive drooling.

FIGURE 30-13 The child with epiglottitis should be administered humidified oxygen and transported in a comfortable position.

Racemic epinephrine is contraindicated. The paramedic should have all intubation equipment available, including an appropriate-sized endotracheal tube. Intubation, however, is contraindicated, unless complete airway obstruction occurs. Transtracheal ventilation may be required. The child should be transported to the hospital as quickly as possible. If total obstruction develops, attempts should be made to ventilate the patient with high pressures. Often this may require depressing the pop-off valve on the bag-valve-mask device. (See Figure 30-14.)

Asthma. Asthma is a common respiratory disease that affects more than 6 million Americans. It occurs usually before age 10 in approximately 50% of the cases, and before age 30 in an additional 33% of cases. There is

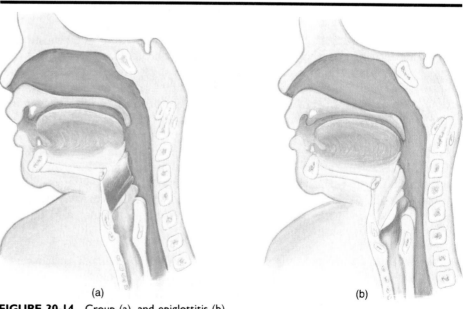

(a) (b)

FIGURE 30-14 Croup (a) and epiglottitis (b).

a family tendency toward the disease and it is often associated with atopic conditions, such as eczema and allergies. Prompt prehospital recognition and treatment are essential as children can die from asthma.

Asthma is characterized by obstruction of the airway due to bronchospasm. In the acute attack, the patient will develop intense bronchospasm, which often is followed by swelling of the mucous membranes lining the bronchioles. Subsequently, there may be plugging of the bronchi by thick mucus, thus further obstructing the airway. As bronchospasm develops, with an associated increase in sputum production, the lungs become progressively hyperinflated since air flow is more restricted on exhalation. This effectively reduces vital capacity and results in decreased gas exchange at the alveoli, resulting in hypoxemia. If allowed to progress untreated, hypoxemia will worsen, and unconsciousness and death may ensue.

Assessment. Asthma can often be differentiated from other pediatric respiratory illnesses by the history. Often, there is a prior history of asthma or reactive airway disease. The child's medications may also be an indicator. Children with asthma often will have an inhaler or will take a theophylline or oral beta agonist preparation.

On physical examination, the child is usually sitting up, leaning forward, and tachypneic. Often, there is an associated unproductive cough. Accessory respiratory muscle usage is usually evident. Wheezing may be heard. However, in a severe attack, the patient may not wheeze at all—this is often an ominous finding. Generally, there is an associated tachycardia, and this should be monitored, since virtually all medications used to treat asthma increase the heart rate.

Management. The primary therapeutic goal in the asthmatic is to correct hypoxia and reverse bronchospasm. First, it is imperative that an airway be established. Supplemental, humidified oxygen should be administered. Subcutaneous epinephrine may be ordered by the medical control physician. In addition, the medical control physician may order the administration of aminophylline. Many paramedic units have the capability of administering nebulized bronchodilator medications, such as albuterol, terbutaline, or isoetharine, and administration of these agents may be requested. If there is a prolonged transport time, the administration of a steroid preparation may be requested by the medical control physician.

Status Asthmaticus. Status asthmaticus is defined as a severe, prolonged asthma attack that cannot be broken by repeated doses of epinephrine. This is a serious medical emergency and prompt recognition, treatment, and transport are required. Often, the child suffering status asthmaticus will have a greatly distended chest from continued air trapping. Breath sounds, and often wheezing, may be absent. The patient is usually exhausted, severely acidotic, and often dehydrated. The management of status asthmaticus is basically the same as asthma. However, the paramedic should recognize that respiratory arrest is imminent, and he or she should be prepared for endotracheal intubation. Transport should be immediate, with aggressive treatment continued enroute.

✱ Status asthmaticus requires immediate transport with treatment administered enroute.

Aspirated Foreign Body. Children, especially 1- to 3-year-olds, are always putting objects into their mouths. These children are at increased risk of aspirating the object, especially when they are running or falling. In addition, many children choke on, or aspirate, food given to them by their parents or other well-meaning adults. Young children have not yet

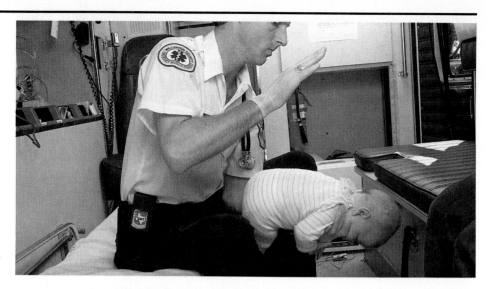

FIGURE 30-15 Attempting to relieve airway obstruction in a baby.

developed coordinated chewing motions in the mouth and pharynx and cannot adequately chew food. Common foods associated with aspiration and airway obstruction in children include chewing gum, hot dogs, grapes, peanuts, and sausages.

Assessment. The child with a suspected aspirated foreign body may present in one of two ways. If the obstruction is complete, the child will not be breathing. If it is partial, the child may exhibit labored breathing, retractions, chest expansion, and cyanosis. A foreign body aspirated into the respiratory tree will often drop until it lodges. Large objects will lodge in the trachea or the mainstem bronchi. Smaller objects may drop to the bronchioles. Often, the food particle will act as a one-way valve, allowing the entry of air, while restricting its exit. This results in hyperexpansion of the affected lung. If severe, tracheal deviation, away from the involved lung, may be noted.

Management. When confronted with the child suspected of aspirating a foreign body, the paramedic should immediately complete the primary survey. If complete obstruction is noted, the paramedic should clear the airway with accepted basic life support techniques. If unsuccessful, the paramedic should visualize the airway with a laryngoscope. If the foreign body is seen, and readily accessible, it can be removed with Magill forceps. If the airway cannot be cleared by routine measures, cricothyroidotomy may be indicated.

If the obstruction is partial, the child should be made comfortable and should be administered humidified oxygen. Intubation equipment should be readily available, since complete airway obstruction can occur. The child should be transported to a hospital, where the foreign body can be removed by fiberoptic bronchoscopy.

PEDIATRIC ADVANCED LIFE SUPPORT (PALS)

Recognition of Respiratory Failure and Shock: Anticipating Cardiopulmonary Arrest

Cardiopulmonary arrest in infants and children is usually not a sudden event. Instead, it is the end result of progressive deterioration in respiratory and cardiac function. Because of this, the goal of pediatric advanced life support is to recognize and prevent cardiopulmonary arrest.

All sick children should undergo a Rapid Cardiopulmonary Assessment. The goal is to answer the question, *"Does this child have pulmonary or circulatory failure that may lead to cardiopulmonary arrest?"* Recognition of the physiologically unstable infant is made by physical examination alone.

Children who should receive the Rapid Cardiopulmonary Assessment include those with:

* The goal of the Rapid Cardiopulmonary Assessment is to answer the question, "Does this child have a pulmonary or circulatory problem that may lead to cardiac arrest?"

❏ Respiratory rate > 60
❏ Heart rate   > 180 or < 80 (under 5 years)
                  > 160 (over 5 years)
❏ Respiratory distress
❏ Trauma
❏ Burns
❏ Cyanosis
❏ Altered level of consciousness
❏ Seizures
❏ Fever with petechiae (small skin hemorrhages)

Rapid Cardiopulmonary Assessment

The Rapid Cardiopulmonary Assessment follows the basic ABCs of CPR and consists of the following procedures:

Airway Patency. The airway should be inspected and determined to be (see Figures 30-16 through 30-18):

1. patent,
2. maintainable with head positioning, suctioning, or airway adjuncts, or
3. unmaintainable and requiring intervention, such as endotracheal intubation or removal of a foreign body

Breathing. Evaluation of breathing includes assessment of (see Figures 30-19 and 30-20):

❏ *Respiratory Rate.* Tachypnea is often the first manifestation of respiratory distress in infants. An infant breathing at a rapid rate will eventually tire. Thus, a decreasing respiratory rate is not necessarily a sign of improvement. A slow respiratory rate in an acutely ill infant or child is an ominous sign.
❏ *Air Entry.* The quality of air entry can be assessed by observing for chest rise, breath sounds, stridor, or wheezing.
  Respiratory Mechanics. Increased work of breathing in the infant and child is evidenced by nasal flaring and use of the accessory respiratory muscles.
❏ *Color.* Cyanosis is a fairly late sign of respiratory failure and is most frequently seen in the mucous membranes of the mouth and the nail beds. Cyanosis of the extremities alone is more likely due to circulatory failure (shock) than respiratory failure.

Circulation. The cardiovascular assessment consists of the following procedures (see Figure 30-21):

❏ *Heart Rate.* Normal heart rates for age were presented earlier in the chapter. Infants develop sinus tachycardia in response to stress. Thus, any tachycardia in an infant or child requires further evaluation to determine the cause.

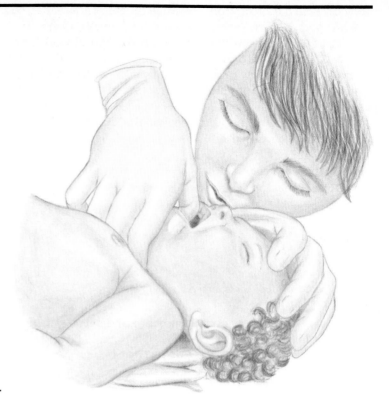

FIGURE 30-16 Opening the airway in a child.

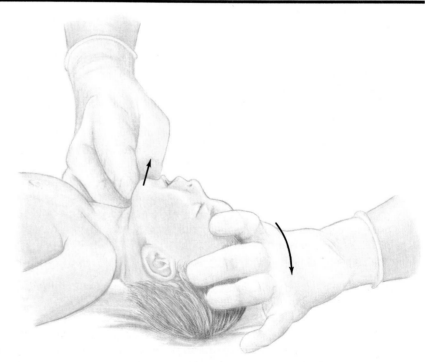

FIGURE 30-17 Chin-lift/Head tilt method.

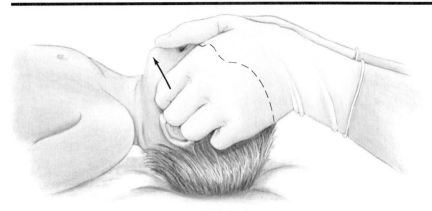

FIGURE 30-18 Jaw-thrust method.

Bradycardia in a distressed infant or child may indicate hypoxia and is an ominous sign of impending cardiac arrest.

❑ *Blood Pressure.* Hypotension is a late and often sudden sign of cardiovascular decompensation. Even mild hypotension should be taken seriously and treated quickly and vigorously, since cardiopulmonary arrest is imminent.

❑ *Peripheral Circulation.* The presence of pulses is a good indicator of the adequacy of end-organ perfusion. The pulse pressure (the difference between the systolic and diastolic blood pressure) narrows as shock develops. Loss of central pulses is an ominous sign.

❑ *End-Organ Perfusion.* The end-organ perfusion is most evident in the skin, kidneys, and brain. Decreased perfusion of the skin is an early sign of shock. A capillary refill time of greater than 2 seconds is indicative of low cardiac output. Impairment of brain perfusion is usually evidenced by a change in mental status. The child may become confused or lethargic. Seizures may occur. Failure of the child to recognize the parents' faces is often an ominous sign. Urine output is directly related to kidney perfusion. Nor-

✱ Decreased perfusion of the skin is an early sign of shock.

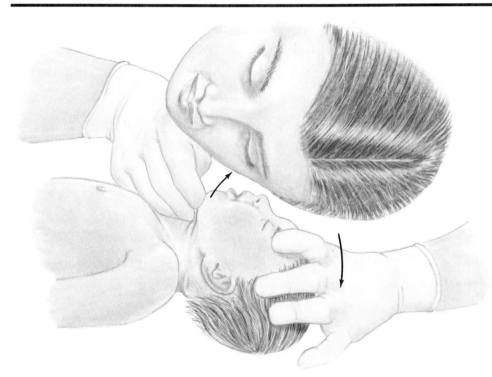

FIGURE 30-19 Assessing the airway.

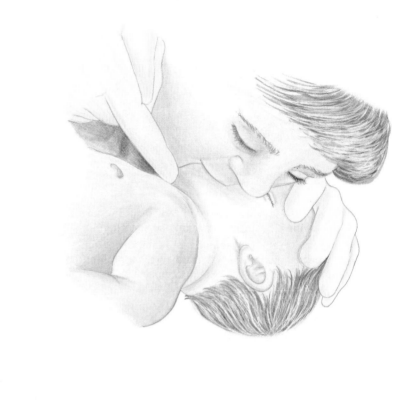

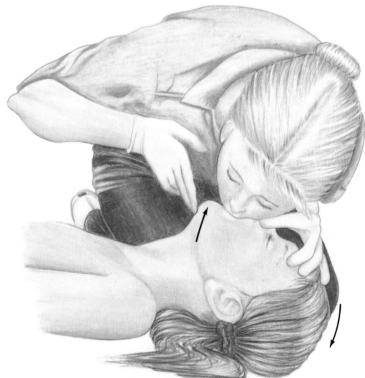

FIGURE 30-20 Artificial ventilations.

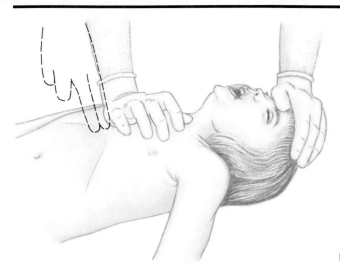

FIGURE 30-21 Hand placement for CPR.

mal urine output is 1–2 mL/kg/hr. Urine flow of less than 1 mL/kg/hr. is an indicator of poor renal perfusion.

The Rapid Cardiopulmonary Assessment should be repeated throughout initial assessment and patient transport. This will aid in determining whether the patient's condition is deteriorating or improving. Any decompensation or change in the patient's status should be immediately treated.

Management of the Critically Ill Infant or Child

Basic Life Support. Basic life support (BLS) is a fundamental emergency skill. A brief review of pediatric BLS is presented in Tables 30-4 through 30-10:

Pediatric Airway Management

The pediatric airway is somewhat different than that of the adult. Important differences include:

- ❏ The larynx is slightly higher in the neck.
- ❏ The epiglottis is U-shaped and extends into the pharynx.
- ❏ The vocal cords are short and concave.
- ❏ The narrowest portion of the airway is at the level of the cricoid cartilage (in children less than 8 years old).

These have several clinical implications in airway management. First, it is slightly more difficult to visualize the airway for endotracheal intubation. Second, the size of the endotracheal tube should be based on size of the cricoid ring, rather than the glottic opening.

Many of the same airway management techniques for adults are applicable in children. There are, however, some differences. First, esophageal obturator airways (EOA's) should not be used in pediatrics because of the variations in airway size in children. Second, use of nasopharyngeal airways in children is discouraged. Young children have rather large adenoidal tissue and insertion of a nasopharyngeal airway can lacerate these tissues, causing bleeding into the airway.

TABLE 30-4 OBSTRUCTED AIRWAY—INFANT CONSCIOUS

Step	Objective	Critical Performance
1. Assessment	Determine airway obstruction.*	Observe breathing difficulties.*
2. Back Blows	Deliver 4 back blows.	Supporting head and neck with one hand, straddle infant face down, head lower than trunk, over your forearm supported on your thigh. Deliver 4 back blows, forcefully, between the shoulder blades with the heel of the hand (3–5 sec).
3. Chest Thrusts	Deliver 4 chest thrusts.	While supporting the head, sandwich infant between your hands and turn on back, with head lower than trunk. Deliver 4 thrusts in the midsternal region in the same manner as external chest compressions, but at a slower rate (3–5 sec).
4. Sequencing	Repeat sequence.	Repeat Steps 2 and 3 until either the foreign body is expelled or the infant becomes unconscious (see below).

Infant with Obstructed Airway Becomes Unconscious

Step	Objective	Critical Performance
5. Call for Help.	Call for help.	Call out "Help!" or, if others respond, activate EMS system.
6. Foreign Body Check	Manual removal of foreign body if one is found (tongue-jaw lift, NOT blind finger sweep).	Keep victim's face up. Place thumb in infant's mouth, over tongue. Lift tongue and jaw forward with fingers wrapped around lower jaw. Look into mouth; remove foreign body ONLY IF VISUALIZED.
7. Breathing Attempt	Ventilate	Open airway with head-tilt/chin-lift. Seal mouth and nose properly. Attempt to ventilate.
8. Back Blows	(Airway is obstructed.) Deliver 4 back blows.	Supporting head and neck with one hand, straddle infant face down, head lower than trunk, over your forearm supported on your thigh. Deliver 4 back blows, forcefully, between the shoulder blades with the heel of the hand (3–5 sec).
9. Chest Thrusts	Deliver 4 chest thrusts.	While supporting the head and neck, sandwich infant between your hands and turn on back, with head lower than trunk. Deliver 4 thrusts in the midsternal region in the same manner as external chest compressions, but at a slower rate (3–5 sec).
10. Foreign Body Check	(Airway remains obstructed.) Manual removal of foreign body if one is found.	Keep victim's face up. Do tongue-jaw lift, but NOT blind finger sweep. Look into mouth, remove foreign body ONLY IF VISUALIZED.
11. Breathing Attempt	Ventilate.	Open airway with head-tilt/chin-lift. Seal mouth and nose properly. Reattempt to ventilate.
12. Sequencing	(Airway remains obstructed.) Repeat sequence.	Repeat Steps 8–11 until successful.†

* This procedure should be initiated in a conscious infant only if the airway obstruction is due to a witnessed or strongly suspected aspiration and if respiratory difficulty is increasing and the cough is ineffective. If the obstruction is caused by airway swelling due to infections, such as epiglottitis or croup, these procedures may be harmful: the infant should be rushed to the nearest ALS facility, allowing the infant to maintain the position of maximum comfort.
† After airway obstruction is cleared, ventilate twice and proceed with CPR as indicated.
(Reproduced with permission of the American Heart Association)

TABLE 30-5 OBSTRUCTED AIRWAY—INFANT UNCONSCIOUS

Step	Objective	Critical Performance
1. Assessment	Determine unresponsiveness. Call for help. Position the infant.	Tap or gently shake shoulder. Call out "Help!" Turn on back as unit, if necessary, supporting head and neck. Place on firm, hard surface.
	Open the airway.	Use head-tilt/chin-lift maneuver to sniffing or neutral position. Do not overextend the head.
	Determine breathlessness.	Maintain open airway. Ear over mouth, observe chest: look, listen, feel for breathing (3–5 sec).
2. Breathing Attempt	Ventilate.	Maintain open airway. Make tight seal on mouth and nose of infant with rescuer's mouth. Attempt to ventilate.
	(Airway is obstructed.) Ventilate.	Reposition infant's head. Seal mouth and nose properly. Reattempt to ventilate.
	(Airway remains obstructed.) Activate EMS system	If someone responded to call for help, send him/her to activate EMS system.
3. Back Blows	Deliver 4 back blows.	Supporting head and neck with one hand, straddle infant face down, head lower than trunk, over your forearm supported on your thigh. Deliver 4 back blows, forcefully, between the shoulder blades with the heel of the hand (3–5 sec).
4. Chest Thrusts	Deliver 4 chest thrusts.	While supporting the head and neck, sandwich infant between your hands and turn on back, with head lower than trunk. Deliver 4 thrusts in the mid-sternal region the same manner as external chest compressions, but at a slower rate (3–5 sec).
5. Foreign Body Check	(Airway remains obstructed.) Manual removal of foreign body if one is found (tongue-jaw lift, NOT blind finger sweep).	Keep victim's face up. Place thumb in infant's mouth, over tongue. Lift tongue and jaw forward with fingers wrapped around lower jaw. Look into mouth; remove foreign body ONLY IF VISUALIZED.
6. Breathing Attempt	Ventilate.	Open airway with head-tilt/chin-lift. Seal mouth and nose properly. Reattempt to ventilate.
7. Sequencing	Repeat sequence.	Repeat Steps 3–6 until successful.*

* After airway obstruction is cleared, ventilate twice and proceed with CPR as indicated.
(Reproduced with permission of the American Heart Association)

TABLE 30-6 OBSTRUCTED AIRWAY—CHILD CONSCIOUS

Step	Objective	Critical Performance
1. Assessment	Determine airway obstruction.*	Ask "Are you choking?" Determine if victim can cough or speak.
2. Heimlich Maneuver	Perform abdominal thrusts (only if victim's cough is ineffective and there is increasing respiratory difficulty.	Stand behind the victim. Wrap arms around victim's waist. Make a fist with one hand and place the thumb side against victim's abdomen, in the midline slightly above the navel and well below the tip of the xiphoid. Grasp fist with the other hand. Press into the victim's abdomen with quick upward thrusts. Each thrust should be distinct and delivered with the intent of relieving the airway obstruction. Repeat thrusts until either the foreign body is expelled or the victim becomes unconscious (see below).
3. Positioning	Position the victim. Call for help.	Turn on back as unit. Place face up, arms by side. Call out "Help!" or if others respond, activate EMS system.
4. Foreign Body Check	Manual removal of foreign body if one is found. DO NOT perform blind finger sweep.	Keep victim's face up. Use tongue-jaw lift to open mouth. Look into mouth; remove foreign body ONLY IF VISUALIZED.
5. Breathing Attempt	Ventilate.	Open airway with head-tilt/chin-lift. Seal mouth and nose properly. Attempt to ventilate.
6. Heimlich Maneuver	(Airway is obstructed.) Perform abdominal thrusts.	Kneel at victim's feet if on the floor, or stand at victim's feet if on a table. Place heel of one hand against victim's abdomen, in the midline slightly above navel and well below tip of xiphoid. Place second hand directly on top of first hand. Press into the abdomen with quick upward thrusts. Perform 6–10 abdominal thrusts.
7. Foreign Body Check	(Airway remains obstructed.) Manual removal of foreign body if one is found. DO NOT perform blind finger sweep.	Keep victim's face up. Use tongue-jaw lift to open mouth. Look into mouth; remove foreign body ONLY IF VISUALIZED.
8. Breathing Attempt	Ventilate.	Open airway with head-tilt/chin-lift. Seal mouth and nose properly. Reattempt to ventilate.
9. Sequencing	(Airway remains obstructed.) Repeat sequence.	Repeat Steps 6–8 until successful.[†]

* This procedure should be initiated in a conscious child only if the airway obstruction is due to a witnessed or strongly suspected aspiration and if respiratory difficulty is increasing and the cough is ineffective. If obstruction is caused by airway swelling due to infection such as epiglottitis or croup, these procedures may be harmful; the child should be rushed to the nearest ALS facility, allowing the child to maintain the position of maximum comfort.
[†] After airway obstruction is cleared, ventilate twice and proceed with CPR as indicated.
(Reproduced with permission of the American Heart Association)

TABLE 30-7   OBSTRUCTED AIRWAY—CHILD UNCONSCIOUS

Step	Objective	Critical Performance
1. Assessment	Determine unresponsiveness.	Tap or gently shake shoulder. Shout "Are you OK?"
	Call for help.	Call out "Help!"
	Position the victim.	Turn on back as unit, if necessary, supporting head and neck (4–10 sec).
	Open the airway.	Use head-tilt/chin-lift maneuver.
	Determine breathlessness.	Maintain open airway. Ear over mouth, observe chest: look, listen, feel for breathing (3–5 sec).
2. Breathing Attempt	Ventilate.	Maintain open airway. Seal mouth and nose properly. Attempt to ventilate.
	(Airway is obstructed.) Ventilate.	Reposition victim's head. Seal mouth and nose properly. Reattempt to ventilate.
	(Airway remains obstructed.) Activate EMS system.	If someone responded to call for help, send him/her to activate EMS system.
3. Heimlich Maneuver	Perform abdominal thrusts.	Kneel at victim's feet if on the floor, or stand at victim's feet if on a table. Place heel of one hand against victim's abdomen in the midline slightly above navel and well below tip of xiphoid. Place second hand directly on top of first hand. Press into the abdomen with quick upward thrusts. Each thrust should be distinct and delivered with the intent of relieving the airway. Perform 6–10 abdominal thrusts.
4. Foreign Body Check	(Airway remains obstructed.) Manual removal of foreign body if one is found. DO NOT perform blind finger sweep.	Keep victim's face up. Use tongue-jaw lift to open mouth. Look into mouth; remove foreign body ONLY IF VISUALIZED.
5. Breathing Attempt	Ventilate.	Open airway with head-tilt/chin-lift maneuver. Seal mouth and nose properly. Reattempt to ventilate.
6. Sequencing	Repeat sequence.	Repeat Steps 3–5 until successful.*

* After airway obstruction is cleared, ventilate twice and proceed with CPR as indicated.
(Reproduced with permission of the American Heart Association)

TABLE 30-8 INFANT CPR

Step	Objective	Critical Performance
1. **A**IRWAY	Assessment: Determine unresponsiveness. Call for help. Position the infant. Open the airway.	Tap or gently shake shoulder. Call out "Help!" Turn on back as unit, supporting head and neck. Place on firm, hard surface. Use head-tilt/chin-lift maneuver to sniffing or neutral position. Do not overextend the head.

2. **B**REATHING	Assessment:
	Determine breathlessness.
	
	Ventilate twice.
		Maintain open airway.
		Ear over mouth, observe chest: look, listen, feel
		   for breathing (3−5 sec).
		Maintain open airway.
		Make tight seal on infant's mouth and nose with
		   rescuer's mouth.
		Ventilate 2 times at 1−1.5 sec./inspiration.
		Observe chest rise.
		Allow deflation between breaths.

3. **C**IRCULATION	Assessment:
	Determine pulselessness.
	Activate EMS system.
	
	Begin chest compressions.
		Feel for brachial pulse (5−10 sec).
		Maintain head-tilt with other hand.
		If someone responded to call for help, send him/
		   her to activate EMS system.
		Total time, Step 1−Activate EMS system:
		   15−35 sec.
		Imagine line between nipples (intermammary
		   line).
		Place 2−3 fingers on sternum, 1 finger's width
		   below intermammary line.
		Equal compression-relaxation.
		Compress vertically, $1/2$ to 1 inches.
		Keep fingers on sternum during upstroke.
		Complete chest relaxation on upstroke.
		Say any helpful mnemonic.
		Compression rate: at least 100/min (5 in 3
		   sec or less).

4. Compression/Ventilation Cycles	Do 10 cycles of 5 compressions and 1 ventilation.	Proper compression/ventilation ratio: 5 compressions to 1 slow ventilation per cycle. Pause for ventilation. Observe chest rise: 1−1.5 sec./inspiration; 10 cycles/45 sec or less.
5. Reassessment	Determine pulselessness.	Feel for brachial pulse (5 sec).* If there is no pulse, go to Step 6.
6. Continue CPR	Ventilate once. Resume compression/ ventilation cycles.	Ventilate 1 time. Observe chest rise: 1−1.5 sec./inspiration. Feel for brachial pulse every few minutes.

* If pulse is present, open airway and check for spontaneous breathing. (a) If breathing is present, maintain open airway and monitor breathing and pulse. (b) If breathing is absent, perform rescue breathing at 20 times/min and monitor pulse. (Reproduced with permission of the American Heart Association)

TABLE 30-9   CHILD CPR, ONE RESCUER

Step	Objective	Critical Performance
1. **A**IRWAY	Assessment. Determine unresponsiveness. Call for help. Position the victim. Open the airway.	Tap or gently shake shoulder. Shout "Are you OK?" Call out "Help!" Turn on back as unit, if necessary, supporting head and neck (4–10 sec). Use head-tilt/chin-lift maneuver.
2. **B**REATHING	Assessment: Determine breathlessness. Ventilate twice.	Maintain open airway. Ear over mouth, observe chest: look, listen, feel for breathing (3–5 sec). Maintain open airway. Seal mouth and nose properly. Ventilate 2 times at 1–1.5 sec./inspiration. Observe chest rise. Allow deflation between breaths.
3. **C**IRCULATION	Assessment: Determine pulselessness. Activate EMS system. Begin chest compressions.	Feel for carotid pulse on near side of victim (5–10 sec). Maintain head-tilt with other hand. If someone responded to call for help, send him/her to activate EMS system. Total time, Step 1—Activate EMS system: 15–35 sec. Rescuer kneels by victim's shoulders. Landmark check prior to initial hand placement.§ Proper hand position throughout. Rescuer's shoulders over victim's sternum. Equal compression-relaxation. Compress 1 to 1½ inches. Keep hand on sternum during upstroke. Complete chest relaxation on upstroke. Say any helpful mnemonic. Compression rate: 80–100/min (5 per 3–4 sec).
4. Compression/Ventilation Cycles	Do 10 cycles of 5 compressions and 1 ventilation.	Proper compression/ventilation ratio: 5 compressions to 1 slow ventilation per cycle. Observe chest rise: 1–1.5 sec./inspiration (10 cycles/60–87 sec).
5. Reassessment†	Determine pulselessness.	Feel for carotid pulse (5 sec).‡ If there is no pulse, go to Step 6.
6. Continue CPR	Ventilate once. Resume compression/ventilation cycles.	Ventilate one time. Observe chest rise: 1–1.5 sec./inspiration. Feel for carotid pulse every few minutes.

* If child is above age of approximately 8 years, the method for adults should be used.
† 2nd rescuer arrives to replace 1st rescuer: (a) 2nd rescuer identifies self by saying "I know CPR. Can I help?" (b) 2nd rescuer then does pulse check in Step 5 and continues with Step 6. (During practice and testing only one rescuer actually ventilates the manikin. The 2nd rescuer simulates ventilation.) (c) 1st rescuer assesses the adequacy of 2nd rescuer's CPR by observing chest rise during ventilations and by checking the pulse during chest compressions.
‡ If pulse is present, open airway and check for spontaneous breathing. (a) If breathing is present, maintain open airway and monitor breathing and pulse. (b) If breathing is absent, perform rescue breathing at 15 times/min and monitor pulse.
§ Thereafter, check hand position visually.
(Reproduced with permission of the American Heart Association)

TABLE 30-10 CHILD CPR, TWO RESCUERS

Step	Objective	Critical Performance
1. **A**IRWAY	**One rescuer (ventilator):** Assessment: Determine unresponsiveness. Position the victim. Open the airway.	Tap or gently shake shoulder. Shout "Are you OK?" Turn on back if necessary (4–10 sec). Use a proper technique to open airway.
2. **B**REATHING	Assessment: Determine breathlessness. Ventilate twice.	Look, listen, and feel (3–5 sec). Observe chest rise: 1–1.5 sec./inspiration.
3. **C**IRCULATION	Assessment: Determine pulselessness. State assessment results. **Other rescuer (compressor):** Get into position for compressions. Locate landmark notch.	Feel for carotid pulse (5–10 sec). Say "No pulse." Hand, shoulders in correct position. Landmark check.
4. Compression/Ventilation Cycles	**Compressor:** Begin chest compressions. **Ventilator:** Ventilate after every 5th compression and check compression effectiveness. (Minimum of 10 cycles.)	Correct ratio compressions/ventilations: 5/1. Compression rate: 80–100/min (5 compressions/ 3–4 sec). Say any helpful mnemonic. Stop compressing for each ventilation. Ventilate 1 time (1–1.5 sec./inspiration). Check pulse occasionally to assess compressions. Time for 10 cycles: 40–53 sec.
5. Call for Switch	**Compressor:** Call for switch when fatigued.	Give clear signal to change. Compressor completes 5th compression. Ventilator completes ventilation after 5th compression.
6. Switch	Simultaneously switch: **Ventilator:** Move to chest. **Compressor:** Move to head.	Move to chest. Become compressor. Get into position for compressions. Locate landmark notch. Move to head. Become ventilator. Check carotid pulse (5 sec). Say "No pulse." Ventilate once (1–1.5 sec./inspiration).[†]
7. Continue CPR	Resume compression/ ventilation cycles.	Resume Step 4.

* (a) If CPR is in progress with one rescuer (layperson), the entrance of the two rescuers occurs after the completion of one rescuer's cycle of 5 compressions and 1 ventilation. The EMS should be activated first. The two new rescuer's start with Step 6. (b) If CPR is in progress with one healthcare provider, the entrance of a second healthcare provider is at the end of a cycle after check for pulse by first rescuer. The new cycle starts with one ventilation by the first rescuer, and the second rescuer becomes the compressor.

[†] During practice and testing only one rescuer actually ventilates the manikin. The other rescuer simulates ventilation.
(Reproduced with permission of the American Heart Association)

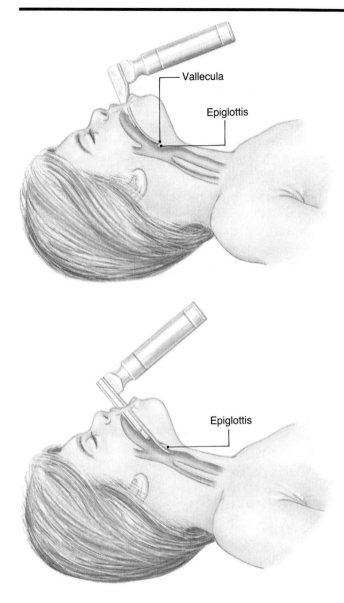

Vallecula

Epiglottis

Epiglottis

FIGURE 30-22 Placement of the laryngoscope in the child.

Finally, there are several special considerations in endotracheal intubation that must be considered. (See Figure 30-22.) As mentioned above, the airway of a child differs from that of an adult. It is, of course, smaller. In addition, it is more flexible, the tongue is relatively larger, and the glottic opening is higher in the neck. As a rule, in children under 8 years of age, uncuffed endotracheal tubes should be used. Cuffed tubes may be used in older children. Table 30-11 illustrates suggested endotracheal tube and suction catheter sizes for age. Intubation should be preceded by adequate ventilation with 100% oxygen. Although either a straight or curved blade may be used, a straight blade is recommended in infants. During intubation the heart rate should be monitored for the presence of dysrhythmia. Indications for intubation include the inability of the paramedic to ventilate the unconscious patient, cardiac or respiratory arrest, the inability of the patient to protect his or her airway, and the need for prolonged artificial ventilation.

✱ As a rule, uncuffed endotracheal tubes should be used in children under 8 years of age.

Ventilation of the Pediatric Patient. The bag-valve-mask (BVM) device is the ideal device for ventilation of the pediatric patient. Pediatric BVMs should not contain pressure pop-off valves, or should contain valves that

TABLE 30-11   Equipment Guidelines According to Age and Weight

Equipment	Age (50th Percentile Weight)					
	Premie (1–2.5 kg)	Neonate (2.5–4.0 kg)	6 Months (7.0 kg)	1–2 Years (10–12 kg)	5 Years (16–18 kg)	8–10 Years (24–30 kg)
Airway–oral	infant (00)	infant small (0)	small (1)	small (2)	medium (3)	medium large (4.5)
Breathing Self-inflating bag	infant	infant	child	child	child	child adult
O₂ ventilation mask	premature	newborn	infant/child	child	child	small adult
Endotracheal tube	2.5–3.0 (uncuffed)	3.0–3.5 (uncuffed)	3.5–4.0 (uncuffed)	4.0–4.5 (uncuffed)	5.0–5.5 (uncuffed)	5.5–6.5 (cuffed)
Laryngoscope blade	0 (straight)	1 (straight)	1 (straight)	1–2 (straight)	2 (straight or curved)	2–3 (straight or curved)
Suction/stylet (F)	6–8/6	8/6	8–10/6	10/6	14/14	14/14
Circulation BP cuff	newborn	newborn	infant	child	child	child adult

Venous access
  Angiocath
  Butterfly needle
  Intracath
  Arm board
	
	22–24
	25
	———
	6″
		
		22–24
		23–25
		———
		6″
			
			22–24
			23–25
			19
			6″–8″
				
				20–22
				23
				19
				8″
					
					18–20
					20–23
					16
					8″–15″
						
						16–20
						18–21
						14
						15

Orogastric tube (F)	5	5–8	8	10	10–12	14–18
Chest tube (F)	10–14	12–18	14–20	14–24	20–32	28–38

(Reproduced with permission of the American Heart Association)

are readily occluded, since ventilation pressures required during pediatric CPR may exceed the limit of the pop-off valve. Also, oxygen-powered breathing devices (demand valves) should not be used in pediatric resuscitation.

Vascular Access and Fluid Therapy.   The intravenous techniques for children are basically the same as for adults. However, there are additional veins in the infant that may be accessed. These include veins of the neck and scalp, as well as of the arms, hands, and feet. The external jugular vein, however, should only be used for life-threatening situations. Commonly used solutions include normal saline and lactated Ringer's. Intravenous infusions in children should be closely monitored, as it is very easy to fluid-overload the pediatric patient. Minidrip administration sets should be routinely used in pediatric cases.

The use of intraosseous infusion has become popular in the pediatric patient. (See Figures 30-23 and 30-24.) This is especially true when large volumes of fluid must be administered, as occurs in hypovolemic shock, and other means of venous access are not available. Certain PALS drugs can be administered intraosseously. These include epinephrine, atropine, dopamine, lidocaine, sodium bicarbonate, and dobutamine. Indications for intraosseous infusion include a child less than 5 years of age, the existence of shock or cardiac arrest, the patient who is comatose, and if attempts at peripheral IV insertion have been unsuccessful.

✱ Always remember the intraosseous route for administering drugs and fluids to the pediatric patient less than 5 years of age when an IV cannot be placed.

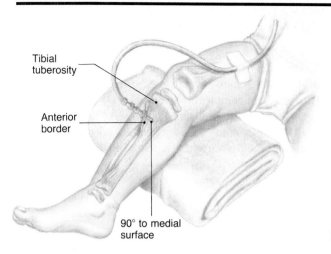

Tibial
tuberosity

Anterior
border

90° to medial
surface

FIGURE 30-23 Intraosseous administration.

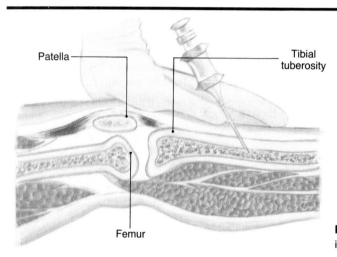

Patella

Tibial
tuberosity

Femur

FIGURE 30-24 Correct needle placement for intraosseous administration.

A standard 16- or 18-gauge needle (either hypodermic or spinal) can be used for intraosseous infusion. The anterior surface of the leg below the knee should be prepped with an antiseptic solution. The needle is then inserted, in a twisting fashion, 1–3 centimeters below the tibial tuberosity. Insertion should be slightly inferior in direction and perpendicular to the skin. Placement of the needle into the marrow cavity can be determined by noting a lack of resistance as the needle passes through the bony cortex, the needle standing upright without support, the ability to aspirate bone marrow into a syringe, or free flow of the infusion without infiltration into the subcutaneous tissues.

The accurate dosing of fluids in children is crucial. Too much fluid can result in heart failure and pulmonary edema. Too little fluid can be ineffective. The initial dosage of fluid in hypovolemic shock should be 20 mL/kg, given over 10 to 20 minutes as soon as IV access is obtained. After the infusion, the child should be reassessed. If perfusion is still diminished, then a second bolus of 20 mL/kg should be administered. A child with hypovolemic shock may require 40–60 mL/Kg, while a child with septic shock may require at least 60–80 mL/kg. Regardless, the most important factor of pediatric fluid therapy is frequent patient reassessment.

Medications.   Cardiopulmonary arrest in children is almost always due to a primary respiratory problem, such as drowning, choking, or smoke inhalation. The major aim in pediatric resuscitation is airway management and ventilation, as well as replacement of intravascular volume, if indicated. In certain cases, medications may be required. The objectives of medication therapy in pediatric cardiac arrest include the following:

- ❏ to correct hypoxemia
- ❏ to increase perfusion pressure during chest compression
- ❏ to stimulate spontaneous or more forceful cardiac contractions
- ❏ to accelerate the heart rate
- ❏ to correct metabolic acidosis
- ❏ to suppress ventricular ectopy.

The dosages of medications must be modified for the pediatric patient. Tables 30-12 through 30-15 illustrate recommended pediatric drug dosage in advanced cardiac life support.

Electrical Therapy.   The initial dosage for electrical defibrillation is 2 joules per kilogram of body weight. If this is unsuccessful, it should be increased to 4 joules per kilogram. If this is unsuccessful, attention should be aimed at correcting hypoxia and acidosis.

SUMMARY

Pediatric emergencies can be stressful for both the paramedic and the family. Most pediatric emergencies result from trauma, ingestion of poisons, respiratory emergencies, or febrile seizure activity. In addition, the paramedic must always be on the lookout for signs and symptoms of child abuse or neglect. The approach and management of pediatric emergencies must be modified for the age and size of the child. Certain skills generally considered routine, such as IV administration and ACLS, become more difficult in the pediatric patient, due to size and other factors. It is important to remember that children are not "small adults." They have special considerations and needs, and must be managed accordingly.

FURTHER READING

AMERICAN HEART ASSOCIATION AND AMERICAN ACADEMY OF PEDIATRICS. *Textbook of Pediatric Advanced Life Support.* Dallas: American Heart Association, 1988.

BEHRMAN, RICHARD, AND V. C. VAUGHN. *Nelson's Textbook of Pediatrics,* Thirteenth Edition. Philadelphia: W.B. Saunders, 1987.

TABLE 30-12 Pediatric Infusion Dosages.

Drug	Dose	How Supplied*	Remarks
Epinephrine hydrochloride	0.01 mg/kg 0.1 mL/kg	1:10,000 (0.1 mg/mL)	Most useful drug in cardiac arrest; 1:1,000 must be diluted.
Sodium bicarbonate	1 mEq/kg 1 mL/kg	1 mEq/mL (8.4% soln)	Infuse slowly and *only* when ventilation is adequate.
Atropine sulfate	0.02 mg/kg 0.2 mL/kg	0.1 mg/mL	Minimum dose of 0.1 mg (1 mL); use for bradycardia after assessing ventilation. Maximum dose: infants and children = 10 mg; adolescents = 2.0 mg
Calcium chloride	20 mg/kg (0.2 mL/kg)	100 mg/mL (10% soln)	Use only for hypo-calcemia, calcium blocker overdose, hyperkalemia or hypermagnesemia; give slowly.
Glucose	0.5–1.0 g/kg	0.5 g/mL $D_{50}W$	Dilute 1:1 with water ($D_{25}W$): dose is then 2–4 mL/kg.
Lidocaine hydrochloride	1 mg/kg	10 mg/mL (1%) 20 mg/mL (2%)	Used for ventricular arrhythmias only.
Bretylium tosylate	5 mg/kg	50 mg/mL	Use if lidocaine is not effective; repeat dose with 10 mg/kg if first dose not effective.
Infusions			
Epinephrine infusion	0.1–1.0 μg/ kg/min	1 mg/mL 1:1,000	Titrate infusion to desired hemo-dynamic effect.
Dopamine hydrochloride infusion	2–20 μg/kg/ min	40 mg/mL	Titrate to desired hemodynamic response.
Dobutamine infusion	5–20 μg/kg/ min	250 mg/vial lyophilized	Titrate to desired hemodynamic response; little vasoconstriction even at high rates.
Isoproterenol infusion	0.1–1.0 μg/ kg/min	1 mg/5 mL	Titrate to desired hemodynamic effect; vasodilator.
Lidocaine infusion	20–50 μg/ kg/min	40 mg/mL (4%)	Use lower infusion dose with shock, liver disease.

* For IV push medications, preparation listed is form available in prefilled syringes.
(Reproduced with permission of the American Heart Association)

TABLE 30-13

Isoproterenol Epinephrine	0.6 × body weight (in kg) is the mg dose added to make 100 mL	Then 1 mL/hr delivers 0.1 μg/kg/min
Dopamine Dobutamine	6 × body weight (in kg) is the mg dose added to make 100 mL	Then 1 mL/hr delivers 1 μg/kg/min

(Reproduced with permission of the American Heart Association)

TABLE 30-14 Resuscitation Medications, by Weight and Age, for Infants and Children 0–10 Years

Age	50th Percentile Weight (kg)	Epinephrine		Atropine		Bicarbonate*	
		mg	mL	mg	mL	mEq	mL
Newborn	3.0	0.03	0.3	0.1	1.0	3.0	6.0
1 Month	4.0	0.04	0.4	0.1	1.0	4.0	8.0
3 Months	5.5	0.055	0.55	0.11	1.1	5.5	11.0
6 Months	7.0	0.07	0.7	0.14	1.4	7.0	7.0
1 Year	10.0	0.10	1.0	0.20	2.0	10.0	10.0
2 Years	12.0	0.12	1.2	0.24	2.4	12.0	12.0
3 Years	14.0	0.14	1.4	0.28	2.8	14.0	14.0
4 Years	16.0	0.16	1.6	0.32	3.2	16.0	16.0
5 Years	18.0	0.18	1.8	0.36	3.6	18.0	18.0
6 Years	20.0	0.20	2.0	0.40	4.0	20.0	20.0
7 Years	22.0	0.22	2.2	0.44	4.4	22.0	22.0
8 Years	25.0	0.25	2.5	0.50	5.0	25.0	25.0
9 Years	28.0	0.28	2.8	0.56	5.6	28.0	28.0
10 Years	34.0	0.34	3.4	0.68	6.8	34.0	34.0

Volume (mL) is based on the following concentrations:
Epinephrine: 1:10,000 (0.1 mg/mL)
Atropine: 0.1 mg/mL
Bicarbonate: ≤ 3 months = 4.2% solution (0.5 mEq/mL)
> 3 months = 8.4% solution (1 mEq/mL)
* The use of bicarbonate in cardiac arrest is controversial. Good ventilation must be established before bicarbonate is used.
(Reproduced with permission of the American Heart Association)

TABLE 30-15 Infusion Medications, by Weight and Age, for Infants and Children 0–10 Years

Add: 100 mL of diluent, 0.6 mg (3 mL)* of **Isoproterenol**
0.6 mg (0.6 mL)* of **epinephrine**
60.0 mg (1.5 mL)* of **dopamine**
60.0 mg (2.4 mL)* of **dobutamine**

Infuse: at 1 mL/kg/hr or according to following table in order

To Give: 0.1 μg/kg/min isoproterenol
0.1 μg/kg/min epinephrine
10 μg/kg/min dopamine
10 μg/kg/min dobutamine

Age	50th Percentile Weight (kg)	Infusion Rate (mL/hr)
Newborn	3	3
1 Month	4	4
3 Months	5.5	5.5
6 Months	7.0	7.0
1 Year	10.0	10.0
2 Years	12.0	12.0
3 Years	14.0	14.0
4 Years	16.0	16.0
5 Years	18.0	18.0
6 Years	20.0	20.0
7 Years	22.0	22.0
8 Years	25.0	25.0
9 Years	28.0	28.0
10 Years	34.0	34.0

These are starting doses. Adjust concentration to dose and fluid tolerance.
* Based on the following concentrations: isoproterenol = 0.2 mg/mL
epinephrine = 1:1000 (1 mg/mL)
dopamine = 40 mg/mL
dobutamine = 25 mg/mL
(Reproduced with permission of the American Heart Association)

TABLE 30-16

	Infant	Child
AIRWAY	Head-tilt/chin-lift	Head-tilt/chin-lift
	Jaw-thrust	Jaw-thrust
BREATHING		
Initial	Two breaths at	Two breaths at
	1.0–1.5 sec/breath	1.0–1.5 sec/breath
Subsequent	20 breaths/minute	15 breaths/minute
CIRCULATION		
Pulse check	Brachial/femoral	Carotid
Compression area	Lower third of sternum	Lower third of sternum
Compressed with	2–3 fingers	Heel of one hand
Depth	0.5–1.0 inch (approx.)	1.0–1.5 inch (approx.)
Rate	At least 100/minute	80–100/minute
Compression: ventilation ratio	5:1 (pause for ventilation)	5:1 (pause for ventilation)
Foreign Body Airway Obstruction	Back blows/chest thrusts	Heimlich maneuver

(Reproduced with permission of the American Heart Association)

31

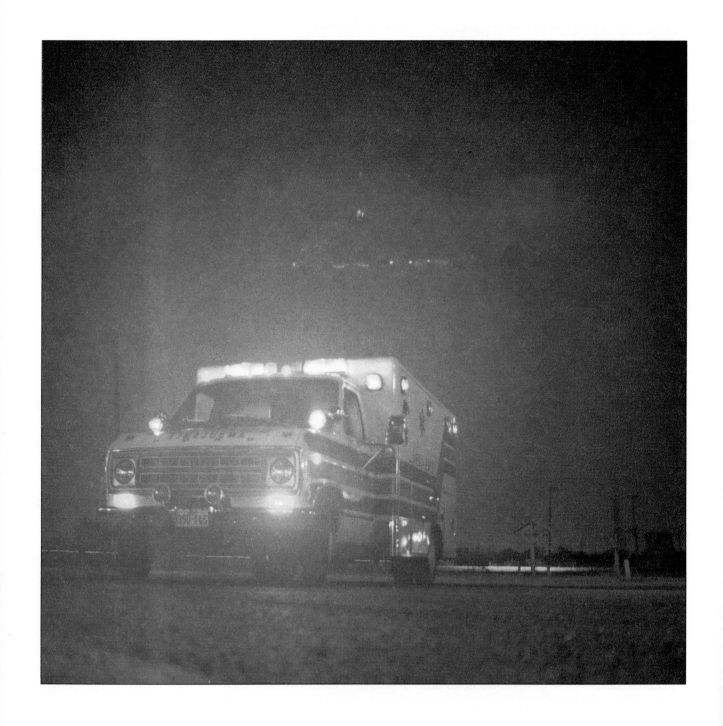

Gynecological Emergencies

Objectives for Chapter 31

Upon completing this chapter, the student should be able to:

1. Identify the location and function of the following organs:
   - ovaries
   - uterus
   - cervix
   - labia
   - fallopian tubes
   - vagina
   - perineum
   - endometrium

2. Describe the stages of the menstrual cycle.

3. Discuss assessment of the gynecological patient.

4. Discuss the recognition and management of pelvic inflammatory disease (PID).

5. Discuss nontraumatic causes of abdominal pain in the female.

6. Discuss the physical and psychological implications of rape and sexual assault and describe prehospital treatment.

CASE STUDY

Unit 38 of Wilmington EMS is dispatched to a local shopping mall. When the paramedics arrive, a mall security guard meets them and takes them to the mall office. There, on the couch, is a morbidly obese female. The patient is in tears and complaining of excruciating lower abdominal pain. The paramedics complete a primary and secondary assessment. The patient's vital signs are stable. Her pulse rate is 100. The tilt test is negative. The pain appears to be in the lower left quadrant, but it is difficult to determine because of the patient's obesity. The paramedics administer oxygen and insert an IV of lactated Ringer's solution. With the help of mall security, they take the patient to the ambulance. She remains stable throughout transport.

In the emergency department, a urine pregnancy test is positive. A pelvic ultrasound examination is carried out, revealing an ectopic pregnancy in the left fallopian tube. The patient is taken to surgery, where her left fallopian tube and the ectopic pregnancy are removed. After the operation, the patient has some respiratory problems as a result of her obesity. She spends 24 hours on the ventilator and is then weaned. She is discharged 5 days later.

INTRODUCTION

■ **gynecology** the branch of medicine that treats disorders of the female reproductive system.

Gynecology is the branch of medicine that deals with the female reproductive tract. Therefore, gynecological emergencies are emergencies that involve the female reproductive tract. Most gynecological emergency patients have either abdominal pain or vaginal bleeding. This chapter discusses the nonpregnant patient. The obstetrical patient is the subject of Chapter 32.

ANATOMY AND PHYSIOLOGY

The female reproductive organs are located entirely within the pelvic cavity, close to the urinary bladder. (See Figure 31-1.) The female reproductive tract consists of the following organs:

❑ *Ovaries.* The ovaries, located at the lateral aspect of the fallopian tubes, are the female gonads. (See Figure 31-2.) Their function is twofold. First, they produce estrogen and progesterone in response to follicle stimulating hormone (FSH) and luteinizing hormone (LH) secreted from the anterior pituitary gland. Second, they produce eggs for reproduction.

❑ *Fallopian Tubes.* The fallopian tubes are hollow tubes that transport the egg from the ovary to the uterus. Fertilization usually occurs in the fallopian tube.

❑ *Uterus.* The uterus is a small, pear-shaped organ that connects with the vagina. The uterus is the organ in which the developing fetus grows. It stretches from a length of about 5 cm, in the nonpregnant state, to a size capable of containing an 8-pound fetus. The upper portion of the uterus is referred to as the *fundus*. The lower portion of the uterus, which extends into the vagina, is referred to as the *cervix*.

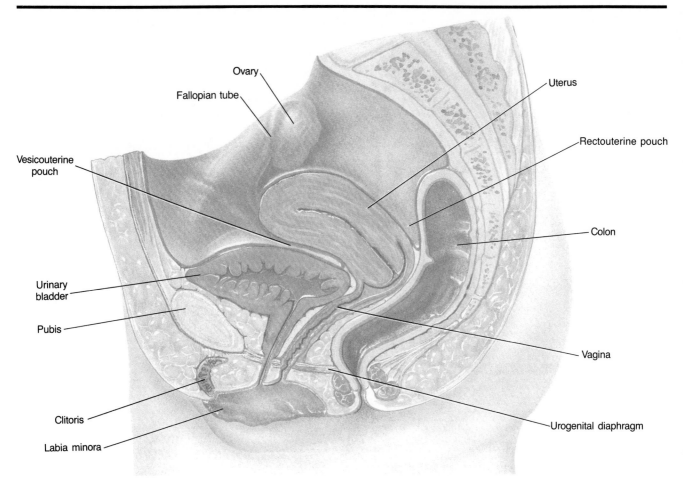

FIGURE 31-1   Cross-sectional anatomy of the female reproductive system.

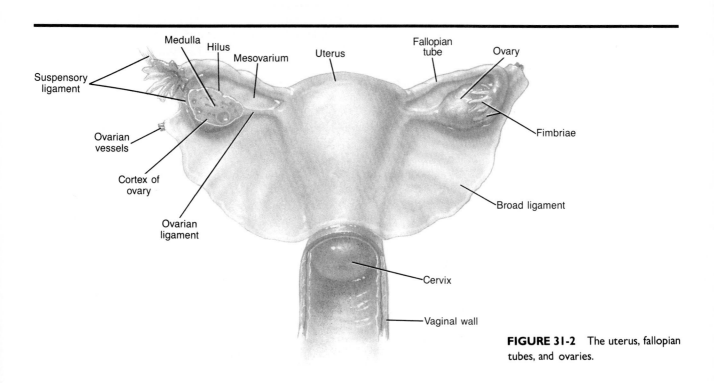

FIGURE 31-2   The uterus, fallopian tubes, and ovaries.

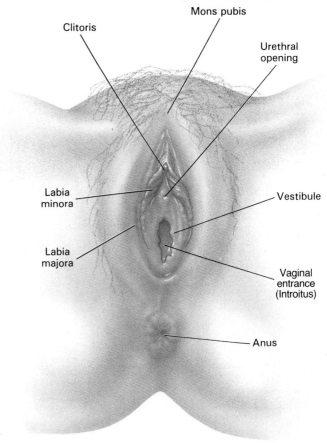

FIGURE 31-3 The vulva.

❏ *Endometrium.* The **endometrium** is the lining of the uterus. Each month, under the influence of estrogen and progesterone, the endometrium is built up in anticipation of implantation of a fertilized ovum. If fertilization does not occur, the lining simply sloughs off. This sloughing off of the uterine lining is referred to as the *menstrual period.*

❏ *Cervix.* The cervix, or "neck" of the uterus, is visible through the vagina. During labor, the cervix dilates from its closed state to a diameter of approximately 10 cm, to allow passage of the baby.

❏ *Vagina.* The vagina is the connection between the uterus and the outside of the body. It is the female sex organ and receives the penis during intercourse.

❏ *Perineum.* The term perineum refers to the area surrounding the vagina and anus. This area is sometimes torn during childbirth.

❏ *Labia.* The labia are the structures that protect the vagina and the urethra. There are two distinct sets of labia. (See Figure 31-3.) The *labia majora* are located laterally. The *labia minora* are more medial. Both sets of labia are subject to injury during trauma to the perineal area, such as occurs with rape.

❏ *Urethra.* The urinary bladder drains through the urethra, which is located superior and anterior to the vagina. In the human female, the urethra is 2–3 cm long. Because the female urethra is so short, the female is more susceptible to bladder infections than the male, since the distance bacteria must travel to cause infection is much less. Females tend to have more frequent bladder infections once they become sexually active.

Menstrual Cycles

The female undergoes a monthly hormonal cycle that prepares the uterus to receive a fertilized egg. A girl's menses, or menstrual periods, usually begin when she is between 12 and 14 years old. The beginning of the menses is termed **menarche.** At first, the periods are irregular. Later they become more regular and predictable.

The menstrual cycle is influenced by estrogen and progesterone, which are produced by the ovaries. In turn, secretion of estrogen and progesterone is controlled by secretion of FSH and LH from the anterior pituitary.

The average menstrual cycle lasts approximately 28 days, although the length varies from one woman to another. What is considered normal is what is normal for the individual woman. Day 1 of the menstrual cycle is the day on which bleeding begins. The menstrual flow usually lasts from 3 to 5 days, and this number also varies from woman to woman.

The first two weeks of the menstrual cycle are dominated by estrogen. Estrogen causes the lining of the uterus to thicken and to become engorged with blood vessels. This is referred to as the *proliferative phase.* At approximately day 14, a sudden surge in LH secretion causes the ovary to release an egg, which matured over the first two weeks of the menstrual cycle. Release of an egg from the ovary is called *ovulation.* The egg is grasped by fine, hairlike structures in the end of the fallopian tube. These structures sweep the egg toward the uterus. If the woman has had sexual intercourse within approximately 24 hours of ovulation, fertilization may take place. If the egg is fertilized, it normally implants in the thickened lining of the uterus, where the fetus subsequently develops. The stage of the menstrual cycle immediately surrounding ovulation is referred to as the *secretory phase.*

If the egg is not fertilized, as normally happens, the woman's estrogen level falls and her uterine lining sloughs away, starting a new menstrual cycle. The interval immediately preceding and including the menstrual period is referred to as the *menstrual phase.* The absence of a menstrual period, especially in a woman whose periods are usually regular and who is sexually active, should raise the suspicion of pregnancy.

Menstrual periods continue to occur until a woman is in her forties or fifties. At that time, they begin to decline in frequency and length, until they ultimately stop. This stoppage of the menstrual cycle is referred to as **menopause.** Occasionally, physicians use the term *surgical menopause,* which means that a woman's periods have stopped because of surgical removal of her uterus, ovaries, or both.

ASSESSMENT OF THE GYNECOLOGICAL PATIENT

Assessment of the gynecological patient should include the standard primary and secondary assessment described earlier in this text. In addition, the paramedic should ask specific questions about the patient's history. Most gynecological patients have lower abdominal pain or discomfort, or vaginal bleeding. If pain is present, it is important to determine its character. Is it sharp or dull? How did the pain start—suddenly or gradually? How long has the pain lasted? Is it persistent or intermittent? Where is the pain located? Does it radiate anywhere? Is there anything that makes the pain better or worse?

Determine if the patient has other medical problems, such as a bladder infection or kidney stones. Quickly gather the obstetric history: The patient should be able relate the number of times she has been pregnant, or her *gravidity*, and the number of pregnancies that have produced a viable infant, or her *parity*. Also question the patient about previous cesarean sections, pelvic surgeries, and dilation and curettage (D&C) procedures.

It is important to document the date of the patient's last menstrual period, commonly abbreviated LMP. Ask whether the period was of a normal length, and if the flow was heavier or lighter than usual. An easy way for a women to estimate menstrual flow is by the number of pads or tampons used. She can easily compare this number to her routine usage. It is also important to inquire how regular the patient's periods tend to be. Ask the patient what form of birth control, if any, she uses, and if she uses it regularly.

With the exception of oral contraceptives ("the pill") and intrauterine devices (IUD), side-effects caused by contraceptives are relatively rare. Oral contraceptives have been associated with hypertension, rare incidents of stroke and heart attack, and possibly pulmonary embolism. IUDs can cause perforation of the uterus, uterine infection, or irregular uterine bleeding. This is especially true for IUDs that have been allowed to remain in place longer than recommended by the manufacturer, generally no more than 2 years.

Any missed or late period should be assumed to be due to pregnancy until proven otherwise. If pregnancy is suspected, inquire about other signs, including breast tenderness, bloating, urinary frequency, or nausea and vomiting. Question the patient about the presence or absence of vaginal discharge. It is helpful to ascertain the color of the discharge and whether there is any associated odor or blood. Also ask the patient about any prior history of trauma to the reproductive tract. Occasionally it is helpful to ascertain whether the patient, if sexually active, has had pain or bleeding during or after sexual intercourse.

In addition to gynecological symptoms, ask the patient about other associated symptoms, such as fever, chills, syncope, diaphoresis, diarrhea, or constipation.

It is important to remember that patients with gynecological complaints may be embarrassed or frightened about discussing these problems. Assess the patient's emotional state. If a patient does not care to discuss her complaint in detail, respect her wishes and transport her to the emergency department, where a more detailed assessment can be completed.

Physical examination of the gynecological patient is limited in the field. Primary and secondary assessment should be completed. Pay particular attention to the abdominal examination. Document and report any masses, distention, guarding, or tenderness. If significant bleeding is reported or evident, it may be necessary to inspect the patient's perineum. Document the character of the discharge, including color, amount, and the presence or absence of clots. DO NOT PERFORM AN INTERNAL VAGINAL EXAM IN THE FIELD.

* In the female patient of childbearing age always document the LMP.

* Do not perform an internal vaginal exam in the field.

GYNECOLOGICAL EMERGENCIES

Gynecological emergencies can be generally divided into two categories, medical and traumatic. Gynecological emergencies of a medical nature are often hard to diagnose in the field. Probably the most common cause of nontraumatic abdominal pain is pelvic inflammatory disease (PID).

Pelvic Inflammatory Disease

Pelvic inflammatory disease is an infection of the female reproductive tract. The organs most commonly involved are the uterus, fallopian tubes, and ovaries. Occasionally, the adjoining structures, such as the peritoneum and intestines, also become involved. The most common causes of PID are gonorrhea and chlamydial infections. In addition, other bacteria, such as staph or strep, can be causative agents. Commonly, gonorrhea or chlamydia progresses undetected in a female until frank PID develops.

PID may be either acute or chronic and, if it is allowed to progress untreated, sepsis may develop. In addition, PID may cause the pelvic organs to "stick together," causing adhesions. Adhesions are a common cause of chronic pelvic pain and cause an increase in the frequency of ectopic pregnancies.

Assessment of the Patient With PID.   The most common complaint of patients with PID is abdominal pain. It is often diffuse and located along the lower abdomen. It may be moderate to severe, which occasionally makes it difficult to distinguish from appendicitis. It may occur with increased intensity either before or after the menstrual period. Often it is made worse by sexual intercourse, as movement of the cervix tends to cause discomfort.

In severe cases, PID may be accompanied by fever, chills, nausea, and vomiting. Occasionally, patients have an associated vaginal discharge, often yellow in color, as well as irregular menses.

Generally, on physical examination, the patient with PID appears acutely ill or toxic. The blood pressure is normal, although the pulse rate may be slightly increased. Fever may or may not be present. Palpation of the lower abdomen generally elicits moderate to severe pain. Occasionally, in severe cases, the abdomen will be tense with obvious rebound tenderness. Such cases may be impossible to distinguish from appendicitis.

Emergency Management of the Patient With PID.   The primary treatment for PID is antibiotics, often administered intravenously over an extended period. In the field, the primary goal is to make the patient as comfortable as possible. Generally, the abdominal pain of PID increases when the patient is walking. The patient should be placed on the ambulance stretcher in the position in which she is most comfortable. She may wish to draw her knees up toward her chest, as this decreases tension on the peritoneum. DO NOT PERFORM A VAGINAL EXAMINATION.

Other Nontramatic Causes of Gynecological Abdominal Pain

Ectopic Pregnancy.   Many different problems with the female reproductive system can cause abdominal pain. One problem that is important for emergency department personnel to rule out is ectopic pregnancy. *Ectopic pregnancy* is the implantation of a growing fetus in a place where it does not belong. The most common site is within the fallopian tubes. This

■ **ectopic pregnancy** the implantation of a developing fetus outside of the uterus, often in a fallopian tube.

✳ Ectopic pregnancy is life-threatening.

is a surgical emergency, because the tube can rupture and massive hemorrhage can occur. Patients with ectopic pregnancy often have one-sided abdominal pain, a late or missed menstrual period, and, occasionally, vaginal bleeding.

Ovarian Cysts.   *Cysts* are fluid-filled pockets. When they develop in the ovary, they can rupture and be a source of abdominal pain. When an egg is released from the ovary, a cyst is often left in its place. Occasionally, cysts develop independent of ovulation.

Appendicitis.   As mentioned previously, appendicitis is very difficult to distinguish from PID or even ectopic pregnancy in the field. Patients with appendicitis usually have abdominal pain that begins around the navel and slowly migrates to the right lower quadrant. The pain may be associated with anorexia, fever, nausea and vomiting, or even shock.

Cystitis.   Bladder infection, or *cystitis,* is a common cause of abdominal pain. The bladder lies anterior to the reproductive organs and, when inflamed, causes pain, generally immediately above the symphysis pubis.

Other Pelvic Infections.   Women who have recently had gynecological surgeries, induced abortions, or miscarriages, or who have recently had babies, can subsequently develop pelvic infections. These infections often present in a manner similar to PID. Therefore, it is important to determine if a woman has recently had any gynecological surgical procedures. An occasional complication of childbirth or gynecological procedures is an infection of the uterine lining. This disorder, *endometritis,* can be quite serious if not quickly treated.

Mittleschmertz.   Occasionally, a woman has a day or two of abdominal pain halfway through her menstrual cycle. The pain, referred to as *mittleschmertz,* is associated with release of the egg from the ovary. The pain is usually self-limited, and treatment is symptomatic.

Management of Patients With Abdominal Pain

Any woman with significant abdominal pain should be treated and transported to the hospital. Administer oxygen, if indicated. Establish an IV with lactated Ringer's or a similar solution, since rupture of an ectopic pregnancy can cause significant, rapid blood loss into the abdomen.

Traumatic Gynecological Emergencies

Most cases of vaginal bleeding result from obstetrical problems or are related to the menstrual period. However, trauma to the vagina and perineum can cause bleeding. Causes of such trauma include straddle injuries (such as may occur with a bicycle), blows to the perineal area, foreign bodies inserted into the vagina, attempts at abortion, lacerations following childbirth, and sexual assault.

Injuries to the external genitalia should be managed by simple pressure over the laceration. In most cases of vaginal bleeding, the source is not readily apparent. If bleeding is severe, start an IV of lactated Ringer's solution in order to maintain intravascular volume. Monitor the patient's vital signs closely. If required, apply antishock trousers. NEVER pack the vagina with any material or dressing, regardless of the severity of the bleeding. Transport the patient to the emergency department rapidly.

Sexual Assault.   Sexual assault is one of the fastest growing crimes in the United States. Unfortunately, it is estimated that more than 60 percent of all sexual assaults are never reported to authorities. Sexual abuse of children is reported even less frequently. There is no "typical victim" of sexual assault. Nobody, from small children to aged adults, is immune.

Sexual assault is sexual contact without the consent of the person assaulted. Definitions may vary from state to state, but as a rule, *rape* is defined as penetration of the vagina of an unwilling female by a male, or of the rectum in a male. In most states, penetration must occur for an act to be classified as rape. Regardless of the legal definition, sexual assault is a crime of violence with serious physical and psychological implications.

Most victims of sexual assault know their assailants. The motivation of the rapist is often unclear. However, humiliation, control of the victim, the desire to inflict pain, or frank aggression, have been implicated as motives.

✱ Psychological and emotional support should be afforded the sexual assault victim.

Assessment of the Victim of Sexual Assault.   Most victims of sexual abuse are female. However, males are not immune, especially male children. As a rule, victims of sexual abuse SHOULD NOT be questioned about the incident in the field. It is not important, from the standpoint of prehospital care, to determine whether penetration took place. Do not inquire about the patient's sexual practices. Even well-intentioned questions may lead to guilt feelings in the patient.

The victim of sexual assault may be withdrawn or hysterical. Some victims use denial, anger, or fear as defense mechanisms. The victim should be approached calmly and professionally. If he or she is incompletely dressed, a cover should be offered. Respect the victim's modesty. Explain all procedures before beginning them. Avoid touching the patient other than to take vital signs or examine other physical injuries. DO NOT examine the genitalia unless there is life-threatening hemorrhage.

Management of the Sexual Assault Patient.   Psychological and emotional support is the most important help the paramedic can offer. Maintain a nonjudgmental attitude and assure the victim of confidentiality. If the victim is female, allow her to be cared for by a female EMT or paramedic (if available), or, if she desires, have a female accompany her to the hospital. (See Figure 31-4.)

Provide a safe environment, such as the back of a well-lit ambulance. Respond to the victim's feelings and respect his or her wishes. Unless the victim has life-threatening injuries, verbally obtain permission to treat before you begin your assessment.

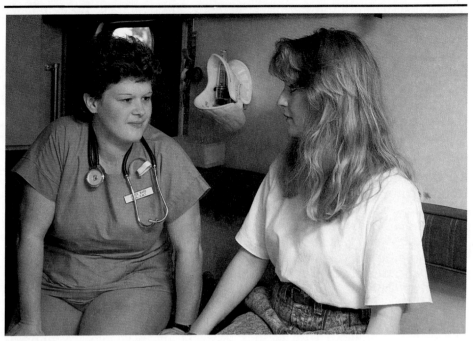

FIGURE 31-4 If possible, have a female EMT or paramedic accompany the victim of alleged sexual assault to the hospital.

Preservation of physical evidence is important. When the patient arrives at the hospital, a physician will complete a sexual assault examination. At that time, various legal physical evidence will be gathered. To protect this evidence, it is important that the paramedic follow these guidelines:

- ❏ Handle clothing as little as possible, if at all.
- ❏ Do not examine the perineal area.
- ❏ Do not use plastic bags for blood-stained articles.
- ❏ Bag each item separately, if they must be bagged.
- ❏ Do not allow the patient to comb her hair or clean her fingernails.
- ❏ Do not allow the patient to change her clothes, bathe, or douche before the medical examination.
- ❏ Do not clean wounds if at all possible.

SUMMARY

Most gynecological emergency patients have either abdominal pain or vaginal bleeding. The patient with abdominal pain should be made comfortable and transported to the emergency department. The management of vaginal bleeding depends on the severity. Minor bleeding should be simply monitored. Severe bleeding should be treated with IV fluids or antishock trousers, if indicated.

For the victim of sexual assault, the paramedic should first be concerned about life-threatening physical injuries. The second most important aspect of management is emotional support. Another important role of the paramedic in treating victims of sexual assault is preservation of physical evidence. As with any type of emergency care, the primary concern is the patient.

FURTHER READING

LANROS, NEDELL E., *Assessment and Intervention in Emergency Nursing, Third Edition.* Norwalk, CT: Appleton and Lange, 1988.

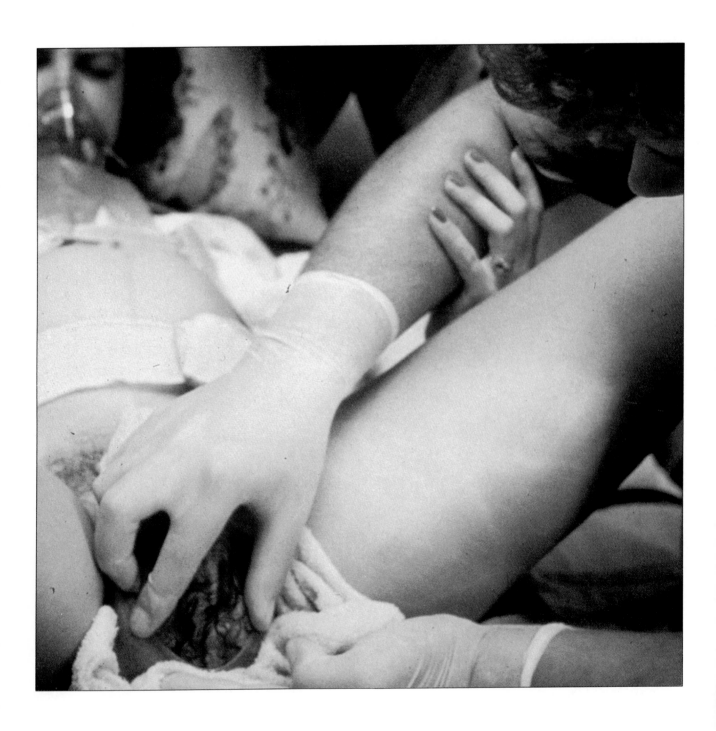

32

Obstetrical Emergencies

Objectives for Chapter 32

Upon completing this chapter, the student should be able to:

1. Identify the normal sites of fertilization and implantation of the fertilized egg.

2. Describe fetal-maternal blood flow and the role of the placenta.

3. Define the following terms:
- antepartum
- natal
- primigravida
- multigravida
- postpartum
- prenatal
- primipara
- multipara

4. Identify the details of the history that should be obtained from an obstetrical patient.

5. Discuss the effects of pregnancy on preexisting conditions such as diabetes, hypertension, and cardiac problems.

6. Define the following:
- spontaneous abortion
- criminal abortion
- therapeutic abortion

7. Describe the management of the patient who has suffered abortion.

8. Describe the pathophysiology and management of:
- ectopic pregnancy
- abruptio placentae
- placenta previa

9. Describe the pathophysiology and prehospital management of the hypertensive disorders of pregnancy.

10. Distinguish between pregnancy-induced hypertension, preeclampsia, and eclampsia.

11. Describe the stages of labor and the length of each stage.

12. List and describe the steps of a normal delivery.

13. Describe the management, during delivery, of a cord that becomes wrapped around the baby's neck.

14. Describe the pathophysiology and management of:
- prolapsed cord
- uterine inversion
- uterine rupture

15. Describe the management of a multiple-birth delivery.

16. Describe the management of a breech presentation.

17. Describe the pathophysiology and management of postpartum hemorrhage.

The members of Fire Station Crew 29 were in the television room when they heard an automobile speed up to the door of the station. The captain looked out and saw an old station wagon parked out front. Beside it was a man yelling, "Help! My wife needs help!"

The whole crew went to help. In the back seat of the station wagon was a pregnant 29-year-old white female. She kept saying, "The baby is coming, the baby is coming!" The ambulance normally based at Station 29 had gone out for gas. The captain notified fire dispatch, and the ambulance was dispatched to return. Meanwhile, the EMTs on the engine determined that this was the patient's sixth pregnancy and that she felt as though she had to move her bowels.

The patient's screams now changed to, "I've got to push, I've got to push." The EMTs checked for crowning. The top of the baby's head could be seen. A pair of gloves and bulb suction were retrieved from the medic box on the engine. Shortly, in the station wagon, the patient delivered a female infant.

At about the time of delivery, the paramedics arrived. They helped the EMT cut the cord and wrap the baby. Apgar scores were 8 at 1 minute and 9 at 5 minutes. The mother received fundal massage, oxygen, and an IV of lactated Ringer's solution. Both mother and daughter were transported to the hospital without incident. The next morning, as the Station 29 crew members were walking to their cars, they saw a stork artfully painted on the window of the car belonging to the EMT who had delivered the baby.

INTRODUCTION

This chapter will address pregnancy and childbirth and the complications associated with them. It is important to remember that childbirth is a natural process and occurs daily. Complications are uncommon, but when they occur, they must be recognized rapidly and managed accordingly.

THE PRENATAL PERIOD

Anatomy and Physiology of the Obstetric Patient

■ **ovulation** the growth and discharge of an egg from the ovary.

Pregnancy is a normal event. It begins with ovulation in the female. **Ovulation** is the growth and discharge of an egg, or *ovum*, from the ovary. The ovum develops under the influence of the hormones estrogen and progesterone. Fourteen days before the beginning of the next menstrual period, the ovum is released from the ovary into the abdominal cavity. It then enters the wide opening of the fallopian tube, where it is transported to the uterus.

If the woman has had intercourse within 24 to 48 hours before ovulation, fertilization may occur in the fallopian tube. *Fertilization* is the combination of the female ovum and the male spermatozoa. (See Figure 32-1.) After fertilization, the ovum begins to divide immediately. The fertilized ovum continues down the fallopian tube to the uterus, where it ultimately

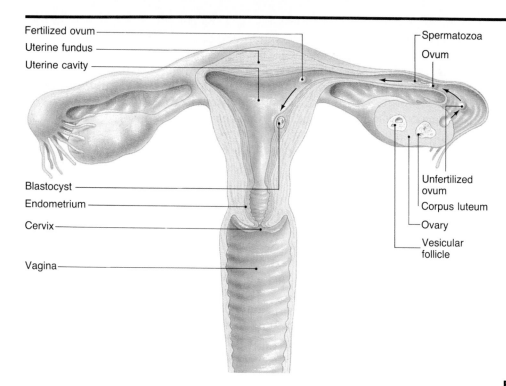

FIGURE 32-1   Fertilization and implantation of the ovum.

attaches itself to the inner lining of the uterus. This process is called *implantation.*

Early in pregnancy, the **placenta** develops. (See Figure 32-2.) The placenta has several important functions for the developing fetus. It provides for the exchange of respiratory gases, transport of nutrients from the mother to the fetus, excretion of wastes, and transfer of heat. In addition, the placenta becomes an active endocrine gland, producing several important hormones.

The placenta is attached to the developing fetus by the **umbilical cord.** This cord normally contains two arteries and one vein. The umbili-

■ **placenta** the organ that supports the fetus during intrauterine development. The placenta is attached to the wall of the uterus and to the umbilical cord.

■ **umbilical cord** structure, containing 2 arteries and 1 vein, which connects the placenta and the fetus.

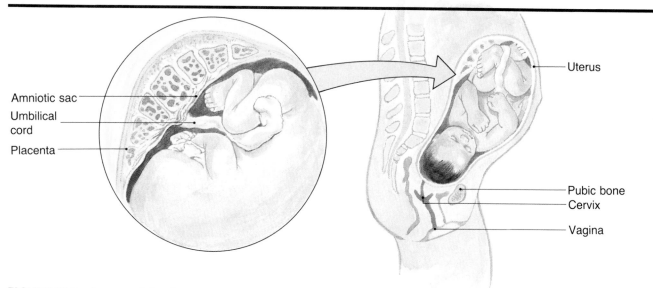

FIGURE 32-2   Anatomy of the placenta.

cal vein transports oxygenated blood toward the fetus, while the umbilical arteries return relatively deoxygenated blood to the placenta.

The **amniotic sac** also develops early in pregnancy. The amniotic sac consists of membranes that surround and protect the developing fetus throughout intrauterine development. Eventually, the amniotic sac will fill with **amniotic fluid,** which cushions the fetus against trauma and provides a stable environment in which the fetus can develop. The volume of amniotic fluid, approximately 1,000 mL, is maintained by the fetus's continual swallowing of fluid as well as continual urination.

Fetal Development.   Fetal development begins immediately after implantation and is quite complex. There are a few developmental milestones that paramedics should be familiar with. First, the normal duration of pregnancy is 40 weeks from the first day of the mother's last menstrual period. This is equal to 10 lunar months or, roughly, 9 calendar months. The time at which fertilization occurs is called *conception*. Conception occurs approximately 14 days after the first day of the last menstrual period. With this knowledge, it is possible to calculate, with fair accuracy, the approximate date the baby should be born. This date is commonly called the due date, or, medically, the **estimated date of confinement (EDC).** The mother is usually told this date on her first prenatal visit.

During normal fetal development, the sex of the infant can usually be determined by the end of the third month. By the end of the fifth month, *fetal heart tones (FHTs)* can be detected by stethoscope, and the mother generally has felt fetal movement. By the end of the sixth month, the baby may be capable of surviving if born prematurely. Fetuses born after the end of the seventh month have an excellent chance of survival. By the middle of the tenth month the baby is considered *term,* or fully developed. (See Figure 32-3.)

Generally, pregnancy is divided into *trimesters*. Each trimester is approximately 13 weeks, or 3 calendar months. Most of the fetus's organ systems develop during the first trimester. Therefore, this is when the fetus is most vulnerable to the development of birth defects.

■ **amniotic sac** the membranes that surround and protect the developing fetus throughout intrauterine development.

■ **amniotic fluid** clear, watery fluid which surrounds and protects the developing fetus.

■ **estimated date of confinement (EDC)** the approximate day the child will be born. This date is usually based on the date of the mother's last menstrual period (LMP).

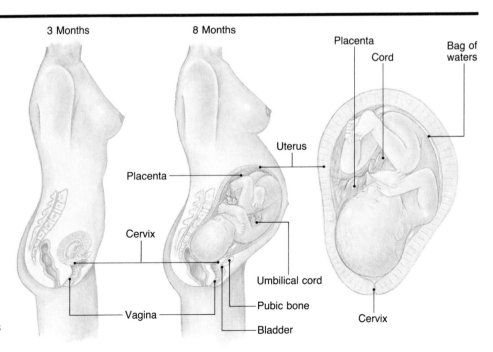

FIGURE 32-3 Uterine changes associated with pregnancy.

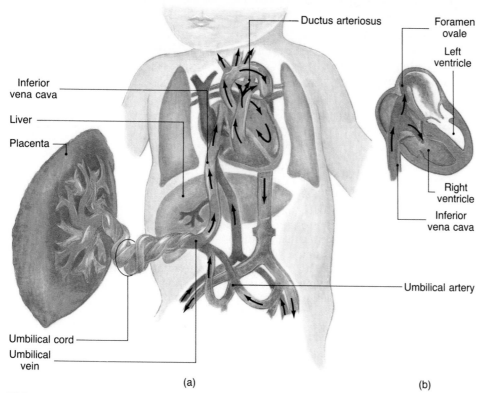

Labels in figure:
- Ductus arteriosus
- Foramen ovale
- Left ventricle
- Inferior vena cava
- Liver
- Placenta
- Right ventricle
- Inferior vena cava
- Umbilical artery
- Umbilical cord
- Umbilical vein

(a)   (b)

FIGURE 32-4   The maternal-fetal circulation.

Fetal Circulation.   The fetus receives its oxygen and nutrients from its mother through the placenta. Thus, while in the uterus, the fetus does not need to use its respiratory system or its gastrointestinal tract. Because of this, the fetal circulation shunts blood around the lungs and gastrointestinal tract.

The infant receives its blood, from the placenta, by means of the umbilical vein. (See Figure 32-4.) The umbilical vein connects directly to the inferior vena cava by a specialized structure called the *ductus venosus.* Blood then travels through the inferior vena cava to the heart. The blood enters the right atrium and passes through the tricuspid valve into the right ventricle. It then exits the right ventricle, through the pulmonic valve, into the pulmonary artery. The fetus's heart has a hole between the right and left atria, termed the *foramen ovale,* which allows mixing of the oxygenated blood in the right atrium with that leaving the left ventricle bound for the aorta.

At this time, the blood is still oxygenated. Once in the pulmonary artery, the blood enters the *ductus arteriosus,* which connects the pulmonary artery with the aorta. The ductus arteriosus causes blood to bypass the lungs. Once in the aorta, blood flow is basically the same as in extrauterine life. Deoxygenated blood containing waste products exits the fetus, after passage through the liver, via the umbilical arteries.

The fetal circulation changes immediately at birth. As soon as the baby takes his or her first breath, the ambient pressure in the lungs decreases dramatically. Because of this pressure change, the ductus arteriosus closes, diverting blood to the lungs. In addition, the ductus venosus closes, stopping blood flow from the placenta. The foramen ovale also closes as a result of pressure changes in the heart which stop blood flow from the right to left atrium.

Obstetric Terminology

The field of obstetrics has its own unique terminology. The paramedic should be familiar with this terminology, as patient documentation and communications with other health care workers, and physicians, often requires it. (See Table 32-1.)

TABLE 32-1 Common Obstetrical Terminology

Term	Meaning
antepartum	the time interval prior to delivery of the fetus
postpartum	the time interval after delivery of the fetus
prenatal	the time interval prior to birth, synonymous with antepartum
natal	literally means birth
gravidity	the number of times a woman has been pregnant
primigravida	a woman who is pregnant for the first time
multigravida	a woman who has been pregnant more than once
nulligravida	a woman who has not been pregnant
parity	the number of times a woman has delivered a viable fetus
primipara	a woman who has delivered her first child
multipara	a woman who has delivered more than one baby
nullipara	a woman who has yet to deliver her first child
grand multiparity	a woman who has delivered at least seven babies

The gravidity and parity of a woman is expressed in the following convention: $G_4 P_2$. "G" refers to the gravidity and "P" refers to the parity.

Assessment of the Obstetrical Patient

The initial approach to the obstetrical patient should be the same as for the nonobstetrical patient, with special attention paid to the developing fetus. Complete the primary and secondary survey quickly. Next, obtain essential obstetric information.

When treating an obstetric patient, obtain information related to the pregnancy, such as the mother's gravidity and parity, the length of gestation, and the estimated date of confinement (EDC), if known. In addition, you should determine whether the patient has had any cesarean sections or any gynecological or obstetrical complications in the past. It is also important to determine whether the patient has had any prenatal care.

If the patient is in pain, try to determine when the pain started and whether its onset was sudden or slow. Also, attempt to determine the character of the pain: its duration, location, and radiation, if any. It is especially important to determine whether the pain is regular.

The presence of vaginal bleeding or spotting is a major concern in an obstetrical patient. In addition, question the patient about the presence of other vaginal discharges.

A general overview of the patient's current state of health is important. Pay particular attention to current medications and drug or medication allergies.

Pregnancy should be highly suspect in a patient who has missed a menstrual period or whose period is late. If she is unsure if she is pregnant, the patient should be questioned about breast tenderness, urinary frequency, and nausea and vomiting. If pregnancy has been confirmed, then specific questions about **prenatal** care are important. Ask the patient whether a sonogram examination was carried out and what it revealed. A sonogram reveals the age of the fetus, the presence of more than one fetus, abnormal presentations, and certain birth defects.

■ **prenatal** means essentially the same thing as "antepartum" and refers to the time period before birth. Health care visits during pregnancy are referred to as "prenatal visits" or "prenatal care."

When confronted with a patient in active labor, the paramedic should assess whether she feels the need to push or has the urge to move her bowels. Determine whether the patient thinks her membranes have ruptured. Patients often sense this as a dribbling of water or, in some cases, a true gush of water.

Physical Examination of the Obstetric Patient.   Physical examination of the obstetric patient is essentially the same as for any emergency patient. However, the paramedic should first estimate the date of the pregnancy by measuring the fundal height. The *fundal height* is the distance from the symphysis pubis to the top of uterine fundus. Each centimeter of fundal height roughly corresponds to a week of gestation. For example, a woman with a fundal height of 24 cm has a gestational age of approximately 24 weeks. If the fundus is just palpable above the symphysis pubis, the pregnancy is about 12–16 weeks gestation. When the uterine fundus reaches the umbilicus, the pregnancy is about 20 weeks. As pregnancy nears term, the fundus is palpable near the xiphoid process.

If fetal movement is felt when the abdomen is palpated, the pregnancy is at least 20 weeks. Fetal heart tones can be heard by stethoscope at approximately 18–20 weeks. The normal fetal heart rate ranges from 140–160 beats per minute.

Generally, vital signs in the pregnant patient should be taken with the patient lying on her left side. As pregnancy progresses, the uterus increases in size. Ultimately, when the patient is supine, the weight of the uterus compresses the inferior vena cava, severely compromising venous blood return from the lower extremities. Turning the patient to her left side alleviates this problem.

Occasionally, it may be helpful to perform orthostatic vital signs. First, the blood pressure and pulse rate are obtained after the patient has rested for five minutes in the left lateral recumbent position. Then the vital signs are repeated with the patient sitting up or standing. A drop in the blood pressure level of 15 mm/Hg or more, or an increase in the pulse rate of 20 beats per minute or more, is considered significant and should be reported and documented. When performing this maneuver, it is always important to be alert for syncope. Also, this procedure should not be performed if the patient is in obvious shock.

The patient should be examined for the presence of a *prolapsed cord,* an umbilical cord that comes out of the uterus ahead of the fetus. This can be accomplished simply by looking at the perineum. If, during the physical examination, the patient reports that she feels the need to push, or if she feels as though she must move her bowels, she should be examined for crowning. **Crowning** is the bulging of the fetal head past the opening of the vagina during a contraction. Crowning is an indication of impending delivery. The patient should be examined for crowning only during a contraction. DO NOT CARRY OUT AN INTERNAL VAGINAL EXAMINATION IN THE FIELD.

■ **crowning** the bulging of the fetal head past the opening of the vagina during a contraction. Crowning is an indication of impending delivery.

Complications of Pregnancy

Pregnancy is a normal process. However, persons who are pregnant are not immune from other health problems. Several factors, including trauma and preexisting health problems, complicate pregnancy.

Trauma.   Paramedics are frequently called to render aid to a pregnant woman who has been in a motor vehicle accident or who has sustained a fall. In pregnancy, syncope occurs frequently. The syncope of pregnancy often results from compression of the inferior vena cava, as described above, or from normal changes in the cardiovascular system associated with pregnancy. Also, the weight of the gravid uterus alters the patient's balance, making her more susceptible to falls.

Pregnant victims of major trauma are more susceptible to life-threatening injury than are nonpregnant victims, because of the increased vascularity of the gravid uterus. Generally, the amniotic fluid cushions the fetus from blunt trauma fairly well. However, in direct abdominal trauma, the pregnant patient may suffer premature separation of the placenta from the uterine wall, premature labor, abortion, uterine rupture, and possibly, fetal death. Fetal death may result from death of the mother, separation of the placenta from the uterine wall, maternal shock, uterine rupture, or fetal head injury. Any pregnant patient who has suffered trauma should be immediately transported to the emergency department and evaluated by a physician.

Medical Conditions in Pregnancy. The pregnant patient is subject to all the medical problems that occur in the nonpregnant state. Abdominal pain is a common complaint. It is often caused by the stretching of the ligaments that support the uterus. However, appendicitis and cholecystitis can also occur. In pregnancy, the abdominal organs are displaced because of the increased mass in the abdomen of the gravid uterus. The pregnant patient with appendicitis may complain of right upper quadrant pain, or even back pain. The symptoms of acute cholecystitis may also differ from those in nonpregnant patients. Any pregnant patient with abdominal pain should be evaluated by a physician.

Pregnancy aggravates many medical conditions. One of the most common is diabetes mellitus. Previously diagnosed diabetes can become unstable during pregnancy. Also, many patients develop diabetes during pregnancy (*gestational diabetes*). Pregnant diabetics cannot be managed with oral drugs, since these tend to cross the placenta and affect the fetus. Therefore, all pregnant diabetics are placed on insulin if their blood sugar levels cannot be controlled by diet alone.

Diabetes also affects the infant. Infants of diabetic mothers, especially those with poorly controlled blood sugar levels, tend to be large. This complicates delivery. Such infants also may have trouble maintaining body temperature after birth and may be subject to hypoglycemia.

Hypertension is also aggravated by pregnancy. Generally, blood pressure is lower in pregnancy than in the nonpregnant state. However, women who were borderline hypertensive before becoming pregnant may become dangerously hypertensive when pregnant. Also, many common blood pressure medications cannot be used during pregnancy. In addition, preeclampsia (discussed later in this chapter) may contribute to maternal hypertension. Persistent hypertension may adversely affect the placenta, thus compromising the fetus as well as placing the mother at increased risk for stroke or renal failure.

During pregnancy, cardiac output increases up to 30 percent. (See Figure 32-5.) Patients who have serious preexisting heart disease may develop congestive heart failure in pregnancy. When confronted by a pregnant patient in obvious heart failure, the paramedic should inquire about preexisting heart disease or murmurs. It is important to be aware, however, that most patients develop a quiet systolic flow murmur during pregnancy. This is caused by increased cardiac output and should be documented on the chart. It is rarely a source of concern.

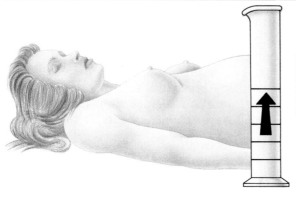

Blood volume usually increases by about 45%. Dilution resulting from the disproportionate increase of plasma volume over the red cell mass is responsible for the so-called "anemia of pregnancy."

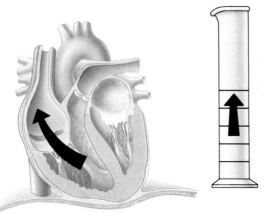

Cardiac output increases by 1.0 to 1.5 L/min during the 1st trimester, reaches 6 to 7 L/min by the late 2nd trimester, and is maintained essentially at this level until delivery.

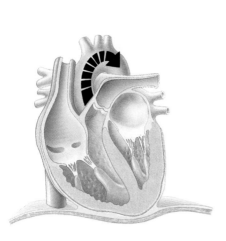

The stroke volume progressively declines to term following a rise early in pregnacy. Heart rate, however, increases by an average of 10 to 15 beats/min.

FIGURE 32-5 The hemodynamic changes of pregnancy

Vaginal Bleeding During Pregnancy. Vaginal bleeding during pregnancy is always a cause for concern. Bleeding in early pregnancy is often caused by spontaneous abortion, ectopic pregnancy, or vaginal trauma. Bleeding in the third trimester is usually caused by abruptio placentae, placenta previa, or trauma to the vagina or cervix. Bleeding can range from simple spotting to life-threatening hemorrhage. Generally, the exact etiology of vaginal bleeding during pregnancy cannot be determined in the field.

Abortion. **Abortion** is the termination of a pregnancy before the fetus is viable, generally considered to be about 20 weeks gestation. The terms "abortion" and "miscarriage" can be used interchangeably. Generally, people think of abortion as termination of pregnancy at maternal request and of miscarriage as an accident of nature. Medically, the term "abortion" refers to both types of fetal loss. Approximately 15 percent of pregnancies result in abortion. Often, abortion results from defects in the fetus or maternal infection. The several classifications of abortion include:

❑ *Spontaneous Abortion.* A spontaneous abortion, commonly called a *miscarriage,* occurs of its own accord. Most spontaneous abortions occur before the twelfth week of pregnancy. Many occur within two weeks after conception and are mistaken for menstrual periods.

❑ *Threatened Abortion.* A threatened abortion is a pregnancy in which the cervix is slightly open and the fetus remains in the uterus and is still alive. In some cases of threatened abortion, the pregnancy can be salvaged.

❑ *Inevitable Abortion.* An inevitable abortion is one in which the fetus has not yet passed from the uterus, but the pregnancy cannot be salvaged.

❑ *Incomplete Abortion.* An incomplete abortion is one in which some, but not all, fetal tissue has been passed. Incomplete abortions are associated with a high incidence of infection.

❑ *Criminal Abortion.* A criminal abortion is an attempt to destroy a fetus by a person who is not licensed or permitted to do so. Criminal abortions are often attempted by amateurs and are rarely done in aseptic surroundings.

❑ *Therapeutic Abortion.* A therapeutic abortion is an abortion in which the pregnancy posed a threat to the mother's health and abortion was judged to be medically indicated.

❑ *Elective Abortion.* An elective abortion is one in which the termination of pregnancy is desired and requested by the mother. Elective abortions during the first and second trimesters of pregnancy have been legal in the United States since 1973. Most elective abortions are performed during the first trimester of pregnancy. However, some clinics perform second-trimester abortions. Second-trimester abortions have a higher complication rate than first-trimester abortions. Third-trimester abortions are generally illegal in this country.

Assessment. Most women who are having abortions have vaginal bleeding. Often, women who have first-trimester miscarriages report passing tissue or excessive clotting. In late first-trimester and second-trimester abortions, a recognizable fetus may be passed. In addition, there will often be significant abdominal cramping and pain. If the abortion was not recent, then frank signs and symptoms of infection may be present.

The physical examination should include orthostatic vital signs, if possible. Examine the external genitalia to determine how much bleeding or tissue is present. Any tissue or large clots should be retained and given to emergency department personnel.

✱ Treat the patient suffering miscarriage as you would any patient at risk for shock.

Management of the Patient Suffering Abortion. The abortion patient should be treated in the same manner as any patient at risk for hypovolemic shock. Administer oxygen and establish an IV of normal saline or lactated Ringer's solution to restore lost fluid volume. If the patient is bleeding severely and shock is impending, establish a second IV and apply antishock trousers.

As mentioned above, any tissue or large clots should be retained and given to emergency department personnel. If the abortion occurs during the late first trimester or later, a fetus may be passed. Often, the placenta does not detach, and the fetus is suspended by the umbilical cord. In such a case, place the umbilical clamps from the OB kit on the cord and cut the cord. Wrap the fetus in linen or other suitable material and transport it to the hospital with the mother.

An abortion is generally a very sad time. Provide emotional support to the parents. Parents who wish to view the fetus should be allowed to do so. Occasionally, parents request baptism of the fetus. This can be performed by making the sign of a cross and stating, "I baptize you in the name of the father, the son, and the holy spirit. Amen."

Ectopic Pregnancy. An *ectopic pregnancy,* the implantation of a fertilized ovum outside of the uterus, occurs once in approximately 200 pregnancies. The most common implantation site is in a fallopian tube. However, the ovum can attach to an ovary or anywhere in the abdominal cavity.

✳ Any female of childbearing age with lower abdominal pain is pregnant and has an ectopic pregnancy until proven otherwise.

An ectopic pregnancy is a medical emergency. The developing fetus can grow so large that it may rupture the fallopian tube, causing extensive bleeding into the pelvis and abdominal cavity. Women can die from the complications of ruptured ectopic pregnancies.

Several predisposing factors can lead to ectopic pregnancy. They include previous pelvic infections, such as PID, pelvic adhesions from prior abdominal surgery, tubal ligations, or the presence of an IUD. All of these tend to scar the fallopian tube, thus preventing transport of the fetus to its normal implantation site in the uterus.

Most patients with ectopic pregnancy have abdominal pain, which may be severe; often, there is associated vaginal bleeding. In 15–20 percent of cases women report shoulder pain, which is probably referred pain. Many patients report a missed period or intermittent spotting over 6–8 weeks. Patients often report pregnancy-associated symptoms, such as breast tenderness, nausea, vomiting, or fatigue. Many patients report a prior history of PID, tubal ligation, previous ectopic pregnancy, or pelvic surgeries.

Assessment of the Patient With Ectopic Pregnancy. The patient with ectopic pregnancy is at risk for the rapid development of shock. Take vital signs frequently and regularly. Orthostatic vital signs may be helpful, unless the patient is in frank shock. The abdominal examination may reveal significant lower quadrant tenderness, often more pronounced on one side than the other. Rebound tenderness or rigidity may be present. Avoid repeated abdominal examination, as this may cause the ectopic pregnancy to rupture. Vaginal bleeding may range from spotting to profuse hemorrhage. Do not perform a vaginal examination in the field.

Management of the Patient With Ectopic Pregnancy. Ectopic pregnancy is difficult to diagnose in the field. However, a patient suspected of suffering ectopic pregnancy should be handled like any patient in shock or at risk of hypovolemic shock. The patient should receive high-flow oxygen and ventilatory support as indicated. Start an IV of lactated Ringer's solution or normal saline. Repeat vital signs regularly. If the patient is in shock, apply antishock trousers. Transport should be rapid, as prompt surgical intervention is required.

Third-trimester Bleeding. Third-trimester bleeding should be attributed to placenta previa or abruptio placentae until proven otherwise, although it can be caused by injury to the vagina or cervix. Abruptio placentae and placenta previa are emergencies which threaten both the mother and the fetus. (See Figure 32-6.)

Abruptio Placentae. *Abruptio placentae* is the premature separation of the placenta from the wall of the uterus. Separation can be either partial or complete. Complete separation almost always results in death of the fetus. Several factors may predispose a patient to abruptio placentae. These include preeclampsia, maternal hypertension, **multiparity,** abdominal trauma, or an extremely short umbilical cord.

When abruptio placentae occurs, blood tends to collect behind the separating placenta. As a result, vaginal blood loss is minimal. If the placenta is not completely separated, it may apply pressure on the bleeding uterine wall. If the placenta separates completely, this pressure is lost and severe hemorrhage can occur quite suddenly.

Assessment of the Patient With Abruptio Placentae. Most frequently, patients suffering abruptio placenta have constant, severe abdominal pain. Often the patient says that the pain "feels like something is tearing." The abdomen is very tender. Vaginal bleeding may range from absent to very heavy; if present, bleeding will be very dark. Occasionally, the patient has a history of placental abruption in previous pregnancies.

■ **multiparity** a woman who has delivered more than one baby.

✱ Third trimester bleeding should be attributed to placenta previa or abruptio placentae until proven otherwise.

Abruptio placentae (premature separation)

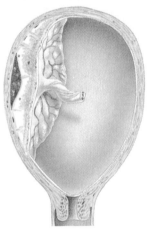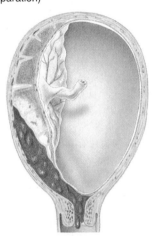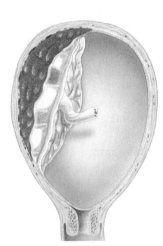

| Partial separation (concealed hemorrhage) | Partial separation (apparent hemorrhage) | Complete separation (concealed hemorrhage) |

Placenta previa (abnormal implantation)

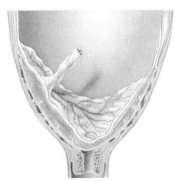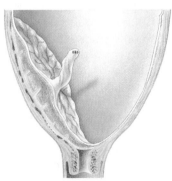

Total placenta previa

Partial placenta previa

FIGURE 32-6 Third trimester bleeding emergencies.

Physical examination will reveal a very tender uterus that may feel tightly contracted. Fetal heart tones may be slow or absent. Do not perform a vaginal examination.

✱ Internal vaginal exams should not be carried out in the prehospital setting.

Management of the Patient With Abruptio Placentae. In abruptio placentae there are two lives at stake. First, administer oxygen at high concentration. The fetus also receives oxygen when it is administered to the mother, unless complete abruption has occurred. Second, establish one or two large-bore IVs with either lactated Ringer's solution or normal saline. Monitor vital signs and fetal heart tones continuously. If shock is impending, apply antishock trousers without inflating the abdominal compartment. Transport the patient rapidly, since definitive treatment is cesarean section, if the fetus is still viable, upon arrival at the emergency department.

Placenta Previa. *Placenta previa* is the attachment of the placenta very low in the uterus so that it partially or completely covers the internal cervical os, or opening. There are three categories of placenta previa: complete, partial, and marginal. *Complete placenta previa* completely covers the internal cervical os and is, fortunately, quite rare. *Partial placenta previa* is partial coverage of the internal cervical os by the placenta. *Marginal placenta previa* occurs when the placenta is adjacent to the cervical os but does not extend over it. Marginal or partial placenta previa occurs in approximately 1 out of every 200 pregnancies. Predisposing factors include multiparity, maternal age greater than 35, and pregnancies in rapid succession.

Implantation of the placenta occurs early in pregnancy. Unless a sonogram is done, placenta previa is usually not detected until the third trimester. At that time, when fetal pressure on the placenta increases, or uterine contractions begin, the cervix **effaces,** or thins out, resulting in placental bleeding. In addition, sexual intercourse or digital vaginal examination can precipitate bleeding from placenta previa.

■ **effacement** the thinning of the cervix during labor.

Assessment of the Patient With Placenta Previa. The patient with placenta previa is usually a multigravida in her third trimester of pregnancy. She may have a history of prior placenta previa or of bleeding early in the current pregnancy. She may report a recent episode of sexual intercourse or vaginal examination just before vaginal bleeding began, or she may not bleed until the onset of labor.

The most common sign of placenta previa is painless, bright red vaginal bleeding. In fact, any painless bleeding in pregnancy is considered placenta previa until proven otherwise. The bleeding may or may not be associated with uterine contractions. The uterus is usually soft, and the fetus may be in an unusual presentation. VAGINAL EXAMINATION SHOULD NEVER BE ATTEMPTED, AS AN EXAMINING FINGER CAN PUNCTURE THE PLACENTA, CAUSING FATAL HEMORRHAGE.

✱ A vaginal examination in a patient with placenta previa can cause a fatal hemorrhage.

Managment of the Patient With Placenta Previa. As with abruptio placentae, there are two lives at stake. Treatment should consist of the following: First, administer oxygen at high concentration. Second, establish one or two large-bore IVs with either lactated Ringer's solution or normal saline. Monitor vital signs and fetal heart tones continuously. If shock is impending, apply antishock trousers without inflating the abdominal compartment. Transport the patient rapidly, since definitive treatment is cesarean section, if the fetus is still viable, upon arrival at the emergency department.

Other Complications of Pregnancy. In addition to the causes of vaginal bleeding described above, there are other complications of pregnancy that the paramedic should be aware of. These include toxemia of pregnancy, the supine-hypotensive syndrome, Braxton-Hicks contractions, and premature labor.

Hypertensive Disorders of Pregnancy. Several pregnancy-associated problems are collectively called *hypertensive disorders of pregnancy* (formerly called "toxemia of pregnancy"). These disorders are characterized by hypertension, weight gain, edema, protein in the urine, and, in late stages, seizures. Hypertensive disorders of pregnancy occur in approximately 5 percent of pregnancies. They are thought to be caused by abnormal vasospasm in the mother, which results in increased blood pressure and other associated symptoms. The hypertensive disorders of pregnancy are generally classified as follows:

❑ *Pregnancy-Induced Hypertension (PIH).* PIH is characterized by a blood pressure of 140/90 level or greater in pregnancy in a patient who was previously normotensive. PIH is the early stage of the disease process. It is important to remember that blood pressure usually drops in pregnancy, and a blood pressure reading of 130/80 may be elevated.

❑ *Preeclampsia.* Preeclamptic patients are those that have hypertension, abnormal weight gain, edema, headache, protein in the urine, epigastric pain, and, occasionally, visual disturbances. If untreated, preeclampsia may progress to the next stage, eclampsia.

✱ Eclampsia is a threat to both the mother's and the baby's life.

❑ *Eclampsia.* Eclampsia is the most serious manifestation of the hypertensive disorders of pregnancy and is characterized by grand mal seizure activity. Eclampsia is often preceded by visual disturbances, such as flashing lights or spots before the eyes. Also, the development of epigastric pain or pain in the right upper abdominal quadrant often indicates impending seizure. Eclampsia can be distinguished from epilepsy by the history and physical appearance of the patient. Patients who become eclamptic are usually edematous and have markedly elevated blood pressure, while epileptics usually have a prior history of seizures and are taking anticonvulsant medications.

The hypertensive disorders of pregnancy tend to occur most often with a woman's first pregnancy. They also appear to occur more frequently in patients with preexisting hypertension. Diabetes mellitus is also associated with an increased incidence of this disease process.

Patients who develop PIH and preeclampsia are at increased risk for cerebral hemorrhage, the development of renal failure, and pulmonary edema. Patients who are preeclamptic have intravascular volume depletion, since a great deal of their body fluid is in the third space. If eclampsia develops, death of the mother and fetus frequently results.

Assessment of the Patient Suffering Hypertensive Disorders of Pregnancy. The history is important when the paramedic encounters a patient suspected of suffering from the hypertensive disorders of pregnancy. Question the patient about excessive weight gain, headaches, visual problems, epigastric or right upper quadrant abdominal pain, apprehension, or seizures.

On physical exam, patients with PIH or preeclampsia are usually markedly edematous. They are often pale and apprehensive. The reflexes are hyperactive. The blood pressure, which is usually elevated, should be taken after the patient has rested for 5 minutes in the left lateral recumbent position.

Management of the Patient With Hypertensive Disorders of Pregnancy. Definitive treatment of the hypertensive disorders of pregnancy is delivery of the fetus. However, in the field, use the following management tactics to prevent dangerously high blood pressures or seizure activity.

PIH. The patient who is pregnant and has elevated blood pressure, without edema or other signs of preeclampsia, should be closely monitored and transported to the hospital. Record the fetal heart tones and the mother's blood pressure level. If the blood pressure is dangerously high, the medical control physician may request the administration of Apresoline or similar antihypertensives which are safe for use in pregnancy.

Preeclampsia. The patient who is hypertensive and shows other signs and symptoms of preeclampsia, such as edema, headaches, and visual disturbances, should be treated quickly. Keep the patient calm, and dim the lights. Place the patient in the left lateral recumbent position and quickly carry out primary and secondary survey. Begin an IV of D5W. Transport the patient rapidly, without lights or sirens. If the transport time is long, the medical control physician may request the administration of magnesium sulfate.

Eclampsia. If the patient has already suffered a seizure or a seizure appears to be imminent, then, in addition to the above measures, administer oxygen and manage the airway appropriately. Administer 5–10 mg Valium intravenously, as ordered by the medical control physician. In addition, the physician may request the administration of magnesium sulfate, especially if transport time is long. It is important to keep calcium chloride available for use as an antidote to magnesium sulfate.

The Supine-Hypotensive Syndrome. The *supine-hypotensive syndrome* usually occurs in the third trimester of pregnancy. The increased mass and weight of the gravid uterus compresses the inferior vena cava when the patient is supine, markedly decreasing blood return to the heart and reducing cardiac output. (See Figure 32-7.) Some patients are predisposed to this problem because of an overall decrease in circulating blood volume or anemia.

Assessment and Management of the Patient With Supine-Hypotensive Syndrome. As mentioned previously, the supine-hypotensive syndrome usually occurs in a patient late in her pregnancy who has been supine for a period of time. Question the patient about prior episodes of a similar nature and about any recent hemorrhage or fluid loss.

The physical examination should be directed at determining whether the patient is volume depleted. If there are no indications of volume depletion, such as decreased skin turgor or thirst, place the patient in the left lateral recumbent position and monitor the fetal heart tones and maternal vital signs frequently.

If there is clinical evidence of volume depletion, administer oxygen and start an IV of normal saline or lactated Ringer's solution. Monitor vital signs, fetal heart tones, and ECG. If there is evidence of shock, apply antishock trousers, inflating only the leg compartments. Transport the patient promptly.

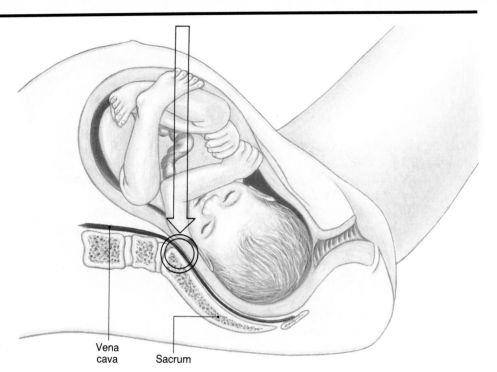

FIGURE 32-7 The supine-hypotensive syndrome results from compression of the inferior vena cava by the gravid uterus.

Vena
cava   Sacrum

Braxton-Hicks Contractions and Preterm Labor. It is occasionally difficult to determine the onset of labor. For many weeks before labor begins, the uterus contracts irregularly, thus conditioning itself for the birth process. As the EDC approaches, these contractions become more frequent. Ultimately, the contractions become stronger and more regular, signaling the onset of labor. *Labor* consists of uterine contractions that change the dilation or effacement of the cervix. The contractions of labor are firm, fairly regular, and quite painful. *Braxton-Hicks contractions,* occasionally called false labor, are generally less intense than labor contractions and do not change the cervix.

It is virtually impossible to distinguish false labor from true labor in the field. Distinguishing the two requires repeated vaginal examinations, over time, to determine whether the cervix is effacing or dilating. This, of course, should not be done in the field. Therefore, all patients with uterine contractions should be transported to the hospital for additional evaluation.

Braxton-Hicks contractions do not require treatment by the paramedic aside from reassurance of the patient and, if necessary, transport for evaluation by a physician. True labor that begins before the 38th week of gestation, referred to as *preterm labor,* may require intervention. Many conditions may lead to preterm labor, including premature rupture of the membranes and abnormalities in the cervix or uterus. In many cases, it is desirable to attempt to stop preterm labor to give the fetus additional time to develop in the uterus.

Assessment of the Patient With Preterm Labor. When confronted by a patient with uterine contractions, first determine the approximate gestational age of the fetus. If it is less than 38 weeks, then preterm labor is suspected. If gestational age is greater than 38 weeks, the patient should be treated as a term patient, as described later in this chapter.

After determining gestational age, obtain a brief obstetrical history. Then question the mother about the urge to push or the need to move her bowels or urinate. She should also be questioned about the status of her membranes. Any sensation of fluid leakage or "gushing" from the vagina should be interpreted as ruptured membranes until proven otherwise. Next, palpate the contractions by placing your hand on the patient's abdomen. Note the intensity and length of the contractions, as well as the interval between contractions.

Management of the Patient With Preterm Labor. Preterm labor, especially if quite early, should be stopped if possible. The process of stopping labor, or *tocolysis,* is frequently practiced in obstetrics. It is, however, infrequently done in the field.

There are three general approaches to tocolysis. The first is to sedate the patient, often with narcotics or barbiturates, and allow her to rest. Often, after a period of rest, the contractions stop on their own. The second approach is to administer a fluid bolus intravenously. The administration of approximately 1 liter of fluid intravenously increases the intravascular fluid volume, thus inhibiting ADH secretion from the posterior pituitary. Since oxytocin and ADH are secreted from the same area of the pituitary, the inhibition of ADH secretion also inhibits oxytocin release, often causing cessation of uterine contractions. Ultimately, if the above methods fail, a beta agonist, such as terbutaline or ritodrine, may be administered to stop labor by inhibiting smooth muscle uterine contraction.

As a rule, tocolysis in the field is limited to sedation and hydration, especially if transport time is long. Paramedics may, however, transport a patient from one medical facility to another with beta agonist administration underway and should therefore be familiar with its use.

✱ The patient with suspected pre-term labor should be transported immediately.

THE PUERPERIUM

The *puerperium* is the time period surrounding birth of the fetus. Childbirth generally occurs in a hospital or similar facility with appropriate equipment. Occasionally, prehospital personnel may be called upon to attend a delivery. Therefore, they should be familiar with the birth process and some of the complications associated with it.

Deliveries

The delivery of the fetus is the culmination of pregnancy. The process by which delivery occurs is **labor.** Labor is generally divided into three stages (see Figure 32-8):

■ **labor** the time and processes that occur during childbirth.

❑ *First Stage.* The first stage of labor begins with the onset of uterine contractions and ends with complete dilation of the cervix. It lasts approximately 8 hours in **nulliparous** women and 5 hours in multiparous women. Contractions may be irregular at first. Later in the first stage, the contractions increase in intensity and the intervals between contractions shorten.

■ **nullipara** a woman who has never delivered a baby.

❑ *Second Stage.* The second stage of labor begins with complete dilation of the cervix and ends with delivery of the fetus. In the nulliparous patient, the second stage lasts approximately 50 minutes; in the multiparous patient, it lasts approximately 20 minutes. Contractions are strong, and each one may last 2 or 3 minutes. Often, the patient feels pain in her lower back, as the fetus descends into the pelvis. The urge to push or "bear down" usually begins in the second stage. The membranes usually rupture at this time, if they have not ruptured previously.

❑ *Third Stage.* The third stage of labor begins with delivery of the fetus and ends with delivery of the placenta. Delivery of the placenta usually occurs within 30 minutes after birth.

First stage: beginning of contractions to full cervical dilation

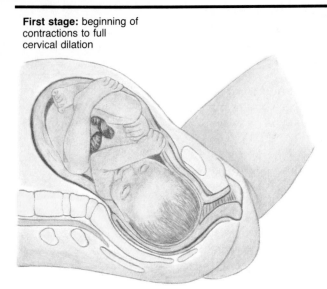

Second stage: baby enters birth canal and is born

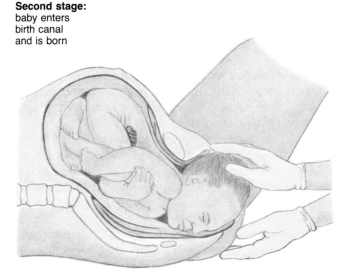

Third stage: delivery of the placenta

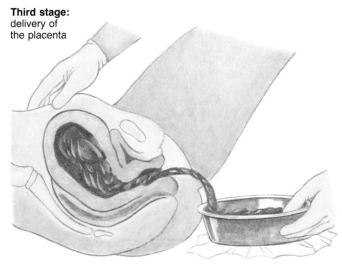

FIGURE 32-8   Stages of labor.

As discussed earlier, labor is painful. The pain begins in the abdomen. Later, as the fetus moves farther down into the pelvis, the pain may extend to the back. The contractions are regular and generally increase in frequency and intensity. The total length of labor averages 6 to 12 hours, with a great deal of individual variation. Labor usually lasts longer in the nulliparous patient than in the multiparous patient.

The uterus and cervix must undergo several changes to facilitate delivery of the fetus. First, the cervix must efface. *Effacement* is the thinning and shortening of the cervix. Early in pregnancy the cervix is quite thick and long, but after complete effacement it is paper thin. Effacement usually begins several days before active labor ensues. Second, the cervix must dilate. *Dilation* is the progressive stretching of the opening of the cervix. The cervix dilates from its closed position to 10 cm, which is considered complete dilation.

When dilation and effacement are complete, the baby's head moves down into the vagina. Late in the second stage of labor, the head can be seen at the opening of the vagina during a contraction. This is termed crowning.

The part of the baby that is born first is termed the *presenting part*. In the majority of cases, this is the head. Occasionally, the buttocks or other parts present first. In the field, the presenting part cannot usually be determined until crowning has occurred, since vaginal examinations should not be performed.

Management of the Patient in Labor

Probably one of the most important decisions paramedics must make with a patient in labor is whether to attempt to deliver the infant at the scene or transport the patient to the hospital. (See Figure 32-9.) There are several factors to take into consideration when making this decision. They include the patient's number of previous pregnancies, the length of labor during the previous pregnancies, the frequency of contractions, the maternal urge to push, and the presence of crowning. Some women have rapid labors and may be completely dilated in a short period of time. Also, as mentioned above, multiparas generally have shorter labors than nulliparas. The maternal urge to push or the presence of crowning indicates that delivery is imminent and the infant should be delivered at the scene or in the ambulance.

However, certain factors should prompt immediate transport, de-

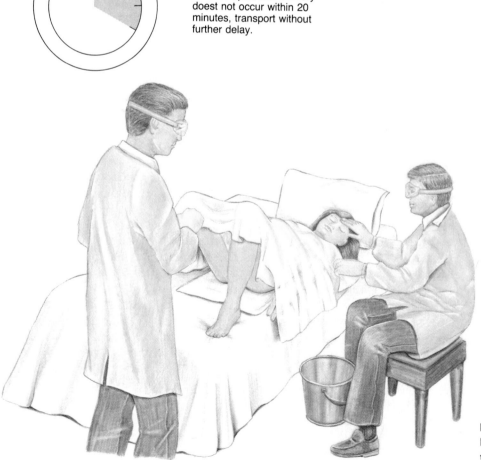

If contractions are 2 to 3 minutes apart and delivery doest not occur within 20 minutes, transport without further delay.

FIGURE 32-9 The decision to deliver at the scene or to attempt transport is often a difficult one.

spite the threat of delivery. These include prior rupture of membranes, since prolonged time between rupture and delivery often leads to fetal infection, abnormal presentation, such as breech or transverse, or fetal distress, as evidenced by fetal bradycardia or meconium staining (the presence of *meconium*, the first fetal stools, in the amniotic fluid).

Unscheduled Field Delivery

✱ Remember, childbirth is a normal event.

If delivery is imminent, equipment and facilities must be quickly prepared. (See Procedure 32-1.) Prepare a delivery area. This should be out of public view, such as in a bedroom or the back of the ambulance. Administer oxygen to the mother. If time permits, establish an IV of lactated Ringer's solution or normal saline. The patient should be placed on her back and, if time permits, draped. Until delivery, the fetal heart rate should be monitored frequently. A drop in the fetal heart rate to less than 90 beats per minute indicates fetal distress and should prompt immediate transport. Coach the mother to breath deeply between contractions and to push with contractions. Prepare the OB equipment and don sterile gloves. As the head crowns, control it with gentle pressure. (See Figures 32-10 through 32-20.) An explosive delivery results in increased tearing of maternal tissue. If the membranes are still intact, rupture them with your fingertips to allow leakage of the amniotic fluid.

If the umbilical cord is around the infant's neck during delivery, gently slip it over the infant's head, if possible. If the cord is too tight to slip over the head, apply two umbilical clamps and cut the cord. As soon as the infant's head is clear of the vagina, instruct the mother not to push, and suction the infant's mouth and nose with the bulb syringe. Then allow the mother to push and support the head as it rotates. Deliver first the anterior shoulder and then the posterior shoulder. The remainder of the body will follow.

Remember to keep the baby at the level of the vagina to prevent over- or undertransfusion of blood from the cord. Never "milk" the cord. Clamp the cord as follows: Supporting the baby, place the first umbilical clamp approximately 10 cm from the baby. Place the second clamp approximately 5 cm above the first. Then carefully cut the umbilical cord between the clamps.

At this point, suction the infant again, using the bulb suction. Then, wipe the infant dry and inspect the cord for bleeding. Wrap the baby in a warm blanket and place it on its side with the head approximately 15 degrees below the torso to facilitate drainage of any aspirated secretions. Note the time of birth.

After birth, the mother's vagina should continue to ooze blood. Do not pull on the umbilical cord. Eventually, the cord will appear to lengthen, which indicates separation of the placenta. The placenta should be delivered and transported with the mother to the hospital. There is no need to delay transport for delivery of the placenta.

At this time, massage the uterine fundus by placing one hand immediately above the symphysis pubis and the other on the uterine fundus. Cup the uterus between the two hands and support it as it is massaged. Continue massage until the uterus assumes a woody hardness. Avoid overmassage.

Following delivery, inspect the mother's perineum for tears. If any tears are present, apply direct pressure. Continuously monitor vital signs. Note the presence of continued hemorrhage and report it to the medical control physician. Following stabilization, transport the mother and infant to the hospital.

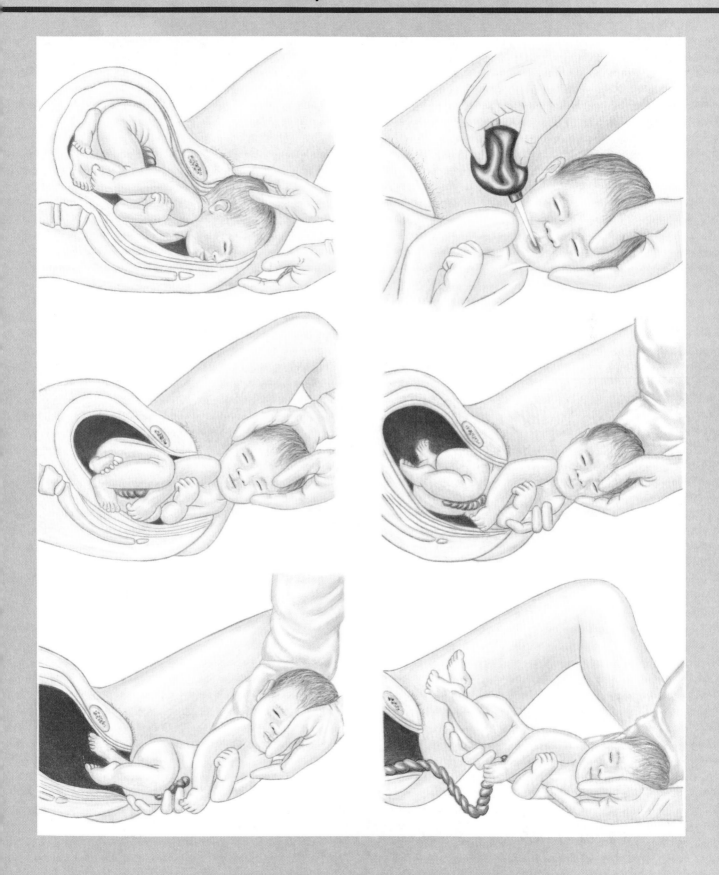

(Photos by Harriette Hartigan/ARTEMIS)

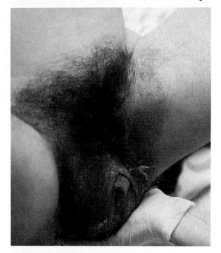

FIGURE 32-10   Crowning.

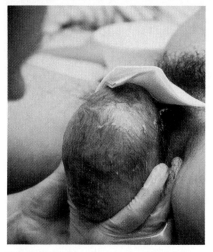

FIGURE 32-11   Delivery of the head.

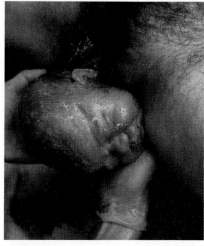

FIGURE 32-12   External rotation of the head.

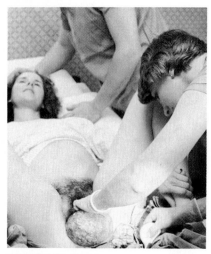

FIGURE 32-13   As soon as possible, suction the mouth, then nose.

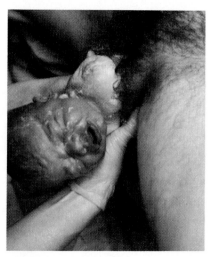

FIGURE 32-14   Delivery of the anterior shoulder.

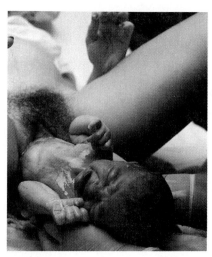

FIGURE 32-15   Complete delivery of the infant.

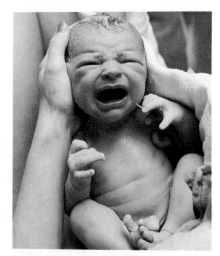

FIGURE 32-16   Dry the infant.

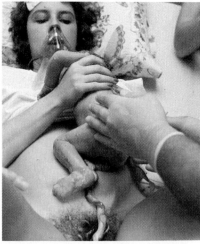

FIGURE 32-17   Place the infant on the mother's stomach.

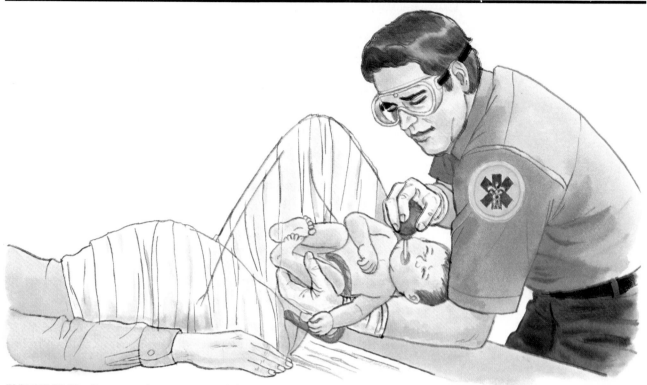

FIGURE 32-18   Re-suction the airway as needed.

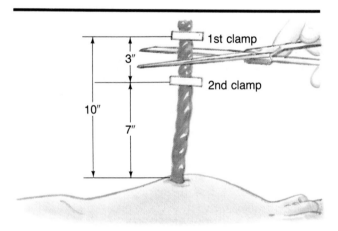

1st clamp

3″

2nd clamp

10″

7″

FIGURE 32-19   Clamp and cut the cord.

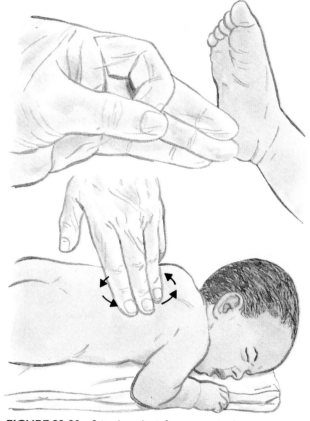

FIGURE 32-20   Stimulate the infant as required.

Complications of Delivery

Most deliveries are uncomplicated. Complications can arise, however, and the paramedic should be prepared to deal with them.

Cephalopelvic Disproportion. *Cephalopelvic disproportion* occurs when the baby's head is too big to pass through the maternal pelvis easily. This may be caused by an oversized baby. Large babies are associated with diabetes, multiparity, or postmaturity. Fetal abnormalities such as hydrocephalus, conjoined twins, or fetal tumors may make vaginal delivery impossible. Women of short stature or women with contracted pelvises are at increased risk for this problem. If cephalopelvic disproportion is not recognized and managed appropriately, fetal demise or uterine rupture may occur.

Cephalopelvic disproportion tends to occur most frequently in the primigravida. There may be strong contractions for an extended period of time. On physical examination, the fetus may feel large. Also, labor generally does not progress. The fetus may be in distress, as evidenced by fetal bradycardia or meconium staining.

The usual management of cephalopelvic disproportion is cesarean section. In the field, the mother should be administered oxygen and an IV of lactated Ringer's or normal saline started. Transport should be immediate and rapid.

Abnormal Presentations. Most babies present head first, or *vertex*. However, approximately 3 percent of deliveries are *breech presentations,* in which the presenting part is the feet or the buttocks. Breech presentations are more common in premature infants and in mothers with uterine abnormalities. Such deliveries carry an increased risk for fetal trauma, anoxia, and cord prolapse.

Delivery of the breech presentation is best accomplished at the hospital, and cesarean section is usually required. However, if field delivery is unavoidable, then the following maneuvers are recommended. First, position the mother with her buttocks at the edge of a firm bed. Ask her to hold her legs in a flexed position. Often she will require assistance in doing this. As the infant delivers, do not pull on the legs, simply support them. Allow the entire body to be delivered with contractions only while you support the infant. (Figure 32-21.)

As the head passes the pubis, apply gentle upward traction until the mouth appears over the perineum. If the head does not deliver, and the baby begins to breathe spontaneously with its face pressed against the vaginal wall, place a gloved hand in the vagina with the palm toward the infant's face. Form a "V" with the index and middle finger on either side of the infant's nose and push the vaginal wall away from the infant's face to allow unrestricted respiration. (Figure 32-22.) If necessary, continue throughout transport.

Other abnormal presentations can complicate delivery. One of the most common is the *occiput posterior position*. Normally, as the infant descends into the pelvis, its face is turned posteriorly. This is important, as extension of the head assists delivery. However, if the baby descends facing forward, or occiput posterior, its passage through the pelvis is delayed. This presentation occurs most frequently in primigravidas. In multigravidas it usually resolves spontaneously.

The presenting part may also be the face or brow, rather than the crown of the head. Occasionally, during these presentations, the face or

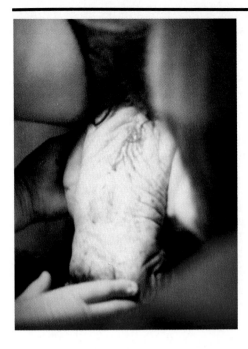

FIGURE 32-21 Breech delivery.

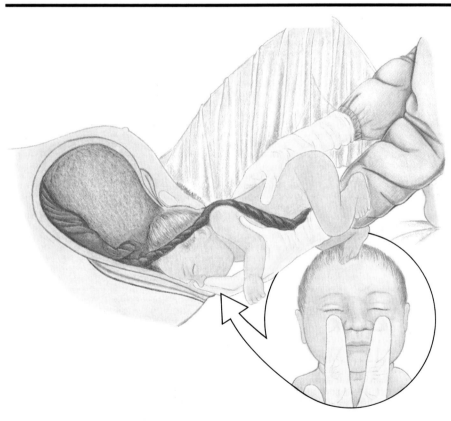

FIGURE 32-22 Placement of the fingers to maintain the airway in a breech birth.

brow can be seen high in the pelvis during a contraction. Usually, vaginal delivery is impossible in these cases.

In addition to head-first and breech presentations, the fetus can lie transversely in the uterus. In such a case, the fetus cannot enter the pelvis for delivery. If the membranes rupture, the umbilical cord can prolapse (see below), or an arm or leg can enter the vagina. Vaginal delivery is impossible.

Early recognition of an abnormal presentation is important. If one is suspected, the mother should be reassured, placed on oxygen, and transported immediately, since forceps or cesarean delivery is often required.

Prolapsed Cord. A *prolapsed cord* occurs when the umbilical cord falls down into the pelvis and is compressed between the fetus and the bony pelvis, shutting off fetal circulation. (Figure 32-23.) This tends to occur most frequently in abnormal presentations, with multiple or premature births, or in conjunction with premature rupture of the membranes. It is a serious emergency, and fetal death will occur quickly without prompt intervention.

If the umbilical cord is seen in the vagina, insert two fingers of a gloved hand to raise the presenting part of the fetus off the cord. At the same time, check the cord for pulsations. Place the mother in Trendelenburg or knee-chest position. (See Figure 32-24.) Administer high-flow oxygen to the mother and transport her immediately, with the fingers continuing to hold the presenting part off the umbilical cord. If assis-

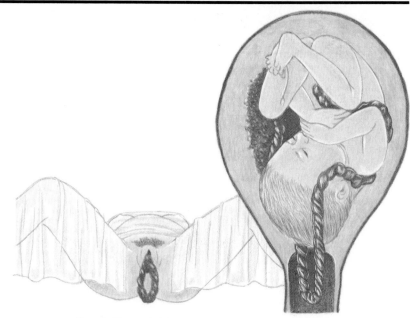

- Elevate hips, administer oxygen and keep warm

- Keep baby's head away from cord

- Do not attempt to push cord back

- Wrap cord in sterile moist towel

- Transport mother to hospital, continuing pressure on baby's head

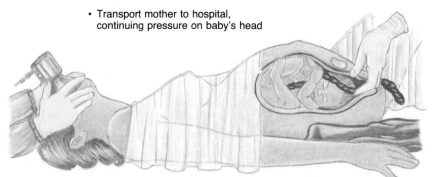

FIGURE 32-23   Prolapsed cord.

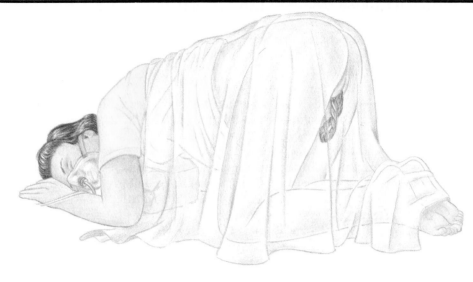

FIGURE 32-24 Patient positioning for prolapsed cord.

tance is available, apply dressings moistened with sterile saline to the exposed cord. DO NOT ATTEMPT TO PUSH THE CORD BACK. Definitive treatment is cesarean section.

Multiple Births. Multiple births are fairly rare. Usually, the mother knows or at least suspects the presence of more than one fetus. Multiple birth should also be suspected if the mother's abdomen remains large after delivery of one baby.

In twin births, labor often begins earlier than expected, and the infants are generally smaller than babies born singly. Usually, one twin presents vertex and the other breech. There may be one or two placentas.

After delivery of the first baby, clamp and cut the cord. Then deliver the second baby.

Precipitous Delivery. A *precipitous delivery* is a delivery that occurs after less than 3 hours of labor. This type of delivery occurs most frequently in the **grand multipara** and is associated with a higher-than-normal incidence of fetal trauma, tearing of the umbilical cord, or maternal lacerations.

The best way to handle precipitous delivery is to be prepared. Do not turn your attention from the mother. Be ready for a rapid delivery and attempt to control the head. Once delivered, the baby may have some difficulty with temperature regulation and should be kept warm.

■ **grand multipara** a woman who has delivered at least seven babies.

Shoulder Dystocia. A *shoulder dystocia* occurs when the infant's shoulders are larger than its head. This occurs most frequently with diabetic and obese mothers and in postmature pregnancies. In shoulder dystocia, labor progresses normally and the head is delivered routinely. However, immediately after the head is delivered, it retracts back into the perineum because the shoulders are trapped between the symphysis pubis and the sacrum ("turtle sign").

If a shoulder dystocia occurs, do not pull on the head. Administer oxygen to the mother and have her drop her buttocks off the end of the bed. Then flex her thighs upward to facilitate delivery and apply firm pressure with an open hand immediately above the symphysis pubis. If delivery does not occur, transport the patient immediately.

Maternal Complications of Labor and Deliver

Several maternal problems can arise during and after delivery. These include postpartum hemorrhage, uterine rupture, uterine inversion, and pulmonary embolism.

■ **postpartum** the time period after delivery of the fetus.

Postpartum Hemorrhage. **Postpartum hemorrhage** is the loss of 500 mL or more blood in the first 24 hours following delivery. It occurs in approximately 5 percent of deliveries. The most common cause of postpartum hemorrhage is *uterine atony,* or lack of uterine muscle tone. This tends to occur most frequently in the multigravida and is most common following multiple births or births of large infants. Uterine atony also occurs after precipitous deliveries and prolonged labors. In addition to uterine atony, postpartum hemorrhage can be caused by placenta previa, abruptio placentae, retained placental parts, clotting disorders in the mother, or vaginal and cervical tears. Occasionally, the uterus fails to return to its normal size during the postpartum period, and postpartum hemorrhage occurs long after the birth.

Assessment of the patient with postpartum hemorrhage should focus on the history and the predisposing factors described above. The paramedic must rely heavily on the clinical appearance of the patient and her vital signs. Often, the uterus will feel boggy and soft on physical examination. Vaginal bleeding is usually obvious.

Management of Postpartum Hemorrhage. When confronted by a patient with postpartum hemorrhage, complete the primary and secondary survey immediately. Administer oxygen and begin fundal massage. Administer one or two large-bore IVs of either normal saline or lactated Ringer's solution. If shock is evident, apply antishock trousers. Never attempt to force delivery of the placenta or pack the vagina with dressings. In severe cases, the medical control physician may request the administration of pitocin.

Uterine Rupture. *Uterine rupture* is the actual tearing, or rupture, of the uterus. It usually occurs during labor or at its onset but can occur before labor with abdominal trauma. During labor, it often results from tetanic uterine contractions or a surgically scarred uterus, such as occurs from previous cesarean section. It can also occur following a prolonged or obstructed labor, as in the case of cephalopelvic disproportion, or in conjunction with abnormal presentations.

The patient with uterine rupture will often be in shock. There may be a history of continuous abdominal pain which has increased in intensity. Labor may have started, then appeared to have stopped when the uterus ruptured. On physical examination there is often profound shock without evidence of external hemorrhage. Fetal heart tones are absent, and the abdomen is often tender and rigid and may exhibit rebound tenderness.

Management is the same as for any patient in shock. Administer oxygen at high concentration. Next, establish one or two large-bore IVs with either lactated Ringer's solution or normal saline. Monitor vital signs and fetal heart tones continuously. If shock is impending, apply antishock trousers without inflating the abdominal compartment. Transport the patient rapidly, since definitive treatment is cesarean section, if the fetus is still viable, with repair or removal of the uterus.

Uterine Inversion. *Uterine inversion,* a rare emergency, occurs when the uterus turns inside out after delivery. When uterine inversion occurs, the supporting ligaments and blood vessels supplying blood to the uterus are torn, usually causing profound shock. Uterine inversion usually results from pulling on the umbilical cord while awaiting delivery of the placenta or from attempts to express the placenta when the uterus is relaxed.

If uterine inversion occurs, the paramedic must act quickly. First, place the patient supine and begin oxygen administration. DO NOT attempt to detach the placenta or pull on the cord. Initiate one or two large-bore IVs of normal saline or lactated Ringer's solution. Make one attempt to replace the uterus: With the palm of the hand, push the fundus of the inverted uterus toward the vagina. If one attempt is unsuccessful, cover the uterus with towels moistened with saline and transport the patient immediately.

Pulmonary Embolism. *Pulmonary embolism* is the presence of a blood clot in the pulmonary vascular system. It can occur after pregnancy, usually as a result of venous thromboembolism. It is one of the most common causes of maternal death and appears to occur more frequently following cesarean section than vaginal delivery.

Pulmonary embolism can also occur at any time during pregnancy. There is usually a sudden onset of dyspnea and often sharp chest pain. On physical examination, the patient may show tachycardia, tachypnea, and, in severe cases, hypotension.

Management of pulmonary embolism consists of administration of high-flow oxygen and IV of D5W TKO. Monitor the patient's ECG and vital signs closely and transport her rapidly.

SUMMARY

Obstetrical emergencies are fairly uncommon. However, all pregnant patients are at risk for developing complications, and it is impossible to predict which ones actually will. It is therefore important to recognize these complications and act accordingly.

FURTHER READING

Cunningham, F. Gary, MacDonald, Paul C., and Gant, Norman F., *Williams Obstetrics, Eighteenth Edition.* Norwalk, CT: Appleton & Lange, 1989.

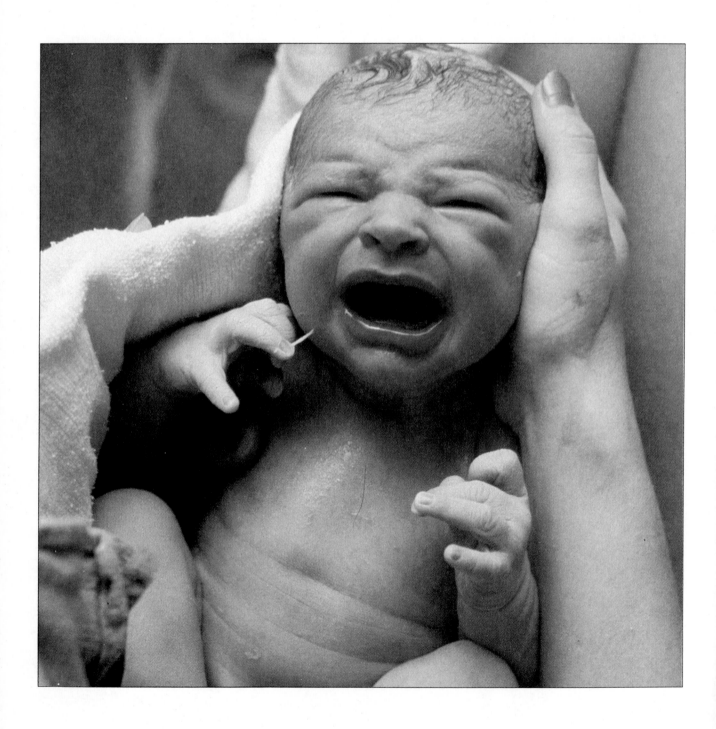

33

Emergency Management of the Neonate

Objectives for Chapter 33

Upon completing this chapter, the student should be able to:

1. Describe the routine care of the newborn.

2. List four means by which heat loss occurs in neonates.

3. Discuss the effects of hypothermia on the neonate.

4. Define the parameters of Apgar scoring and the numerical values used.

5. Describe and explain the significance of the inverted-pyramid approach to neonatal resuscitation.

6. Describe two methods of stimulating a distressed neonate.

7. Describe the appropriate administration of oxygen to a neonate.

8. Describe methods and problems in ventilating the distressed infant.

9. Describe the technique and rates used in cardiac massage in the neonate.

10. Explain the significance of meconium staining.

11. Describe the indications and procedure for endotracheal intubation of a distressed neonate.

12. List drugs and fluids used in neonatal resuscitation and give the correct dosages.

The paramedics of Bell County General Hospital were dispatched to assist a woman in labor. Upon arrival, they found a 24-year-old female who was about to deliver her baby. The paramedics quickly determined that there is not enough time to transport the patient to the hospital and they prepared for delivery.

The delivery was uneventful. However, the baby remained blue and limp, even after the paramedics suctioned the airway. The paramedics quickly moved the infant to the side of the bed where the light was better. There the baby was dried, again suctioned, and stimulated. He still remained blue and limp. Supplemental "blow by" oxygen was delivered, yet the neonate's heart rate remained at less than 100.

The paramedics grabbed the bag-valve-mask unit and applied artificial ventilation. Almost immediately, the infant "pinked up" and began to cry. Using the pulse oximeter, the paramedics determined oxygen saturation to be 95 percent. Next, they wrapped the infant in a blanket with its head covered and gave it to the mother to hold. They continued the "blow by" oxygen as the mother and infant were transported. The 5-minute Apgar score was 9. The baby went home from the hospital the day after the mother.

INTRODUCTION

After a neonate is delivered, the paramedic has two patients to manage: the mother and the baby. This chapter describes care of the neonate and discusses the special needs of the distressed neonate and the premature neonate. It also addresses neonatal transport.

■ **neonate** an infant from the time of birth to one month of age.

A **neonate** is an infant less than one month of age. (See Figure 33-1.) The following discussion is primarily concerned with the newborn neonate.

ROUTINE CARE OF THE NEWBORN

Establishment of the Airway

The neonate requires attention immediately after birth. One of the first steps in caring for the neonate is airway management. During delivery, fluid is forced out of the baby's lungs, into the oropharynx, and out the nose and mouth. This fluid drainage is independent of gravity. As soon as the neonate's head is delivered, the mouth and then the nose should be suctioned with a bulb suction. Suctioning should be repeated upon delivery of the body.

■ **DeLee trap suction** a suction device which contains a suction trap connected to a suction catheter. The negative pressure which powers it can come either from the mouth of the operator or, preferably, from an external vacuum source.

The neonate should be maintained at the same level as the mother's vagina, with its head approximately 15 degrees below its torso. This facilitates the drainage of secretions and helps prevent aspiration. If there appears to be a large amount of secretions, a **DeLee suction trap**, attached to a suction source, should be used. Both the nose and mouth should be repeatedly suctioned until clear.

The neonate should take its first breath within a few seconds after delivery. The timing of the first breath is unrelated to the cutting of the

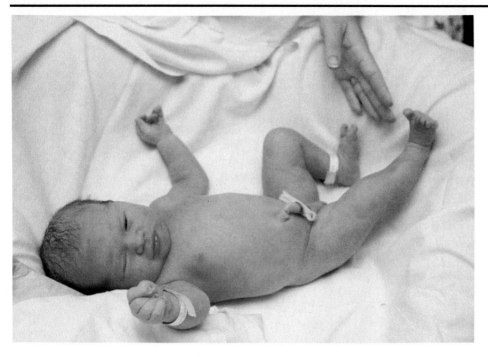

FIGURE 33-1 Term neonate.

umbilical cord. The factors that impel the baby's first breath include mild acidosis, initiation of the stretch reflexes in the lung, hypoxia, and hypothermia. (See Figure 33-2.)

If the neonate does not cry immediately, stimulate it by gently rubbing its back. Vigorous spanking or rubbing is seldom necessary.

Heat Loss in the Neonate

Heat loss is one of the most important risks to the neonate. Heat loss can occur through evaporation, convection, conduction, or radiation. Most heat loss in the neonate occurs through *evaporation*. The neonate is born wet, and the amniotic fluid quickly evaporates, thus cooling the neonate. Immediately after birth, the neonate's core temperature can drop 1 degree C. from its birth temperature of 38 degrees.

Loss of heat can also occur through *convection,* depending on the temperature of the room and air movement around the neonate. *Conduction* can occur through surfaces in contact with the neonate. In addition, the neonate can lose heat through *radiation* to colder objects nearby.

Heat loss should be prevented. (See Figure 33-3.) Dry the neonate immediately to prevent evaporative cooling. The *ambient temperature,* the temperature in the delivery room or ambulance, should be at least 23–24 degrees C. (74–76 degrees F). To prevent drafts, make sure all doors and windows are closed. Discard the towel used to dry the neonate and swaddle the neonate in a warm, dry receiving blanket or other suitable material. In colder areas, place well-insulated hot-water bottles or rubber gloves filled with warm water around the neonate to help maintain a warm body temperature.

Cutting the Umbilical Cord

After the neonate's airway has been stabilized and heat loss has been prevented, clamp and cut the umbilical cord. Maintaining the baby at the same level as the vagina, as described above, prevents transfusion of

✱ Heat loss is a major risk to the neonate.

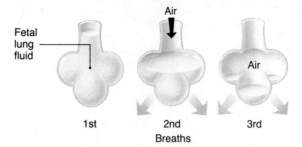

Air

Fetal lung fluid

Air

1st   2nd   3rd
Breaths

Following birth, the lungs expand as they are filled with air. The fetal lung fluid gradually leaves the alveoli.

Arterioles dilate and blood flow increases

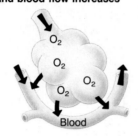

O_2
O_2
O_2
O_2
Blood

At the same time as the lungs are expanding and the fetal lung fluid is clearing, the arterioles in the lung begin to open, allowing a considerable increase in the amount of blood flowing through the lungs.

Pulmonary blood flow increases

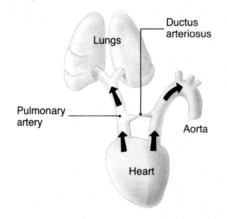

Ductus arteriosus

Lungs

Pulmonary artery

Aorta

Heart

Blood previously diverted through the ductus arteriosus flows through the lungs where it picks up oxygen to transport to tissues throughout the body. Soon there is no need for the ductus, and it eventually closes.

FIGURE 33-2 Hemodynamic changes in the neonate at birth.

✳ Never "milk" the umbilical cord during a delivery.

blood. Do not "milk" or strip the umbilical cord, since this increases blood viscosity, or *polycythemia*. Polycythemia can cause cardiopulmonary problems and can contribute to excessive red blood cell destruction, which may lead to hyperbilirubinemia (an increased level of bilirubin in the blood, causing jaundice).

Apply the umbilical clamps within 30–45 seconds after birth. Place the first clamp approximately 10 cm from the neonate. Place the second clamp approximately 5 cm farther away from the neonate than the first clamp. Then cut the cord between the two clamps. After the cord is cut, inspect it periodically to be sure that there is no additional bleeding.

Assessment of the Neonate

Assess the neonate immediately after birth. Ideally, if two paramedics are available, one should attend the mother and the other the neonate.

Obtain vital signs quickly. The neonate's respiratory rate should average 40–60 breaths per minute. If asphyxia is present, begin resuscitation at once. Next, check the heart rate. The heart rate is normally 150–

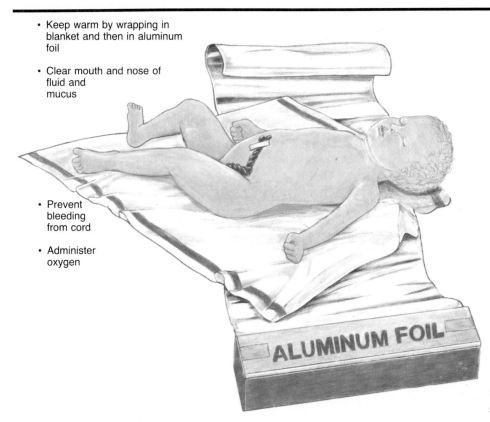

- Keep warm by wrapping in blanket and then in aluminum foil

- Clear mouth and nose of fluid and mucus

- Prevent bleeding from cord

- Administer oxygen

ALUMINUM FOIL

FIGURE 33-3 The paramedic should keep the infant warm.

180 beats per minute at birth, slowing to 130–140 beats per minute shortly thereafter. A pulse rate of less than 100 beats per minute indicates distress and requires emergency intervention. The skin color should be evaluated as well. Some cyanosis of the extremities is common immediately after birth. However, cyanosis of the central part of the body is abnormal, as is persistent peripheral cyanosis.

The APGAR Score

As soon as possible, the neonate should be assigned an **APGAR score.** Ideally, this is done at 1 and 5 minutes after birth. However, if the neonate is not breathing, DO NOT withhold resuscitation until after the APGAR score is determined.

The APGAR scoring system helps to differentiate those neonates who need only routine care from those who need greater assistance and also predicts long-term survival. It was developed in 1952 by Dr. Virginia Apgar, an anesthesiologist. The parameters included in APGAR scoring are heart rate, respiratory effort, muscle tone, response to stimulation, and color. A score of 0, 1, or 2 is given for each parameter. The minimum total score is 0 and the maximum is 10. (See Table 33-1.) A score of 7–10 indicates an active and vigorous neonate that requires only routine care. A score of 4–6 indicates a moderately depressed neonate that requires oxygenation and stimulation. Severely depressed neonates, those with APGAR scores of less than 4, require immediate resuscitation. By repeating the APGAR score at 1 and 5 minutes, it is possible to determine whether intervention has caused a change in the neonate's status.

■ **APGAR scoring** a numerical system of rating the condition of a newborn. It evaluates the neonate's heart rate, respiratory rate, muscle tone, reflex irritability, and color.

✳ Never delay resuscitation to determine the APGAR score.

TABLE 33-1   The APGAR Scoring Method

Sign	0	1	2	Score	
				1 min	5 min
Heart rate	Absent	Below 100	Over 100		
Respiration (effort)	Absent	Slow and irregular	Normal; crying		
Muscle tone	Limp	Some flexion— extremities	Active; good motion in extremities		
Irritability	No response	Crying; some motion	Crying; vigorous		
Skin color	Bluish or paleness	Pink or typical new-born color; hands and feet are blue	Pink or typical newborn color; entire body		
			TOTAL SCORE =		

THE PREMATURE NEONATE

The *premature neonate* is one that weighs less than 2500 g (5.5 pounds) or that is born before the 38th week of gestation. (See Figure 33-4.) Premature neonates are at risk for hypothermia, hypoglycemia, volume depletion, several respiratory problems, and, in some cases, cardiovascular problems related to hypoxia.

Premature neonates are more susceptible to heat loss than full-term neonates for the following reasons:

1. The premature neonate tends to lose heat more readily than the term neonate, because of its relatively large body surface as compared to its weight.

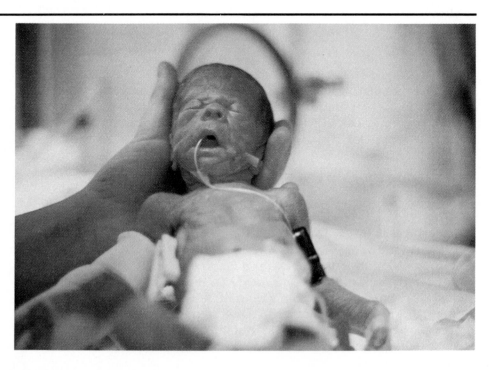

FIGURE 33-4 The premature neonate.

2. The premature neonate has not sufficiently developed the control mechanisms needed to regulate body temperature.

3. The premature neonate has smaller subcutaneous stores of insulating fat.

4. Neonates cannot shiver and must maintain body temperature through other mechanisms.

As with full-term neonates, keep the airway clear. If the premature neonate shows signs or symptoms of respiratory distress, administer supplemental oxygen and, if necessary, carry out ventilation (see below). Monitor the umbilical cord for bleeding. If possible, transport the neonate to a facility with a neonatal intensive care unit (NICU).

NEONATAL DISTRESS

The neonate in distress may be either full-term or premature. The presence of fetal **meconium** at birth indicates the possibility of fetal respiratory distress. If the neonate is simply meconium stained, then distress may have been remote. If, however, there is particulate meconium, then it is likely that distress has recently occurred, and the neonate should be managed accordingly. If the neonate has aspirated meconium, severe lung inflammation and pneumonia may develop. If meconium is visible during delivery, do not induce respiratory effort until the meconium is removed from the trachea by suctioning under direct visualization with the laryngoscope. (See Figure 33-5.) Report the presence of meconium to the medical control physician.

The most common problems in the period immediately after birth involve the airway and ventilation. Resuscitation of the neonate primarily consists of ventilation and oxygenation. The use of IV fluids, drugs, or cardiac equipment is usually not indicated. Suctioning, drying, and stimulating the distressed neonate are particularly important.

The single most important indicator of neonatal distress is fetal heart rate. The neonate has a relatively fixed stroke volume; thus cardiac output is directly related to heart rate. Bradycardia, as caused by hypoxia, causes decreased cardiac output and, ultimately, poor perfusion. A pulse rate of less than 60 beats per minute in a distressed neonate indicates that CPR should be initiated. The paramedic should monitor the heart rate manually.

Each EMS unit should contain a neonatal resuscitation kit that includes the following supplies:

❑ Bag-valve-mask unit
❑ Bulb syringe
❑ DeLee suction trap
❑ Laryngoscope with size 0 and size 1 blades
❑ Uncuffed endotracheal tubes (2.5, 3.0, 3.5) with appropriate suction catheters
❑ Endotracheal tube stylet
❑ Umbilical catheter and 10 mL syringe
❑ Three-way stopcock
❑ 20 mL syringe and 8 french feeding tube for gastric suction
❑ Dextrostix

■ **meconium** dark-green material found in the intestine of the full-term neonate. It can be expelled from the intestine into the amniotic fluid during periods of fetal distress.

✳ The presence of meconium indicates the fetal distress either recently or some time in the past.

When head is delivered

As soon as the baby's head is delivered (prior to delivery of the shoulders) *the mouth, oropharynx, and hypopharynx should be thoroughly suctioned,* using a 10 Fr. DeLee suction catheter or other flexible suction catheter. Any catheter used should be no smaller than a 10 Fr.

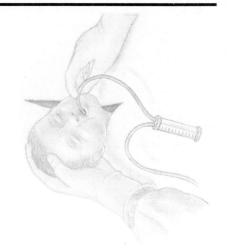

Following delivery

After delivery of the infant, the trachea should be intubated and any residual meconium removed from the lower airway.

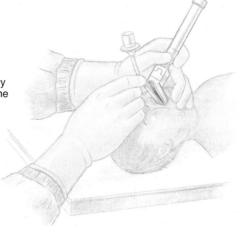

FIGURE 33-5 Management of the infant with meconium staining.

- ❑ Assorted syringes and needles
- ❑ Towels (sterile)
- ❑ Medications:
    - ❑ Pediatric sodium bicarbonate (10 mEq in 10 mL)
    - ❑ Atropine sulfate
    - ❑ Epinephrine 1:10,000
    - ❑ Neonatal Narcan
    - ❑ Volume expander (lactated Ringer's solution or saline)
    - ❑ 10% dextrose in water

Resuscitation of the Distressed Neonate

The vast majority of neonates do not require resuscitation beyond stimulation, maintenance of the airway, and maintenance of body temperature. Unfortunately, it is difficult to predict which neonates will require resuscitation. The inverted pyramid illustrates the relative frequency with which various steps in neonatal resuscitation are required. (See Figure 33-6.) Procedure 33-1 illustrates the steps involved in resuscitating a neonate.

Step 1: Drying, Warming, Positioning, Suction, and Tactile Stimulation. The first step in resuscitation involves drying, warming, positioning, suction-

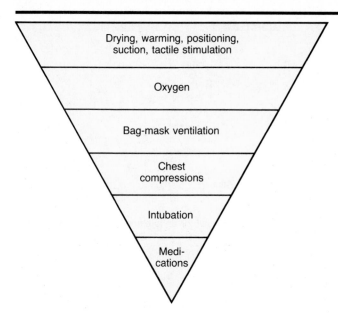

Drying, warming, positioning, suction, tactile stimulation

Oxygen

Bag-mask ventilation

Chest compressions

Intubation

Medi-cations

FIGURE 33-6 The Inverted Pyramid for resuscitation of the distressed neonate.

ing, and stimulating the neonate. (See Figure 33-7.) Immediately upon delivery, minimize heat loss by drying the neonate. Next, place the neonate in a warm, dry blanket. Make sure the environment is warm and free of drafts.

After it is dry, place the neonate on its back with its head slightly below its body and its neck slightly extended. This facilitates drainage of secretions and fluid from the lungs. Place a small blanket, folded to a 2 cm thickness, under the neonate's shoulders to help maintain this position. (See Figure 33-8.)

Next, suction the neonate again, using a bulb syringe or DeLee suction trap. Deep suctioning can cause a vagal response and result in bradycardia. Because of this, suctioning should last no longer than 10 seconds. If meconium is present, the airway should be visualized with a laryngoscope and the meconium suctioned, preferably with a DeLee suction trap. (See Figure 33-9.) If there is a great deal of meconium, place an endotracheal tube and suction the entire tube. (Procedure 33-2.) Next, stimulate the neonate by slapping the soles of its feet and rubbing its back.

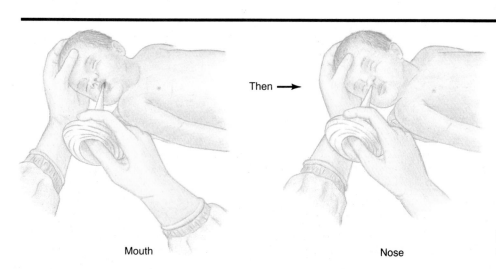

Mouth   Then →   Nose

FIGURE 33-7 Suctioning the mouth, then nose.

CORRECT

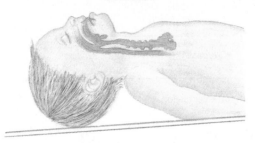

Neck slightly extended

Care should be taken to prevent hyperextension or underextension of the neck since either may decrease air entry.

INCORRECT

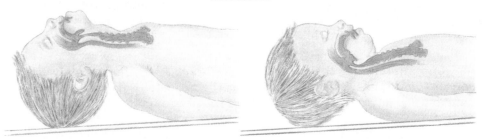

Neck hyperextended   Neck underextended

FIGURE 33-8   Positioning the neonate to open the airway.

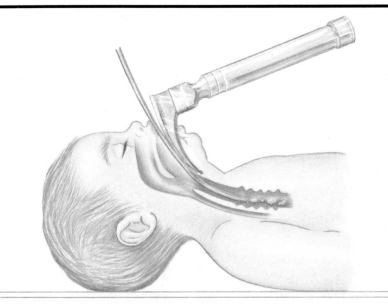

FIGURE 33-9   Tracheal suctioning is important in cases of meconium staining.

1. Ventilate with 100% oxygen for 15-30 seconds

2. Evaluate heart rate.

3. Initiate chest compressions if:
   *HR less than 60, or between 60 and 80 and **not** increasing.*

4. Evaluate heart rate:
   Below 80— Continue chest compressions.

80 or above—
Discontinue chest compressions

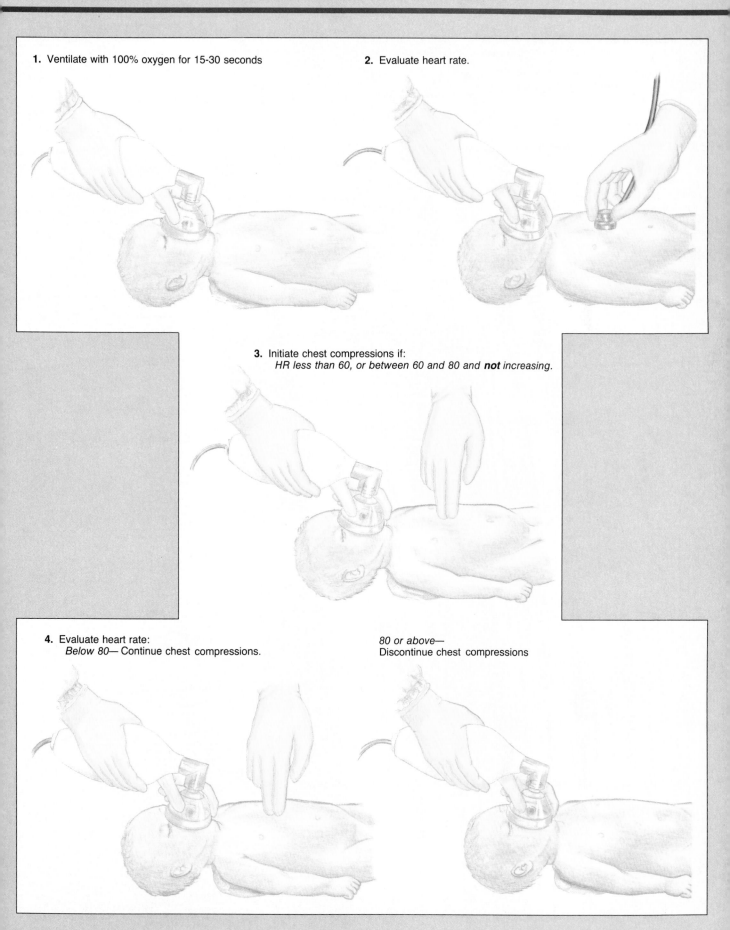

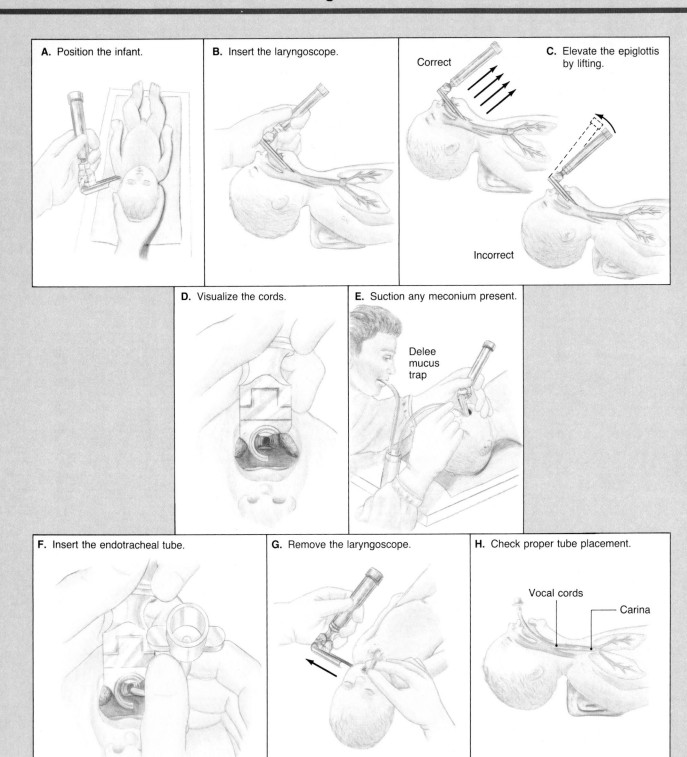

A. Position the infant.

B. Insert the laryngoscope.

C. Elevate the epiglottis by lifting.

Correct

Incorrect

D. Visualize the cords.

E. Suction any meconium present.

Delee mucus trap

F. Insert the endotracheal tube.

G. Remove the laryngoscope.

H. Check proper tube placement.

Vocal cords

Carina

Assessment. After carrying out the maneuvers described above, assess the neonate. Assessment should include the following parameters:

- ❑ *Respiratory effort.* The rate and depth of the neonate's breathing should increase immediately with tactile stimulation. If the respiratory response is appropriate, evaluate the heart rate next. If the respiratory rate is inappropriate, begin positive-pressure ventilation (see Step 3).

- ❑ *Heart rate.* The heart rate is a critical component of neonatal resuscitation. Check the heart rate by listening to the apical area of the heart with a stethoscope, feeling the pulse by lightly grasping the umbilical cord, or feeling either the brachial or femoral pulse. If the heart rate is greater than 100 and spontaneous respirations are present, continue the assessment. If the heart rate is less than 100, begin positive-pressure ventilation immediately (see Step 3).

- ❑ *Color.* A neonate may be cyanotic despite a heart rate greater than 100 and spontaneous respirations. If you note *central cyanosis,* or cyanosis of the chest and abdomen, in a neonate with adequate ventilation and a pulse rate greater than 100, administer supplemental oxygen (see Step 2). Neonates with peripheral cyanosis do not usually need supplemental oxygen unless the cyanosis is prolonged.

- ❑ *Apgar score.* As described previously, if resuscitation is not required, obtain 1- and 5-minute Apgar scores.

Step 2: Supplemental Oxygen. If central cyanosis is present or the adequacy of ventilation is uncertain, administer supplemental oxygen by blowing oxygen across the neonate's face. (See Figure 33-10.) If possible, the oxygen should be warmed. Continue oxygen administration until the neonate's color has improved throughout. Although oxygen toxicity is a concern, this condition is usually associated with prolonged usage over several days. Administration in the field will not cause problems. NEVER DEPRIVE A NEONATE OF OXYGEN IN THE PREHOSPITAL SETTING FOR FEAR OF TOXICITY.

✳ Never deprive a neonate of oxygen in the prehospital setting for fear of toxicity.

Step 3: Ventilation. Begin positive-pressure ventilation if any of the following conditions are present:

1. heart rate < 100

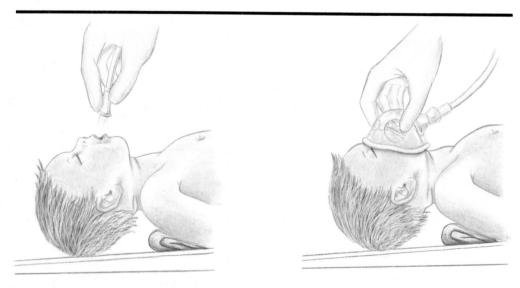

Tubing   Mask

FIGURE 33-10 Oxygen administration for the neonate.

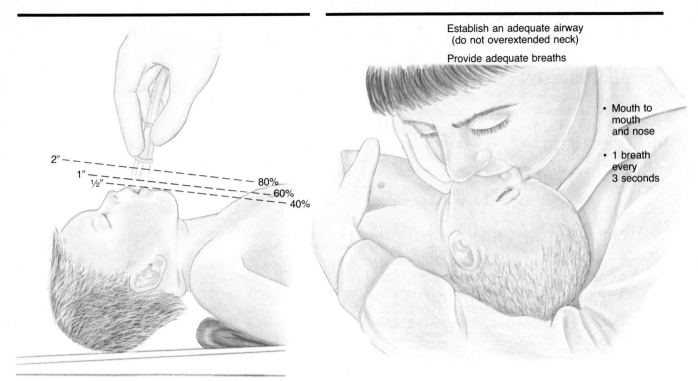

FIGURE 33-11 Guidelines for estimating oxygen concentration.

FIGURE 33-12 Mouth-to-mouth and nose ventilations should be attempted if steps 1 and 2 fail.

Labels in Figure 33-11: 2", 1", ½", 80%, 60%, 40%

Labels in Figure 33-12: Establish an adequate airway (do not overextended neck); Provide adequate breaths; • Mouth to mouth and nose; • 1 breath every 3 seconds

2. apnea

3. persistent central cyanosis after administration of supplemental oxygen

A ventilatory rate of 40–60 breaths per minute is usually adequate. (See Figures 33-11 and 33-12.) A bag-valve-mask unit is the device of choice. The initial pressures required to ventilate a neonate may be as high as 60 cm/H$_2$O. If the bag-valve-mask unit has a pop-off pressure valve, you may have to depress it to ensure adequate ventilation.

Endotracheal intubation should be carried out if any of the following conditions are present:

1. The bag-valve-mask unit does not work.

2. Tracheal suctioning is required (for example, for thick meconium).

3. Prolonged ventilation will be required.

The endotracheal tube should be uncuffed. Ensure proper placement by noting symmetrical chest wall motion and equal breath sounds.

Step 4: Chest Compressions. Chest compressions should be initiated if either of these conditions exists:

1. The heart rate is < 60; OR

2. The heart rate is between 60 and 80 and does not increase despite 30 seconds of positive-pressure ventilation and supplemental oxygenation.

Perform chest compressions by encircling the neonate's chest and placing both of your fingers on the lower one-third of the sternum. (See Figure 33-13.) If the neonate is large, use two-finger compressions. Regardless of the method, the sternum should be compressed 1.5–2.0 cm at

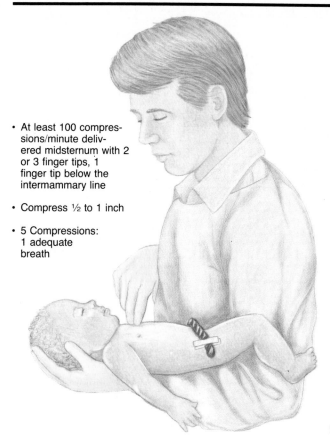

- At least 100 compressions/minute delivered midsternum with 2 or 3 finger tips, 1 finger tip below the intermammary line

- Compress ½ to 1 inch

- 5 Compressions: 1 adequate breath

FIGURE 33-13   Chest compressions in the distressed neonate.

a rate of 120 times per minute. Compressions should always be accompanied by positive-pressure ventilation. Reassess the neonate periodically. Discontinue compressions if the spontaneous heart rate exceeds 80 per minute.

Step 5: Medications and Fluids.   Most cardiopulmonary arrests in neonates result from hypoxia. Because of this, initial therapy consists of ventilation and oxygenation. However, when these measures fail, fluid and medications should be administered.

Fluids and drugs can be administered most readily through the umbilical vein. The umbilical cord contains three vessels, two arteries and one vein. The vein is larger than the arteries and has a thinner wall. To establish venous access, trim the umbilical cord with a scalpel blade to 1 cm above the abdomen. Insert a 5 french umbilical catheter into the umbilical vein. Connect the catheter to a three-way stopcock and fill it with saline. Insert the catheter until the tip is just below the skin and you note free flow of blood. If the catheter is inserted too far, it may become wedged against the liver and it will not function. After it is in place, secure the catheter with umbilical tape.

If an umbilical vein catheter cannot be placed, many medications can be given via the endotracheal tube. These include atropine, epinephrine, lidocaine, and naloxone. Table 33-2 lists recommended medications and doses for the neonate. Fluid therapy should consist of 10 mL/kg of saline or lactated Ringer's solution given by syringe over a 10-minute period.

Continue all resuscitative measures until the neonate is resuscitated or until the emergency department staff assumes care.

TABLE 33-2 Medications for Neonatal Resuscitation

Medication	Concentration to Administer	Preparation	Dosage/Route*	Total Dose/Infant		Rate/Precautions
Epinephrine	1:10,000	1 mL	0.1–0.3 mL/kg I.V. or I.T.	*weight*	*total mL's*	Give rapidly
				1 kg	0.1–0.3 mL	
				2 kg	0.2–0.6 mL	
				3 kg	0.3–0.9 mL	
				4 kg	0.4–1.2 mL	
Volume Expanders	Whole Blood 5% Albumin Normal Saline Ringer's Lactate	40 mL	10 mL/kg I.V.	*weight*	*total mL's*	Give over 5–10 min
				1 kg	10 mL	
				2 kg	20 mL	
				3 kg	30 mL	
				4 kg	40 mL	
Sodium Bicarbonate	0.5 mEq/mL (4.2% solution)	20 mL or two 10-mL prefilled syringes	2 mEq/kg I.V.	*weight*	*total dose* / *total mL's*	Give *slowly*, over at least 2 min
				1 kg	2 mEq / 4 mL	Give only if infant being effectively ventilated
				2 kg	4 mEq / 8 mL	
				3 kg	6 mEq / 12 mL	
				4 kg	8 mEq / 16 mL	
Narcan Neonatal	0.02 mg/mL	2 mL	0.5 mL/kg I.V., I.M., S.Q., I.T.	*weight*	*total mL's*	Give rapidly
				1 kg	0.5 mL	
				2 kg	1.0 mL	
				3 kg	1.5 mL	
				4 kg	2.0 mL	
Dopamine	$6 \times \dfrac{weight \text{ (kg)} \times desired\ dose\ (mcg/kg/min)}{desired\ fluid\ (mL/hr)} = \dfrac{mg\ of\ dopamine}{per\ 100\ mL\ of\ solution}$		Begin at 5 mcg/kg/min (may increase to 20 mcg/kg/min if necessary) I.V.	*weight*	*total mcg/min*	Give as continuous infusion using an infusion pump
				1 kg	5–20 mcg/min	Monitor HR and BP closely
				2 kg	10–40 mcg/min	Seek consultation
				3 kg	15–60 mcg/min	
				4 kg	20–80 mcg/min	

From: *Textbook of Neonatal Resuscitation* © 1987, American Heart Association.

* I.M.–Intramuscular
I.T.–Intratracheal
I.V.–Intravenous
S.Q.–Subcutaneous

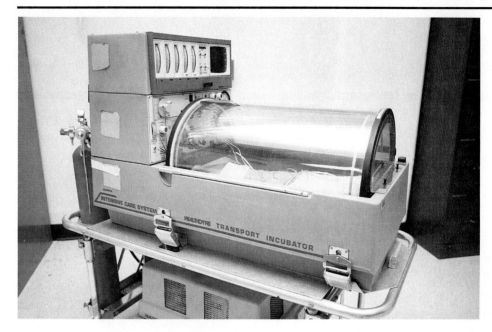

FIGURE 33-14 Neonatal transport isolette.

NEONATAL TRANSPORT

Paramedics are frequently called upon to transport a high-risk neonate from a facility where stabilization has occurred to a neonatal intensive care unit (NICU). The trip may be across the street or across the state. Usually, a pediatric nurse, respiratory therapist, and, often, a physician accompany the neonate. During transport, it is important to maintain body temperature, control oxygen administration, and maintain ventilatory support. Often, a transport isolette with its own heat, light, and oxygen source is available. (See Figure 33-14.) Usually in such cases, intravenous medications are being infused through the umbilical vein and the umbilical artery is catheterized as well.

If a self-contained isolette is not available for transport, it is important to keep the ambulance warm. Wrap the neonate in several blankets and place hot-water bottles containing water heated to less than 40 degrees C. (104 degrees F.) near, but not touching, the neonate. Do not use chemical heat packs to keep the neonate warm.

SUMMARY

After a woman gives birth, the paramedic must care for two patients. The neonate has several special needs. The most important is protection of the airway and support of ventilation. Next, the neonate should be kept warm. If a neonate becomes distressed, then ventilatory support, stimulation, and, if required, CPR should be initiated. Distressed neonates should be transported to a facility with an NICU if possible.

FURTHER READING

AMERICAN HEART ASSOCIATION AND AMERICAN ACADEMY OF PEDIATRICS, *Textbook of Neonatal Resuscitation.* Dallas, TX: American Heart Association, 1987.

AMERICAN HEART ASSOCIATION AND AMERICAN ACADEMY OF PEDIATRICS, *Textbook of Pediatric Advanced Life Support.* Dallas, TX: American Heart Association, 1988.

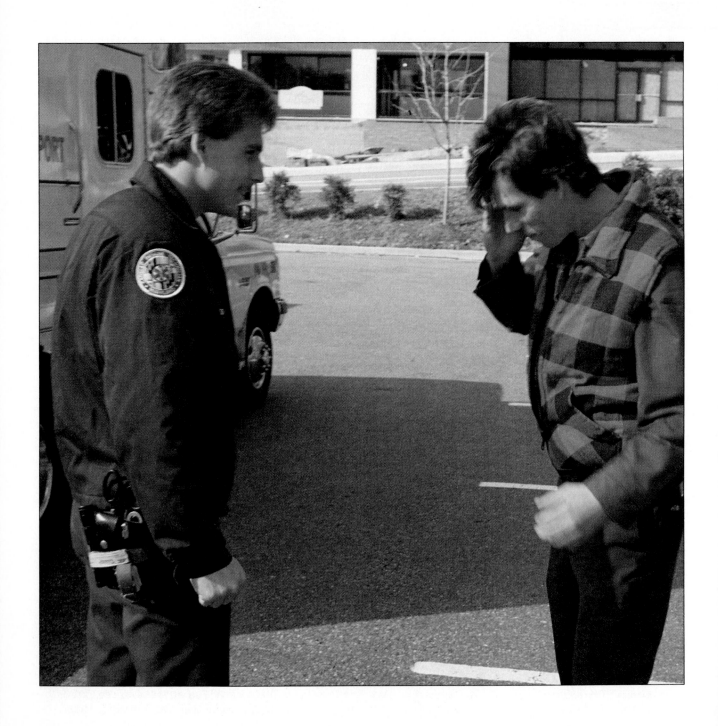

34

Behavioral and Psychiatric Emergencies

Objectives for Chapter 34

Upon completing this chapter, the student should be able to:

1. Define the term behavioral emergency.

2. Describe verbal communication techniques useful in managing the emotionally disturbed patient.

3. List factors associated with increased risk of suicide.

4. Describe the use of open-ended versus closed-ended questions.

5. Define and briefly describe the management of the following conditions:

- anxiety
- suicide
- mania
- depression
- schizophrenia
- behavioral problems in the elderly
- behavioral problems in children

6. Describe the indications and procedure for restraining a violent patient.

7. Discuss the role of drugs and alcohol in behavioral emergencies.

8. List physical problems which can be manifested as psychiatric problems.

CASE STUDY

On Saturday night, paramedics were dispatched to an address some distance from the station. They pulled up to a small frame house and were met at the door by a middle-aged woman. She said, "I'm sick of this. Just get him out of here." She pointed to a poorly dressed young man seated in front of a television. He was wearing his socks on his hands, and his gaze was fixed on the television screen. However, the television was not tuned to a station; there was only static coming from the television's speaker.

The paramedics attempted a primary and secondary survey, but the patient did not acknowledge their presence. The mother stated that the young man was a patient of the mental health center but had missed his last two appointments. She showed the paramedics two empty pill bottles, one for haloperidol (Haldol) and the other unlabeled. She told them that her son had not taken his medicine in over 3 weeks and that he had been sitting in front of the television for 2 days.

One of the paramedics turned the television off and knelt beside the patient. The patient immediately stopped staring at the television and looked at the paramedic. Finally, the patient spoke. The paramedics learned that the patient had been "receiving messages from extraterrestrial beings" through the television. These beings had given him various instructions. His most recent directive was to lead the people of Australia "out of their bondage."

The patient was oriented only to person. He denied taking any medications. He would stop, in mid-conversation, to listen to his hallucinations. Evidently, he could still receive messages through the television even when it was turned off. The paramedics asked if he wanted to go to the hospital. He said, "Sure, let's go," got up, grabbed a pack of cigarettes, and headed for the ambulance with the paramedics behind him. Seated in the back of the ambulance, one paramedic positioned himself near the door and learned more about the patient's television messages on the way to the hospital.

When the patient arrived at the hospital, two nurses recognized him. He had a long history of schizophrenia, and this was just one of many "breaks." The patient did well when he was taking his medication.

INTRODUCTION

The emergency department and the EMS system are now the most common points of entry by disturbed persons into the mental health system. There are several reasons for this. First, over the last 10 years there has been a trend to *deinstitutionalize* the mentally ill. These patients, formerly confined to mental hospitals, now receive care through community centers and other facilities. Second, drug and substance abuse, a major problem in our society, is a frequent cause of behavioral and psychiatric crises. These patients are not generally enrolled in the mental health system. They enter the health care system through EMS, either seeking help or because of a drug-related accident or illness.

UNDERSTANDING BEHAVIORAL EMERGENCIES

A *behavioral emergency* is an intrapsychic, environmental, situational, or organic alteration that results in behavior that cannot be tolerated by the patient or others and requires immediate attention.

Intrapsychic Causes

Intrapsychic causes of altered behavior are those that arise from problems within the person. Such behavior usually results from an acute stage of an underlying psychiatric condition. A wide range of behavior can be manifested, such as:

- depression
- withdrawal
- catatonia
- violence
- suicidal acts
- homicidal acts
- paranoid reactions
- phobias
- hysterical conversion
- disorientation and disorganization

In the field, behavioral emergencies resulting from intrapsychic causes are less common than those resulting from other causes, such as alcohol or drug abuse.

Interpersonal/Environmental Causes

Interpersonal and environmental causes of behavioral emergencies result from reactions to stimuli outside the person. They often result from overwhelming and stressful incidents, such as the death of a loved one, rape, or a disaster. The change in behavior can frequently be linked to a specific incident or series of incidents. The range of behavior manifested is broad, and a patient's specific symptoms are often related to the type of incident that precipitated them.

Organic Causes

An *organic cause* of altered behavior results from a disturbance in the patient's physical or biochemical state. Such disturbances include drugs, alcohol, trauma, illness, and dementia. The area of the brain affected by the disturbance determines the type of behavior change seen.

Substance abuse is the pathological use of a substance to the point that it significantly interferes with a person's normal activities. Alcohol abuse, a common problem, often complicates an underlying medical or behavioral condition. Alcohol is a CNS depressant, and alcohol abuse should be suspected in any patient who has a breath odor of ethanol, slurred speech, or unsteady gait, or who is slow to respond to questions. In addition, evidence of recent alcohol consumption often appears in the form of empty cans or bottles or reports from friends or bystanders.

Drug abuse can result from the frequent use of either street or prescription drugs. Because of the wide variety of drugs abused today and the wide variety of clinical symptoms, the drug abuser is often much more difficult to evaluate than the alcohol abuser. Assessment of the patient suspected of drug abuse should include routine examination of the vital signs and pupillary reaction. There is often physical evidence of abuse, such as prescription bottles, drug paraphernalia, or needle tracks. The behavior of the substance-abuse patient can include withdrawal, suicidal or homicidal actions, violent behavior, or hysteria.

Trauma can also result in alterations in a patient's behavior. Causative factors include increased intracranial pressure, decreased circulation to the brain, or hypoxia resulting from hypoperfusion.

Medical illnesses can also have behavioral manifestations. The diabetic may exhibit confusion, slurred speech, and unsteady gait, particularly with hypoglycemia. Because of this, diabetics are occasionally thought to be drunk, and in such cases medical care is not summoned until coma ensues. Various electrolyte imbalances can result in a behavior change, often manifested as confusion, violence, and extreme anxiety.

Dementia results from actual damage to brain cells. It is often associated with aging and thus occurs most frequently in the elderly, in whom it is referred to as *organic brain syndrome. Alzheimer's disease* is a progressive degenerative disease that attacks the brain and results in impaired memory, thinking, and behavior. It affects approximately 2.5 million American adults and is present in approximately 25 percent of persons age 85 and older. Signs of dementia often include impairment or loss of memory and impaired judgment, often complicated by poor eyesight and hearing. The onset of dementia is usually slow and gradual.

It is important to consider the possibility of organic disease in *ALL* behavioral emergencies. Thus physical assessment of patients with aberrant behavior is the same as for all other patients. Physical assessment is extremely important, as it may uncover unsuspected causes of the altered behavior, such as drugs.

ASSESSMENT OF BEHAVIORAL EMERGENCIES

Behavioral emergencies are stressful for paramedics and other public safety personnel, because of the feeling of uncertainty which often exists at the scene. It is often difficult to determine the cause of the crisis. In addition, in the past, paramedic education has not covered behavioral problems thoroughly, and because of this, the paramedic may feel unprepared. Also, there are few prehospital protocols for behavioral emergencies, since these situations do not lend themselves to a structured approach.

✱ Always evaluate the scene for danger before you leave the vehicle.

Emergency medical providers may be injured at the scene of behavioral emergencies. Therefore, it is important to evaluate the scene for possible danger before leaving the vehicle. Paramedics cannot render aid if they become victims. Unless you are adequately trained, avoid the following situations:

❑ a patient with a weapon
❑ riot scenes
❑ fire scenes
❑ hostage situations
❑ radioactive sites

If the potential danger is minimal, then observe the scene for evidence of what has happened. This includes evidence of violence, substance abuse, or suicide attempt.

The paramedic should perform primary and secondary assessments in addition to gathering information necessary for immediate management of life-threatening conditions. Sources of information should include observation of the patient, statements volunteered by the patient, information gained from interviewing the patient, and information obtained from family members, bystanders, and first responders. A systematic approach to assessment is critical. The information obtained should include:

- precipitating situation or problem
- patient's current life situation
- patient's recent medical and psychiatric history
- patient's past medical and psychiatric history
- patient's mental status
- patient's affect and physical signs
- patient's behavior

From the assessment, the paramedic should draw conclusions about the possible cause of the behavioral change.

Interviewing Techniques

The interview is the most important part of assessing the behavioral emergency patient. The interview should be organized and logical. Use of a formal checklist is not practical, however. Only short interviews should be conducted in the field, and the situation should dictate the interview's scope. Gather only information that is critical to prehospital management and transportation of the patient, unless the patient volunteers more.

The interview should be open-ended, although both direct and indirect questions may be asked. Allow the patient to take the lead in the interview, unless you are afraid that essential information will be lost or the patient is depressed, minimally responsive, or suicidal. If the patient is reluctant to answer certain questions, do not press, as the patient may withdraw completely and provide no information. Be prepared to spend whatever time is required to obtain information, unless the patient's physical condition requires immediate transport or he is endangering himself or someone else. Above all, do not make judgments about the patient's behavior or answers.

The following guidelines will make the interview most effective:

- Remove the patient from the crisis situation and exclude the disturbing person or objects.
- Communicate self-confidence as well as honesty, firmness, and a reasonable attitude about issues important to the patient and the situation.
- It is not necessary either to agree or disagree if the patient distorts reality.
- Simply understand that these distortions are real for the patient.
- Encourage the patient to sit down and relax.
- Encourage the patient to speak in his or her own words, and appear interested in his or her statements.
- Interrupt the patient as little as possible, unless you must redirect a disorganized, rambling communication.
- Do not be afraid of long silent periods. Remain relaxed and attentive.
- If the patient begins to cry or laugh, do not interrupt the display of emotion by talking.

- Encourage the patient to relate his or her story. Nod your head and say things like, "I see, tell me more."
- Use the interview to build a sense of structure if the patient views the situation as chaotic and unexplainable or if the patient's thoughts are disorganized.
- Do not argue with the patient.
- If you must ask questions to keep the interview moving, avoid closed-ended questions (those that can be answered simply "yes" or "no").
- Position yourself so as not to intimidate the patient. Look as though you are at ease.
- Do not shout at a disturbed patient.
- Do not touch a patient without the patient's permission.
- Do not judge the patient's actions or statements. Let the patient understand that you are a neutral party.
- Do not lie or be dishonest.
- Do not place patient between yourself and the exit.

GENERAL MANAGEMENT AND INTERVENTION TECHNIQUES FOR BEHAVIORAL EMERGENCIES

The paramedic's attitude is the single most important factor in dealing with the disturbed patient. Communicate warmth, sensitivity, and compassion. (See Figure 34-1.) The patient must take you seriously. Intervene only to the extent that you feel competent, and be aware of your own professional limitations.

The following are general guidelines for managing behavioral emergencies:

1. Before intervening, assess the risk to your own safety.
2. Give first priority to life-threatening injuries.
3. Take command of the situation.

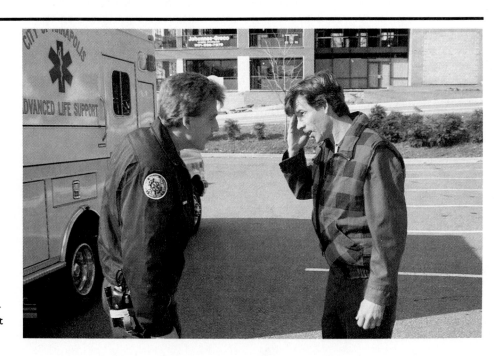

FIGURE 34-1 The psychotic patient should be dealt with in a quiet and reassuring manner.

4. Assign bystanders to perform some tasks when appropriate.

5. Accept the patient's feelings. Do not tell the patient how to feel.

6. Display a calm, reassuring attitude to calm the patient.

7. Avoid severe anxiety reactions in family members, friends, and bystanders by good management. Have appropriate authorities remove unnecessary persons from the scene.

8. Have familiar persons provide support to the patient as necessary.

9. To avoid heightening the patient's anxiety, develop some rapport with the patient before carrying out a physical examination. Maintain privacy, professionalism, and efficiency.

10. If the patient is anxious or confused, explain all procedures carefully.

Some emotionally disturbed patients are transported under police arrest. If this happens, remember that you are acting as an agent of the police. If possible, a police officer should accompany the patient in the ambulance. This is good practice for both safety and medical-legal reasons.

SPECIFIC PSYCHIATRIC DISORDERS

The psychiatric and behavioral emergencies that paramedics most often encounter fall into the following categories:

- ❑ depressive disorders
- ❑ suicidal patients
- ❑ anxiety disorders
- ❑ manic disorders
- ❑ schizophrenic disorders
- ❑ paranoid disorders
- ❑ disorders of age (delirium and dementia)
- ❑ alcohol and substance abuse or dependence

Depression

Depression is a common psychiatric disorder. It affects over 20 percent of the population and accounts for the majority of psychiatric referrals. **Depression** is a mood disorder characterized by feelings of helplessness and hopelessness. Typically, the patient loses interest and pleasure in his or her usual activities. Depressed patients cry easily. They exhibit behavioral and physical changes, such as appetite changes, weight loss or gain, insomnia, low energy level and malaise, feelings of worthlessness or inappropriate guilt, and, in many cases, recurrent thoughts of death or suicide.

■ **depression** a mood disorder characterized by hopelessness and malaise.

Management. Depressed patients should receive supportive care. Encourage them and allow them to talk, and be sure to question such patients about thoughts of suicide. Remember that depression often has an organic cause, such as organic brain syndrome, hypothyroidism, or chronic corticosteroid usage. The seriously depressed patient should be transported to the hospital.

Suicide

Suicide is a frequent cause of death in the United States today. It is quite prevalent in the 15–24 age group. After age 24, the incidence drops, until age 40, when it again begins to rise. Women attempt suicide more frequently than men, yet men are more successful, accounting for 70 percent of all suicides. Men tend to use highly lethal suicide methods, such as guns, carbon monoxide asphyxiation, or hanging. Women tend to use less violent methods, such as pills or wrist lacerations.

Stress is related to suicidal behavior. The paramedic should try to evaluate the stress from the patient's point of view. If the patient's stress level is high, then the suicide potential is high. Any person who has attempted suicide, threatened suicide, revealed self-destructive thoughts, or who shows symptoms of a severe depression should be transported to the hospital for psychiatric evaluation.

When confronted by a patient who is possibly suicidal, assess the suicide potential by evaluating the risk factors. Suicide risk factors include:

❑ Previous attempts (80 percent of persons who successfully commit suicide have made a previous attempt).
❑ Depression (suicide is 500 times more common among patients who are severely depressed than those who are not).
❑ Age (incidence is high during ages 15–24 years; over age 40 the incidence begins to increase again).
❑ Alcohol or drug abuse.
❑ Divorced or widowed (5 times higher rate than among other groups).
❑ Giving away personal belongings, especially those the patient cherishes.
❑ Living alone.
❑ The presence of psychosis with depression (for example, suicidal or destructive thoughts, or hallucinations about killing or death).
❑ Homosexuality (homosexuals who are depressed, aging, alcoholic, HIV-infected).
❑ Major separation trauma (mate, loved one, job, money).
❑ Major physical stresses (surgery, childbirth, sleep deprivation).
❑ Loss of independence (disabling illness).
❑ Lack of goals and plans for the future.
❑ Suicide of same-sexed parent.
❑ Has a plan for committing suicide.

If you suspect suicide potential, do not hesitate to discuss your concerns with the patient. Ask such questions as:

1. How do you feel about life?
2. Do you have any thoughts about killing yourself?
3. Have you ever tried to kill yourself?

It is important to evaluate the lethality of the suicide plan (for example, a gun versus a few pills). The more lethal the plan, the higher the risk. In addition, determine whether the patient has immediate access to the suicide device (is there a gun in the house?). Also determine how specific the plan is. A well-organized, well-thought-out suicide plan is much more dangerous than a vague plan. Finally, determine if the patient has made a prior attempt.

Management. The first priority in the management of a suicidal patient is to protect the patient from self-harm. To do this, the paramedic must gain access to the patient. This may require breaking in, if the patient is unconscious and can be seen. If the patient is armed, consider him to be homicidal as well as suicidal and do not approach.

If you can approach the patient, emergency care, if indicated, has the highest priority. Conduct a brief interview to assess the situation and determine the need for further action. Do not leave the suicidal patient alone. Use physical restraints if necessary. Administer haloperidol (Haldol) if ordered by the medical control physician. ALL SUICIDAL PATIENTS SHOULD BE TRANSPORTED TO THE HOSPITAL.

Anxiety Disorders

Anxiety is a normal response to stress. However, it can build to such a point that it overwhelms the patient, who then feels helpless and becomes unable to function normally. Typically, these patients develop an acute onset of intense terror, accompanied by a feeling of impending doom. The patient subsequently fears loss of control. This is what is referred to as an *anxiety disorder,* or "panic attack." Typical manifestations of an anxiety disorder include:

- ❑ hyperventilation
- ❑ fear of going crazy, dying, or losing control
- ❑ somatic complaints, such as chest discomfort, palpitations, headache, dyspnea, choking or smothering, faintness, syncope, or vertigo
- ❑ feelings of unreality
- ❑ trembling and sweating
- ❑ urinary frequency and diarrhea

Management. The management of the patient suffering an anxiety disorder is primarily supportive. Look for physical causes for the patient's symptoms before attributing them purely to anxiety. Allow the patient to talk, and provide gentle reassurance while transporting him or her to the hospital.

Manic Disorders

Mania and manic disorders can be thought of as the opposite of severe depression. Mania appears frequently in *bipolar disorder,* also called *manic-depressive disorder,* which results in tremendous swings in mood. Manic patients appear "high." Mania is characterized by an elevated and expansive mood. Patients have a marked increase in activity, either social, work, or sexual, and a decreased need for sleep. In addition, patients are physically restless and speak garrulously. They are unable to concentrate or complete tasks. They may have a sense of inflated self-esteem, to a point that they become delusional. The manic phase of the bipolar disorder can last weeks or months. Other disorders are also associated with mania. One of the most common is abuse of stimulant drugs, such as cocaine, amphetamines, or PCP.

■ **mania** a mood characterized by great excitement and activity.

Management. The management of mania depends on whether the patient is violent. If the patient is not violent, he or she should be "talked down." Sit down at the patient's eye level and talk matter-of-factly. Avoid discussing the delusional symptoms. Try to determine from the patient or family members what medications, if any, the patient is taking. Lithium is commonly used for the treatment of mania. If the patient takes this medication or has done so in the past, suspect bipolar disorder. However, if the patient has never been on medication for mania, or if the family reports that this is the first time the patient has behaved in this way, suspect drug abuse. Transport the patient to the emergency department for additional evaluation. The medical control physician may request the administration of haloperidol (Haldol) or another antipsychotic drug if the patient is at risk of self-harm or of harming others.

Schizophrenia

■ **schizophrenia** a group of mental disorders characterized by disturbances in thought, mood, and behavior.

Schizophrenia is a disease characterized by deterioration from a previous level of functioning. The onset of this disease usually occurs in late adolescence or early adulthood. Often patients first develop symptoms of schizophrenia during adolescence. This is often preceded by a period of social withdrawal, poor hygiene, blunted affect, and disturbed communications.

The signs and symptoms of schizophrenia are varied, but there are several characteristic findings. These include:

■ **hallucination** a sense perception that has no basis in reality. For example, hearing voices when no one is present.

❑ *Hallucinations.* Most schizophrenic patients suffer **hallucinations.** These may be either auditory or visual. The patient may hear voices or see people or things that are not there. Often the hallucinations are persecutory.

❑ *Delusions.* Schizophrenics often cannot distinguish reality from fiction. They suffer various **delusions.** Some are persecutory, while others have religious overtones. Some patients have delusions of grandeur, in which they imagine themselves to be rich, important, or powerful.

■ **delusion** a false belief that a patient firmly maintains despite overwhelming evidence to the contrary.

❑ *Altered thought.* Schizophrenics suffer from altered thought processes. The patients cannot reason abstractly and thought is concrete.

❑ *Inappropriate affect.* The patient's **affect,** or emotional state, is generally inappropriate. The patient may laugh or cry at inappropriate times.

■ **affect** a patient's appearance as perceived by the rescuer.

❑ *Disorganization.* The schizophrenic is disorganized in thought and dress. Clothing is inappropriate or, on some occasions, absent.

Schizophrenic symptoms must be present for over 6 months before the diagnosis can be made. Patients with schizophrenic symptoms of less than 6 months duration are referred to as *schizophreniform.* Schizophrenia has several forms. *Catatonic schizophrenia* is a rare disorder. It is manifested by a catatonic stupor, which is a marked decrease in the patient's reactivity to his or her environment. The patient becomes detached from the environment. These patients may take and maintain a rigid and bizarre posture for hours at a time. *Paranoid schizophrenia* is characterized by persecutory delusions, grandiose delusions, delusional jealousy, or hallucinations with persecutory or grandiose content. These patients often feel that someone, often the KGB or CIA, is after them. This paranoia often results from the patient's feeling of self-importance. Some paranoid schizophrenics become delusional and believe that they are someone whom they are not, such as Jesus Christ or Napoleon. Another form of schizophrenia, *undifferentiated schizophrenia,* includes patients who do not fit into other categories.

Management. The management of the schizophrenic depends on the situation. If the patient is nonviolent, transportation is all that is required. However, if the patient is delusional to such a degree that he or she poses a threat to others, antipsychotic medication is indicated.

BEHAVIORAL EMERGENCIES IN THE AGED

Chronological age is not an adequate indication of a patient's mental or physical status. Problems usually associated with aging can occur at any age. Common physical problems associated with the elderly include organic brain syndrome, chronic illness, and diminished eyesight and hearing. Depression, which is common in the elderly, is often mistaken for dementia.

When confronted with an elderly person in a crisis, the paramedic should do the following:

- ❑ Assess the patient's ability to communicate.
- ❑ Provide continual reassurance.
- ❑ Compensate for the patient's loss of sight and hearing with reassuring physical contact.
- ❑ Treat the patient with respect. Call the patient by name and title, such as "Mrs. Jones." Avoid such terms as "dear," "honey," and "babe."
- ❑ Avoid administering medication.
- ❑ Describe what you are going to do before you do it.
- ❑ Take your time. Do not convey the impression that you are in a hurry.
- ❑ Allow family members and friends to remain with the patient if possible.

CRISIS IN THE PEDIATRIC PATIENT

Behavioral emergencies are not limited to adults. Children also have behavioral crises. The child's developmental stage will affect his or her behavior. When confronted with an emotionally distraught or disruptive child, follow these guidelines:

- ❑ Avoid separating a young child from his or her mother.
- ❑ Attempt to prevent the child from seeing things that will increase his or her distress.
- ❑ Make all explanations brief and simple, and repeat them often.
- ❑ Be calm and speak slowly.
- ❑ Identify yourself by giving both your name and your function.
- ❑ Be truthful with the child. Telling the truth will develop trust.
- ❑ Encourage the child to help with his or her care.
- ❑ Reassure the child by carrying out all interventions gently.
- ❑ Do not discourage the child from crying or showing emotion.
- ❑ If you must be separated from the child, introduce the person who will assume responsibility for care.
- ❑ Allow the child to keep a favorite blanket or toy.
- ❑ Do not leave the child alone, even for a short period.

CONTROLLING THE VIOLENT SITUATION

Paramedics occasionally encounter severely disturbed patients who pose a threat to themselves or others. In most jurisdictions these patients may be hospitalized against their will, at least until they have been examined by a psychiatrist. Paramedics must be familiar with appropriate mental health laws in the state and city in which they work.

If, after the assessment is complete, the patient appears to be homicidal, do not attempt restraint. If the patient is armed, move everyone out of range and summon law enforcement officials. Avoid heroic efforts. If, however, the patient is not armed and you must contain his or her violent behavior, you may use "reasonable force" in restraining the patient. Before beginning this, seek police authorization. There should be at least four persons available to restrain the patient, and all must understand

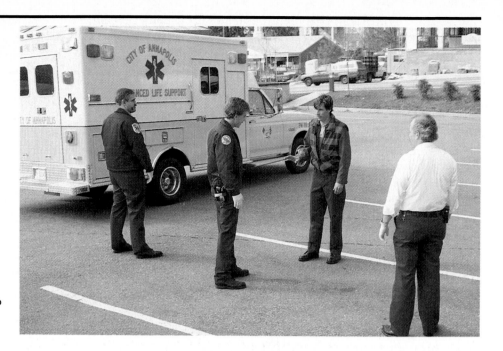

FIGURE 34-2 If it is necessary to restrain the patient, make sure you have adequate assistance.

the plan of restraint. (See Figure 34-2.) Use only the amount of force necessary to restrain the patient. Do not be overzealous.

Methods of Restraint

There are many techniques and devices for restraining the violent patient. Before restraining a person, first consider the normal range of motion of the major joints. The arms cannot flail backwards, the legs cannot kick backwards, and the spinal column cannot double over backwards. Also, consider the power of each major muscle group. For example, the flexor muscles of the arm are much stronger than the extensor muscles. Whenever possible, position the patient so that his or her strength and range of motion are limited.

Paramedics should become familiar with the restraint devices used in their EMS systems. Commercial leather restraints are available, but restraints can be improvised from common materials. Examples include:

❏ Small towels, cravats, or triangular bandages can be wrapped around a wrist or ankle and secured with strong tape to the cot.
❏ Webbed straps, ordinarily used with spine boards, can be used as restraints.
❏ Roll bandage (Kling) can be used to restrict movement of the extremities and thus restrain the patient.

When it becomes necessary to restrain a patient, do not attempt to hold him for a long period. This sets up a confrontation and aggravates the situation. It also restricts the paramedic's activities, because the paramedic will be too busy holding the patient to treat him. Continuous restraint also requires more than one paramedic or assistant per patient.

The sequence of actions required to restrain an unarmed patient is as follows:

1. Make certain you have adequate assistance, since this will reduce the likelihood of injury to both the patient and the paramedic.
2. Offer the patient one final opportunity to cooperate. (See Figure 34-3.)

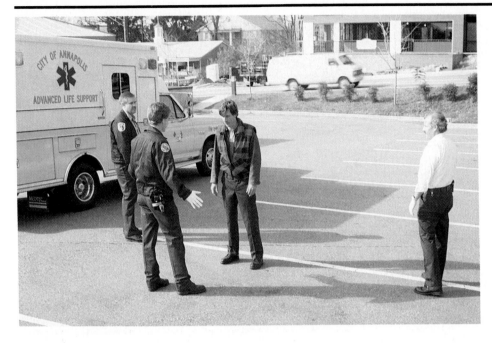

FIGURE 34-3 Offer the patient a final opportunity to cooperate and encircle the patient.

3. If the patient does not respond to this request, at least two persons should move swiftly towards him. The patient cannot focus on both paramedics at once. (See Figure 34-4.) Also, swiftness minimizes the accuracy of a potential kick or blow. At this time, one paramedic should continue talking with the patient.

4. Both paramedics should cautiously move closer and behind the patient. They should not assume that they are in control at this point, as the patient can still kick, bend forward, bite, spit, and jerk about.

5. If the patient does calm down, you may elect to transport without restraints. In this case, continue to reassure the patient. The patient should lie down, and a paramedic should be positioned between the patient and the doors of the ambulance. If the patient becomes dangerous en route, apply restraints.

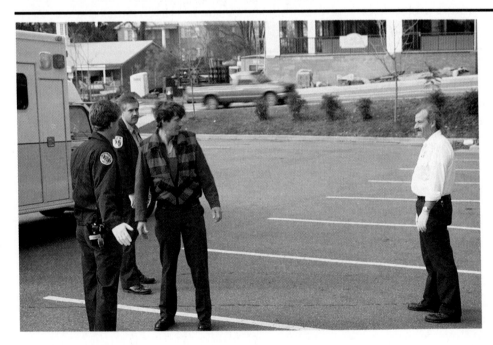

FIGURE 34-4 The patient cannot keep his eye on more than one person at a time. Two of the paramedics should rush the patient at the same time.

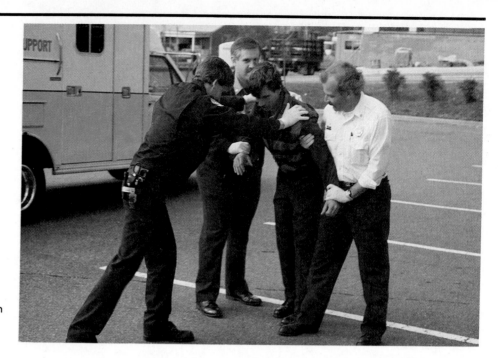

FIGURE 34-5 If necessary, "take down" the patient by placing a leg in front of of the patient's leg and bringing the patient forward.

6. If the patient continues to resist, the paramedics near the patient should position their inside legs in front of the patient's leg and force the patient forward into a prone position. (See Figure 34-5.) The prone position prevents the patient from using the strong abdominal muscles to sit up. Therefore, the arms are more easily restrained and the legs can kick less effectively. (See Figure 34-6.) Also, biting and spitting are effectively controlled.

7. Continue to reassure the patient. Both paramedics should maintain a good grip on the patient's outstretched arm, while leaning their weight on the patient's back.

Positioning and Restraining Patient for Transport

Once the patient is subdued, he should be positioned prone or on the side. (See Figure 34-7.) This dramatically reduces resistance and allows continued assessment and maintenance of the airway. Adjust the cot to its

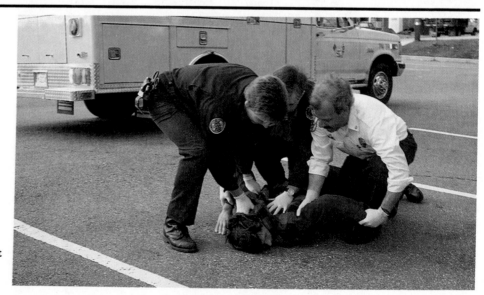

FIGURE 34-6 Maintain the patient on his stomach so that he cannot kick.

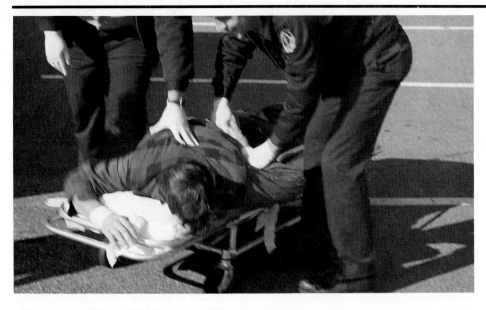

FIGURE 34-7 Place the patient on the stretcher face down and restrain as directed.

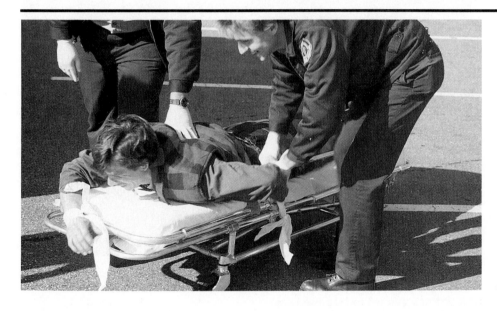

FIGURE 34-8 Secure the arms and legs.

lowest position to improve stability, avoid lifting, and shorten the distance should the patient fall. Do not allow the patient's large muscle groups to work together. For example, restrain one arm at the patient's side and the other above the patient's head. Place a webbed strap across the patient's lumbar region, but do not tighten it too tightly. After applying restraints to the ankles and securing the cot, secure the ankle restraints to one another. (See Figures 34-8, 34-9, and 34-10.) Do not remove the restraints until there are enough personnel present to control the patient.

Methods of Avoiding Injury to the Paramedic

The following precautions can help the paramedic avoid injury:

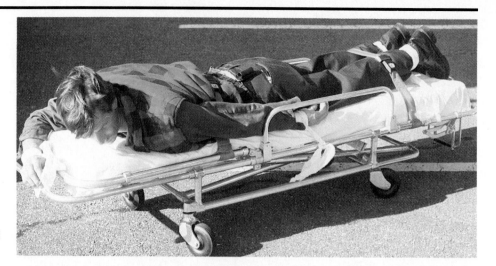

FIGURE 34-9 Patient prepared for transport.

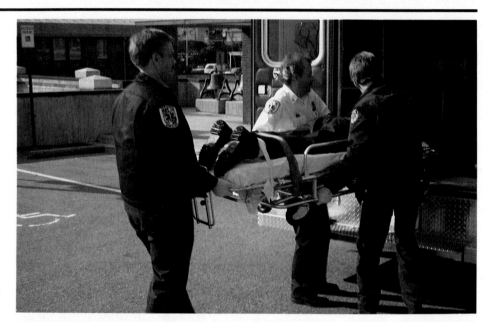

FIGURE 34-10 Transport with adequate assistance.

In a room with a hostile patient:

☐ Remain at a safe distance.
☐ Do not allow the patient to block your exit.
☐ Keep furniture between you and the patient.
☐ Do not make threatening statements.
☐ If there are two paramedics, they should stand apart from each other, at equal distance from the patient.
☐ Do not allow a single paramedic to remain alone with the patient.

For protection against thrown objects:

☐ Hold a folded blanket in front of your arm while holding the bottom of the blanket to the floor with your foot.
☐ Hold the blanket away from your body.
☐ Use the same blanket to wrap the violent patient.

SUMMARY

Paramedics do not see society at its best. Many calls are purely behavioral emergencies, although there is a strong behavioral component to every emergency. Most behavioral emergencies encountered in the field require little more than reassurance to the patient. However, violent or suicidal patients require aggressive therapy. Each patient should be treated on an individual basis as the presenting signs and symptoms dictate.

FURTHER READING

GEORGE, JAMES E., *Law and Emergency Care*. Saint Louis, MO: C.V. Mosby, 1980.

KAPLAN, HAROLD I., AND SADLOCK, BENJAMIN J., *Modern Synopsis of Comprehensive Textbook of Psychiatry/III*. Third Edition (Revised). Baltimore, MD: Williams and Wilkins, 1987.

Glossary

abandonment the termination of a health care provider-patient relationship, without assurance that an equal or greater level of care will continue.

abdomen portion of the body located between the thorax and the pelvis; the superior portion of the abdominopelvic cavity.

abdominal cavity the anterior body cavity located between the diaphragm and the pelvis.

abduct to draw away from the midline.

abduction movement of a body part or extremity away from the midline.

aberrant wandering or deviating from the normal or usual course. In psychiatry it usually refers to behavior that is abnormal.

aberrant conduction conduction of the electrical impulse through the heart's conductive system in an abnormal fashion.

ABO system system of blood typing based on the presence of proteins on the surface of the red blood cells.

abortion the termination of pregnancy before the twentieth week of gestation. The term "abortion" refers to miscarriages and induced abortions. Generally, however, "abortion" is used for elective termination of pregnancy and *miscarriage* for the loss of a fetus, before 20 weeks, by natural means.

abrasion scraping or abrading away of the superficial layers of the skin. An open soft tissue injury.

absolute refractory period the period of the cardiac cycle when stimulation will not produce any depolarization whatsoever.

absorb to take into the body.

acceleration the rate at which speed or velocity increases.

acid a chemical substance which liberates hydrogen ions (H^+) when in solution.

acidosis a state where the pH is lower than normal due to an increased hydrogen ion concentration.

acquired immune deficiency syndrome (AIDS) fatal illness caused by infection with the Human Immunodeficiency Virus (HIV). It destroys the ability of the immune system to fight infection and patients die from overwhelming infection.

action potential the stimulation of myocardial cells, as evidenced by a change in the membrane electrical charge, which subsequently is spread across the myocardium.

active transport biochemical process where a substance is moved across a cell membrane against a gradient, using energy.

acute having a rapid onset and a short course.

acute myocardial infarction death and subsequent necrosis of the heart muscle caused by inadequate blood supply.

addiction the physical or psychological dependence on a substance.

adduction movement of a body part or extremity toward the midline.

adrenergic see sympathomimetic.

affect a patient's appearance as perceived by the rescuer.

afferent fibers carrying impulses toward the center of the body. Sensory nerves send messages toward the brain and are thus afferent.

afterload the pressure or resistance against which the heart must pump.

aggravate to worsen or increase in severity.

agonist a drug or other substance that causes a physiological response.

air embolism presence of an air bubble in the circulatory system.

alarm term used by the fire service to identify groups of fire apparatus and personnel called to assist on-scene personnel at major events. Each alarm brings a given amount of personnel and apparatus to the scene.

albumin protein found in all animal tissues that

constitutes one of the major proteins in human blood.

alkali a strong base, a substance which liberates hydroxyl ions (OH⁻) when in solution.

alkalosis a state where the pH is higher than normal due to a decreased hydrogen ion concentration.

allergic reaction hypersensitivity to a given antigen. A reaction more pronounced than would occur in the general population.

alleviate to reduce or eliminate. It usually refers to a problem or discomforting feeling.

allied health term used to describe ancillary health care professionals, apart from physicians and nurses, such as paramedics, respiratory therapists, and physical therapists.

alpha radiation lowest level of nuclear radiation. A weak source of energy, it is stopped by clothing or the first layer of skin.

ALS Advanced Life Support. EMS personnel trained to use intravenous therapy, drug therapy, intubation, and defibrillation.

alveoli one of the millions of microscopic chambers in the lung. It is where the gases of respiration are exchanged.

Alzheimer's disease a progressive, degenerative disease that attacks the brain and results in impaired memory, thinking, and behavior. It affects an estimated 2.5 million adults.

ambient surrounding on all sides.

amniotic fluid clear, watery fluid which surrounds and protects the developing fetus.

amniotic sac the membranes that surround and protect the developing fetus throughout intrauterine development.

amphetamine substance which acts on the central nervous system as a stimulant.

amputation severance, removal or detachment, either partial or complete, of a body part.

anaphylaxis an acute, generalized, and violent antigen-antibody reaction which may be rapidly fatal.

anastomosis a communication between two or more vessels.

anatomy the study of body structure.

aneurysm the ballooning of an arterial wall, resulting from a defect or weakness in the wall.

angina pectoris chest pain, most often due to periodic cardiac ischemia either from coronary artery blockage or spasm.

anion a negatively charged ion. It is attracted to the positive pole of an electrode (anode), hence the name.

anisocoria pupils of unequal size.

anorexia lack or loss of appetite.

antagonist a drug or other substance which blocks a physiological response or that blocks the action of another drug or substance.

antepartum refers to the time interval prior to delivery of the fetus.

antiadrenergic see sympatholytic.

antibiotics medications effective in inhibiting the growth or killing of bacteria. They have no impact on viruses.

antibodies proteins, produced by plasma cells, released in response to an antigen. Antibodies bind to antigens to facilitate their removal by scavenger cells such as macrophages and neutrophils.

anticholinergic see parasympatholytic.

antidote substance which neutralizes a poison or the effects of a poison.

antigen any substance capable of inducing an immune response.

anxiety anxiety is an emotional state caused by stress. It is characterized by increase in sympathetic nervous system tone.

aortic dissection a degeneration of the wall of the aorta.

APGAR scoring a numerical system of rating the condition of a newborn. It evaluates the neonate's heart rate, respiratory rate, muscle tone, reflex irritability, and color.

apnea the absence of breathing.

Apothecary's system an antiquated system of weights and measures used widely in early medicine.

apparatus term used to describe rescue vehicles that respond to emergencies.

arachnoid web-like in appearance.

arachnoid membrane middle layer of the meninges.

arrhythmia the absence of cardiac electrical activity, often used interchangeably with dysrhythmia.

arteriosclerosis a thickening, loss of elasticity, and hardening of the walls of the arteries from calcium.

arterio-venous malformation an abnormal link between an artery and a vein.

articulate to join together and permit motion.

arytenoid folds cupped or ladle-shaped tissues found posterior to the vocal cords.

ascites accumulation of fluid within the peritoneal cavity.

asphyxia a decrease in the amount of oxygen and an increase in the amount of carbon dioxide as a result of some interference with respiration.

assault an action that places a person in immediate fear of bodily harm.

atelectasis collapse of the alveoli of the lung.

atherosclerosis a progressive, degenerative disease of the medium-sized and large arteries.

atopy patients with a group of diseases of an allergic nature. Included in these are: asthma, eczema, and allergic rhinitis. These diseases have a strong hereditary component.

attenuated diluted or weakened. Applied to organisms that are weakened so as not to be infectious, so that they can be administered to provoke an immune response.

audiovestibular system the organs and structures of the inner ear associated with hearing and balance.

auscultation the process of listening to the internal organs; usually associated with use of a stethoscope.

automaticity the capability of self-depolarization. Refers to pacemaker cells of the heart.

autonomic dysfunction an abnormality of the involuntary aspect of the nervous system.

autonomic nervous system part of the nervous system controlling involuntary bodily functions. It is divided into the sympathetic and the parasympathetic divisions.

autotransfuse to cause the displacement of the patient's blood from one region to another.

avulsion forceful tearing away or separation of body tissue. The avulsion may be partial or complete.

axial loading places the forces of trauma along the axis of the spine and may result in compression fractures.

bacteria small, unicellular organisms present throughout the environment. They are capable of life independent of other organisms.

band a group of radio frequencies close together on the electromagnetic spectrum.

barbiturates organic compounds derived from barbituric acid which depress the central nervous system, respirations, heart rate, and decrease blood pressure.

battery the unlawful touching of a person without his or her consent.

Battle's sign a black-and-blue discoloration over the mastoid process (just behind the ear), characteristic of a basilar skull fracture.

benzodiazepines general term to describe a group of tranquilizing drugs with similar chemical structures.

beta radiation medium-strength radiation stopped with light clothing or the uppermost layer of skin.

bilateral periorbital ecchymosis a black-and-blue discoloration of the area surrounding the eyes. It is associated with a basilar skull fracture.

bile a yellow to green viscous fluid secreted by the liver and stored in the gall bladder. It is secreted into the small bowel, aids in digestion of fats, and gives the stool its normal coloration.

biochemistry the study of chemical events occurring within a living organism.

biophysics the application of the principles of physics to body mechanics.

biotelemetry the process of transmitting physiologi-cal data, such as an electrocardiogram, over distance, usually by radio.

Biot's respirations breathing pattern characterized by irregular periods of apnea and hyperpnea associated with increased intracranial pressure.

blood brain barrier a protective mechanism that selectively allows the entry of only a limited number of compounds into the brain.

bradycardia a heart rate less than 60.

brain the largest portion of the central nervous system, contained within the cranial vault.

brainstem that part of the brain which connects the cerebral hemispheres with the spinal cord. It is comprised of the medulla oblongata, the pons, and the midbrain.

bronchiolitis viral infection of the medium-sized airways occurring most frequently during the first year of life.

bruit the sound of turbulent blood flow through a vessel, often associated with atherosclerotic disease.

buffer substance which neutralizes or weakens a strong acid or base.

bundle branch block a kind of interventricular heart block where conduction through either the right of left bundle branches is blocked or delayed.

bundle of Kent an accessory AV conduction pathway that is thought to be responsible for the ECG findings of pre-excitation syndrome.

burnout occurs when the coping mechanisms no longer buffer the stressors of the job. It can compromise personal health and well-being.

calculus a stone, usually formed of crystalline urinary salts.

cancellous having a latticework structure, as in the spongy tissue of the bone.

cancellous bone spongy bone tissue found at the distal and proximal ends of the long bones.

cannulated to have a tube inserted into a body duct or cavity.

capillary refill diagnostic sign for evaluating peripheral circulation. A capillary bed, such as the fingernail, is compressed. The time taken for color to return to the bed is the capillary refill time, usually 2 seconds or less.

cardiac contractile force the force generated by the heart during each contraction.

cardiac cycle the period of time from the end of one cardiac contraction until the end of the next.

cardiac output the amount of blood pumped by the heart in 1 minute.

cardiogenic shock the inability of the heart to meet the metabolic needs of the body, resulting in inadequate tissue perfusion.

cardiology the study of the heart and related diseases.

cardiovascular disease diseases affecting the heart, peripheral blood vessels, or both.

cardioversion the passage of a current through the heart during a specific part of the cardiac cycle to terminate certain dysrhythmias.

carina the point at which the trachea bifurcates into the right and left mainstem bronchi.

cartilage connective tissue providing the articular surfaces of the skeletal system.

cataracts medical condition where the lens of the eye loses its clearness.

catecholamines class of hormones which act upon the autonomic nervous system. They include epinephrine, norepinephrine, and similar compounds.

cation a positively charged ion. It is attracted to the negative pole of an electrode (cathode), hence the name.

cauda equina terminal portion of the spinal cord which is shaped much like the tail of a horse (Cauda Equina is Latin for "tail of a horse.")

caudally of, at, or near the foot end of the body.

cavitation formation of a partial vacuum, and subsequent cavity, within a liquid. This describes the action of a high-velocity projectile on the human body, which is 60% water.

cell the basic unit of life and the fundamental element of which an organism, such as the human body, is composed.

cell membrane structure which surrounds the cell. It plays a major role in maintaining the internal environment of the cell.

cephalic toward the head end of the body.

cerebellum portion of the brain located dorsally to the pons and medulla oblongata. It plays an important role in the fine control of voluntary muscular movements.

cerebrospinal fluid watery, clear fluid which acts as a cushion, protecting the brain and spinal cord from physical impact. The cerebrospinal fluid also serves as an accessory circulatory system for the central nervous system.

cerebrum the largest part of the brain. It consists of two hemispheres separated by a deep longitudinal fissure. The cerebrum is the seat of consciousness and the center of the higher mental functions, such as memory, learning, reasoning, judgment, intelligence, and the emotions.

certification the process by which an agency or association grants recognition to an individual who has met its qualifications.

Cheyne-Stokes respirations breathing pattern characterized by progressive increase in the rate and volume of respirations that later gradually subsides. Usually associated with a disturbance in the respiratory center of the brain.

cholinergic see parasympathomimetic.

chronic of long duration.

chronotrope a drug or other substance which affects the heart rate.

chronotropy pertaining to heart rate.

ciliated having hair-like processes projecting from the cells which propel mucus.

circumferential encircling or around the complete exterior.

civil law the division of the legal system that deals with non-criminal issues and conflicts between two parties.

clonic alternating contraction and relaxation of muscles.

clubbing the enlargement of the distal fingers and toes, often due to chronic respiratory or cardiovascular disease.

cochlea snail-shaped structure within the inner ear containing the receptors for hearing.

colloid osmotic pressure pressure generated by the presence of colloids in the vascular system or in the interstitial spaces.

coma a state of unconsciousness from which the patient cannot be aroused.

command post a fixed location where the incident commander is located. Typically a vehicle with radio communications, it is often staffed by a number of other agency representatives to provide support and coordination in the rescue effort.

compensated shock a hemodynamic insult to the body in which the body responds effectively. Signs and symptoms are limited, and the human system functions normally.

compensatory pause the pause following an ectopic beat where the SA node is unaffected and the cadence of the heart is not interrupted.

computer-aided-dispatch enhanced dispatch system in which computerized data is used to assist dispatchers in selection and routing of emergency equipment and resources.

concussion a transient period of unconsciousness. In most cases, the unconsciousness will be followed by a complete return of function.

conduction moving electrons, ions, heat, or sound waves through a conductor or conducting medium.

consent the granting of permission to treat, as by a patient to a health care provider.

contiguous in contact or closely associated.

contralateral relating to the opposite side of the body.

contrecoup occurring on the opposite side. An injury to the brain opposite the site of the impact.

contusion closed wound in which the skin is unbroken, although damage has occurred to the immediate tissue beneath.

convection transferring of heat via currents in liquids or gases.

convulsion a sudden, violent, uncontrollable contraction of a group of muscles.

COPD Chronic Obstructive Pulmonary Disease, characterized by a decreased ability of the lungs to perform the function of ventilation.

corrosive substances acids, alkalis, or antiseptics.

cranium vault-like portion of the skull containing the brain.

crepitation a grating sensation, felt or heard in such conditions as subcutaneous emphysema or bone fracture.

cribiform plate thin, sharp plate in the central cranium.

cricothyroid membrane the membrane located between the cricoid and thyroid cartilages of the larynx.

criminal law the division of the legal system that deals with wrongs against society or its members.

critical/immediate category a triage term used to describe critically injured patients requiring immediate transportation.

critical incident stress stress reaction commonly experienced by emergency personnel after a large or particularly stressful emergency response.

critical incident stress debriefing a meeting of rescue workers after a stressful event to allow open discussion of their emotions and feelings.

croup laryngotracheobronchitis, a common viral infection of young children resulting in edema of the subglottic tissues, characterized by barking cough and inspiratory stridor.

crowning the bulging of the fetal head, past the opening of the vagina, during a contraction. Crowning is an indication of impending delivery.

Cullen's sign a bluish discoloration of the area around the umbilicus, caused by intra-abdominal hemorrhage.

CVA (cerebrovascular accident) an interruption of blood flow, from either ischemic or hemorrhagic lesions, to a portion of the brain, resulting in damage or destruction of brain tissue. CVA is referred to as "stroke" by the lay person.

cyanosis bluish discoloration of the skin due to an increase in carboxyhemoglobin in the blood and directly related to poor ventilation.

cystic medial necrosis a death and degeneration of part of the wall of an artery.

cytoplasm material within the cell that provides for structure, support, and certain biochemical functions.

dead/nonsalvageable a triage term used to describe patients who are obviously dead or who have mortal wounds.

deceleration the rate at which speed decreases.

decerebrate posture sustained contraction of the extensor muscles resulting from a lesion in the brainstem. The patient presents with stiff and extended extremities and retracted head.

decoder a device that receives and recognizes unique codes or tones sent over the air.

decompensated shock a continuing hemodynamic insult to the body in which the compensatory mechanisms break down. The signs and symptoms become very pronounced, and the patient moves rapidly toward death.

decompression sickness condition, commonly known as "the bends," in which nitrogen bubbles develop within the tissues due to a rapid reduction of air pressure after a diver comes to the surface following exposure to compressed air.

decorticate posture characteristic posture of a patient with a lesion at or above the upper brainstem. He or she presents with the arms flexed, fists clenched, and legs extended.

defense mechanisms adaptive functions of the personality that help an individual adjust to stressful situations.

defibrillation the passage of a DC electrical current through a fibrillating heart to depolarize a "critical mass" of myocardial cells, allowing them to depolarize uniformly, resulting in an organized rhythm.

dehydration an abnormal decrease in total body water.

delay category a triage term used to describe injured patients who do not have immediate life-threatening injuries, and who can wait a period of time for definitive treatment and transportation.

DeLee trap suction a suction device which contains a suction trap connected to a suction catheter. The negative pressure which powers it can be either from the mouth of the operator or from an external vacuum source.

delegation of authority the granting of privileges by a physician to a non-physician to perform well-delineated skills and procedures.

delirium tremens (DTs) disorder found in habitual and excessive users of alcoholic beverages after cessation of drinking for 48–72 hours. Patients experience visual, tactile, and auditory hallucinations.

delusion a false belief that the patient firmly maintains despite overwhelming evidence to the contrary.

dementia a deterioration of mental status.

depression a mood disorder characterized by hopelessness and malaise.

dermatomes areas of the skin innervated by spinal nerves.

dermis true skin, also called the corium. It is the layer of tissue producing the epidermis, and housing structures, blood vessels, and nerves normally associated with the skin.

diabetes mellitus endocrine disorder characterized by inadequate insulin production by the beta cells of the islets of Langerhans of the pancreas.

dialysate physiologic solution used in renal dialysis.

dialysis process of exchanging various biochemical substances across a semipermeable membrane to remove toxic substances.

diaphysis hollow shaft of the long bones.

diastole the period of time when the myocardium is relaxed and cardiac filling and coronary perfusion occur.

diffusion the movement of solutes (substances dissolved in a solution) from an area of greater concentration to an area of lesser concentration.

direct medical control communications between EMS field personnel and a medical control physician during an emergency run, also called "on-line medical control."

disentanglement the process of freeing a patient from wreckage to allow for proper care, removal, and transfer.

dislocation displacement of a long bone or other structure from its normal anatomical location.

dispatch term used to describe the dispatch center for emergency services. Also called "alarm headquarters" by the fire service.

diuretic a medication which stimulates the kidneys to excrete water.

diverticula small, finger-like pouches on the colon associated with degeneration of the muscular layer of the organ.

diverticulosis the presence of bleeding from small pouches on the colon, which tend to develop with age.

division used by some agencies in place of the term "sector" to describe a group of rescuers working for a supervisor. The supervisor is commonly called a "divisional officer."

doll's eye reflex the eyes turning as the head is turned. An unnatural response, indicative of severe CNS dysfunction.

drug a chemical agent used in diagnosis, treatment, and prevention of disease.

duodenum first part of the small bowel. About 10 inches in length, it receives the secretions of the liver and the pancreas.

duplex transmissions method of radio transmission in which simultaneous transmission and reception occur using two frequencies.

dura mater tough layer of the meninges firmly attached to the interior of the skull.

dysconjugate gaze failure of the eyes to rotate simultaneously in the same direction.

dyspnea difficult or labored breathing.

dysrhythmia any deviation from the normal electrical rhythm of the heart.

ecchymosis blue-black discoloration of the skin due to leakage of blood into the tissues.

ECG an electrocardiogram (ECG) is a graphic recording of the electrical activities of the heart.

ectopic beats cardiac depolarization resulting from depolarization of cells in the heart which are not a part of the heart's normal pacemaker.

ectopic pregnancy the implantation of a developing fetus outside of the uterus, often in a fallopian tube.

eczema skin disorder seen commonly in allergic patients.

effacement the thinning of the cervix during labor.

efferent fibers carrying conducted impulses away from the brain or spinal cord to the periphery.

effusion the escape of fluid, normally from the vascular space, into a cavity (e.g. pleural effusion).

electrocardiogram (ECG) the graphic recording of the heart's electrical activity. It may be displayed either on paper or on an oscilloscope.

electrolytes chemical substances that dissociate into charged particles when placed in water.

emboli a clot or other particle brought by the blood from another vessel and forced into a smaller one.

emergency medical dispatcher person responsible for assignment of emergency medical resources to a medical emergency.

emergency medical services a complex health care system that provides immediate, on-scene patient care to those suffering sudden illness and injury.

EMS System a comprehensive approach to providing emergency medical services.

EMT-Basic a person, currently certified, who has successfully completed the U.S. Department of Transportation (USDOT) National Standard Curriculum for EMT-Basic.

EMT-Intermediate a person, currently certified, who has successfully completed the USDOT National Standard Curriculum for EMT-I.

EMT-Paramedic a person, currently certified, who has successfully completed the USDOT National Standard Curriculum for EMT-P.

encoder a device for generating unique codes or tones that are recognized by another radio's decoder.

endocrine gland gland that secretes hormones directly into the blood.

endometrium the inner lining of the uterus where the fertilized egg implants.

energy the capacity to do work in the strict physical sense.

enzyme biochemical catalyst which speeds chemical reactions. The enzyme itself does not normally change during the process.

epidermis outermost layer of the skin comprised of dead or dying cells.

epidural hematoma accumulation of blood between the dura mater and the cranium.

epigastrium portion of the abdomen immediately below the xiphoid process.

epiglottitis bacterial infection of the epiglottis, usually occurring in children older than age 4. A serious medical emergency.

epilepsy paroxysmal disturbances of neurological function usually resulting from disturbance of electrical activity in the brain.

epiphysis ends of the long bone, including the epiphyseal or growth plate, and support structures underlying the joint.

erythema general reddening of the skin due to dilation of the superficial capillaries.

eschar hard, leathery product of deep third-degree burn. It consists of dead and denatured skin.

esophageal varices an abnormal dilation of veins in the lower esophagus, a common complication of cirrhosis of the liver.

estimated date of confinement (EDC) the approximate day a child will be born. This date is usually based on the date of the last menstrual period (LMP).

ethics the rules, standards, and morals governing the activities of a group or profession.

evaporation change from liquid to a gaseous state.

excursion extent of movement of a body part, such as the chest during respiration.

extracellular fluid portion of the body's fluid outside the body's cells.

extravasation the leakage of fluid or medication outside a blood vessel.

extrication the use of force to free a patient from entrapment.

extrication officer title of an individual who supervises all personnel and activities related to an extrication process.

facilitated diffusion biochemical process where a substance is selectively transported across a semipermeable membrane using "helper proteins."

fibrosis the formation of fiber-like connective tissue, also called "scar tissue," in an organ.

FiO₂ the concentration of oxygen in inspired air.

flail chest a defect in the chest wall which allows for free movement of a segment. Breathing will cause paradoxical chest wall motion.

fontanelles areas in the infant skull where bones have not yet fused. Posterior and anterior fontanelles are present at birth.

fracture disruption of the bone tissue. Types of fractures include: comminuted, greenstick, impacted, linear, oblique, spiral, and transverse.

frostbite localized freezing of a body area.

fungi class of organisms containing the yeast and molds.

gag reflex the act of retching or striving to vomit, a normal reflex triggered by touching the soft palate or the throat.

gamma radiation powerful electromagnetic radiation emitted by radioactive substances. It is stronger than alpha or beta radiation.

gastritis an inflammation of the lining of the stomach.

genitalia reproductive organs of either the male or the female.

geriatric abuse a syndrome in which an elderly person has received serious physical or psychological injury.

geriatrics the study and treatment of diseases of the old.

Glasgow Coma Scale tool used in evaluating and quantifying the degree of coma by determining the best motor, verbal, and eye-opening response to standardized stimuli.

glaucoma medical condition where the pressure within the eye increases.

glottis the slit-like opening between the vocal cords.

Golden Hour the first hour following a serious accident. Studies have shown that patients who receive definitive care within the first hour have an increased chance of survival.

grand mal form of seizure characterized by tonic-clonic muscle contractions. It may occur with or without coma.

grand multiparity a woman who has delivered at least seven babies.

gravidity the number of times a woman has been pregnant.

gray matter the gray portions of the central nervous system which include the cerebral cortex, basal ganglia, and nuclei of the brain, as well as the gray columns of the spinal cord.

Grey Turner's sign the ecchymotic discoloration of the flanks and umbilical region, associated with intra-abdominal hemorrhage, often of pancreatic origin.

guarding voluntary or involuntary contraction of the abdominal muscles in response to severe abdominal pain.

gynecology the branch of medicine that treats disorders of the female reproductive system.

half-life time required for half of the nuclei of a radioactive substance to lose activity by undergoing radioactive decay.

hallucination a sense perception that has no basis in reality. For example, hearing voices when no one is present.

hallucinogen drug which produces hallucinations.

haversian canals small perforations of the bones through which the blood vessels and nerves travel into the bone itself.

hazard zone an area of rescue operations that poses a significant threat to rescuers.

heat cramps acute painful spasms of the voluntary muscles following strenuous activity in a hot environment without adequate fluid or salt intake.

heat exhaustion acute reaction to heat exposure. Blood pools in the vessels as the body attempts to give off excessive heat. It can lead to collapse due to inadequate blood return to the heart.

heat stroke acute, dangerous reaction to heat exposure, characterized by a body temperature usually above 106 degrees F (41.1 degrees C). The body ceases to perspire.

hematemesis vomiting of blood.

hematocrit the percentage of the blood consisting of the red blood cells, or erythrocytes (usually 35–45 percent).

hematoma collection of blood beneath the skin or trapped within a body compartment.

hematuria presence of blood in the urine.

hemodialysis a medical procedure whereby waste products and fluid, normally excreted by the kidneys, are removed by a machine.

hemoglobin an iron-containing compound, found within the red blood cell, that is responsible for the transport and delivery of oxygen to the body cells.

hemoptysis expectoration of blood from the respiratory tree.

hemothorax blood within the pleural cavity.

Hertz a measurement of radio frequency, one cycle per second.

histamine a chemical released by mast cells and basophils upon stimulation. It is one of the most powerful vasodilators known and a major mediator of anaphylaxis.

homeostasis the body's natural tendency to keep the internal environment constant.

hormone chemical substance released by a gland that controls or affects other glands or body systems.

hydrolytic splits compounds when in the presence of water.

hypercarbia an increased level of carbon dioxide in the blood.

hyperpyrexia elevation of body temperature above 106 degrees F (41.1 degrees C).

hypertension a common disorder characterized by elevation of the blood pressure persistently exceeding 140/90 mmHg.

hypertensive emergency an acute elevation of blood pressure which requires the blood pressure to be lowered within one hour, characterized by end-organ changes such as hypertensive encephalopathy, renal failure, or blindness.

hypertensive encephalopathy a complication of hypertension indicated by severe headache, nausea, vomiting, and altered mental status. Neurological symptoms may include blindness, muscle twitches, inability to speak, weakness, and paralysis.

hypertensive urgency an acute elevation of blood pressure which requires the blood pressure to be lowered in 24 hours, usually unaccompanied by end-organ changes.

hyperthermia unusually high body temperature.

hypertonic a state where a solution has a higher solute concentration on one side of a semipermeable membrane compared to the other side.

hypertonic phase phase of a seizure when muscles are in a state of greater than normal tension or of incomplete relaxation.

hypertrophy an increase in the size or bulk of an organ.

hyperventilation an increased rate or depth of breathing; it often results in an abnormal lowering of carbon dioxide in the system.

hypoglycemia complication of diabetes characterized by low levels of blood glucose. This often occurs from too high a dose of insulin or from inadequate food intake following a normal insulin dose. Sometimes called insulin shock, hypoglycemia is a true medical emergency.

hypoglycemic seizure seizure that can occur when blood glucose levels fall dangerously low, seriously altering the brain's energy supply.

hypothalamus portion of the diencephalon producing neurosecretions important in the control of certain metabolic activities including body temperature regulation.

hypothermia having a body temperature below normal.

hypotonic a state where a solution has a lower solute concentration on one side of a semipermeable membrane compared to the other side.

hypoventilation a reduced rate or depth of breathing, often resulting in an abnormal rise of carbon dioxide in the system.

hypoxemia reduction in the oxygen content in the arterial blood or in the PaO_2.

hypoxia state in which insufficient oxygen is available to meet the oxygen requirements of the cells.

ileum third and longest portion of the small bowel. It is approximately 12 feet in length and extends from the jejunum to the ileo-cecal valve.

immunity the state of being resistant to noxious substances or organisms due to previous exposure to the same or similar organisms.

Immunoglobulin E (IgE) antibody responsible for mediating allergic and anaphylactic reactions.

impact forceful contact or collision. It is the forceful exchange of energy that results frequently in trauma.

incident commander the individual in charge of and responsible for all activities at an incident when the incident command system is in effect.

incident command system a management program designed for controlling, directing, and coordinating emergency response resources. It applies in managing fires, hazardous materials, and mass casualty incidents, as well as during other rescue operations. Major components of the system include the incident commander and subdivided subordinate management team of sectors or divisions.

incision very smooth or surgical laceration, frequently caused by a knife or scalpel.

indirect medical control the establishment of system policies and procedures, such as treatment protocols and case reviews. Also called "off-line medical control."

inertia the tendency of an object to remain at rest or to remain in motion unless acted upon by an external force.

ingestion the entrance of a substance into the body through the gastrointestinal tract.

inhalation the entrance of a substance into the body through the respiratory tract.

injection the entrance of a substance into the body through a break in the skin.

inotrope a drug or other substance which affects the contractile force of the heart.

inotropy pertaining to cardiac contractile force.

insertion attachment of a muscle to the bone that moves when the muscle contracts.

inspection the physical assessment skill of visually examining a patient.

insulin pancreatic hormone needed to transport simple sugars form the interstitial spaces into the cells.

integumentary system skin, consisting of the epidermis and dermis.

intercalated disc specialized band of tissue inserted between myocardial cells which increases the rate in which the action potential is spread from cell to cell.

intercostal muscles muscles between the rib which serve to expand the chest.

interpolated beat a PVC that falls between two sinus beats without effectively interrupting the rhythm.

interstitial fluid portion of the body fluid found outside the body's cells, yet not within the circulatory system. Interstitial fluid is that fluid found within the interstitial space between the cells.

intervener physician a licensed physician, professionally unrelated to patients on the scene, who attempts to assist paramedic field crews.

intracellular fluid portion of the body fluid inside the body's cells.

intracerebral hemorrhage bleeding directly into the tissue of the brain.

intracranial pressure pressure exerted on the brain by the blood and cerebrospinal fluid.

intractable resistant to cure, relief, or control.

intrathoracic within the thoracic cage.

intravascular fluid portion of the body's fluid outside the body's cells and within the circulatory system.

intubation to pass a tube into an opening of the body.

ion a charged particle.

ionization the process of changing a substance into separate charged particles (ions).

ionizing radiation electromagnetic radiation (e.g. X-ray) or particulate radiation (e.g. alpha particles, beta particles, and neutrons) capable of producing ions by direct or secondary processes.

ipsilateral on, or referring to, the same side.

iris pigmented portion of the eye. It is the muscular area that constricts or dilates to change the size of the pupil.

ischemic colitis an inflammation of the colon due to impaired or decreased blood supply.

isotonic a state where solutions on opposite sides of a semipermeable membrane are in equal concentration.

J wave ECG deflection found at the junction of the QRS complex and the ST segment. It is associated with hypothermia and seen at core temperatures below 32°, most commonly in leads II and V.

Jacksonian seizure a form of seizure localized to one part or one group of muscles.

jejunum second portion of the small bowel. It is approximately 8 feet in length and is located between the duodenum and the ileum.

ketoacidosis complication of diabetes due to decreased insulin secretion or intake. It is characterized by high levels of glucose in the blood, metabolic acidosis, and, in advanced stages, coma. Ketoacidosis is often called diabetic coma.

kinetic energy the energy an object has while it is in motion. It is related to the object's velocity and mass.

kinetics the branch of dynamics that deals with motion, taking into consideration mass and force.

Korsakoff's syndrome psychosis characterized by disorientation, muttering delirium, insomnia, delusions, and hallucinations. Symptoms include painful extremities, bilateral wrist drop (rarely), bilateral foot drop (frequently), and pain or pressure over the long nerves.

Kussmaul respirations a very deep, gasping respiratory pattern, found in diabetic coma.

kyphosis exaggeration in the normal posterior curvature of the spine.

labor the time and processes that occur during childbirth.

laceration open wound, normally a tear with jagged borders.

lacrimal ducts passageways carrying the lacrimal fluid (tears) from the lacrimal glands to the eye.

landing zone an area or sector designated as a landing point for helicopters.

laryngospasm a spasm of the vocal folds that may occlude the airway. It is a protective mechanism to prevent aspiration of foreign bodies into the airway.

libel the act of injuring a person's name, character, or reputation by false or malicious writings.

licensure the process by which a governmental agency grants permission to engage in a given occupation to an applicant who has attained the degree of competency required to ensure the public's protection.

ligament connective tissue connecting bone to bone and holding the joints together. The ligaments will stretch to allow joint movement.

litigation the act or process of carrying on a lawsuit.

living will a written request to withhold heroic life support measures from a patient with a terminal condition. A living will is usually executed before the patient becomes ill or injured and is used to express that person's wishes.

logarithm mathematical concept that eases calculation of large numbers. The log of a number is the exponent of the power to which a given base must be raised to equal that number. For example, the log of 100 is 2 ($100 = 10^2$), and the log of 1,000 is 3 ($1,000 = 10^3$).

lumen opening or space within a needle, artery, vein, or other hollow vessel.

lymphatic system a complex network of small thin vessels, valves, ducts, lymph nodes, and organs which helps to protect and maintain the fluid environment of the body and plays a major role in fighting disease. The lymph is restored to the regular circulation by the thoracic duct and the lymphatic duct.

malaise discomfort or uneasiness often associated with disease.

Mallory-Weiss tear a tear in the lower esophagus which is often caused by severe and prolonged retching.

mammalian diving reflex (diving reflex) a complex cardiovascular reflex, resulting from submersion of the face and nose in water, which constricts blood flow everywhere except to the brain. It decreases cardiac output and rate, and produces stable or slightly increased arterial blood pressure.

mania a mood characerized by increased excitement and activity; madness.

maxillary having to do with, or related to, the maxilla, the bone of the upper jaw.

McGill forceps instrument used in airway management for reaching into the oropharynx to manipulate a foreign body, endotracheal tube, or similar item.

mechanism of injury the actual forces that caused the patient's injuries.

meconium dark, green material found in the intestine of the full-term neonate. It can be expelled from the intestine into the amniotic fluid during periods of fetal distress.

mediastinum central cavity within the thorax containing the heart, great vessels, trachea, and esophagus.

medical director a physician who, by experience or training, handles the clinical and patient care aspects of the EMS system.

medical terminology the language and terms of medicine, based mostly on Latin and Greek.

medulla the central portion of an organ.

medulla oblongata the lower portion of the brainstem.

melena black, tarry feces due to gastrointestinal bleeding.

menarche the onset of menses, usually occurring between ages 12 and 14.

Ménière's disease a disease of the inner ear characterized by vertigo, nerve deafness, and roaring or buzzing in the ear.

meninges membranes covering and protecting the brain and spinal cord. They consist of the pia mater, arachnoid membrane, and dura mater.

meningitis infection of the lining of the brain and spinal cord, most commonly by bacteria or viruses.

menopause the cessation of menses and the end of a woman's reproductive life.

mesentery double fold of peritoneum that supports the major portion of the small bowel, suspending it from the posterior abdominal wall.

metaphysis growth zone of the bone, active during the developmental stages of youth. It is located between the epiphysis and the diaphysis.

metric system a system of weights and measures widely used in science and medicine and based on a base unit of 10.

midbrain the portion of the brain connecting the pons and cerebellum with the cerebral hemispheres.

milliliter unit for measuring volume; 1/1,000 of a liter.

minute volume (V_{min}) the amount of air inhaled and exhaled in one minute; it equals the respiratory rate times the tidal volume.

mitochondria organelle responsible for provision of cellular energy.

modulator a device that transforms electrical energy into sound waves.

morality the principles of right and wrong as governed by individual conscience.

motion the process of changing place; movement.

mucus a thick, slippery secretion that functions as a lubricant and protects various surfaces.

mucus membrane a membrane lining many of the body cavities that handle air transport, usually containing small mucus secreting glands.

multigravida a woman who has been pregnant more than once.

multiparity a woman who has delivered more than one baby.

multiplex transmissions method of radio transmissions in which voice and other data can be transmitted simultaniously by use of multiple frequencies.

nasal flaring excessive widening of the nares with respiration.

natal literally means birth.

National Standard Curriculum paramedic training curriculum published by the United States Department of Transportation, widely used as the standard guidelines for paramedic education.

negligence a deviation from an accepted standard of care. It is synonymous with malpractice in the context of medical care.

neonate an infant from the time of birth to one month of age.

nerve conduction velocity the rate at which a nervous impulse is conducted along a nerve.

neurilemma thin, fibrous sheath surrounding the peripheral nerve fiber.

neuron the nerve cell, the fundamental unit of the nervous system.

neurotransmitter a substance that is released from the axon terminal of a presynaptic neuron on excitation which travels across the synaptic cleft to either excite or inhibit the target cell. Examples include: acetylcholine, norepinephrine, and dopamine.

noncompensatory pause the pause following an ectopic beat where the SA node is depolarized and the underlying cadence of the heart is interrupted.

nucleus cellular organelle which contains the genetic material (DNA).

nulligravida a woman who has never been pregnant.

nullipara a woman who has never delivered a baby.

oblique having a slanted position or direction.

odontoid process finger-like projection of the second cervical vertebra, around which the first cervical vertebra rotates.

off-line medical control see indirect medical control.

on-line medical control see direct medical control.

omentum sheet of peritoneum and fat tissue, covering and protecting the anterior surface of the interior abdomen.

organ a group of tissues with a common function.

organelles specialized structures within the cell which provide for cellular needs.

organism a group of organ systems; the functional unit of life.

origin attachment of a muscle to a bone that does not move (or experiences the least movement) when the muscle contracts.

orthopnea dyspnea while lying supine.

osmosis the movement of a solvent (water) across a semipermeable membrane from an area of lesser (solute) concentration to an area of greater (solute) concentration. Osmosis is a form of diffusion.

osteoporosis softening of bone tissue due to the loss of essential minerals, principally calcium.

overdose a dose of a drug in excess of that usually prescribed. It can potentially adversely affect the patient's health.

overhydration an excess of total body water.

ovulation the growth and discharge of an egg from the ovary.

packaging the completion of emergency care procedures needed for transferring a patient from the scene to an ambulance.

palpation the physical assessment skill of examining a patient by touch.

palpitation a sensation that the heart is pounding or racing.

paradoxical breathing an asymmetrical chest wall movement caused by a defect (e.g. flail chest) which lessens respiratory efficiency.

paradoxical movement moving in a fashion opposite to that expected. It is often seen in flail chest injuries where the flail segment moves in an opposite direction compared to the rest of the chest.

paraplegia paralysis involving the lower extremities. Usually related to injury or lesion to the spinal cord.

parasympathetic nervous system division of the autonomic nervous system that is responsible for controlling vegetative functions.

parasympatholytic a drug or other substance that blocks or inhibits the actions of the parasympathetic nervous system (also called anticholinergic).

parasympathomimetic a drug or other substance which causes effects like those of the parasympathetic nervous system (also called cholinergic).

parenchyma the principal or essential parts of an organ.

parenteral drugs drugs administered into the body without going through the digestive tract.

parietal pleura fine fibrous sheath covering the interior of the thorax.

parity the number of times a woman has delivered a fetus which has aged enough to be viable.

paroxysmal nocturnal dyspnea (PND) a sudden episode of difficult breathing occurring after lying down, most commonly caused by left heart failure.

pediatrics that branch of medicine dealing with the health care needs of infants and children.

peptic ulcer disease injury to the mucus lining of the upper part of the gastrointestinal tract due to stomach acids, digestive enzymes, and other chemicals.

percussion the act of striking an object or area to elicit a sound or vibration.

perfusion fluid passing through an organ or a part of the body.

pericardial tamponade filling of the pericardial sac with fluid which limits the filling of the heart.

pericardium two-layered sac surrounding the heart.

periosteum the exterior covering of a bone.

peripheral vascular resistance the resistance to blood flow due to the peripheral blood vessels. This pressure must be overcome for the heart to pump blood effectively.

peristalsis wavelike muscular motion of the esophagus and bowel which moves food through them.

peritoneum serous membrane covering the viscera of the abdomen and lining the interior of the abdominal cavity.

petit mal seizure form of seizure where consciousness may or may not be lost.

pH scientific method of expressing the acidity or alkalinity of a solution. It is the logarithm of the hydrogen ion concentration divided by one. The higher the pH, the more alkaline the solution. The lower the pH, the more acidic the solution.

pharmacodynamics the study of a drug's action upon the body.

pharmacokinetics the study of how drugs enter the body, reach their site of action, and are eventually eliminated.

pharmacology the study of drugs and how they affect the body.

phonation the process of generating speech and other sounds.

physiology the study of body function.

pia mater inner and most delicate layer of the meninges. It covers the convolutions of the brain and spinal cord.

placenta the organ that supports the fetus during intrauterine development. The placenta is attached to the wall of the uterus and to the umbilical cord.

plasma the fluid portion of the blood consisting of serum and protein substances in solution.

pleura a membrane covering the lungs, and lining the thoracic cavity.

pneumomediastinum the presence of air in the mediastinum.

Poiseuille's law a law of physiology that states that blood flow through a vessel is directly proportional to the diameter of the vessel to the fourth power.

poison control center information center staffed by trained personnel which provides up-tp-date toxicological information.

poisoning taking any substance into the body that interferes with normal physiological functions.

polycythemia an excess of red blood cells.

pons process of tissue which connects two or more parts of an organ.

portal system circulatory system that collects blood from parts of the abdominal viscera and transports it to the liver.

postpartum the time period after delivery of the fetus.

prefix one or more syllables affixed to the beginning of a word to modify its meaning.

preload the pressure within the ventricles at the end of diastole, commonly called the "end-diastolic volume."

prenatal means essentially the same as "antepartum" and refers to the time period before birth. Health care visits during pregnancy referred to as "prenatal visits" or "prenatal care."

presacral edema an accumulation of fluid in the sacral area in the recumbent patient, usually related to congestive heart failure.

priapism a painful, prolonged erection of the penis due to spinal injury or disease process. (It may occur in sickle cell anemia.)

primary assessment first aspect of the patient assessment, designed to determine any immediate threats to the patient's life. It assesses airway, breathing, and circulation, and looks for significant hemorrhage.

primary treatment patient treatment that targets three life-threatening medical problems: breathing trouble, hemorrhaging, and circulation trouble.

primary ventricular fibrillation ventricular fibrillation due to a problem occurring within the heart itself, such as acute myocardial infarction.

primigravida a woman who is pregnant for the first time.

primiparity a woman who has delivered her first child.

Prinzmetal's angina variant of angina caused by vasospasm of the coronary arteries and not blockage *per se*.

professional a person who exhibits the conduct or qualities that characterize a practitioner in a particular field or occupation.

profile the size and shape of a projectile as it contacts a target.

pronation turning of the palm or foot downward or backward.

protocols a set of policies and procedures for all components of an EMS system.

proximate cause a legal concept describing a person who, through his or her actions, does something that produces an effect. In current usage, it literally means that a person was the immediate causative factor in a civil or criminal wrong.

psychomotor mental processes which cause, or are associated with, physical activity.

psychosis any major mental disorder of organic or emotional origin. It is usually evidenced by derangement of the personality or loss of contact with reality.

pulmonary embolism blood clot or other thrombus in the pulmonary circulation which adversely affects oxygenation of the blood.

pulse oximetry assessment modality that measures the oxygen saturation level of the blood through a noninvasive sensor placed on a finger or ear lobe.

puncture specific soft-tissue injury involving a deep, narrow wound to the skin and underlying organs. It carries an increased danger of infection.

pyrexia above normal body temperature, fever.

pyrogen any substance capable of causing a fever.

quadriplegia paralysis of all four extremities, usually related to a high spinal injury or lesion in the spinal cord.

radiation emission of rays in all directions from a common center. Ionizing radiation is that which either directly or indirectly induces ionization of radiation-absorbing material.

radio an electronic device that transmits sound waves and telemetry over distances using electromagnetic waves.

rales abnormal breath sound due to the presence of fluids in the smaller airways.

rebound tenderness tenderness on release of the examiner's hands, allowing the patient's abdominal wall to return to its normal position. Rebound tenderness is associated with peritoneal irritation.

reciprocity the process by which an agency grants certification or licensure to an individual who has comparable certification or licensure from another agency.

recompression the restoration of pressure, often used in the treatment of diving emergencies so that a patient can be slowly decompressed.

refractory a disorder or condition that resists treatment.

refractory period the period of time when myocardial cells have not completely repolarized and cannot be stimulated again.

relative refractory period the period of the cardiac cycle when a sufficiently strong stimulus may produce depolarization.

repeater a radio base station modified to retransmit a radio broadcast so that the range of the broadcast can increase.

repolarization the return of the muscle cell to its pre-excitation resting state.

res ipsa loquitur a Latin phrase meaning "the thing speaks for itself," used in negligence proceedings.

rescue to free from confinement or danger.

research diligent and scientific study, investigation, and experimentation in order to establish facts and determine their significance.

resource term applied to all personnel, vehicles, apparatus, equipment, and medical supplies that may respond to an emergency incident.

respiration the exchange of gases between a living organism and the environment.

resting potential the normal electrical state of cardiac cells.

reticular activating system the system responsible for consciousness. A series of nervous tissues keeping the human system in a state of consciousness.

retraction the act of drawing back or inward.

retroperitoneal behind the peritoneum. The organs within this space include the kidneys, spleen, and part of the pancreas.

Reye's Syndrome illness of uncertain etiology that results in alteration of mental function in children. Often associated with viral infections and the use of aspirin.

rhonchi abnormal breath sound due to the presence of fluid or mucous in the larger airways.

roentgen unit for describing exposure dose of radiation.

root word a word to which a suffix, prefix, or both, is affixed.

safety officer a person with the knowledge and authority to intervene in unsafe rescue situations who makes the "go-no go" decision for the rescue operation.

scapula large, flat, and irregular bone located in the posterior shoulder which articulates with the humerus.

schizophrenia a group of mental disorders characterized by disturbances in thought, mood, and behavior.

SCUBA abbreviation for Self Contained Underwater Breathing Apparatus.

sebaceous glands glands within the dermis that secrete sebum.

sebum fatty secretions of the sebaceous gland. It helps keep the skin pliable and waterproof.

secondary assessment part of the physical assessment process where detailed historical and physical findings are evaluated in order to determine the patient's medical or traumatic problem.

secondary ventricular fibrillation ventricular fibrillation due to a problem elsewhere in the body which secondarily affects the heart (e.g. electrolyte abnormalities, hypoxia, hypovolemia).

sector a component of the incident command system that is subordinate to an incident commander. A group of rescuers working for a supervisor within the sector. The supervisor is commonly referred to as the "sector officer."

sector officer the person supervising a group of rescuers. The sector officer is subordinate to the incident commander, and receives direction from the incident commander.

sector vest a vest worn by sector or divisional officers and their aides to identify persons with incident management responsibilities. They are typically bright-colored and bear titles.

seizure a disorder of the nervous system due to a sudden, excessive, disorderly discharge of brain neurons.

Seldinger technique a technique for guiding a larger catheter into a vein previously entered with a small catheter, using a wire dilator.

semicircular canals the three rings of the inner ear. They sense the motion of the head and provide positional sense for the body.

semipermeable membrane specialized biological membrane, such as that which encloses the body's cells, which allows the passage of certain substances and restricts the passage of others.

senescence the process of growing old.

senile dementia general term used to describe an abnormal decline in mental functioning seen in the elderly.

septicemia the presence of an infectious agent, usually bacteria, within the bloodstream.

septum a wall that divides a chamber into two cavities.

shock a state of inadequate tissue perfusion.

simplex communications method of radio transmission in which both transmission and reception occur on the same frequency.

size-up to quickly assess a particular situation, determine the nature and extent of the emergency scene, and decide what resources will be needed to resolve the emergency.

slander the act of injuring a person's name, character, or reputation by false or malicious spoken words.

snoring upper airway noise caused by partial obstruction of the airway by the tongue or similar materials.

spinal foramen the opening in the vertebra through which the spinal cord passes.

spondylolysis a degeneration of the vertebral body.

staging the collection of vehicles at a central location for distribution as needed at a major incident scene.

staging sector the component of the incident command system that is responsible for managing a staging area.

standing orders paramedic field interventions that are completed before contacting the medical control physician.

Starling's Law of the Heart law of physiology which states the more the myocardium is stretched, up to a certain amount, the more forceful the subsequent contraction will be.

START the acronym for Simple Triage And Rapid Treatment. The START program describes a rapid method of triaging large numbers of patients at an emergency incident.

status epilepticus act of having two or more seizures in succession without intervening periods of consciousness.

sternocleidomastoid muscle of the lateral neck and anterior thorax attaching at the mastoid, clavicle, and sternum. It serves as an accessory muscle of respiration and lifts the sternum and anterior chest during deep respiration.

stimulus (pl. stimuli) any factor or input into the sensory system that causes an action or response.

Stokes-Adams syndrome a series of symptoms resulting from heart block, most commonly syncope, which results from decreased blood flow to the brain caused by a sudden increase in cardiac output.

stress a nonspecific mental or physical strain. It is always present to some degree in everyone.

stressor a stressor is any agent or situation that causes stress.

stridor high pitched "crowing" sound, caused by restriction of the upper airway.

stroke an interruption of blood flow—from emboli, thrombus, or hemorrhage—to an area of the brain.

stroke volume The amount of blood ejected by the heart in one cardiac contraction.

subcutaneous emphysema the presence of air within the subcutaneous tissues, often associated with pneumothorax.

subdural hematoma collection of blood directly beneath the dura mater.

subluxation incomplete dislocation of a joint. The surfaces remain in contact while the joint is somewhat deformed.

sudden death death within 1 hour after the onset of symptoms.

sudden infant death syndrome (SIDS) illness of unknown etiology that occurs during the first year of life.

suffix one or more syllables affixed to the end of a word to modify its meaning.

supination turning of the palm or foot upward or forward.

supply sector the title for a sector within the incident command system that is responsible for obtaining and distributing additional supplies at a major incident. A sector officer is assigned as the supervisor.

surface absorption the entrance of a substance into the body directly through the skin.

surfactant a compound secreted by cells in the lungs which contributes to the elastic properties of the pulmonary tissues.

sutures pseudojoints which join the various bones of the skull to form the cranium.

sympathetic nervous system division of the autonomic nervous system that prepares the body for stressful situations.

sympathetic stimulation a stimulus which triggers the sympathetic nervous system, increasing heart rate and blood pressure, as well as other actions of the sympathetic nervous system.

sympatholytic a drug or other substance which blocks the actions of the sympathetic nervous system (also called antiadrenergic).

sympathomimetic a drug or other substance which causes effects like those of the sympathetic nervous system (also called adrenergic).

syncope a transient loss of consciousness, caused by inadequate blood flow to the brain.

syncytium group of cardiac muscle cells which physiologically function as a unit.

synovial having to do with, or relating to, the lubrication of a joint.

systole the period of the cardiac cycle when the myocardium is contracting.

tachycardia a heart rate greater than 100.

tachypnea rapid respirations.

tactile fremitus vibratory tremors felt through the chest by palpation.

Ten-code system radio code system published by the Association of Public Safety Communications Officers that uses the number "10" followed by another code number.

tendon band of connective tissue that attaches muscle to bone.

tension pneumothorax buildup of air under pressure within the thorax. By compressing the lung, it severely reduces the effectiveness of respiration.

tentorium extension of the dura mater separating the cerebrum from the cerebellum.

thermal gradient the difference in temperature between the environment and the body.

thermogenesis the production of heat, especially within the body.

thyrotoxicosis toxic condition characterized by tachycardia, nervous symptoms, and rapid metabolism due to hyperactivity of the thyroid gland.

TIA (transient ischemic attack) temporary interruption of the blood supply to the brain.

tiered response a type of EMS system where BLS-level vehicles are initially dispatched to all calls unless ALS-level care is needed.

tilt test a drop in the systolic blood pressure of 15 mmHg, or an increase in the pulse rate of 15 beats per minute when a patient is moved from a supine to a seated position is considered positive and suggestive of relative hypovolemia. Also called "orthostatic vital signs."

tissue a group of cells which, together, have a common function or purpose.

titration estimation of the appropriate dosage by slowly changing the rate of administration.

tonic phase the phase of a seizure characterized by tension or contraction of muscles.

tonicity the number of particles present per unit volume.

tort law a branch of civil law concerning civil wrongs between two parties.

toxicology medical and biological science that studies the detection, chemistry, pharmacological actions, and antidotes of toxic substances.

toxins poisonous chemicals secreted by bacteria, or released following destruction of the bacteria.

tracheal tugging retraction of the tissues of the neck due to airway obstruction or dyspnea.

transfer of command a process of transferring of command responsibilities from one individual to another. Commonly a formal process of face-to-face communication, followed by a briefing on the situation, and then a radio announcement to a dispatch center that a certain individual has now assumed command of the incident. The transfer of command process also applies to the transfer of sector or division responsibilities.

transient ischemic attack reversible interruption of blood flow to the brain. Often seen as a precursor to major stroke.

transportation the act of moving a patient from the scene into the ambulance, or from the ambulance into the emergency department.

transportation sector the title for a sector within the incident command system that is responsible for obtaining and coordinating all patient transportation. A sector officer is asssigned as a supervisor.

trauma a physical injury or wound caused by external force or violence.

trauma center hospital that has the capability of caring for the acutely injured patient. Trauma centers must meet strict criteria to use this designation.

traumatic asphyxia compression of the chest due to a crush injury. It limits chest expansion yet tamponades hemorrhage.

treatment sector the title for a sector within the incident command system that is responsible for collecting and treating patients in a centralized treatment area. A sector officer is assigned as a supervisor.

triage the act of sorting patients by the severity of their injuries.

triage sector the title for a sector within the incident command system that is responsible for triaging all patients. A sector officer is assigned as a supervisor.

tunica adventitia outer fibrous layer of the blood vessels. It maintains their maximum size.

tunica intima interior layer of the blood vessels. It is smooth, and provides for the free flow of blood.

tunica media the middle, muscular layer of the blood vessel. It controls the vessel lumen size.

umbilical cord structure containing 2 arteries and 1 vein which connects the placenta and the fetus.

umbilicus the navel, the remnant of the umbilical cord.

Universal Precautions set of procedures and precautions published by the Centers for Disease Control to assist health care personnel in protecting themselves from infectious disease.

untoward an unexpected reaction, usually associated with the administration of a drug.

uremia toxic condition caused by the retention of nitrogen-based substances (urea) in the blood, normally excreted by the kidneys.

urticaria name given the raised areas that occur on the skin associated with vasodilation due to histamine release. Commonly referred to as "hives."

vallecula the depression between the epiglottis and the base of the tongue.

Valsalva's maneuver forced exhalation against a closed glottis. This maneuver increases the intra-abdominal and intra-thoracic pressure, causing slowing of the pulse.

varicosities an abnormal dilation and distention of a vein.

velocity a rate of motion in a particular direction in relation to time.

vertigo loss of positional sensation and the perception that the horizon and all points of reference are moving.

vesicular breath sounds heard in the normal lung.

viruses microscopic organisms smaller than the bacteria, which require the assistance of another organism for their survival. Viruses are a common cause of human disease.

visceral pleura fine lining covering the lungs. With the parietal pleura, it forms the seal holding the lungs to the interior of the thoracic cage.

vitreous humor clear, watery fluid filling the posterior chamber of the eye. It is responsible for giving the eye its sperical shape.

voting a process by which the repeater station receiving the strongest incoming signal is chosen to rebroadcast the signal.

water the universal solvent. Approximately 60 percent of the weight of the human body is due to water.

watt a fundamental unit of electrical power.

Wernicke's syndrome condition characterized by loss of memory and disorientation, associated with chronic alcohol intake and a diet deficient in thiamine.

wheezing whistling-type breath sound associated with narrowing or spasm of the smaller airways.

white matter nervous tissue composed of white nerve fibers.

Wolff-Parkinson-White a disorder of the heart characterized by early contraction of part of the heart muscle.

Index

intravascular fluid, 273
intravenous fluid therapy, 303–5
intravenous bolus (*ill.*), 334
Intropin (*see* dopamine)
intubation, (*see* endotracheal intubation)
intubation, digital, 427
ionizing radiation, 841
ipecac, syrup of, 366, 786–87
iris, anatomy of, 411
irreversible shock, 294
islets of Langerhans, 709
isoproterenol, 340
Isoptin (*see* verapamil)
isotonic, 276
Isuprel (*see* isoproterenol)

J waves, 835
jaw lift, 214
jaw thrust, 213–14
jaw-thrust without head-tilt, 214
jejunum, 447
jugular venous distention, 172

Kent, bundle of, 658
kidney stone, 750, 760
kinetic energy, 376
kinetics of trauma, 373, 376
Korsakoff's psychosis, 735
Kreb's cycle, 293
Kussmaul respirations, 175, 712–13

labetalol, 345
laceration, 500
lactated Ringer's, 284
laryngeal edema (in burn trauma), 508
laryngoscope, 228–30
    MacIntosh blade, 228–29
    Miller-Abbott blade, 228–29
laryngospasm, 174, 208
laryngotracheobronchitis, 888–89
Lasix (*see* furosemide)
law, 38
    abandonment, 42
    assault and battery, 43
    Boyle's, 845
    consent, 42
    criminal, definition of, 38
    definition of, 38
    do not resuscitate, 40
    drugs, 317–18
    Good Samaritan, 39–40
    Henry's, 845
    libel, 43
    living will, 40
    medical liability, 43–45
    medical practice acts, 39
    negligence, 41
    Newton's, 376
    Poiseuille's, 543, 586
    proximate cause, 41
    refusal of care, 43
    res ipsa loquitur, 41
    slander, 43
    Starling's Law of the Heart, 588
left ventricular failure, 671–73
    prehospital management, 673
Levophed (*see* norepinephrine)
lice, 815

lidocaine, 346
ligaments, 477
ligamentum arteriosum, 445
ligamentum teres, 455
litigation, 38
living wills, 40
loading, axial, 415

magnesium, 276
magnesium sulfate, 365, 939
Mallory-Weiss tear, 866
maneuver, Sellick's, 227
    Valsalva's, 862
manic disorders, 982–83
mannitol, 437
marijuana, 795
marine animal stings, 794
mask, nonrebreather, 260
    simple face, 259–60
    venturi, 260–61
mass casualty, 32
mater, dura, 407, 720
    pia, 407, 720
McGill forceps, 173, 231
measles, 816
mechanism of injury, 159, 374
meconium, 961
mediastinum, 445
medical dictionary, 114
medical liability, 43–45
medical control, 20
    direct, 20
    indirect, 20–21
        off-line (*see* medical control, indirect)
        on-line (*see* medical control, direct)
        protocols, 21
        standing orders, 22
medical practice acts, 39
medical terminology, 114–22
    abbreviations, 122–27
medication allergies, 192
medulla oblongata, 722
melena, 867
membrane, semipermeable, 276
membranes (*ill.*), 136
menarche, 917
Ménière's disease, 864
meninges, 403, 720
meningitis, 807, 886–87
menopause, 917
menstruation, 917
mesentery, 448
metabolic acidosis, 287
metabolic alkalosis, 287
metaphysis, 475
methylprednisolone, 777
metric system, 326–27
    conversions, 327–28
microNEFRIN (*see* racemic epinephrine)
midbrain, 722
minute volume, 205, 557
miscarriage (*see* abortion)
mittelschmerz, 766, 920
modified jaw-thrust, 426
monitoring, cardiac, 185–86
    electrocardiogram, 689–95
morphine, 353
mouth-to-mouth, 262
mouth-to-nose, 262
mucous membrane, 201
multiple casualty incident, overview, 82–83

mumps, 816
muscular system (*ill.*), 138
musculoskeletal system (*ill.*), 137–38
mutual aid, 32
myocardial infarction, 667
    in-hospital management, 671
    prehospital management, 669–70
        drugs used in, 670
    signs and symptoms, 668–69
    subendocardial, 667
    sudden death, 668
    transmural, 667

Nagel, Dr. Eugene, 4
naloxone, 367
Narcan (*see* naloxone)
narcotics, 795, 797
nasal cannula, 258–59
nasal flaring, 559
nasopharyngeal airway, 215
nasotracheal intubation, 238–39
    advantages, 240–41
    blind, 241
National Registry of Emergency Medical Technicians, 12
National Standard Curriculum, 10
near-drowning, 837
neck, anatomy of, 412
needle decompression, 468
negligence, 41
neonatal resuscitation (*table*), 970
neonate, 875, 956
    distress, 961
    premature, 960
    resuscitation of, 962–71
    routine care of, 956–58
    transport, 971
nervous system, 718; *ill.,* 141–42
    autonomic, 324–25
    pathophysiology and management, 730
neurogenic shock, 295
neurological assessment, 180–81
    Glasgow Coma Scale, 181–82
neuron, 719
neurotransmitter, 719
nifedipine, 357
nines, rule of, 505
nitroglycerin, 356
Nitrolingual Spray (*see* nitroglycerin)
Nitronox, 354, 465, 492
Nitrostat (*see* nitroglycerin)
nitrous oxide, 354
node, atrioventricular (AV), 593
    sinoatrial (SA), 593
non-compensatory pause, 619
nonrebreather mask, 260
norepinephrine, 339
norepinephrine (neurotransmitter), 719
normal saline, 284
Normodyne (*see* labetalol)
nuclear radiation (*see* radiation)

Oath of Geneva, 5
obstetrical terminology, 930
obstruction, airway, 206
    child consciousness (*table*), 900
    child unconsciousness (*table*), 901
    infant unconscious (*table*), 899
    infant conscious (*table*), 898

Self-instructional Workbook for
PARAMEDIC EMERGENCY CARE

The **Self-instructional Workbook for Paramedic Emergency Care** is prepared to help you improve your performance in class, on examinations, and ultimately in providing care to the ill or injured patient. The workbook will help you identify the important principles presented in **Paramedic Emergency Care** and direct you to review any material you don't truly understand. The workbook addresses each case study presented in PEC and explains why certain aspects of care were offered. Self-examinations test your reading comprehension and prepare you for the tests within your training course and for your state examination.

The workbook also includes several special projects which help in learning the knowledge base which is prehospital emergency medicine. These projects include: ambulance report forms, crossword puzzles, EKG exercises, pharmacology math, etc. The workbook contains drug flash cards which can be detached and used to help review and memorize drug dosages, indications, contraindications and routes.

All examinations, crossword puzzles and special projects are keyed in the back of the workbook. This will help you determine your progress immediately. The page reference is given with each answer so you can review the text pages where the content is presented.

Special Features:

Learning Objective Review   Each chapter of the workbook begins with a short review of the object of each learning objective.

Case Study Review   The workbook reviews the case study beginning each chapter of the text. It identifies principles and special considerations of care.

Reading Self-exam   Each chapter contains 10 to 45 questions which test the student's comprehension. Answers and page references are provided.

Ambulance Report Form   The workbook enhances the information given by the case study and then asks the student to record the appropriate information on an ambulance report form. A report form key is found in the workbook key.

Drug Math Worksheets   The drug math worksheets provide the students with practice working with drug dosages and the math required to calculate flow rates and administer medications in the field.

Emergency Drug Cards   The workbook contains perforated 3 by 5 cards which present the emergency drug name, description, indications, precautions and dosage.

EKG Rhythm Strips   The workbook contains two EKG exercises which are designed to help practice the process of EKG interpretation.